CONCISE PATHOLOGY

FOR EXAM PREPARATION

Fourth Edition

CONCISE PATHOLOGY

FOR EXAM PREPARATION

GEETIKA KHANNA BHATTACHARYA, MD (Pathology)
Director Professor & Laboratory In-Charge
CIO Laboratory
Vardhman Mahavir Medical College and
Safdarjung Hospital
New Delhi, India

ELSEVIER

ELSEVIER

RELX India Pvt. Ltd.
Registered Office: 818, 8th Floor, Indraprakash Building, 21, Barakhamba Road, New Delhi 110001
Corporate Office: 14th Floor, Building No. 10B, DLF Cyber City, Phase II, Gurgaon-122002, Haryana, India

Concise Pathology for Exam Preparation, 4th Edition, Geetika Khanna Bhattacharya

ISBN: 978-81-312-6133-0
e-book ISBN: 978-81-312-6134-7

First Printed in India 2021, Reprinted 2021, 2023

Content Strategist - Education Solutions: Arvind KoulContent *Project Manager:* Goldy Bhatnagar
Sr Production Executive: Dhan Singh
*Sr Graphic Designer:*Milind Majgaonkar

Typeset by Thomson Digital
Printed and bound at Balaji Art, Mumbai.

Dedicated to Shriya and Elaina

Preface to the Fourth Edition

The enthusiastic response to the previous editions, suggestions received from the student community, the newer learning points now incorporated in standard textbooks and the introduction of the competence learning focus in the recent times, have all necessitated the fourth edition of this book. This edition has been thoroughly updated and revised in accordance with the new competency-based MBBS curriculum of Pathology. It continues to be structured in a question-answer format that incorporates information in a concise manner with bulleted points, for rapid review. The content has been re-organized and divided into four sections, namely, General Pathology, Haematology, Clinical Pathology and Laboratory Medicine, and Systemic Pathology. Key points and named entities (important cells, inclusions, clinical terms, and syndromes) have been given in bold for easy recapitulation for the MBBS viva voice (oral examination) and also the postgraduate entrance examination. Numerous flowcharts and schematic diagrams (approximately 350 in number), micro- and gross-photographs, X-rays, clinical pictures (approximately 300 in number), have been added to reinforce understanding of the subject, particularly for the 'visual learner'. Hand-drawn diagrams have been introduced, in addition to photomicrographs, to enable prescribed competence in practicals. Special effort has been made to include clinical information in the chapters to accentuate the relevance of each section to actual patient situations. At the same time, every effort has been made to restrict the increase in number of pages, so that students are not overloaded with information.

In addition, complimentary access to full e-book, chapter-wise image bank and online university exam-patterned MCQs have been provided.

The main objectives of this book remain the same:

- To allow a quick self-assessment and revision before the examination.
- To highlight the 'must know' areas (the areas covered in this book are the ones that are frequently referred to/ stressed upon by examiners, and are also relevant to the student from knowledge point of view. Proficiency in these topics will aid students' in understanding their clinical subjects in the coming years).
- To enable students to learn and present their knowledge in a format that is easy to appreciate and assess during an examination.

I am certain that this edition will be more useful and convenient when compared to earlier ones and will find greater acceptability among the undergraduate pathology students.

I would be grateful for any criticism or suggestions, which would help make this book better in any way. Suggestions and comments from teachers and students can be e-mailed at gtka0612@gmail.com.

Geetika Khanna Bhattacharya

Preface to the First Edition

As an examiner and teacher, one often encounters students who have read extensively and have grasped the basic concepts of pathology from their textbooks, but are unable to organize or prioritize this succinctly into the type of answers the examiners expect and appreciate, thus, preventing them from achieving good results/scores in their assessments. The need for a revision or reference manual, which enables students to understand the nuances of key principles of pathology and express them efficiently in the limited time that is usually available to them, thus became obvious.

This book has been written with the following objectives:

- To allow a quick self-assessment and revision before the examination.
- To highlight the areas that need focus (must know areas) and are relevant to the student from both knowledge and examination point of view. (The areas covered in this book are the ones that are frequently referred to/stressed upon by examiners. Also, proficiency in these topics will aid the students in understanding their clinical subjects in the coming years.)
- To enable students to learn and present their knowledge in a format that is easy to appreciate and assess, in the limited time available, during an examination. This book has been primarily written for the discerning undergraduate (MBBS, BDS and Nursing); however, some topics are covered more extensively, and may benefit the postgraduate as well. I welcome any criticism and suggestions that would contribute towards the enhancement of this book.

Geetika Khanna Bhattacharya
Professor, Pathology
CIO Laboratory,
Vardhman Mahavir Medical College (VMMC) and
Safdarjung Hospital
New Delhi, India

Acknowledgements

I am immensely humbled by the enthusiastic reception of the earlier editions of this title. Making a book like this is a labour of love, and its veritable acceptance is heart-warming. I am forever grateful to my students for their overwhelming response, their insights and suggestions, all of which I have tried to incorporate into this new and improved edition.

I would not have been able to complete this arduous project without the tremendous patience of my daughter, who has designed the cover of the book and contributed to the illustration process of the figures in it. I am also thankful for the valued support and guidance of my husband, the blessings of my mother, and the constant encouragement and motivation bestowed upon me, by my brother.

I would like to offer my sincere appreciation to my friends, particularly Dr Sonal Sharma, for her constant and generous help. Big thanks to Dr Sumathi Muralidhar and Dr Amita Malik for contributing to the images and to my departmental staff for their unquestioning support and cooperation.

I am extremely thankful to my publisher, RELX India Pvt. Ltd., particularly Arvind Koul (Content Strategist), Shabina Nasim (Head of Content Project Management) and Goldy Bhatnagar (Content Project Manager), for overseeing this project with great commitment and efficiency while also continuing to concede to request for changes and amendments till the very last minute. As always, it has been an absolute pleasure working with them. A special shout out to Goldy Bhatnagar, for all the late nights she kept to maintain the timeline despite several roadblocks. But most importantly, I continue to be indebted to the authors of the various publications and reference books that have contributed to taking the science forward and that I have consulted during the compilation of this book. I regret being unable to acknowledge them all, individually.

Contents

SECTION I

GENERAL PATHOLOGY

Cellular Responses to Injury

1

Q. Define pathology. (PA1.1, 1.2)

Ans. Pathology is the branch of medical science that deals with the study of morphologic (structural) changes caused by disease in cells, tissues, organs, body fluids or whole body (autopsy pathology). It is derived from the words logos (study) and pathos (suffering) and is concerned with the study of the nature and causes of diseases. Diseases may, in turn, be defined as an abnormal variation in structure or function of any part of the body.

Q. Describe the history and evolution of pathology. (PA1.3)

Ans. Historical perspectives of pathology:

- **Hippocrates (460–370 BC)** considered the **father of modern medicine**, was a major influence on Greek and later Roman medical evolution. He proposed the 'humoural theory' of disease (also called the 'doctrine of four humours'), which assumed that health in a human body was the consequence of balance between these four humours (blood, phlegm, black bile and yellow bile) and the external environment. Any disturbance in this balance would result in disease. Hippocrates gave a fairly accurate description of pathological conditions such as wound healing, tumours, haemorrhoids, malaria and tuberculosis.
- **Cornelius Celsus (about 30BC–38 AD),** was a well-read literary figure, who though not a physician, authored '*De Re Medicina*', which was considered one of the best sources of medical knowledge in the Roman world.
- **Galen (129–201 AD),** while carrying out dissection of animals (pigs and monkeys), came to realize the importance of structures such as the recurrent nerve and the urinary system. He was the first to describe the 'crab-like growth of cancer' and 'bloodletting'. Although still disputed, he is thought to have added a 'fifth sign of inflammation', namely 'loss of function'.
- **Avicenna (980–1037 AD)** was a physician whose major work the 'Canon Medicinae' was based on the doctrines of Galen and Aristotle, and remained until the fifteenth century the best single work in medicine.
- **Bologna** carried out post mortem dissections as early as **1270 AD** for the purpose of understanding normal human anatomy and pathology of disease. Dissections became increasingly common in the coming centuries mostly attempting to substantiate the theories of Galen.
- At the end of the fifteenth century, the Florentine physician, **Antonio Benivieni (1443–1502)**, described the findings of some of the autopsies he performed on his patients. His findings were published in ***'De Abditis Nonnullis ac Mirandis Morborum et Sanationum Causis'*** (About the Hidden Causes of Disease).
- **Giovanni Morgagni (1682–1771)** described the findings of more than 600 autopsies, and methodically correlated his pathological findings with the clinical features exhibited by the patients prior to their demise. His works were published in 1761.
- Almost 20,000 autopsies were performed by Viennese pathologist **Carl Rokitansky (1804–78)** who is also said to have supervised an additional 60,000, in his lifetime.
- **Jean Fernel (1497–1558)** classified diseases into 'general' and 'special' He was the first to summarize the signs and symptoms of individual diseases, as we do to presently. He also diagnosed at autopsy a case of acute appendicitis, and was one of the first to suggest the syphilitic origin of some aneurysms.
- **William Harvey (1578–1657)** explained the circulation of blood and the function of the heart and made important observations on ventricular rupture and left-sided hypertrophy in a patient with aortic valve insufficiency.
- **Antony van Leeuwenhoek (1632–1723),** was a Dutch scientist commonly known as the 'Father of Microbiology'. He is best known for his contributions towards the microscopy and microbiology. He was the first to observe and describe single celled organisms.
- The invention of the first real microscope only took place in the 16–17th century by **Rudolf Virchow (1821–1902),** generally recognized to be the father of microscopic pathology, realized the importance of microscopy in pathology and used it extensively in his autopsies.
- Over a period of time, development of technology has led to introduction of new research techniques, such as electron microscopy, immunological techniques (immunohistochemistry and immunofluorescence) and molecular pathology, which have lead to expansion of pathology into a subject with many sub-specialties and branches.

Q. Define and classify disease.

Ans. Disease is defined as the state in which an individual exhibit anatomical, functional, or biochemical deviation from normal. Based on origin, a disease may be classified as follows:

1. **Developmental**
   (a) Genetic
   (b) Congenital

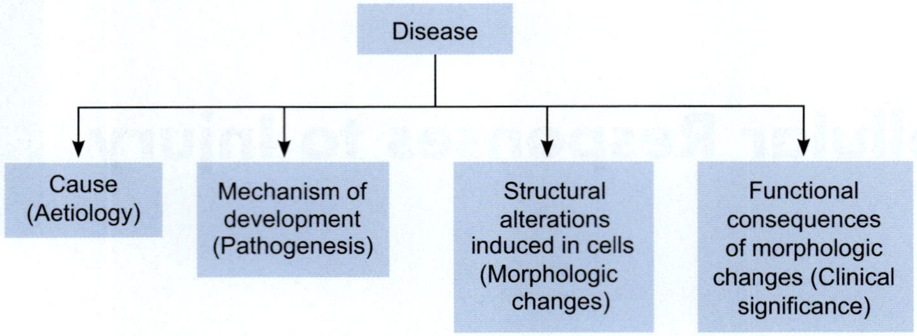

Flowchart 1.1 Four major aspects of a disease that form the core of pathology.

2. **Acquired**
   - (a) Inflammatory: Infectious or immune in origin.
   - (b) Neoplastic: Benign and malignant (cancerous) tumours.
   - (c) Degenerative: Ageing and wear- and tear-related diseases.
   - (d) Metabolic: Diseases related to metabolic disorders.
   - (e) Iatrogenic: Induced by therapy, for example drugs, radiation, etc.

Q. What are the four aspects of a disease that form the core of pathology? (PA1.1, 1.2)

Ans. A disease is studied under the following four headings (Flowchart 1.1).

1. **Aetiology:** This means the 'cause of the disease'. When the cause of a disease is known it is called **primary aetiology;** in case it is unknown it is called **idiopathic**. There are two major classes of **aetiologic factors: genetic** and **acquired**. The latter includes infectious, nutritional, chemical, physical, etc. A large number of diseases are multifactorial in origin.
2. **Pathogenesis:** Pathogenesis means the underlying mechanisms through which the cause operates to produce the pathological and clinical manifestations. It depicts the sequence of events that occur in the cell/tissue after the initial exposure to the injurious agent to the development of the signs and symptoms. In the present scenario 'pathogenesis' gives us information on how the disease evolves at the cellular or molecular level and therefore aids in deciding the therapeutic targets and modalities.
3. **Morphologic changes:** These include the structural alterations in cells or tissues that occur following the disease. The structural changes in the organ can be seen with the naked eye or only under the microscope. Those changes that can be seen with the naked eye are called **gross morphologic changes** and those that are seen under the microscope are called **microscopic changes**.
4. **Functional derangements and clinical significance:** The morphologic changes in the tissue influence its normal function. The change in normal or physiologic functions determines the clinical features (symptoms and signs).

Q. Enumerate and write briefly on different branches of pathology. (PA1.1, 1.2)

Ans. Pathology is a diverse field of medicine with several subareas or branches (Flowchart 1.2). These include:

1. **General pathology:** This deals with understanding of the general mechanisms of injury in cells and tissues, as well as the body's responses to these injurious stimuli. This includes cellular adaptation to injury, necrosis, inflammation, wound healing and neoplasia. General pathology is a broad term that encompasses both **anatomical** and **clinical** pathology.
   - (a) **Anatomical pathology:** Anatomic pathology is a specialty that is concerned with the study of changes in the structure of tissues and organs as a consequence of disease. This includes the study of biopsy specimens (biopsy pathology) as well as postmortem examination (autopsy pathology). A tissue diagnosis is an essential prerequisite prior to starting treatment protocols involving surgery and/or radiation and/or drugs. Anatomic pathology is itself divided into the following sub specialties:
     - (i) **Surgical pathology:** The essential components of surgical pathology include:
       - ***Gross examination:*** Naked eye examination of diseased tissues, sometimes aided with a magnifying glass. Gross examination includes examination of the **weight, size, shape, colour, consistency, texture surface and edges/margins of the lesion.**
       - ***Microscopic examination:*** Also called 'histopathological examination', its methodology involves processing of tissue to prepare sections, which are then stained and examined under the microscope (***histochemistry***). ***Immunohistochemistry*** is a specialized histopathological technique in which antibodies are used for localization of specific proteins to aid to the diagnosis and classification of cancers. ***Molecular pathology techniques*** also contribute to diagnosing diseases, both neoplastic and non-neoplastic.
     - (ii) **Cytopathology:** This branch of pathology deals with the study of dispersed cells as well as tissue fragments spread and stained on glass slides. It is based on the principle that diseased tissue (tissue affected by inflammation or neoplasia) looses intercellular cohesion leading to easy dispersion when aspirated. The main cytopathology specimens include material obtained from fine needle

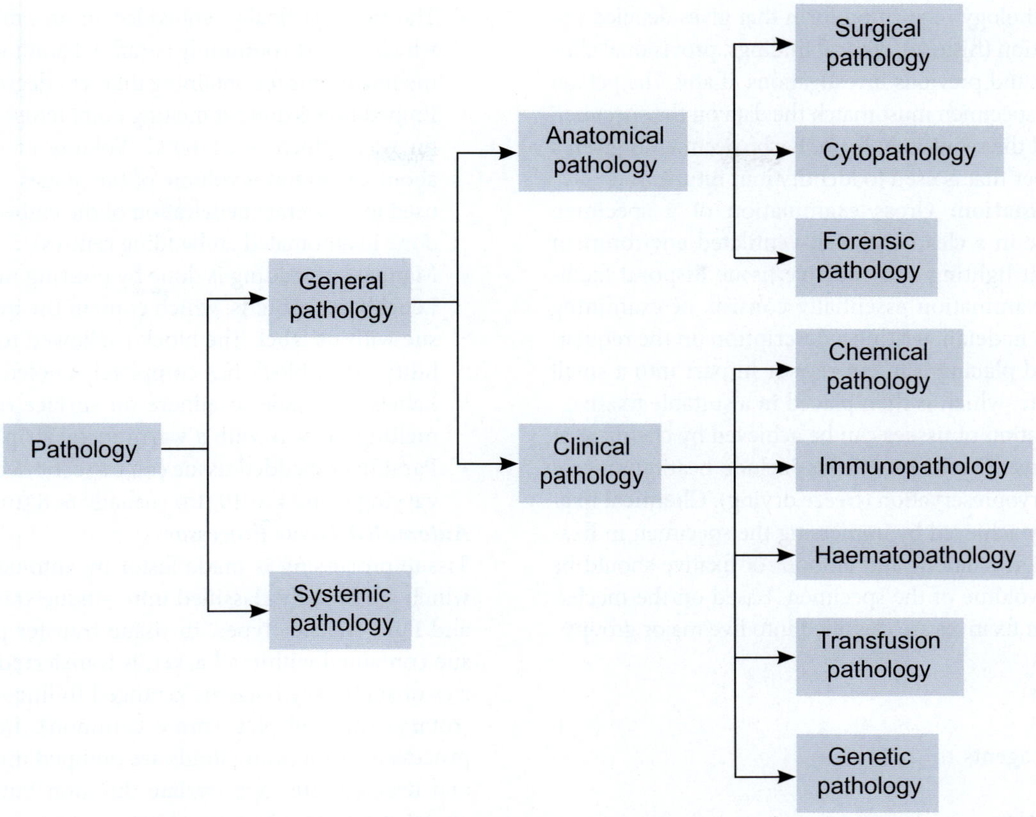

Flowchart 1.2 Branches of pathology.

aspiration (FNA) and body fluid smears (exfoliative cytology). Cytopathology is mainly used for diagnosis and prevention of cancer.

(iii) **Forensic pathology:** It is a branch of pathology concerned with determining the cause, mechanism or manner of death by means of an autopsy. The autopsy is performed by a trained pathologist who collects and examines tissue specimens to arrive at conclusions. Forensic pathologists are frequently asked to confirm the age and identity of a cadaver as well as opine regarding the cause and circumstances of death in medico legal cases.

(b) **Clinical pathology:** It involves diagnosing a disease through the laboratory analysis of bodily fluids and/or tissues. It is therefore also referred to as ***laboratory medicine.*** The main subspecialties of clinical pathology include:

(i) **Chemical pathology (clinical chemistry):** The qualitative and quantitative analysis of various components of bodily fluids such as the blood or urine, for example electrolytes, enzymes, hormones, proteins, lipids, tumour (cancer) markers and drugs (both therapeutic and illicit) is called chemical pathology.

(ii) **Immunopathology:** It refers to the study of disorders of the immune system including hypersensitivities (allergies), immunodeficiencies, autoimmunity and organ-transplant rejection.

(iii) **Haematopathology:** This entails study of diseases of blood and the approach to their diagnosis, for example anaemia, leukaemia, lymphoma, coagulation or bleeding disorders, etc.

(iv) **Transfusion medicine:** This subspeciality of pathology involves typing and compatibility testing on blood and blood products for transfusion purposes.

(v) **Genetic pathology:** This includes three main branches—***cytogenetics*** (which involves the microscopic analysis of numerical and structural chromosomal abnormalities, such as an increase or reduction in the number of chromosomes or a translocation of a part of one chromosome to another), ***molecular genetics*** (analysis of structure and function of genes at the molecular level) and ***biochemical genetics*** (evaluation of molecular aspects of genetic evolution, mutation, gene action and regulation).

2. **Systemic pathology:** Systemic pathology is concerned with the specific responses of specialized organs and tissues to abnormal stimuli. It involves the study of the cause and mechanism of development (pathogenesis) of disease, as well as the host response, specific to a particular organ system, for example cardiovascular, gastrointestinal, etc.

Q. Write briefly on the various routine and special techniques in histopathology. (PA1.1, 1.2)

Ans. Histopathological diagnosis of disease includes the following sequential steps:

1. **Specimen receiving:** All tissue specimens received in surgical pathology laboratory should be accompanied with a properly

filled histopathology requisition form that gives detailed patient information (history), clinical findings, provisional clinical diagnosis and previous investigations, if any. The person accessing the specimen must match the data on the specimen container and the requisition form. Each specimen is given a unique number that is used to identify it in future.

2. **Gross examination:** Gross examination of a specimen must be done in a clean and well-ventilated environment with sufficient lighting and effective tissue disposal facilities. Gross examination essentially consists of examining the specimen in detail, writing a description on the requisition form and placing it in entirety or in part into a small plastic cassette, which is then placed in a suitable fixative.
3. **Fixation:** Fixation of tissues can be achieved by chemical or physical means. **Physical methods** include heating, microwaving and cryopreservation (freeze drying). **Chemical fixation** is usually achieved by immersing the specimen in fixative (immersion fixation) and amount of fixative should be 10–20 times volume of the specimen. Based on the mechanism of action fixatives are classified into five major groups:
   - Aldehydes
   - Mercurials
   - Alcohols
   - Oxidizing agents
   - Picrates

   Aims of Fixation
   - Fixation confers stability to the tissue (prevents autolysis) and hardens it to enable easy handling.
   - It halts bacterial putrefaction.
   - Some fixatives enhance later staining techniques.
4. **Tissue processing**
   - In order to cut thin sections of any tissue, it should be of a particular consistency and hardness. This can be achieved by infiltrating and surrounding the tissue with a medium, which is similar in density to the tissue. Paraffin wax (a polycrystalline mixture of solid hydrocarbons produced during the refining of coal and mineral oils) is the most commonly used followed by colloidin, nitrocellulose and various types of resins. This process is called 'tissue processing' and it can be divided into various sub-stages, for example dehydration, clearing, impregnation and embedding.
   - Tissue processing can be done manually or by automation.
   - Dehydration and clearing are the most important steps in this process.
   - Tissue fixed in aqueous solutions cannot be directly infiltrated with paraffin. First, water from the tissues must be removed by dehydration. Tissue is dehydrated by using increasing strength of alcohol, for example 50%, 70%, 90% and 100%. The duration for which tissues are kept in solutions of different concentrations of alcohol varies depending on the size and type of the tissue, and the fixative used. Other dehydrants can also be used but they have some disadvantages, for example acetone is inflammable and dioxane has toxic fumes.
   - As paraffin wax is not alcohol soluble, alcohol is replaced with a substance in which wax is soluble. This step is called clearing. Agents used for clearing of tissue include xylene, chloroform, benzene, carbon tetrachloride or toluene.
   - The tissue is finally embedded in an embedding agent, which is most commonly paraffin. Paraffins have different melting points for obtaining different degrees of hardness. Embedding is done at melting point temperature of paraffin wax, which is 54–60°C. Volume of wax should be about 25–30 times volume of the tissues. Vacuum can be used to accelerate penetration of the embedding agent (as done in automated embedding centres).
   - Manual embedding is done by pouring molten wax into Leuckhart's moulds, which contain the impregnated tissue with its label. The block is allowed to settle and solidify. After block has completely cooled it is trimmed. Labels are made to adhere on surface of the block by melting the wax with a warm metal strip.
   - Paraffin embedded tissue can be sectioned at a thickness varying from 4 to 10 μm (usually 6–8 μm).

   Automated Tissue Processor

   Tissue processing is made faster by automated machines, which are broadly classified into—tissue-transfer (Fig. 1.1) and fluid-transfer types. In tissue-transfer processors, tissue contained within a basket, is transferred through a series of stationary reagents arranged in line or in a circular (rotary) carousel plan (more common). In fluid-transfer processors, processing fluids are pumped into the chamber and drained after appropriate duration but the tissue remains stationary. Agitation hastens processing.
5. **Sectioning**: Once the tissue has been embedded, it must be cut into sections with appropriate thickness (ensuring that only a single layer of cells makes up the section). This is achieved with an instrument called a 'microtome'. Microtomes are mechanical devices used for cutting uniform sections of tissue of desired thickness. Most frequently used microtome in histopathology laboratories is a rotary microtome (Fig. 1.2). It can cut a large number of sections at a time, particularly serial sections).

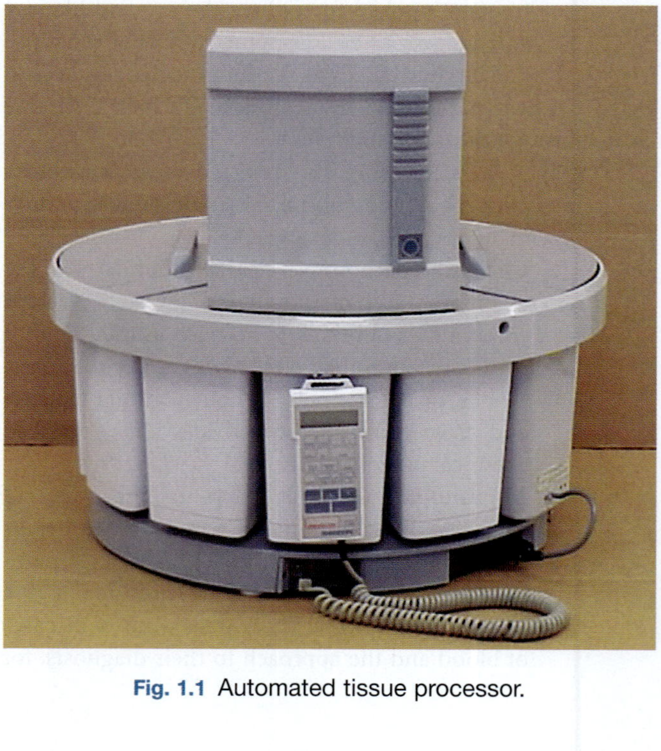

Fig. 1.1 Automated tissue processor.

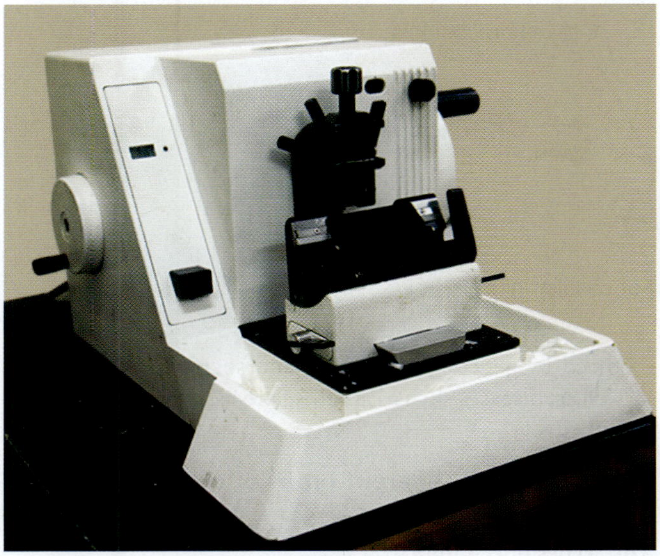

Fig. 1.2 Rotary microtome.

A diamond pencil is needed to write identification details like name or specific number. An adhesive (albumin, gelatin, starch, resin and poly-L-lysine) is smeared on to the slides so that the sections stick well to the slides. It is important to have a properly fixed and embedded block to prevent artifacts during sectioning. Common artifacts include tearing, serrations, holes, folding, etc.

6. **Staining:** Water-soluble dyes will not penetrate the sections till the paraffin wax is taken out of them. Therefore, before any staining can be done, the sections are 'deparaffinized' by running them through xylene to alcohols to water. The staining process makes use of a variety of dyes that have been chosen for their ability to stain various cellular components of tissue. The routine stain is that of haematoxylin and eosin (H&E). Other stains are referred to as 'special stains' because they are employed in specific situations according to the diagnostic need.

   Haematoxylin is a natural dye extracted by boiling wood of the logwood tree (*Haematoxylin campechianum*). It comes as a brownish tan powder, which is poorly soluble in water and somewhat more soluble in ethyl alcohol. The dye becomes active by conversion to haematin, which can be obtained by oxidizing crude haematoxylin. Oxidation can be carried out naturally by exposure to light and air for 6 weeks to several months (ripening). It can also be achieved much faster by adding a wide variety of oxidizing agents, the two most common being sodium iodate and mercuric oxide. The addition of glycerin to several formulae is said to guard against over-oxidation and to retard fungal growth.

   Eosin is red, acidic dye used to stain cell cytoplasm, collagen and muscle fibres. Structures that stain readily with eosin are termed eosinophilic. It has two main forms—Eosin Y and B, and is most often used as a counter stain to haematoxylin in haematoxylin and eosin (H&E) staining.

H&E Staining

Procedure: The first step involves staining of nuclei to a blue colour with a haematoxylin solution. The second step is counterstaining with a xanthene dye, for example eosin Y, eosin B, or erythrosin B. In this process cytoplasm, collagen, keratin and erythrocytes stain red.

Steps

- Deparaffinize sections.
- Hydrate in graded alcohols (absolute alcohol, followed by 95% and 70% alcohol).
- Wash briefly in distilled water.
- Stain in Harris haematoxylin solution for 2–5 min.
- Rinse in running tap water.
- Differentiate in 1% HCl in 70% alcohol for 30 s.
- Rinse in running tap water.
- Most haematoxylin solutions, which stain regressively, require differentiation, that is, treatment with an acid reagent to remove excess stain from tissue section. The tissue section is subsequently treated with an alkaline solution to neutralize acid and restore a blue colour to the tissue. This process is called blueing and can be achieved by treating tissue section with either ammonia vapour, 2.5% ammonium hydroxide for 2 min, running tap water for 10 min, or Scott's tap water substitute (TWS) for 2 min.
- Counterstain in eosin–phloxine B solution (or eosin Y solution) for 30 s–1 min.
- Dehydrate through 95% and absolute alcohol.
- Clear in two changes of xylene, 5 min each.
- Mount with xylene-based mounting medium.

Q. Define homeostasis.

Ans. Homeostasis (from Greek: hómoios, 'similar' and stásis,'standing still,' defined by Claude Bernard) is the property of a system, either open or closed, that regulates its internal environment and tends to maintain a stable, constant state. Human homeostasis is defined as the ability of the human cell to handle the normal physiologic demands, maintaining a steady state.

Q. Define cellular adaptation. (PA 2.6).

Ans. Excessive physiologic stress or pathologic stimuli bring about reversible functional and morphologic changes, pushing a normal cell into an altered, but steady state called cellular adaptation (Flowchart 1.3).

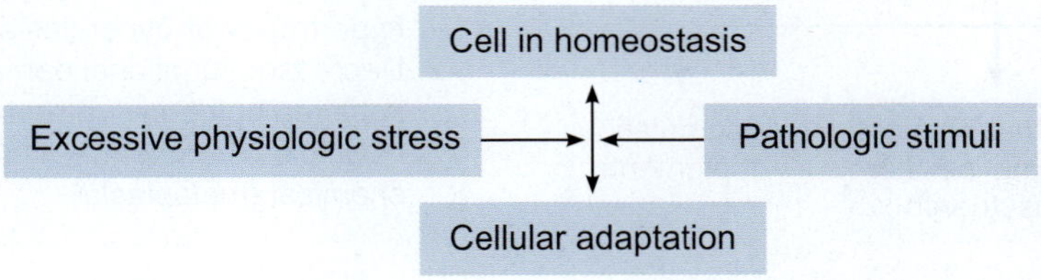

FLOWCHART 1.3 Evolution of cellular adaptation.

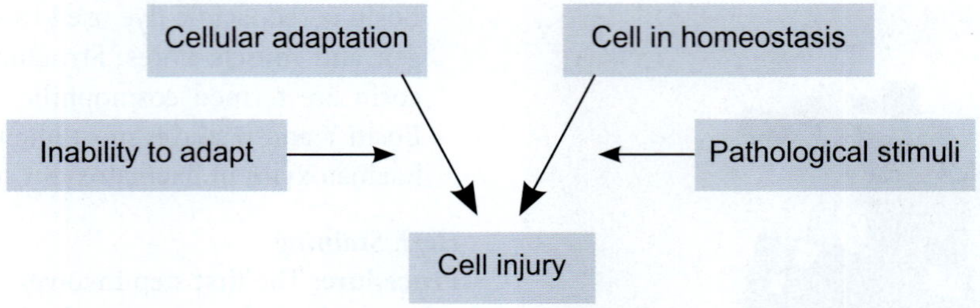

Flowchart 1.4 Evolution of cellular injury.

Q. Define cell injury. (PA2.1)

Ans. When the cell cannot adapt anymore or when the limits of adaptive response to a stimulus are exceeded, a sequence of events labelled *cell injury* follows (Flowchart 1.4).

Q. Enumerate the various cellular responses to injury. (PA2.1)

Ans. Cellular responses to injury may manifest as:

1. **Cellular adaptations:** Adaptive response may be in the form of **atrophy** (decrease in cell size and metabolic activity), **hypertrophy** (increase in size of the cell), **hyperplasia** (increase in number and functional activity of the cell), and **metaplasia** (a change in the phenotype of the cell).
2. **Cell injury:** This includes subcellular alterations (residual effects of cell injury) in various organelles due to **sublethal/chronic, reversible,** and **irreversible injury**. **Cell death** (by necrosis or apoptosis) is the result of progressive injury. Nutrient deprivation triggers an adaptive cellular response labelled **autophagy** that may also result in cell death.
3. **Intracellular accumulations (Flowchart 1.5):** Intracellular accumulations include accumulation of:
   (a) Normal cellular constituents in excess
   (b) Abnormal substances
   (c) Pigments
4. **Pathological calcification:** This refers to abnormal tissue deposition of calcium salts together with small amounts of iron, magnesium and mineral salts. There are two types of calcification—**dystrophic** and **metastatic**. The former occurs in the absence of any abnormalities in the calcium metabolism, whereas, the latter is invariably associated with hypercalcaemia.
5. **Cell ageing:** Represents progressive accumulation over the years of sublethal injury that may either lead to cell death or inadequate response of the cell to injury. Ageing is influenced by genetic factors, diet and social environment, as well as, diseases such as atherosclerosis, diabetes and osteoarthritis.

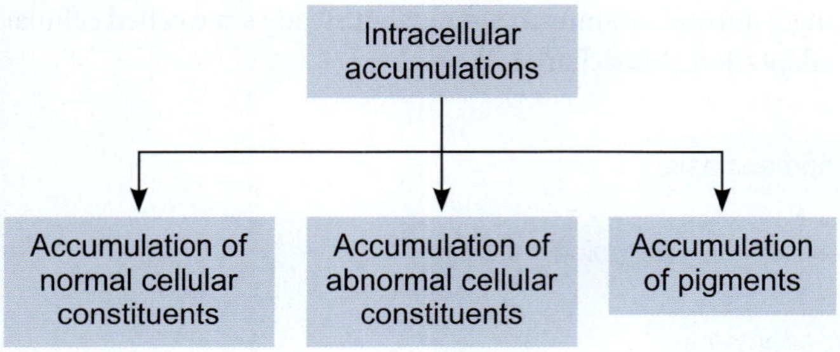

Flowchart 1.5 Intracellular accumulations.

Q. What are the different types of cell injury? (PA2.1)

Ans. Types of cell injury:

1. **Reversible**: If the structural and functional changes, induced by an injurious stimulus, *can* revert to normal on removal of the same, it is called reversible injury.
2. **Irreversible**: If the structural and functional changes, induced by an injurious stimulus, *cannot* be reversed even after removal of the same, it is called irreversible injury.

Q. Enumerate and describe in brief different types of cellular adaptations. (PA2.6)

Ans. Cellular adaptations occur as a response to persistent non-lethal injurious stimuli and may manifest as cellular hypertrophy, hyperplasia, atrophy or metaplasia (Flowchart 1.6).

Hyperplasia

Definition

Increase in number of cells in an organ or tissue leading to increased size/mass of the tissue or organ that may result in its gross enlargement (Fig. 1.3A–B). *Hyperplasia takes place in cells, which are capable of synthesizing DNA.* In non-dividing cells, only hypertrophy occurs. Hyperplasia and hypertrophy often occur together. Hyperplasia basically occurs as a result of increased recruitment of cells from G0 phase of the cell cycle. It is important to remember that unregulated and persistent hyperplasia can eventually lead to neoplasia.

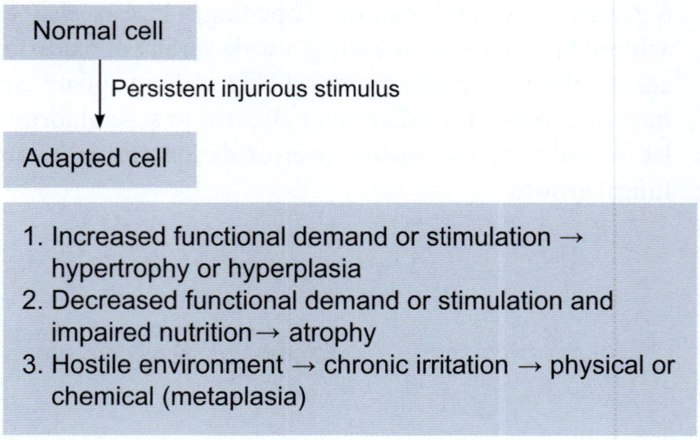

Flowchart 1.6 Adaptive responses to cell injury.

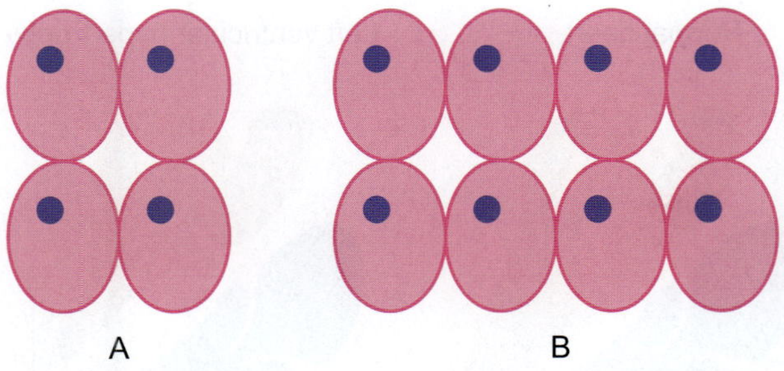

Fig. 1.3 Mechanism of hyperpasia. (A) Normal number of cells and (B) increased number of cells.

Mechanism

1. Hyperplasia occurs due to production of transcription factors that turn on cellular genes including genes encoding growth factors, receptors for growth factors, and cell cycle regulators, leading to increased local production of growth factors, increased level of growth factor receptors, and activation of intracellular signalling pathways.
2. In hormonal hyperplasia, hormones themselves act as growth factors and trigger transcription of genes.
3. In compensatory hyperplasia, there is proliferation of remaining cells and development of new cells from stem cells. Compensatory hyperplasia occurs when a part of an organ or contralateral organ is destroyed or removed, such as hyperplasia of nephrons of the other kidney which occurs following unilateral nephrectomy or regeneration of liver which occurs following partial hepatectomy.

Types

1. Physiologic hyperplasia
   (a) *Hormonal hyperplasia:* Hormonal stimulation increases the functional capacity of the tissue when needed, for example breast and uterus in puberty, pregnancy and lactation.
   (b) *Compensatory hyperplasia:* Increase in tissue mass after damage or partial resection, for example regeneration of liver after partial hepatectomy.
2. Pathologic hyperplasia: Hyperplasia due to excessive hormonal stimulation or excessive effects of growth factors on target cells, for example *endometrial hyperplasia* (occurs when balance between progesterone and oestrogen is disturbed; Fig. 1.4), *benign nodular prostatic hyperplasia* or *NHP* (occurs due to androgen excess; Fig. 1.5), epithelial hyperplasia in breast, exuberant granulation tissue formation in a wound, and pseudoeitheliomatous hyperplasia seen in non-healing ulcers.

Hypertrophy

Definition

Increase in size of the cell due to increased synthesis of structural components and not due to cellular swelling is known as hypertrophy. Non-dividing cells, for example myocardial fibres, undergo hypertrophy only. Dividing cells (stable cells, quiescent cells) undergo both hyperplasia and hypertrophy.

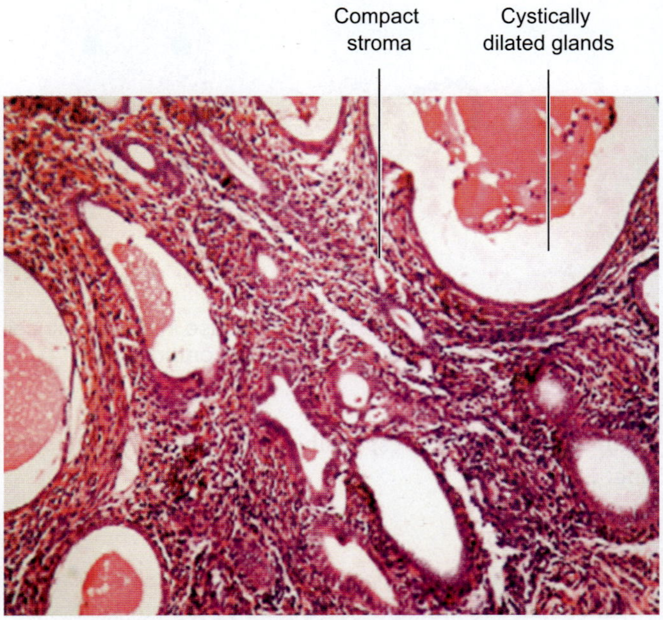

Fig. 1.4 Cystic hyperplasia endometrium showing crowded, dilated glands lined by columnar epithelium (H&E; 100×).

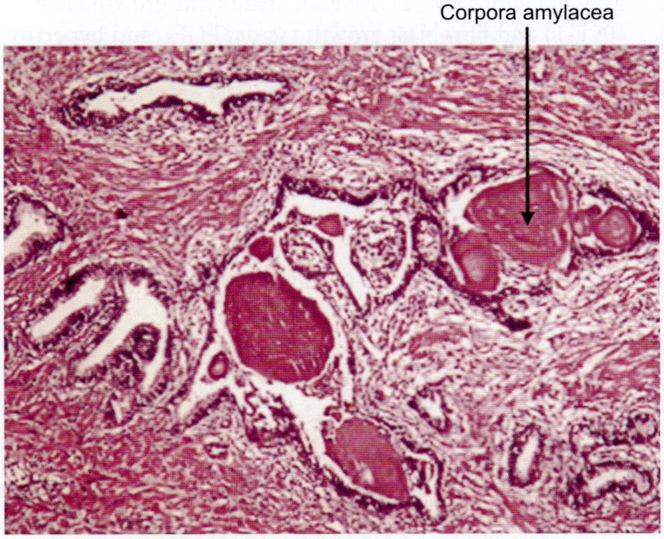

Fig. 1.5 Nodular hyperplasia prostate showing hyperplastic glands containing corpora amylacea (H&E; 100×).

Mechanism

Induction of genes stimulates synthesis of cellular proteins (Fig. 1.6A–C), for example genes encoding transcription factors, growth factors and vasoactive agents. In the heart, increased workload (mechanical stretch), growth factors (transforming growth factor-beta and Insulin-like growth factor-1) and alfa-adrenergic hormones activate signal transduction pathways (phosphoinositide-3-kinase/AKT pathway and downstream signalling of G-protein coupled receptors), which in turn activate transcription factors like GATA4 (critical transcription factor for proper mammalian cardiac development and essential for survival of the embryo), NFAT (nuclear factor of activated T cells) and MEF 2 (myocyte enhancer 2). They work together to increase

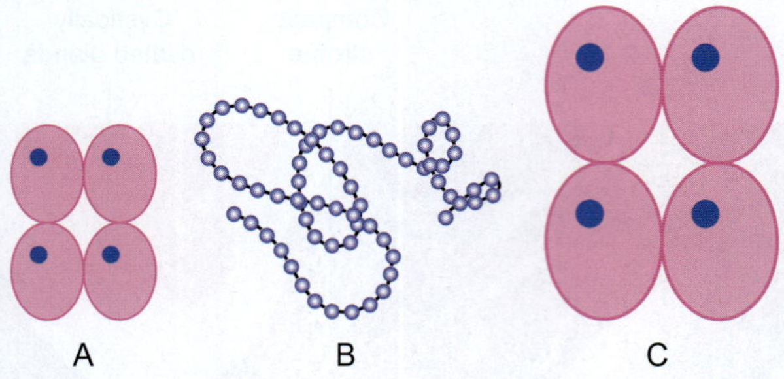

Fig. 1.6 Mechanism of hypertrophy. Increase in size of the cell due to increased synthesis of structural components.

synthesis of proteins responsible for cardiac hypertrophy (Fig. 1.7).

Types

1. *Physiological hypertrophy*: This occurs due to increased functional demand and stimulation by growth factors and hormones, for example uterine enlargement in pregnancy and breast hypertrophy during lactation.
2. *Pathological hypertrophy*: Growth factors like 'transforming growth factor-beta (TGF-beta), insulin like growth factor-1 (IGF-1) and fibroblast growth factor (FGF)' and hypertrophy agonists like 'alfa adrenergic agonists, nitric oxide, endothelin-1, angiotensin II and bradykinin' are involved in pathological hypertrophy. Examples include:
   (a) Hypertrophy of cardiac muscle in systemic hypertension and aortic valve stenosis (chronic haemodynamic overload) leading to left ventricular hypertrophy (Fig. 1.8).

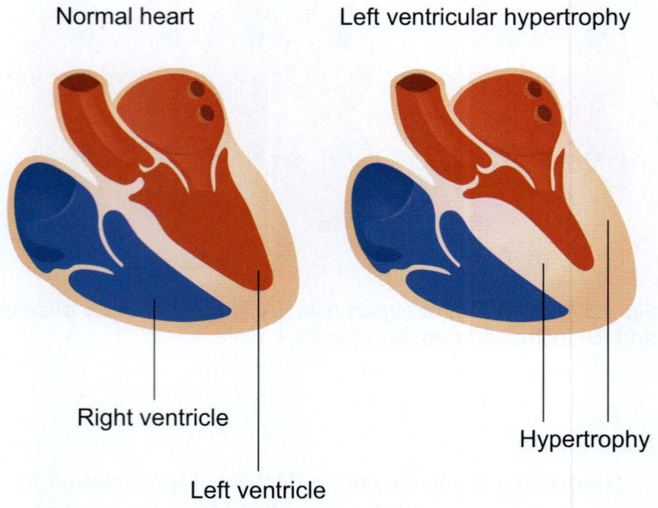

Fig. 1.8 Pathological hypertrophy left ventricle.

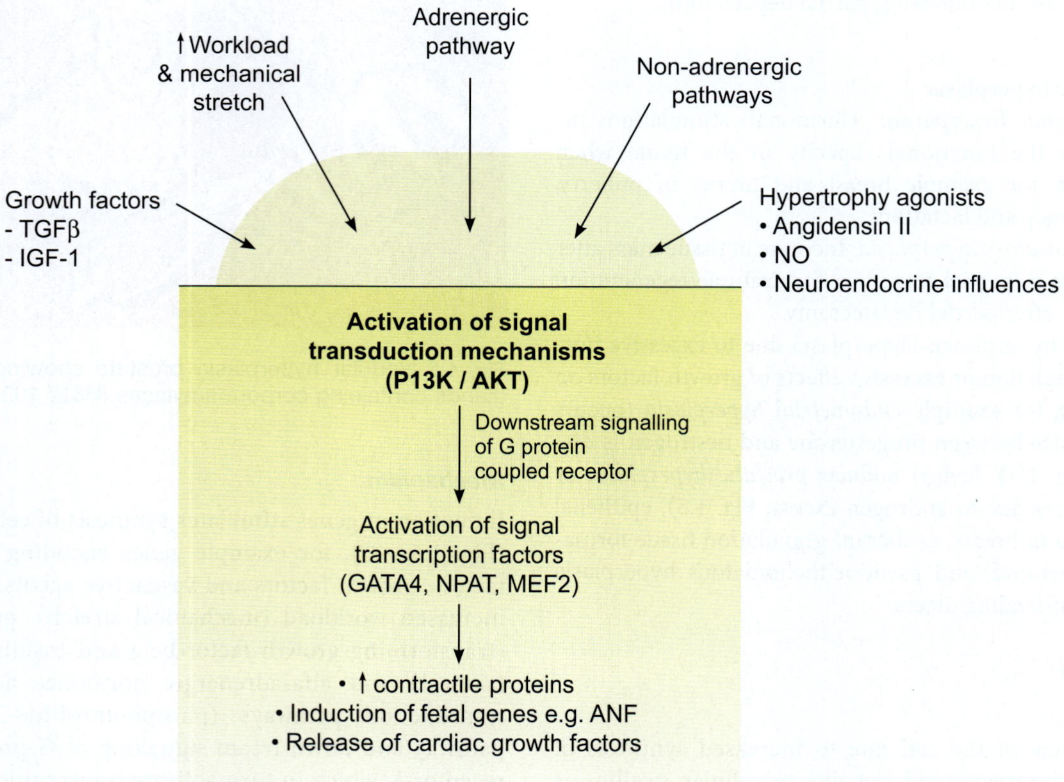

Fig. 1.7 Mechanisms of cardiac hypertrophy.

(b) Compensatory hypertrophy, which occurs when an organ or tissue is called upon to do additional work or to perform the work of destroyed tissue or of a paired organ.

Atrophy

Definition

A decrease in size of a body organ, tissue or cell along with decreased function, owing to disease, injury or lack of use.

Mechanism

Atrophy is the result of decreased protein synthesis or increased protein degradation. Protein degradation is mediated by:

- Lysosomal acid hydrolases, which degrade endocytosed proteins (taken up from extracellular environment, cell surface as well as some cellular components).
- Ubiquitin-proteasome pathway, which causes degradation of many cytosolic and nuclear proteins.

Types

1. *Physiological atrophy*: Common during early development, for example atrophy of notochord or thyroglossal duct during foetal development and uterus after parturition.
2. *Pathological atrophy*:
   (a) Decreased workload due to immobilization and prolonged functional inactivity leads to **disuse atrophy**.
   (b) Loss of innervation or denervation of muscle leading to it's wasting (**denervation atrophy**), as seen in polio and motor neuron disease (Fig. 1.9).
   (c) Diminished blood supply as seen in atherosclerosis can cause **ischaemic atrophy**.
   (d) Nutritional deficiency, for example marasmus and cancer cachexia are associated with the use of skeletal muscle as a source of energy and lead to **nutritional atrophy**.

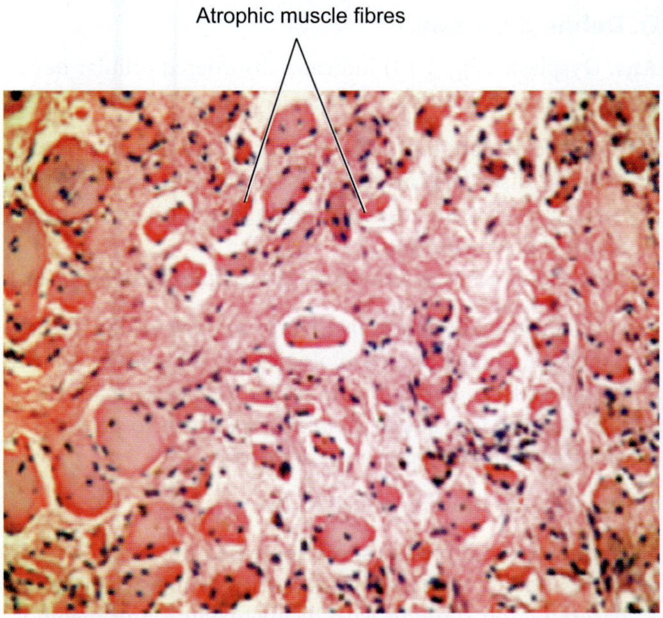

Fig. 1.9 Photomicrograph showing muscle atrophy (H&E; 100×).

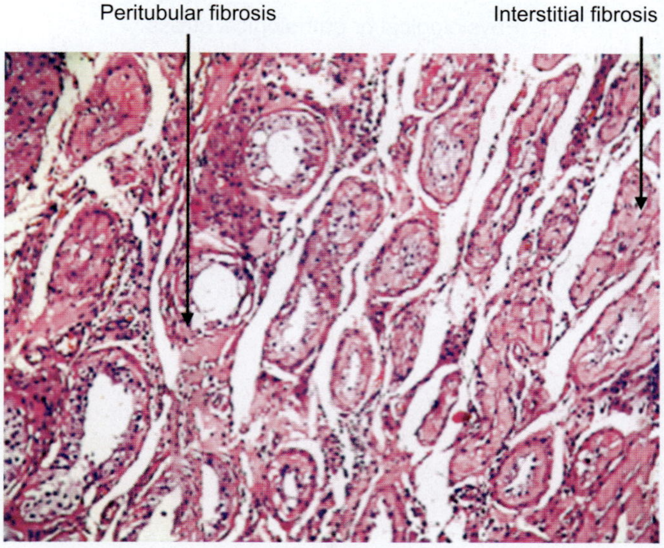

Fig. 1.10 Atrophic testis showing marked loss of germ cells within the tubules, with peritubular and interstitial fibrosis (H&E; 100×).

   (e) Loss of endocrine stimulation after menopause induces **endocrine atrophy** of reproductive organs.
   (f) **Senile atrophy** is an ageing-associated cell loss, which is typically seen in tissues containing permanent cells, for example brain and heart or testes (Fig. 1.10).
   (g) Compression as in benign tumours, cysts, etc. may cause atrophy of surrounding tissue (**pressure atrophy**).

Metaplasia

Definition

Reversible change in which there is replacement of one adult/differentiated cell type (epithelial or mesenchymal) by another adult/differentiated cell type.

Mechanism

Metaplasia usually results from reprogramming or altered differentiation of stem cells in normal epithelial tissue, or undifferentiated mesenchymal cells present in connective tissue (Fig. 1.11). The stem cells are nudged along a different pathway of differentiation by cytokines, growth factors,

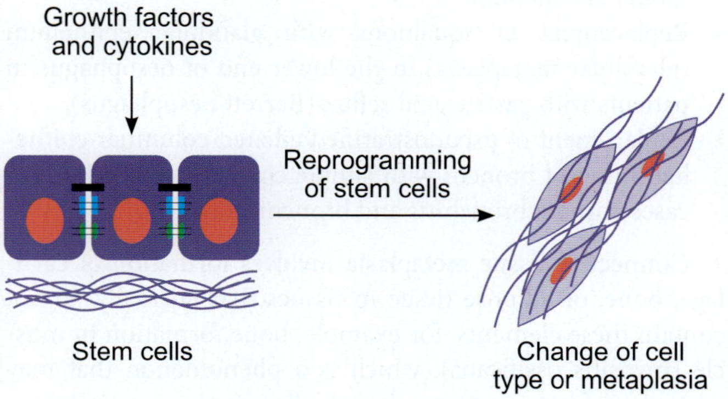

Fig. 1.11 Mechanism of metaplasia

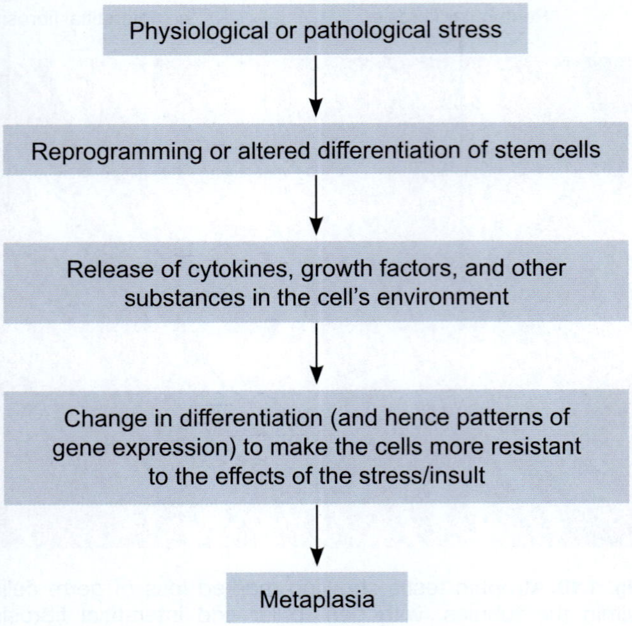

Flowchart 1.7 Evolution of metaplasia.

and other substances in the cell's environment. Such a change in differentiation (and hence patterns of gene expression) makes the cells more resistant to the effects of the insult (Flowchart 1.7). It is usually a reversible phenomenon. Metaplasia can be epithelial or connective tissue (mesenchymal).

Examples of Metaplasia

Epithelial metaplasia is more common than connective tissue metaplasia. The following are the examples of epithelial metaplasia:

- Columnar to squamous change (squamous metaplasia) in respiratory tract in response to chronic irritation (smoking) and vitamin A deficiency.
- Squamous metaplasia of the endocervical mucosa (Fig. 1.12 A and B) due to chronic infection or irritation (prolapse of the uterus).
- Squamous metaplasia of the columnar epithelial cells of salivary gland ducts due to stones.
- Squamous metaplasia of the transitional epithelium of the bladder due to stones or infection with the parasite *Schistosoma haematobium.*
- Replacement of squamous with glandular epithelium (glandular metaplasia) in the lower end of oesophagus in patients with gastric acid reflux (Barrett oesophagus).
- Replacement of pseudostratified ciliated columnar epithelial lining of bronchi with simple columnar epithelium in cases chronic bronchitis and bronchiectasis.

Connective tissue metaplasia involves formation of cartilage, bone, or adipose tissue in tissues that normally do not contain these elements, for example, bone formation in muscle (myositis ossificans), which is a phenomenon that may occur after fractures. Osseous metaplasia is also seen in laryngeal and bronchial cartilage of the elderly.

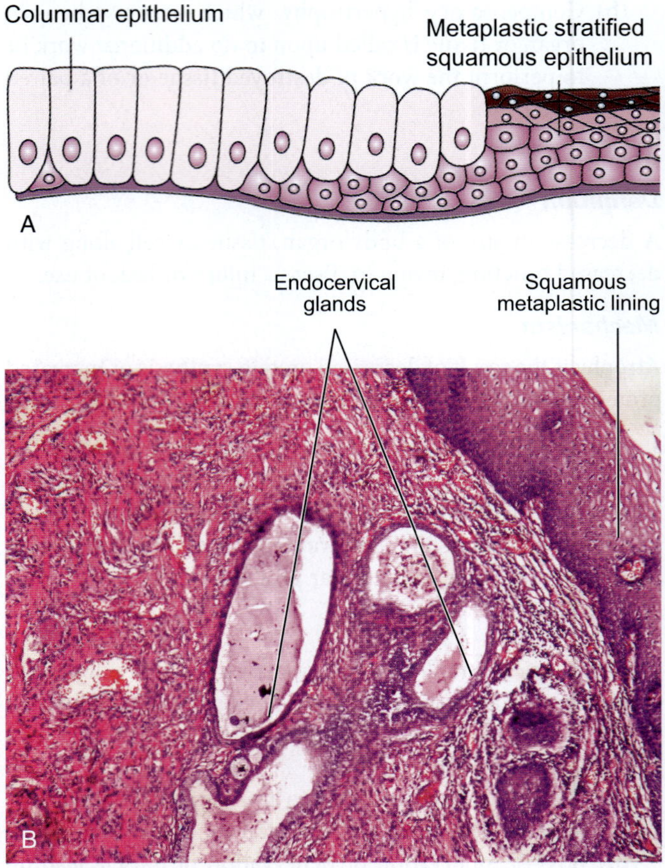

Fig. 1.12 (A) Schematic representation of squamous metaplasia in endocervical mucosa. (B). Photomicrograph from cervix showing squamous metaplasia of the endocervical mucosa (H&E; 100×).

Note: The factors that predispose to metaplasia, if persistent, may eventually lead to induction of cancer in metaplastic epithelium, eg, metaplasia from squamous to columnar epithelium in *Barrett's oesophagus may progress to adenocarcinoma oesophagus.*

Q. Define dysplasia.

Ans. Dysplasia (Fig. 1.13) indicates disordered cellular development characterized by:

- Loss of orientation of cells with respect to one another, for example disorderly arrangement of the cells from basal to surface layer as in stratified squamous epithelium ***(architectural disorientation).***
- Lack of uniformity of individual cells ***(cellular pleomorphism).***

Dysplasia is usually caused by diverse cellular insults, including physical, chemical, and biological. It is typically seen in epithelial cells and may be reversible (at least in its early/milder stage). More severe dysplasia is known to progress to carcinoma in situ and invasive carcinoma.

Dysplastic cells are characterized by:

- Accelerated cell proliferation (increased mitoses).
- Nuclear abnormalities, such as hyperchromasia (increased basophilia on staining with haematoxylin), and pleomorphism (altered nuclear size and nuclear shape).

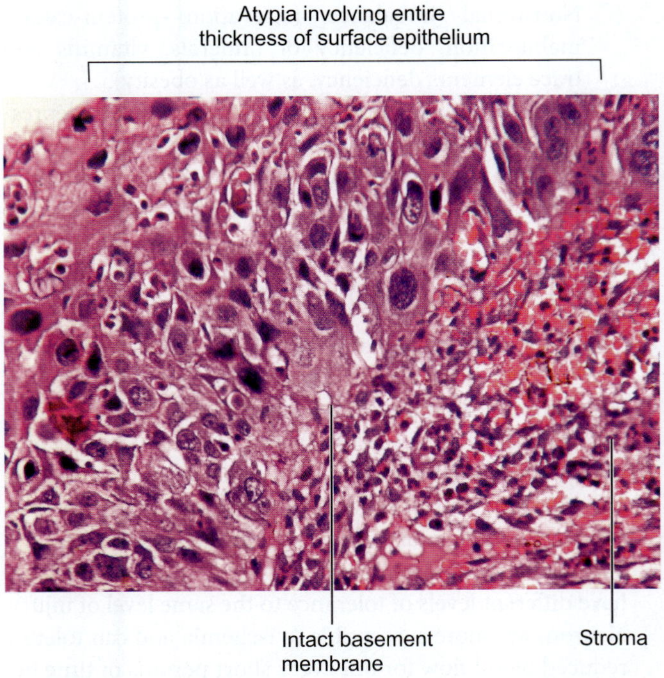

Fig. 1.13 Stratified squamous epithelium showing severe dysplastic changes (H&E; 200×). The epithelium shows diffuse atypia and loss of maturation.

- Increased nuclear cytoplasmic ratio.
- Loss of polarity and disorderly arrangement of cells from basal to surface layer in stratified epithelium.

Dysplasia is the earliest recognized form of a precancerous lesion. It can be low grade or high grade depending on the cellular and architectural features. Low-grade dysplasia (atypical cells involve one-third thickness from the basal layer to the surface layer) is low risk and rarely transforms into high-grade dysplasia, or frank malignancy. High-grade dysplasia (atypical cells involve two-third thickness from the basal layer to the surface layer) carries a higher risk for progression toward malignant transformation.

Carcinoma in situ, literally means 'cancer in place'. It indicates that the entire thickness of the epithelium is showing dysplastic changes; however, the lesion is still localized and has not invaded past the basement membrane into the subepthelial stroma (Fig. 1.14).

Invasive carcinoma is the final step in this sequence. It indicates that the malignant cells have invaded beyond the basement membrane and have the potential to metastasize (spread to other parts of the body).

In 1988, the Bethesda system (TBS) was introduced by the National Cancer Society (NCI) of the United States for reporting Papanicoloau smears (cervical and vaginal cytology). The recommendations were subsequently revised in 1991 and 2001. TBS recommended a 2-tiered reporting system for squamous intraepithelial lesions (SILs): low-grade SIL (LSIL) and high-grade SIL (HSIL) taking into account the role of human papilloma virus in cervical cancer. It also introduced TBS terminology of 'atypical squamous cells of undetermined significance' (ASCUS) and 'atypical glandular cells of undetermined significance' (AGUS). A diagnosis of 'LSIL or LGSIL' indicates mild dysplasia (cervical intraepithelial neoplasia or CIN 1), more than likely caused by a human papilloma progresses to HSIL or invasive malignancy. Therefore, most cases of LSIL results can be managed with a simple 'watch and wait' policy. In the cases with a likelihood of progression to more severe dysplasia, the lesion is managed more aggressively by performing a colposcopy with biopsy. Treatment involves removal of the affected tissue, which can be accomplished by loop electrosurgical excision procedure (LEEP), cryosurgery, cone biopsy, or laser ablation.

'High-grade squamous intraepithelial lesion (HSIL or HGSIL)' indicates moderate or severe cervical intraepithelial neoplasia (corresponding to CIN 2 or 3 or carcinoma in situ). In some cases these lesions can lead to invasive cervical cancer, if not followed and treated appropriately (about 20%). Thus HSIL must be followed by an immediate colposcopy with biopsy to sample or remove the dysplastic tissue. HSIL treatment involves the removal of the affected cells by LEEP, cryotherapy, cautery, or laser ablation.

Q. Differentiate between metaplasia and dysplasia.

Ans. Differences between metaplasia and dysplasia are shown in Table 1.1.

Q. Write briefly on aetiopathogenesis and biochemical basis of cell injury. (PA2.1, 2.2)

Ans. Cell injury includes subcellular alterations (residual effects of cell injury) in various organelles due to sublethal or chronic, reversible, as well as irreversible injury. Progressive

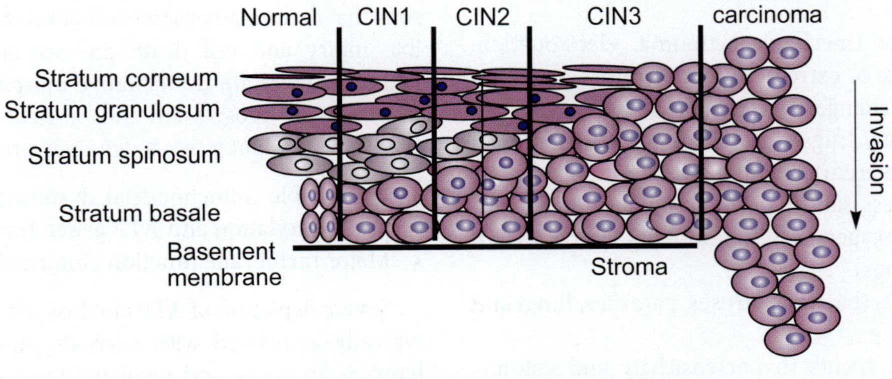

Fig. 1.14 Spectrum of histopathological changes in dysplasia.

Table 1.1 Differences between metaplasia and dysplasia

Features	Metaplasia	Dysplasia
Definition	Replacement of one adult epithelial or mesenchymal cell type by another	Disordered cellular development characterized by: 1. Loss of orientation of cells with respect to one another 2. Lack of uniformity of individual cells
Types	Squamous, columnar (epithelial) and osseous, cartilaginous (mesenchymal)	Epithelial only
Cellular pleomorphism	Mature cellular development; no pleomorphism	Disordered cellular development due to aberrant/delayed maturation or differentiation; pleomorphism present
Natural history	Reversible on withdrawal of stimulus	May regress on withdrawal of inciting stimulus or progress to higher grades of dysplasia or carcinoma in situ

injury eventually leads to cell death (by necrosis or apoptosis). Nutrient deprivation triggers an adaptive cellular response labelled autophagy that may also result in cell death.

Causes of Cell Injury

Cell injury can result due to the following causes:

1. **Genetic:**
   (a) Development defects (errors in morphogenesis).
   (b) Cytogenetic defects (chromosomal abnormalities).
   (c) Single gene defects (Mendelian disorders).
   (d) Multifactorial inheritance disorders.
2. **Acquired:**
   (a) Hypoxia/ischaemia (deficiency of oxygen due to impaired or obstructed blood supply, decreased oxygen carrying capacity of red cells as in blood loss, anaemia, carbon monoxide poisoning, heart disease, lung abnormalities). Chronic hypoxia leads to cellular adaptive response like atrophy whereas acute hypoxia leads to cell injury usually leading to cell death.
   (b) Physical agents (mechanical trauma, electrocution, thermal damage or extremes of temperature, radiation injury, sudden changes in atmospheric pressure).
   (c) Chemical agents/drugs (insecticides, pesticides, arsenic, asbestos, mercury, cyanide, acids and alkalis, air pollutants, excess salt, hypertonic glucose, high concentrations of oxygen, alcohol, smoking, narcotics and therapeutic drugs).
   (d) Microbial agents (bacteria, viruses, parasites, fungi and rickettsiae).
   (e) Immunological agents (hypersensitivity and autoimmunity).
   (f) Nutritional imbalance (starvation—protein-calorie malnutrition, deficiency of minerals, vitamins and trace elements deficiency, as well as obesity).
   (g) Psychological factors (mental stress, anxiety, depression, schizophrenia, psychosis, neurosis).
   (h) Idiopathic (cause of injury is unknown).
   (i) Ageing (impaired ability of cells to replicate and repair).

Mechanism of Cell Injury

The cellular responses to pathological stimuli depend on:

- Type, duration and severity of injury: Cellular responses may vary depending on the degree of insult and its duration. Small doses of an injurious stimulus like a chemical toxin or brief periods of reduced blood supply may induce reversible injury, whereas large doses of the same or more prolonged ischemia might result either in instantaneous cell death or in slow, irreversible injury ultimately leading to cell death.
- Type, status and adaptability of target cell: Different tissues have different levels of tolerance to the same level of injury. Neurons are more susceptible to ischemia and can tolerate reduced blood flow for only very short periods of time before they are damaged irreversibly. On the other hand, muscle cells can survive without any morphological changes with similar deprivation. The cell's nutritional and hormonal status and its metabolic needs are important in its response to injury. Genetic variations affecting the activity of hepatic enzymes that convert chemicals and drugs to toxic by-products may affect the response of cells to them. This forms the basis for identifying genetic polymorphisms that affect the cell's response to injurious agents.

Targets of Injurious Stimuli

The most important targets of injurious stimuli are:

(a) *Aerobic* respiration [involving mitochondrial oxidative phosphorylation and production of adenosine triphosphate (ATP)]
(b) *Cell membrane*
(c) *Protein synthesis*
(d) *Cytoskeleton*
(e) *Genetic apparatus*

The cellular alterations associated with reversible injury mostly revert back to normal, if the injurious stimulus abates. Sustained or severe injury, however, causes cells to reach a 'point of no return', that is, 'irreversible injury' and 'cell death'. The reasons that determine progression of reversible injury to irreversible injury and cell death are not adequately understood. Although there are no definitive morphologic or biochemical indicators of progression into a state of irreversibility, two events are thought to most definitely predict irreversibility:

- Irreversible mitochondrial dysfunction (lack of oxidative phosphorylation and ATP generation).
- Major membrane function abnormality.

Severe depletion of ATP and loss of membrane integrity are typically associated with necrosis. Apoptosis, on the other hand, is an active and regulated process not associated with ATP depletion.

Role of Mitochondria in Cell Injury

Mitochondria are responsible for cellular respiration and the production of ATP which in turn is responsible for vital functions of the cell including:

1. Maintenance of cellular osmolarity
2. Membrane transport
3. Protein synthesis

Biochemical Basis of Cell Injury

Cell injury leads to the following biochemical changes:

1. ***ATP depletion:*** ATP is generated in two ways:
   (a) Oxidative phosphorylation of ADP in mitochondria (major pathway).
   (b) Glycolysis (generation of ATP in the absence of oxygen using glucose derived from glycogen).

   ATP is required for:
   (i) Membrane transport
   (ii) Protein synthesis
   (iii) Lipogenesis
   (iv) Phospholipid turnover

   ATP depletion results in dysfunction of all of the aforementioned mechanisms. There is deranged activity of the energy-dependent sodium pump responsible for membrane transport, which results in increase in intracellular sodium and efflux of potassium. This sodium gain is accompanied by iso-osmotic gain of water, which causes cellular swelling and dilatation of endoplasmic reticulum (ER). To compensate for the ATP depletion, there is an increase in anaerobic glycolysis in an attempt to maintain the cell's energy sources. This results in depletion of intracellular glycogen stores and lactic acid accumulation, which in turn leads to decreased intracellular pH and reduced activity of many cellular enzymes.
2. ***Oxygen and oxygen-derived free radical-mediated damage:*** Reactive oxygen species (ROS) are chemically active species containing oxygen. Examples include peroxides, superoxide, hydroxyl radical and singlet oxygen. ROS are normally formed as a natural by-product of metabolism of oxygen. Environmental stress (e.g. UV or heat exposure) or other injurious stimuli, however, causes marked increase in ROS levels, which can result in damage to the cell. Cumulatively, this is known as **'oxidative stress'.**
3. ***Loss of calcium homeostasis:*** Normal cytosolic free calcium levels are very low, and most intracellular calcium is sequestered in the ER and mitochondria. Cell injury leads to failure of the Ca^{2+} pump, which results in influx of Ca^{2+} across cell membrane, and increased release of calcium from mitochondria and endoplasmic reticulum. Increased cytosolic calcium causes activation of numerous cellular enzymes (phospholipases, proteases, endonuclease and caspases). Mitochondrial damage also accelerates generation of ROS as well as formation of permeability transition pores in the mitochondrial membrane. The latter causes loss of mitochondrial membrane potential and pH changes which lead to further depletion of ATP and eventually cellular necrosis. Also, there is leakage of mitochondrial pro-apoptotic proteins and Cytochrome C and into the cytosol, which initiates apoptosis.

Q. Describe the sequence of events occurring in reversible and irreversible injury. (PA2.1)

Ans: Cell injury is of the following types:

1. ***Reversible:***
   (a) If the structural and functional changes, induced by an injurious stimulus, can revert back to normal on removal of the same, it is called reversible injury (Flowchart 1.8A).
   (b) The hallmarks of reversible injury are decreased oxidative phosphorylation, ATP depletion, and cellular swelling caused by changes in ion concentrations and water influx.
   (c) It is histologically characterized by pallor, hydropic change, vacuolar degeneration, plasma membrane blebbing and blunting, villous distortion, accumulation of myelin figures, mitochondrial swelling, distortion of microvilli, loosening of intercellular attachments, dilatation of the endoplasmic reticulum, and nuclear disaggregation.
   (d) Examples of reversible cell injury include cloudy swelling, vacuolar degeneration, hydropic and fatty change.
2. ***Irreversible:***
   (a) If the structural and functional changes, induced by an injurious stimulus, cannot be reversed even after removal of the same, it is called irreversible injury (Flowchart 1.8 B).
   (b) If the damage persists, the injury becomes irreversible and may progress to cell death. Irreversible injury is histologically characterized by further mitochondrial and ER swelling followed by lysis, dispersal and destruction of ribosomes, defects in protein synthesis, cytoskeletal, and DNA damage.
   (c) Due to low oxygen levels there is a decrease in the aerobic respiration and the cell switches to anaerobic respiration (glycolytic pathway) for generation of ATP, which leads to depletion of glycogen and increase in lactic acid.
   (d) Depleted levels of ATP also interfere with generation of phospholipids from cellular fatty acids, which are necessary for repair and regeneration of the plasma membrane. There is leakage of enzymes across the damaged plasma membrane and lysosomal membranes.
   (e) Extracellular calcium enters the cell and intracellular calcium stores are released, resulting in the activation of catabolic enzymes. Further damage to cell membrane takes place and there is continued loss of proteins, essential coenzymes, and ribonucleic acids from the hyper-permeable plasma membrane. Loss of metabolites essential for ATP generation further depletes ATP levels.

Essential differences between reversible and irreversible injury are tabulated in Table 1.2. Sequence of events occurring in reversible and irreversible injury has been depicted in Flowcharts 1.8 A–B, and Fig. 1.15, respectively.

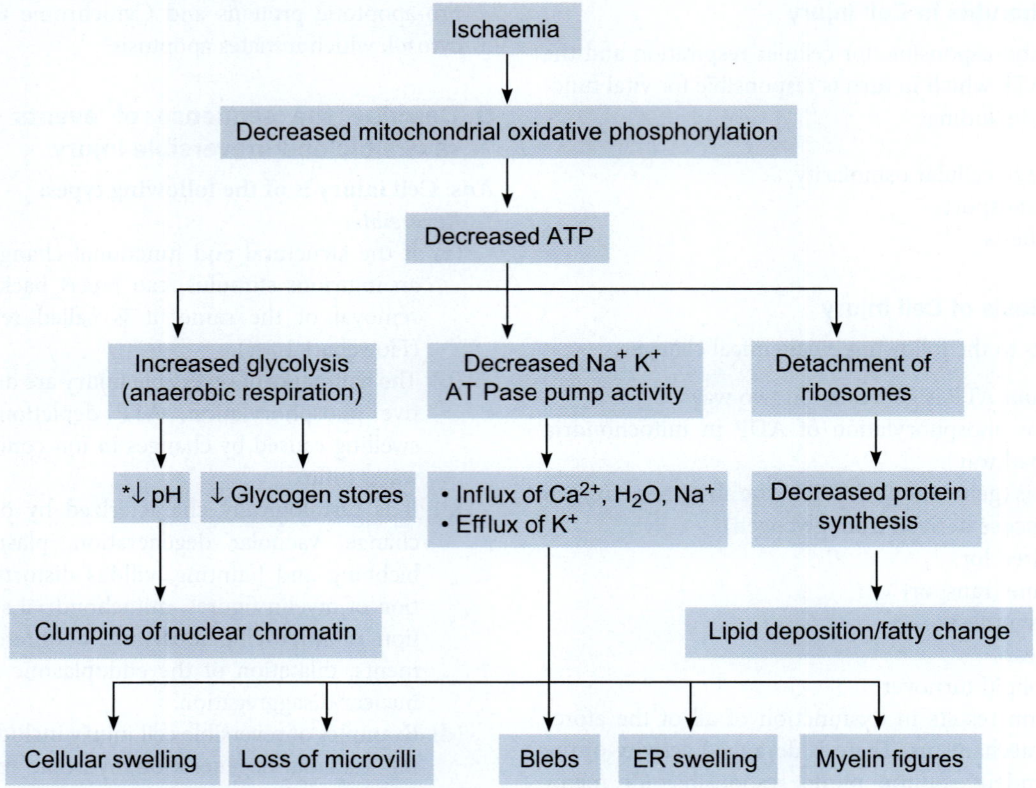

Flowchart 1.8 (A) Sequence of events in reversible injury.

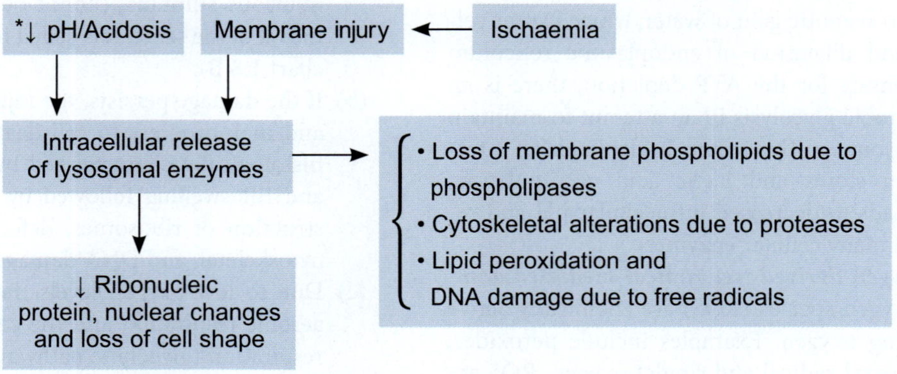

Flowchart 1.8 (B) Sequence of events in irreversible injury.

Q. Write briefly on free radical-mediated cell injury. (PA2.1)

Ans. Free radicals are chemical species with an unpaired electron in their outer orbit. They are natural by-products of chemical processes involved in metabolism. Normally, they are rapidly destroyed after production, as they are highly unstable. Excess of free radicals is the result of increased production or inefficient removal. When present in excess free radicals can react with inorganic and organic molecules (proteins, lipids and carbohydrates), which are mainly present in membranes and nucleic acids and cause cellular damage.

Salient Features of Free Radicals

- They have unpaired electrons in the outer orbit.
- They are highly reactive species.
- They are self-propagating and non-specific in nature.
- They are damaging to organic and inorganic molecules.

Mechanism of Generation of Free Radicals

Free radicals can be generated in the following ways:

1. **Reduction of molecular oxygen (O_2):** Reduction of molecular oxygen produces superoxide ($\cdot O^{-2}$):

$$O_2 + e^- \rightarrow \cdot O^{-2}$$

Dismutation of superoxide produces hydrogen peroxide (H_2O_2):

$$2H^+ + \cdot O^-$$

$$2 + \cdot O^{2-} \rightarrow H_2O_2 + O_2$$

Hydrogen peroxide may be partially reduced to hydroxyl radical (OH) or fully reduced to water:

$$H_2O_2 + e^- \rightarrow HO^- + \cdot OH$$

$$2H_2O_2 \rightarrow 2H_2O + O_2$$

2. **Ionizing radiation:** Water comprises almost 60% of the human body. Ionizing radiation, for example, UV and X-rays can interact with water to generate harmful intermediates

Table 1.2 Differences between reversible and irreversible cell injury

Features	Reversible injury	Irreversible injury
Definition	If the structural and functional changes, induced by an injurious stimulus, *can* revert to normal on removal of the same, it is called reversible injury	If the structural and functional changes, induced by an injurious stimulus, *cannot* be reversed even after removal of the same, it is called irreversible injury
Cell membrane		
Blebbing, blunting, distortion, loss of microvilli	Present	Present; more prominent than reversible injury
Defects	Absent	Present
Endoplasmic reticulum	Shows swelling only	Shows swelling and lysis
Ribosomes	Dispersed	Dispersed and destroyed
Lysosomes	Autophagy of organelles by lysosomes, no rupture	Rupture of lysosomes and autolysis of cell
Mitochondria	Swelling, small amorphous densities present	Swelling, large densities present
Nucleus	Clumping of nuclear chromatin	Pyknosis, karyolysis or karyorrhexis
Myelin figures (large intracellular whorled phospholipid bodies)	May be present	Mostly present
Calcification	Absent	Dystrophic calcification may be seen

(radiolysis). During this process, water loses an electron and becomes highly reactive. Following which it is sequentially converted to hydroxyl radicals (·OH), hydrogen peroxide (H_2O_2), superoxide radical ($\cdot O^{2-}$), and ultimately oxygen (O_2).

3. **Enzymatic metabolism of exogenous chemicals/drugs:** Hepatic metabolism of the solvent carbon tetrachloride (CCl_4) by mixed oxidases produces the free radical CCl_3.
4. **Transition metals:** Iron (Fenton reaction) as well as copper can catalyse the formation of ROS. Normally, these reactive metals are kept in check by binding of their ions to storage and transport proteins such as transferrin, ferritin, lactoferrin and ceruloplasmin, thereby decreasing the formation of ROS.
5. **Nitric oxide (NO):** Acts as a free radical and can be converted to highly reactive peroxynitrite anion ($ONOO^-$) as well as NO_2 and NO_3^-.

Pathways of Free Radical Production

Chemical reactions leading to the endogenous production of free radicals:

1. $O_2 \rightarrow O_2^{\cdot -}$ (superoxide anion)

2. $2O_2^{\cdot -} + 2H^+ \xrightarrow{\text{Superoxide dismutase}} H_2O_2 + O_2$ (hydrogen peroxide)

3. $H_2O \xrightarrow{\text{Radiation}} H\cdot + OH^-$ (hydroxyl radical)

4. $Fe^{++} + H_2O_2 \xrightarrow{\text{Fenton reaction}} Fe^{+++} + OH\cdot + OH^-$ (hydroxyl radical)

5. $H_2O_2 + O_2^{\cdot} \xrightarrow{\text{Haber-Weiss reaction}} OH^{\cdot} + OH^- + O_2$ (hydroxyl radical)

6. $CCl_4 \xrightarrow{\text{Cytochrome P450}} CCl_3^{\cdot}$

Endogenous Sources of Free Radicals

- Synthesis of leukotrienes and prostaglandins and lipid peroxidation in the plasma.
- Cytochrome P450 mediated reactions in ER.
- Electron transport in mitochondria.
- Xanthine oxidase, aldehyde oxidase, and reactions involving divalent metals like Cu^{++}, Fe^{++} in the cytoplasm.
- Oxidases in peroxisomes.

Effects of Free Radicals

Free radicals react with inorganic and organic molecules (proteins, lipids, carbohydrates), which are mainly present in membranes and nucleic acids. They have the following effects:

- **Lipid peroxidation:** Lipid and free radical interactions produce peroxides (initiation). Peroxides are reactive and unstable species, which start a chain reaction of lipid peroxidation (propagation). In some cases, the chain reaction is terminated by antioxidants.
- **Modification of proteins by oxidation:** Oxidation of amino acid residue side chain leads to formation of protein-protein cross-linkages, and oxidation of the protein backbone results in protein fragmentation.
- **DNA lesions:** Free radicals attack thymine and other nucleotides of nuclear and mitochondrial DNA to produce single stranded breaks in DNA.

Removal/Neutralization of Free Radicals

Free radicals are inherently unstable and usually decay spontaneously. Inactivation/neutralization of free radicals to minimize injury can also be induced by:

- **Antioxidants,** for example, vitamins A, C, E, and β-carotene.

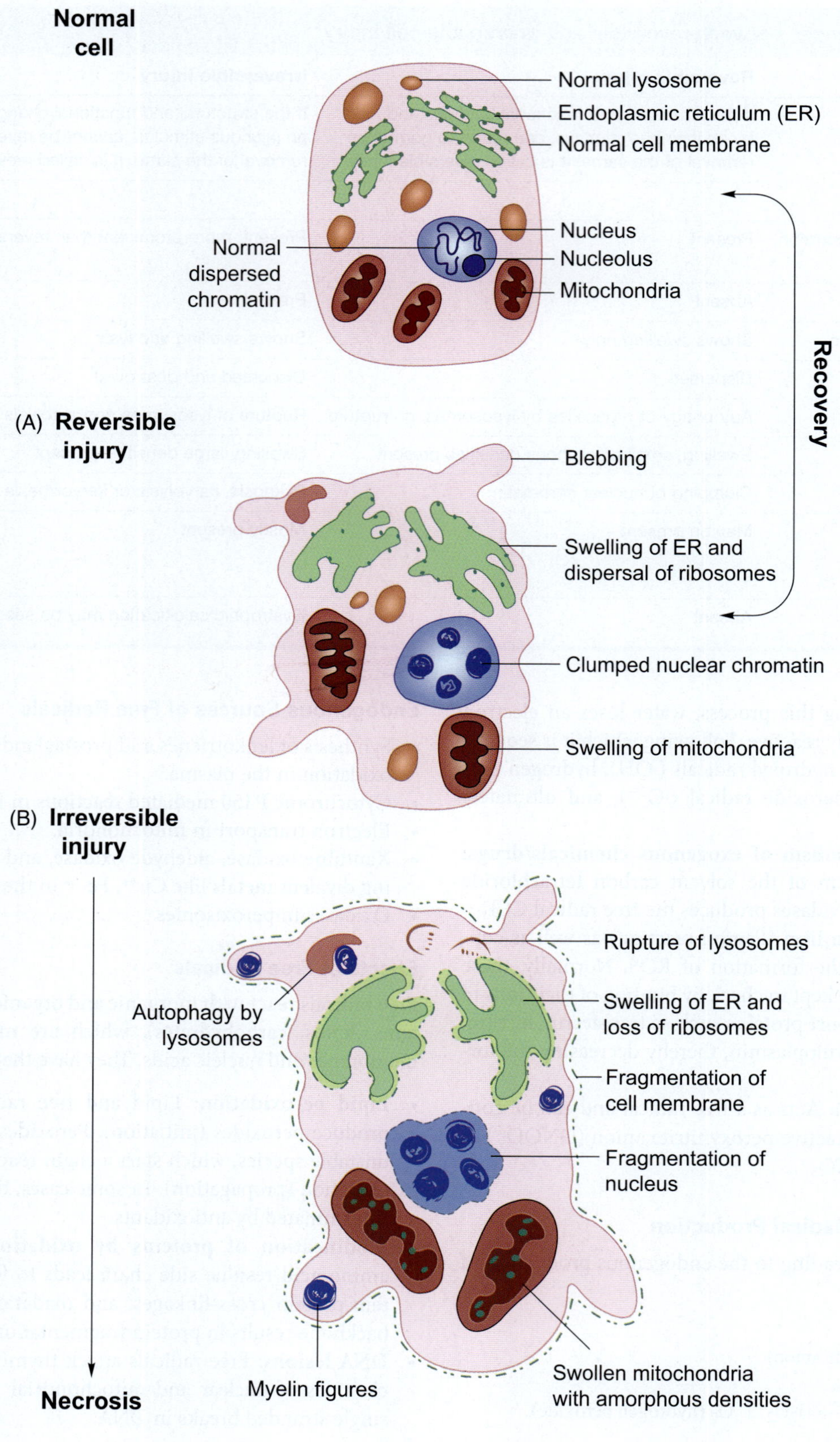

Fig. 1.15 Normal cell and morphological changes in (A) reversible and (B) irreversible injury.

- **Iron- and copper-binding proteins,** for example transferrin, ferritin, lactoferrin and ceruloplasmin (they decrease free metal form by binding to it).
- **Enzymes,** for example catalase, superoxide dismutase and glutathione peroxidase catalyse free radical breakdown in the following ways:

$$1.\ 2H + 2O_2^{\cdot} \xrightarrow{\text{Superoxide dismutase}} H_2O_2 + O_2$$

$$2.\ 2OH^{\cdot} + 2GSH \xrightarrow{\text{Glutathione peroxidase}} 2H_2O + GSSG$$

$$3.\ 2H_2O_2 \xrightarrow{\text{Catalase}} O_2 + 2H_2O$$

Q. Write briefly on reperfusion injury.

Ans. Reperfusion injury is defined as the tissue damage caused by reestablishment of circulation after a period of ischemia or hypoxia. Normally, it is understood that reversible injury should get better with reperfusion; however, reperfusion itself can sometimes be a cause of cell injury. Restoration of circulation in ischemic tissues results in microvascular injury, which manifests as increased permeability of capillaries and arterioles. Endothelial cells get activated to produce ROS in the presence of increased oxygen.

Nitric oxide production is reduced, and this initiates an inflammatory response, which entails release of interleukins as well as generation of free radicals by infiltrating neutrophils in response to tissue damage. ROS also turn on redox signalling to initiate apoptosis. The restored blood flow therefore damages cellular proteins, DNA and the plasma membrane. WBCs also adhere to the endothelium of small capillaries, obstructing them, and leading to more ischaemia. Activation of the complement system may also contribute to ischemia–reperfusion injury.

Q. Write briefly on antioxidants.

Ans. Antioxidants are the substances, which inhibit oxidation of proteins, carbohydrates, lipids and DNA (also called 'free radical scavengers'). Oxidative stress is a result of an imbalance between reactive oxygen species (ROS) and antioxidant mechanisms. Antioxidants reduce or retard ageing, carcinogenesis, diabetes, liver disease, kidney disease, cardiovascular disease, neurodegenerative disorders by decreasing oxidative stress. Fruits and vegetables contain a large amount of flavonoids and antioxidant supplements that contribute to protection against different health problems.

Antioxidant Types

1. **Enzymatic antioxidants: Superoxide dismutase (SOD)** catalyses the dismutation of $O_2^{\cdot} -$ to O_2 with remarkable efficiency by successive oxidation and reduction of the transition metal ion and to the less-reactive species H_2O_2. **Catalase** is present in the cells of plants, animals and aerobic bacteria. It is an enzyme located in a cell organelle called the peroxisome and promotes the conversion of hydrogen peroxide to water and molecular oxygen. **GPx enzymes** (glutathione peroxidase) in presence of tripeptide glutathione (GSH) add two electrons to reduce peroxides. GPx decomposes peroxides to water (or alcohol) while simultaneously oxidizing GSH. The antioxidant properties of these enzymes allow them to eliminate peroxides as potential substrates for the Fenton reaction.
2. **Non-enzymatic antioxidants: Exogenous non-enzymatic antioxidants** include **Vitamin C, vitamin A** and **sulfhydryl containing compounds like cysteine** and **glutathione. Vitamin C** is a powerful antioxidant that works in aqueous environments of the body; Vitamin C associates with **Vitamin E** to regenerate α-tocopherol from α-tocopherol radicals in membranes and lipoproteins. **Endogenous non-enzymatic antioxidants** include **storage and transport proteins such as transferrin, ferritin** and **ceruloplasmin** which bind to reactive metals like iron and copper and stop them from catalysing reactions that give rise to ROS.

Q. Define necrosis and describe its various morphological patterns.

Ans. Disturbances of the external environment beyond the limits of homeostasis lead to premature cell death, which is called *necrosis*. Necrosis may be caused by ischaemia, infection, poisoning, etc., and is invariably pathological. It usually precipitates an inflammatory response and is accompanied by cell swelling, lysis and lysosomal leakage (Flowchart 1.9). Self-digestion of cells by enzymes liberated from its own lysosomes on the other hand is labelled *autolysis* (Table 1.3). **The morphological features of necrosis vary with its type. Changes common to most types include:**

1. **Cytoplasmic changes (Fig. 1.16A)**
   (a) **Increased eosinophilia of the cytoplasm**, due to
      (i) loss of normal cytoplasmic basophilia caused by the loss of RNA and
      (ii) denaturation of cytoplasmic proteins which then bind strongly to the dye eosin.
   (b) **Glassy homogenous cytoplasm** due to loss of glycogen.
   (c) **Swelling and vacuolation of the cytoplasm** which occurs after enzymatic digestion has started.
   (d) **Cellular and organelle swelling** which eventually lead to **discontinuities in cell and organelle membranes and ultimately rupture.**

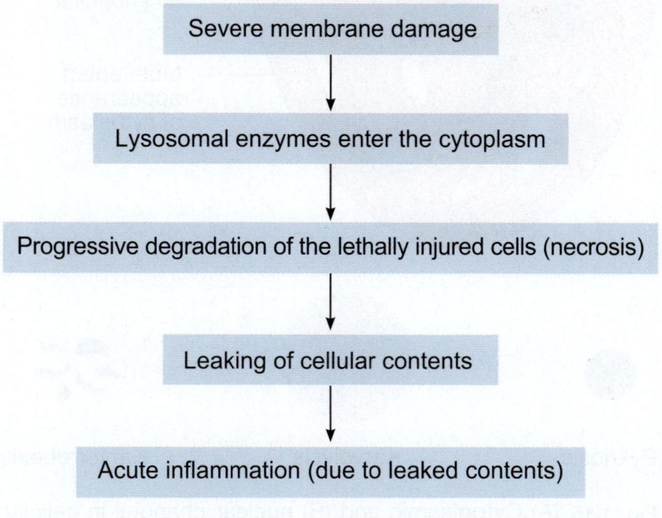

Flowchart 1.9 Sequence of events in cellular necrosis.

Table 1.3 Differences between autolysis and necrosis

Features	Autolysis	Necrosis
Definition	Self-digestion of cells by enzymes liberated from its own lysosomes	Spectrum of morphologic changes that follow cell death in living tissue, resulting from the progressive degradative action of enzymes on lethally injured cells
Reaction	• In *living tissue*, inflammatory cells may be present	• Presence of inflammatory cells
	• In *post-mortem* cases, there is complete absence of inflammatory cells	• Does not occur post-mortem
Calcification	Absent	Dystrophic calcification may be present

(e) **Formation of myelin figures** (phospholipid masses derived from damaged cell membranes).

2. **Nuclear changes (Fig. 1.16**B)

The changes in nucleus appear in one of the following three patterns:

(a) Nuclear shrinkage and increased basophilia **(pyknosis).**

(b) Nuclear fragmentation **(karyorrhexis).**

(c) Loss or fading of basophilia due to DNase activity **(karyolysis).**

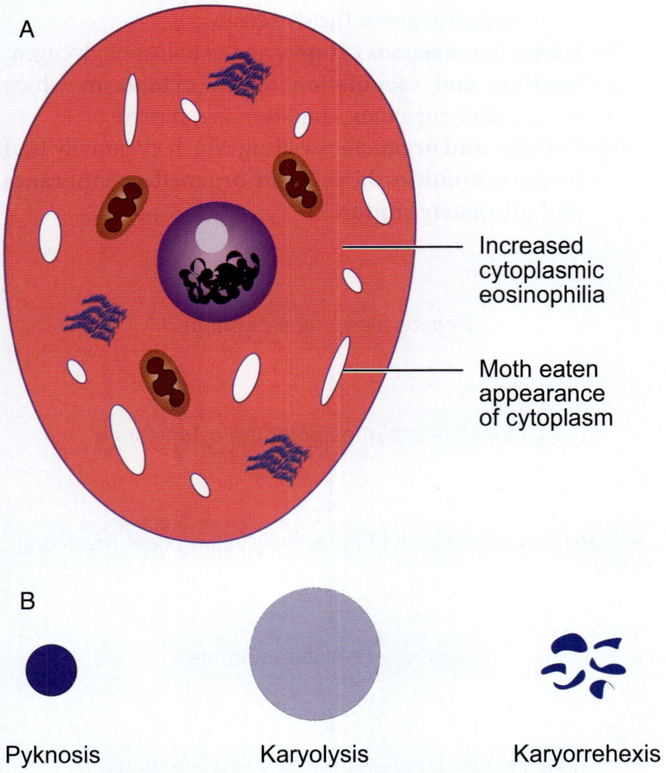

Fig. 1.16 (A) Cytoplasmic and (B) nuclear changes in cellular necrosis.

Decreased pH

↓

Denaturation of structural as well as enzymatic proteins

↓

Lack of enzymatic proteins blocks proteolysis

↓

Preservation of basic architecture of cell/tissue

Flowchart 1.10 Mechanism of evolution of coagulative necrosis.

Morphological Patterns of Necrosis Include

1. **Coagulative necrosis**

(a) It is **the most common pattern** of necrosis and is **caused by ischaemic injury** resulting in hypoxic death of cells in all tissues **except the brain**.

(b) There is **preservation of the basic architectural outlines** and type of tissue can be recognized but cellular details are lost.

(c) Cell injury leads to increasing intracellular acidosis, which denatures not only structural proteins but also enzymatic proteins, and so blocks the proteolysis of the cell, thereby preventing loss of architecture of the tissue (Flowchart 1.10).

(d) On *gross examination*, the affected area (area of infarction) is often wedge-shaped (with the apex pointing to focus of vascular occlusion), dry, pale in colour and firm in texture.

(e) *Microscopically*, increased eosinophilia of the cytoplasm and decreased basophilia of the nucleus are observed. Myocardial infarction is an excellent example in which acidophilic, coagulated anucleate myocardial cells are seen in the infarcted zone (Fig. 1.17).

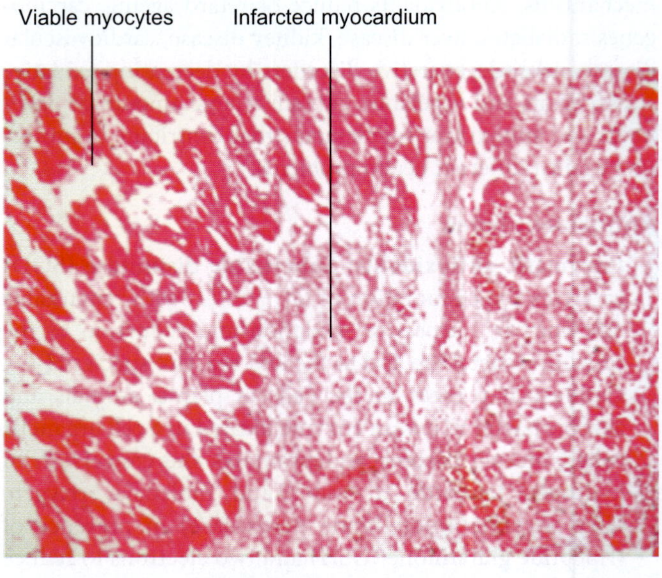

Fig. 1.17 Infarcted myocardium surrounded by viable cardiac myocytes (H&E; 100×).

Table 1.4 Differences between coagulative and liquefactive necrosis

Features	Coagulative necrosis	Liquefactive necrosis
Cause	Hypoxic/ischaemic injury in all tissues except in brain, for example myocardial, renal or placental infarction	• Bacterial and fungal infections • Hypoxic injury in brain
Tissue architecture	Tissue architecture is preserved; the basic outline of cell is intact, although cytoplasmic and nuclear details are lost	Both cell outline and intracellular details are lost; tissue architecture is not preserved
Pathogenesis	Due to intracellular acidosis, structural as well as enzymatic proteins are denatured and proteolysis is blocked; dead cells are removed by fragmentation and phagocytosis	Hydrolytic enzymes from bacteria and fungi as well as inflammatory cells cause complete digestion of dead cells and formation of pus (lysis)
Morphology	Conversion of cells into acidophilic, coagulated, anucleate units	No cellular outline/tissue architecture recognized

2. **Liquefactive necrosis** (colliquative necrosis)
   (a) This occurs in situations in which **enzymatic breakdown is more prominent than protein denaturation** unlike coagulative necrosis (Table 1.4).
   (b) It is usually associated with **bacterial or fungal infections** because microbes stimulate the accumulation of leukocytes and liberation of enzymes from these cells.
   (c) The **organ–cellular architecture is lost**, and the tissue is digested and converted into a liquefied mass, which appears creamy yellow in colour and is called '**pus**'.
   (d) Liquefactive necrosis is **most commonly seen in organs that have a high-fat and low-protein content** (e.g. the brain), **or those with a high-enzymatic content** (e.g. the pancreas), and **typically causes gangrene of intestine** (Fig. 1.18) and **limbs** and **hypoxic death in brain.**
   (e) Lack of a proper collagenous connective tissue framework in an organ also aids to this type of necrosis.
   (f) The mechanism of evolution of liquefactive necrosis is shown in Flowchart 1.11.
3. **Gangrenous necrosis**
   (a) This is a clinical term, not a specific pattern of necrosis.
   (b) It is usually used in context of the lower limbs, which have lost their blood supply and have undergone necrosis, initially coagulative (dry gangrene), and later liquefactive due to secondary bacterial infection and immigrating leukocytes (wet gangrene) (Table 1.6).
   (c) Mechanism of evolution of gangrenous necrosis is shown in Flowchart 1.11.
4. **Caseous necrosis**
   (a) This type of necrosis is typically associated with **tuberculous infection.**
   (b) On *gross examination*, the necrotic areas appear cheesy white (caseous). Microscopically, the debris appears amorphous, eosinophilic and granular (Fig. 1.19), and is surrounded by a distinct inflammatory reaction called granulomatous reaction.

Bacterial infection and accumulation of inflammatory cells
↓ Release of enzymes
Autolysis and heterolysis

Flowchart 1.11 Mechanism of evolution of liquefactive necrosis.

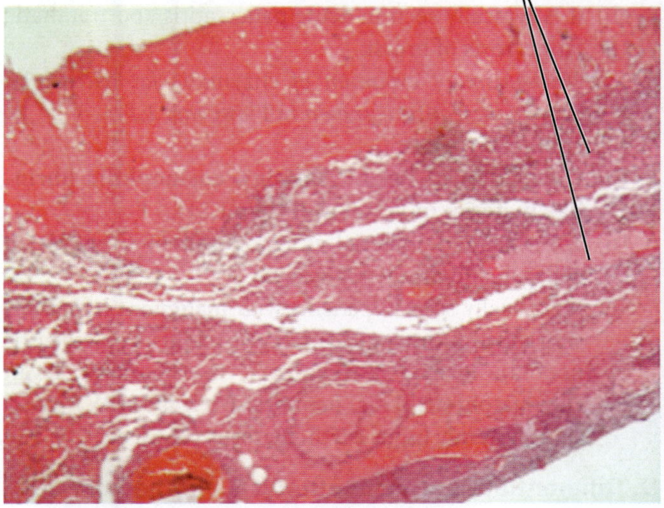

Fig. 1.18 Liquefactive necrosis/gangrene of intestine (H&E; 100×).

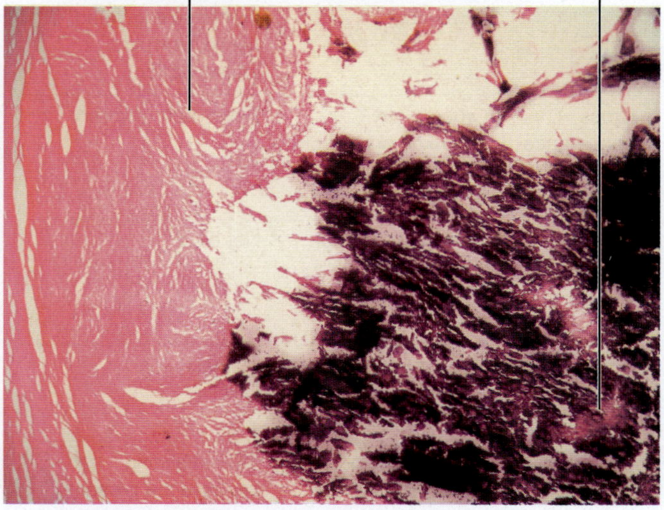

Fig. 1.19 Section from a lymph node showing amorphous, eosinophilic and granular debris (caseous necrosis) surrounded by a granulomatous reaction composed of Langhans giant cells and chronic inflammatory cells (H&E; 100×).

Table 1.5 Differences between coagulative and caseous necrosis

Features	Coagulative necrosis	Caseous necrosis
Cause	Hypoxia	Tuberculous infection of lymph nodes, lungs, skin, etc.
Pathogenesis	Due to intracellular acidosis, structural as well as enzymatic proteins are denatured and proteolysis is blocked	Delayed hypersensitivity reaction to *mycobacterial* capsular antigens
Gross	Affected tissue is firm in texture	Cheesy white appearance
Tissue architecture	Preserved	Completely obliterated

(c) **Tissue architecture is completely obliterated unlike coagulative necrosis** (Table 1.5). Dystrophic calcification may be seen (Table 1.6).

5. **Enzymatic fat necrosis**
   (a) It refers to a focal area of fat destruction that converts adipocytes to necrotic cells with shadowy outlines and basophilic calcium deposits, surrounded by an inflammatory reaction (Fig. 1.20).

Table 1.6 Differences between dry and wet gangrene

Features	Dry gangrene	Wet gangrene
Cause	Mainly arterial occlusion (coagulative necrosis)	More in venous occlusion; obstruction invariably followed by secondary bacterial infection (liquefactive necrosis)
Distribution	Limbs (atherosclerotic narrowing)	More common in bowel (seen in obstruction due to strangulated hernia, volvulus, intussception)
Gross appearance	Organ is dry, shrunken and black (due to deposition of iron sulphide)	Moist, soft, swollen
Line of demarcation	Present at junction between healthy and gangrenous parts	Not clear
Putrefaction	Limited (no infection and less blood supply)	Marked
Presence of bacteria	Absent, little or no septicaemia	Overwhelming septicaemia present
Spread	Slow	Rapid
Prognosis	Better	Poor

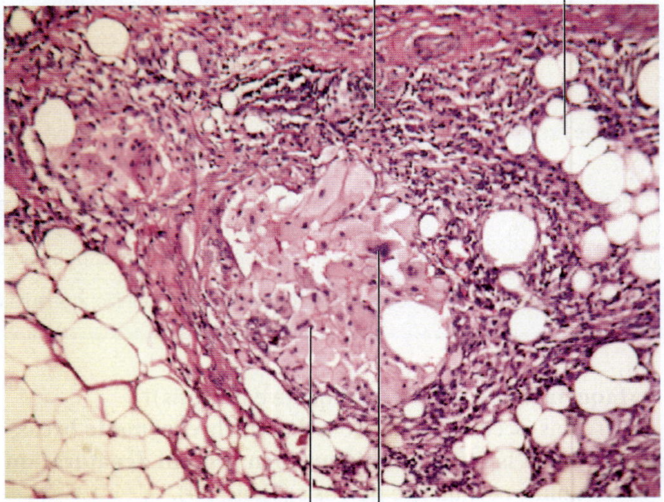

Fig. 1.20 Fat necrosis in the breast showing disruption of normal adipocytes and accumulation of lipid-laden foamy histiocytes with a multinucleate giant cell (H&E; 200×).

Release of activated pancreatic lipases into pancreas and peritoneal cavity

↓

Focal areas of destruction of fat and release of fatty acids

↓

Released fatty acids combine with calcium (saponification)

↓

Chalky white areas

Flowchart 1.12 Mechanism of evolution of enzymatic fat necrosis.

   (b) It is typically seen in acute pancreatitis and traumatic fat necrosis of breast.
   (c) *Mechanism of evolution of enzymatic fat necrosis in acute pancreatitis is shown in Flowchart 1.12.*

6. **Fibrinoid necrosis**
   (a) **Deposition of bright, smudgy, eosinophilic fibrin-like material in vessel wall** (Fig. 1.21).
   (b) The fibrinoid material is composed of degenerated collagen and ground substance.
   (c) It is usually seen in patients with **malignant hypertension** and **immunological injury** (vasculitis—polyarteritis nodosa). It may also be seen in **rheumatic fever, rheumatoid arthritis, hepatitis B virus (HBV) infection, systemic lupus erythematosus (SLE)**, etc.

Q. Differentiate between autolysis and necrosis.

Ans. Differences between autolysis and necrosis are shown in Table 1.3.

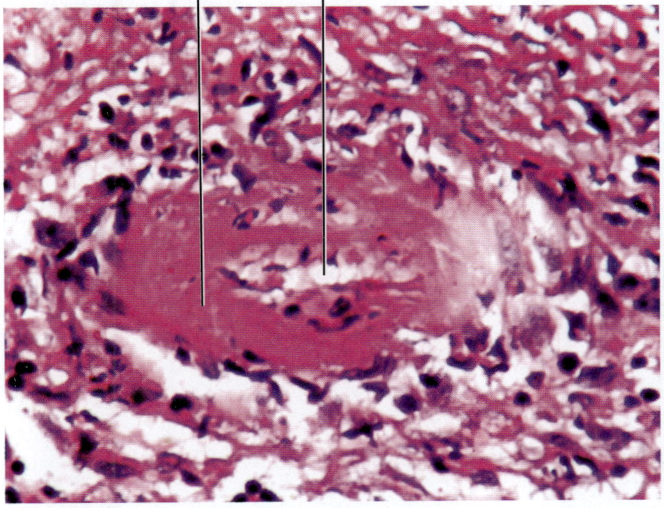

Fig. 1.21 Fibrinoid necrosis of vessel wall seen as bright pink smudgy deposits (H&E; 200×).

Q. Differentiate between coagulative and liquefactive necrosis.

Ans. Differences between coagulative and liquefactive necrosis are shown in Table 1.4.

Q. Differentiate between coagulative and caseous necrosis.

Ans. Differences between coagulative and caseous necrosis are shown in Table 1.5.

Q. Differentiate between dry and wet gangrene.

Ans. Differences between dry and wet gangrene are shown in Table 1.6.

Q. What are the types of cell death?

Ans. Cell death is primarily categorized into **programmed cell death (PCD)** or **non-PCD based on their signal dependency. PCD** can be further categorized as **apoptotic cell death** or **non-apoptotic cell death. Programmed apoptosis** consists of **apoptosis,** as well as **anoikis** (a form of programmed cell death that occurs in anchorage-dependent cells when they detach from the surrounding extracellular matrix). Multiple mechanisms and phenotypes compose programmed non-apoptotic cell death, including vacuole-presenting cell death **(autophagy, entosis, methuosis and paraptosis)**, mitochondrial-dependent cell death **(mitoptosis and parthanatos)**, iron-dependent cell death **(ferroptosis)**, immune-reactive cell death **(pyroptosis and NETosis)**, as well as other types, such as **necroptosis** (shares aspects of both necrosis and apoptosis). **Necrosis represents a form of non-programmed cell death.**

Apoptosis can be **intrinsic apoptosis** (RCD initiated by stresses of the extracellular or intracellular microenvironment, demarcated by MOMP, and precipitated by executioner caspases, mainly CASP3); **extrinsic apoptosis** (variant of RCD initiated by stresses from the extracellular microenvironment detected by plasma membrane receptors, propagated by CASP8 and precipitated by executioner caspases, mainly CASP3). **Non-apoptotic PCD** is lacelled **"caspase-independent programmed cell-death"** which is as efficient as apoptosis and can function as either backup mechanisms or the main type of PCD. **Anoikis** is almost identical to apoptosis except in its induction.

Q. Define apoptosis and describe its morphology, biochemical basis and underlying mechanism. (PA2.7)

Ans. Apoptosis is a form of genetically programmed cell death designed to eliminate unwanted host cells through activation of a coordinated series of events. It occurs in physiological and pathological conditions, in contrast with necrosis, which is always pathological (Table 1.7).

- **Physiological apoptosis**
  - During development/embryogenesis (implantation and organogenesis).

Table 1.7 Differences between apoptosis and necrosis

Features	Apoptosis	Necrosis
Definition	Programmed and coordinated cell death, which eliminates unwanted/ harmful cells or removes cells damaged beyond repair	Spectrum of morphologic changes that follow cell death in living tissue, largely resulting from the progressive degradative action of enzymes on lethally injured cells
Causes	May be physiological or pathological	Always pathological, eg, hypoxia, toxins
Involves	Single or small groups of cells	Large groups of cells
Inflammation	Absent	Present
Cellular change	Cell shrinkage	Cell swelling
Cell membrane	Bleb formation	Membrane disruption
Nucleus	Chromatin condensation followed by fragmentation	Nuclear pyknosis, karyolysis and karyorrhexis
Removal of cell	Phagocytosis of apoptotic bodies by macrophages	Enzymatic digestion or phagocytosis of cell debris by macrophages
Lysosomes/ other organelles	Intact	Hydrolytic enzyme release due to rupture
Mechanism	Genetically coordinated	Due to ATP depletion, free radicals, mitochondrial damage, etc.
Agarose gel electrophoresis	Stepladder DNA pattern	Diffuse DNA pattern

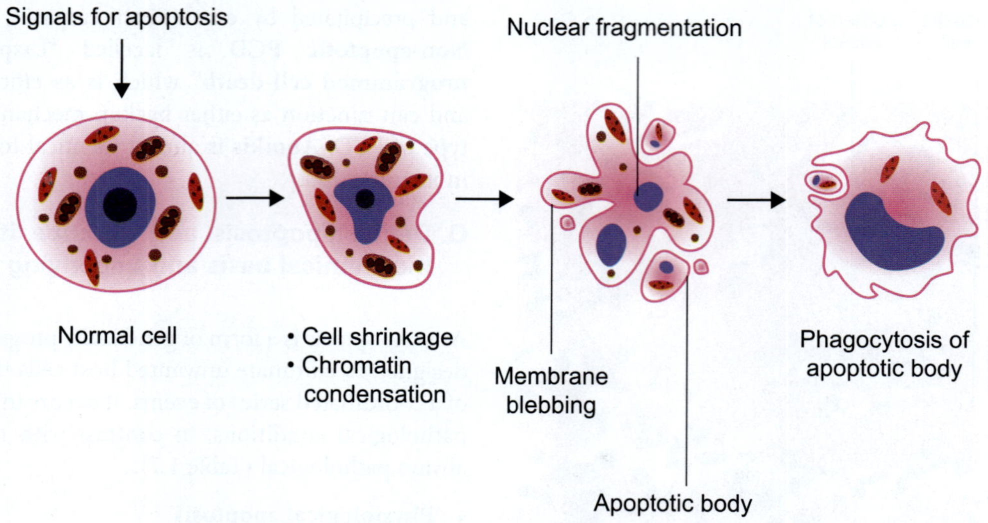

Fig. 1.22 Sequence of morphological changes in apoptosis.

- Hormone-dependent involution (regression of lactational changes in breast and prostatic atrophy).
- Cell deletion in proliferating cell population such as intestinal crypt epithelia.
- Apoptosis of immune T and B cells as in clonal deletion or cell death induced by cytotoxic T cells.
- Cell ageing.

- **Pathological apoptosis**
  - Cellular damage by diseases/noxious agents, for example councilman bodies in hepatitis.
  - Pathological atrophy in parenchymal organs after duct obstruction, for example salivary gland and pancreas.
  - Pathological atrophy in hormone-dependent organs, for example prostate.
  - Cell death in the tumours.
  - Low doses of thermal injury, radiation and anticancer drugs.

Sequence of Morphological Changes in Apoptosis (Fig. 1.22)

1. Cell shrinkage (increased density of the cytoplasm with tightly packed organelles).
2. Chromatin condensation under the nuclear membrane followed by nuclear fragmentation.
3. Formation of cytoplasmic blebs followed by fragmentation into apoptotic bodies (surface blebbing followed by fragmentation into membrane-bound apoptotic bodies).
4. Phagocytosis of apoptotic bodies (ingestion by macrophages followed by lysosomal degradation).

Sequence of Biochemical Events in Apoptosis

1. **Protein cleavage by proteolytic enzymes**

Activation of caspases (family of cysteine proteases having a unique ability to cleave after aspartic acid residues)
↓
Protein hydrolysis → Cleavage or breakup of nuclear scaffold
Protein hydrolysis → Cleavage or breakup of cytoskeletal proteins

2. **Protein cross-linkage**

Activation of transglutaminases
↓
Cross-linking of cytoplasmic proteins leading to covalently linked shrunken cells
↓
Easy breakdown into apoptotic bodies

3. **DNA condensation and breakdown**

DNA breakdown into large pieces (50–300 kb)
↓
Internucleosomal cleavage by endonucleases forming oligonucleosomes (180–200 bp) visualized on agarose gel electrophoresis as DNA ladders

4. **Recognition of dying cells by phagocytes**

Flip-flop of apoptotic cell
↓
Phosphatidylserine and thrombospondin flip on the external surface from the inner layers
↓
Easy recognition and phagocytosis of the apoptotic cell

Mechanism of Apoptosis

Apoptosis is the end point of an energy-dependent cascade of molecular events having four steps.

1. **Initiation of apoptosis by activation of signalling pathways:** There are a number of mechanisms through which apoptosis can be induced in cells. The sensitivity of cells to any of these stimuli can vary depending on a number of

factors, such as the expression of pro- and antiapoptotic proteins, for example, the Bcl-2 proteins or the inhibitor of apoptosis proteins (IAP), the severity of the stimulus, and the stage of the cell cycle. In some cases the apoptotic stimuli comprise extrinsic signals, such as the binding of death-inducing ligands to cell surface receptors called death receptors. These ligands can either be soluble factors or can be expressed on the surface of cells, such as cytotoxic T lymphocytes. In other cases apoptosis can be initiated following intrinsic signals that are produced following cellular stress. Cellular stress may occur from exposure to radiation or chemicals, or to viral infection. It might also be a consequence of growth factor deprivation or oxidative stress caused by free radicals. In general intrinsic signals initiate apoptosis via the involvement of the mitochondria. The relative ratios of the various Bcl-2 proteins can often determine how much cellular stress is necessary to induce apoptosis.

There are two main signalling pathways in apoptosis:

(a) Extrinsic/death receptor-initiated pathway (Flowchart 1.13): involves extracellular or transmembrane signals, which may be *positive* (leading to initiation) or *negative* (opposing initiation). Extrinsic pathway is mainly initiated by engagement of plasma membrane death receptors on cells. Death receptors are members of the tumour necrosis factor (TNF)-receptor family that contains a cytoplasmic domain called death domain because it delivers signals for apoptosis. Important death receptors include TNFR1 and a related protein called Fas (also called CD 95). The ligand for Fas is Fas ligand (Fas L), which is expressed on T cells.

(b) Intrinsic/mitochondrial pathway (the major mechanism of apoptosis; Flowchart 1.14).

2. **Control and integration:** Commitment or abortion of lethal signals is controlled byBCL2 family of proteins which include 'antiapoptotic proteins' (BCL2, BCLXL and MCL1); 'proapoptotic proteins' (BAX and BAK); and 'BCL2 sensor proteins' (BAD, BIM, Puma, Noxa). Also, the cytoplasm of normal cells contains inhibitors of apoptosis (IAP) which are neutralized by proapoptotic factors.
3. **Execution phase:** Proteolytic cascade involving *execution caspases* (caspases 3 and 6). *Caspase 3* also converts a cytoplasmic DNase into an active form by cleaving the inhibitor of this enzyme (this DNase induces internucleosomal cleavage of DNA; Fig. 1.23).

Extracellular signals
- Injuries: radiation, toxins and free radicals
- Withdrawal of growth factors, hormones or cytokines
- Receptor–ligand interactions (Fas–Fas ligand, TNF–TNF receptor)

↓

Act on intracellular regulatory molecules

OR

A Physicochemical agents like heat, radiation, viruses, xenobiotics and glucocorticoids directly bind to nuclear receptors

Binding of Fas L to Fas (receptor–ligand interactions)

↓

Three or more molecules of Fas are brought together

↓

The cytoplasmic domain of three Fas molecules forms a binding site for an adapter protein FADD (Fas-associated death domain)

↓

FADD binds inactive Caspase-8

↓

B Activation of Caspase-8 and initiation of caspase cascade

Flowchart 1.13 Extrinsic/death receptor-initiated pathway.

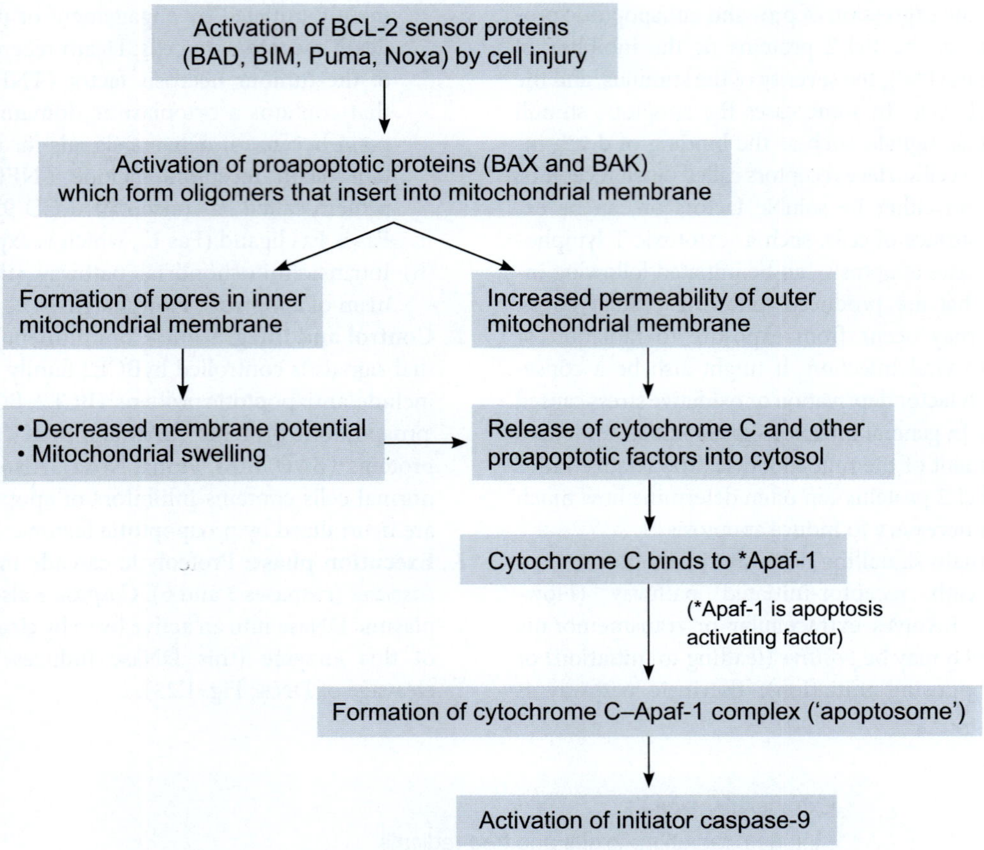

Flowchart 1.14 Intrinsic/mitochondrial pathway.

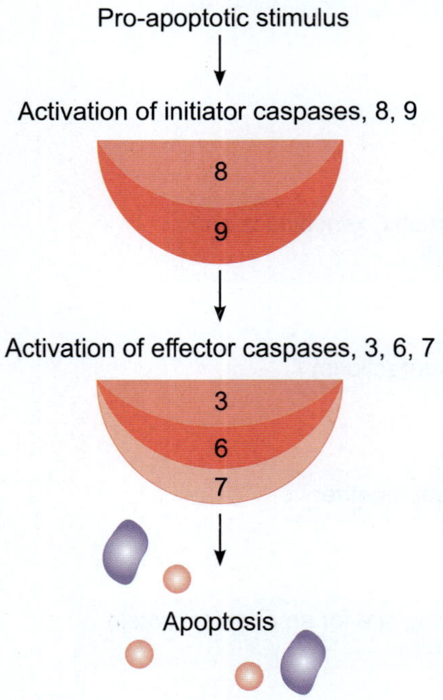

Fig. 1.23 The caspase cascade.

4. **Removal of dead cells:** Early recognition and removal by macrophages. Removal is aided by:
   (a) Expression of phosphatidylserine: in normal cells phosphatidylserine is present in the inner leaflet of the plasma membrane; during apoptosis there is turning out of the phosphatidylserine so that it is expressed on the outer membrane and is easily recognized by the macrophage.
   (b) Secretion of soluble factors by apoptotic cells, for example thrombospondin, which recruit macrophages.
   (c) Coating of apoptotic cells by natural antibodies and proteins of the complement system, which are easily recognized by macrophage receptors.

Q. Differentiate between apoptosis and necrosis. (PA2.7)

Ans. Differences between apoptosis and necrosis are shown in Table 1.7.

Q. Enumerate the disorders associated with apoptosis. (PA2.7)

Ans. Disorders associated with apoptosis:

1. Disorders associated with decreased apoptosis: cancer, autoimmunity.
2. Disorders associated with increased apoptosis:
   (a) Neurodegenerative diseases (Alzheimer, Huntington, Parkinson).
   (b) Ischaemic injury in stroke and myocardial infarction.
   (c) Death of virus-infected cells as in AIDS.

Q. Write briefly about diagnosis of apoptosis. (PA2.7)

Ans. Diagnosis of apoptosis:

1. Stepladder pattern on agarose gel electrophoresis.
2. Terminal deoxynucleotidyl transferase biotin-dUTP nick end labelling (TUNEL) technique for in vivo detection.
3. H&E, Feulgen and acridine orange staining of apoptotic cells.

4. Measurement of cytosolic cytochrome c and activated caspase levels.
5. Expression of phosphatidylserine on the outer leaflet of the plasma membrane by apoptotic cells enables their recognition by using the dye Annexin V.

Q. Classify intracellular accumulations and write briefly about them. (PA2.3)

Ans. In some metabolic derangements, cells may accumulate large amounts of various substances, which may be native, normal constituents of the cell or aberrant, abnormal substances. These may remain inert or cause varying degrees of cellular injury. The substances may get deposited in the cytosol (usually within lysosomes) or in the nucleus. They may be synthesized by the affected cells or produced elsewhere. Based on the origin of the accumulating substance, intracellular accumulations are classified into three types:

1. A normal cellular constituent accumulated in excess, such as water, lipids, proteins, and carbohydrates. The normal substance may accumulate as a result of either overproduction or inadequate metabolization/removal, which may result from genetic or acquired defects in its packaging, transport or secretion, or defect in an enzyme, which is responsible for degradation of the metabolite. These disorders are therefore sometimes referred to as 'storage diseases'.
2. An abnormal substance (coal dust, minerals or products of infectious agents, or by-products of abnormal metabolism) may get deposited in the cell because the cell is not equipped with the enzymes to degrade neither the substance nor the ability to transport it to other sites.
3. Pigments may deposit in the cell due to overproduction or aberrant metabolism.

I. Accumulation of Normal Cellular Constituent in Excess

1. **Water**
   (a) **Cloudy swelling**
   (i) A form of **reversible injury**, cloudy swelling is also called **granular degeneration** (named so because of the presence of prominent protein granules in the cytoplasm).
   (ii) It is characterized by intracytoplasmic accumulation of water due to abnormal ionic and fluid homeostasis.
   (iii) It commonly affects hepatocytes, renal tubular cells (Fig. 1.24) and myocardium
   Gross pathology: The affected organ is enlarged, soft and pale (pallor is due to mechanical compression of capillaries by retained water).
   Microscopy: Cells are swollen, full of proteinaceous granules (thought to be fragmented mitochondrial proteins or products of disturbed protein metabolism), and have frayed cell margins. Nuclei are normal in early stages, but could later appear faint or intensely staining.

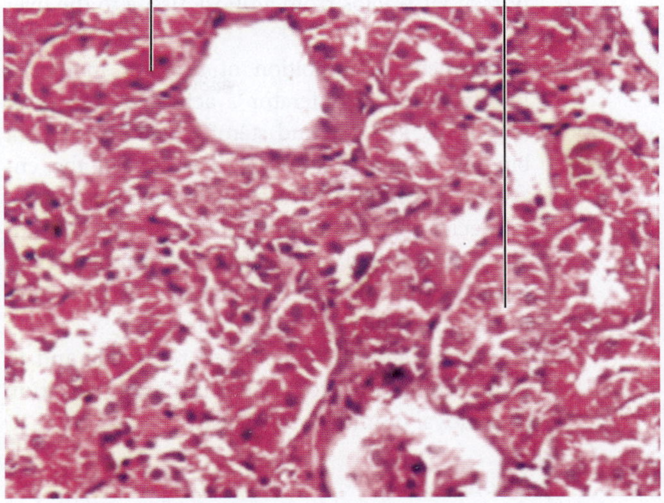

Fig. 1.24 Section from cloudy swelling kidney showing tubules lined by swollen cells with frayed margins and increased granularity (H&E; 200×).

   (b) **Hydropic/vacuolar degeneration**
   (i) This is an extension of changes seen in cloudy swelling.
   (ii) Affected cells are ballooned, pale, watery and vacuolated.
   (iii) Vacuoles coalesce and push nucleus towards the periphery.
   (iv) Cell bursts and nucleus undergoes karyorrhexis/lysis.
2. **Fat:** Abnormal accumulation of triglycerides in the cytosol of parenchymal cells is called fatty change (steatosis). It mainly affects **liver** and **heart** but can also be seen in muscle and kidney.
   (a) **Fatty change liver**
   (i) Fatty liver can range from fatty liver alone (steatosis) to fatty liver associated with inflammation (steatohepatitis).
   (ii) This condition can occur with the use of alcohol (alcohol-related fatty liver) or in the absence of alcohol [non-alcoholic fatty liver disease (NAFLD)]. If steatohepatitis is present but a history of alcohol use is not, the condition is termed non-alcoholic steatohepatitis (NASH).
   (iii) Fatty change in the liver results from excessive accumulation of lipids within hepatocytes. Simple fatty liver is believed to be benign, but NASH can progress to cirrhosis and can be associated with hepatocellular carcinoma.
   (iv) The main risk factors for simple fatty liver (NAFLD) and NASH are obesity, diabetes, high triglyceride levels, or a high-fat diet.
   (v) Defects in fat metabolism are responsible for pathogenesis of fatty liver. The main cause of fatty liver is an imbalance in energy consumption and

its combustion resulting in lipid storage or peripheral resistance to insulin, whereby the transport of fatty acids from adipose tissue to the liver is increased.

(vi) Impairment or inhibition of receptor molecules [peroxisome proliferator activated receptor (PPAR)-α, PPAR-γ, and sterol regulatory element binding protein (SREBP1)] that control the enzymes responsible for the oxidation and synthesis of fatty acids appears to contribute toward fat accumulation. In addition, alcoholism is known to damage mitochondria and other cellular structures, further impairing cellular energy mechanism.

(vii) Hepatic steatosis is considered reversible and to some extent non-progressive, if there is cessation or removal of underlying cause.

Causes

(i) Alcohol abuse
(ii) Starvation/malnutrition
(iii) Diabetes mellitus
(iv) Obesity
(v) Hepatotoxins like CCl_4, ether, aflatoxins, etc.
(vi) Certain drugs like steroids, tetracyclines, aspirin (Reye syndrome in infants), methotrexate, halothane, etc.
(vii) Hypoxia in anaemia and cardiac failure
(viii) Late pregnancy
(ix) Chronic illness like tuberculosis

Note: Alcohol abuse and diabetes (usually with obesity) are the most common causes of fatty liver.

***Mechanism of fatty change* (*Flowchart 1.15*):**
Under normal circumstances lipids enter the hepatocytes in three ways:

(i) From diet as 'chylomicrons' (triglycerides and phospholipids).
(ii) From peripheral adipose tissue as 'free fatty acids'.
(iii) From acetate present in liver cells (intrahepatic synthesis).

Most of the free fatty acids are esterified to triglycerides by α-glycerophosphate. Some are converted to cholesterol, phospholipids and ketones. Intrahepatic triglycerides are also converted to lipoproteins, which are then released into the circulation. Excess accumulation of triglycerides may result from defects at any step from the entry of free fatty acids to the exit of lipoproteins. In starvation, diabetes, and chronic alcoholism, there is an increase in generation of free fatty acids (1); in hypoxia, toxin exposure, and chronic alcoholism, there is a reduction in free fatty acid oxidation (2,3). In chronic alcoholism there is an increase in esterification of free fatty acids into triglycerides (4) and in starvation and malnutrition, there is a reduced exit of triglycerides from the hepatocytes due to deficiency of lipid binding apoproteins (lipids form complexes with apoproteins to form lipoproteins; 5), all leading to fatty change.

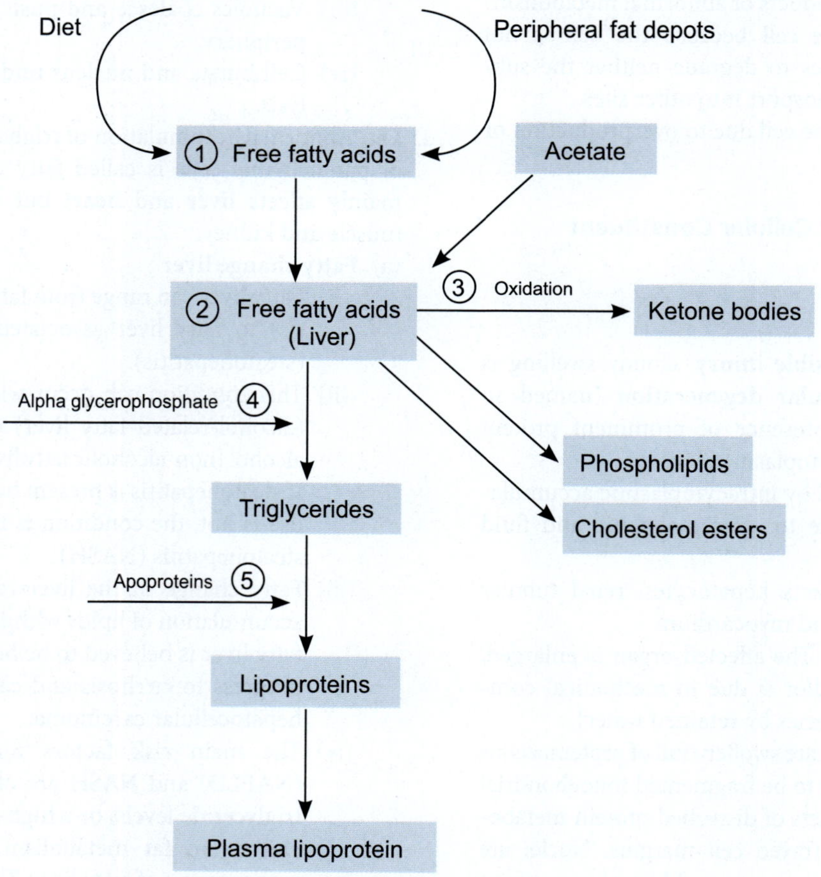

Flowchart 1.15 Mechanism of development of fatty liver.

Therefore, the main pathophysiological mechanisms underlying fatty change can be summarized as:

(i) Decreased mitochondrial fatty acid β-oxidation.

(ii) Increased endogenous fatty acid synthesis or enhanced delivery of fatty acids to the liver.

(iii) Deficient incorporation or export of triglycerides as very low-density lipoprotein.

Pathology

Gross: With diffuse involvement, organ appears enlarged (may weigh up to 3–5 kg), pale, soft, yellow and greasy. Focal fatty change may be seen as yellow mottling on cut surface.

Microscopy (See Fig. 1.25; Flowchart 1.16)

Microscopically, the hepatocytes appear swollen and show vacuoles in the cytoplasm (steps involving alcohol and xylene during tissue processing dissolves the fat; thus fat containing areas appear as clear spaces). To confirm that the clearing is due to fat, frozen sectioning is done and the section is stained with oil red-O and Sudan IV stains, which give orange-red and black colours, respectively. The evolution of microscopic changes of fatty liver can be divided into two stages.

(i) ***Early stage:*** Small fat vacuoles in the cytoplasm around the nucleus.

(ii) ***Late stage:*** The vacuoles coalesce to create cleared spaces that displace the nucleus to the cell periphery. Occasionally, contiguous cells rupture to form fatty cysts.

(b) **Fatty change heart:**

(i) Fatty degeneration of heart is usually due to prolonged hypoxia, as in severe anaemia, and diphtherial myocarditis. Lipid is found in myocardium as small droplets.

(ii) Two patterns may be observed:

- Prolonged moderate hypoxia: causes focal intracellular deposits of fat that create grossly yellow bands of myocardium alternating with darker red-brown normal myocardium (**tigered effect**).
- Profound hypoxia or myocarditis: affects myocytes uniformly.

3. **Carbohydrates:** Accumulation of carbohydrates is seen in conditions like glycogenosis and mucinous degeneration (Fig. 1.26). Intracellular deposits of glycogen can be seen in poorly controlled diabetes mellitus in renal tubules, cardiac muscle and β cells of the islets of Langerhans.
4. **Proteins:** Proteins can accumulate as:

(a) **Colloid droplets:** Normally, in the kidney, minute amounts of albumin filtered through the glomerulus are reabsorbed by pinocytosis in the proximal convoluted tubules. In disorders with heavy protein leakage across the glomerular filter, for example nephrotic syndrome, the protein appears as pink, hyaline

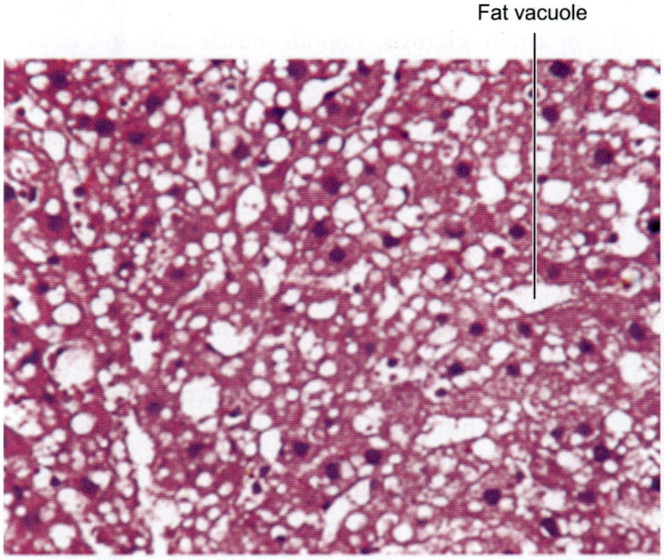

Fig. 1.25 Hepatocytes showing fatty change. The fat vacuole has pushed the nucleus into the peripherally displaced cytoplasm (H&E; 200×).

Liver liposomes (diffuse minute membrane-bound inclusions)
↓
Microvesicular fatty change (small vacuoles around the nucleus)
↓
Macrovesicular fatty change (vacuoles coalesce to form larger vacuoles, pushing the nucleus to the periphery)
↓
Rupture of contiguous cells
↓
Formation of fatty cysts

Flowchart 1.16 Sequence of events in the evolution of fatty liver.

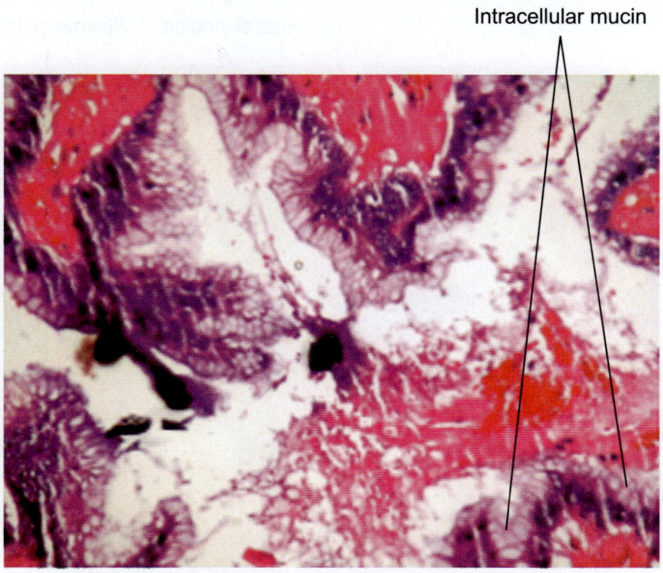

Fig. 1.26 Intracellular (epithelial) mucin in a benign mucinous tumour of the ovary (H&E; 400×).

cytoplasmic reabsorption droplets in proximal renal tubules. If the proteinuria reverses, the protein droplets are metabolized and disappear.

(b) **Russell bodies:** Active synthesis of immunoglobulins leads to excessive amounts of secretory protein in plasma cells causing huge distension of endoplasmic reticulum (ER), which appear as large eosinophilic inclusions (Fig. 1.27A and B).

(c) **Accumulation of misfolded proteins:** Defective secretion and transport of proteins, as in α-1 antitrypsin deficiency, results in accumulation of misfolded protein in ER causing ER stress as well as loss of protein function inducing emphysema and cirrhosis.

(d) **Mallory body, or 'alcoholic hyalin':** This is an eosinophilic cytoplasmic inclusion seen in liver cells. It is usually seen in association with alcoholic liver disease and is composed of aggregates of intermediate filaments.

(e) **Neurofibrillary tangles:** Found in Alzheimer disease, these are aggregated protein inclusions that contain microtubule-associated proteins and neurofilaments (indicating disruption of the neuronal cytoskeleton).

5. **Cholesterol and cholesterol esters**

Normally, the cellular metabolism is under tight control to ensure normal cell membrane synthesis without significant intracellular accumulation of cholesterol and cholesterol esters. Accumulation results in the event of several pathologic processes (e.g. hereditary and acquired hyperlipidemic syndromes), especially in the macrophages.

(a) Macrophages in contact with the lipid debris of necrotic cells or oxidized forms of lipoproteins may get filled with the lipid, imparting a foamy appearance to their cytoplasm (foam cells are polygonal cells with foamy cytoplasm and small, hyperchromatic, central nucleus).

(b) In **atherosclerosis**, smooth muscle cells and macrophages are filled with lipid vacuoles containing cholesterol and cholesteryl esters.

(c) **Xanthomas** are defined as aggregates of foamy macrophages present in the subepithelial connective tissue of skin or in tendons.

(d) **Cholesterolosis** (Fig. 1.28) is an intracellular accumulation of lipids (cholesterol). When cholesterol is excess in bile, it passes into the lamina propria where it is phagocytosed by macrophages. These cholesterol-containing macrophages may aggregate and enlarge the mucosal folds, producing yellow micropolyps, 1–2 mm in size. This contrasts with the normal pinkish-red colour of the surrounding mucosa and is labelled **'strawberry gallbladder'.**

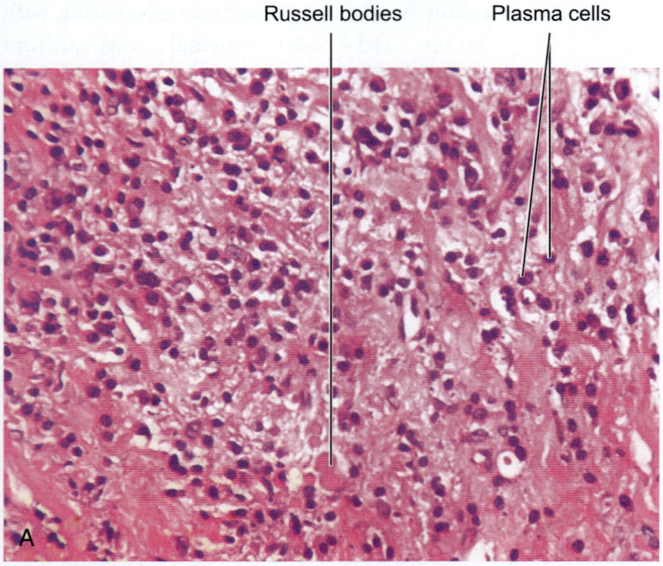

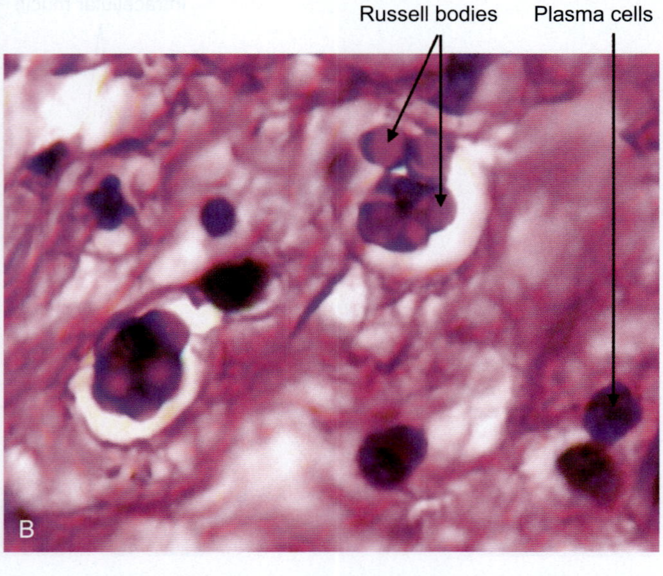

Fig. 1.27 (A) Sheets of plasma cells showing intracellular and extracellular Russell bodies, which are seen as pink globular structures (H&E; 200×). (B) Russell bodies (H&E; 400×).

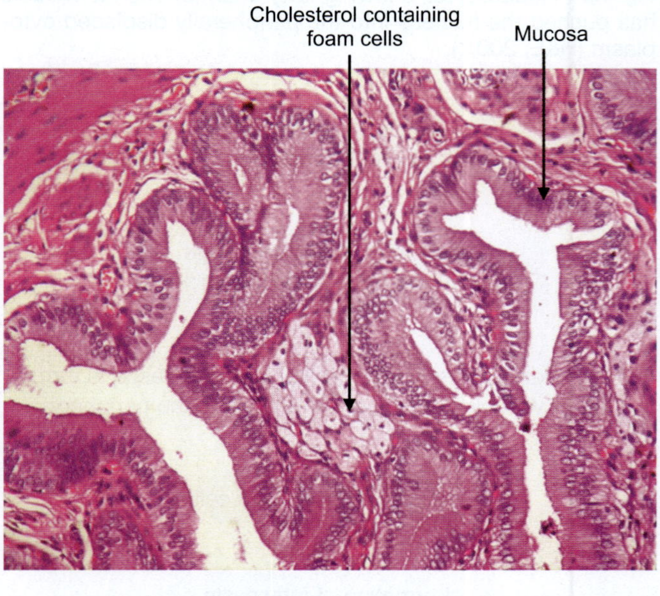

Fig. 1.28 Cholesterolosis gall bladder showing cholesterol-containing macrophages aggregating and enlarging the mucosal folds, and producing yellow micropolyps 1–2 mm in size (H&E; 200×).

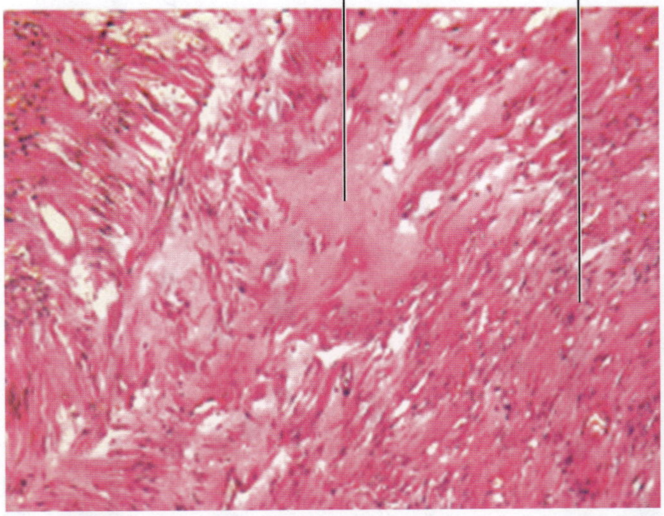

Fig. 1.29 Hyaline degeneration in a leiomyoma showing extracellular deposits of hyaline between whorls of smooth muscle cells (H&E; 200×).

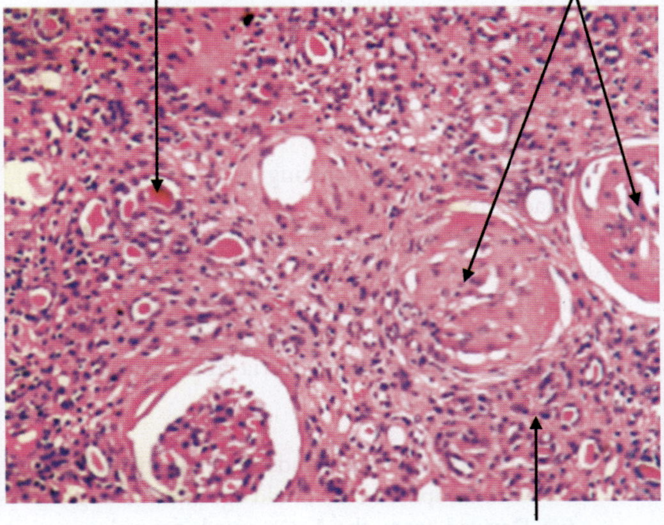

Fig. 1.30 Hyaline deposits in glomeruli in chronic pyelonephritis (H&E; 200×).

II. Accumulation of Abnormal Cellular Constituents

Hyaline change (derived from Hyalos glass) is defined as deposition of a glassy, homogenous, eosinophilic material resulting from a variety of heterogeneous pathologic conditions. Hyaline may be:

(a) **Intracellular:** when it is seen within epithelial cells, for example:
 (i) ***Hyaline droplets:*** Observed in proximal convoluted tubules due to excessive reabsorption of plasma proteins.
 (ii) ***Hyaline degeneration:*** Hyaline deposits in voluntary muscle, for example degeneration of rectus abdominis.
 (iii) ***Mallory's hyaline:*** Aggregates of intermediate filaments seen in hepatocytes in alcoholic injury.
 (iv) ***Hyaline inclusions:*** Nuclear and cytoplasmic inclusions seen in viral infections.
 (v) ***Russell bodies:*** Excessive immunoglobulins in endoplasmic reticulum of plasma cells.

(b) **Extracellular:** Seen in connective tissue, for example hyaline degeneration in leiomyomas (Fig. 1.29), hyaline arteriosclerosis and hyalinization of glomeruli in chronic glomerulonephritis (Fig. 1.30).

III. Accumulation of Pigments

Pigment refers to material that has colour and can be seen without staining. In pathology, pigments play an important role in the diagnosis of diseases such as gout, jaundice, melanomas, albinism and haemorrhage. In a section of tissue, the term pigment refers to a material that has colour and can be seen without staining. It can either be normal or pathological, and is usually identified by its colour, size and shape, or by chemical testing. Pigments can be classified as:

1. **Endogenous pigments**
 (a) **Melanin**
  (i) Non-haemoglobin-derived brown-black pigment (Fig. 1.31).

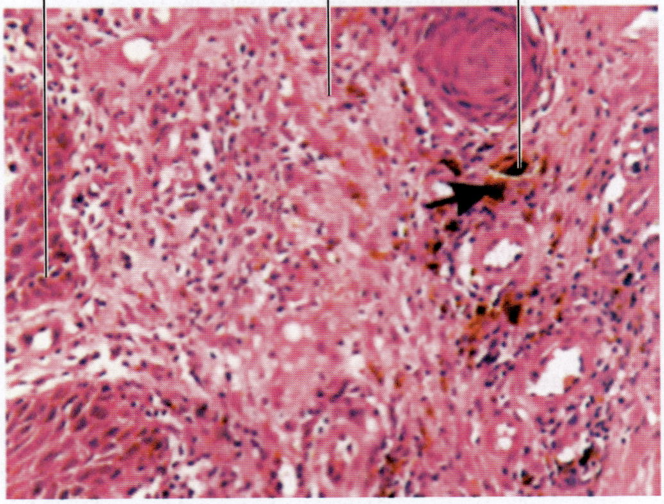

Fig. 1.31 Melanin deposits in the upper dermis (H&E; 200×).

  (ii) Normally present in skin, hair, choroids, meninges and adrenal medulla.
  (iii) Synthesized by melanocytes and dendritic cells.

Disorders of pigmentation involving melanin

- ***Hyperpigmentation***
  - Addison disease.
  - Adrenogenital syndrome.
  - Chloasma/melasma.
  - Chronic arsenical poisoning (raindrop pigmentation)
  - Linea nigra (a hyperpigmented line found on the abdomen during pregnancy).
  - Café-au-lait spots (neurofibromatosis, Albright syndrome).
  - Perioral pigmentation in Peutz–Jeghers syndrome.
  - Melanocytic tumours/nevi.

- Dermatopathic lymphadenitis.
- Acanthosis nigricans (pigmentation of intertriginous areas associated with hyperinsulinemia).

- ***Hypopigmentation:***
  - Albinism
  - Vitiligo
  - Leprosy
  - Post-inflammatory scarring
  - Radiation dermatitis

Staining characteristics of melanin: Can be bleached with hydrogen peroxide and stained with *Masson–Fontana argentaffin stain;* this forms the basis of differentiation of melanin from melanin lookalikes, for example homogentisic acid seen in alkaptonuria and carbon seen in anthracosis.

(b) **Lipofuscin**

(i) Lipid-derived wear and tear pigment (associated with atrophied cells of old age and wasting).

(ii) Derived from the Latin word 'fuscus', meaning brown.

(iii) Sometimes called **'residual bodies'** (collection of indigestible material in the lysosomes after intracellular lipid peroxidation of polyunsaturated lipids of subcellular membranes).

(iv) Yellow-brown, insoluble, granular, intracytoplasmic (perinuclear in location; Fig. 1.32).

(v) Seen in *myocardium*, *hepatocytes*, *Leydig cells* and *neurons.*

(vi) Due to the brown colour and association with atrophy, lipofuscin deposition is also called 'brown atrophy'.

Staining characteristics of lipofuscin

- *Acid fast* (AFB positive).
- *Autofluorescent.*
- Stains positive with *fat stains.*
- Reduces ferricyanide to ferrocyanide (*Schmorl reaction*).

(c) **Haemosiderin**

(i) Golden-yellow to brown, crystalline granular pigment, which stains with **Prussian blue stain** (colourless potassium ferrocyanide combines with ferric irons of haemosiderin to form a deep blue ferric ferrocyanide; Fig. 1.33).

(ii) **Haemosiderosis** is defined as the presence of stainable iron in tissue. Iron is stored in the tissue in two main forms—ferritin (iron complexed with apoferritin) and haemosiderin (aggregates of ferritin). Based on distribution of deposited iron, haemosiderosis may be classified as:

Localized: deposits in macrophages, fibroblasts, endothelial and alveolar cells secondary to haemorrhage in tissues, for example bruise, black eye, brown induration of lung and infarction.

Generalized: deposits in reticuloendothelial cells (liver, spleen, bone marrow) or parenchymal organs (liver, pancreas, kidney, heart) secondary to haemolytic disorders, blood transfusions, parenteral iron therapy, idiopathic haemosiderosis and Bantu disease.

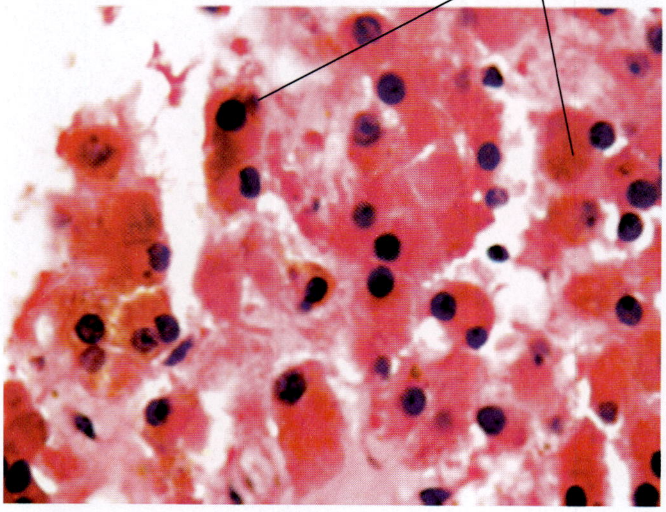

Fig. 1.32 Lipofuscin in Leydig cells in a section from testicular atrophy (H&E; 400×).

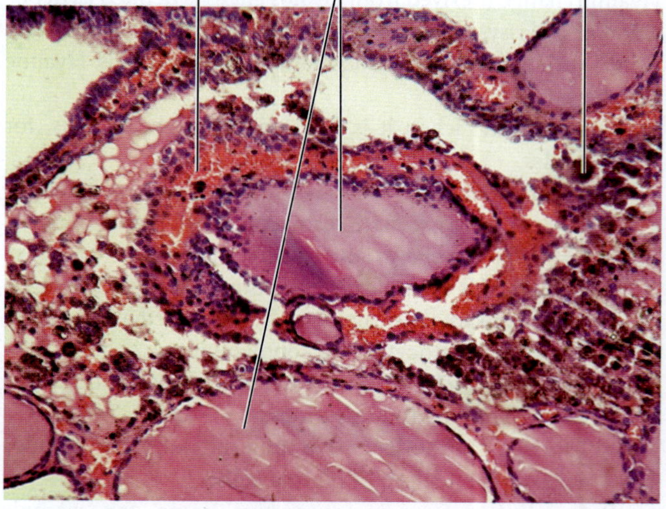

Fig. 1.33 Haemosiderin deposits in a multinodular goiter (H&E; 100×).

(iii) Severe progressive iron overload leading to fibrosis and organ failure is called *haemochromatosis.*

(d) **Acid haematin (haemozoin)**

(i) Haemoprotein-derived brown-black pigment seen in malaria.

(ii) Does not stain with Prussian blue (because iron is in ferric form).

(e) **Bilirubin**

(i) Major pigment found in bile (Fig. 1.34), stains with *Gmelin reaction* (oxidation by concentrated nitric acid to red/blue-green products) and *Stein's technique* (oxidation by iodine to form a green biliverdin pigment).

(ii) Derived from haemoglobin but contains no iron.

(iii) Excess of this pigment in tissues causes *jaundice.*

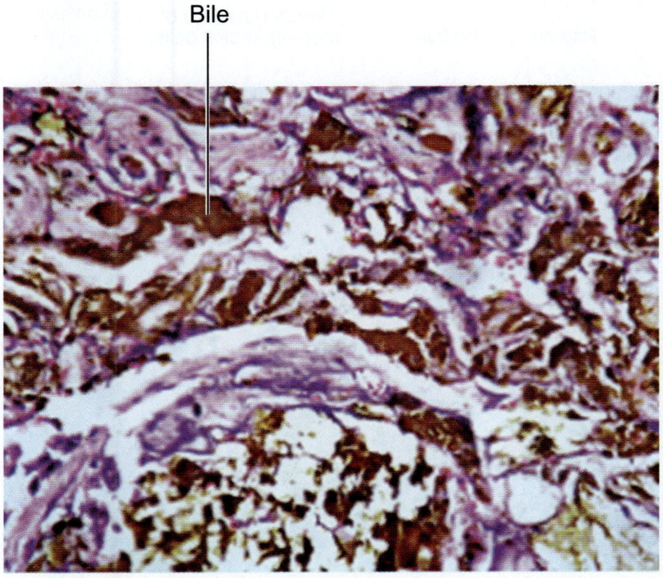

Fig. 1.34 Bile pigment in a section from liver (H&E; 200×).

(f) **Porphyrins**

(i) Porphyria is a group of diseases in which there is excessive production of chemicals called 'porphyrins'.

(ii) It affects the skin and/or nervous system.

(iii) Acute porphyria presents with waxing and waning episodes of abdominal pain, chest pain, vomiting, confusion, constipation, fever and seizures. The patient also has skin blisters or itching, which generally occur with sunlight exposure.

(iv) It is an inherited disease resulting from a mutation in one of the genes coding for enzymes involved in haeme synthesis. It may be autosomal dominant or autosomal recessive in inheritance.

(v) Enzyme deficiency leads to accumulation of large amounts of intermediates in the body, which include porphyrin precursors and porphyrins (delta-aminolevulinic acid, porphobilinogen, uroporphyrin, coproporphyrin and protoporphyrin). The intermediates initially accumulate in the liver or the bone marrow and then appear in blood. They are excreted from the body in urine and faeces. Urine from some porphyria patients may be reddish in colour due to the presence of excess porphyrins and related substances in the urine, and may darken after exposure to light.

(vi) Porphyrias are classified into several types:

- *Acute porphyrias:*
  - ALA-D porphyria—autosomal recessive
  - Acute intermittent porphyria—autosomal dominant
  - Hereditary coproporphyria—autosomal dominant
  - Variegate porphyria—autosomal dominant
- *Non-acute porphyrias:*
  - Congenital erythropoietic porphyria—autosomal recessive
  - Porphyria cutanea tarda—complex genetic transmission
  - Erythropoietic protoporphyria—autosomal dominant

The clinicopathological features of various porphyrias are summarized in Table 1.8.

2. **Exogenous pigments**

(a) **Inhaled pigments:** The most common inhaled pigment is carbon; others include silica, iron, and asbestos. Inhaled carbon is taken up by alveolar macrophages and may settle in the lungs or may be carried by lymphatics

Table 1.8 Clinicopathological features of various porphyrias

Acute intermittent porphyria	Abdominal pain is the most common complaint followed by generalized weakness, vomiting, confusion, tachycardia, fluctuating blood pressure, urinary retention, psychosis, hallucinations and seizures. Porphobilinogen levels are increased. Photosensitivity is absent.
Mixed or variegate porphyria	Variegate porphyria is characterized by lesions in the skin which exhibit slow healing and usually leave pigmented or slightly depressed scars. Photosensitivity, abdominal pain and neurological manifestations are prominent manifestations.
Hereditary coproporphyria	Coproporphyrin levels are high making the patient sensitive to sunlight, patients with HCP present with acute attacks of abdominal pain, vomiting, diarrhea, neuropsychiatric manifestations, hypertension and seizures, as well as increased skin fragility, bullous lesions after exposure to sunlight and increased scarring.
Protoporphyria	Some degree of photosensitivity and skin lesions are seen. The lesions generally subside in 12–24 h and heal without prominent scarring or pigmentation. Hepatobiliary dysfunction may be seen.
Porphyria cutanea tarda	This is the most common porphyria. In porphyria cutanea tarda, exposed skin shows abnormalities similar to those found in variegate porphyria. Most patients have hepatobiliary dysfunction in the form of haemosiderosis, cirrhosis, and sometimes hepatocellular carcinoma
Congenital erythropoietic porphyria	This is a very rare disease, which manifests immediately after birth with passage of dark urine and photosensitivity with skin lesions. These may be accompanied by brownish pigmentation of teeth, increased hair growth, and pronounced scarring. Rare cases with loss of digits and cartilage from ears or nose may be noted.
ALA-D porphyria	ALA-D porphyria involves the nervous system and/or the skin. The disease usually manifests after puberty, more often in women with severe abdominal pain, nausea, vomiting, tachycardia and hypertension, confusion, seizures, and the passing of ALA (delta-aminolevulinic acid) in the urine.

to hilar lymph nodes. Collections of carbon blacken pulmonary parenchyma (**anthracosis**). Excessive accumulations of carbon, as seen in polluted urban areas, may result in emphysema or coal workers' pneumoconiosis.

(b) **Ingested pigments:** Chronic ingestion of metals can cause the following conditions:
   (i) ***Argyria:*** Due to chronic ingestion of silver, causes brownish pigmentation of skin, bowel and kidney.
   (ii) ***Chronic lead poisoning:*** Lead interferes with a number of body functions primarily affecting the central nervous, haematopoietic, hepatic and renal. Acute toxicity is usually due to occupational exposure and is rare. Chronic toxicity on the other hand is much more common. Weakness of extensor muscles (e.g. foot drop, wrist drop), delirium and hallucinations, and blue pigmentation on teeth at gum line are common manifestations of chronic lead poisoning.
   (iii) ***Melanosis coli:*** Pigmentation of colon associated with prolonged ingestion of cathartics.
   (iv) ***Carotenemia:*** Yellow-red discoloration of skin caused by ingestion of carrots.

(c) **Injected pigments:** These include India ink, cinnabar, carbon, etc. used in tattooing. They are ingested by macrophages that reside permanently in the connective tissue.

Q. Write briefly on pathologic calcification. (PA2.5)

Ans. Pathologic calcification is defined as abnormal deposition of calcium salts together with smaller amounts of iron, magnesium and mineral salt forms.

Types

1. **Dystrophic calcification:** Deposition of calcium in dead tissue, for example areas of necrosis (coagulative/liquefactive/caseous/enzymatic fat), atheromas/focal intimal injuries in aorta and larger arteries or ageing heart valves. Dystrophic calcification occurs despite normal calcium metabolism.
2. **Metastatic calcification:** Deposition of calcium in viable tissue, for example blood vessels, kidneys, lungs and gastric mucosa. Metastatic calcification has the same morphology and pathogenesis as dystrophic calcification; however, it is always seen in a background of deranged calcium metabolism (hypercalcaemia). Causes of metastatic calcification include:
   (a) Hyperparathyroidism and hyperthyroidism.
   (b) Vitamin-D intoxication.
   (c) Systemic sarcoidosis (macrophages activate vitamin D precursor).
   (d) Milk–alkali syndrome (excessive calcium ingestion with antacids and milk).
   (e) 'Williams syndrome' or idiopathic hypercalcaemia of infancy (hypersensitivity to vitamin D).
   (f) Renal failure (causes retention of phosphate leading to secondary hyperparathyroidism).
   (g) Increased bone catabolism associated with disseminated bone tumours.

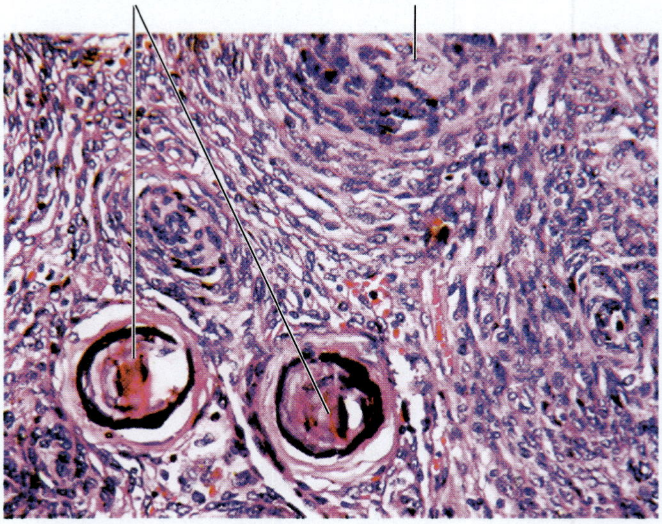

Fig. 1.35 Dystrophic calcification (psammoma bodies) in a meningioma (H&E; 200×).

Pathogenesis

Pathological calcification has two major phases:

- **Initiation:** may occur in:
  - Extracellular sites in membrane-bound vesicles 200 nm in size. Calcium is concentrated in these vesicles due to its affinity for acidic phospholipids.
  - Intracellular sites in mitochondria.
- **Propagation:** involves the formation of crystals of calcium hydroxyapatite.

Morphology

Gross pathology

Appears as fine white granules or clumps of gritty deposits.

Microscopy

- Seen on Haematoxylin and Eosin (H&E) sections as intracellular or extracellular basophilic amorphous granular deposits.
- Sometimes single necrotic cells act as seeds which get encrusted with lamellar mineral deposits (**'psammoma body'**) labelled so due to resemblance to grains of sand and commonly seen in some papillary cancers, for example thyroid and meningiomas (Fig. 1.35).
- Calcium and iron salts may gather about long slender spicules of asbestos in lung, creating beaded, dumb-bell forms called '**asbestos bodies**'.

Q. Differentiate between dystrophic and metastatic calcification. (PA2.5)

Ans. Differences between dystrophic and metastatic calcification are shown in Table 1.9.

Q. Define cell ageing. Enumerate the biochemical and morphological alterations that occur during ageing. (PA2.7)

Ans. Cell ageing is defined as loss of functional capacity and progressive decline in proliferative capacity, which ends in cell death. Most scientists now agree that ageing is, at least in part,

Table 1.9 Differences between dystrophic and metastatic calcification

Features	Dystrophic calcification	Metastatic calcification
Definition	Deposits of calcium salts in dead and degenerated tissue	Deposits of calcium salts in viable tissue
Calcium metabolism	Normal	Deranged
Serum calcium level	Normal	Increased
Sites of deposition	Necrosis, infarcts, thrombi, haematomas, dead parasites, old scars, atheromas	Blood vessels, kidneys, lungs and gastric mucosa

the result of accumulating damage to the molecules—such as proteins, lipids, and nucleic acids (DNA and RNA)—that make up our cells. Reactive oxygen species (ROS) are thought to have a substantial role in damaging biological molecules by stealing their electrons. Normally, an oxygen molecule (O_2) is reduced by transfer of four electrons to H_2 to get converted into two molecules of water. But if an oxygen molecule only takes up one or two electrons, the result is one of a group of highly unstable molecules (ROS) which can mutate genes, damage the lipids that make up cell membranes, and break the cellular proteins, thereby causing cellular injury in multiple and overlapping ways.

Factors Affecting Cellular Ageing

- Genetic factors
- Social conditions
- Diet and antioxidants
- Lifestyle diseases such as atherosclerosis, ischaemic heart disease, diabetes mellitus and hypertension
- Age-related diseases, for example osteoarthritis

Morphological Changes in Senescent Cells

- Irregular and abnormal lobation of nuclei
- Pleomorphic and vacuolated mitochondria
- Dilatation and distortion of endoplasmic reticulum
- Disruption of Golgi apparatus

Indicators of Declining Cell Function

- Decreased oxidative phosphorylation
- Decreased synthesis of structural and enzymatic proteins and cell receptors
- Decreased capacity for uptake of nutrients
- Reduced repair of chromosomal damage

Senescence Related Changes in the Organ Systems

- Immune system: Reduced IgG response and increased frequency of infections is typical. T cells take longer to replenish in older people, and their ability to function declines.
- Heart and blood vessels: Thickening of heart muscle is common as a response to the thickening of the arteries (arteries usually stiffen with age, making it more difficult for the heart to pump blood through them).
- Lungs: The maximum capacity of the lungs may decrease to as much as 40% of normal.
- Brain: As the brain ages, some of the neural pathways seem to become less efficient.
- Urinary system: Efficiency of the kidneys reduces with age. The total capacity of the bladder declines and tissue may atrophy, causing incontinence.
- Body fat: Body fat increases until middle age and then weight typically begins to decrease.
- Musculoskeletal system: Muscle tone declines with age; though regular exercise can slow this decline. Bones begin to lose density by about age 35.
- Sight and hearing: Difficulty in vision may ensue consequent to age-related cataracts and vascular changes in retina. Hearing impairment due to otosclerosis is common.

Theories of Cell Ageing

Cell ageing is considered to be multifactorial in origin. The following hypotheses have been put forward to explain the cellular basis of ageing:

1. ***Endogenous molecular program of cellular senescence***
   (a) Normally, DNA damage is repaired by DNA repair enzymes.
   (b) Accumulation of DNA damage due to defective DNA repair mechanisms induces ageing.
   (c) Activation of senescence-inducing apoptotic genes (on chromosomes 1 and 4) and induction of growth inhibitors also contribute to cell ageing.
   (d) Telomeres are critical for stabilization of terminal portion of chromosomes and anchoring them to nuclear matrix. They are a kind of molecular cap that protects the ends of the chromosomes from damage. Telomere DNA has over 1000 bases, with the sequence TTAGG that repeats over and over. De novo synthesis of telomeres is regulated by an enzyme called telomerase. In order to divide, a normal cell has to replicate the entire DNA in its chromosomes. But normal cells have difficulty in copying the last few bases on the telomere.
   (e) As a result, the telomere shortens with each round of DNA replication and cell division. As a cell ages, the telomere keeps shortening until it reaches a finite length. At that point, cells stop dividing. This halt in growth is triggered by a gene called p53, which is activated in response to DNA damage. A telomere that becomes too short no longer protects the chromosome from DNA damage. When the damage takes place, p53 responds by stopping cell replication and forcing it into senescence. In response to DNA damage (including shortened telomeres), cells either age or self-destruct (apoptosis, programmed cell death), if the damage cannot be easily repaired. As a telomere gets too short, the finite cell growth prevents DNA damaged cell growth that could lead to development of abnormal cells and cancer.

Free radical injury

↓

Covalent modification of intracellular and extracellular proteins, lipids and nucleic acids

↓

Declining function of proteasomes (proteolytic machine that eliminates abnormal or unwanted intracellular proteins)

↓

Accumulation of damaged cellular organelles

↓

Cell ageing

Flowchart 1.17 Exogenous influences in cellular ageing.

2. ***Exogenous influences***
   (a) Extensive observations suggest that DNA damage accumulates with age and that this may be due to an increase in production of free radicals and a decline in DNA repair capacity with age. Mutation or disrupted expression of genes that increase DNA damage often results in premature ageing. In contrast, interventions that enhance resistance to oxidative stress and reduce DNA damage contribute toward longevity.
   (b) Cellular macromolecules are constantly exposed to both extrinsic and intrinsic damages in the form of UV irradiation, toxic environmental agents, and ROS. ROS are produced during normal cellular metabolism, and when their production exceeds the capacity of detoxification, they can cause oxidative damage (Flowchart 1.17). Progressive and irreversible accumulation of oxidative damage contributes to impaired physiological function, thus contributing to increased incidence of disease.

Factors That Reduce Cellular Ageing

1. Caloric and dietary protein restriction inhibits **mTOR activity** (TOR is a nutrient sensitive central controller of cell growth); but also **IGF-1** (activation of which causes upregulation of cell growth and metabolism leading to increased DNA replication and therefore increased frequency of errors in replication), two mechanisms implicated in ageing. Specifically, reducing leucine intake is sufficient to inhibit mTOR activity, achievable through reducing animal food consumption).
2. Mediterranean diet.
3. The amount/duration of sleep.
4. Physical exercise.
5. Avoidance of chronic stress.

Q. Write briefly on heat shock proteins.

Ans: These proteins were initially called heat shock proteins (HSP) because they were found in fruit fly larvae after slight elevation of temperature. They are induced by a large variety of stimuli besides heat shock itself, namely UV radiation, bacterial products, viral infections, parasite toxins, alcohol overload of the endoplasmic reticulum, etc.

They are essential to cell survival in species subjected to injury. Their function is necessary for the homeostasis of the living cell, and becomes especially important in disease, when our cells have to cope with a stressful environment.

- There are two main families of HSP, namely HSP 60 and 70 (Table 1.10). These are involved in intracellular protein folding and translocation, as well as targeting of proteins to their final destination, and are therefore called 'chaperones' or 'chaperonins'. Their levels have been found to increase in stress.
- Ubiquitin is a small HSP critical to protein degradation (proteins are degraded in cellular incinerators called 'proteasomes', when denatured beyond repair). It is universally or ubiquitously present in cells. It has been found to be involved in a variety of degenerative diseases like Alzheimer disease, Parkinsonism, and Creutzfeldt–Jakob disease.

Table 1.10 Major families of molecular chaperones

Chaperone families	Major functions of chaperone families
Small HSP (e.g. Hsp27)	1. Prevents the aggregation of other proteins by collecting protein 'garbage' or irreversibly damaged proteins
HSP60 family	2. Assists in protein folding and refolding
HSP70 family	3. Assists in protein folding and refolding
HSP90 family	4. Promotes the maturation, structural maintenance, and regulation of specific target proteins involved in cell cycle and signal transduction; prevents the aggregation of other proteins by collecting damaged protein
HSP100 family	5. Responsible for degradation of irreversibly damaged proteins, promotion of proteolysis of specific cellular substrates, and regulation of transcription

HSP, Heat shock proteins.

Acute Inflammation

2

Q. Define inflammation. (PA4.1)

Ans. Inflammation is a complex reaction to injury that comprises 'vascular responses' and 'migration and activation of leukocytes'. It basically starts as the body's defence reaction, but may turn potentially harmful.

Q. What are the different stimuli for acute inflammation? (PA4.1)

Ans. Stimuli for acute inflammation include:

1. **Physical agents**: heat, radiation, electrocution and mechanical trauma (blunt/penetrating/crush injuries).
2. **Chemical agents**: organic and inorganic poisons, acids and alkalies, insecticides and pesticides.
3. **Infectious agents**: bacteria, viruses, fungi and parasites.
4. **Immunological agents**: autoimmunity, hypersensitivity reactions.
5. **Ischaemia:** infarction of cardiac muscle (myocardial infarction).

Q. What are the cardinal signs of inflammation? (PA4.1)

Ans. Cardinal signs of inflammation are as follows:

1. Rubor (redness)
2. Tumour (swelling)
3. Calor (heat)
4. Dolour (pain)

(1–4) Proposed by Celsus in the first century AD

5. Functio laesa (loss of function)–added later by Virchow

Q. What are the different types of inflammation? (PA4.1)

Ans. Inflammation can be acute or chronic:

1. **Acute:** Transient process, which occurs within minutes of injury, lasts for hours or days and represents the early body reaction. It is usually followed by repair, a process by which tissue is restored to its original state as far as possible.
2. **Chronic:** It occurs when the causative agent of acute inflammation persists for a long time. Fibrosis and tissue necrosis usually accompany chronic inflammation.

Differences between acute and chronic inflammation are listed in Table 2.1.

Q. What are the major components of acute inflammation? (PA4.1)

Ans. There are two major components of acute inflammation:

1. **Vascular events**
   (a) Alterations in vascular calibre that lead to an increase in blood flow.
   (b) Structural changes in microvasculature, which permit plasma proteins and leukocytes to leave the circulation.
2. **Cellular events:** Immigration of leukocytes from microcirculation and their accumulation in the focus of injury.

Q. Enumerate and describe the different pattern recognition receptors in acute inflammation. (PA4.1)

Ans. Mammalian immunity is of two types: **innate and acquired immunity**. The innate immune system is the first line of host defence against pathogens and is mediated by macrophages and dendritic cells (DCs). Acquired immunity is involved in the late phase of infection and is also responsible for generation of immunological memory. Acquired immunity is specific and develops by clonal selection from a large spectrum of lymphocytes bearing antigen specific receptors that are generated via a mechanism generally known as gene rearrangement. The innate immune response was originally thought to be completely non-specific, but now it is known that it is able to discriminate between self-antigens and a variety of pathogens. Innate system recognizes microorganisms via few germline-encoded **pattern-recognition receptors (PRRs)** unlike the large number of rearranged receptors utilized by the acquired immune system. PRRs recognize microbial components, known as **pathogen-associated molecular patterns (PAMPs)** that are essential for the survival of the microorganism and are therefore difficult for the microorganism to alter. PAMPs that have been identified so far are proteins (e.g. bacterial flagellin), nucleic acids (e.g. viral ssRNA) or glycans (e.g. bacterial lipopolysaccharide (LPS). Different PRRs react with specific PAMPs and activate specific signalling pathways in an attempt eliminate the pathogen. The PRRs are divided into four families:

- Toll-like receptors (**TLR**).
- Nucleotide-binding oligomerization domain-like receptors (**NLR**).
- C-type lectin receptors (**CLR**).
- RIG-1 like receptors (**RLR**) (Fig. 2.1).

Table 2.1 Comparison between acute and chronic inflammation

Feature	Acute	Chronic
Causative agents	Physical (heat, radiation and mechanical trauma) Chemical agents (organic and inorganic poisons) Infectious agents (bacteria, viruses and parasites) Immunological agents (hypersensitivity reactions)	Persistent acute inflammation due to non-degradable pathogens Persistent foreign bodies Autoimmune reactions
Major cells involved	Mainly neutrophils; also eosinophils and basophils	Mononuclear cells (monocytes, macrophages, lymphocytes, plasma cells) and fibroblasts
Primary mediators	Vasoactive amines, eicosanoids	Interferon gamma (IFN-γ) and other cytokines, growth factors, reactive oxygen species and hydrolytic enzymes
Onset	Immediate/rapid	Insidious/delayed
Duration	Few days	Up to many months or years
Outcomes	Resolution, fibrosis and chronic inflammation	Tissue destruction and scarring
Cardinal signs and systemic manifestations	Pain (dolour) Heat (calor) Redness (rubor) Swelling (tumour) Loss of function (functio leasa)	Absence of any cardinal signs Patient is asymptomatic or presents with low-grade fever, lethargy, loss of appetite and weight loss Patient may also present with high-grade fever
Oedema	Present	Absent
Angiogenesis	Absent	Present
Tissue destruction	Absent	Present
Attempts at repair	Absent	Present
Fibrosis	Absent	Present

TLRs as Pattern-Recognition Receptors

"Toll" was the founding member of the TLR family, which is now known to have 12 identified members in mammals till date. TLRs are transmembrane glycoproteins having extracellular domains containing leucine-rich-repeat (LRR) motifs and a cytoplasmic signalling domain homologous to that of the interleukin 1 receptor (IL-1R), termed the Toll/IL-1R homology (TIR) domain. TLRs are expressed on immune cells (macrophages, DCs, B cells), as well as non-immune cells (T cells, fibroblasts and epithelial cells) and can be further divided into several subfamilies, each of which recognizes related PAMPs. TLR expression changes in response to variation in pathogens, cytokine levels and environmental stresses.

Based on differential staining characteristics of their cell walls, bacteria are classified into Gram-positive and -negative organisms. Some of the cell-wall components stimulate immune cells and serve as PAMPs, recognized by individual TLRs. LPS, an endotoxin, is one of the most potent immunostimulants. The lipid portion of LPS termed "lipid A" is responsible for most of the pathogenic phenomena associated with Gram-negative bacterial infection such as endotoxin shock. LPS liberated from Gram-negative bacteria associates with LPS binding protein (LBP), an acute-phase protein present in the bloodstream, and then binds to CD14, a glycosylphosphatidylinositol (GPI) linked protein expressed on the cell surface of phagocytes. Stimulation of TLRs by microbial products leads to the activation of signalling pathways that result in the expression of antimicrobial genes and inflammatory cytokines.

In addition to TLRs, pattern recognition receptors (PRRs) also include complement receptors, scavenger receptors, and C-type lectin receptors, all of which participate in innate immunity. Innate immune recognition operates not only at the membrane level, but also during the process of phagocytosis (TLR 3, TLR 7/8, TLR 9 and TLR 13 and/or C receptors and Fcγ receptors). If microbes survive the intraphagosomal activity and escape into the cytosol, then cytosolic recognition systems like the retinoic acid-inducible gene-I (RIG-I)-like

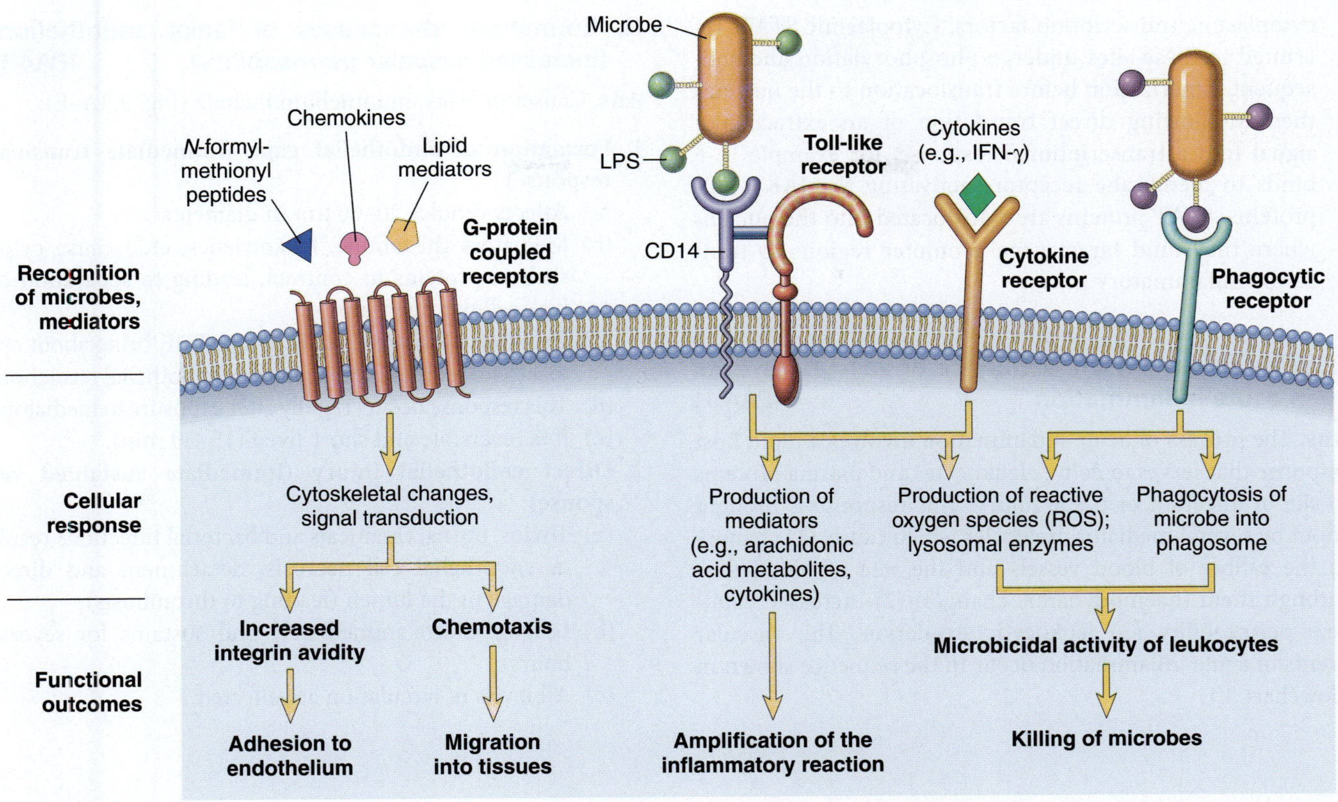

Fig. 2.1 Pattern recognition receptors in acute inflammation. (*Source*: *Robbins Basic Pathology, Tenth Edition*: Vinay Kumar, Abul K. Abbas, Jon C. Aster, Fig. 3.6, Page 66, Elsevier Inc., 2018.)

receptors (RLRs), nucleotide-binding oligomerization domain, leucine-rich repeat-containing protein receptors (NLRs), the family of absent in melanoma (AIM)-like receptors (ALRs), along with a number of cytosolic DNA sensors are at the cell's disposal for intracytosolic recognition of microorganisms or molecules released as a consequence of their damage (damage-associated molecular patterns or DAMPs), for example DNA breakdown products (uric acid), mitochondrial breakdown products (ATP), and DNA itself when it is released into the cytosol. The cytosolic sensors activate a cytosolic complex labelled **"the inflammasome"** which induces the release of IL-1, which in turn activates phagocytosis to destroy damage associated products.

Q. Write briefly on the various pathways involved in inflammation. (PA4.1)

Ans. Inflammatory stimuli activate intracellular signalling pathways that then initiate production of inflammatory mediators. Microbial products and cytokines such as interleukin-1β (IL-1β), interleukin-6 (IL-6), and tumour necrosis factor-α (TNF-α), mediate inflammation through interaction with the TLRs, IL-1 receptor (IL-1R), IL-6 receptor (IL-6R) and the TNF receptor (TNFR). Receptor activation triggers the following intracellular signalling pathways:

1. **NF-κB pathway:** NF-κB is a transcription factor that plays important roles in inflammatory, immune response and apoptosis. NF-κB activity is induced by microbial products, inflammatory cytokines and enzymes. Under physiological conditions, IκB proteins present in the cytoplasm inhibit NF-κB. PRRs activate IκB kinase (IKK) which regulates NF-κB pathway activation through IκB phosphorylation. IκB phosphorylation results in its degradation and release of NF-κB for nuclear translocation and gene transcription activation. This pathway regulates pro-inflammatory cytokine production and inflammatory cell recruitment, which contribute to the inflammatory response.
2. **MAPK pathway:** MAPKs are a family of serine/threonine protein kinases that regulate inflammatory cytokines (such as IL-1, TNF-α and IL-6), which in turn controls cellular proliferation, differentiation and apoptosis. Each MAPK signalling pathway comprises at least three components: a MAPK, a MAPK kinase (MAPKK) and a MAPK kinase kinase (MAPKKK). MAPKKKs phosphorylate and activate MAPKKs, which in turn phosphorylate and activate MAPKs. Activation of the MAPKs leads to phosphorylation and activation of p38 transcription factors present in the cytoplasm or nucleus, which initiates the inflammatory response.
3. **JAK-STAT pathway:** The JAK-STAT pathway involves a signalling mechanism through which extracellular factors (cytokines, growth factors, interferons, leptin and growth hormone) can control gene expression. Receptor-associated JAKs are activated by ligands and phosphorylate one other; creating docking sites for STATs, which are latent,

cytoplasmic transcription factors. Cytoplasmic STATs recruited to these sites undergo phosphorylation and subsequent dimerization before translocation to the nucleus; thereby allowing direct translation of an extracellular signal into a transcriptional response, for example IL-6 binds to membrane receptors activating the JAK-STAT proteins. STAT proteins are translocated into the nucleus where they bind target gene promoter regions to transcribe inflammatory genes.

Q. Write briefly on the sequence of vascular events in acute inflammation. (PA4.1)

Ans. The process of acute inflammation involves a rapid host response that serves to deliver leukocytes and plasma proteins to site of infection or tissue injury. This response is brought about by several mediator molecules which cause: (1) changes in the calibre of blood vessels and the rate of blood flow through them (haemodynamic changes) (2) increased capillary permeability (3) leukocytic exudation. The vascular events in acute inflammation occur in the sequence shown in Flowchart 2.1.

Q. Enumerate the causes of leaky endothelium (increased vascular permeability). (PA4.1)

Ans. Causes of leaky endothelium include (Fig. 2.2A–E):

1. **Formation of endothelial gaps (immediate transient response)**
   (a) Affects venules 20–60 μm in diameter.
   (b) Mediators (histamine, leukotrienes, etc.) cause cytoskeletal proteins to contract, leading to separation of intercellular junctions.
   (c) Cytokine mediators, like IL-1 and TNF, bring about cytoskeletal reorganization, causing endothelial retraction.
   (d) This response occurs rapidly after exposure to mediators.
   (e) It is reversible and short-lived (15–30 min).
2. **Direct endothelial injury (immediate sustained response)**
   (a) Toxins, burns, chemicals and bacterial infections result in endothelial cell necrosis, detachment and direct damage in the lumen (leading to thrombosis).
   (b) Leakage starts immediately and sustains for several hours.
   (c) All levels of circulation are affected.

Immediate transient vasoconstriction of arterioles

↓ Histamine, prostaglandins, PAF, kinins and NO

Persistent progressive vasodilatation of arterioles

↓

Opening of new capillary beds (local heat and redness)

↓

Increased blood volume in microcirculation elevating the hydrostatic pressure

↓

Transudation of fluid into the extracellular space

↓ Further injury and release of histamine, leukotrienes, PAF, and kinins

Increased vascular permeability and escape of exudate into the interstitium (hallmark of acute inflammation)

↓

Stasis

↓

Leucocytic margination or peripheral orientation of WBCs along the endothelial surface (neutrophils stick to the endothelium and migrate through vascular wall into the interstitial tissue. RBCs are smaller, move faster and are oriented centrally)

Flowchart 2.1 Vascular events in acute inflammation.

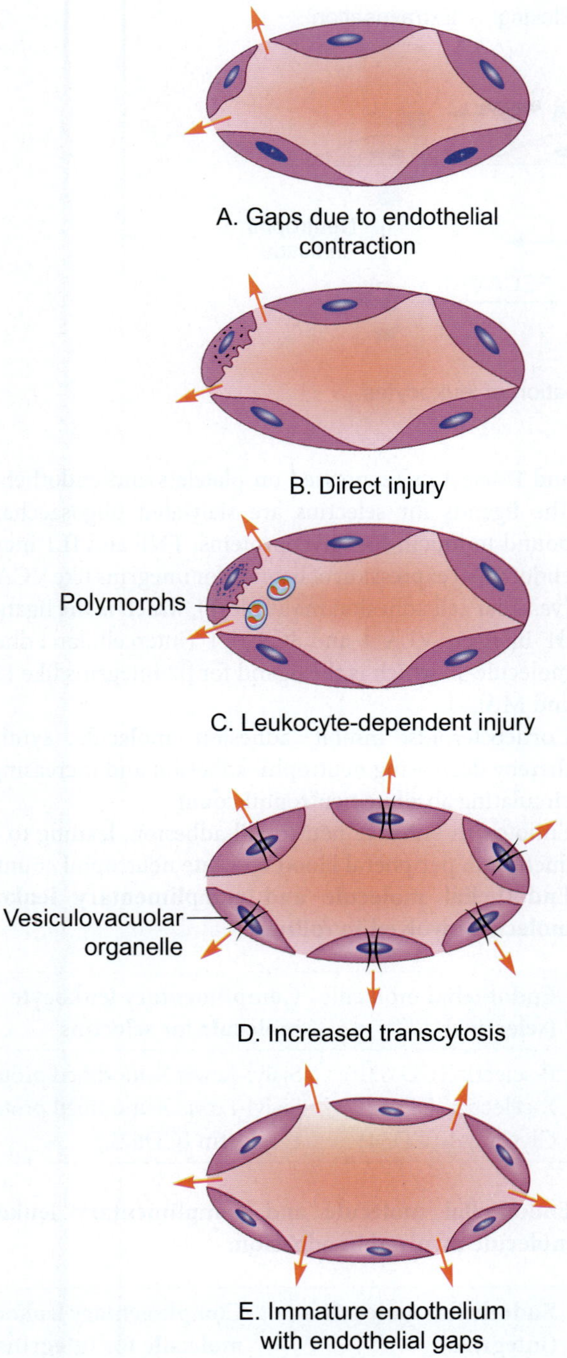

Fig. 2.2 Causes of leaky endothelium. (A) Gaps due to endothelial contraction. (B) Direct injury. (C) Leukocyte dependant injury. (D) Increased transcytosis. (E) Immature endothelium with endothelial gaps.

3. **Delayed prolonged leakage**
   (a) Begins after a delay of 2–12 h, lasts for several hours or even days.
   (b) Involves venules and capillaries.
   (c) Caused by thermal injury, X-rays, UV radiation and bacterial toxins, which lead to delayed endothelial damage by apoptosis or cause endothelial retraction by releasing cytokines.
4. **Leukocyte-mediated endothelial injury**
   (a) Leukocytes adhere to endothelium, release toxic oxygen species and proteolytic enzymes, which cause endothelial injury and increased permeability.
   (b) Largely restricted to venules, pulmonary and glomerular capillaries where leukocytes adhere for prolonged periods.
5. **Increased transcytosis across the endothelial cytoplasm**
   (a) Occurs across interconnected channels made of vesicles and vacuoles called vesiculovacuolar organelles.
   (b) Certain factors, for example vascular endothelial growth factor (VEGF), appear to cause vascular leakage by increasing the number and size of the vascular channels.
6. **Leakage from new blood vessels**
   New vessels formed during angiogenesis remain leaky until endothelial cells mature and form intracellular junctions.

Q. Write briefly on the cellular events involved in acute inflammation. (PA4.1)

Ans. The journey of leukocytes from the vessel lumen to the tissue involves many steps that are controlled by adhesion molecules and cytokines called chemokines. The sequence of cellular events is as follows:

1. **Extravasation of leukocytes**-movement of leukocytes from vessel lumen to the interstitial space (Flowchart 2.2; Fig. 2.3).
2. **Leukocytic recruitment to the site of injury/extravasation** which entails the following events:
   (a) **Luminal events** (events occurring in the vascular lumen):
      (i) **Margination** (peripheral orientation of leukocytes): The two main mechanisms that bring about margination are—rouleaux formation and—dilation of post-capillary venules. Release of increased amounts of fibrinogen (an acute phase protein) in response to cytokines secreted near the site of inflammation induces rouleaux formation, which pushes the

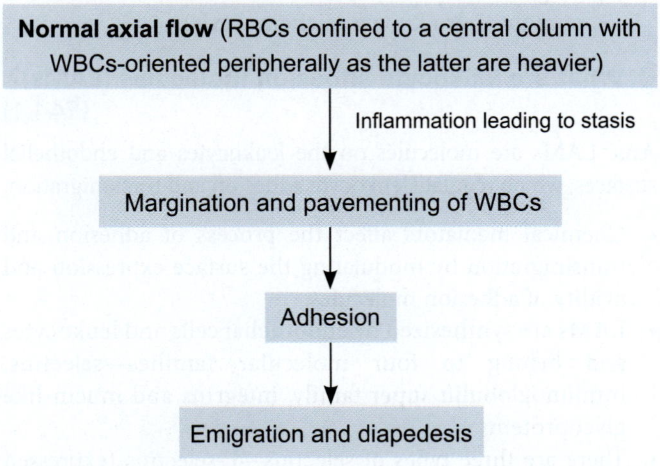

Flowchart 2.2 Sequence of cellular events in acute inflammation.

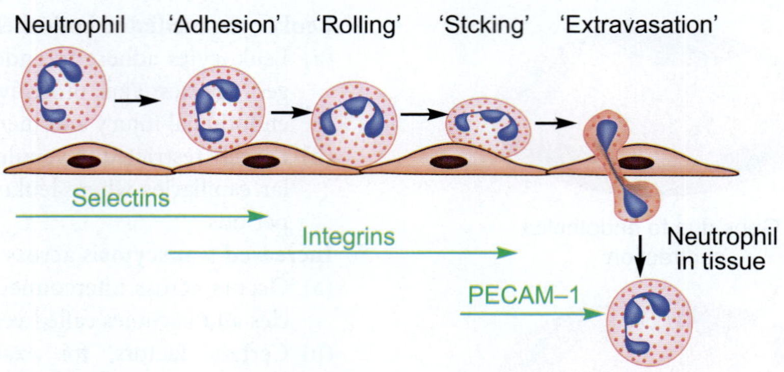

Fig. 2.3 Mechanism of extravasation of leukocytes.

neutrophils against endothelium of the venules. Dilation of post-capillary venues due to inflammatory mediators slows down the velocity of blood flow in these areas, causing neutrophils to marginate against the endothelium of the venules.

(ii) **Rolling** (weak attachment of leukocytes to endothelium, detachment and binding again, causing a rolling movement mediated by **Selectin family** of adhesion molecules and its complementary ligands), **pavementing or adhesion** (activation of leukocytes and firm binding of leukocytes to endothelium mediated by **integrins** and corresponding ligands). The chemical mediators involved in inducing selectins include tumour necrosis factor (TNF), Interleukin-1 (IL-1) and chemokines. TNF and IL-1 also increase the expression of ligands for integrins on leukocytes. Chemokines (chemoattractant cytokines) are responsible for leukocyte activation and transformation of low affinity leukocytic integrins to high affinity integrins.

(b) **Transmigration across the endothelium (emigration or diapedesis):** Emigration is facilitated by focal dissolution of the exposed basement membrane by leukocyte-derived collagenase. This is facilitated by members of the immunoglobulin superfamily - CD31 or -platelet endothelial cell adhesion molecule (PECAM-1).

(c) **Migration** in interstitial tissue towards a chemotactic stimulus (also known as **chemotaxis**).

Q. What are leukocyte adhesion molecules (LAMs)? (PA4.1)

Ans. LAMs are molecules on the leukocytes and endothelial surfaces, which regulate leukocyte adhesion and transmigration.

- Chemical mediators affect the process of adhesion and transmigration by modulating the surface expression and avidity of adhesion molecules.
- LAMs are synthesized by endothelial cells and leukocytes and belong to four molecular families—selectins, immunoglobulin super family, integrins and mucin-like glycoproteins.
- There are three types of selectins—L-selectins (expressed on leukocytes); E-selectins (expressed on endothelial cells) and P-selectins (expressed on platelets and endothelium). The ligands for selectins are sialylated oligosaccharides bound to mucin-like glycoproteins. TNF and IL1 increase endothelial expression of ligands for integrins like VCAM-1 (vascular cell adhesion molecule-1), which is the ligand for β1 integrin VLA-4 and ICAM-1 (intercellular adhesion molecule-1) which is the ligand for β2 integrins like LFA-1 and MAC-1.
- Corticosteroids inhibit adhesion molecule synthesis, thereby decreasing neutrophil adhesion and increasing the circulating absolute neutrophil count.
- Endotoxins enhance neutrophil adhesion, leading to a reduction in peripheral blood absolute neutrophil count.
- **Endothelial molecule and complimentary leukocyte molecule involved in rolling:**

Endothelial molecule (selectins)	Complimentary leukocyte molecule for selectins
P-selectin (CD 62P)	Sialyl-Lewis X-modified proteins
E-selectin (CD 62E)	Sialyl-Lewis X-modified proteins
GlyCam-1 (CD34)	L-selectin (CD62L)

- **Endothelial molecule and complimentary leukocyte molecule involved in adhesion:**

Endothelial molecule (integrins)	Complimentary leukocyte molecule for integrins
ICAM-1 (immunoglobulin family)	CD 11b/CD18 (β2) integrin (LFA-1, MAC-1)
VCAM-1 (immunoglobulin family)	VLA-4 (β1) integrin
GlyCam-1 (CD34)	L-selectin (CD62L)

- CD31 or platelet endothelial cell adhesion molecule-1 (PECAM-1) is the molecule involved in diapedesis.
- **There are three main types LAM deficiencies:**
  - **LAM deficiency type 1** (integrin defects which present with recurrent bacterial infections, usually *Staphylococcus aureus* and gram-negative enteric bacteria. There is sustained leukocytosis due to the absence of leukocyte margination and the patient gives a history of delayed umbilical stump separation).

- **LAM deficiency type II** (selectin defects which manifest with recurrent infections, Bombay phenotype and mental retardation).
- **LAM deficiency type III** (mutations in the gene FERMT3 leading to impaired integrin activation resulting in recurrent infections, leukocytosis and petechial haemorrhage).

Q. Write briefly on chemotaxis. (PA4.1)

Ans. Chemotaxis is defined as locomotion oriented along a chemical gradient. All granulocytes, monocytes and to some extent lymphocytes exhibit directed movement to the area of injury, which is facilitated by chemotactic agents (chemoattractants).

Chemoattractants

1. **Exogenous**—bacterial products.
2. **Endogenous**—C3a, C5a, leukotrienes (mainly LTB-4) and cytokines (mainly IL-6).

Mechanism of Chemotaxis (Flowchart 2.3; Fig. 2.4)

- Neutrophils have numerous receptors, namely, ones for complement, cytokines (Interleukins and IFN-γ), chemokines, lectins, and other proteins. They also express receptors for endothelium and Fc receptors for opsonin.
- In leukocytes, the cellular polarity during chemotaxis is regulated by activities of small Rho guanosine triphosphatases (Rho GTPases) and the phosphoinositide 3-kinases (PI3Ks).
- In neutrophils, lipid products of PI3Ks are the main regulators for activation of Rho GTPases. They accumulate asymmetrically to the plasma membrane at the leading edge of polarized cells.
- The signal that regulates chemotactic movement is initiated by Gi protein-coupled receptors on the cell surface that bind specific chemoattractants.
- The Gi proteins belong to a family of heterotrimeric G proteins, which consist of three subunits: α, β and γ.
- The α subunits contain GTPase activity. Ligand-bound receptors promote the exchange of GDP with GTP on the α subunits, and the GTP-bound forms of Gα subunits are subsequently dissociated from the βγ subunits.
- While the α subunits of the Gi proteins inhibit adenylyl cyclases, the Gβγ subunits can regulate a number of effectors, including phospholipase (PLC) β2/3, phosphatidylinositide 3

Binding of chemoattractants to specific transmembrane G protein–coupled receptors (GPCRs) on the surface of leukocytes

↓

Recruitment of G protein due to signals from GPCRs

↓

Activation of phospholipase C (PLC), phosphoinositol 3 kinase (PI3K) and protein tyrosine kinases (effector molecules)

↓

PLC + PI3K act on membrane phospholipids

↓

Generation of lipid second messengers

↓

↑ Cytosolic calcium

↓

Activation of GTPases and numerous kinases

↓

Polymerization of actin

↓

Locomotion

Flowchart 2.3 Mechanism of chemotaxis.

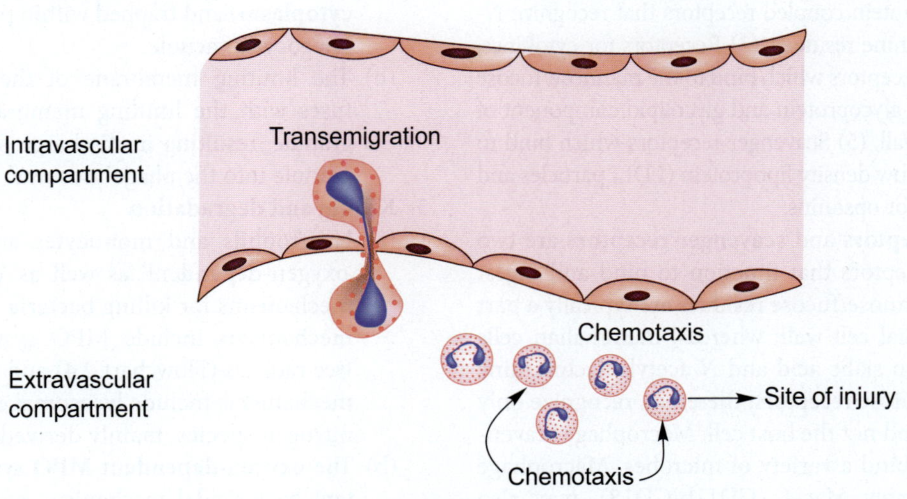

Fig. 2.4 Mechanism of chemotaxis.

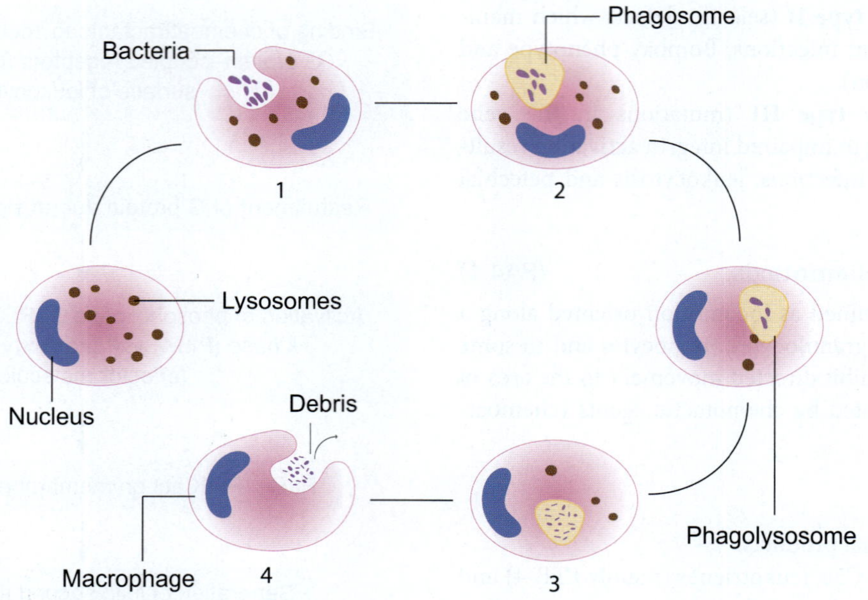

Fig. 2.5 Mechanism of phagocytosis. (1) Engulfment, (2) Phagosome formation, (3) Killing and digestion, (4) Egestion of debris.

(PI3K)γ, ion channels, G protein-coupled receptor kinases and some subtypes of adenylyl cyclases.

Q. Write briefly on phagocytosis. (PA4.1)

Ans. Phagocytosis is defined as leukocytic engulfment of microorganisms, foreign particles and cellular debris. The two most important phagocytic cells are:

1. Polymorphs
2. Circulating monocytes or macrophages

Steps in Phagocytosis (Fig. 2.5)

1. **Recognition and attachment**
   (a) Typically, phagocytosis is initiated by recognition of the microorganisms and particles by receptors expressed on the leukocyte surface. Leukocytes express several receptors including (1) Receptors for microbial products like TLRs, (2) G protein coupled receptors that recognize *N*-formyl methionine residues, (3) Receptors for cytokines, (4) Mannose receptors which bind to the mannose/fucose residues of the glycoprotein and glycolipid component of bacterial cell wall, (5) Scavenger receptors which bind to microbes and low density lipoprotein (LDL) particles and (6) Receptors for opsonins.
   (b) **Mannose receptors** and **scavenger receptors** are two important receptors that function to bind and ingest microbes. Mannose/fucose residues are typically a part of the microbial cell wall; whereas, mammalian cells instead contain sialic acid and *N*-acetylgalactosamine residues. Mannose receptors, therefore, recognize only the microbe and not the host cell. Macrophage scavenger receptors bind a variety of microbes. Macrophage integrins, notably Mac-1 (CD11b/CD18), may also bind microbes for phagocytosis.
   (c) The efficiency of phagocytosis is greatly enhanced by **opsonization** of bacteria (or foreign material).
   (d) The process of coating of a particle, such as a microbe, to target it for phagocytosis is called **opsonization** and the substances that do this are called **opsonins.** Phagocytes express high-affinity receptors for opsonins.
   (e) Major opsonins are **'IgG antibodies'**, **'C3b breakdown products of complement'** and **plasma carbohydrate-binding lectins called 'collectins'**, which bind to the microbial cell wall sugar groups.
   (f) Leukocytes express **receptors for opsonins** that facilitate phagocytosis of the coated microbes, for example **Fc receptor for IgG (FcγRI), complement receptors 1 and 3 (CR1 and 3) for complement fragments** and **C1q for the collectins.**
2. **Engulfment**
   (a) Bacteria are engulfed by **pseudopodia** (**extensions of cytoplasm**) and trapped within phagosomes forming a phagocytic vacuole.
   (b) The limiting membrane of the phagocytic vacuole fuses with the limiting membrane of the lysosomal granule, resulting in discharge of the contents of the granule into the phagolysosome.
3. **Killing and degradation**
   (a) Neutrophils and monocytes are armed with both 'oxygen-dependent' as well as 'oxygen-independent' mechanisms for killing bacteria. 'Oxygen-dependent' mechanisms include MPO system and O_2-derived free radicals (Flowchart 2.4) and 'oxygen-independent' mechanisms include lysosomal enzymes and reactive nitrogen species, mainly derived from nitric oxide.
   (b) The **oxygen-dependent MPO system** is the most potent bactericidal mechanism available to neutrophils and monocytes.

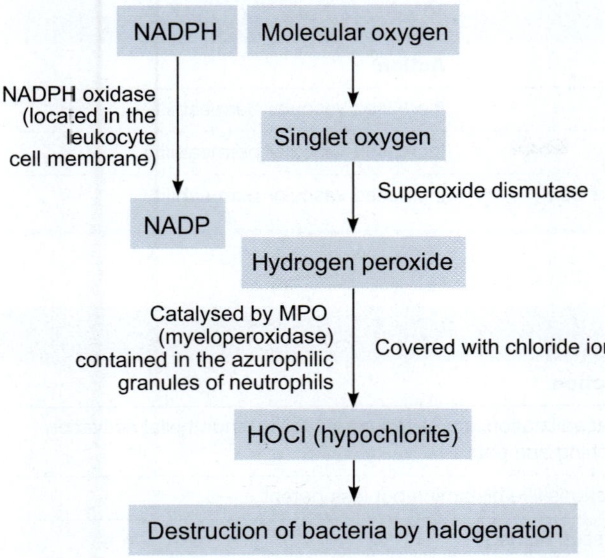

Flowchart 2.4 Mechanism of killing by MPO–H_2O_2–halide system.

Other constituents of leukocyte granules, which are also capable of killing microorganisms include:

- ***Bactericidal/permeability-increasing substances*** (cause phospholipase activation and degradation of phospholipids).
- ***Lysozymes*** (causes degradation of bacterial coat oligosaccharides).
- ***Major basic protein*** (important eosinophilic granule constituent, which is toxic to parasites).
- ***Defensins*** (peptides that kill microbes by creating holes in their membranes).
- ***Neutrophil extracellular taps or NETs*** (Extracellular fibrillary networks consisting a viscous meshwork of nuclear chromatin of neutrophils that trap the microbe at the site of infection by fibrils and prevent their spread). The nuclear chromatin in the NETs, which includes histones and associated DNA, has been found in blood in cases of sepsis; and is also thought to be a source of nuclear antigens in autoimmune diseases.

Q. Enumerate the defects in leukocyte functions. (PA4.1)

Ans. Defects in leukocyte functions may be:

1. **Genetic**
   (a) **Chediak–Higashi syndrome:**
   - This is an autosomal recessive disorder of lysosomal granules; in which there is impaired fusion of lysosomes with phagosomes to form phagolysosomes.
   - It arises from a mutation of a lysosomal trafficking regulator protein (LYST) which leads to a decrease in phagocytosis resulting in disruption of protein synthesis as well as the storage and secretory function of lysosomal granules in WBCs, further resulting in defective WBCs with abnormal function and enlarged vesicles (giant granules).
   - Also present is neutropenia and deficiency in serotonin and adenosine-phosphate-containing granules in platelets causing impaired platelet aggregation, leading to prolonged bleeding time.
   - Patients are therefore susceptible to infections and often present with additional manifestations of oculo-cutaneous albinism (due to pathological aggregation of melanosomes) with hypo-pigmentation of hair, skin and eyes and also nerve defects.

   (b) **Chronic granulomatous disease of childhood:**
   - X-linked/autosomal recessive disease characterized by mutations in any one of the five components of the nicotinamide adenine dinucleotide phosphate (NADPH) oxidase in phagocytes.
   - This enzyme generates superoxide and is essential for intracellular killing of pathogens by phagocytes (oxidative burst).
   - CGD is a primary immunodeficiency that leads to recurrent or persistent intracellular bacterial and fungal infections and to granuloma formation. As the neutrophil defence is inadequate/low a macrophage rich granulomatous inflammation tries to contain the infection.
   - Patients with CGD are susceptible to severe and recurrent infections due to catalase-positive organisms and organisms resistant to non-oxidative killing.
   - The first manifestations of CGD appear during the first year of life in the form of infections, dermatitis, colitis, and a failure to thrive. Cutaneous disease occurs in 60%–70% of patients.
   - The nitroblue tetrazolium (NBT) dye test is used to diagnose CGD (Neutrophils in patients with CGD are unable to reduce oxidized NBT to insoluble blue formazan).

   (c) **Myeloperoxidase deficiency:** Reduced microbial killing due to absent MPO–H_2O_2 system.
2. **Acquired**
   (a) **Defective chemotaxis**: thermal injury, diabetes, malignancy, sepsis and immunodeficiencies.
   (b) **Defective adhesion:** haemodialysis and diabetes.
   (c) **Defective phagocytosis and microbicidal activity**: leukaemia, anaemia, sepsis, diabetes, neonates and malnutrition.

Q. Enumerate the chemical mediators of inflammation. (PA4.2)

Ans. Chemical mediators of inflammation may be plasma derived or cell derived.

- **Plasma-derived** mediators are mainly produced in the liver; circulate in precursor form and must be activated. These include three interdependent systems, namely, (1) Complement system, (2) Kinins, and (3) Clotting system (Table 2.2).
- **Cell-derived** mediators are synthesized de novo or are preformed and stored in intracellular granules and need to be secreted. These include vasoactive amines, arachidonic acid metabolites, cytokines, chemokines, platelet activating factor, nitric oxide, neuropeptides and lysosomal constituents of leukocytes (Table 2.3).

Table 2.2 Plasma-derived mediators

Sources	Mediator	Action
Clotting and fibrinolytic system	Fibrin split products	Increased vascular permeability
Kinin system	Kinin/bradykinin	Increased vascular permeability
Complement system	Anaphylatoxins, C3a, C4a and C5a	Increased vascular permeability

Table 2.3 Cell-derived mediators

Sources	Mediator	Action
Mast cells, basophils and platelets	Histamine[a]	Vasodilatation, increased permeability, endothelial activation, itching and pain
Platelets and enterochromaffin cells	Serotonin[a]	Actions like histamine but less potent
Neutrophils and macrophages	Lysosomal enzymes[a]	Tissue damage
All leukocytes and endothelial cells	Platelet-activating factor[b]	Increased vascular permeability
All leukocytes	Leukotrienes[b] (slow reacting substances of anaphylaxis)	**LTC4, LTD4 and LTE4** • Increased permeability of vessels • Smooth muscle contraction • Vasoconstriction • Bronchoconstriction **LTB4** • Chemotaxis • Cell adherence
All leukocytes, platelets and endothelial cells	Prostaglandins[b]	**PGD2 and PGE2** • Vasodilatation • Bronchodilatation • Increased permeability of vessels
		PGF2α • Vasodilatation • Bronchoconstriction **TXA2** • Vasoconstriction • Bronchoconstriction • Platelet aggregation **PGI2** • Vasodilatation • Bronchodilatation • Inhibition of platelet aggregation
Lymphocytes, macrophages and endothelial cells	Cytokines[b]	Increased leukocyte adhesion, thrombosis, fibroblastic proliferation and acute phase reaction (increased secretion of **IL8** chemotactic for neutrophils, **PF4** chemotactic for neutrophils, monocytes and eosinophils, **MCP-1** chemotactic for monocytes and **eotaxin** chemotactic for eosinophils)
Macrophages	Nitric oxide[b]	Vasodilatation, antiplatelet effect and microbicidal action
Neutrophils and macrophages	Oxygen-derived free radicals	Endothelial damage and increased vascular permeability

[a]Preformed mediators.
[b]Newly synthesized mediators.

- **Production of active mediators** is triggered by microbial products or by host proteins, such as proteins of the complement, kinin and coagulation systems that are themselves activated by microbes and damaged tissue.
- Most mediators act by binding to specific receptors on target cells; one mediator can stimulate release of other mediators.
- Once activated and released from the cells, most of these mediators are short-lived.
- The **various mechanisms underlying their action** include:
- Receptor–ligand interactions.
- Direct enzymatic activity.
- Oxidative damage.

Q. Enumerate the steps involved in generation of arachidonic acid metabolites. (PA4.2)

Ans. Steps involved in generation of arachidonic acid metabolites and their role in inflammation are summarized in Flowchart 2.5.

- There are two types of cyclooxygenases–COX-1 and COX-2. It was earlier thought that COX-1 are responsible for the production of prostaglandins that are involved in both inflammation and homoeostasis (fluid and electrolyte balance and cytoprotection of gastrointestinal tract or GIT), whereas COX-2 generate prostaglandins that are only involved in inflammation. The role of COX-2 inhibitors has therefore been explored as anti-inflammatory agents. It has now been found that COX-2 may not be completely selective and may also play a role in homoeostasis and also COX-2 inhibitors may increase the risk of cardiovascular and cerebrovascular events as they decrease endothelial production of Prostacyclin-I-2 (vasodilator and inhibitor of platelet aggregation).
- Lipoxygenase is not affected by non-steroidal antiinflammatory drugs (NSAIDs). Inhibitors of this enzyme may be helpful in asthma as they inhibit production of leukotrienes.

Q. Write briefly on platelet-derived factor (PAF). (PA4.2)

Ans. PAF is a bioactive phospholipid-derived mediator, which has multiple inflammatory effects. It is also known as AGEPC (acetyl-glyceryl-ether-phosphorylcholine) and mediates its effects via a single G protein–coupled receptor. It is regulated by a family of inactivating PAF acetyl hydrolases. The PAF signalling cascade consists of PAF and PAF-like lipids (PAF-LL) that are ligands for a G-protein coupled receptor, the PAF receptor (PAFR). Engagement of the PAFR by PAF or PAF-LL triggers a variety of intracellular signalling cascades that initiate or amplify inflammatory and thrombotic events.

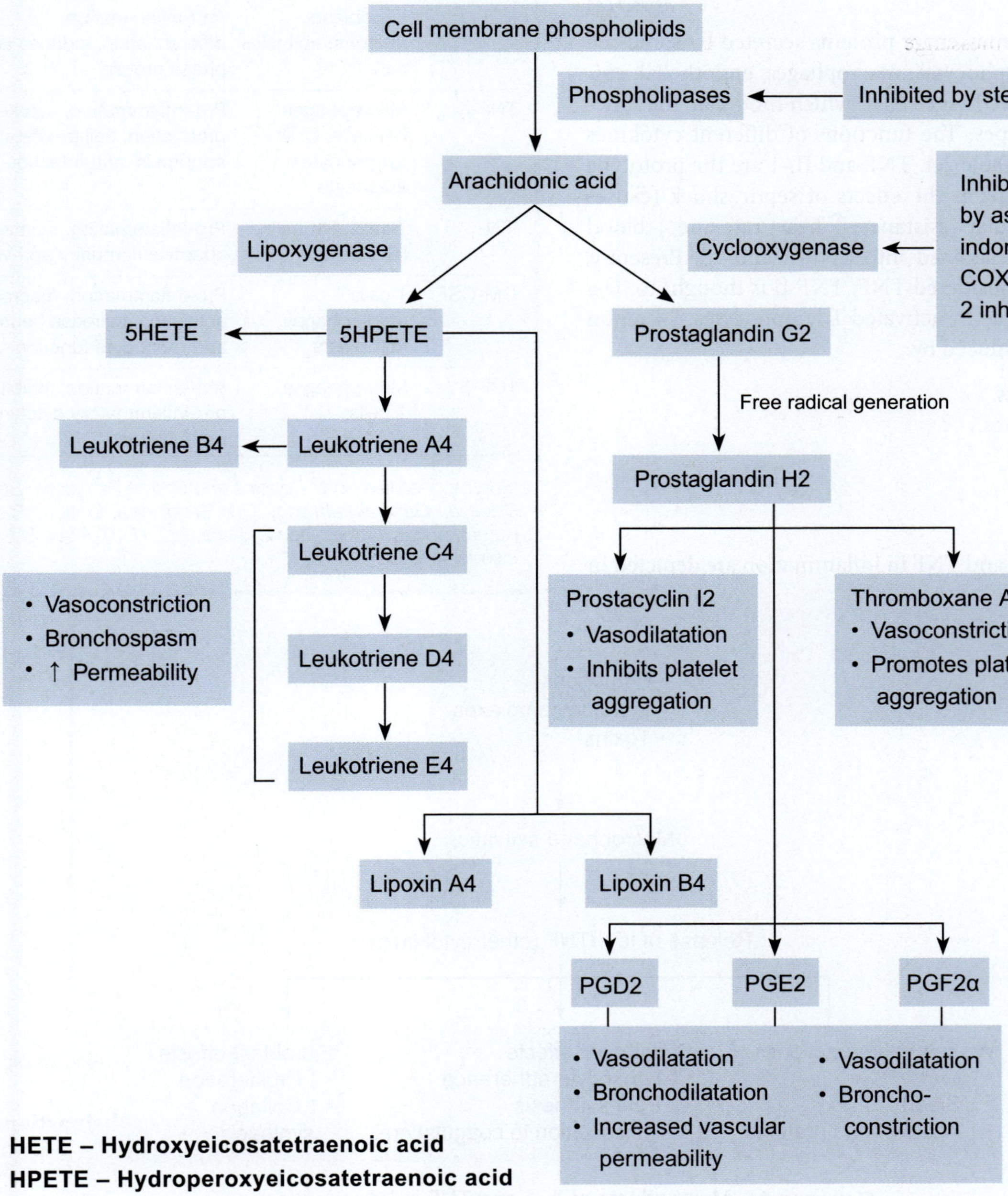

Flowchart 2.5 Generation of arachidonic acid metabolites and their role in inflammation.

- **Sources**
  - Endothelial cells
  - Platelets
  - Neutrophils, basophils and monocytes
- **Actions/effects**
  - Vasoconstriction/vasodilatation and increased vascular permeability.
  - Bronchospasm/bronchconstriction.
  - Activation of neutrophils (induces extrusion of neutrophil extracellular traps), monocytes, and platelets.
  - Enhanced endothelial-leukocyte, platelet-leukocyte, and platelet-endothelial cell interactions.
  - Platelet aggregation and degranulation.
  - Increased chemotaxis and leukocytic degranulation.
  - Increase in oxidative burst.
  - Enhanced synthesis of mediators, for example eicosanoids.

Q. What are cytokines? Describe their role in inflammation. (PA4.2)

Ans. Cytokines are messenger proteins secreted by some cell types (activated lymphocytes, macrophages, endothelial, epithelial and connective tissue cells), which modulate the function of other cell types. The functions of different cytokines are summarised in Table 2.4. TNF and IL-1 are the prototype cytokines. TNF mediates the effects of septic shock (causes hypotension, ↓ vascular resistance, ↑ heart rate and ↓ blood pH). It was earlier classified into TNF-α and -β. Presently, TNF-α is actually considered TNF; TNF-β is thought to be a lymphotoxin produced by activated T lymphocytes. Secretion of TNF and IL1 is induced by:

- Bacterial products.
- Immune complexes.
- Toxins.
- Cytokines.
- Physical injury.

Major effects of IL-1 and TNF in inflammation are depicted in Flowchart 2.6.

Table 2.4 Summary of cytokines and their functions

Cytokine	Main sources	Function
IL-1β	Macrophages, monocytes	Pro-inflammation, proliferation, apoptosis, differentiation
IL-4	Th-cells	Anti-inflammation, T-cell and B-cell proliferation, B-cell differentiation
IL-6	Macrophages, T-cells, adipocyte	Pro-inflammation, differentiation, cytokine production
IL-8	Macrophages, epithelial cells, endothelial cells	Pro-inflammation, chemotaxis, angiogenesis
IL-10	Monocytes, T-cells, B-cells	Anti-inflammation, inhibition of the pro-inflammatory cytokines
IL-12	Dendritic cells, macrophages, neutrophils	Pro-inflammation, cell differentiation, activates NK cell
IL-11	Fibroblasts, neurons, epithelial cells	Anti-inflammation, differentiation, induces acute phase protein
TNF-α	Macrophages, NK cells, CD4 + lymphocytes, adipocyte	Pro-inflammation, cytokine production, cell proliferation, apoptosis, anti-infection
IFN-γ	T-cells, NK cells, NKT cells	Pro-inflammation, innate, adaptive immunity anti-viral
GM-CSF	T-cells, macrophages, fibroblasts	Pro-inflammation, macrophage activation, increase neutrophil and monocyte function
TGF-β	Macrophages, T cells	Anti-inflammation, inhibition of pro-inflammatory cytokine production

(*Source*: Modified from: *Robbins and Cotran Pathologic Basis of Disease - General Pathology,* First Bangladesh Edition: Vinay Kumar, Abul K. Abbas, Jon C. Aster, Fig. 17-37, Page 802, Elsevier Inc., 2017.)

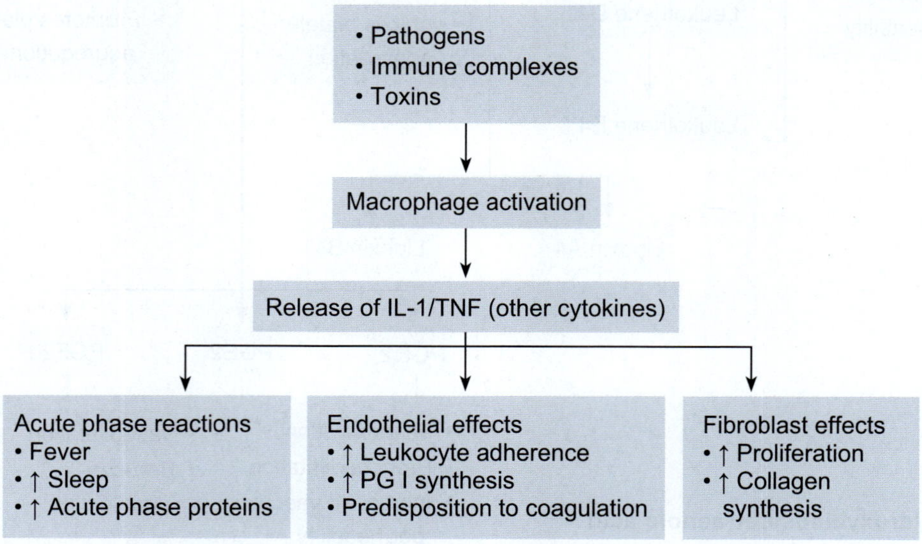

Flowchart 2.6 Major effects of IL-1 and TNF in inflammation.

Interferon gamma (IFNγ) is a dimerized soluble cytokine that has antiviral, immunoregulatory, and anti-tumour properties. This interferon was originally called macrophage-activating factor, and is especially important in the maintenance of chronic inflammation. IFNγ is produced predominantly by natural killer (NK) and natural killer T (NKT) cells as part of the innate immune response, and by CD4 Th1 and CD8 cytotoxic T lymphocyte (CTL) effector T cells once antigen-specific immunity develops. IFNγ has the following actions:

- Promotion of NK cell activity.
- Increased antigen presentation and lysosome activity of macrophages.
- Activation of inducible nitric oxide synthase (iNOS).
- Increased production of IgG2a and IgG3 from activated plasma B cells.
- Increased expression of class I MHC molecules as well as class II MHC on antigen-presenting cells.
- Increased leukocytic adhesion and migration.

Q. Write briefly on chemokines. (PA4.2)

Ans. Chemokines are a family of small, 8–10 kD proteins that act primarily as chemoattractants for specific leukocytes. They bind to seven transmembrane G protein–coupled receptors. There are 40 different types of chemokines and 20 different types of chemokine receptors. Chemokines are classified into four groups based on the arrangement of conserved cysteine residues in the proteins, namely,

1. **CXC chemokines or α-chemokines**
   (a) One amino acid residue separates first two conserved cysteine residues.
   (b) Typical example is IL8. IL8 is secreted by macrophages and endothelial cells and primarily acts on neutrophils (activation and chemotaxis of neutrophils).
2. **CC chemokines or β-chemokines**
   (a) Two conserved cysteine residues are located adjacent to each other.
   (b) Include MCP-1, eotaxin, MIP-α and RANTES (regulated and normal T cell expressed and secreted).
   (c) Chemotactic for monocytes, eosinophils, basophils and lymphocytes (not neutrophils).
3. **C chemokines or γ-chemokines:** Lack first and third (two of four) cysteines, for example lymphotactin specific for lymphocytes.
4. **CX_3C chemokines:** Three amino acid residues between two cysteines, for example fractalkine.

Q. Write briefly on nitrous oxide (NO). (PA4.2)

Ans. NO (also called endothelium-derived relaxing factor) is a soluble gas produced by endothelial cells (eNOS), macrophages (iNOS) and neurons (nNOS).

- Of these isoforms, eNOS is constitutively expressed (activated rapidly by increase in calcium).
- iNOS is induced when macrophages are activated by cytokines (TNF, γIFN).
- NO is synthesized from L-arginine by NOS (nitric oxide synthase).
- Acts in a paracrine manner via cyclic GMP.
- Causes vasodilatation, ↓ platelet aggregation, ↓ platelet adhesion, ↓ mast cell-induced inflammation.
- Regulates leukocyte recruitment and microbicidal activity.

Q. Write briefly on neuropeptides. (PA4.2)

Ans. Neuropeptides are small proteins such as substance P and neurokinin A that transmit pain signals, regulate vessel tone and modulate vascular permeability. They are secreted by nerve fibres in lungs, GIT and leukocytes.

Q. Write briefly on the 'complement system'. (PA4.2)

Ans. Complement was first discovered as a **heat-labile component of normal plasma** that was found to **add to** or **augment the opsonization of bacteria by antibodies** and **facilitate bacterial killing.** The name derives from the fact that this system was found to 'complement' the antibacterial activity of the antibody.

- Complement system is an **important part of the innate** and **adaptive immune responses.**
- It is constituted by a **collection of 30 different proteins,** which include serum and cell surface proteins as well as cell membrane receptors.
- The complement proteins, in their precursor zymogen forms, are **widely distributed throughout body fluids and tissues without any adverse effect.** They are activated at sites of infection or injury, however, to trigger a series of potent inflammatory events. Their action occurs via **three pathways**:

1. **Classical pathway** (Flowchart 2.7)
2. **Alternative pathway** (Flowchart 2.8)
3. **Mannose-binding lectin pathway or MBL–MASP** (MBL-associated serine proteases; homologous to the classical pathway; Flowchart 2.9):

Effector Functions of Complement Proteins

- **C3b and its cleavage products** are potent effector proteins in opsonization and phagocytosis by neutrophils and macrophages.
- C3a and C5a are majorly involved in leukocyte activation and chemotaxis of neutrophils, monocytes, eosinophils and basophils. They also induce vasodilatation and increase permeability of the capillary beds by increasing histamine release from mast cells. C5a, in addition, activates the lipooxygenase pathway of arachidonic acid metabolism in neutrophils and monocytes, thereby augmenting the release of chemical mediators.
- The **early complement components** (C1q, C3) break down and eliminate apoptotic cells and the antigen-antibody complexes from the body, failure of which can lead to immune complex diseases.
- **Killing of microbes through direct lysis is mediated by the MAC, C5b-9** (Complement-mediated lysis can cause serious disorders such as Rh disease, immune haemolytic anaemia and immune thrombocytopenic purpura).
- **Complement promotes antibody formation through breakdown products.** Breakdown of C3b generates a fragment (C3d) that binds to antigens to aid in their uptake by antigen-presenting cells and B cells.
- Complement proteins also **protect against pathogens by inducing innate and adaptive immunity**.

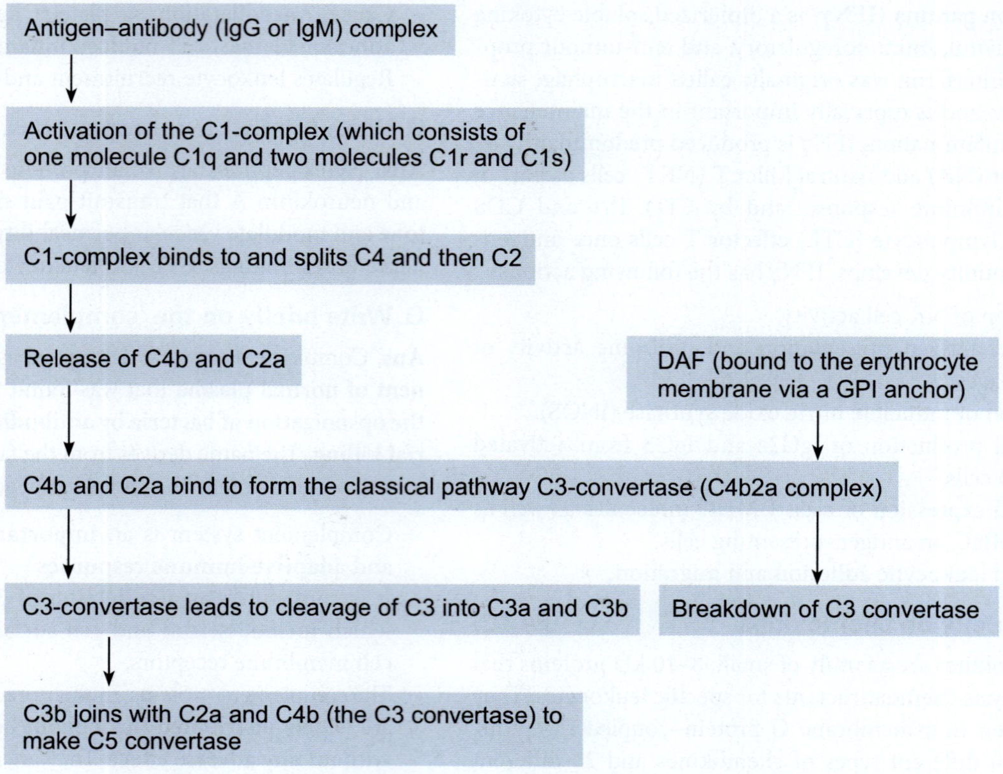

Flowchart 2.7 Classical pathway of complement activation.

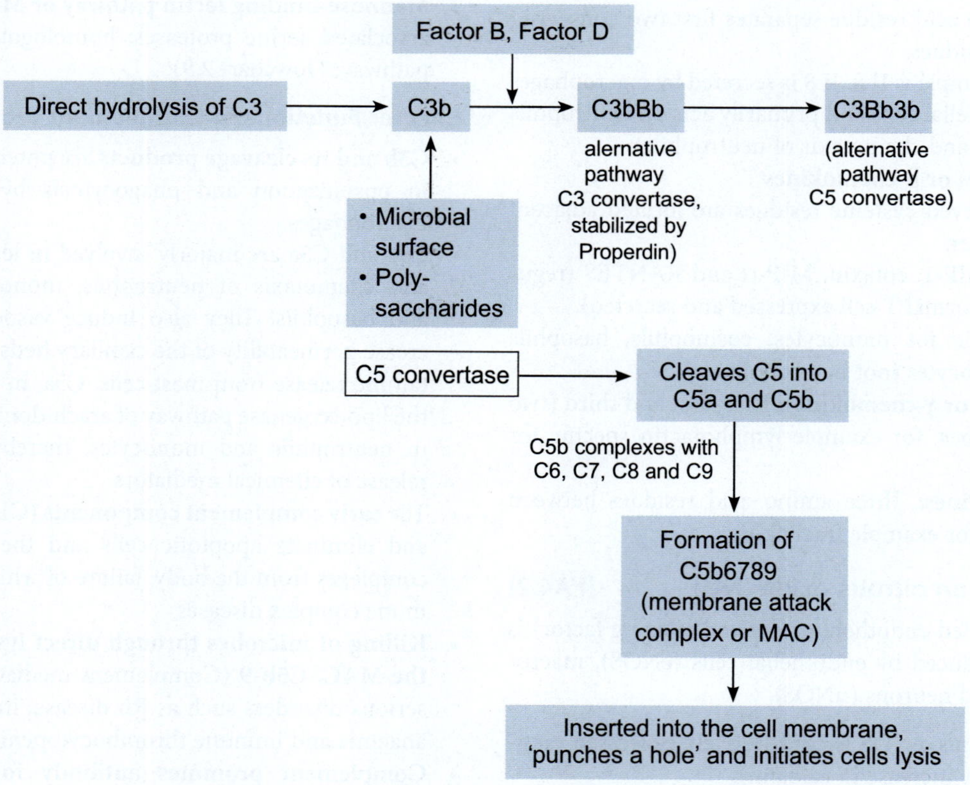

Flowchart 2.8 Alternative pathway of complement activation.

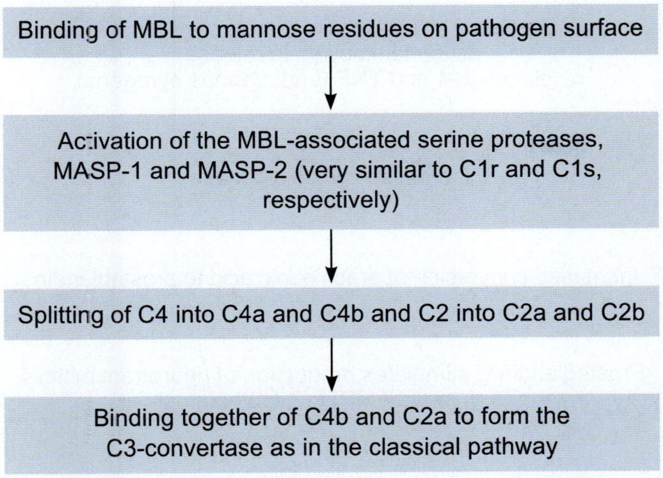

Flowchart 2.9 Complement activation by MBL–MASP pathway.

Q. Enumerate the steps involved in activation of kinin and clotting systems. (PA4.2)

Ans. Factor XII (Hageman factor) is a protein that circulates in the inactive form. It undergoes conformational changes and gets activated on exposure to negatively charged surfaces such as basement membranes, proteolytic enzymes, bacterial lipopolysaccharide and foreign materials. When activated, it is able to further activate three plasma systems involved in inflammation: the kinin system, fibrinolysis system and coagulation system (Flowchart 2.10).

1. **Kinin system:** Kinins are potent inflammatory agents formed in plasma and tissue by the action of serine proteases **kallikreins** on specific plasma glycoproteins termed **kininogens**. Kinins are rapidly inactivated by **kininases**, and therefore have rapid and short-lived functions. The most significant function of kinins is their ability to amplify inflammatory responses by stimulating local tissue and inflammatory cells to generate additional mediators, including prostanoids, cytokines (especially tumour necrosis factor and interleukins), nitric oxide and tachykinins. The kinin system eventually generates proteins like **bradykinin**, which has the following functions:
   (a) Smooth muscle contraction.
   (b) Vasodilatation.
   (c) Increased vascular permeability.
   (d) Generation of pain.
2. **Clotting/coagulation system:** The coagulation proteins undergo a complex interplay of reactions resulting in the conversion of soluble fibrinogen to insoluble fibrin strands. Natural anticoagulants are anti-inflammatory in nature, they bring down the levels of cytokines, facilitate the

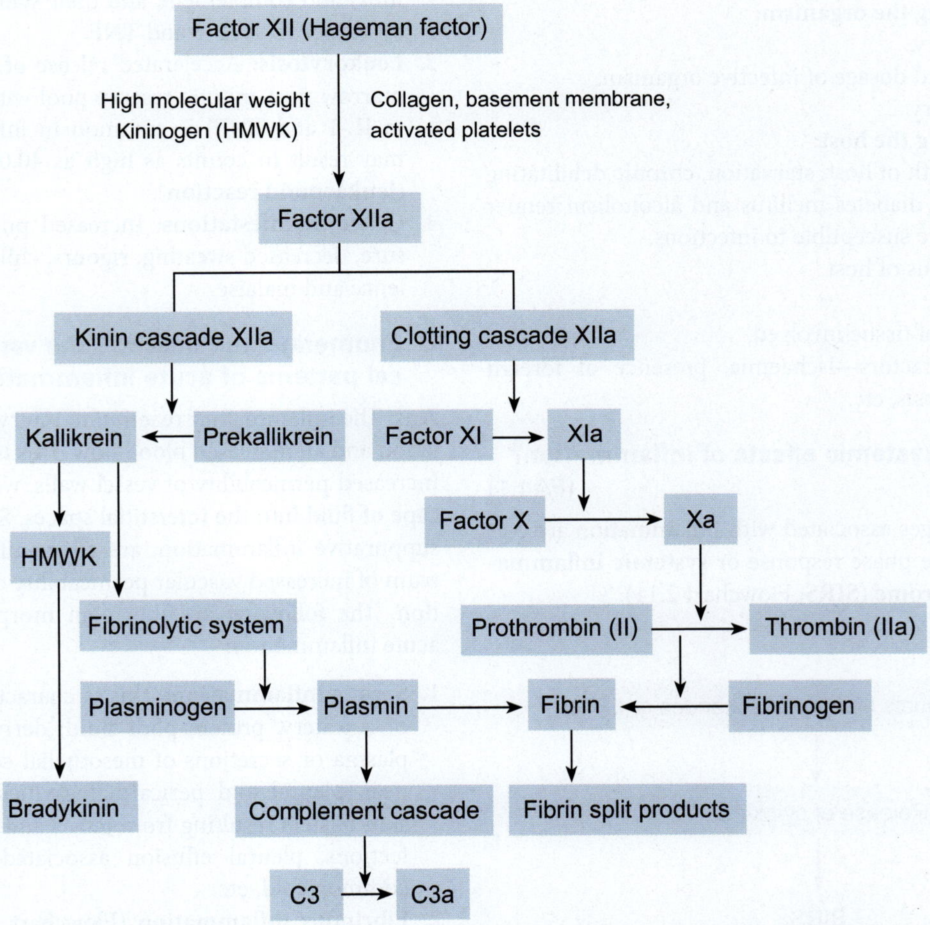

Flowchart 2.10 Interrelationship of four plasma-derived systems (Hageman factor XII of the clotting system plays a key role in the interaction of these systems).

neutralisation of some inflammatory mediators and minimise endothelial cell dysfunction by rendering the cells less responsive to inflammatory mediators. Hence, downregulation of anticoagulant pathways not only promotes thrombosis but also amplifies the inflammatory process. Inflammatory signalling is mainly mediated via thrombin and protease-activated receptors (PARs).

3. **Fibrinolytic system:** The fibrinolytic system is activated simultaneously with the coagulation cascade and functions to maintain the fluidity of blood during coagulation. It also serves in clot lysis once tissue repair begins. When a clot is formed, plasminogen is incorporated and then converted to plasmin by tissue plasminogen activator (tPA) and fragments of factor XII. Endothelial cells release tPA in response to thrombin. Plasmin degrades fibrin and fibrinogen into small fibrin degradation products (FDPs), converts C3 to C3a and activates factor XII. FDPs are anticoagulant in nature because they compete with fibrinogen for thrombin; they are normally cleared by the monocyte-macrophage system.

Q. Enumerate the factors determining variation in inflammatory response of different individuals. (PA4.1)

Ans. Factors determining variation in individual inflammatory responses are as follows:

1. **Factors involving the organism:**
   (a) Type of injury.
   (b) Virulence and dosage of infective organism.
   (c) Portal of entry.
2. **Factors involving the host:**
   (a) General health of host; starvation, chronic debilitating diseases like diabetes mellitus and alcoholism render the host more susceptible to infections.
   (b) Immune status of host.
   (c) Neutropenia.
   (d) Site or type of tissue involved.
   (e) Local host factors—ischaemia, presence of foreign bodies, necrosis, etc.

Q. What are the systemic effects of inflammation? (PA4.1)

Ans. Systemic changes associated with inflammation are collectively called acute phase response or **systemic inflammatory response syndrome** (**SIRS**; Flowchart 2.11).

Bacterial products (lipopolysaccharides or LPS)
↓
Release of cytokines
↓
SIRS

Flowchart 2.11 Systemic inflammatory response syndrome.

Bacterial products (exogenous pyrogens) act on leukocytes to release cytokines IL-1 and TNF (endogenous pyrogens)
↓
Increased cyclooxygenase
↓
Increased conversion of arachidonic acid to prostaglandins
↓
Prostaglandin E stimulates production of neurotransmitters (e.g. cyclic AMP) in hypothalamus
↓
Resetting of the temperature at a higher level

Flowchart 2.12 Mechanism of development of fever in SIRS.

Manifestations of SIRS include:

1. **Fever:** The mechanism underlying development of fever is depicted in Flowchart 2.12.
2. **Release of acute phase proteins:** Acute phase proteins/reactants, for example C reactive protein (CRP), fibrinogen and serum amyloid A (SAA) protein, are mostly synthesized in the liver. They bind to the cell wall (act as opsonins) and complement, and their synthesis is regulated by cytokines IL-1, IL-6 and TNF.
3. **Leukocytosis:** Accelerated release of cells from the bone marrow post-mitotic reserve pool with a shift to left (due to IL-1 and TNF) is common in inflammation and this may result in counts as high as 40,000–100,000 cells/μL (**leukaemoid reaction**).
4. **Other manifestations:** Increased pulse and blood pressure, decreased sweating, rigours, chills, anorexia, somnolence and malaise.

Q. Enumerate and describe the various morphological patterns of acute inflammation. (PA4.4)

Ans. The inflammatory reaction to injury begins with vasodilation and an increased blood flow. This is accompanied by an increased permeability of vessel walls, which leads to the escape of fluid into the interstitial spaces. Serous, fibrinous and suppurative inflammation, are all manifestations of a spectrum of increased vascular permeability caused by inflammation. The following are the main morphologic patterns of acute inflammation:

1. **Serous inflammation:** This is characterized by collection of a watery, protein-poor fluid; derived from either the plasma or secretions of mesothelial cells that line peritoneal, pleural and pericardial cavities. Examples include skin blisters resulting from burns and scalding or viral infections, pleural effusion associated with tuberculosis, common cold, etc.
2. **Fibrinous inflammation** (Flowchart 2.13; Fig. 2.6): This type of inflammation occurs as a consequence of more severe injuries, with greater vascular permeability allowing

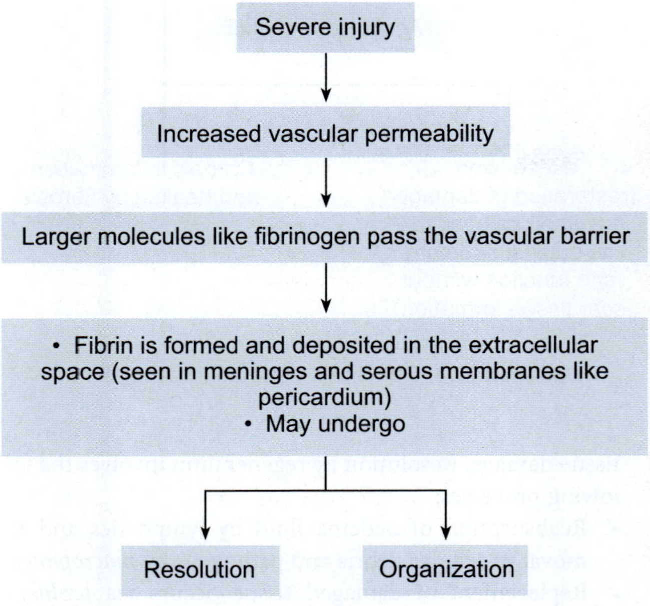

Flowchart 2.13 Pathogenesis and outcomes of fibrinous inflammation.

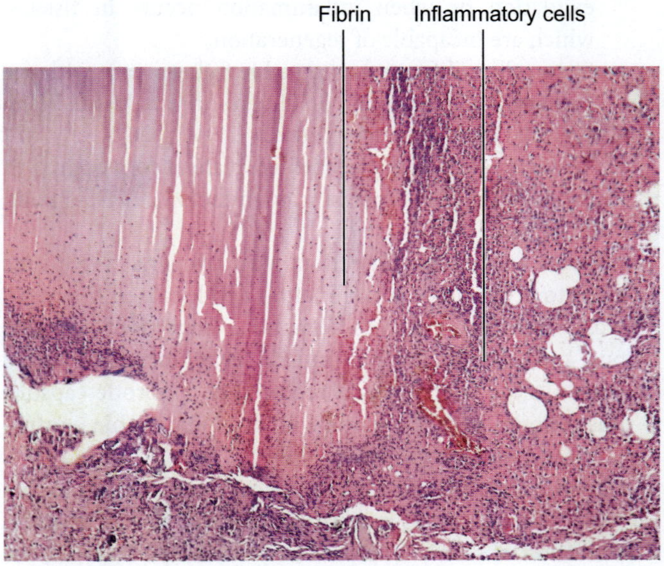

Fig. 2.6 Fibrinous inflammation composed of pink fibrinous deposits and acute and chronic inflammatory cells (H&E; 100×).

larger molecules (fibrinogen) to pass the endothelial barrier. Fibrinous inflammation may resolve completely or organize. Organization is commonly seen in serous cavities, where the fibrinous exudate converts into a scar between serous membranes, limiting their function. During inflammation of the intestine (pseudomembranous colitis), pseudomembrane can form. Other examples of fibrinous inflammation include 'bread and butter' pericarditis seen in acute rheumatic fever and fibrinous pleuritis.

3. **Suppurative inflammation**
   - Involves production of large amount of pus or purulent exudates comprising neutrophils, necrotic cells and oedema fluid. The pus may collect locally to form an

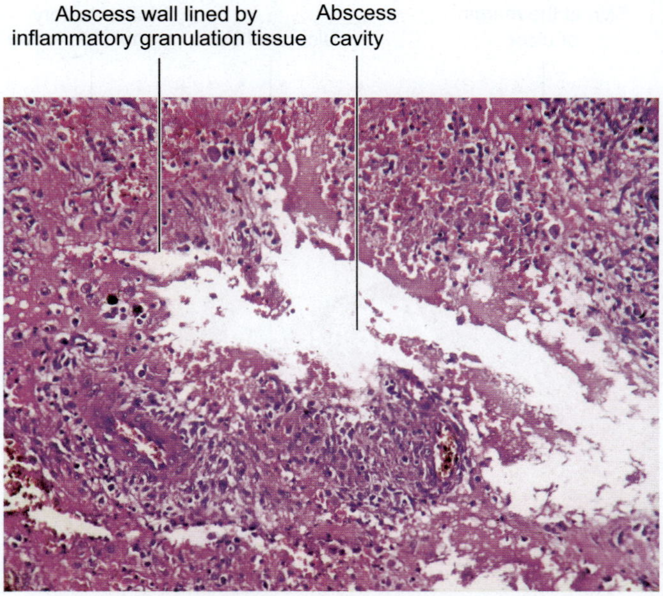

Fig. 2.7 Abscess showing a large central necrotic cavity rimmed by a layer of preserved neutrophils and surrounded by a zone of dilated vessels and proliferating fibroblasts (H&E; 100×).

abscess (abscesses, typically have a large central necrotic cavity rimmed by a layer of preserved neutrophils and may be surrounded by a zone of dilated vessels and proliferating fibroblasts; Fig. 2.7).
   - Occurs secondary to infections with pyogenic (pus-producing organisms), for example staphylococci.
4. **Phlegmonous inflammation: A phlegmon** is a localized area of acute inflammation of the soft tissue (subcutaneous tissue, muscle) and sometimes visceral tissue (pancreas, intestine and appendix). It may result from inflammation related to a bacterial infection or non-infectious causes (e.g. pancreatitis). A phlegmon may progress to a well-formed **abscess** if untreated. Histopathology shows diffuse infiltration of neutrophils and tissue necrosis.
5. **Catarrhal inflammation:** Acute inflammation of the mucous membranes resulting in excessive mucous production. It is characterized by increased blood flow to the mucosal vessels, edema of the interstitial tissue, enlargement and hypersecretion of the secretory epithelial cells. Catarrhal inflammation may result from hypersensitivity reactions, bacterial and viral infections and physical and chemical tissue injury.
6. **Membranous inflammation:** This type of inflammation involves formation of a membrane over the epithelial surfaces. The membrane is constituted by fibrin, desquamated epithelial and inflammatory cells, for example membrane formation is pharyngitis associated with *Corynebacterium diphtheriae*.

Q. Define cellulitis. (PA4.1)

Ans. Cellulitis is acute inflammatory process of the dermis and/or subcutis due to an infection. It presents with swelling, increased local temperature, tenderness and erythema.

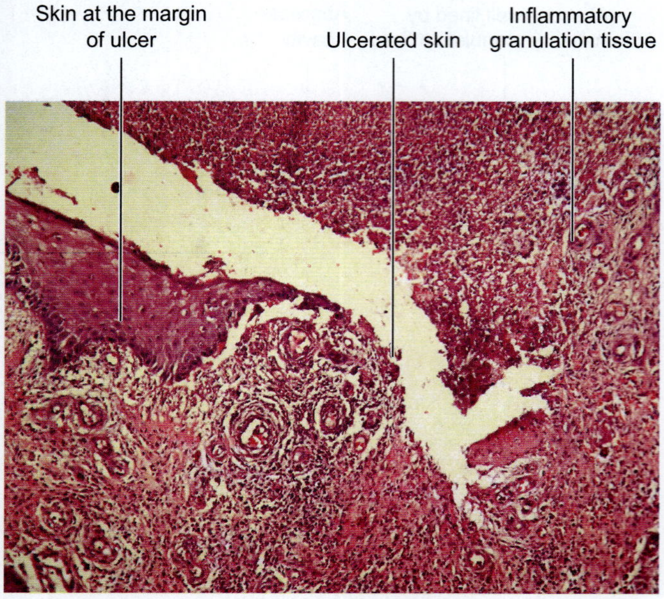

Fig. 2.8 Ulcer showing discontinuity in the lining epithelium with underlying inflammatory granulation tissue (H&E; 100×).

Q. Define an ulcer. (PA4.1)

Ans. An ulcer is a local defect, or excavation on the surface of an organ or tissue that results due to sloughing of inflammatory necrotic material. During the acute stage, there is intense polymorphonuclear infiltration and vascular dilatation (Fig. 2.8). With chronicity, the base and margins of the ulcer develop fibroblastic proliferation, scarring and infiltration by chronic inflammatory cells.

Q. What are the possible outcomes of acute inflammation? (PA4.1)

Ans. Resolution processes work at re-instating tissue homeostasis by cessation of tissue infiltration by neutrophils, apoptosis of already present neutrophils, and down regulation of chemokines and cytokines, which initiates healing. Acute inflammation can have the following outcomes (Flowchart 2.14):

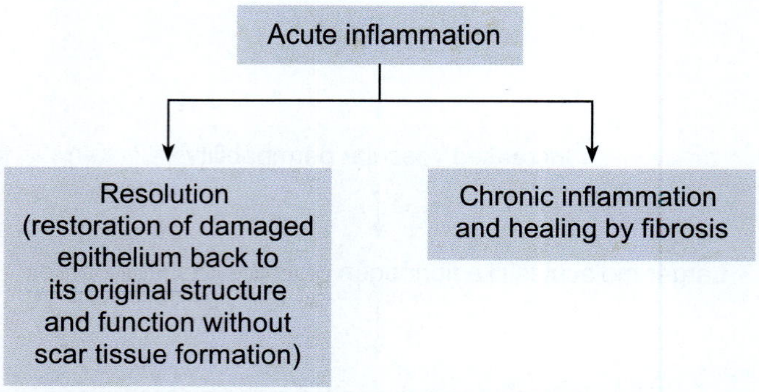

Flowchart 2.14 Outcomes of acute inflammation.

1. **Resolution with regeneration:** Resolution means complete return of the tissue architecture to its original self and occur when the injury is short lived and mild with minimal tissue damage. Resolution by regeneration involves the following processes:
   - Reabsorption of oedema fluid by lymphatics and removal of cellular debris and pathogens by *macrophages.*
   - Replacement of damaged tissue occurs via *proliferation* of *stem cells* mediated by Il-10 and transforming growth factor beta (TGF-beta).
2. **Organization/resolution with scarring**
   - This occurs when there is significant tissue damage and exudation or when inflammation occurs in tissues, which are incapable of regeneration.
   - Stem cell proliferation is not able to keep pace with the damage and destruction leading to original tissue being replaced by fibrotic scar tissue.
   - This is mediated by cytokines like platelet derived growth factor (PDGF), fibroblast growth factor-2 (FGF-2) and TGF-beta.
3. **Abscess formation:** Infection with pyogenic organisms leads to active acute inflammation and localised tissue *necrosis* resulting in abscess formation. The abscess contains pus and gets walled off initially by granulation tissue, which in the later stages is replaced by a fibrotic capsule. Pus contains **necrotic tissue** with **dead and viable neutrophils** and **dead pathogens.**
4. **Chronic inflammation:** Persistence of causative factor results in persistent antigen presentation to *T-helper* cells and activation of *CD4+ Th cells.* This is mediated by cytokines like IL-1, TNF, IL-12 and IL-6.

Chronic Inflammation 3

Q. Define chronic inflammation. (PA4.3)

Ans. Inflammation of **prolonged duration (lasting weeks or months)** is labelled chronic inflammation. It is characterized by three simultaneously ongoing components:

1. **Active inflammation**
2. **Tissue destruction**
3. **Attempts at repair**

Chronic inflammation is differentiated from acute inflammation based on the absence of the cardinal signs of acute inflammation (redness, swelling, pain and increased temperature), as well as active vascular and cellular changes (hyperemia, exudation and neutrophil emigration). As the former is insidious in onset and of a longer duration, it is invariably accompanied by tissue manifestations of the immune response, repair, necrosis and fibrosis. The amount of fibrosis in the tissues is a function of the duration of chronic inflammation. Typically, chronic inflammation is **low grade** and associated with an **asymptomatic clinical response**. It has the following characteristics:

- Follows a solitary acute inflammatory reaction that fails to subside.
- Occurs without a clinically apparent acute phase.
- Results from repeated episodes of acute inflammation.
- Coexists with acute inflammation (acute on chronic inflammation).

Q. Write briefly on the pathophysiology/causes of "chronic inflammation". (PA4.3)

Ans. Chronic inflammation can result from the following:

1. **Persistent infections**, such as tuberculosis, syphilis, infections due to certain viruses, fungi and parasites. Typically, organisms leading to chronic inflammation.
   (a) Are of low toxicity.
   (b) Evoke an immune response called delayed hypersensitivity.
   (c) Are characterized by a specific inflammatory response called a **granulomatous** reaction.

   Failure of eliminating the agents causing the above infections (*Mycobacterium tuberculosis*, protozoa, fungi and other parasites) that can resist host defenses and remain in the tissue for an extended period gives rise to chronic inflammation.
2. **Prolonged exposure to low levels of potentially toxic agents/irritants/foreign materials which are not eliminated by enzymatic breakdown or phagocytosis:**
   Exogenous—Industrial chemicals like Silica dust → Silicosis
   Endogenous—Toxic lipid components → Atherosclerosis.
3. **Autoimmunity:** Immune reaction against one's own antigens can result in chronic tissue damage and diseases such as rheumatoid arthritis, systemic lupus erythematosus (SLE).
4. **Recurrent episodes of acute inflammation:** Recurrent bouts of acute inflammation can lead to chronic inflammation. However, in some cases, chronic inflammation is an independent response and not a sequel to acute inflammation, for example diseases such as tuberculosis and rheumatoid arthritis.
5. **Persistent elevation of inflammatory and biochemical inducers:** Inflammatory and biochemical substances causing oxidative stress and mitochondrial dysfunction such as excess of free radical molecules, advanced glycation end products (AGEs), uric acid (urate) crystals, oxidized lipoproteins, homocysteine and others can induce chronic inflammatory changes.
6. **Chronic inflammatory diseases** are the most significant cause of death in the world and include conditions such as stroke, allergies and chronic respiratory diseases, cardiovascular disorders, arthritis and joint diseases, cancer, obesity and diabetes.

Q. What are the symptoms of chronic inflammation? (PA4.3)

Ans. Some of the common signs and symptoms that develop during chronic inflammation are listed below:

- Body pain
- Fever
- Constant fatigue and insomnia
- Depression, anxiety and mood disorders
- Gastrointestinal complications such as constipation, diarrhoea and acid reflux
- Weight gain
- Frequent infections

Q. Enumerate the laboratory tests for chronic inflammation.

Ans. Laboratory tests undertaken to assess patients for chronic inflammation are usually useful when the inflammation occurs in association with another medical conditions. These include:

- Serum protein electrophoresis, which shows concomitant hypoalbuminemia and polyclonal increase in all gamma globulins (polyclonal gammopathy).

- High-sensitivity C-reactive protein (hsCRP) and fibrinogen levels when increased indicate inflammation; however, they are not specific markers for chronic inflammation and are also elevated in acute inflammation (normal serum level for hsCRP is <0.55 mg/L in men and <1.0 mg/L in women; normal level of fibrinogen is 200–300 mg/dL). hs-CRP is often used to assess increased cardiovascular disease (CVD) risk. Increased plasma hs-CRP level is now considered as a CVD risk factor much like dyslipidemia and metabolic syndrome.
- Increased levels of SAA (Serum Amyloid A) also indicate chronic inflammation.
- Levels of pro-inflammatory cytokines such as TNF-alpha, IL-1beta, IL-6 and IL-8 can be estimated to diagnose chronic inflammation but are not cost effective enough to be used for routine purposes.

Q. Write briefly on the role of inflammation in carcinogenensis. (PA4.3)

Ans. Inflammation is closely associated with an increased production of ROS and RNOS, which can damage DNA. Chronic inflammation is, therefore, an ongoing process that can increase mutations and increase the risk for carcinogenesis. Activated macrophages are a major source of ROS and have been found to be a component of the tumour microenvironment of breast cancer where they facilitate tumour growth. Obesity, which increases chronic inflammation, is now recognized as a major cancer risk factor. An association has been found between CRP levels and cancer. Aging is another major risk factor for cancer and age-related sterile chronic inflammation (in the absence of infection termed inflamm-aging) is thought to be an underlying aetiological factor. Gut microbiota is thought to become more pro-inflammatory with aging and contribute to systemic chronic inflammation.

Q. Write briefly on the morphological features of "chronic inflammation". (PA4.3, 4.4)

Ans. Most of the features of acute inflammation continue as the inflammation becomes chronic, including vasodilation, increase in blood flow, increased capillary permeability and migration of neutrophils into the infected tissue through the capillary wall (diapedesis). The hallmark of chronic inflammation is a decrease in the number of short-lived neutrophils and infiltration by inflammatory cells such as macrophages, lymphocytes and plasma cells in the tissue site, producing inflammatory cytokines, growth factors, enzymes and hence contributing to the progression of tissue damage and secondary repair including fibrosis. To summarize, the three morphological hallmarks of chronic inflammation are as follows:

1. Infiltration by *mononuclear cells* (lymphocytes, macrophages and plasma cells).
2. *Tissue destruction* due to persistent offending agent/inflammation.
3. *Healing* by connective tissue replacement of damaged tissue includes proliferation of blood vessels (angiogenesis and fibrosis).

Overview of chronic inflammation is represented in Flowchart 3.1.

Morphological types of chronic inflammation

- ***Non-specific chronic inflammation:*** This is characterized by formation of non-specific granulation tissue comprising mononuclear inflammatory cells (lymphocytes, macrophages, plasma cells), proliferating fibroblasts, connective tissue, blood vessels and epithelial cells. Examples of chronic inflammation include chronic cholecycitis (inflammation of the gall bladder; Fig. 3.1), chronic gastritis

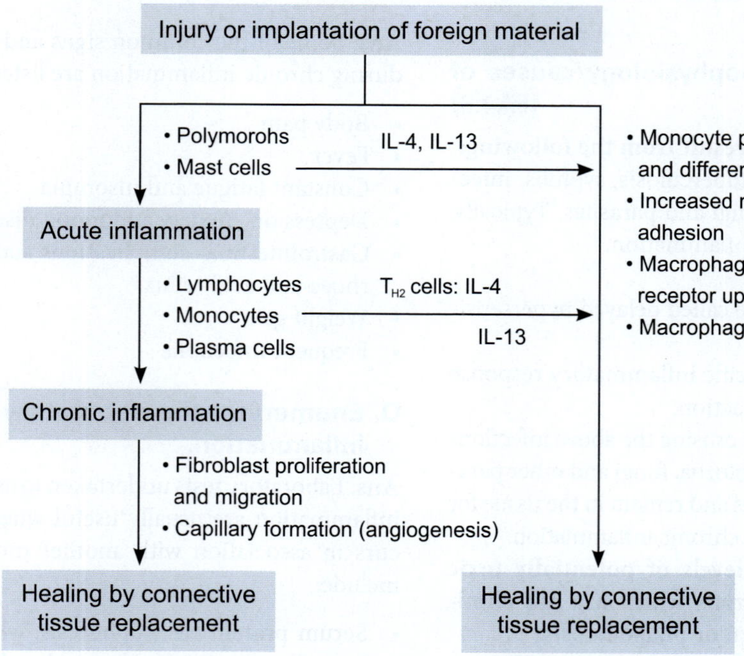

Flowchart 3.1 Overview of chronic inflammation.

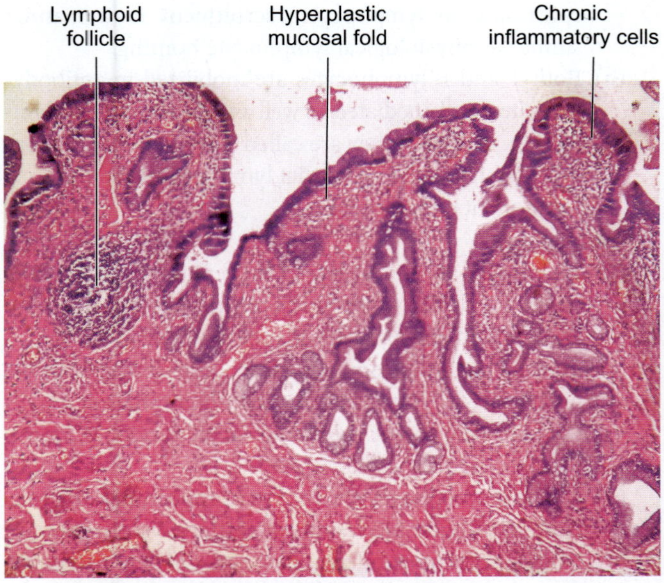

Fig. 3.1 Section from gall bladder showing mucosal hypertrophy and infiltration of the wall by chronic non-specific inflammatory cells (H&E; 100×).

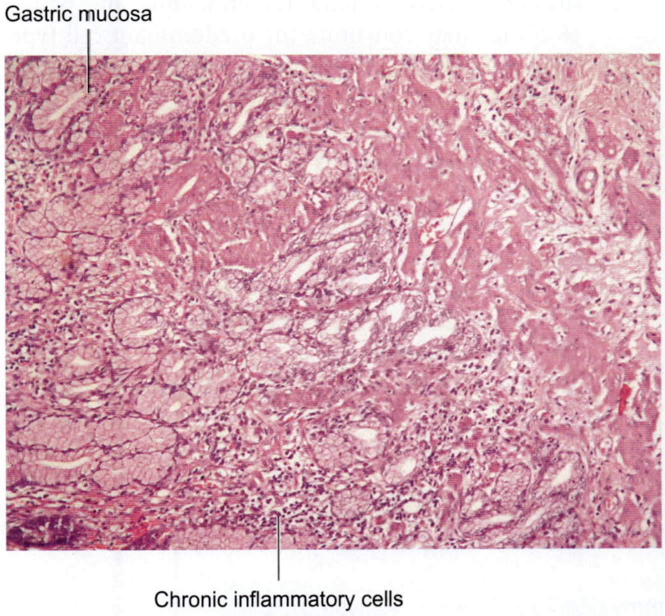

Fig. 3.2 Section from chronic gastritis showing gastric mucosa infiltrated by chronic non-specific inflammatory cells (H&E; 100×).

(inflammation of the stomach; Fig. 3.2), chronic cervicitis (inflammation of the cervix; Fig. 3.3) and chronic osteomyelitis (inflammation of bone; Fig. 3.4).

- ***Granulomatous inflammation:*** This is a specific type of chronic inflammation characterized by the presence of distinct nodular lesions or granulomas which are composed of aggregates of activated macrophages or its derived cell called epithelioid cells usually surrounded by lymphocytes. The macrophages or epithelioid cells inside the granulomas often coalesce to form Langhans giant cells or foreign body giant cells.

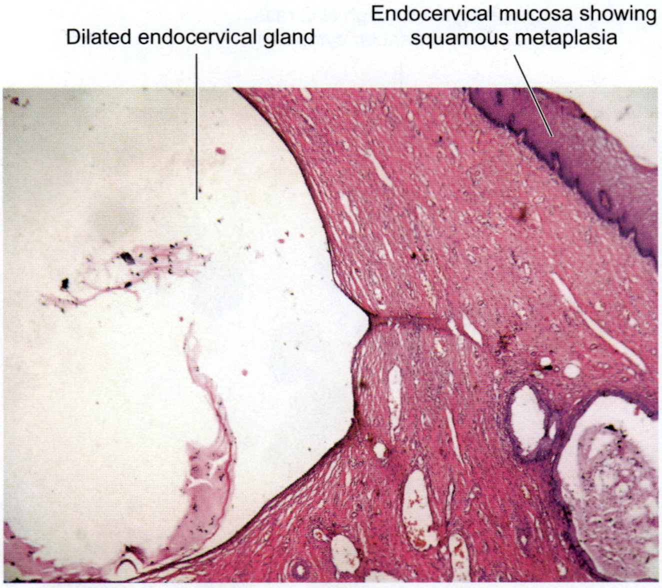

Fig. 3.3 Section from chronic cervicitis with squamous metaplasia. The cervical stroma shows chronic inflammation and the mucosa overlying the glands shows replacement of normal glandular mucosa by stratified squamous epithelium (H&E; 100×).

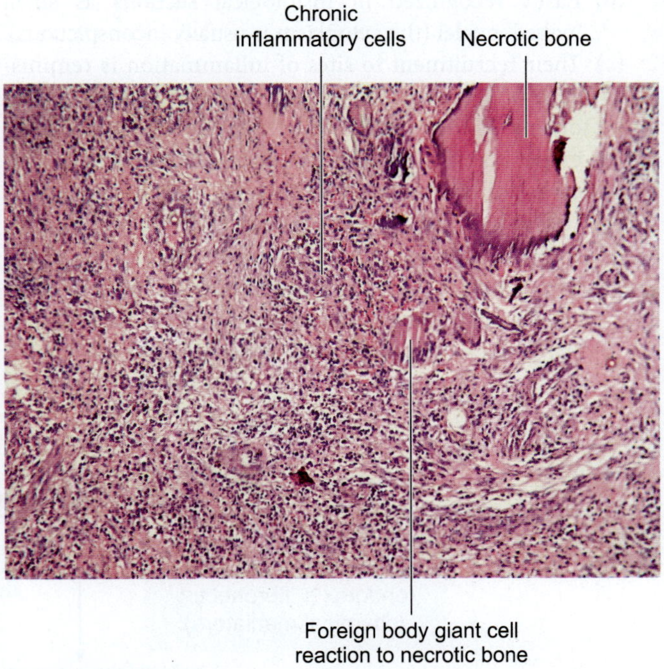

Fig. 3.4 Section from chronic osteomyelitis showing dead bone surrounded by chronic non-specific inflammation and an occasional foreign body giant cell (H&E; 100×).

Q. Write briefly on the cells involved in chronic inflammation. (PA4.3)

Ans. The cells involved in chronic inflammation include:

1. **Lymphocytes**
   (a) Vary in size from 7 to 9 μm in diameter, and are the second most common white blood cell type. They have a round deeply staining nucleus surrounded by a relatively thin rim of cytoplasm (Fig. 3.5).

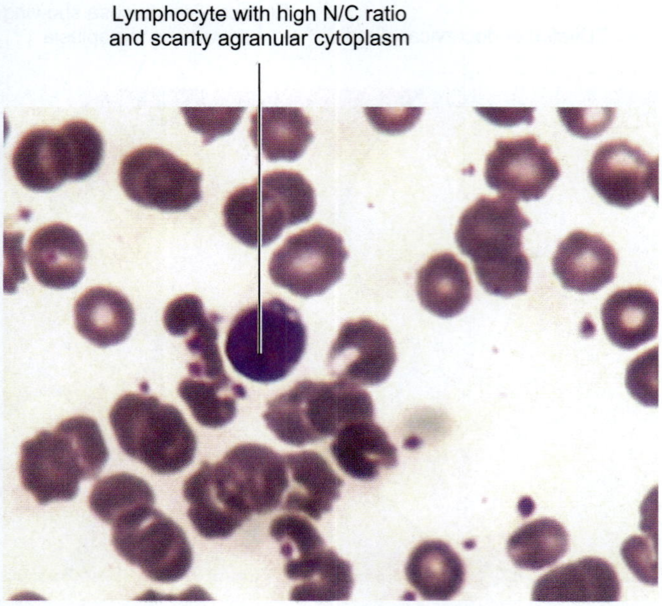

Fig. 3.5 A small lymphocyte showing scanty basophilic, agranular cytoplasm; high N:C ratio and clumped nuclear chromatin (Leishman; 400×).

(b) Easily recognized in histological sections as small 'naked' nuclei (the cytoplasm is usually inconspicuous).

(c) Their recruitment to sites of inflammation is reminiscent of lymphocyte homing to peripheral lymphoid organs. Under physiological conditions, lymphocytes express certain homing receptors which adhere to vascular addressin expressed on high endothelial venules (HEVs), initiating a lymphocyte migration process composed of sequential adhesive interactions. It has been found that in chronic inflammation too HEV-like vessels are induced, despite the fact that the inflamed site is not originally lymphoid tissue, and these vessels contribute to lymphocyte recruitment in a manner similar to physiological lymphocyte homing.

(d) Both T and B lymphocytes are mobilized in antibody-mediated, cell-mediated as well as non-immune inflammation. Although they are called 'chronic inflammatory cells' but it is to be noted that lymphocytes are a normal component of some tissues.

2. **Macrophages**

(a) Monocytes are the largest of the leukocytes, constitute about 5% of the white blood cell population and have an indented kidney/bean shaped nucleus.

(b) They are derived from haematopoietic stem cells in the bone marrow. Mononuclear cell differentiation entails the following stages: mononuclear stem cells → monoblast → monocyte/macrophage.

(c) Tissue macrophages are diverse in appearance and may contain indigestible residue in tertiary lysosomes.

(d) Macrophages have different names in different tissues, for example **'sinus histiocytes' in lymph node, 'osteoclasts' in bone, 'microglia' in central nervous system, 'Kupffer cells' in liver**, mesangial cells in the glomerulus, Langerhans' cells in the skin and **'alveolar macrophages' in lung.**

(e) Monocytes begin to emigrate into extravascular tissues quite early in acute inflammation, and within 48 h they may constitute the predominant cell type. They bring about phagocytosis, initiate tissue repair, secrete mediators of inflammation and influence lymphocyte function (interact with lymphocytes in chronic inflammation as shown in Flowchart 3.2 and Fig. 3.6).

(f) Three ways in which macrophages accumulate in the site of injury are:

(i) Continuous recruitment from the circulation mediated by chemotactic factors.

(ii) Continuous cell division.

(iii) Prolonged survival and immobilization.

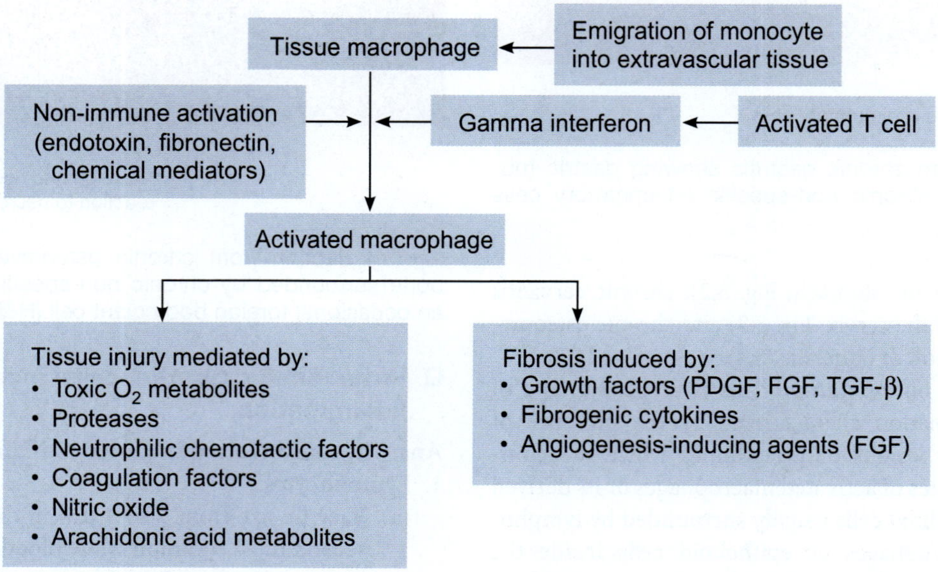

Flowchart 3.2 Interactions of macrophages with lymphocytes in chronic inflammation.

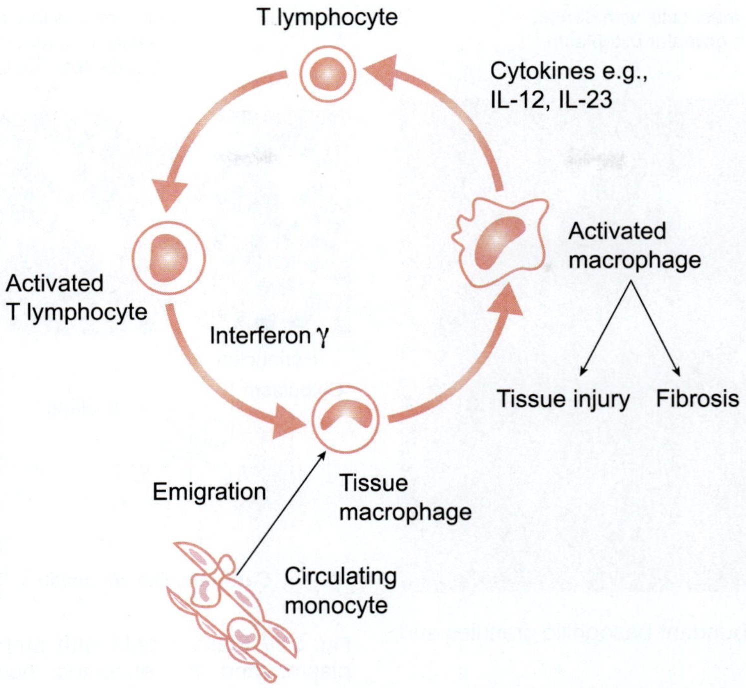

Fig. 3.6 Macrophage lymphocyte interaction in chronic inflammation.

(g) The chief role of macrophages in chronic inflammation is phagocytosis. In addition, macrophages release important inflammatory mediators which include:
  (i) Proteases (like collagenases and elastases).
  (ii) Plasminogen activator (activates fibrinolytic system).
  (iii) Complement products.
  (iv) Chemotactic agents for other leukocytes.
  (v) Growth factors for fibroblasts and blood vessels.
  (vi) Cytokines like IL-1 and TNF.
  (vii) Oxygen-derived free radicals.

(h) Different macrophage populations serve distinct functions—some may be important for microbial killing and inflammation, and others for repair. Macrophages are the cells chiefly responsible for tissue destruction (one of the hallmarks of chronic inflammation). The ongoing tissue destruction can itself activate the inflammatory cascade, so that features of both acute and chronic inflammation may coexist in certain circumstances.

(i) Fibrocytes are mesenchymal cells that arise from monocyte precursors. They have both the inflammatory characteristics of macrophages and the tissue remodelling properties of fibroblasts.

3. **Eosinophil** (Fig. 3.7)
  (a) They are 12–17 μm in diameter and have large bright red, or reddish-purple granules. Eosinophils are recruited from the blood to participate in IgE-mediated immune reactions and parasitic infections.
  (b) Eotaxin, derived from leukocytes and epithelial cells, is a chemokine for eosinophils.
  (c) Eosinophils contain 'major basic protein' in their granules, which is toxic to parasites and mammalian epithelial cells. Recruitment and extravasation from blood is driven by the same factors which are responsible for extravasation of neutrophils and by **eotaxin** (chemokine derived from leukocytes and epithelial cells which is specific for eosinophils).

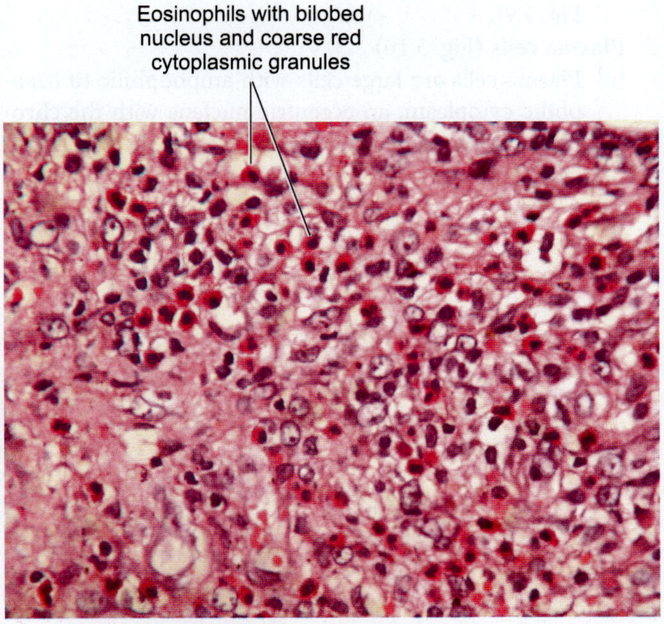

Fig. 3.7 Section showing numerous eosinophils with bilobed nuclei and coarse red granules (H&E; 200×).

4. **Mast cells** (Fig. 3.8)
  (a) Widely present in connective tissue, mast cells are irregularly-shaped cells with a round and single nucleus, and a dense granular cytoplasm, the granules often obscuring the nucleus and other organelles.
  (b) Participate in both acute and chronic inflammatory cells.
  (c) Express on their surface the receptor that binds to the Fc portion of IgE antibody to degranulate mast cells

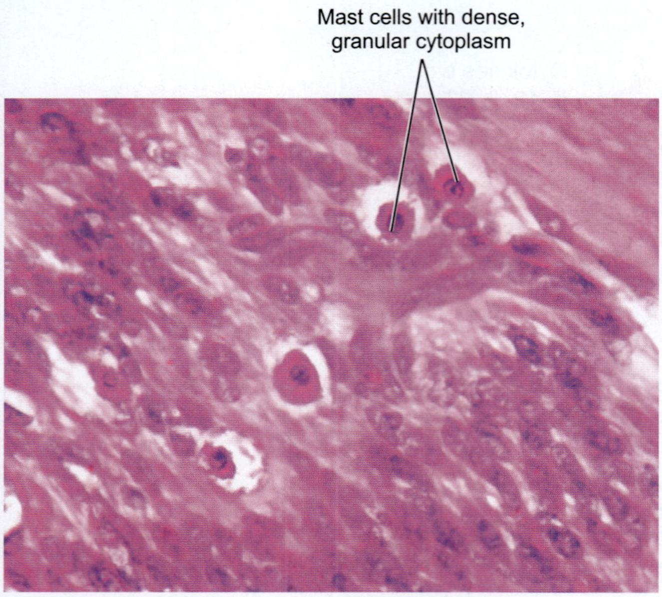

Fig. 3.8 Mast cells showing abundant basophilic granules and round nuclei.

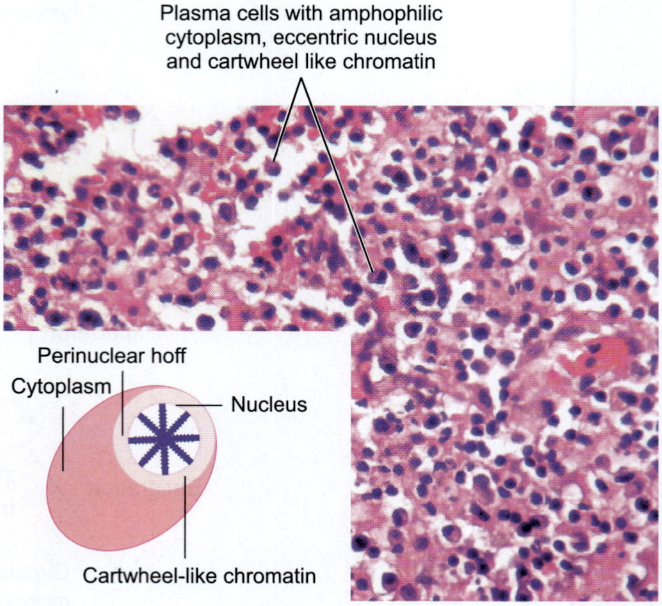

Fig. 3.10 Plasma cells with amphophilic to basophilic cytoplasm, and an eccentric nucleus with heterochromatin arranged in a characteristic cart wheel or clock-face arrangement and pale perinuclear zone (H&E; 100×).

and release mediators (histamines and prostaglandins; Fig. 3.9).

5. **Plasma cells** (Fig. 3.10)
   (a) Plasma cells are large cells with amphophilic to basophilic cytoplasm, an eccentric nucleus with the chromatin arranged in a characteristic cart-wheel or clock-face pattern.
   (b) Their cytoplasm contains a pale perinuclear zone that on electron microscopy shows an extensive Golgi apparatus and centrioles.
   (c) Plasma cells have abundant rough endoplasmic reticulum coupled with a well-developed Golgi apparatus,

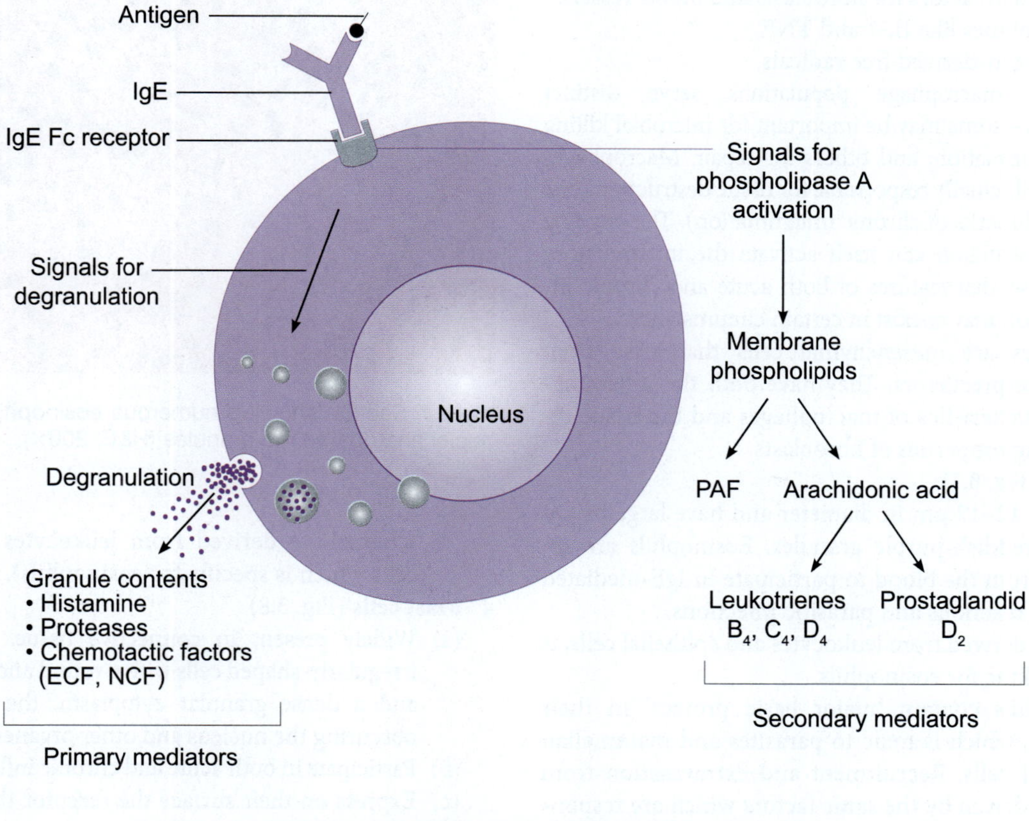

Fig. 3.9 Mediators released from mast cells.

which together are responsible for immunoglobulin secretion.

6. **Neutrophils**
Although neutrophils have been classically associated with acute inflammation, they may sometimes be seen in chronic inflammation as well (recruited by mediators produced by activated macrophages and lymphocytes), for example chronic osteomyelitis (bacterial infection of bone). This is labelled 'acute on chronic inflammation'.

Q. What is an activated macrophage? (PA4.3)

Ans. An activated macrophage has the following salient features:

- Increased cell size.
- Increased level of lysosomal enzymes.
- Active metabolism.
- Greater ability to phagocytose and kill.
- Secretion of a large variety of biologically active products.

Q. What is granulomatous inflammation? Enumerate the causes of granulomatous diseases. (PA4.3)

Ans. Granulomatous inflammation is a distinctive pattern of chronic inflammatory reaction characterized by the presence of granulomas. A granuloma is a microscopic aggregation of activated macrophages, which transform into epithelioid (epithelial like) cells. **Epithelioid cells have scanty to moderate, ill defined, pale pink cytoplasm, and a slipper-shaped vesicular nucleus.** These are surrounded by a collar of mononuclear cells (lymphocytes and plasma cells). Necrosis may or may not be present. Older granulomas have an enclosing **rim of fibroblasts** and **connective tissue**. Epithelioid cells fuse to form **'giant cells'** 40–50 μm in size with 20 or more nuclei arranged peripherally like a horseshoe (**Langhans giant cells, typical of tuberculous inflammation**) or haphazardly as in **foreign body giant cells**.

Types of Granulomas (Table 3.1)

1. **Infectious granulomas**
   (a) **Tuberculosis** (PA19.2, 19.3) (prototype of granulomatous disease): Caused by *Mycobacterium tuberculosis*, tuberculosis is associated with the formation of caseating granulomas (granulomas showing presence of central granular debris with loss of all cellular detail and higher positivity for acid fast bacilli; Fig. 3.11) or non-caseating granulomas (absence of caseation and low positivity for acid fast bacilli).
   (b) **Leprosy:** Caused by *Mycobacterium leprae.* Non-caseating granulomas are typically seen with or without acid fast lepra bacilli in the macrophages.
   (c) **Syphilis:** Cauesd by *Treponema pallidum.* **Gumma** formation is the disease hallmark. Gumma is histopathologically characterized by a central necrotic area without loss of cellular outline; plasma cell infiltrate with a wall of histiocytes.
   (d) **Cat scratch disease:** Cauesd by a Gram-negative bacillus. It typically shows rounded or stellate granulomas containing central granular debris and large number of neutrophils.

Table 3.1 Types of granulomas

1. **Infectious granulomas**
   (a) **Bacterial**
      (i) Tuberculosis (Mycobacterium tuberculosis)
      (ii) Leprosy (Mycobacterium leprae)
      (iii) Granuloma inguinale (donovanosis caused by C. donovani)
      (iv) Brucellosis (Mediterranean fever caused by Brucells abortus)
      (v) Cat scratch disease (Bartonella henselae)
      (vi) Actinomycosis (bacterial)
   (b) **Fungal**
      (i) Aspergillus spp.
      (ii) Mucorales
      (iii) Pneumocystis jiroveci
      (iv) Blastomycosis (Blastomyces dermatitiduis)
      (v) Cryptococcosis (Cryptococcus neoformans)
      (vi) Histoplasmosis (Histoplasma capsulatum)
      (vii) Coccidioidomycosis (Coccidioides immitis)
   (c) **Parasitic**
      (i) Schistosomiasis (Bilharziasis)
      (ii) Echinococcosis (Echinococcus granulosus)
   (d) **Spirochetal:** Syphilis (*Treponema pallidum*)
2. **Non-infectious or immune granulomas**
   (a) **Inorganic metals and dusts**
      (i) Silicosis
      (ii) Berylliosis
      (iii) Pneumoconiosis
      (iv) Asbestosis
   (b) **Miscellaneous**
      (i) Sarcoidosis
      (ii) Crohn's disease
   (c) **Autoimmune**
      (i) Rheumatoid nodule
      (ii) Granuloma annulare
      (iii) Necrobiosis lipoidica
      (iv) Granulomatosis with polyangiitis
3. **Foreign body granulomas:** Talc, starch, suture, wood splinters, metal, glass, hyaluronic acid, injectable fillers

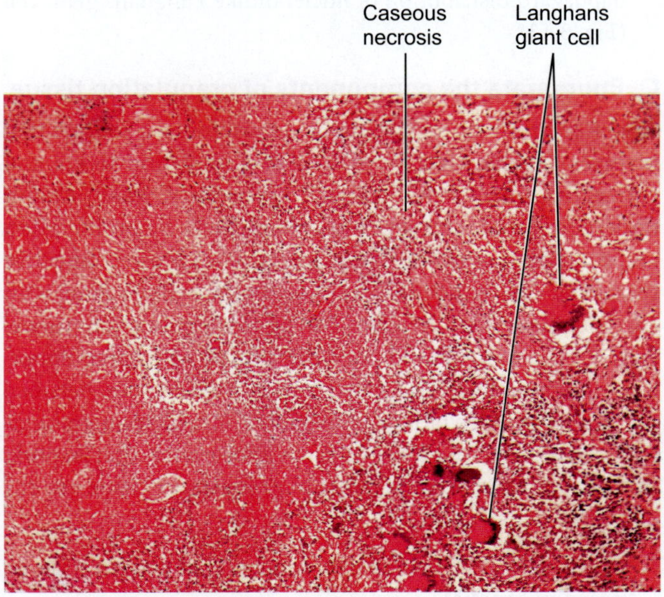

Fig. 3.11 Section showing widespread caseous necrosis with scattered Langhans giant cells (H&E; 100×).

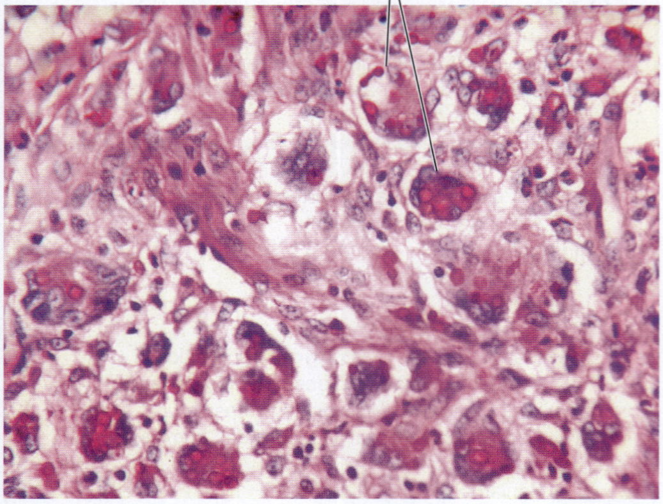

Fig. 3.12 A PAS stained section showing a suppurative granuloma with presence of fungal spores in the giant cells (PAS; 400×). *PAS*, Periodic acid–Schiff.

(e) **Deep fungal infections:** Fungal granulomas are caused by organisms like *histoplasma* and *blastomyces* and are typically suppurative (granulomas with neutrophilic inflammation; Fig. 3.12).

2. **Non-infectious or immune granulomas:** Granulomas form in response to persistent presence of non-degradable or particulate material, which incites an immune response. These are usually non-caseating epithelioid cell granulomas. Examples include sarcoidosis and hypersensitivity pneumonitis.
3. **Foreign body granulomas:** Formed as a response to foreign bodies like talc, suture, and intravenous drugs. The foreign material can be identified in the center of the granuloma or within the foreign body giant cells, which have a haphazard distribution of nuclei unlike Langhans giant cell (Fig. 3.13).

Q. Enumerate the components of granulation tissue.

Ans. Repair by connective tissue deposition is a process that involves angiogenesis, formation of granulation tissue and connective tissue remodelling. Tissue injury, which cannot undergo repair by regeneration alone, heals by proliferation and migration of fibroblasts, deposition of loose connective tissue and capillary proliferation. All of the above along with chronic inflammatory cells constitute 'granulation tissue' (Fig. 3.14) which should not be confused with 'granulomatous inflammation' described earlier (differences between the two entities are tabulated in Table 3.2). The term granulation tissue is derived from its gross appearance, that is, pink, soft and granular. Components of granulation tissue are enlisted as:

1. Newly formed blood vessels (endothelial proliferation or neoangiogenesis).
2. Chronic inflammatory cells.
3. Proliferating fibroblasts.

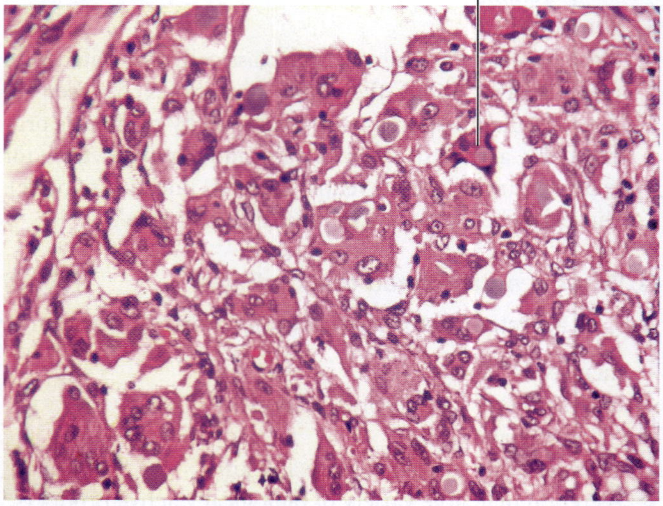

Fig. 3.13 H&E stained section showing a foreign body giant cell reaction to oil droplets (400×).

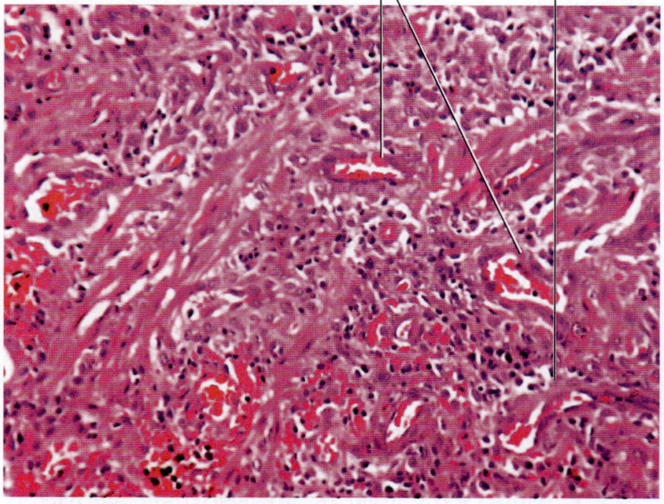

Fig. 3.14 Section showing granulation tissue composed of numerous variable sized capillaries in an oedematous background with scattered plasma cells, lymphocytes, histiocytes and fibroblasts (H&E; 200×).

4. Extracellular matrix which in comparison to ordinary extracellular matrix is more cellular and more vascular.

Q. Enumerate the different types of giant cells. (PA4.3)

Ans. Types of giant cells:

1. **Langhans giant cell**
   (a) Named after Theodor Langhans, a German pathologist.
   (b) Formed when epithelioid cells or macrophages fuse together.
   (c) Its nuclei are arranged in a horseshoe shape around the periphery of the cell (Fig. 3.15).

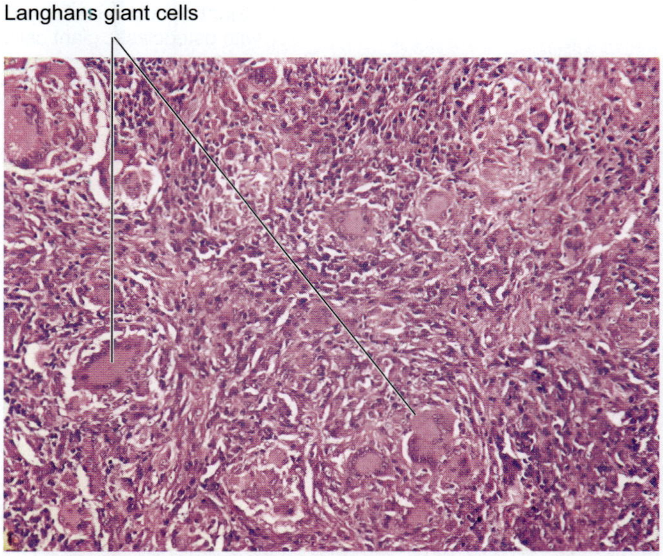

Fig. 3.15 Tuberculous lymphadenitis showing numerous multinucleate Langhans giant cells with nuclei arranged in a horseshoe shape pattern in the periphery of the cell (H&E; 200×).

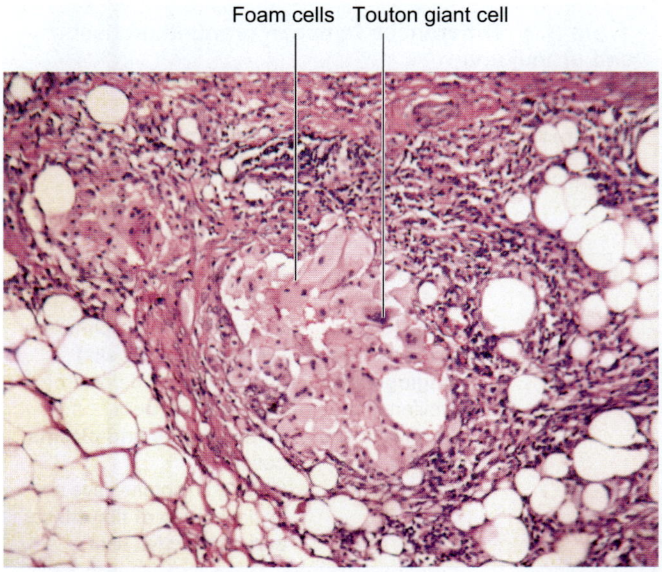

Fig. 3.16 Xanthogranulomatous inflammation showing multinucleate giant cells with foamy cytoplasm (H&E; 200×).

(d) Not exclusive to a tuberculous pathology and can be seen in many other granulomatous diseases.

2. **Touton giant cell**
   (a) Seen in lipid-laden lesions like fat necrosis, xanthomas and xanthogranulomas.
   (b) Formed by fusion of epithelioid macrophages like Langhans giant cell, however, in these, the nuclei form a ring and are surrounded by foamy cytoplasm (Fig. 3.16).
   (c) Touton cells develop when the stimulus to cell fusion is accompanied also by a factor stimulating lipid uptake, which is missing in the development of the other two giant cell 'types'.

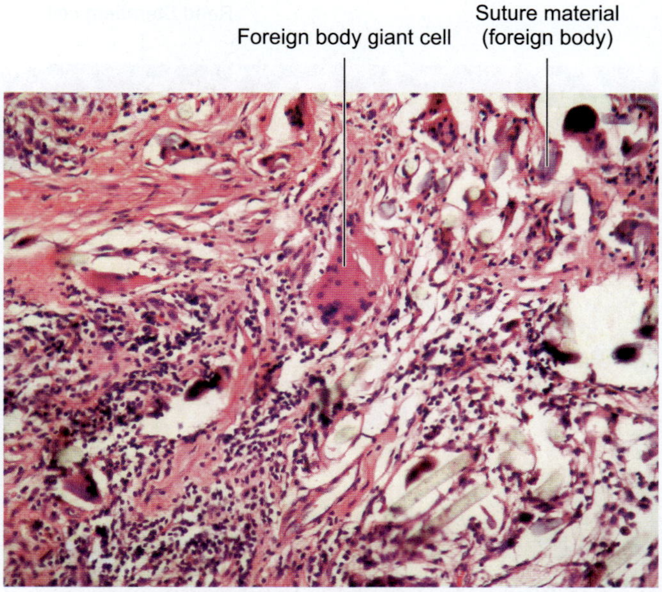

Fig. 3.17 Section showing foreign body granulomatous reaction to wood splinters. Giant cells surrounding the foreign body contain many nuclei which are arranged centrally in an overlapping and haphazard fashion (H&E; 200×).

3. **Foreign body giant cells**
   (a) Foreign body giant cells are also formed when epithelioid macrophages fuse together; however, their nuclei are arranged ion a haphazard manner (Fig. 3.17).
   (b) Develop as a reaction to the presence of a foreign substance (e.g. talc, sutures or vegetable matter).
4. **Giant cells associated with viral diseases:** Viruses, such as *Morbillivirus* (measles causing paramyxovirus), herpes simplex, herpes zoster and papilloma virus can cause abnormal cell division in the epidermal cells, to give rise to cells which are much larger than normal and have multiple nuclei (Fig. 3.18).

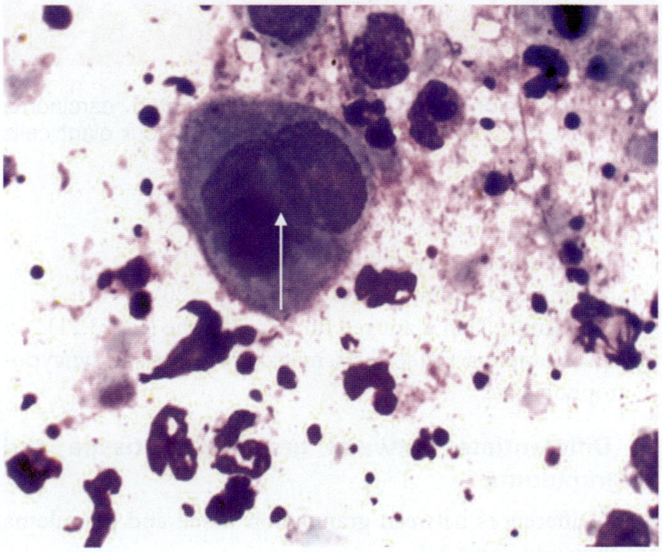

Fig. 3.18 Smear from a herpetic ulcer showing a massively enlarged multinucleate cell (Giemsa; 400×).

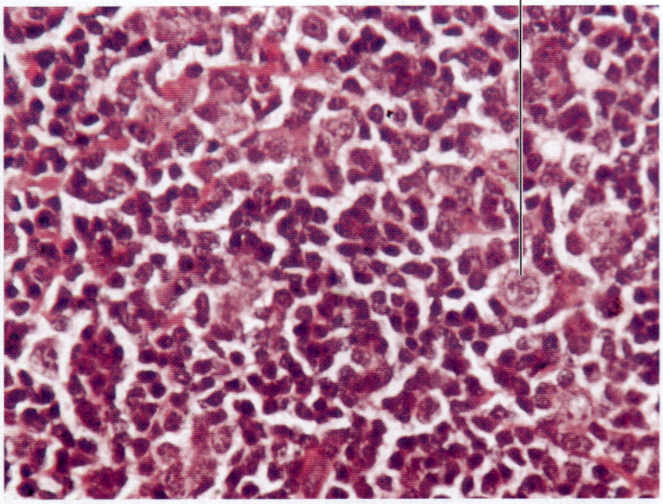

Fig. 3.19 Section from Hodgkin lymphoma showing typical binucleate RS cells with mirror image nuclei having prominent nucleoli (**Owl's eye appearance;** H&E; 400×).

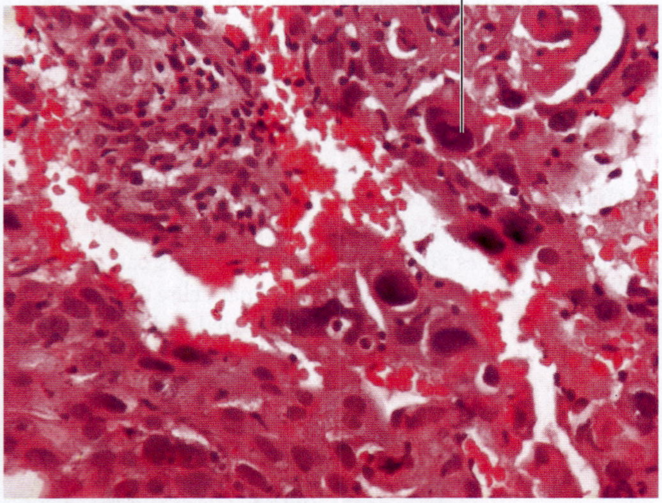

Fig. 3.20 Section from a poorly differentiated carcinoma showing anaplastic, bizarre multinucleate tumour giant cells (H&E; 400×).

5. **Tumour giant cells:** These include:
   (a) Reed–Sternberg cell (Fig. 3.19).
   (b) Anaplastic tumour giant cells (Fig. 3.20).
   (c) Giant cells in giant cell tumour of bone (Fig. 3.21).
6. **Miscellaneous:** Osteoclasts, megakaryocytes and syncytiotrophoblastic.

Q. Differentiate between granulation tissue and granuloma.

Ans. Differences between granulation tissue and granuloma are shown in Table 3.2.

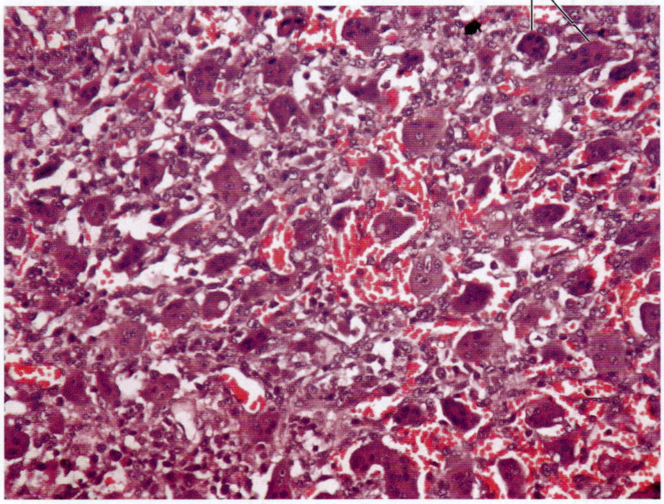

Fig. 3.21 Section from a giant cell tumour of bone showing multinucleate giant cells with numerous haphazardly arranged nuclei lying in the neoplastic stroma (H&E; 200×).

Table 3.2 Differences between granulation tissue and granuloma

Features	Granulation tissue	Granuloma
Component of	Healing and repair	Chronic inflammation; occurs due to delayed hypersensitivity response
Definition	Tissue composed of newly formed blood vessels **(angiogenesis),** proliferating fibroblasts and chronic inflammatory cells	Microscopic aggregation of macrophages that are transformed into epithelium like **(epithelioid cells)** surrounded by a collar of mononuclear cells **(lymphocytes and plasma cells)** Older granulomas have an enclosing **rim of fibroblasts and connective tissue**
Giant cells	Not seen	Epithelioid cells fuse to form '**Langhans giant cells**' 40–50 μm in size with 20 or more nuclei arranged peripherally
Remodelling (maturation and reorganization of fibrous tissue)	Seen	Not seen
Growth factors	Angiogenic and fibrogenic growth factors involved, for example PDGF, FGF, TNF and VEGF	Involvement of cytokines like IL-1, IL-12 and γIFN

Healing and Repair

4

Q. Define repair. (PA5.1)

Ans. Repair is defined as restoration of tissue architecture and function after injury, and occurs in two ways:

1. **Regeneration:** An injured cell is said to have regenerated when it returns to normal after replacement of all the damaged components. Tissues with high proliferative capacity, such as the haematopoietic system and the epithelia of the skin, renew themselves continuously and can regenerate after injury, as long as the *stem cells* of these tissues are not destroyed. Tissue injury of mild and moderate degree generally heals by regeneration.
2. **Healing with scar formation:** If the individual tissue is incapable of complete restoration to original state or if the supporting structures [extracellular matrix (ECM) components] are severely damaged, repair occurs by laying down of connective tissue. This is termed as healing with scar formation. Chronic inflammation stimulates scar formation because of local production of growth factors (GFs) and cytokines that promote fibroblast proliferation and collagen synthesis.

Q. Define fibrosis. (PA5.1)

Ans. A term used to describe extensive deposition of collagen that occurs in parenchymal organs as a consequence of chronic inflammation. Fibrosis develops in a tissue space by organization of the inflammatory exudate occupying the tissue space.

Q. Write briefly on cell cycle.

Ans. During differentiation, mammalian cells alternate between a phase of division (**mitosis**) and a resting phase (**interphase**). The sequence of events that control DNA replication and mitosis and, hence, cellular proliferation is labelled cell cycle (Fig. 4.1).

Phases of Cell Cycle

Interphase is supposedly a resting stage between cell divisions; however, it is actually a period of several essential activities, which are a prerequisite for making the next mitosis possible, for example synthesis of RNA and protein production. Interphase lasts about 12–24 h in mammalian tissue and can be divided into four phases: Gap 0 (G_0), Gap 1 (G_1), S (synthesis phase) and Gap 2 (G_2). Human genome is doubled in the **S phase**, and **halved** during **M phase**. The period between M and S phase is called **G_1**; and that between S and M phases is called **G_2**. So, the cell cycle consists of:

- **G_0 (resting phase)**: When a cell leaves the cell cycle and quits dividing, it is said to be in G_0 phase. This may be a transient phase or indefinite as in the case of a permanent cell that has reached the end stage of its development and will not divide (e.g. cardiac myocytes or neurons).
- **G_1 (presynthetic growth phase)**: In this phase, cells enlarge due to production of RNA and synthesis of proteins. G_1 checkpoint is an important controlling mechanism that ensures adequate preparation for DNA synthesis.
- **S (synthetic phase)**: Synthesis of DNA and duplication of the centrosome takes place in this phase.
- **G_2 (premitotic growth phase)**: The cell continues to grow and produce new proteins like G_1 phase. Another checkpoint (G_2 checkpoint) toward the end of G_2 phase determines whether the cell is adequately prepared to proceed to the M phase and divide or not.
- **M phase (mitotic phase)**: After protein synthesis and enlargement, the cell enters a phase of division to give rise to two similar daughter cells. Mitosis lasts only 1–2 h. As in both G_1 and G_2, the mitotic phase also has a checkpoint (called metaphase checkpoint) that ensures the readiness of the cell to complete cell division.

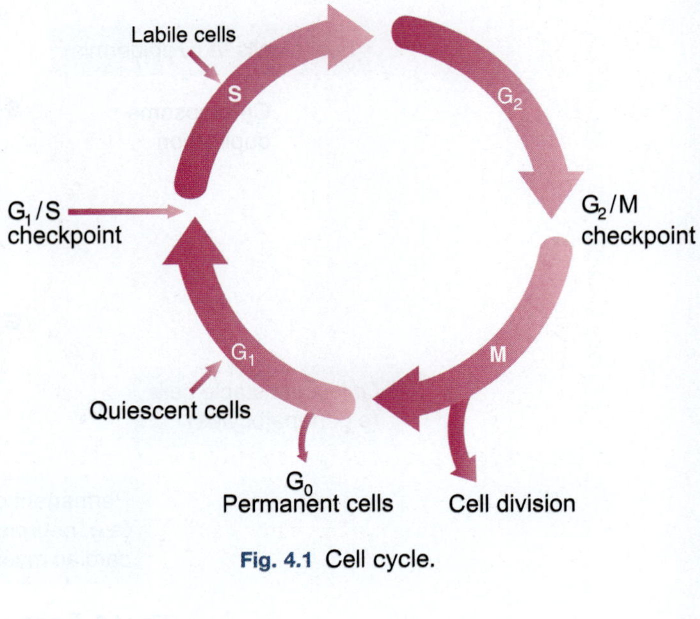

Fig. 4.1 Cell cycle.

Control of the Cell Cycle

Progression of the cell cycle is tightly regulated by the following proteins:

- **Cyclins:** These are classified as *G1 cyclins* (D cyclins), *S-phase cyclins* (cyclins E and A) and *mitotic cyclins* (B cyclins). Their levels vary corresponding to the different phases of cell cycle (cyclins are named so because of the cyclical nature of their production and degradation during cell cycle).
- **Cyclin-dependent kinases (CDKs):** These cyclin-associated enzymes include a G_1 CDK (CDK4), an S-phase CDK (CDK2) and an M-phase CDK (CDK1). Their cellular levels are relatively stable and they get activated on binding to the appropriate cyclin.

Steps in the Cell Cycle

1. The binding of G_1-cyclins to CDKs is an indication to the cell to initiate chromosomal replication. CDKs activated by combining with cyclins initiate the cell cycle by phosphorylating proteins such as retinoblastoma (RB) susceptibility protein, which normally prevents cells from replicating by forming a tight, inactive complex with the transcription factor E2F. Phosphorylation releases RB, activating E2F, which in turn stimulates transcription.
2. The cyclin–CDK complexes are tightly regulated by *CDK inhibitors (CDKIs)*, which themselves are inhibited by other growth factors. CDKIs include several families. One family comprising p21 (CDKN1A), p27 (CDKN1B), and p57 (CDKN1C) inhibits multiple CDKs. Another family comprising p15 (CDKN2B), p16 (CDKN2A), p18 (CDKN2C) and p19 (CDKN2D) has selective effects on cyclins CDK4 and CDK6.
3. The G_1/S checkpoint ensures the integrity of DNA before replication; whereas, the G_2/M checkpoint does the same after replication. These checkpoints monitor whether the cell is prepared enough to enter mitosis. When there is DNA damage, the activation of checkpoints delays the cell cycle and triggers DNA repair mechanisms. If DNA damage is too severe to be repaired, the cells are eliminated by apoptosis.
4. Increased levels of cyclin A bound to CDK2 initiates DNA duplication in the nucleus.
5. The levels of mitotic or B cyclins rise in the M phase and the M-phase promoting factor (the complex of mitotic B cyclins with the M-phase CDK or CDK1) initiates the formation of the mitotic spindle, condensation of the chromatin as well as dissolution of the nuclear envelope.

Q. Classify different types of mammalian cells. (PA5.1)

Ans. Cells are divided into three groups based on their ability to repair themselves (Fig. 4.2):

1. **Labile/continuously dividing cells:** Cells which replenish their damaged/injured counterparts by continuous division and maturation of cells from the stem cell pool, for example surface epithelial cells (skin, oral cavity, vagina and cervix), haematopoietic cells in bone marrow and columnar epithelium of GIT.
2. **Stable/quiescent cells (facultative mitotic cells):** Cells of this type are in G_0 stage of cell cycle, and do not replicate actively in their normal state; however, they are capable of proliferating in response to loss of tissue mass, for example parenchymal cells of solid organs (liver, kidneys and pancreas), endothelial cells, fibroblasts, smooth muscle cells, chondrocytes and osteocytes.
3. **Permanent/non-dividing cells:** Terminally differentiated cells, which are non-proliferative and incapable of regenerating, for example neurons, skeletal muscle and cardiac muscle cells.

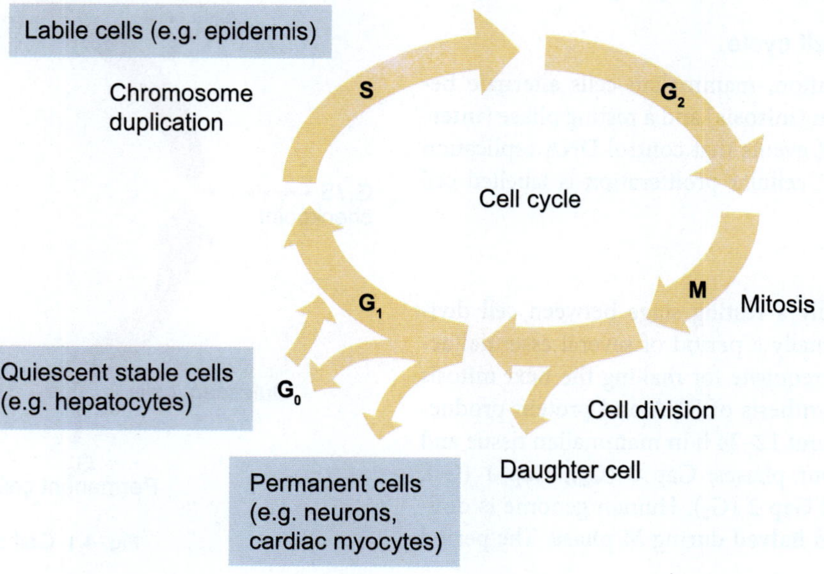

Fig. 4.2 Types of mammalian cells.

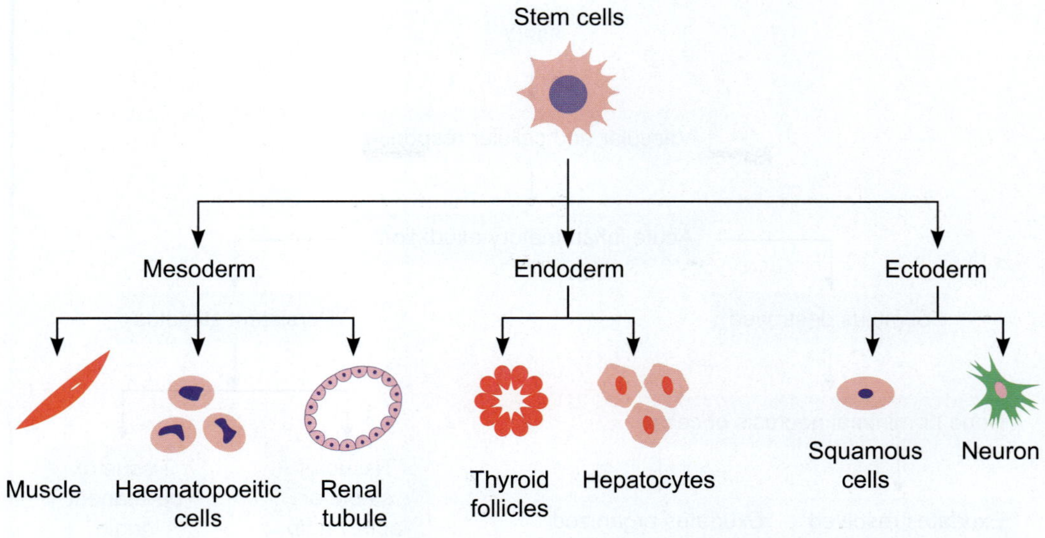

Fig. 4.3 Differentiation pathways of stem cells.

Q. What are stem cells? (PA5.1)

Ans. Stem cells are cells with **self-renewal capacity**. They are also characterized by **asymmetric replication** (a property of stem cells by virtue of which, after every cell cycle, some of the daughter cells retain their self-renewal capacity while the others enter a differentiation pathway, and are converted into a mature non-dividing population; Fig. 4.3). Stem cells may be:

- **Embryonic stem cells**: Stem cells that are isolated from embryos are called **embryonic stem cell (ES)**. These are the most undifferentiated stem cells located in the inner cell mass of the blastocyst. They can give rise to any type of cell in the body and are therefore also called **totipotent stem cells.** Embryonic stem cells are the source of origin of all the three germ layers.
- **Adult stem cells** have a markedly restricted differentiation capacity and are usually lineage specific. Adult stem cells located outside the bone marrow and in the tissue are generally referred to as **tissue stem cells**, for example **liver stem cells** which differentiate into hepatocytes and biliary cells. Tissue stem cells are located within a protected microenvironment called '**stem cell niches**'. **Neural tissue stem cells** are located in the subventricular area and dentate gyrus; and can generate neurons, astrocytes and oligodendrocytes. They have a potential role in neurodegenerative diseases and spinal cord injuries. **Skin stem cells** are found in the hair follicle bulge and **corneal stem cells** are present in the limbus. Corneal stem cells are present mainly in the limbus and can contribute to repair of damaged conjunctiva and corneal opacities. **Islet cell stem cells** are being explored for patients of Type 1 diabetes. The most elaborately studied stem cells are **haematopoietic stem cells** as well as **stromal cells located in the bone marrow**. The former are capable of differentiating into various blood cell lineages, while the latter, also called mesenchymal stem cells, are multipotent and can differentiate into a variety of stromal cells (chondrocytes, osteocytes, adipocytes and myocytes). Haematopoietic stem cells can be clinically used to replace depleted marrow cells (following chemotherapy for leukaemia) or provide normal cells to overcome red cell defects (sickle cell disease). Marrow stromal cells (mesenchymal stem cells) can be used clinically to provide stromal cellular scaffolding for tissue regeneration.

Totipotent stem cell
↓
Pluripotent stem cell
↓
Multipotent stem cell
↓
Lineage-committed stem cells
↓
Differentiated cells

Flowchart 4.1 Evolution and maturation of stem cells.

The evolution and maturation of stem cells is depicted in Flowchart 4.1.

Q. Enumerate the sequence of events involved in reparative response following an injury.

Ans. Pathways of reparative response following injury are shown in Flowchart 4.2.

Q. Enumerate the growth factors and cytokines involved in regeneration and wound healing.

Ans. Growth factors (GFs) are mostly proteins that prolong survival and induce proliferation of specific cells (Table 4.1). They bind to specific receptors and deliver signals that

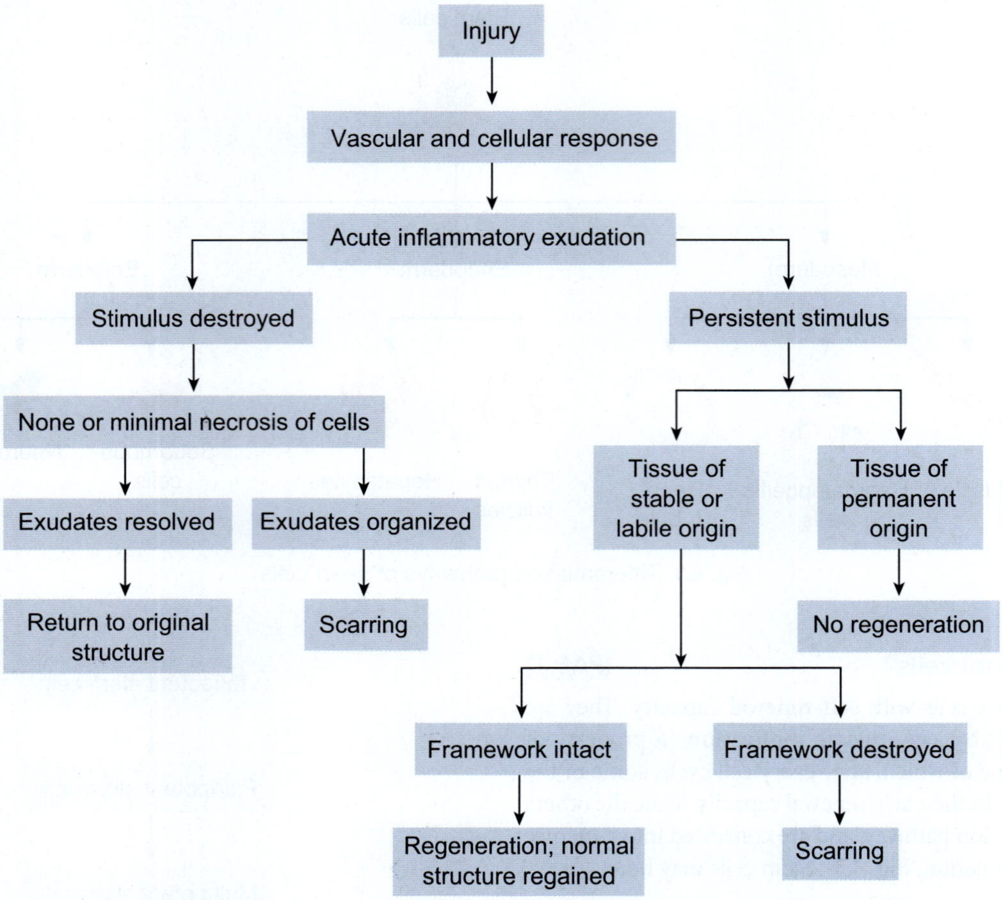

Flowchart 4.2 Pathways of reparative response following injury.

stimulate expression of genes whose products induce growth. They have the following functions:

1. Cell cycle activation (by direct stimulation or removal of blocks that inhibit cell cycle).
2. Prevention of apoptosis.
3. Enhanced synthesis of cellular proteins.

Q. What are the different signalling mechanisms in cell growth? Write briefly on receptors and signalling pathways involved in healing and repair. (PA5.1)

Ans. Growth factors (GFs) act by binding to specific receptors, which deliver signals to target cells. Signalling may be:

1. **Autocrine** (GFs act on the same cells that secrete them, for example HGF).
2. **Paracrine** (GFs act on cells adjacent to the cells that secrete them, for example produced by macrophages and action on fibroblasts).
3. **Endocrine** (produced by endocrine cells and carried in the blood stream to distant target cells, for example hormones).

Receptors and Signalling Pathways

- Binding of a ligand to its receptor triggers a series of intracellular signals that induce transcription factor activation or repression leading to different cellular events.
- Receptors can be on the surface of the target cells, in the cytoplasm or in the nucleus.

Signal transduction can originate from three types of receptors:

1. **Receptors with intrinsic tyrosine kinase activity** (Flowchart 4.3): These are dimeric transmembrane molecules having.
   (a) An extracellular ligand-binding domain.
   (b) Transmembrane region.
   (c) A cytoplasmic tail with tyrosine kinase activity.
   Example: An important pathway stimulated by Rous sarcoma virus (RAS) activation is the mitogen-activated protein (MAP) kinase cascade, which is involved in the intracellular signalling of many growth factors, for example Insulin, EGF, TGF-α, HGF, PDGF and VEGF.
2. **Seven transmembrane G protein–coupled receptors** (Flowchart 4.4): Polypeptides containing seven transmembrane α-helical segments (traverse the plasma membrane 7 times). *Examples*: Vasopressin, histamine, serotonin, glucagon and chemokines.
3. **Receptors lacking intrinsic tyrosine kinase activity:** Receptors can transmit extracellular signals to nucleus by activating Janus kinases (JAKs), which activate cytoplasmic transcription factors STATs (signal transducers and activators of transcription), which in turn enter the nucleus and activate gene transcription.

Table 4.1 Growth factors and cytokines involved in regeneration and wound healing

Type of growth factor	Symbol	Receptor	Sources	Functions
Epidermal growth factor	EGF	EGFR1 (ERBB1)	Platelets, macrophages, salivary glands, keratinocytes, etc.	Mitogenic for keratinocytes and fibroblasts; stimulates keratinocyte migration and granulation tissue formation
Fibroblast growth factor (FGF) family	FGF	FGFRs (1-4)	Platelets and macrophages	Wound repair. angiogenesis
Transforming growth factor-α	TGF-α	ERB B2 (HER-2 or HER-2/Neu)	Activated macrophages, T lymphocytes, keratinocytes, etc.	Similar to EGF; stimulates replication of hepatocytes and many epithelial cells
Hepatocyte growth factor/ scatter factor	HGF/SF	c-MET	Mesenchymal cells	Enhances proliferation of epithelial and endothelial cells
Vascular endothelial cell growth factor (isoforms A, B, C and D)	VEGF	VEGFR-1, VEGFR-2 and VEGFR-3	Mesenchymal cells	Increases vascular permeability; mitogenic for endothelial cells
Platelet-derived growth factor (isoforms A, B, C and D)	PDGF	PDGFR α and β	Platelets, macrophages, endothelial cells, keratinocytes, smooth muscle cells	Chemotactic for neutrophils, macrophages and smooth muscle cells; stimulates production of matrix metalloproteinases (MMPs), fibronectin, stimulates angiogenesis
Tumour necrosis factor	TNF	TNF-R	Macrophages, mast cells, T lymphocytes	Activates macrophages; regulates other cytokines
Interleukins	ILs	IL-R	Macrophages, mast cells, lymphocytes and many tissues	Chemotactic, angiogenic; regulate other cytokines
Transforming growth factor-β (TGF-β isoforms - TGF-β1, TGF-β2 and TGF-β3)	TGF-β	TGF-β receptors (types I and II)	Platelets, T lymphocytes, macrophages, endothelial cells	Chemotactic, angiogenic, mitogenic for fibroblasts, stimulates wound contraction, and matrix deposition
Interferons	IFN-α	Interferon receptors	Lymphocytes and fibroblasts	Activate macrophages, inhibit fibroblast proliferation, regulate other cytokines

FGF, Fibroblast growth factor; HGF, hepatocyte growth factor; MMPs, matrix metalloproteinases; TGF, transforming growth factor; VEGF, vascular endothelial growth factor.

Ligand binding
↓
Dimerization and phosphorylation of receptor subunits
↓
Activation of the receptor tyrosine kinase
↓
Activation of intracellular proteins like RAS, phosphatidylinositol 3-kinase (PI 3-kinase), phospholipase Cγ (PLC-γ)
↓
Entry into cell cycle/induction of transcription

Flowchart 4.3 Signal transduction mediated by receptors with intrinsic tyrosine kinase activity.

Examples: Receptors for cytokines like IL-2, IL-3, interferons, granulocyte monocyte-colony stimulating factor (GM-CSF) and growth hormone.

Note: All ligands do not induce stimulatory signals, growth inhibitory signals are also generated, for example TGF-β binding with its receptor phosphorylates some intracellular proteins, which in turn increase the synthesis of CDK inhibitors and block the activity of transcription factors and cell cycle progression.

Signalling initiated by ligand binding and conformational change in receptors
↓
Receptors associate with intracellular G proteins that contain GDP
↓
Exchange of GTP with GDP resulting in activation of the proteins
↓
Activation of cyclic AMP and inositol 1,4,5 triphosphate, which releases calcium from endoplasmic reticulum

Flowchart 4.4 Signal transduction mediated by seven transmembrane G protein–coupled receptors.

4. **Nuclear receptors:** Lipid soluble ligands (steroid hormones, thyroid hormone, vitamin D and retinoids) can diffuse into the cell to interact with intracellular proteins forming a receptor–ligand complex which in turn binds to the inactive receptor located in the nucleus to activate it.

Activated receptor binds to the specific DNA sequences known as hormone response elements on target genes or transcription factor.

Example: A group of receptors called peroxisome proliferator-activated receptors (PPARs) involved in inflammation and atherosclerosis.

Q. Write briefly on extracellular matrix (ECM) and cell–matrix interactions. (PA5.1)

Ans. Tissue repair depends on

1. Growth factor activity.
2. Interaction between cells and ECM components.

ECM is a constantly changing macromolecular complex, which assembles into a network that surrounds and supports the cells. It has the following functions:

1. Provides support and anchorage for cells, segregates tissues from one another and regulates intercellular communication.
2. Sequesters growth factors and serves as a reservoir for them (e.g., FGF and HGF; allows rapid deployment of growth factors after injury for regeneration).
3. Provides a substrate for cell adhesion.
4. Sequesters water to provide turgor to soft tissues.
5. Sequesters minerals to provide rigidity to bone.
6. Regulates proliferation and controls cell growth, movement and differentiation (by signalling through cellular receptors of integrin family).

ECM Exists in Two Different Forms

1. **Interstitial matrix:** Synthesized by mesenchymal cells, this randomly fills up the space between cells and supporting vascular and smooth muscle structures.
2. **Basement membrane:** The interstitial matrix organizes itself around epithelial, endothelial and smooth muscle cells to form a meshwork, which anchors down the above cells to loose connective tissue underneath. This meshwork is called 'basement membrane'. Its major components are amorphous non-fibrillar type IV collagen and laminin.

Components of ECM

- **Fibrous structural proteins** such as collagens and elastins for tensile strength and recoil.
- **Water hydrated gels** such as proteoglycans and hyaluronate for resilience and lubrication.
- **Adhesive glycoproteins** that connect the matrix elements to one another and to cells.

Fibrous Structural Proteins

1. **Fibrillar and non-fibrillar collagen**
   (a) Collagen provides the extracellular framework of most tissues in the body. All collagen types have a triple helical structure. Three separate polypeptide chains are braided into a rope-like triple helix.
   (b) Collagen proteins are rich in hydroxyproline and hydroxylysine.
   (c) Thirty different types are known.
   (d) Some types (I, II, III and V) form fibrils by virtue of lateral cross-linking of the triple helices.
   (e) Cross-linking is the result of covalent bonding catalysed by the enzyme lysyl oxidase in the presence of vitamin C.
   (f) Nonfibrillar collagens form the basement membrane (type IV collagen) or are components of structures like intervertebral discs (type IX collagen) or dermoepidermal junction (type VII collagen).
2. **Elastin**
   (a) Gives elasticity to tissues, allowing them to stretch when needed and then return to their original state.
   (b) Especially important in walls of large vessels, lungs, uterus, skin and ligaments.
   (c) Elastins are synthesized by fibroblasts and smooth muscle cells.
   (d) Morphologically, consist of a central core of elastin surrounded by a meshwork of a fibrillar glycoprotein.

Water Hydrated Gels

1. Provide compressibility to the tissue and serve as reservoirs of growth factors.
2. Proteoglycans are comprised of long polysaccharides called glycosaminoglycans (heparan sulphate and dermatan sulphate) linked to a protein backbone.
3. Hyaluronan is comprised of disaccharide repeats without any protein core.

Adhesive Glycoproteins and Adhesion Receptors

Structurally diverse molecules that are involved in cell-to-cell adhesion, linkage between cells and ECM and binding between ECM components include.

1. **Fibronectin** (main constituent of interstitial matrix): a protein that connects cells with collagen fibres in the ECM, allowing cells to move through the ECM. Fibronectins bind collagen and cell surface integrins, facilitating cell movement.
2. **Laminin** (main component of basement membrane): assists in cell adhesion and binds cells to other ECM components such as type IV collagen and heparin sulphate.
3. **Adhesion receptors** are also known as **cell adhesion molecules or CAMs;** CAMs are grouped into four categories, namely, immunoglobulins, cadherins, selectins and integrins. These proteins function as transmembrane receptors. As receptors, CAMs can bind to similar or different molecules in other cells, providing for interaction between the same cells (homotypic interaction) or different cell types (heterotypic interaction). *Selectins* are involved in leukocyte/endothelial interactions; *integrins* bind to ECM proteins, such as fibronectin, laminin, and osteopontin; *fibronectin* binds to collagen, fibrin, proteoglycans, and cell surface receptors; and *laminin* has binding domains for both ECM and cell surface receptors.

Q. Write briefly on cell and tissue regeneration.

Ans. The ability to regenerate is dependent on the type of cell.

- **Labile tissues** undergo continuous renewal.
- In **stable tissues,** tissue regeneration occurs but is a limited process (with the exception of liver). Pancreas, adrenals, kidneys, thyroid and lungs have limited regenerative capacity; however, as much as 40%–60% of the liver may

regenerate subsequent to its loss. Regeneration is dependent on many variables, for example, growth factors, inhibitors, signal transduction pathways, transcription factors and ECM proteins.

- TNF and IL-6 stimulate transition of the cells from G_0 to G_1 phase of cell cycle and HGF and EGF family of factors help in progression through the rest of the cell cycle. FGF and TGF-α are mitogenic for hepatocytes. Most epithelial cells share a common receptor (EGFR—epidermal growth factor receptor) with intrinsic tyrosine kinase activity.

Q. Write briefly on repair by connective tissue deposition. (PA5.1)

Ans. Repair by connective tissue deposition occurs when:

- There is severe injury so that parenchymal tissue as well as connective tissue framework of the organ is destroyed.
- Non-dividing cells are injured.

Repair begins within 24 hours; by 3–7 days, a special type of tissue called granulation tissue (so-called because of the pink, soft and granular-gross appearance) is formed. Repair by connective tissue deposition consists of four main stages:

1. Formation of new blood vessels (angiogenesis).
2. Migration and proliferation of fibroblasts.
3. Deposition of ECM.
4. Remodelling of fibrous tissue.

Q. Write briefly on angiogenesis. (PA5.1)

Ans. Two processes assemble blood vessels (Fig. 4.4):

1. **Vasculogenesis:** Involves formation of primitive vascular structures from angioblasts [endothelial precursor cells (EPCs)] in a manner resembling embryonal development of the vascular system. EPCs can be recruited from the bone marrow into tissues to initiate ngiogenesis. EPCs may contribute to the neovascularization of ischemic organs, wounds and tumours. The number of circulating EPCs increases greatly in patients with ischemic conditions,

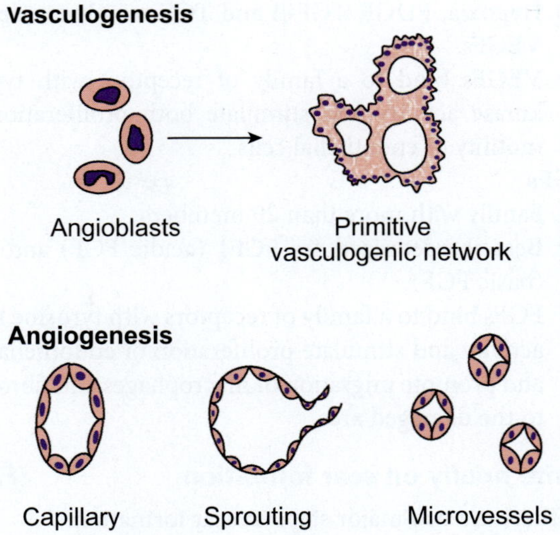

Fig. 4.4 Mechanism of formation of new blood vessels.

suggesting that EPCs may influence vascular function and determine the risk of cardiovascular diseases.

2. **Angiogenesis:** Neovascularization in which pre-existing vessels send out capillary sprouts to produce new vessels with or without pericytes and smooth muscle cells (mostly seen during repair of damaged tissue).

Steps in angiogenesis are shown in Flowchart 4.5.

New vessels formed are leaky due to incompletely formed inter-endothelial junctions. Structural ECM proteins participate in the process of vessel formation through interactions with integrin receptors. Non-structural proteins contribute to angiogenesis by destabilizing cell–ECM interactions to facilitate continued cell migration or degrade the ECM to permit remodelling and ingrowth of vessels.

Growth Factors Involved in Angiogenesis

1. **VEGFs**
   (a) Family of growth factors that include VEGF isoforms—A, B, C, D.

Activation of receptors on endothelial cells in pre-existing vessels by angiogenic growth factors

↓

Release of endothelial proteases that degrade the basement membrane to allow endothelial cells to escape from the original (parent) vessel wall into the surrounding matrix

↓

Migration of endothelial cells towards area of angiogenic stimulus

↓

Proliferation of endothelial cells behind the migrating cells

↓

Remodelling of endothelial cells into capillary tubes

↓

Recruitment of pericytes and smooth muscle cells to form mature vessels

Flowchart 4.5 Steps in angiogenesis.

   (b) Hypoxia, PDGF, TGF-β and TGF-α induce release of VEGFs.
   (c) VEGFs bind to a family of receptors with tyrosine kinase activity and stimulate both proliferation and motility of endothelial cells.
2. **FGFs**
   (a) Family with more than 20 members.
   (b) Best characterized are FGF1 (acidic FGF) and FGF2 (basic FGF).
   (c) FGFs bind to a family of receptors with tyrosine kinase activity and stimulate proliferation of endothelial cells and promote migration of macrophages and fibroblasts to the damaged area.

Q. Write briefly on scar formation. (PA5.1)

Ans. There are two major steps in scar formation:

1. Migration of fibroblasts to the damaged area followed by proliferation.
2. Deposition of ECM by the same cells, which involves the following events:
   (a) Recruitment and stimulation of fibroblasts, which is driven by many growth factors, for example, PDGF, FGF2, TGF-β (elaborated by endothelium and macrophages).
   (b) Macrophages clear extracellular debris and fibrin and also elaborate a host of mediators that induce fibroblast proliferation and ECM production.
   (c) As healing progresses, the number of proliferating fibroblasts and new vessels decrease and collagen synthesis and ECM deposition increases.
   (d) **Decreased collagen degradation rather than increased collagen synthesis is responsible for net collagen accumulation.**
   (e) Ultimately, the granulation tissue scaffold is converted into scar tissue composed of fibroblasts, dense collagen, fragments of elastic tissue and other ECM components.

Q. Write briefly on healing by primary or first intention. (PA5.1)

Ans. Primary union is seen in incised wounds with opposed edges (clean and uninfected wound).

- The incision space/defect fills with blood and fibrin, which subsequently clots and gets dehydrated to form a scab.
- Within 24 h, neutrophils appear along the edges of the incision. The edges then proliferate and migrate under the scab to form a thin continuous epithelial layer.
- By day 5, the incision space is filled with granulation tissue and collagen fibres, which now bridge the incision.
- During the 2nd week, there is continued accumulation of collagen fibres and a connective tissue scar forms by the end of 1 month.

The sequence of events in healing by primary intention are summarized in Flowchart 4.6 and Fig. 4.5A.

Wound

↓

- Filled with blood clot and inflammatory cells
- Neutrophils appear at the margin of the wound

} Day 1

↓

- Neutrophils largely replaced by macrophages
- Granulation tissue formation begins and infiltrates the incision space
- Collagen fibres form at the margins of the incision and are laid down vertically
- Thickening of the epithelial layer due to epithelial cell proliferation and migration of epithelial cells along incised margins

} Day 3

↓

- Incisional space is filled with granulation tissue
- Neovascularization is at its peak
- Collagen fibres become abundant and bridge the incisional gap
- Epidermis regains its normal thickness
- Differentiation of surface cells yields mature epidermal architecture

} Day 5

↓

- Continued accumulation of collagen and proliferation of fibroblasts
- Regression of vessels and blanching

} Day 7

↓

- Scar tissue formation by the end of the first month
- Gradual gain in tensile strength overtime

Flowchart 4.6 Sequence of events in healing by primary or first intention.

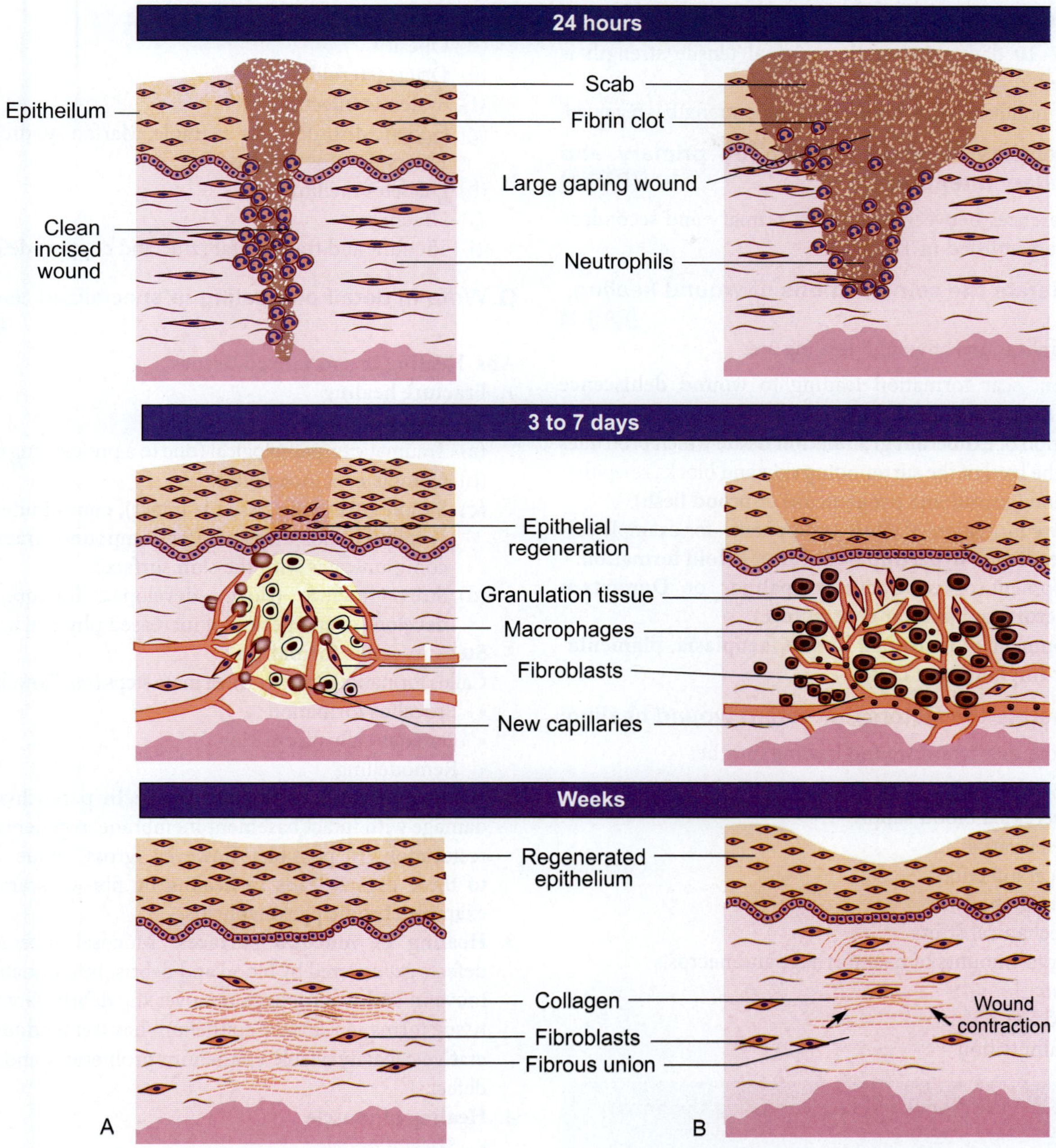

Fig. 4.5 Healing by (A) primary and (B) secondary intentions.

Q. Write briefly on healing by secondary intention. (PA5.1)

Ans. Secondary union unlike primary union is seen in open wounds with separated edges, extensive loss of cells and large defects. The wound gets filled with a large blood clot, necrotic debris and exudate. This is typically followed by an intense inflammatory reaction, laying down of large amounts of granulation tissue, formation of epithelial spurs at the margins of the wound, and a substantial scar with thinning of epidermis (Fig. 4.5B). ***Exuberant granulation tissue*** is characterized by formation of a large mass of granulation tissue that protrudes from the wound and prevents/slows re-epithelialization. It is also referred to as '***proud flesh***'. ***Keloid formation*** is an aberrant wound healing resulting in excessive collagenization leading to the formation of bulging scars. '***Wound contraction***' is pathognomonic of healing by secondary intention. It is mediated by myofibroblasts and aids in decreasing the gap between the dermal edges of the wound.

Characteristic Features of Healing by Secondary Intention

- Associated with large defects filled with blood clots, necrotic debris and exudate.
- Inflammatory reaction is more intense.
- Large amounts of granulation tissue are deposited.
- There is formation of epithelial spurs from margins of the wound.
- Typically demonstrates 'wound contraction' which is mediated by myofibroblasts and aids in decreasing the gap between the dermal edges of the large wound.
- Substantial scar formation and thinning of the epidermis is seen.

Regaining Wound Strength

- After 7–10 days, 10% of the original tensile strength is regained.
- After 3 months, 80% of the original tensile strength is regained.

Q. Differentiate between healing by primary and secondary intention. (PA5.1)

Ans. Differences between healing by primary and secondary intention are enlisted in Table 4.2.

Q. Enumerate the complications of wound healing. (PA5.1)

Ans. Complications of wound healing are:

1. Deficient scar formation leading to **wound dehiscence (rupture)** or **ulceration.**
2. Formation of **exuberant granulation tissue** which protrudes above the level of the surrounding skin and blocks re-epithelialization (**granuloma pyogenicum** or **proud flesh**).
3. Excessive formation of repair components, for example collagen leading to **hypertrophied scar** or **keloid formation.**
4. Development of **contractures (palmar** or **Dupuytren contracture** and **plantar contracture).**
5. Development of **incisional hernia, neoplasia, pigmentation** or **implantation cysts.**

Q. Enumerate the factors that retard wound healing.

Ans. Factors that retard wound healing may be:

1. ***Local***
   (a) Decreased blood supply
   (b) Denervation
   (c) Local infection
   (d) Foreign body
   (e) Mechanical stress
   (f) Large amounts of haemorrhage and necrosis
2. ***Systemic***
   (a) Old age
   (b) Malnutrition
   (c) Anaemia
   (d) Obesity
   (e) Drugs (steroids)
   (f) Systemic infection
   (g) Genetic disorders, for example, Marfan syndrome and Ehlers–Danlos disease
   (h) Diabetes mellitus
   (i) Uraemia
   (j) Vitamin and trace metal (zinc and copper) deficiency

Table 4.2 Differences between healing by primary and secondary intention

Features	Healing by primary intention	Healing by secondary intention
Nature of wound	Seen in incised wounds with well opposed edges (clean and uninfected wound)	Seen in large, open, infected wounds with separated edges; associated with extensive loss of cells
Amount of fibrin and blood	Filled with moderate amount of fibrin and blood	Filled with a large blood clot and necrotic debris and exudate
Inflammatory reaction	Less intense	More intense
Amount of granulation tissue	Less granulation tissue	Extensive granulation tissue
Wound contraction	Wound contraction is not seen	Wound contraction is seen
Complications	Less common	More common

Q. Write in detail on healing in specialized tissues. (PA5.1)

Ans. Healing in specialized tissues

1. **Fracture healing**
   Types of fracture
   (a) Traumatic or pathological (due to a pre-existing disease).
   (b) Complete or incomplete.
   (c) Simple (overlying tissue is intact), comminuted (bone is splintered or displaced) or compound (fracture site communicates with the skin surface).
   (d) Stress fracture (slowly developed fracture, which develops over a period of increased physical activity).
   Steps in callus formation
   Callus formation involves three main steps (see Flowchart 4.7):
   - Procallus formation
   - Osseous callus formation
   - Remodelling
2. **Healing of solid epithelial organs:** In parenchymal cell damage with intact basement membrane, regeneration and restoration is possible; however, gross tissue damage to these organs leads to healing by fibrous scarring, for example chronic pyelonephritis.
3. **Healing of mucosal surfaces:** Mucosal ulceration or defects get covered by blood and debris. Inflammatory cells move in and macrophage removes the debris. Granulation tissue forms. As surface epithelium has tremendous regenerative capacity, viable epithelium proliferates and fills the defect.
4. **Healing of muscle**
   - *Skeletal muscle*
     - Cut ends of the injured skeletal muscle are held together by connective tissue and the gap created is filled with fibrin and inflammatory cells (neutrophils and macrophages).
     - If the muscle sheath is intact, sarcolemmal tubes appear along endomysium and restore muscle fibres, for example, Zenker degeneration of the muscle in typhoid. Various growth factors, including IGF-1, beta FGF, and nerve growth factor (NGF), can improve muscle regeneration.
     - If the muscle sheath is damaged, a disorganized multinucleated mass and scar composed of fibrovascular tissue forms, for example Volkmann ischemic contracture.
   - *Smooth muscle*
     - Smooth muscle regenerates from a type of stem cell called a **pericyte,** which is found in some closely apposed small blood vessels. Pericytes allow smooth

Formation of a haematoma due to bleeding from torn blood vessels

↓

Loose meshwork formed by blood fills the fracture gap

↓

Local inflammatory response

↓

Exudation of fibrin, polymorphs and macrophages at the site of fracture

↓

Ingrowth of granulation tissue (begins with neovascularization)

↓

The degranulated platelets and inflammatory cells secrete mediators that activate osteoprogenitor cells in the periosteum, medullary cavity and surrounding soft tissue

↓

Soft tissue callus or procallus formation (end of the first week)

↓

Osteoprogenitor cells lay down collagen as well as osteoid matrix in granulation tissue

↓

- Calcification of osteoid (woven bone callus)
- Deposition of fibrocartilage and hyaline cartilage

↓

Woven bone is cleared away by osteoclasts and the calcified cartilage disintegrates; in its place lamellar bone with haversian system is laid down

↓

Remodelling of bone
(realignment and mechanical chopping of bone; development of medullary canal)

↓

Compact bone formation

Flowchart 4.7 Steps in callus formation.

muscle cells to regenerate and repair much more readily than skeletal and cardiac muscle tissue. Similar to skeletal muscle tissue, cardiac muscle does not regenerate to a great extent. Dead cardiac muscle tissue is replaced by scar tissue, which cannot contract.

5. **Healing of liver:** Hepatocytes have a high regenerative capacity. If the connective tissue framework of the liver remains intact, injury to hepatocytes ends with complete regeneration and restitution. However, if the connective tissue framework of the liver is damaged, fibrosis ensues.
6. **Healing of kidneys:** Tubular epithelial cells regenerate completely if tubular cell damage occurs but the basement membrane remains intact. Glomerular damage, however, usually results in scarring.

Q. Enumerate the complications of fracture healing. (PA5.1)

Ans. Complications of fracture healing:

1. **Fibrous union** (inadequate immobilization permits constant movement at the fracture site so that the normal constituents of callus do not form; callus is comprised of only fibrous tissue and cartilage).
2. **Non-union.**
3. **Delayed union.**
4. **Pseudoarthrosis** (if a non-union allows too much motion along the fracture gap; the central portion of the callus undergoes cystic degeneration and its luminal surface becomes lined by synovial-like cells creating a false joint called pseudoarthrosis).

5 Haemodynamic Disorders, Thrombosis and Shock

Q. Define oedema. Write briefly on its types. (PA6.1)

Ans. Oedema is defined as abnormal and excessive accumulation of fluid in interstitial tissue spaces and serous cavities. Approximately, 60% of body weight is water—two-thirds of which is intracellular and one-third extracellular. The extracellular space is divided into interstitial and intravascular compartments. Bulk of the extracellular water is formed by interstitial fluid and only 5% of the body's water is present as blood plasma. If the net influx of fluid exceeds the lymphatic drainage, the excessive volume of fluid may accumulate either within the interstitial matrix (**interstitial oedema**) or in the serous body cavities (**effusion**).

Examples of Oedema/Effusion

- Periorbital oedema
- Dependent oedema
- Generalized oedema or anasarca
- Hydrothorax or pleural effusion
- Hydropericardium or pericardial effusion
- Hydroperitoneum or ascites

Oedema causes a palpable swelling and may be the result of either too much pressure or too little protein within the blood vessels.

Classification of Oedema

- ***Localized*** or ***generalized oedema***, based on the distribution and extent of involvement. Localized oedema is limited to a small area, for example an organ (organ-specific oedema) or a limb (elephantiasis, oedema due to venous obstruction as seen in deep vein thrombosis, allergic laryngeal oedema as seen in anaphylaxis and localized inflammatory oedema). Generalized oedema, on the other hand, may involve the entire body (oedema due to congestive cardiac failure, nephrotic syndrome and nutritional deficiency). Differences between generalized and localized oedema are tabulated in Table 5.1.
- ***Transudative*** or ***exudative oedema/effusion***, based on the composition of the fluid.

Consequences of Oedema

Oedema may compromise cellular function in the following ways:

- Due to expansion of the interstitial space, there is an increase in the diffusion distance for oxygen and other nutrients, which hampers cellular metabolism, for example impaired gas exchange due to pulmonary oedema.
- Expansion of the interstitial space also interferes with the removal of toxic by-products of cellular metabolism.
- Persistent and severe subcutaneous oedema may delay wound healing.
- Severe cerebral oedema there may induce herniation of the cerebral matter and also compress cerebral vasculature.

Q. Enumerate the differences between exudate and transudate.

Ans. Differences between exudate and transudate are tabulated in Table 5.2.

Q. What are the factors affecting fluid balance across capillaries? (PA6.1)

Ans. Under normal circumstances, the following factors influence the fluid balance across capillaries (Fig. 5.1):

1. Plasma colloid oncotic pressure (which tends to drive water and salts into the vessels).
2. Capillary hydrostatic pressure (which tends to drive water and salts out of the vessels into the interstitial space).
3. Lymphatic drainage (which tends to drain the interstitial space).
4. Sodium balance (sodium retention increases hydrostatic pressure and causes a dilutional decrease in the colloid osmotic pressure).

Table 5.1 Differences between generalized and localized oedema

Causes	Generalized	Localized
1. Acute	• Acute **cardiac failure** • Acute renal insufficiency	• **Acute inflammation** • Burns • Anaphylaxis • Trauma • Thrombosis
2. Chronic	• Chronic cardiac insufficiency • Chronic renal insufficiency • Chronic malnutrition	• Elephantiasis and oedema due to venous obstruction as seen in deep vein thrombosis
Distribution	Involves large areas or entire body	Limited to a small area (organ specific)

Table 5.2 Differences between exudate and transudate

Features	Exudate	Transudate
Definition	Oedema associated with increased vascular permeability	Filtrate of blood or plasma; no increase in vascular permeability observed
Nature	Inflammatory oedema	Non-inflammatory oedema
Protein content	1. High (more than 4 g/dL) 2. Has high fibrinogen and tendency to coagulate	1. Low (less than 3 g/dL) 2. Mainly albumin, low fibrinogen
Specific gravity	High (more than 1.018)	Low (less than 1.015)
pH	>7.3	<7.3
LDH	High Fluid LDH/serum LDH ratio is >0.6	Low Fluid LDH/serum LDH ratio is <0.6
Cells	Highly cellular; rich in polymorphs	Few, mainly mesothelial cells
Example	Pus seen in pyogenic infections	Fluid in congestive cardiac failure

Normally, at the arteriolar end of the capillary bed, the hydrostatic pressure exceeds the plasma oncotic (colloid osmotic) pressure pushing the water and electrolytes out from the vessels into the interstitial tissue. At the venous end of the capillary bed, osmotic pressure is more than the hydrostatic pressure and hence the fluid is reabsorbed from the interstitial tissue into the vessels at this end. The interstitial fluid is drained by the lymph vessels and this eventually returns to the veins via the thoracic duct. Oedema is the result of increased movement of fluid from the vasculature to the interstitium and occurs when there are:

1. Abnormalities in the hydrostatic and oncotic pressures acting across the vessel walls.
2. Alterations in the endothelial wall structure.
3. Alterations in the lymphatic outflow system.

Q. What are the pathophysiologic categories of oedema? (PA6.1)

Ans. Intravascular alterations resulting in oedema include an increase in capillary hydrostatic pressure and/or a decrease in plasma oncotic pressure, the latter correlating with hypoalbuminemia. As the interstitial fluid pressure increases, lymphatic tissues remove much of the excess volume via thoracic duct; if the limit of lymphatic tissues to remove excess volume is exceeded, tissue oedema results. Important pathophysiologic categories of oedema are enumerated as follows:

1. **Oedema due to increased hydrostatic pressure:** Hydrostatic pressure of capillaries is the force that tends to drive fluid through capillary wall into interstitial space. A rise in hydrostatic pressure at venular end of a capillary to a level more than plasma oncotic pressure results in oedema. Increased hydrostatic pressure may be due to:
   (a) ***Impaired venous return:***
      (i) Congestive heart failure
      (ii) Constrictive pericarditis
      (iii) Ascites (liver cirrhosis)
      (iv) Venous obstruction
      (v) Thrombosis
      (vi) External pressure due to a mass
   (b) ***Arteriolar dilatation:***
      (i) Heat
      (ii) Neurohumoural dysregulation
2. **Oedema due to reduced plasma oncotic pressure:** Normally, plasma oncotic pressure is exerted by plasma proteins and drives fluid into the vessels. Reduced oncotic pressure causes increased movement of fluid into interstitial space. Decreased plasma oncotic pressure may be due to:
   (a) Protein-losing glomerulopathies (nephrotic syndrome)
   (b) Liver cirrhosis (ascites)
   (c) Malnutrition (famine oedema)
   (d) Protein-losing gastroenteropathies
3. **Oedema due to lymphatic obstruction:** Normally, interstitial fluid escapes via lymphatic system. Lymphatic obstruction causes accumulation of fluid in interstitial spaces. Lymphatic obstruction may be due to the following causes:
   (a) Inflammatory
   (b) Neoplastic
   (c) Postsurgical

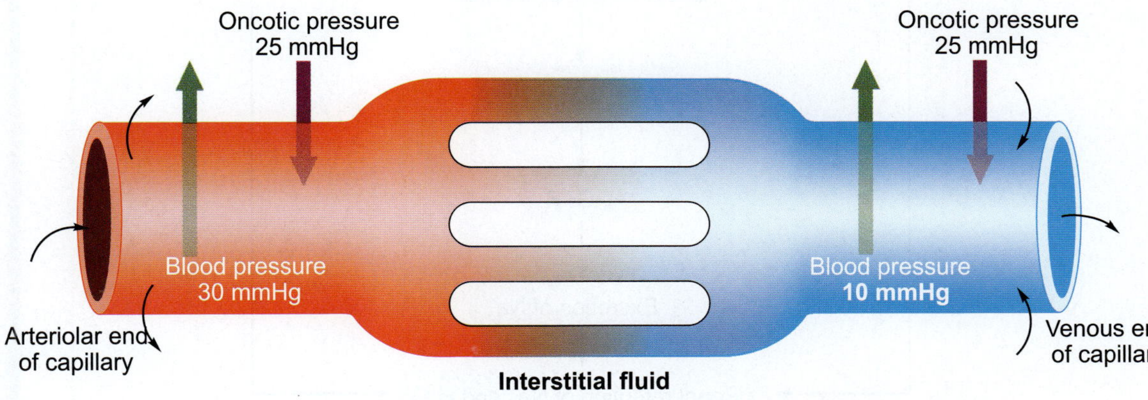

Fig. 5.1 Factors affecting fluid balance across capillaries.

(d) Postirradiation
(e) Due to congenital absence of lymphatics
(f) Recurrent infections (recurrent erysipelas, leprosy, syphilis, filariasis)

4. **Oedema due to sodium retention:** Increased sodium retention is invariably associated with water retention, which leads to increased plasma volume as well as hydrostatic pressure. Dilutional effect on albumin leads to decreased plasma colloid oncotic pressure. Causes of sodium retention include the following:
(a) Excessive salt intake with renal insufficiency.
(b) Increased tubular reabsorption of sodium.
(c) Renal hypoperfusion.
(d) Increased renin–angiotensin–aldosterone secretion.
5. **Oedema due to inflammation:** Endothelial lining may be injured by toxins and their products, for example histamine, anoxia, venoms, drugs and chemicals. Endothelial damage leads to increased vascular permeability and leakage of plasma proteins into the interstitial tissue resulting in oedema.

Q. Write briefly on normal regulatory mechanisms responsible for maintaining sodium and water balance. (PA6.1)

Ans. Eighty percent of sodium is reabsorbed by proximal convoluted tubule under the influence of intrinsic and extrinsic renal mechanisms (Flowchart 5.1). Antidiuretic hormone (ADH) secretion and perception of thirst are primary regulatory factors in regulating water balance. The renin–angiotensin–aldosterone system is the most important hormonal system involved in regulation of sodium. Angiotensin II is the most potent naturally occurring vasoconstrictor and its presser action is mainly attributed to peripheral arteriolar vasoconstriction. It stimulates the adrenal cortex to secrete aldosterone that promotes renal reabsorption of sodium and water. Blood concentration of sodium is regulated by four main mechanisms:

- Release of aldosterone from activation of renin–angiotensin system.
- Increase in proximal tubular reabsorption of sodium due to reduction in glomerular filtration rate (GFR), which is caused by reduced blood flow.
- Release of atriopeptin hormone, which increases GFR and inhibits sodium reabsorption.
- Natriuretic peptides secreted by atrial and ventricular myocardium (considered the endogenous inhibitors of the renin–angiotensin system) cause sodium excretion and diuresis, and induce vasodilatation.

Q. Write briefly on the pathogenesis of oedema.

Ans. Oedema or expansion of interstitial fluid compartment is initiated by an imbalance of Starling forces operating between plasma and the interstitium. It occurs most commonly in response to congestive heart failure, cirrhosis, and nephrotic syndrome. In all of these conditions, due to a disturbance of the circulatory homeostasis, the renal effector mechanisms that tend to conserve sodium are exaggerated (Flowchart 5.2).

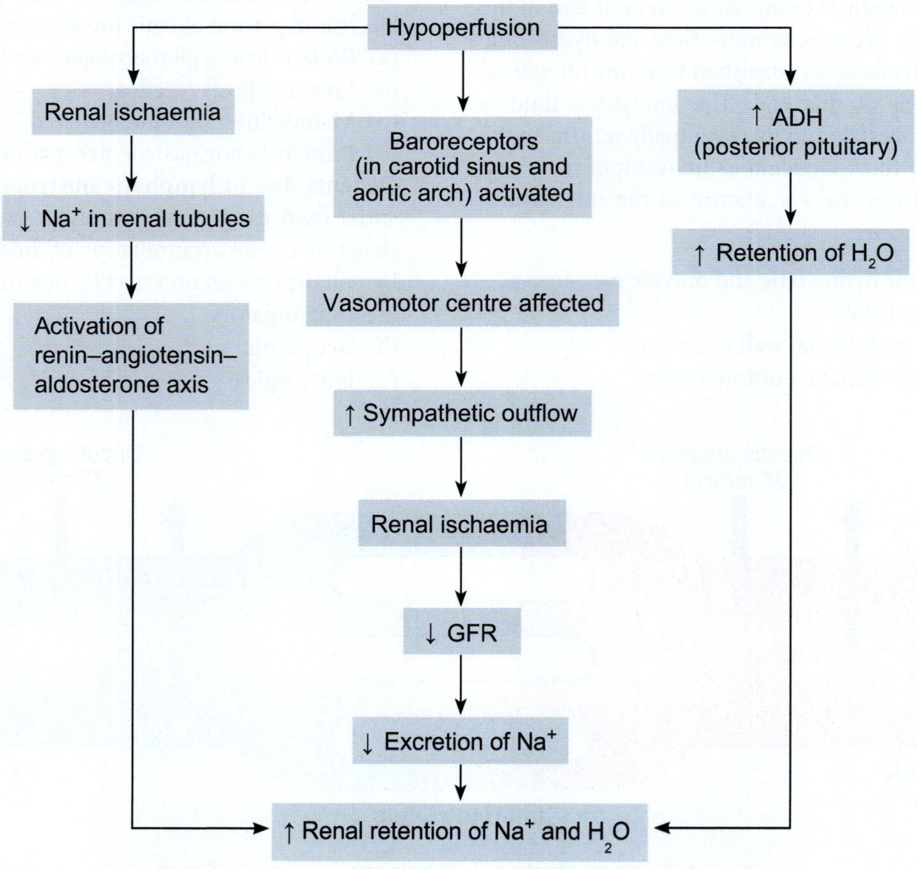

Flowchart 5.1 Normal regulatory mechanisms responsible for maintaining sodium and water balance.

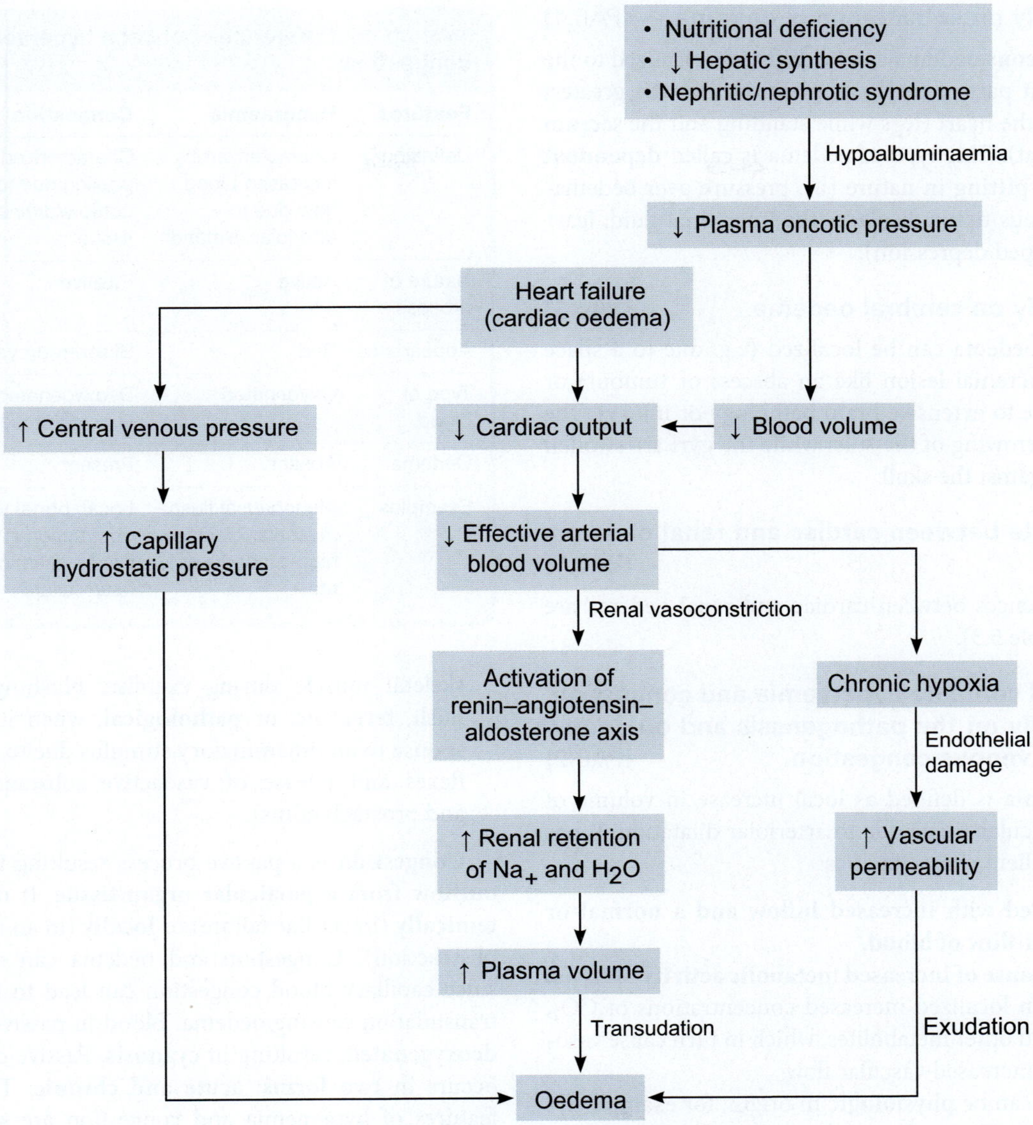

Flowchart 5.2 Pathogenesis of oedema.

Q. Write briefly on renal oedema. (PA6.1)

Ans. Oedema due to renal dysfunction typically appears first in loose connective tissue, for example the eyelids (periorbital oedema).

- Causes of renal oedema include **nephrotic syndrome, glomerulonephritis** (acute glomerulonephritis, rapidly progressive glomerulonephritis) and **acute tubular injury**.
- Nephrotic syndrome is characterized by persistent and heavy proteinuria causing a reduced plasma oncotic pressure leading to generalized severe oedema. Also, a reduction in the effective plasma volume causes activation of the renin–angiotensin–aldosterone mechanism, thereby causing retention of sodium and water or oedema.
- Nephritic oedema is mainly due to excessive reabsorption of sodium and water in the renal tubules and not due to protein loss. It is milder as compared to nephrotic oedema.
- In acute tubular injury, which is due to shock or toxic chemicals, tubules lose their capacity for selective renal concentration of the glomerular filtrate resulting in increased reabsorption and oliguria.

Q. Write briefly on cardiac oedema. (PA6.1)

Ans. Cardiac oedema is mostly a manifestation of congestive heart failure, and occurs due to activation of a series of mechanisms that increase venous capillary pressure, promote sodium and water retention by the kidneys and expansion of the extracellular fluid. These mechanisms, in concert with abnormal Starling forces, such as increased venous capillary pressure and decreased plasma oncotic pressure, promote fluid extravasation and oedema formation (See Flowchart 5.2).

Q. Write briefly on pulmonary oedema. (PA6.1)

Ans. Defined as fluid accumulation in the air spaces and parenchyma of the lungs, pulmonary oedema may lead to respiratory failure due to impaired gas exchange. It is mainly of the following two types:

1. **Cardiogenic pulmonary oedema** (caused by congestive cardiac failure or left ventricular failure which lead to inadequate removal of blood from the pulmonary circulation).
2. **Non-cardiogenic pulmonary oedema** (caused by injury to lung parenchyma or vasculature of the lung).

Q. Write briefly on subcutaneous oedema. (PA6.1)

Ans. Subcutaneous oedema can be diffuse or localized to the most dependent part of the body positioned at the greatest distance below the heart (legs while standing and the sacrum while recumbent). This type of oedema is called **dependent oedema** and is **pitting** in nature (i.e. pressure over oedematous subcutaneous tissue displaces the interstitial fluid, leaving a finger-shaped depression).

Q. Write briefly on cerebral oedema. (PA6.1)

Ans. Cerebral oedema can be localized (e.g. due to a space occupying intracranial lesion like an abscess or tumour) or generalized (due to extensive brain pathology or injury). The latter causes narrowing of the sulci while the gyri are swollen and flattened against the skull.

Q. Differentiate between cardiac and renal oedema. (PA6.1)

Ans. The differences between cardiac and renal oedema are tabulated in Table 5.3).

Q. Define and compare hyperaemia and congestion. Write briefly on the pathogenesis and outcomes of chronic venous congestion. (PA6.2)

Ans. Hyperaemia is defined as local increase in volume of blood in a particular tissue due to arteriolar dilatation. It has the following salient characteristics:

- It is associated with **increased inflow and a normal or decreased outflow of blood.**
- It **occurs because of increased metabolic activity of tissue** that results in localized increased concentrations of CO_2, lactic acid and other metabolites, which in turn cause vasodilation and increased vascular flow.
- Hyperaemia can be **physiologic** in origin, for example hyperaemia of the skin to dissipate heat, increased blood flow to the gastrointestinal tract after a meal, increased inflow in skeletal muscle during exercise, blushing, menopausal flush, fever, etc. or **pathological**, when it occurs in response to an inflammatory stimulus due to neurogenic reflexes and release of vasoactive substances (histamine and prostaglandins).

Table 5.3 Contrasting features of cardiac and renal oedema

Features	Cardiac oedema	Renal oedema
Causes	CHF and right-sided heart failure	Nephritic and nephrotic syndrome/acute tubular injury/necrosis
Mechanism	Decreased cardiac output	Hypoalbuminemia and decreased plasma oncotic pressure
Clinical	• Dependent oedema, the distribution of which changes with posture • Mainly pedal or sacral; later generalized	First observed around face, eyes, ankle and genitalia
Serum albumin	Normal	Decreased
Proteinuria	Absent	Present

Table 5.4 Differences between hyperaemia and congestion

Features	Hyperaemia	Congestion
Definition	Characterized by increased blood flow due to arteriolar dilatation	Characterized by blood pooling due to impaired outflow/drainage from tissue
Nature of process	Active	Passive
Appearance	Red	Bluish-red/cyanosed
Type of blood	Oxygenated	Deoxygenated; tissue hypoxia present
Oedema	Absent	Present
Examples	Menopausal flush, muscular exercise, high-grade fever, etc.	Local: portal venous obstruction in cirrhosis of liver; systemic: right-sided heart failure

Congestion is a passive process resulting from **impaired outflow from a particular organ/tissue**. It may occur **systemically** (in cardiac failure) or **locally** (in an isolated venous obstruction). Congestion and oedema can occur together since capillary blood congestion can lead to increased fluid transudation causing oedema. Blood in passive congestion is **deoxygenated**, resulting in **cyanosis**. Passive congestion also occurs in **two forms**: **acute and chronic**. The contrasting features of hyperaemia and congestion are summarized in Table 5.4.

In **acute congestion**, the blood is contained inside the dilated veins and capillaries. This condition is usually without serious consequences, however, in the scenario of rapid accumulation of blood, there may be hypoxia and mechanical compression of the surrounding tissue leading to necrosis. In **chronic passive congestion**, prolonged ischaemia/hypoxia may be accompanied by loss of parenchymal cells, which are usually replaced by fibrosis. **The pathogenesis and outcomes of chronic venous congestion are depicted in Flowchart 5.3A and B.**

Q. Write briefly on the pathogenesis and clinicopathological features of pulmonary congestion. (PA6.2)

Ans. Pulmonary congestion is defined as accumulation of fluid within the pulmonary interstitium as well as alveoli. It may be classified into 'acute or chronic' types based on duration.

Acute Pulmonary Congestion

This may be **cardiogenic** or **non-cardiogenic** in origin. Most common cause of carcinogenic oedema is left ventricular failure. Non-cardiogenic oedema is caused by injury to lung parenchyma or vasculature of the lung.

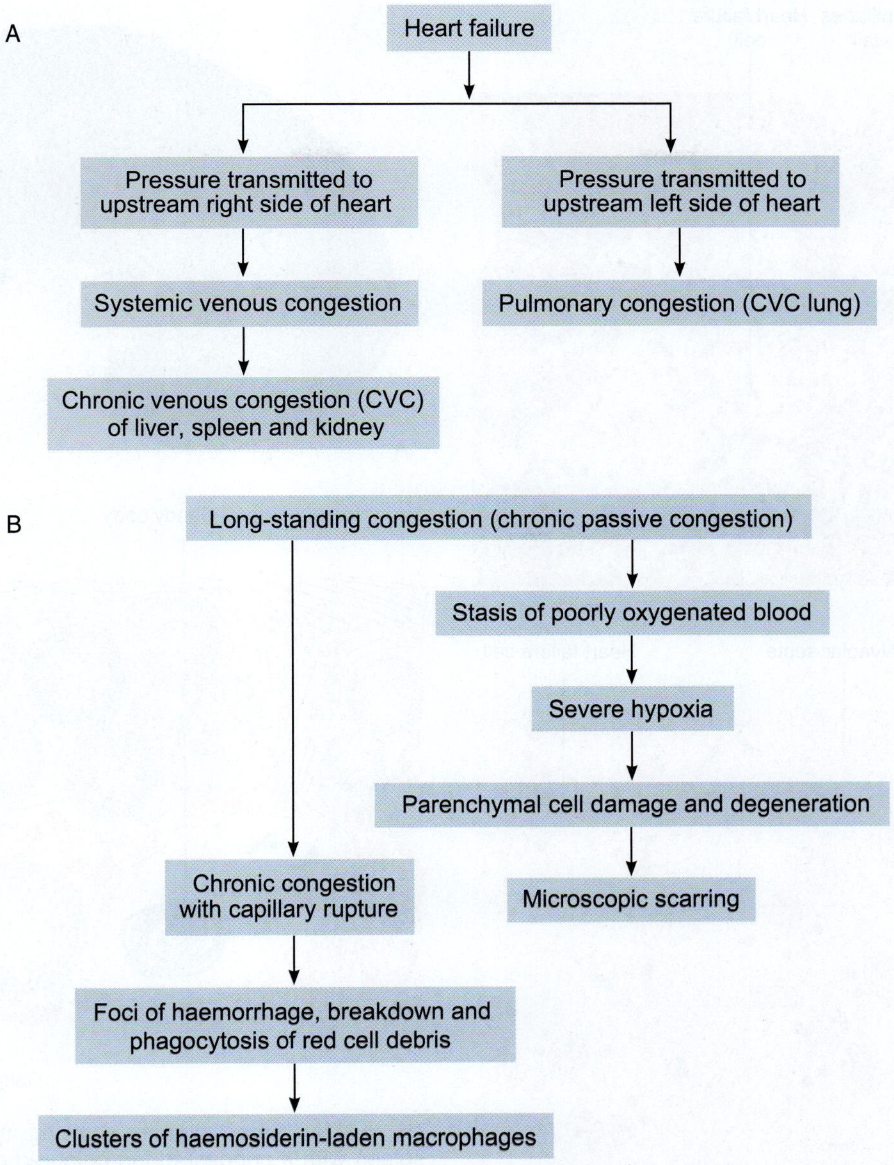

Flowchart 5.3 (A) Pathogenesis of chronic venous congestion (CVC). (B) Outcomes of long-standing congestion.

Gross Morphology

Lungs are enlarged; cut section shows frothy, bloodstained fluid (air in combination with oedema fluid and red cells).

Microscopic Features

The main histopathological features of acute pulmonary congestion are:

- Alveolar septal oedema
- Engorged septal capillaries
- Focal intra-alveolar haemorrhages

Chronic Venous Congestion (CVC) Lung/Brown Induration (Fig. 5.2A and B)

Long-standing pulmonary venous congestion occurs due to left-sided heart failure caused by rheumatic mitral stenosis, coronary artery disease and hypertension. This results in reduced outflow of blood from lungs and increased pulmonary venous pressure.

Gross Morphology

- The lungs are heavier and firmer than normal.
- Cut surface is dark brown in colour (**brown induration**) with oozing of frothy, blood-tinged material.

Microscopic Features

- Dilatation and congestion of septal capillaries with widening of alveolar septa due to interstitial oedema.
- Pulmonary oedema due to movement of fluid from the congested vessels to alveolar spaces.
- Intra-alveolar haemorrhage (due to rupture of congested alveolar capillaries).
- RBC breakdown, which produces haemosiderin, which in turn is taken up by alveolar macrophages. These haemosiderin-laden macrophages present in alveolar lumina are called **heart failure cells** (siderophages).
- Fibrosis and thickening of alveolar septae in the later stages.

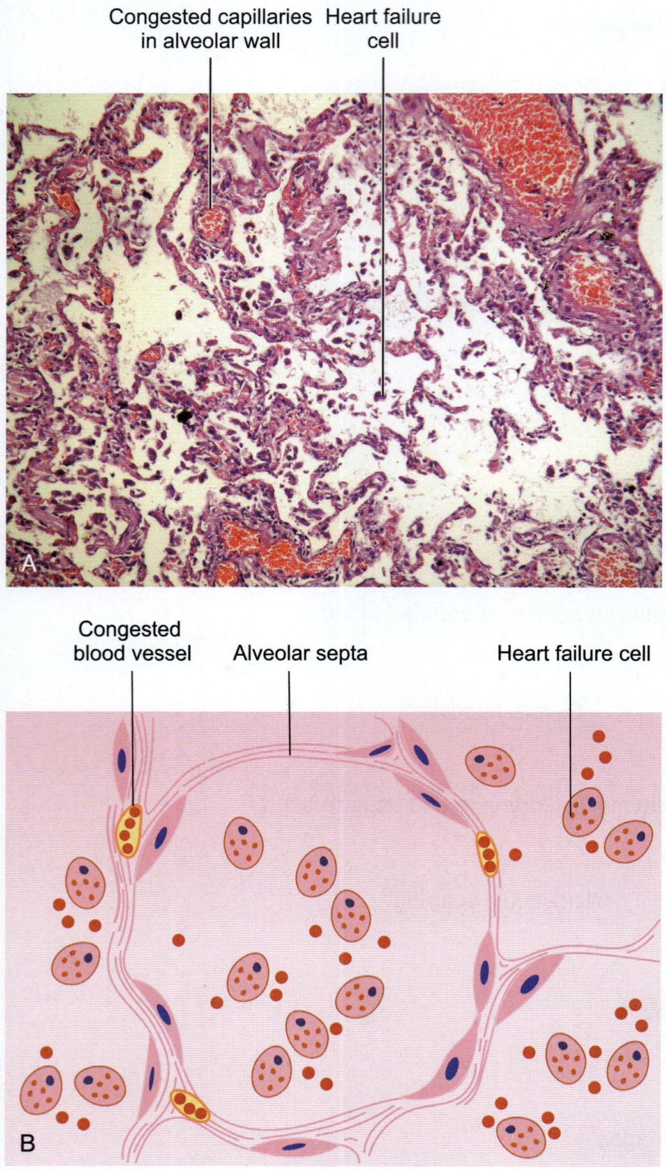

Fig. 5.2 (A and B) Photomicrograph and schematic representation of CVC lung showing congested and widened alveolar septae with haemosiderin- laden macrophages in the alveolar spaces (H&E; 200×).

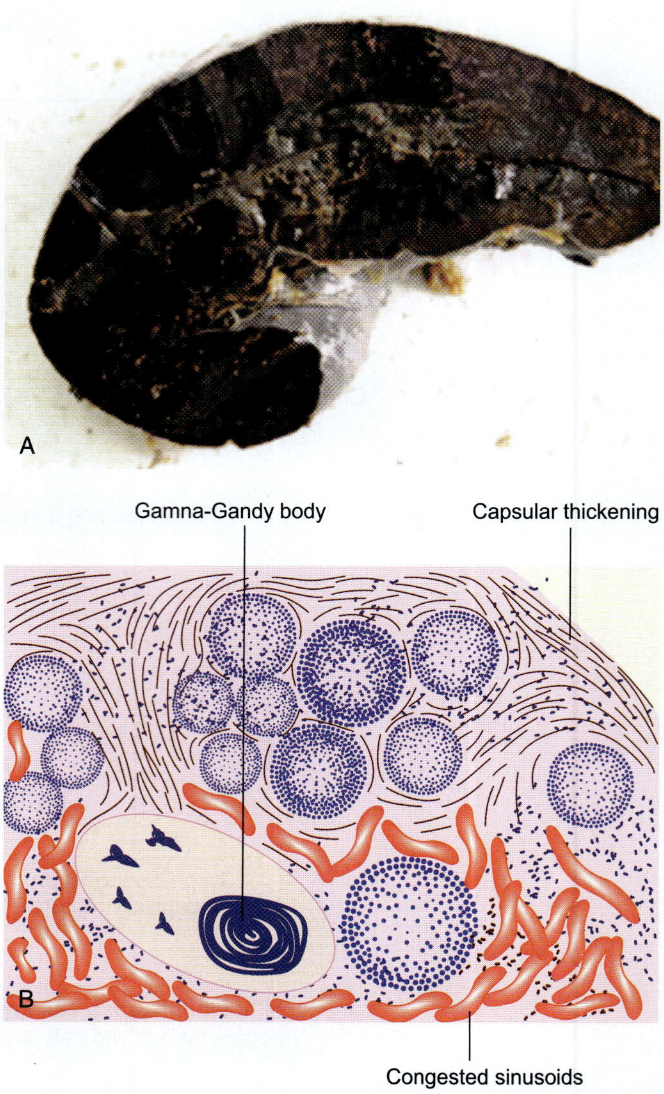

Fig. 5.3 (A) Gross picture showing an enlarged cyanotic spleen with a congested tan coloured cut surface. (B) Schematic diagram showing dilated and congested sinusoids with fibrosis and Gamna-Gandy bodies.

Q. Write briefly on the pathogenesis and clinicopathological features of congestive splenomegaly. (PA6.2)

Ans. Long-term venous outflow obstruction leads to congestive splenomegaly (splenic enlargement and congestion). Causes include portal hypertension (due to thrombosis of hepatic veins; also called to **Budd-Chiari syndrome,** cirrhosis, congestive heart failure or stenosis/thrombosis/inflammation of the portal or splenic veins). Hypersplenism describes splenomegaly together with increased removal/destruction of platelets and/or other blood cells by the spleen.

Gross Morphology (Fig. 5.3A)

- Enlarged, tense and cyanotic spleen with thickening and fibrosis of capsule.
- In the early stages, weighs about 150–250 g, while in the later stages may weigh up to 1000 g.

Microscopic Features (Fig. 5.3B)

1. Hyperplasia of splenic macrophages in the red pulp.
2. Congestion of red pulp and sinusoids with sinusoidal dilatation ultimately causing haemorrhages.
3. Organization of haemorrhage results in formation of siderofibrotic nodules (**Gamna-Gandy bodies** containing haemosiderin and calcium salts).

Q. Write briefly on the pathogenesis and clinicopathological features of hepatic congestion. (PA6.2)

Ans. Congestive hepatopathy refers to hepatic manifestations attributable to right-sided heart failure, Budd-Chiari syndrome, hepatic sinusoidal obstruction syndrome, hepatic infarction and ischaemic hepatitis. Passive congestion often coexists with reduced cardiac output.

Acute hepatic congestion is characterized by:

- Dilated, distended central vein and sinusoids.
- Central hepatocyte degeneration.

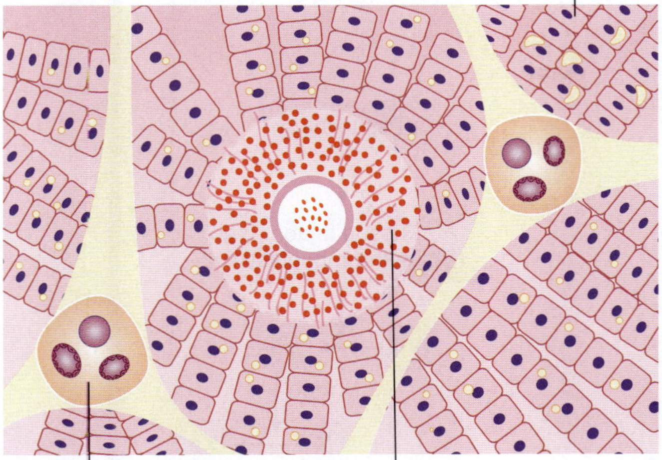

Fig. 5.4 Schematic representation of a section from liver showing congestion and degenerative changes in the centrilobular zone of liver with the peripheral zone showing fatty change.

- Fatty change in periportal hepatocytes (periportal hepatocytes experience less hypoxia because of proximity to hepatic arterioles, and therefore develop fatty change only).

In **chronic passive congestion** of liver (Fig. 5.4), the central region of hepatocytic lobules appears grossly red-brown and slightly depressed with surrounding zones of uncongested liver (***nutmeg appearance***). Central portion of hepatocytes being least perfused, undergoes centrilobular necrosis with loss or drop out of hepatocytes. Severe long-standing congestion may lead to grossly evident hepatic fibrosis (***cardiac cirrhosis***).

Q. Define and describe types of haemorrhage. Write in detail on haemostasis. (PA6.2)

Ans. Extravasation of red cells due to vessel rupture is called haemorrhage.

- It may be external (**external haemorrhage**) or enclosed within the tissue (when it is called a **haematoma**).
- The blood loss may be caused by trauma, bleeding diathesis, leukaemia, scurvy, vasculitis, aneurysmal rupture, inflammatory pathology, neoplastic invasion, etc.
- Haematoma may be insignificant (**bruise**) or large enough to cause fatality, for example **a large retroperitoneal haematoma** or an **internal (visceral) haematoma**.
- Minute 1–2 mm haemorrhages into the skin, mucous membranes or serosal surfaces are denoted as **petechiae** (typically seen with locally increased intravascular pressure, low platelet counts and defective platelet function).
- Larger >3 mm haemorrhages are called **purpura** (associated with the same disorders as petechiae and also occur secondary to trauma, vasculitis or increased vascular fragility).
- Still larger >1–2 cm subcutaneous haematomas or bruises are called **ecchymoses** (generally seen after trauma).
- Accumulation of blood in body cavities may be called **haemothorax, haemopericardium, haemoperitoneum** and **haemarthrosis (joints)** depending on the cavity involved.

Q. Write briefly on haemostasis. (PA6.4)

Ans. Haemostasis is the mechanism, which maintains the integrity of the circulatory system after vascular damage. Normal haemostatic mechanism of the body has three components:

1. **Vascular component:** This involves a reflex spasm of the injured vessel (vasoconstriction), which minimizes the blood loss. The intact vascular endothelium of blood vessels acts as a barrier between circulating platelets and the highly thrombogenic sub-endothelial collagen. The endothelial cells express and release a variety of molecules and substances that inhibit coagulation or limit clotting once it is triggered by the degradation of thrombin or other activated clotting factors. Healthy endothelium releases tissue factor pathway inhibitor (TFPI) into the circulation. Thrombomodulin on the intact endothelial surface binds thrombin and activates protein C which together with protein S inactivates clotting factors Va and VIIIa. Circulating antithrombin (AT) and heparin like molecules (heparin cofactor II or HCII) when bound to heparin proteoglycan on the normal vascular endothelial glycocalyx inhibit thrombin and coagulation factors Xa and IXa. A disintegrin and metalloprotease with a thrombospondin type 1 motif member 13 (ADAMTS-13) that is secreted by hepatic and vascular endothelial cells cleaves large vWF multimers at the endothelial surface and thereby disrupting platelet adhesion. Some of the principal endothelial-derived coagulation inhibitors as well as prothrombotic molecules are listed in Table 5.5.

Table 5.5 List of main endothelial derived coagulation inhibitors and prothrombotic molecules

Anticoagulant	Procoagulant
Thrombin (low concentration)	Thrombin (high concentration)
NO	vWF (binds platelets to ECM)
PGI2	Thrombin
Thrombomodulin (binds thrombin and activates protein C)	Tissue factor expression (activates the external coagulation cascade)
Heparin sulphate	VCAM-1
u-PA and t-PA release	Altered CD39/CD73 expression
C-terminal ADAMTS-18	Endothelin
EPCR	PAI-1
Release of TFPI	ADAMTS-13

ADAMTS, A disintegrin and metalloprotease; *CD39 and 73*, cluster of differentiation 39 and 73; *EPCR*, endothelial protein C receptor; *NO*, nitric oxide; *PAI-1*, plasminogen activator inhibitor 1; *PGI2*, prostacycline; *TFPI*, tissue factor pathway inhibitor; *t-PA*, tissue plasminogen activator; *u-PA*, urokinase; *VCAM-1*, vascular cell adhesion molecule 1; *vWF*, von Willebrand factor.

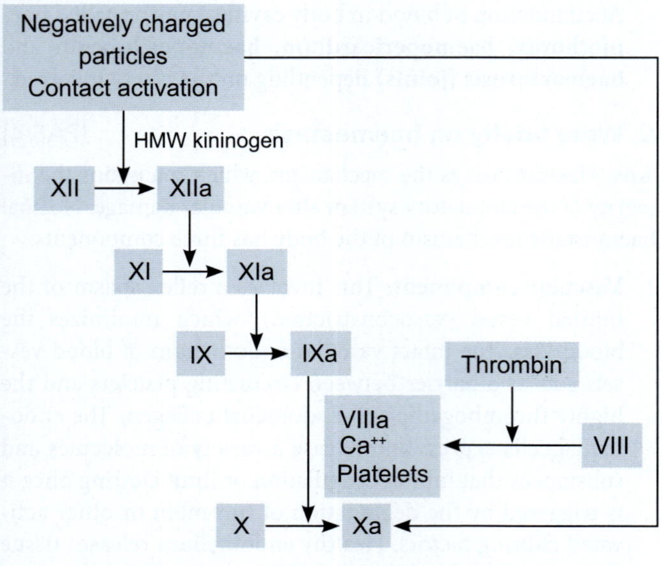

Flowchart 5.4 Intrinsic pathway of coagulation.

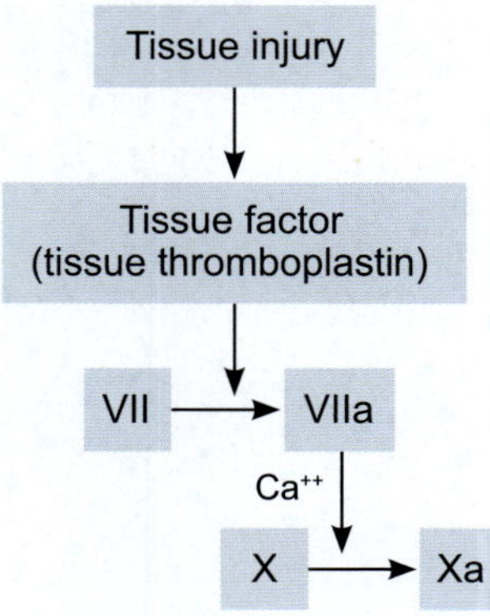

Flowchart 5.5 Extrinsic pathways of coagulation.

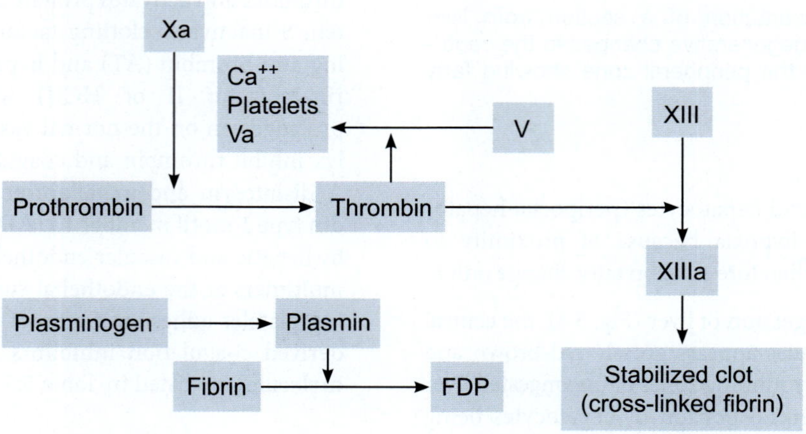

Flowchart 5.6 Common pathways of coagulation.

2. **Platelet component:** Platelets are anucleate discoid structures derived from marrow megakaryocytes. The cytoplasm of platelets contains three major types of storage granules:
   (a) Alpha granules containing a variety of proteins like fibrinogen and von Willebrand factor.
   (b) Dense granules containing serotonin, ADP and calcium.
   (c) Lysosomal granules containing acid hydrolases.

   Following vessel constriction, platelets adhere to the vessel wall and also aggregate to form a platelet plug, which seals off the vascular breach and arrests haemorrhage (**primary haemostasis**). This is followed by activation of the coagulation cascade and fibrin deposition (**secondary haemostasis**).
3. **Components of the coagulation cascade:** Coagulation cascade includes three pathways, namely, the **intrinsic** (Flowchart 5.4), **extrinsic** and the **common pathways** (Flowcharts 5.5 and 5.6). Intrinsic pathway is assessed in vitro by the activated partial thromboplastin time (aPTT). Extrinsic pathway is assessed by the prothrombin time (PT). The coagulation factors involved in the different pathways are tabulated in Table 5.6.

Table 5.6 Coagulation factors

I	Fibrinogen
II	Prothrombin
V	Proaccelerin
VII	Proconvertin
VIII	Anti-haemophilic factor
IX	Christmas factor
X	Stuart-Prower factor
XI	Plasma Thromboplastin antecedent
XII	Hageman factor
XIII	Fibrin stabilizing factor

Prekallikrein: Fletcher factor; HMW kininogen: Fitzgerald factor

Regulation of Coagulation System

Inhibitors of Coagulation

The natural inhibitors of coagulation include:

- Anti-thrombin III
- α-macroglobulin
- Heparin cofactor II
- Protein C and protein S

Fibrinolytic System

The physiological function of the fibrinolytic system is to digest deposits of fibrin (thrombi). Plasminogen activator (PA) converts plasminogen to plasmin. Two types of plasminogen activators are identified - Tissue type PA (derived from leukocytes and endothelial cells) and Urokinase which is plasma derived. Plasminogen activator inhibitor-1 (PAI-1), also known as endothelial PAI, is a serine protease inhibitor (serpin). It functions as the principal inhibitor of tissue- or urokinase-type plasminogen activator, and hence fibrinolysis.

Q. Write briefly on the factors contributing to thrombus formation (What is Virchow's triad? Enlist its components). (PA6.4)

Ans. Thrombosis is the process of formation of a solid mass in the circulation constituted by platelets, fibrin and other entrapped blood elements. Vessel wall injury induces rapid recruitment of the circulating platelets to the site of injury, where they initiate formation of a thrombus. There are three major contributors to thrombus formation which constitute the so called **"Virchow's triad" (Fig. 5.5)**:

1. **Endothelial injury, which may be secondary to:**
   (a) Myocardial infarction
   (b) Ulcerated atherosclerotic plaques
   (c) Cardiac surgery
   (d) Myocarditis
   (e) Infected valve disease
   (f) Prosthetic valves
   (g) Radiation injury

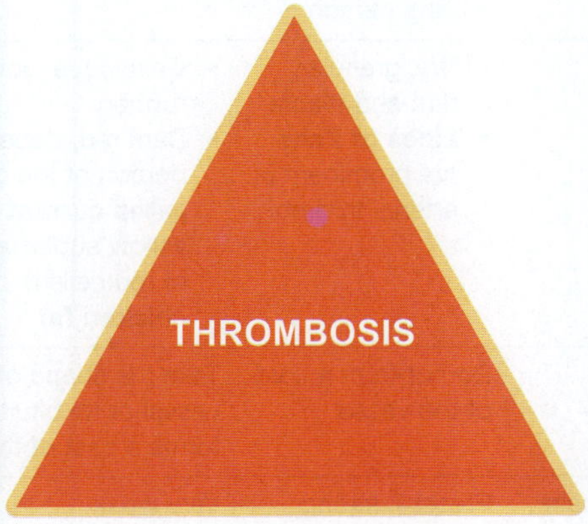

Fig. 5.5 Virchow's triad.

   (h) Chemical agents (smoking, hypercholesterolaemia, homocysteineamia, bacterial toxins and endotoxins)
2. **Alteration in normal blood flow (stasis or turbulence): Stasis** is typically seen in hyperviscosity syndromes and polycythemia; whereas, **turbulence** is commonly associated with hypertension. Alterations in normal flow result in:
   (a) Disruption of laminar flow.
   (b) Decreased hepatic clearance of activated coagulation factors.
   (c) Damage to endothelium.
3. **Conditions predisposing to hypercoagulability:**
   (a) Genetic
      (i) Deficiency of antithrombotic factors like AT III, proteins C and S, methylene tetrahydrofolate reductase (MTHFR) gene mutation and defects in fibrinolysis.
      (ii) Increased prothrombotic factors as in Factor V mutation/factor V Leiden (activated protein C resistance); prothrombin G20210A mutation (excessive levels of prothrombin); high levels of factors VII, XI, IX, VIII, von Willebrand factor and fibrinogen and homocysteinuria.
   (b) Acquired
      (i) **Venous stasis:** Prolonged immobilization and congestive cardiac failure.
      (ii) **Increased platelet activation:** Cancers, acute leukaemias, myeloproliferative disorders, paroxysmal nocturnal haemoglobinuria, prosthetic cardiac valves, atrial fibrillation, myocardial infarction and thrombotic thrombocytopenic purpura.
      (iii) **Increased hepatic synthesis of coagulation factors or reduced anticoagulant synthesis:** Oral contraceptives, pregnancy, etc.
      (iv) **Antiphospholipid syndrome.**
      (v) **Tissue injury:** Surgery, fracture and extensive burns.

Q. Write briefly on the morphology of a thrombus. (PA6.2)

Ans. Thrombi are grey-white, friable, tangled strands of fibrin and platelets, which may form anywhere in the cardiovascular system, as in cardiac chambers, arteries and veins and capillaries.

General Features of Thrombi

- Different sizes and shapes of thrombi may be seen, dictated by:
  - Site of origin.
  - Circumstances leading to their development.
- **Cardiac thrombi** mostly develop in the regions of turbulence and at sites of endocardial injury (atrial appendages, endocardial surface of a myocardial infarct and cardiac valves). Thrombi forming on heart valves are called **vegetations**. They are usually seen in mitral and aortic valves.
- **Thrombi in cardiac chambers** or **aorta** show the presence of laminations or **lines of Zahn** (paler layers of fibrin and platelets alternating with darker layers of RBCs).

- **Thrombi in smaller arteries** or **veins** do not show lines of Zahn.
- **Mural thrombi** are attached to one wall of an underlying structure, usually capacious lumina of heart chambers and aorta without actually completely occluding the lumen.
- **Arterial thrombi** are usually occlusive when they involve smaller- or medium-sized vessels; large vessels, for example iliac and common carotid tend to have mural thrombi.
- **Venous thrombi (phlebothrombosis)** are invariably occlusive and contain a large RBC component, because these are formed in a relatively static environment. These are also called **red** or **stasis thrombi**. They can be found in the veins of the lower extremity (deep leg veins, varicose veins, popliteal, femoral and iliac veins), pulmonary veins, superior and inferior vena cavae, hepatic and portal veins, mesenteric and renal veins. Other features of venous thrombi are as follows:
  - Lines of Zahn are not well developed.
  - Mostly affect veins of lower extremity (90% cases).
  - May be confused with post-mortem clots.
  - Always have a point of attachment to the underlying structure, firmest at the point of origin.
- Contraction of a thrombus gives way to a slit-like lumen, which restores blood flow leading to propagation of the thrombus upstream and downstream.
- Morphologically a thrombus shows the following layers:
  - Platelets adhering to the endothelium or endocardium.
  - Fibrin meshwork.
  - Red blood cells entrapped within the fibrin meshwork.

Q. Differentiate between arterial and venous thrombi. (PA6.4)

Ans. Differences between arterial and venous thrombi are tabulated in Table 5.7.

Q. Differentiate between antemortem and post-mortem clot. (PA6.4)

Ans. Differences between antemortem and post-mortem clot are tabulated in Table 5.8.

Q. Write briefly on fate of a thrombus. (PA6.4)

Ans. A thrombus may undergo the following changes (Fig. 5.6):

1. ***Propagation*** (accumulation of additional platelets and fibrin leading to progression and increase in size; a mural thrombus may progress to become occlusive).
2. ***Embolization*** (propagating tail fragments are poorly attached to the wall and may give rise to emboli; arterial emboli usually travel to the kidneys and venous thrombi lodge in the pulmonary circulation).
3. ***Dissolution*** (fibrinolysis usually on the first or second day; fresh thrombi are more susceptible to lysis than old thrombi).
4. ***Organization and recanalization*** (ingrowth of endothelial cells, smooth muscle and fibroblasts and formation of new channels).

Table 5.7 Differences between arterial and venous thrombi

Features	Arterial thrombi	Venous thrombi
Sites	Common in coronary, cerebral, iliac and femoral arteries (vessels with active blood flow)	Superficial varicose veins and deep veins of leg, for example femoral and iliac veins (vessels with less active blood flow)
Pathogenesis	Due to endothelial injury (as in atherosclerosis or turbulent blood flow)	Due to venous stasis
Progression	Grows in a retrograde direction from point of attachment	Extends in the direction of blood flow
Occlusion	Do not occlude lumen completely	Invariably occlusive
Gross	Grey-white, friable, prominent lines of Zahn	Dark red with fibrin strands; lines of Zahn less prominent or absent
Microscopy	Lines of Zahn show paler layers of fibrin and platelets alternating with darker layers of RBCs	Constituted by more of RBCs and less of fibrin
Complications	Ischaemia/infarction of vital organs	Embolism, oedema, ulceration

Table 5.8 Differences between antemortem and post-mortem clot

Features	Antemortem clots/thrombi	Post-mortem clots
Origin	Formed as part of normal haemostasis or pathological derangement of clotting pathway in a living person	Form in a dead person due to sedimentation and settling down of blood components
Gross	• Dry, granular, firm and friable • **Lines of Zahn** are prominent in arterial thrombi	• Gelatinous, soft and rubbery • Dark red, dependent portion of the clot is called **currant jelly** and yellow supernatant, free of red cells is called **chicken fat**
Shape	Do not form a cast of the vessel	Take the shape of the vessel or its bifurcation forms a cast of the vessel
Attachment to vessel wall	Present; strong	Very weak
Location	Anywhere in the body	In dependent parts of the body

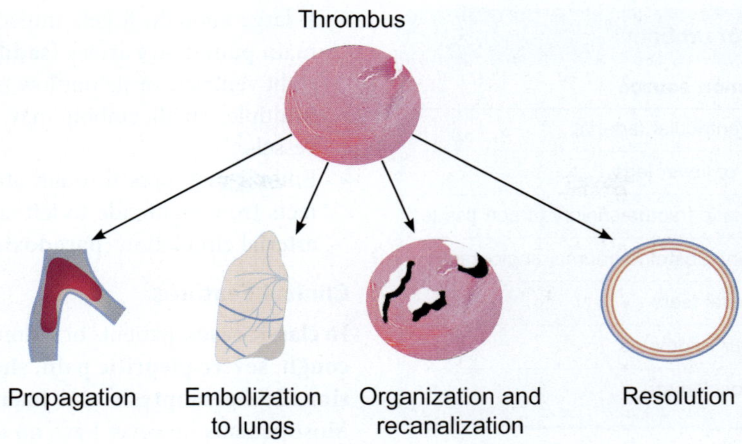

Fig. 5.6 Fate of a thrombus.

5. ***Inflammation and fibrosis*** (central liquefaction, bacterial seeding and influx of inflammatory cells; the liquefaction and infection sometimes make the adjacent vessel wall weak and result in formation of an aneurysm).

Sequence of events in evolution of a thrombus (Flowchart 5.7).

Q. Classify emboli. (PA6.5)

Ans. Emboli are classified based on:

1. **Physical state of emboli**
   (a) Solid: Atheromatous, thromboemboli and tumour emboli.

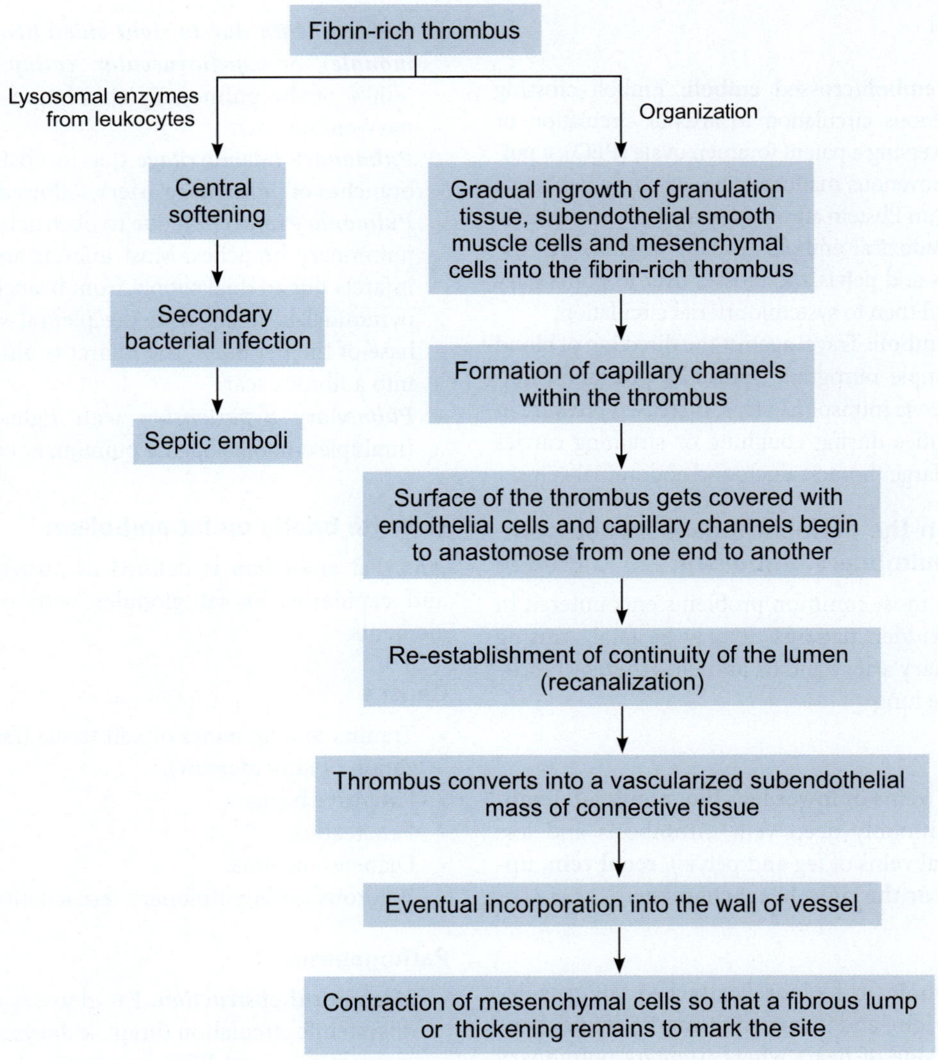

Flowchart 5.7 Sequence of events in evolution of a thrombus.

Table 5.9 Site of origin of emboli

Type of embolism	Common source
Systemic/cardiac	Left ventricular (arterial)
Pulmonary	Veins of lower legs
Fat	Traumatic fractures/injury to soft tissue
Air	Surgery, obstetric trauma, angiography
Amniotic fluid	Placental tears
Tumour embolism	Tumour fragments
Atheromatous emboli	Atherosclerosis

   (b) Liquid: Fat, bone marrow and amniotic fluid emboli.
   (c) Gaseous: Air emboli (seen in decompression sickness).
2. **Site of origin (Table 5.9)**
   (a) Cardiac emboli (left side of heart).
   (b) Arterial emboli (atheromas and aneurysms).
   (c) Venous emboli (deep vein thrombosis).
   (d) Lymphatic emboli (tumour emboli).
3. **Presence or absence of secondary infection**
   (a) Sterile/bland emboli.
   (b) Septic emboli.
4. **Flow**
   (a) **Paradoxical emboli/crossed emboli:** Emboli crossing over from venous circulation to arterial circulation or vice-versa traversing a patent foramen ovale (PFO), a pulmonary arteriovenous malformation, a ventricular septal defect (VSD), an Ebstein anomaly, or a patent ductus arteriosus. A paradoxical embolus usually originates in the deep leg veins and pelvis and crosses over to pulmonary circulation and then to systemic arterial circulation.
   (b) **Retrograde emboli:** Travel against the direction of blood flow, for example retrograde spread of prostatic carcinoma to spine via intraspinal veins. Increased pressure in the body cavities during coughing or straining carries emboli from large thoracic ducts and abdominal veins.

Q. Write briefly on the aetiopathogenesis and complications of pulmonary embolism. (PA6.5)

Ans. It is one of the most common problems encountered in hospitalized or bedridden patients. It may be fatal, causing occlusion of pulmonary artery and its branches thereby blocking blood flow to the lung.

Sources

Thrombi from **large veins of lower legs like popliteal, femoral, iliac** (most commonly deep vein thrombosis and less commonly superficial veins of leg and pelvis), **renal vein, upper extremity veins or the right heart chamber**.

Pathogenesis

- Thrombus as a whole, or its loosely attached tail, gets detached from its origin, and is carried through venous channels to the right side of heart where it enters pulmonary circulation.
- If large enough, it gets impacted at the bifurcation of the main pulmonary artery (**saddle embolus**) or lodges in the right ventricle or its outflow tract.
- Multiple, small emboli may occlude smaller pulmonary vessels.
- Emboli may pass through atrial or ventricular septal defects from right side to left side of the heart to enter into arterial circulation (**paradoxical emboli**).

Clinical Features

In classic cases, patients of pulmonary embolism present with **cough, severe pleuritic pain, shortness of breath, and occasionally haemoptysis and haemorrhagic pleural effusion.** Most patients however have no obvious symptoms at presentation. When symptomatic, the symptoms may vary from a sudden haemodynamic collapse to gradually progressive dyspnea. The diagnosis of pulmonary embolism should be suspected in patients who have respiratory symptoms unexplained by an alternative diagnosis.

Sequelae and Complications

Most emboli remain silent and undergo resolution, organization and incorporation into the wall of the vessel.

Others may cause:

- ***Sudden death due to right-sided heart failure*** (***cor pulmonale***) or ***cardiovascular collapse*** (obstruction of >60% of the pulmonary circulation or massive pulmonary embolism).
- ***Pulmonary haemorrhage*** due to obstruction of terminal branches of pulmonary artery followed by their rupture.
- ***Pulmonary infarction*** due to obstruction of end-arteriolar pulmonary branches. Most infarcts are red/haemorrhagic infarcts due to dual supply from bronchial artery. They are pyramidal is shape with the pleural surface forming the base of the pyramid. The infarct is ultimately transformed into a fibrous scar.
- ***Pulmonary hypertension*** with right-sided heart failure (multiple emboli clogging pulmonary capillary circulation).

Q. Write briefly on fat embolism. (PA6.5)

Ans. Fat embolism is defined as obstruction of arterioles and capillaries by fat globules with or without marrow elements.

Causes

- Trauma to long bones or soft tissue (fracture with embolization of fatty marrow).
- Extensive burns.
- Pancreatitis.
- Diabetes mellitus.
- Vigorous cardiopulmonary resuscitation.

Pathogenesis

- ***Mechanical obstruction***: Fat globules occlude pulmonary or systemic circulation (brain, kidneys and other organs) to cause platelet and RBC aggregation leading to hypoxia of that tissue/organ. These micro globules can be demonstrated

Breakdown of fat globules into free fatty acids

↓

Toxic injury to endothelium by free fatty acids

↓

Platelet activation and recruitment of granulocytes

↓

Production of free radicals, proteases and eicosanoids

↓

Vascular damage

Flowchart 5.8 Biochemical basis of cellular injury in fat embolism.

on frozen sections stained with fat stains (Sudan III, Oil Red O and osmic acid).
- *Biochemical injury* (See Flowchart 5.8).

Clinical Features

Most cases are asymptomatic. In symptomatic patients clinical manifestations appear within 1–3 days of trauma and include:

- Tachypnoea, dyspnoea and tachycardia (**pulmonary insufficiency**).
- Irritability, restlessness, delirium and coma (**neurological effects**).
- Diffuse petechial rash in non-dependent areas (due to thrombocytopaenia resulting from **platelet consumption**).
- Anaemia (**due to aggregation of RBCs** and **microangiopathic haemolysis**).

Sequelae and Complications

- Embolization to brain causing cerebral oedema, haemorrhage and infarcts.
- Embolization to kidneys and other organs.
- Acute respiratory distress syndrome due to impaction of numerous fat globules in the microvasculature of lungs.

Q. Write briefly on systemic thromboembolism. (PA6.5)

Ans. Systemic thromboembolism is a condition in which emboli occlude systemic arterial circulation. Majority of systemic emboli originate from intracardiac mural thrombi (two-thirds from left ventricular wall infarcts; one-fourth from left atrial dilatation and fibrillation and the remaining from aortic aneurysms, atheromas, valvular vegetations and paradoxical emboli). About 10%–15% are of ambiguous origin. Venous emboli mostly travel to the lungs; arterial emboli travel to different sites, most commonly lower extremities or brain.

Consequences of Arterial Embolization

1. Embolization to arteries of the extremities can lead to gangrene (usually affects lower limbs).
2. Mesenteric embolisation can produce bowel infarction.
3. Embolization the kidneys can produce renal infarcts.
4. Embolization the spleen can produce splenic infarcts.
5. Embolization the brain produces ischemic necrosis leading to a stroke.

Q. Write briefly on amniotic fluid embolism. (PA6.5)

Ans. Amniotic fluid embolism is a cause of maternal morbidity during labour and immediate postpartum period, and has a mortality of up to 20%–40%.

Pathogenesis

Caused by infusion of amniotic fluid with all its contents (foetal cells and debris) into maternal circulation due to tears in placental membrane or rupture of uterine vessels.

Clinical Findings

- Sudden respiratory distress.
- Deep cyanosis.
- Hypotensive shock.
- Seizures, convulsions, coma and death.

Microscopic Features

- Pulmonary microcirculation shows foetal skin, squamous cells, lanugo hair and fat from vernix caseosa, mucin from foetal respiratory tract or GIT.
- There is pulmonary oedema and diffuse alveolar damage and haemorrhage.

Causes of Death

- Mechanical blockage of pulmonary circulation.
- DIC.
- Anaphylactic reaction to amniotic fluid.
- Haemorrhage (if the patient survives the initial phase, she may bleed extensively due to disseminated intravascular coagulation or DIC).

Q. Write briefly on air embolism. (PA6.5)

Ans. Air bubbles in the circulation can obstruct vascular flow and cause ischaemic injury.

Causes

Air can be sucked into the arterial and venous circulation in the following conditions:

- Operative procedures (surgery in the head and neck and cardiothoracic regions or obstetric manipulations).
- Trauma, particularly penetrating chest wall injury.
- Decompression sickness.
- Intravenous infusions.
- Angiography/arteriography.

Arterial air embolism can also be associated with a paradoxical embolus that can travel to the arterial circulation from the venous side across a patent foramen ovale or arteriovenous shunts.

Decompression Sickness or Caisson Disease

- ***Acute decompression sickness or Caisson disease*** occurs in individuals exposed to sudden changes in atmospheric pressure, for example scuba and deep-sea divers. When air is breathed at high pressure, large amounts of gas particularly nitrogen, dissolves in blood and tissue. If the diver rapidly ascents from water (depressurizes), the nitrogen bubbles out of the blood to form gas emboli. These bubbles lodge in the blood vessels of muscles and joints causing "bends" and induce oedema, and haemorrhage in lungs causing respiratory distress or "chokes".

- ***Chronic decompression sickness*** is seen in workers of pressurized vessels used in bridge construction and may cause multiple foci of avascular necrosis in femur, tibia and humerus.

Q. Define and classify infarcts. (PA6.6)

Ans.

Definition

An infarct is an area of ischaemic coagulative necrosis caused by occlusion of arterial supply or venous drainage.

Salient Features

- Almost all infarcts result from thromboembolic events affecting arterial circulation.
- Others may result from vasospasm, twisting of vessels (testicular torsion or bowel volvulus), vascular compression (by oedema, entrapment in a hernial sac or tumour), and traumatic vessel rupture.
- Venous thrombosis usually results in venous congestion; can, however, cause infarction in rare instances (as in organs with a single venous outflow channel, for example testes and ovaries).

Classification

Infarcts are classified on the basis of the following:

1. **Colour (amount of haemorrhage)**
   (a) Red or haemorrhagic infarcts
   (b) White or anaemic infarcts
2. **Presence or absence of microbial infection**
   (a) Septic infarcts
   (b) Bland infarcts

Q. Differentiate between red and white infarcts. (PA6.6)

Ans. Differences between red/haemorrhagic and white/pale/anaemic infarcts are tabulated in Table 5.10.

Q. Write briefly on renal infarcts. (PA6.7)

Ans. Renal infarction results from interruption of the normal blood supply to part of, or to the whole kidney.

Causes

- Thromboembolism (from heart valves, ventricular or atrial thrombi, aorta).
- Aortic and renal artery dissection.
- Fibromuscular dysplasia.
- Vasculitis.
- Iatrogenic (e.g. during angiography).
- Malignant hypertension.

Morphology

Gross

- Are often multiple and pale in appearance.
- May be bilateral.
- Usually have a wedge-shaped base resting under the capsule with the apex towards medulla. A narrow rim of renal tissue under the capsule is spared because its blood supply is derived from capsular vessels.

Microscopy

Affected area shows coagulative necrosis due to hypoxia.

Q. Write briefly on pulmonary infarcts. (PA6.6)

Ans. Since lung has a second blood supply through the bronchial arteries, occlusion of a pulmonary artery does not usually produce tissue necrosis. However, pulmonary infarction is fairly common, as an embolus arising in any part of systemic circulation has to pass through the lungs. Infarction is common in a congested lung as in chronic passive venous congestion,

Table 5.10 Differences between red/haemorrhagic and white/pale/anaemic infarcts

Features	Red infarct	White infarct
Organs involved	Spongy organs like lung and gastrointestinal tract	Solid organs, like heart, spleen and kidney
Cause	*Venous occlusion* Seen in: (a) Loose tissues that allow collection of blood or tissues with dual blood supply (lungs, GIT). Haemorrhage seeps into such an infarct when flow is re-established. (b) Tissues that were previously congested due to sluggish venous outflow. (c) When blood flow is re-established in a site with previous arterial occlusion, for example after coronary angioplasty?	*Arterial obstruction* Seen in (a) Solid organs where the solidity of the tissue prevents haemorrhage that can seep through from adjoining capillaries and (b) Tissues with end arterial circulation
Morphology	Congested and red due to haemorrhage; turns brown and firm with time but never appears pale. Haemosiderin-laden macrophages are present in large numbers.	Becomes progressively pale
Margins	Not sharply defined	Sharply defined
Oedema	Present	Absent

hypostatic congestion as seen in postoperative and post-natal period. In the above conditions, when a branch of pulmonary artery is blocked, the supply from the bronchial arteries is insufficient to prevent damage in the obstructed area due to an already increased pulmonary circulatory pressure.

Morphology

Gross

- Lung infarcts may be solitary or multiple and are seen as coagulated, firm, variable sized, wedge-shaped areas that are usually peripheral in location.
- The infarcted area is dark red in colour and has a well-defined outline.
- Lung infarcts are hemorrhagic because—though the pulmonary artery carrying most of the blood and oxygen is cut off (usually by thromboemboli)—the bronchial arteries from the systemic circulation continue to perfuse the lungs.

Microscopy (Fig. 5.7)

- The affected area shows preserved outline of the alveoli, though cellular/nuclear details are lost.
- Tissue appears coagulated and anucleate and the alveoli are filled with fibrin and red cells.
- Cytoplasmic eosinophilia is increased.

Q. Write briefly on splenic infarcts. (PA6.7)

Ans. Several factors predispose to splenic vein thrombosis such as infections (infectious mononucleosis, cytomegalovirus infection, and malaria); inherited clotting disorders (factor deficiencies and antiphospholipid syndrome); and malignancies (pancreatic cancer and metastasis). Splenic vein obstruction sometimes results from emboli from distant organs as in atrial fibrillation, patent foramen ovale, an atheroma or endocarditis. Other causes of splenic infarction include haematological disorders like myeloproliferative disorders and sickle cell anaemia, abdominal trauma, aortic dissection, torsion of the splenic artery or compression of the artery by a tumour.

Morphology

Gross (Fig. 5.8A)

Infarction generally results in a wedge-shaped area of necrosis, with the apex closest to the occlusion and the base at the periphery of the organ.

Microscopy (Fig. 5.8B)

- The infarcted area shows coagulative necrosis (tissue architecture is maintained but cellular details are lost).
- The margins become better defined with time due to development of a narrow rim of congestion and inflammation at the edge of the lesion.

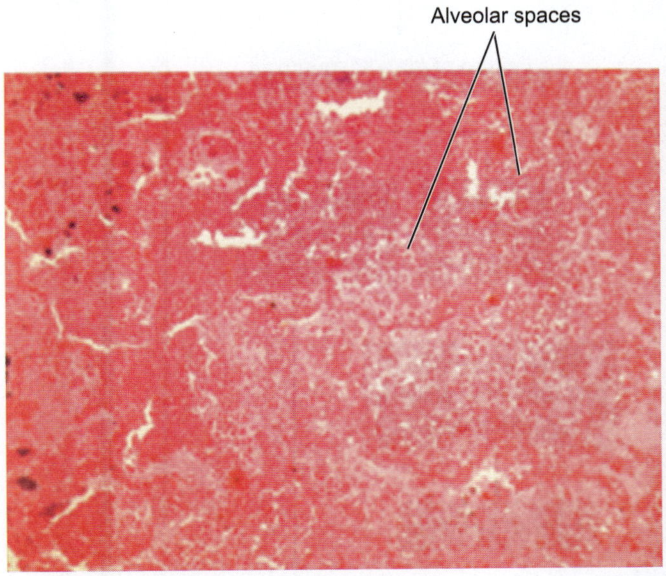

Fig. 5.7 Haemorrhagic infarct lung showing preservation of lung architecture with loss of nuclear details. The alveolar spaces are filled with fibrin and red cells (H&E; 200×).

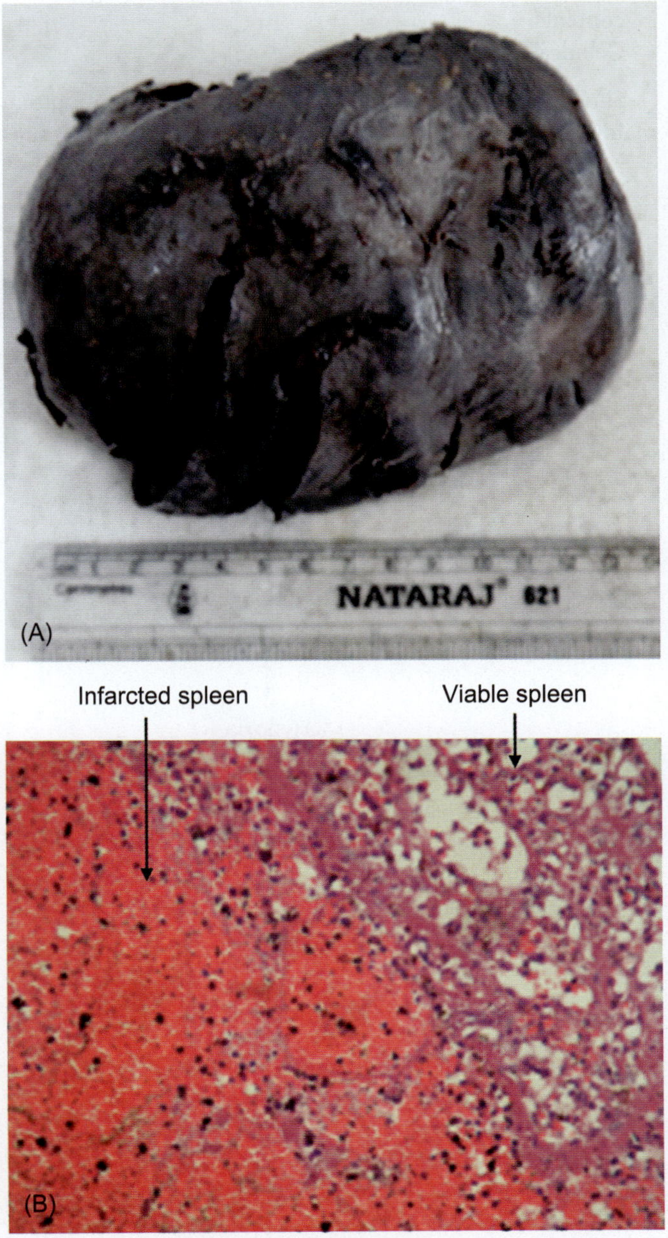

Fig. 5.8 (A) Gross specimen of traumatic laceration and infarction spleen. (B) Section showing the junction of viable *(on the right)* and infarcted area *(on the left)* in spleen.

- Since relatively few extravasated red blood cells are lysed, the resulting haemosiderosis is limited and results in a progressively more pale area of infarction with time.

Q. Define and classify shock. Describe its pathogenesis and clinical presentation. (PA6.3)

Ans. Shock is defined as a clinical state of cardiovascular collapse characterized by the inadequate perfusion of the cells and tissues resulting in hypotension and cellular hypoxia. If uncompensated, it may lead to impaired cellular metabolism and death. Decreased tissue O_2 delivery leads to a shift towards anaerobic metabolism, leading to lactic acidosis. Initially, effects are reversible. Eventually the following cellular changes are seen:

- Membrane pump dysfunction and inadequate regulation of intracellular pH.
- Cellular swelling, membrane damage and leakage of cell contents.
- Cell death.

Shock can occur secondary to decreased cardiac output, maldistribution of circulating blood and defect in the substrate utilization at the cellular and sub-cellular levels. The most common cause of shock is circulatory failure, which manifests mainly as hypotension.

Aetiology and Classification

1. **Hypovolaemic shock:** This form of shock denotes a clinical state of cardiovascular collapse typified by a decrease in the effective circulating blood volume (Flowchart 5.9). Decreased circulating blood volume leads to decreased diastolic filling of the heart, which in turn results in inadequate tissue perfusion.

   Causes
   (a) Severe haemorrhage (post trauma and surgery).
   (b) Fluid loss (severe burns, crush injuries, vomiting and severe diarrhoea).
   (c) Excessive diuretics.
   (d) Acute pancreatitis.

   The clinical presentation of hemorrhagic shock is dependant on the amount of blood lost. Correlation of amount of blood loss and clinical manifestations in hypovolaemic shock is summarized in Table 5.11.

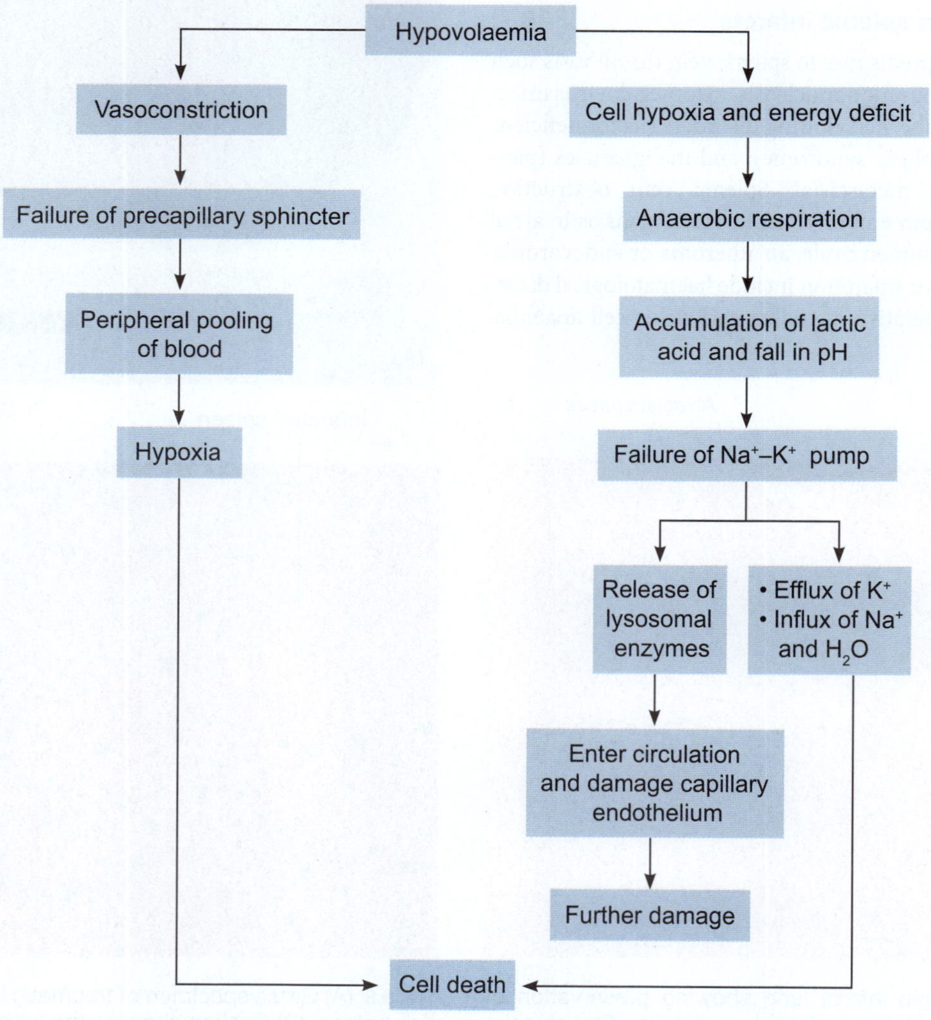

Flowchart 5.9 Pathogenesis of hypovolaemic shock.

Table 5.11 Correlation of amount of blood loss and clinical manifestations in hypovolaemic shock

Haemorrhage class	Blood loss	Clinical manifestations
I	<15% (0.75 L)	Increased heart rate, normal blood pressure
II	15%–30% (0.75–1.5 L)	Increased heart rate, mild lowering of blood pressure
III	30%–40% (1.5–2 L)	Very rapid heart rate, low blood pressure, confusion
IV	>40% (>2 L)	Critical blood pressure and heart rate

2. **Cardiogenic shock:** This type of shock results from failure of myocardial pump. Acute circulatory failure with sudden fall in cardiac output causes reduced effective circulating blood volume. This in turn reduces supply of oxygen to the cells and tissue results in anoxia.

   Causes

   (a) Deficient emptying
      (i) Myocardial infarction
      (ii) Rupture of the heart
      (iii) Cardiac arrhythmias
      (iv) Cardiomyopathies
   (b) Deficient filling
      Cardiac tamponade
   (c) Obstruction to outflow
      (i) Pulmonary embolism
      (ii) Ball valve thrombus
      (iii) Dissecting aortic aneurysm
3. **Neurogenic shock:** Occurs due to loss of vascular tone and peripheral pooling of blood following anaesthesia or spinal cord injury. Emotional shock **(vasovagal syncope)** results from a strong parasympathetic stimulation of the heart, which causes vasodilation and pooling of blood in skeletal muscles and in the viscera.
4. **Anaphylactic shock:** Occurs when an allergic response triggers a quick release of mast cell mediators in large quantities (histamine, prostaglandins and leukotrienes) leading to systemic vasodilatation (associated with hypotension), increased vascular permeability and bronchoconstriction (leading to difficulty in breathing). Anaphylactic shock can lead to death in a matter of minutes if left untreated.
5. **Septic shock:** Occurs when there is widespread endothelial injury and activation due to
   (a) Severe bacterial infections
      (i) Predominantly Gram-positive infections (*staphylococcus aureus, streptococci* and *pneumococci*).
      (ii) Gram-negative infections (*E. coli, Proteus, Klebsiella* and *Pseudomonas*).
   (b) Fungal or rickettsial sepsis.
   (c) Super antigens (polyclonal T lymphocyte activators that induce release of high levels of cytokines that lead to vasodilatation, hypotension and shock).

Pathogenesis of Septic Shock (Flowchart 5.10)

Sepsis is defined as life-threatening organ dysfunction due to dysregulated host response to infection. **Septic shock** occurs in some patients of sepsis when infectious microorganisms in the bloodstream induce a profound inflammatory response causing haemodynamic decompensation and metabolic abnormalities that are associated with increased mortality. **It is defined by persisting hypotension requiring vasopressors to maintain a mean arterial pressure of 65 mm Hg or higher and a serum lactate level greater than18 mg/dL despite adequate volume resuscitation. Proinflammatory mediators** are released causing **activation of leukocytes** and **endothelial cells**, along with the activation of the **coagulation pathway.** The prominent inflammatory response is driven primarily by the cytokines **tumour necrosis factor alpha (TNF-α)** and **interleukin-1 (IL-1)**, along with a number of other mediators including **high-mobility group box 1 (HMGB1) protein.** The development of septic shock is associated with the following abnormalities:

Immunologic Abnormalities

- The following families of **pattern recognition receptors** are involved in the initiation of the sepsis response:
  - Toll-like receptors (TLRs).
  - Nucleotide-oligomerization domain leucine-rich repeat proteins.
  - Cytoplasmic caspase activation and recruiting domain helicases.
- Various bacterial cell-wall components **lipopolysaccharide or LPS (Gram-negative bacteria), peptidoglycan (Gram-positive and Gram-negative bacteria), and lipoteichoic acid (Gram-positive bacteria)** engage with the pattern recognition receptors to activate innate immunity by inducing synthesis of cytokines, for example TNF and ILs, especially IL-1, IL-10, interferon gamma, IL-12, macrophage migration inhibition factor (MIF or MMIF), HMGB1, granulocyte colony-stimulating factor (G-CSF), granulocyte macrophage colony-stimulating factor (GM-CSF), prostaglandins and PAF.
- The most toxic component of Gram-negative bacteria is the lipid A moiety of LPS, which leads to cytokine induction via lipoteichoic acid.
- Gram-positive bacteria may secrete superantigen cytotoxins that bind directly to the major histocompatibility complex (MHC) molecules and T-cell receptors, leading to massive cytokine production.
- The cytokines released also activate the **coagulation pathway** (which results in generation of capillary microthrombi and ischaemic organ damage); **complement system** (which contributes to the clearance of the infecting microorganisms but probably also enhances the tissue damage); and the **Kinin system** (which generates bradykinin).
- There is **elevation in the levels of acute inflammatory markers like C-reactive protein** and **procalcitonin.**
- Hypotension, the cardinal manifestation of sepsis, occurs via induction of **nitric oxide** (NO).
- **Endothelial activation** causes endothelial injury and increased vascular permeability leading to oedema and

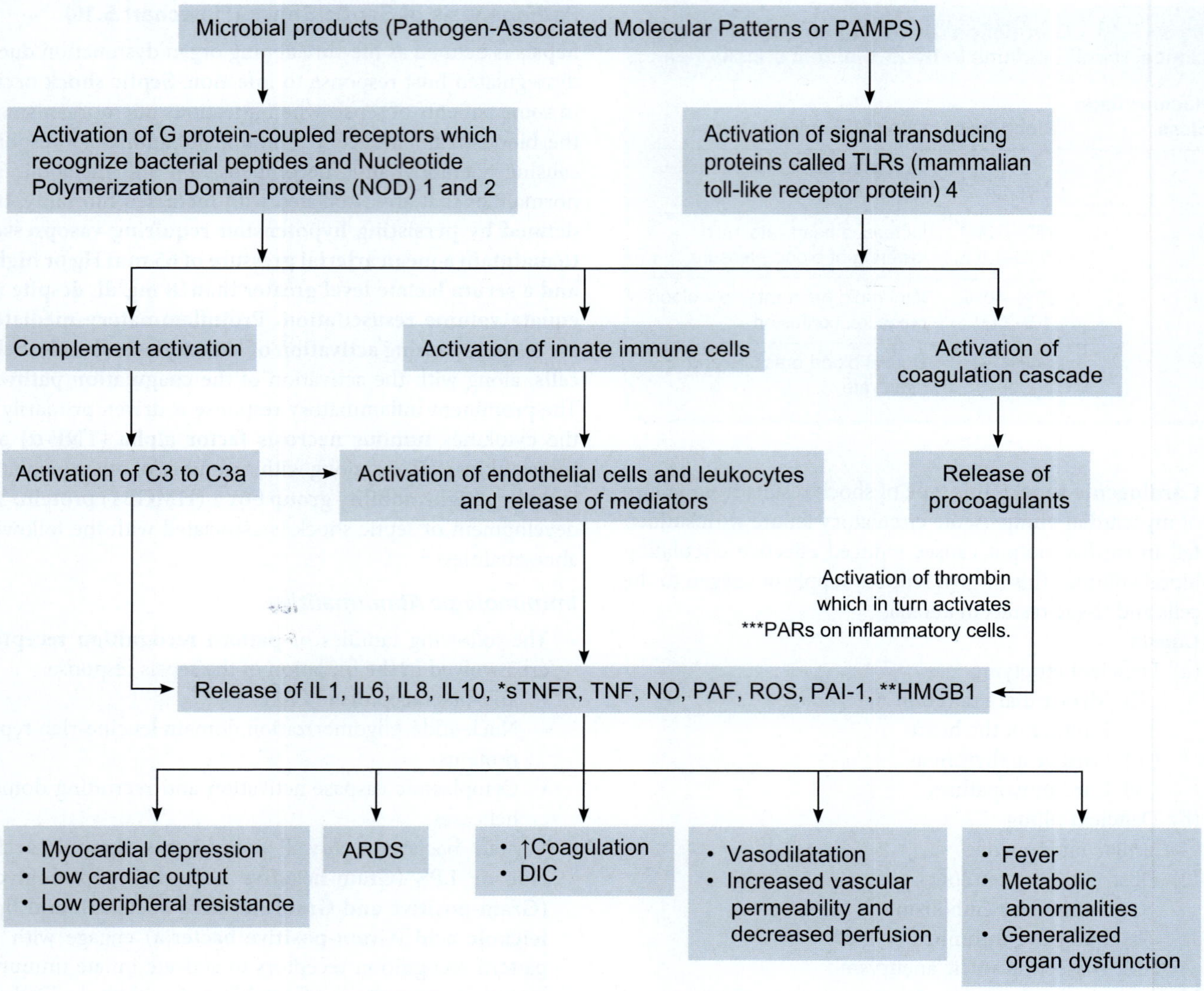

***sTNFR—Soluble TNF receptor**
****HMGB1—High mobility group box 1 protein**
*****PARs—Protease-activated receptors**

Flowchart 5.10 Pathogenesis of septic shock.

exudate formation as well as dysregulation of NO, C3a, C5a and PAF.

- **Mitochondrial dysfunction** is associated with excessive generation of peroxynitrates and reactive oxygen species (ROS) in combination with glutathione depletion contributing to tissue damage and organ dysfunction.
- There is a growing belief that sepsis involves both a **hyper-inflammatory state (proinflammatory Th1response)** and a **state of immunosuppression (antiinflammatory Th2 response)**, which may culminate in a worse prognosis and a greater predisposition to other nosocomial infections.

Abnormalities of Coagulation and Fibrinolysis

- An imbalance of homeostatic mechanisms leads to **disseminated intravascular coagulopathy (DIC)** and **microvascular thrombosis,** causing organ dysfunction and death.
- Inflammatory mediators cause **direct injury to the vascular endothelium,** which release **tissue factor (TF)**, triggering the **extrinsic coagulation cascade** and accelerating thrombin production. Microbial products can also activate factor XII to initiate **intrinsic coagulation cascade.**
- **Endotoxins increase the activity of inhibitors of fibrinolysis**—namely, plasminogen activator inhibitor (PAI-1) and thrombin-activatable fibrinolysis inhibitor (TAFI).
- Levels of protein C and endogenous activated protein C (APC) are also decreased in sepsis.
- The imbalance among inflammation, coagulation, and fibrinolysis results in widespread coagulopathy and microvascular thrombosis and suppressed fibrinolysis, ultimately leading to multiple organ dysfunction (MOD) and death.

Circulatory Abnormalities

- Septic shock is characterized by profound vasodilation (predominantly arterial) and shunting of blood from vital organs to non-vital tissues (distributive shock).
- Vasodilation occurs due to activation of adenosine triphosphate (ATP)-sensitive potassium channels in vascular smooth muscle cells by lactic acidosis and activation of NO synthase.
- Potassium efflux results in decreased calcium influx, and vascular smooth muscle relaxation, which can be refractory to endogenous norepinephrine and epinephrine that are released during shock.
- Due to hypoxia, intracellular aerobic respiration is replaced by anaerobic glycolysis, which in turn causes metabolic acidosis reducing the tissue pH. This leads to arteriolar dilatation and peripheral pooling of blood.
- Reduced peripheral arterial vascular tone if not adequately compensated by a rise in cardiac output may result in hypotension and shock. The performance of the heart, is usually depressed due to release of myocardial depressant substances, coronary blood flow abnormalities, pulmonary hypertension, various cytokines, NO, and beta-receptor downregulation.
- Release of vasodilating substances (e.g. NO and prostacyclin) and vasoconstricting substances (e.g. endothelin) affect regional blood flow. Increased systemic microvascular permeability also develops resulting in oedema of various organs (e.g. the lung microcirculation) and to the development of ARDS.

Accelerated Apoptosis (Programmed Cell Death)

Another important mechanism playing a role in the development of acute organ dysfunction in septic shock is apoptosis (programmed cell death). Accelerated apoptosis is a pivotal pathogenic event in this disease. In addition, certain genetic polymorphisms are becoming recognized as major determinants of susceptibility to infection, as well as risk of death from septic shock.

Stages of Shock

1. **Non-progressive (initial, compensated and reversible) shock:**
   (a) The body makes an attempt to maintain adequate cerebral and coronary blood supply by redistributing blood so that vital organs (brain and heart) are perfused and oxygenated. Cardiac output and systemic vascular resistance (peripheral vasoconstriction) work to keep BP within normal.
   (b) Activation of neurohumoral mechanisms leads to widespread vasoconstriction and fluid conservation by the kidney. These include:
      (i) Activation of baroreceptors and chemoreceptors.
      (ii) Activation of renin–angiotensin–aldosterone system.
      (iii) ADH release.
      (iv) Release of catecholamines.
      (v) Vascular autoregulation—in response to hypoxia and acidosis, regional blood flow to the heart and brain preserved by vasodilatation of coronary and cerebral circulation.
   (c) On examination patient demonstrates tachycardia, decreased pulses, cool extremities, oliguria, mild lactic acidosis.
2. **Progressive decompensated shock:** If the underlying cause is not corrected or the patient has pre-existing cardiovascular disease, persistence of shock leads to
   (a) Pulmonary hypoperfusion and tachypnoea.
   (b) Tissue anoxia initiating anaerobic glycolysis leading to lactic acidosis and ineffective vasomotor response causing peripheral pooling and vasodilatation.
3. **Decompensated (irreversible) shock:** *Widespread cell injury leads to*
   (a) Progressive decrease in blood pressure due to decrease in cardiac output.
   (b) Metabolic acidosis.
   (c) Adult respiratory distress syndrome (ARDS).
   (d) Ischaemic cell death of brain, heart and kidney.

Causes of Irreversibility

- Widespread vasoconstriction starts as a compensatory mechanism but its persistence causes anoxia of tissue.
- Anoxic damage to the endothelial lining causes increased vascular permeability.
- Myocardial ischaemia induces release of myocardial depressant factor (MDF), which causes decreased coronary blood flow.
- Cerebral ischaemia causes depression of vasomotor centre.
- Normally, vasodepressor material (VDM) produced by spleen and skeletal muscle is inactivated in liver. In severe hypoxia of liver, no inactivation of VDM takes place, inducing leading to peripheral vasodilatation.
- Release of TNF.
- Hypercoagulability of blood.

Morphologic Changes in Shock

Morphologic changes in shock are due to hypoxia resulting in degeneration and necrosis in various organs.

Major organs affected are brain, heart, lungs and kidneys. Adrenals, GIT and liver are also affected.

1. **Hypoxic encephalopathy**
   (a) Neurons more prone to hypoxic damage.
   (b) Cytoplasm of affected neurons becomes intensely eosinophilic and the nucleus pyknotic.
   (c) Dead and dying nerve cells are replaced by gliosis.
2. **Heart**
   (a) Heart is more vulnerable to the effects of hypoxia than any other organ.
   (b) Subepicardial and subendocardial regions show haemorrhage and necrosis.
   (c) Zonal lesions (contraction bands in the myocytes near the intercalated disc) and distortion of myofilaments may be seen.

3. **Lung**
Because of dual blood supply, lungs are generally not affected by hypovolaemic shock. In septic shock, lungs may manifest with ARDS (shock lung) or show the following features:
   (a) Diffuse alveolar damage.
   (b) Interstitial lymphocytic infiltrate and oedema.
   (c) Formation of alveolar hyaline membrane, and thickening and fibrosis of alveolar septae.
   (d) Presence of microthrombi in pulmonary microvasculature.
4. **Kidney**
   (a) Shock may lead to irreversible renal injury resulting in anuria and death.
   (b) Kidney is swollen and may show acute tubular necrosis and brown tubular casts. The latter are seen in cases of extensive muscle damage due to intravascular haemolysis.
5. **Adrenals**
   (a) Stress response in shock releases aldosterone, glucocorticoids and catecholamines.
   (b) Active adrenal cells utilize stored lipids for the synthesis of steroids.
   (c) Adrenal haemorrhages may be seen in severe shock.
6. **Haemorrhagic gastroenteropathy**
   (a) Multifocal superficial ulcers are seen.
   (b) Adjoining bowel mucosa is oedematous and haemorrhagic.
   (c) Microscopy reveals mucosal and mural infarction.
7. **Liver**
   (a) Liver is usually enlarged and shows a mottled cut surface.
   (b) Sections show focal (centrilobular) necrosis and fatty change.
8. **Other organs**
   (a) Necrotic foci may be seen in lymph node, spleen and pancreas.
   (b) Patients may succumb to septicaemia due to altered immune status.

Clinical Features of Shock

- Hypotension.
- Cold clammy skin.
- Rapid, thready pulse.
- Shallow and sighing respiration.
- Pale face, sunken eyes and weakness.
- Uncontrolled sepsis—warm skin due to vasodilatation.
- Urinary output less than 30 mL/h.

Diseases of Immune System

6

Q. Write briefly on the human immune system. (PA9.1)

Ans. The **human immune system** is a complex network of signals, which controls responses to antigenic stimulation and protects us from diseases. The components of the immune system are:

- **Antigen-specific** (recognize and act against particular antigens).
- **Systemic** (elicit a response which affects the entire body and is not confined to the initial affected site).
- **Have memory** (recognize and mount an even stronger attack to the same antigen the next time).

The functions of the immune system are:

- To provide resistance against invading pathogens (viruses, bacteria, parasites, etc.) and foreign material (e.g. transplanted organ).
- To remove 'worn-out' cells (e.g. aged cells or tissue debris from site of injury or disease).
- To provide primary defence against cancer.

Inappropriate immune responses may manifest as:

- Allergies.
- Autoimmune diseases.

An **antigen** is a substance (usually a protein) that evokes the production of **antibodies**. An **epitope**, also known as **'antigenic determinant'**, is the part of an antigen that is recognized by the immune system, specifically by antibodies, B cells or T cells.

An **antibody** is a Y-shaped protein (Fig. 6.1) on the surface of B cells that is secreted into the blood or lymph in response to an antigenic stimulus, such as a pathogen, or a transplanted organ. It binds to a specific antigen and neutralizes it. Antibodies are basically **glycoproteins,** which belong to the **immunoglobulin superfamily**. Antibodies (immunoglobulins) have two basic structural units—each with **two large heavy chains** and **two small light chains.** The amino acid sequence in the tips of the 'Y' varies greatly among different antibodies and is labelled the **'variable region'.** It is composed of 110–130 amino acids, which give the antibody its specificity for binding antigen. The variable region includes the ends of the light and heavy chains. Digestion with the protease papain cleaves antibody molecules into three fragments. Two fragments are identical and contain the antigen-binding activity. These are termed the **'Fab fragments' (for fragment antigen binding)**. The other fragment contains no antigen-binding activity but was originally observed to crystallize readily, and for this reason was named the **'Fc fragment' (for Fragment crystallizable).** The **constant region** determines the mechanism used to destroy the antigen.

Antibodies are divided into five major classes: IgM, IgG, IgA, IgD and IgE, based on their constant region structure. IgMs have mu-chains; IgAs have alpha-chains; IgEs have epsilon-chains and IgDs have delta-chains. Differences in heavy chain polypeptides determine the function of different immunoglobulins. The polypeptide protein sequences responsible for these differences are found primarily in the Fc fragment. While there are five different types of heavy chains, there are only two main types of light chains: kappa (κ) and lambda (λ). Each antibody binds to a specific antigen. The antigenic substance may be from the external environment or from within the body.

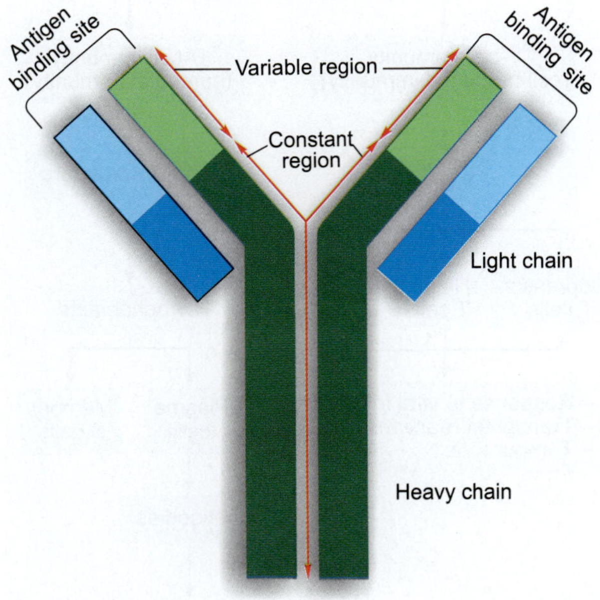

Fig. 6.1 Structure of an immunoglobulin molecule.

Q. What are the different immune responses of the body? (PA9.1)

Ans. The immune responses of the body are classified into two types (Flowchart 6.1):

1. **Natural or innate**
   (a) This is the **initial, non-specific** immune response of the body. Despite the **generalized nature of the response**, it is considered a critical component of the immune system, as defects in it often result in major consequences.
   (b) The main components of the innate immune system are **(1) physical epithelial barriers like skin and mucosal surfaces, (2) granulocytes and macrophages** which use pattern recognition receptors (PAMPs; see Chapters 3 and 5) to sense microbes, **(3) dendritic cells** that present antigens to T cells and produce interferon alfa which prevents viral replication, **(4) a special class of lymphocytes called a natural killer (NK) cells,** that provide defence against viral infections and intracellular pathogens **(5) circulating plasma proteins** (C-reactive protein and mannose binding lectin**), and (6) chemical barriers present in different bodily secretions** (saliva, tears, nasal secretions and sweat contain lysozyme, an enzyme that destroys Gram-positive bacterial cell walls causing cell lysis; vaginal secretions are acidic; spermine and zinc in semen destroy some pathogens and lactoperoxidase is a powerful enzyme found in mother's milk).
   (c) Pathogens are also prevented from entering the respiratory tract by **ciliary action of the tiny nostril hair and the coughing and sneezing reflexes. The flushing actions of tears, saliva and urine also force out pathogens, as does the sloughing off of skin.**
   (d) The **complement system** has several important functions in innate immunity and consists of at least 20 serum glycoproteins, which are activated in a cascade sequence, meaning that activation of a single molecule will lead to thousands of molecules being generated and therefore amplification of the response.
2. **Acquired or adaptive**
   (a) The **adaptive immune system** is the second line of defence against pathogens that are able to evade or overcome innate immune defences. This is an **antigen-specific** immune response.
   (b) There are two types of adaptive immune responses: **humoural immunity**, mediated by antibodies produced by B lymphocytes and **cell-mediated immunity** (CMI), mediated by T lymphocytes.
   (c) The T and B cells of the adaptive immune response are responsible for **long-term memory**. Upon secondary exposure to a specific antigen, the cells of the adaptive immune response exert their effects in a stronger and quicker way than the natural or innate response.

Q. Differentiate between innate and adaptive immunity. (PA9.1)

Ans. Difference between innate and adaptive immunity are tabulated in Table 6.1.

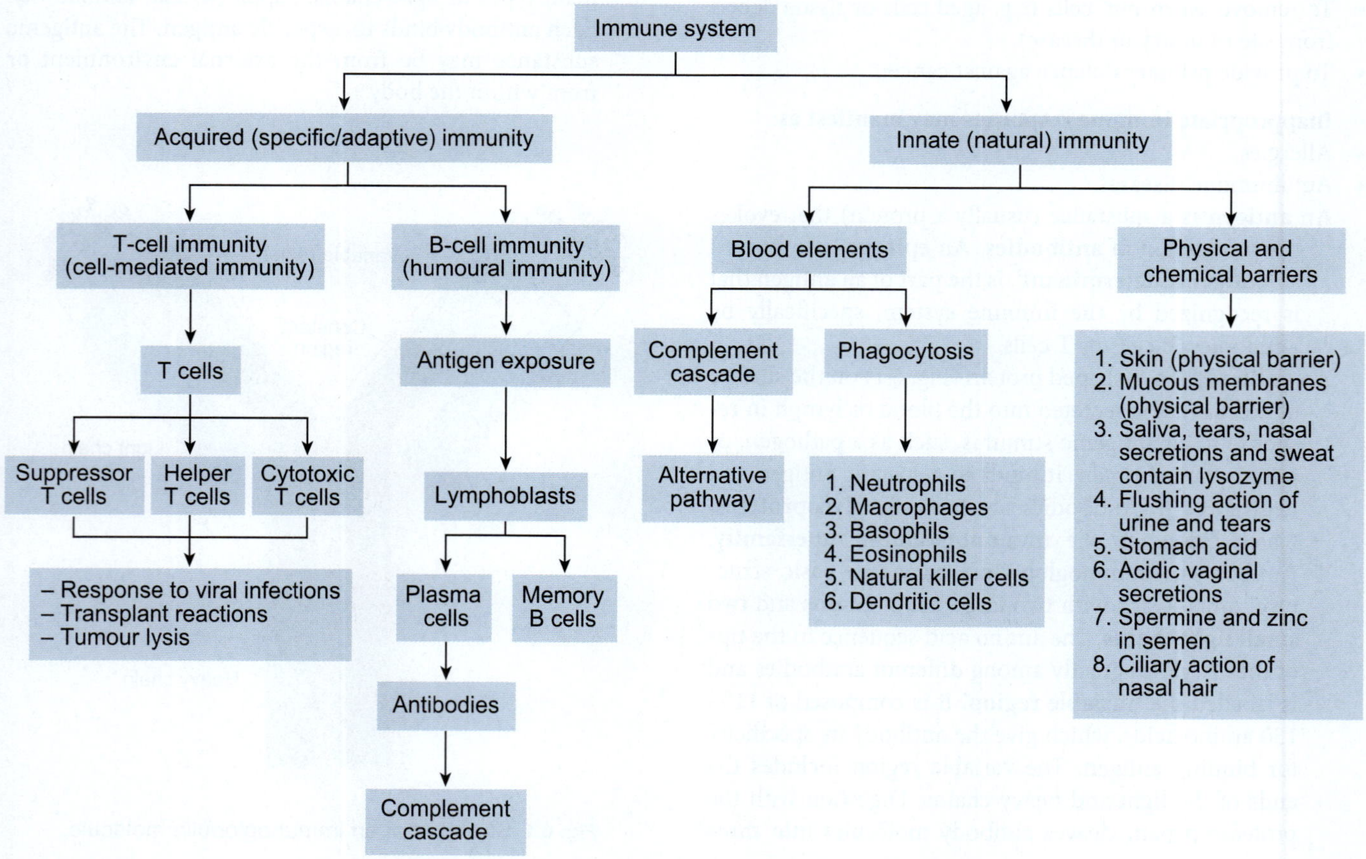

Flowchart 6.1 Types of immune responses.

Table 6.1 Difference between innate and adaptive immunity

S.No.	Characteristics	Innate Immunity	Adaptive Immunity
1	Origin	Present at birth	Induced in response to exposure to a foreign substance/antigen
2	Specificity	Non-specific, generalized response to broad categories of pathogens (bacteria, viruses, fungi, parasites)	Specific response to specific agents
3	Onset	Rapid	Slow (1–2 weeks)
4	Potency	Limited	High
5	Time span	Once activated the immunity remains throughout the life	Can be lifelong or short
6	Inheritance	Inherited from parents and passed to offspring	Cannot be inherited
7	Memory	Reacts with equal potency after every exposure to a specific pathogen; no memory	Adaptive system can remember the specific pathogens which it has encountered before and its response becomes more potent after every exposure
8	Allergic reaction	None	Immediate and delayed hypersensitivity
9	Works against	Microbes	Microbial and non-microbial agents
10	Complement system activation	Alternative and lectin pathways	Classical pathway
11	Components	Anatomic and physiological barriers (skin, mucous membranes), phagocytic leukocytes, dendritic cells, natural killer cells, and plasma proteins	Humoural immunity: B cells (mature into plasma cells which secrete antibodies) Cellular immunity: T cells which mature into effector helper and cytotoxic T cells

Q. What are the functions of the immune system?

Ans. The immune system has several functions, most important of which is self-recognition and non-self recognition. Other functions of the immune system include:

- Providing resistance against invading pathogens (viruses, bacteria, parasites, etc.) and foreign material (e.g. transplanted organ).
- Removing 'worn-out' cells (e.g. aged cells or tissue debris from site of injury or disease).
- Providing primary defense against cancer.

When the process of self-recognition breaks down and the immune system begins to attack self-antigens, the condition is labelled as *autoimmunity*. Examples of autoimmune diseases include systemic lupus erythematosus (SLE), rheumatoid arthritis (RA) and diabetes mellitus (DM).

Q. Write briefly on the cells of immune system. (PA9.1)

Ans. Cells of the immune system include the following:

Naive Lymphocytes

Lymphocytes express specific receptors for antigens. Their maturation takes place before exposure to this antigen. This is referred to as 'clonal selection'. Lymphocytes of the same specificity are said to belong to the same clone and express the same antigen receptors. Naive lymphocytes are those, which have not been expose to the antigen. After antigen exposure naive lymphocytes transform into either **effector T cells** or **Memory T cells**. All lymphocytes originate from a common lymphoid progenitor cell (Fig. 6.2) before differentiating into their distinct type. The maturation of B cells occurs in the bursa of Fabricius (in birds) and in the Gut Associated Lymphoid Tissue (GALT) located in the Peyer's patches of the intestine (in mammals). The cells that migrate to and mature in the thymus form the T cells. After maturation, the lymphocytes enter the circulation and peripheral lymphoid organs. Lymphocytes are divided into two main types:

1. **Large granular lymphocytes**—these are part of the innate immune system, also called natural killer or NK cells.
2. **Small lymphocytes**—these are part of the acquired immune system and are further classified into:
   - T cells and
   - B cells.

T Lymphocytes

- **Thymus-derived** cells, which are mediators of CMI.
- Mature T cells constitute **60%–70% of circulating lymphocytes** and are also present in the **paracortical region of lymph node** and **periarteriolar sheath of the spleen**.
- Each T cell is genetically programmed to recognize a specific cell-bound antigen by means of an **antigen-specific T cell receptor (TCR)**.
- In **95% T cells**, 'TCR' consists of a disulphide linkage made up of **α and β polypeptide chains**. In **5% T cells**, the disulphide linkage is made up of **γ and δ polypeptide chains**.

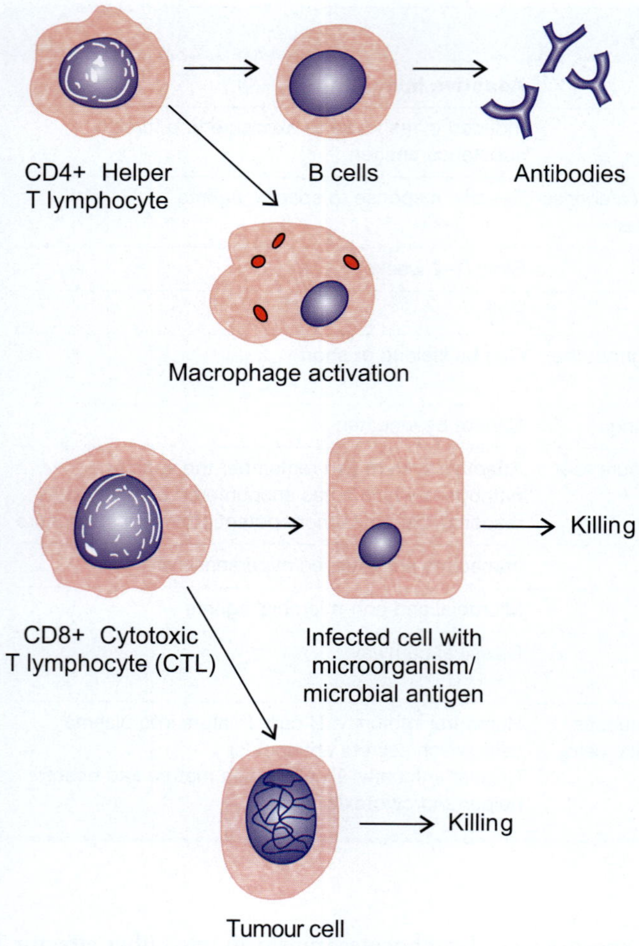

Fig. 6.2 T lymphocyte and its subsets.

The αβ TCR recognizes peptide antigens presented by major histocompatibility antigens. The γδ TCR recognizes peptides, lipids and small molecules without the need for antigen presentation by major histocompatibility antigens. γδ cells are present in the epithelial surfaces (skin, mucosa, GIT) and mainly protect from microbes entering through epithelial surfaces.

- A subset of T cells expresses markers that are also found on **NK cells (NK-T cells)**. The NK-T cells recognize glycolipids displayed by major histocompatibility complex (MHC) like molecule CD1 and their function is inadequately defined.
- 'TCR diversity' is generated by somatic rearrangement of genes coding for α, β and γ, δ chains.
- The enzyme in developing lymphocytes that mediates rearrangement of TCR is the product of RAG1 and RAG2 (recombination activating genes). Inherited defects in RAG proteins results in failure to generate mature lymphocytes.
- Each TCR is non-covalently linked to five polypeptide chains, which form the CD3 complex and ζ-chain dimer (TCR complex). CD3 complex and ζ-chain dimer, are identical in all T cells.
- In addition to CD3 proteins, T cells express a variety of other molecules, that is CD4, CD8, CD2, CD11a, CD28, CD40 and integrins.
- CD4 is expressed in 60% of mature CD3+ T cells and CD8 is expressed in 30% of mature CD3+ T cells.

Table 6.2 CD markers used to identify leukocytes

Type of cell	CD markers
Stem cells	CD34+, CD31−, CD117
All leukocytes	CD45+ (Leukocyte Common Antigen)
Granulocytic lineage	CD45+, CD11b, CD15+, CD24+, CD114+, CD182+
Monocytic lineage	CD4, CD45+, CD14+, CD114+, CD11a, CD11b, CD91+, CD16+
T lymphocyte	CD45+, CD3+
T helper cell	CD45+, CD3+, CD4+
T regulatory cell	CD4, CD25, FOXP3
Cytotoxic T cell	CD45+, CD3+, CD8+
B lymphocyte	CD45+, CD10, CD19+, CD20+, CD21(EBV receptor), CD23, CD79a
Platelets	CD45+, CD61+
NK cells	CD16+, CD56+, CD3−

- Leukocyte cell surface molecules that provide targets for classification based on immunophenotypic identification are called cluster designation markers (CD molecules). Various CD markers used to identify leukocytes are summarised in Table 6.2 given below.
- **T cells are classified into two main groups:**
  - **Conventional adaptive T cells**—Include **'Helper T cells'**, **'cytotoxic T cells'**, **'memory T cells'**, and **'regulatory T cells'. Memory T cells** persist long-term after an infection resolves and upon re-exposure to the same antigen, quickly expand to large numbers of effector T cells, thus providing the immune system with 'memory' against past infections. **Regulatory T cells** are crucial for the maintenance of immunological tolerance by suppressing autoreactive T cells that escaped the process of negative selection in the thymus.
  - **Innate like T cells (ILCs)**—Include **'Natural killer (NK) cells'**, **'mucosal associated invariant T (MAIT) cells'** and **'Gamma delta T cells'. MAIT cells** are associated with blood, liver, lungs and gut mucosa; and **Gamma delta T cells** represent a small subset of T cells, which possess a γδ TCR rather than the αβ TCR on the cell surface and are found mostly in the gut mucosa within intraepithelial lymphocytes. ILCs lack TCRs but generate cytokines similar to T lymphocytes (different subsets produce IFN-γ, IL-5, IL-17, and IL-22). Their functions include:
    - Early defence against infections.
    - Elimination of stressed cells.
    - Influencing differentiation of T lymphocytes.

B Lymphocytes

- **Mediators of humoural immunity** which make antibodies against soluble antigens.
- Derived from progenitor B cells (Fig. 6.3) produced in the **bone marrow** (named B cells because they were found to be derived from a lymphoid organ called **bursa of Fabricius in chickens.**

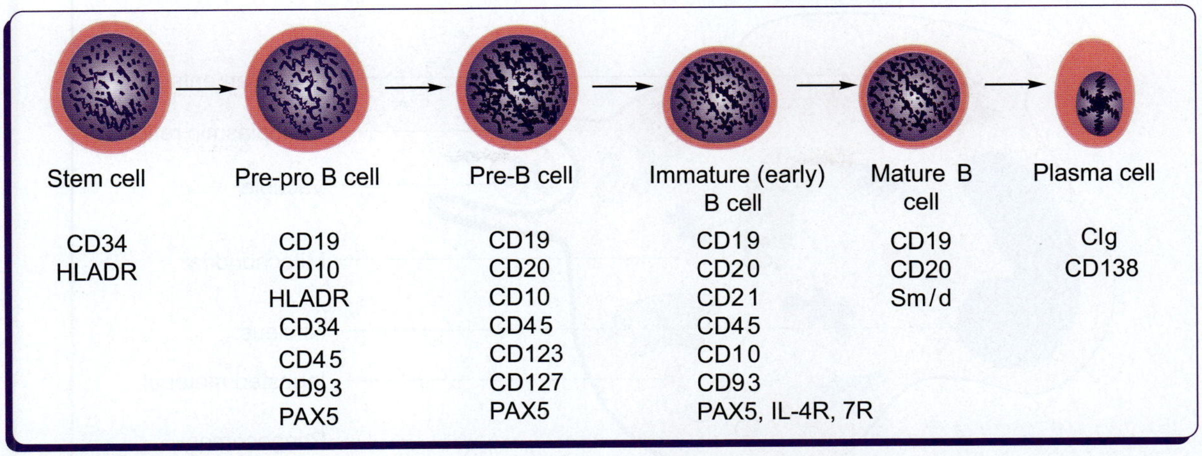

Fig. 6.3 Ontogeny of B lymphocyte.

- Constitute **10%–20% of circulating lymphocytes**. Also present in **lymph nodes (superficial cortex), spleen (white pulp), tonsils, bone narrow** and **mucosa-associated lymphoid tissue (gastrointestinal tract)**.
- Naïve B cells recognize antigens and in the presence of helper T cells differentiate into two types: **plasma B cells (synthesize immunoglobulins)** and **memory B cells (remain in secondary lymphoid organs as memory cells**; already activated by antigen; they produce quicker responses on later exposure to the same antigen).
- B cells recognize antigen via **BCR complex**. Each BCR has a unique antigen specificity derived from an RAG-mediated rearrangement of Ig genes. Analysis of Ig gene rearrangement is useful in the identification of monoclonal B cell tumours. Components of BCR complex include:
  - Membrane-bound surface antibodies (IgM and IgD which are the antigen-binding components).
  - Igα and Igβ (required for signal transduction).
  - Complement receptor CD21 (EBV receptor).
  - Fc receptor.
  - CD40 (member of TNF family).

Dendritic Cells (DCs)

- Dendritic cells are immune cells whose main function is to process antigen material and present it to other cells of the immune system. They initiate T cell responses against protein antigens; express high levels of MHC molecules and possess receptors for pathogens (like TLRs and lectins).
- They grow branched projections, the dendrites, which give the cell its name (Fig. 6.4).
- DCs arise from a CD34+ haematopoietic precursor that gives rise to myeloid (MP) and lymphoid (LP) precursors. MP differentiate into monocyte, macrophage and DC precursors (MDP), which will give rise to monocytes and to the common DC precursors (CDP). CDP can differentiate into plasmacytoid DC (pDC) or the preclassical DC (pre-cDC). Pre-cDC are the progenitors of the two major cDC sub-populations named cDC1 and cDC2. In blood, DCs constitute a rare cell population that can be broadly divided into two subtypes , namely, CD123+CD11c− DCs, called plasmacytoid DCs (pDCs), and CD123−CD11c+ cells, called classical DCs or myeloid DCs (cDC).

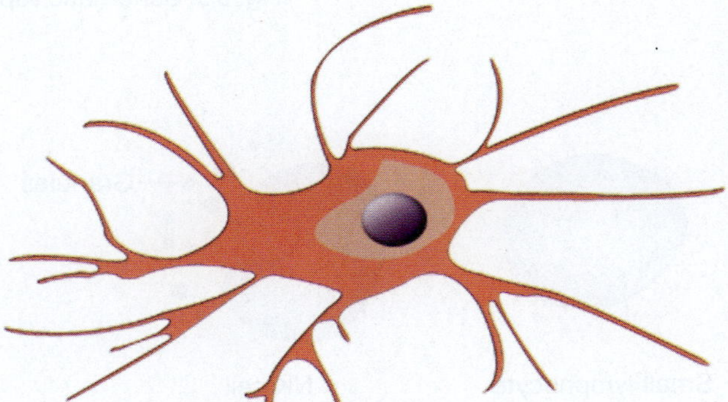

Fig. 6.4 Schematic representation of a dendritic cell, showing its branched projections (dendrites).

- Follicular dendritic cells (FDC) are located in the germinal centres of lymphoid follicles in the lymph nodes and spleen, FDC is another type of cell with dendritic morphology. These cells bear antigens to Fc portion of IgG and complement proteins, and thus augment secondary antibody responses. CD markers include CD21, CD23 and CD35.

Macrophages

- Process and present antigens to immunocompetent T cells (T cells cannot be activated by soluble antigens and antigen presentation essential for induction of CMI).
- Macrophages are important effector cells in delayed hypersensitivity and humoural immunity.
- A macrophage has abundant cytoplasm and an eccentric nucleus. The cytoplasm has many mitochondria, microtubules and microfilaments. The Golgi apparatus is well developed and numerous microcytotic vesicles are evident at or near the cell surface (Fig. 6.5).

NK (Natural Killer) Cells

- Constitute10%–15% of circulating lymphocytes.
- Belong to the group of innate lymphoid cells differentiated from the common lymphoid progenitor, the other two being B and T lymphocytes.

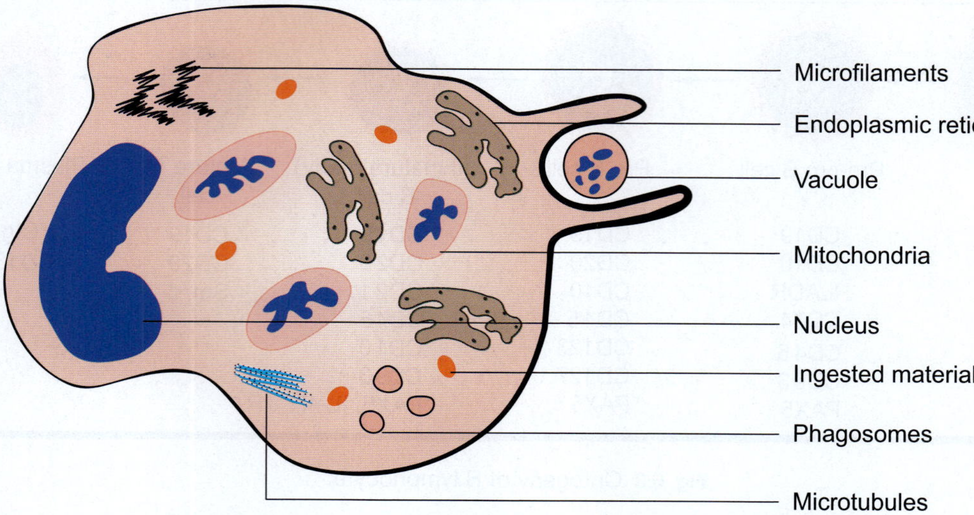

Fig. 6.5 Schematic representation of a macrophage.

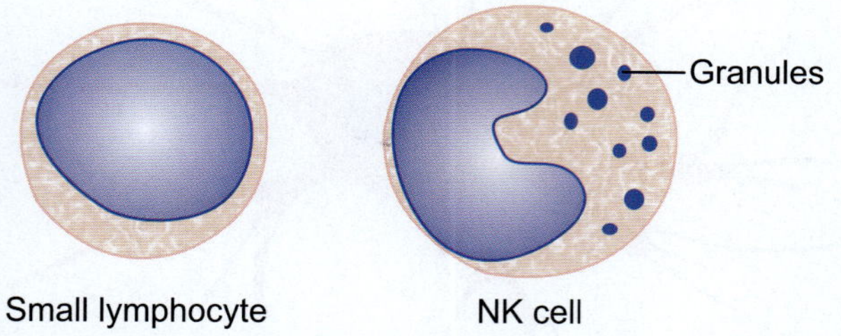

Fig. 6.6 Schematic representation of a NK cell showing its large size, abundant cytoplasm, and azurophilic granules (a small lymphocyte is also shown for comparison).

- Also called large granular lymphocytes (larger than small lymphocytes and have abundant azurophilic granules (Fig. 6.6).
- Lack TCR or BCR. Are negative for the T and B cell markers. Express CD2, CD16 (Fc receptor for IgG) and CD56.
- Secrete TNF-α, IFN-γ and GMCSF that help NK cells communicate with other cells of immune system.
- CD 16 aids in type II hypersensitivity (antibody-dependent cell-mediated cytotoxicity or ADCC) by conferring on NK cells the ability to kill infected cells and tumour cells without prior exposure or activation by them (thereby providing defence against viral infections and intracellular pathogens). NK cells also play a role in the adaptive immune response and have anti tumour activity.
- The function of CD 56 is not clear.
- NK cell activity is regulated by stimulatory (NKG2D) and inhibitory (killer cell immunoglobulin-like receptors and CD94 family of lectin receptors) influences. These MHC-independent receptors use an alternate pathway to induce apoptosis in infected cells. NK cell activation is dependant on the balance of inhibitory and activating receptor stimulation.
- NK cells differ from natural killer T cells (NKTs) by origin and by effector functions; NKT cells may promote NK cell activity by secreting interferon gamma.

Q. Enumerate the differences between T lymphocytes and B lymphocytes. (PA9.1)

Ans. Differences between T and B lymphocytes are shown in Table 6.3).

Q. Write briefly on HLA complex. (PA9.3)

Ans. HLA complex (Fig. 6.7) is a set of multiple genes located on *chromosome 6* that encodes the major histocompatibility complex (MHC) antigens in humans. MHC comprises cell surface proteins, which regulate the human immune system. HLA genes are highly polymorphic, and each gene may have many different alleles, resulting in extreme variation in the human MHC and therefore marked genetic diversity such that no two individuals have the same set of MHC molecules. The immune system uses the HLAs to differentiate self-cells and non-self cells. Any cell displaying some other HLA type is recognised as foreign ('non-self') and is rejected by the body's immune system. This concept underlies transplant rejection. HLA binds peptide fragments of foreign proteins for presentation to appropriate antigen-presenting cell, and has the following components:

- HLAs corresponding to **MHC class I** (**A**, **B** and **C**) present peptides coming from intracellular proteins, which are produced when the latter are broken down in the proteasomes. These MHC–peptide complexes are recognized by cytotoxic T cells (killer T cells) with the help of the co-receptor CD8. Class I proteins are expressed on the surfaces of nearly all cells. MHC class I proteins also include β2-microglobulin, which unlike the HLA proteins is encoded by a gene on chromosome 15.
- HLAs corresponding to **MHC class II** (**DP**, **DM, DO, DQ** and **DR**) present antigens from outside of the cell to T-lymphocytes. These extracellular peptides are taken into the cell with the help of endosomes. The MHC–peptide complexes are recognized by helper T cells with the help of the CD4 co-receptor. These antigens stimulate the multiplication of T-helper cells, which in turn stimulate

Table 6.3 Differences between T lymphocytes and B lymphocytes

Features	T cell	B cell
Origin	Stem cells in bone marrow → thymus	Stem cells in bone marrow → secondary lymphoid organs
Life span	• Blasts: several days • Small T cells: months to years	• Blasts: several days • Small B cells: <1 month
Location 1. Lymph node 2. Spleen 3. Peyer's patches	 Para/deep cortex Periarteriolar sheath Perifollicular zone	 Germinal centre, superficial cortex Germinal centre, red pulp Follicular centre
Percentage population in 1. Blood 2. Bone marrow 3. Lymph node	 80% Rare 85%	 20% Numerous 15%
Surface markers 1. TCR Ag receptor 2. Surface Ig 3. Fc receptor 4. Complement receptor 5. CD markers	 Present Absent Absent Absent • T (helper): CD4,3,7,2 • T (suppressor): CD8,3,7,2	 Absent Present Present Present CD19,21,23
Functions	1. CMI via cytotoxic T cells 2. Delayed hypersensitivity via CD4+ T cells	1. Precursors of plasma cells 2. Contribute to humoural immunity by synthesizing specific antibodies (Igs)

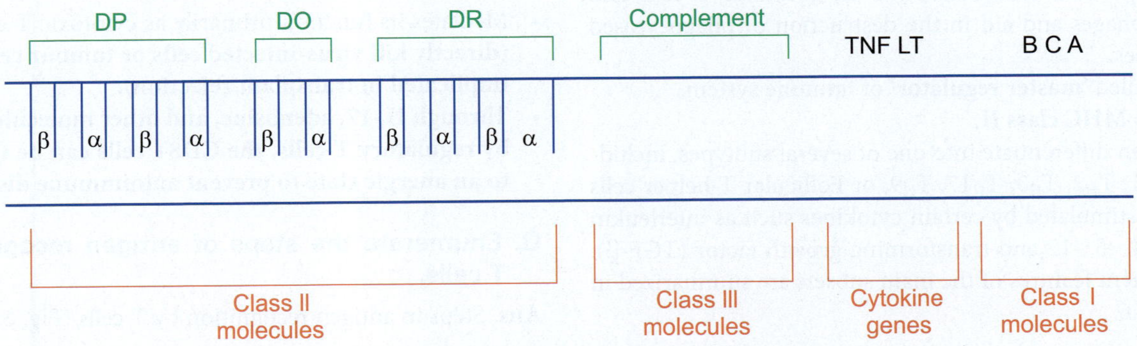

Fig. 6.7 Components of HLA complex.

antibody-producing B cells to produce antibodies to that specific antigen. Self-antigens are suppressed by suppressor T cells. Class II proteins are expressed only on B cells, macrophages and dendritic cells.

- HLAs corresponding to **MHC class III** encode components of the complement system.

Roles of HLA Complex

HLA complex has diverse roles in the human body:

1. **Role in disease:** HLA has been found to be associated with a growing number of diseases (Table 6.4). These include:
   (a) Inflammatory diseases like postinfectious arthropathy and ulcerative colitis.
   (b) Inherited errors of metabolism, like 21-hydroxylase deficiency.
   (c) Autoimmune diseases, like endocrinopathies, type 1 diabetes, celiac disease, ankylosing spondylitis, SLE, myasthenia gravis and Sjögren syndrome. People with certain HLA antigens are more likely to develop certain autoimmune diseases, and HLA typing in autoimmunity is being increasingly used as a tool in diagnosis.

Table 6.4 Association of diseases with HLA

Disease	HLA allele	Disease	HLA allele
Acute anterior uveitis	B27	**Chronic active hepatitis**	DR3
Ankylosing spondylitis	B27	**Primary Sjögren syndrome**	DR3
Postgonococcal arthritis	B27	**Insulin-dependent DM**	DR3, DR4, DR3/DR4
Rheumatoid arthritis	DR4	**21-hydroxylase deficiency**	BW47

2. **Role in graft rejection:** If the immune system recognizes a 'non-self' antigen, it rejects the tissue bearing those antigens. This forms the basis of transplant rejection. Because of the importance of HLA in transplantation, the HLA loci are some of the most frequently typed by serology and PCR.
3. **Role in cancer:** Some HLA-mediated diseases are directly involved in the promotion of cancer; for example, gluten-sensitive enteropathy is associated with increased prevalence of enteropathy-associated T cell lymphoma, and DR3-DQ2 homozygotes comprise the highest risk group.

Q. Differentiate between MHC class I and class II. (PA9.3)

Ans. Differences between MHC class I and class II are shown in Table 6.5.

Table 6.5 Differences between MHC class I and class II

Features	MHC I	MHC II
Location	Present on all nucleated cells and platelets	Found on antigen-presenting cells–macrophages, dendritic cells and activated T and B cells
Constituted by	Alpha chains (α1, α2, α3) and β2 microglobulin	Alpha chains (α1, α2) and beta chains (β1, β2)
Genes coding region	HLA-A, HLA-B, HLA-C	HLA-D (DP, DQ, DR)
Antigen presentation in association with	CD8+ T cells	CD4+ T cells
Functions	Graft rejection, lysis of virus-infected cells and tumour cells	Graft-versus-host response and immunologic reactions involving CD4+ T cells

Q. Enumerate the characteristics of CD4+ and CD8+ T lymphocytes. (PA9.1)

Ans. CD4+ T lymphocyte

- Expressed on 60% of mature T cells (normal CD4 to CD8 ratio is 2:1).
- Called '**helper T cells**' because they secrete cytokines that help B cells mature into memory B cells and plasma cells which produce antibodies, activate cytotoxic T cells and macrophages and aid in the destruction of phagocytosed microbes.
- Also called '**master regulator**' of immune system.
- Bind to **MHC class II.**
- They can differentiate into one of several subtypes, including T_H1, T_H2, T_H3, T_H17, T_H9, or Follicular T-helper cells (TFH) stimulated by certain cytokines such as interleukin IL-2, -4, -6, -12 and transforming growth factor (TGF-β). The salient features of the main subsets are summarized in Table 6.6.

CD8+ T lymphocyte

- Expressed on 30% of mature T cells.
- Binds to **MHC class I.**
- Mediates its function primarily as cytotoxic T cell or CTL **(directly kill virus-infected cells or tumour cells and are implicated in transplant rejection).**
- **Through IL-17, adenosine, and other molecules secreted by regulatory T cells, the CD8+ cells can be inactivated to an anergic state to prevent autoimmune diseases.**

Q. Enumerate the steps of antigen recognition by T cells. (PA9.1)

Ans. Steps in antigen recognition by T cells (Fig. 6.8):

Table 6.6 Subsets of helper T cells

Features	T_H 1 cells	T_H 2 cells	T_H 17 cells	Th9	Tfh
Cytokines/transcription factors that induce this subset	Tbet (IFN-γ and IL-12)	GATA3 (IL-4)	RORγt (TGF-β, IL-6, IL-1 and IL-23)	IRF4, PU.1	BCL-6
Cytokines produced by this subset	IFN-γ	IL-4, 5 and 13	IL-17 and IL-22	IL-9	IL-21, IL-4
Function	Responsible for delayed hypersensitivity, macrophage activation and synthesis of IgG; provide defence against intracellular microbes.	Responsible for synthesis of other classes of antibodies mainly IgA and IgE; important for host defense against large extracellular pathogens (helminthic parasites) and are responsible for allergic responses.	Release IL17, which is a recruiter of neutrophils and monocytes and is important in defence against extracellular bacteria and fungi.	Defence against helminths (parasitic worms); supports CD4 + T-cell expansion and survival; recruits mast cells	Help B cells produce antibody
Role in disease	Autoimmune and chronic inflammatory diseases	Allergies	Autoimmune and chronic inflammatory diseases	Multiple Sclerosis	Asthma and other allergic diseases

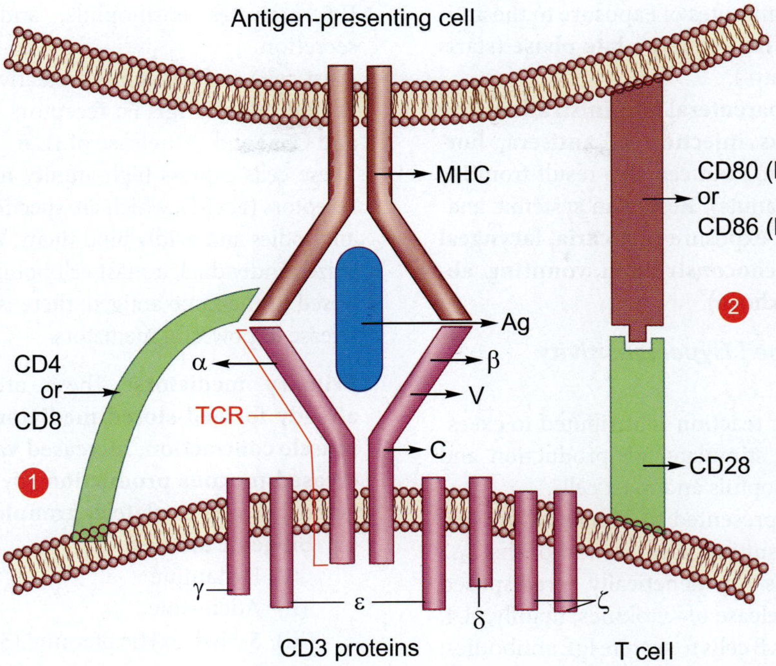

Fig. 6.8 Antigen recognition by T cells (signals 1 and 2).

CD4+ T Cells

- TCR recognizes peptide fragment bound to MHC class II.
- CD4 binds to non-polymorphic portion of MHC class II.
- TCR and MHC-bound antigen provides *signal 1* for T cell activation.
- CD28+costimulatory molecules (B7-1 and B7-2) on antigen-presenting cell provide *signal 2*.

CD8+ T Cells

- Recognition of antigen in association with MHC class I.
- Also need signals 1 and 2 like CD4+ T cells.

Q. Differentiate between helper and suppressor T cells. (PA9.1)

Ans. Differences between helper and suppressor T cells are shown in Table 6.7.

Q. Define hypersensitivity and write in detail on type I hypersensitivity. (PA9.2)

Ans. Hypersensitivity is defined as an **excessive** and **potentially harmful reaction** to an **endogenous** or **exogenous antigen**. It occurs in a **previously sensitized individual** when the balance between the effecter and control immune mechanisms gets disturbed. It is usually associated with **inheritance of susceptibility genes (both HLA and non-HLA)**. HS is classified into **four types** based on the underlying immune mechanism.

Type I Hypersensitivity

Definition

An immunologic reaction, **developing within minutes after combination of an antigen with antibody bound on mast cells or basophils, in already sensitized individuals**. Most reactions are caused due to an **exaggerated T_H2 response and are mediated by IgE antibody**. Based on the **portal of entry** type I hypersensitivity is classified into **two types**:

1. **Local (atopy):** Occurs when the antigen is **confined to a particular site. Manifests with skin allergy, hives, nasal and conjunctival discharge, hay fever, bronchial asthma and allergic gastroenteritis**. May have two distinct phases,

Table 6.7 Differences between helper and suppressor T cells

Features	Helper/inducer T cells	Suppressor/ cytotoxic T lymphocytes
Type	• CD4-positive • CD8-negative	• CD8-positive • CD4-negative
Percentage of peripheral T cells	60%	30%
Antigen recognition in association with	HLA class II	HLA class I
Functions	Release lymphokines and activate macrophages and B cells, responsible for delayed hypersensitivity	Cytotoxicity mediated by pore formation and release of granzymes. Also Fas/FasL-dependent killing
Subsets	T_H1, T_H17, T_H9 and Tfh	TN, naive T cells; T_{SCM}, stem cell memory T cells; T_{CM}, central memory T cells; T_{EFF}, effector T cells; T_{EM}, effector memory cells

immediate (occurs within minutes of exposure to the antigen and subsides in a few hours) and a **late phase** (starts 2–24 h later and lasts for days).

2. **Systemic:** Mostly follows **parenteral administration (bee venom or an intravenous injection of antisera, hormones, enzymes, drugs**, etc.) but can also result from **ingestion** of the allergen (peanuts). Results in systemic anaphylaxis within minutes of exposure **(urticaria, laryngeal oedema, pulmonary bronchoconstriction, vomiting, abdominal cramps and diarrhoea)**.

Mechanism Underlying Type I Hypersensitivity (Flowchart 6.2)

- Immediate hypersensitivity reaction is attributed to excessive T_H2 responses which stimulate IgE production and sensitize and activate eosinophils and mast cells.
- The sensitising antigen is presented to T cells by antigen presenting cells (APCs) resulting in activation of the T_H2 subset of CD4+ T cells in genetically predisposed individuals. This induces release of cytokines, mainly, IL4, IL5 and IL13. IL4 stimulates B cells to secrete IgE antibodies; IL5 activates eosinophils, and IL13 induces mucus secretion.
- Mast cells and basophils are activated by (1) cross-linking of high-affinity IgE Fc receptors, (2) anaphylatoxins (C3a and C5a) and (3) release of IL-8.
- These cells express high-affinity receptors called Fc-epsilon receptors (FceRI), which are specific for the Fc portion of IgE antibodies and avidly bind them. When in a previously sensitized individual, a mast cell bound to IgE antibodies is exposed to the same antigen; there is activation of the cell and release of powerful mediators.

1. **Primary mediators:** These are immediately released **already formed stored mediators** which induce **smooth muscle contraction, increased vascular permeability, increased mucous production** (by nasal, bronchial, gastric glands) as well as **platelet granule release**. They include:
   (a) **Biogenic amines**
      (i) Histamine
      (ii) Adenosine
      (iii) 5-Hydroxytryptamine (5HT)

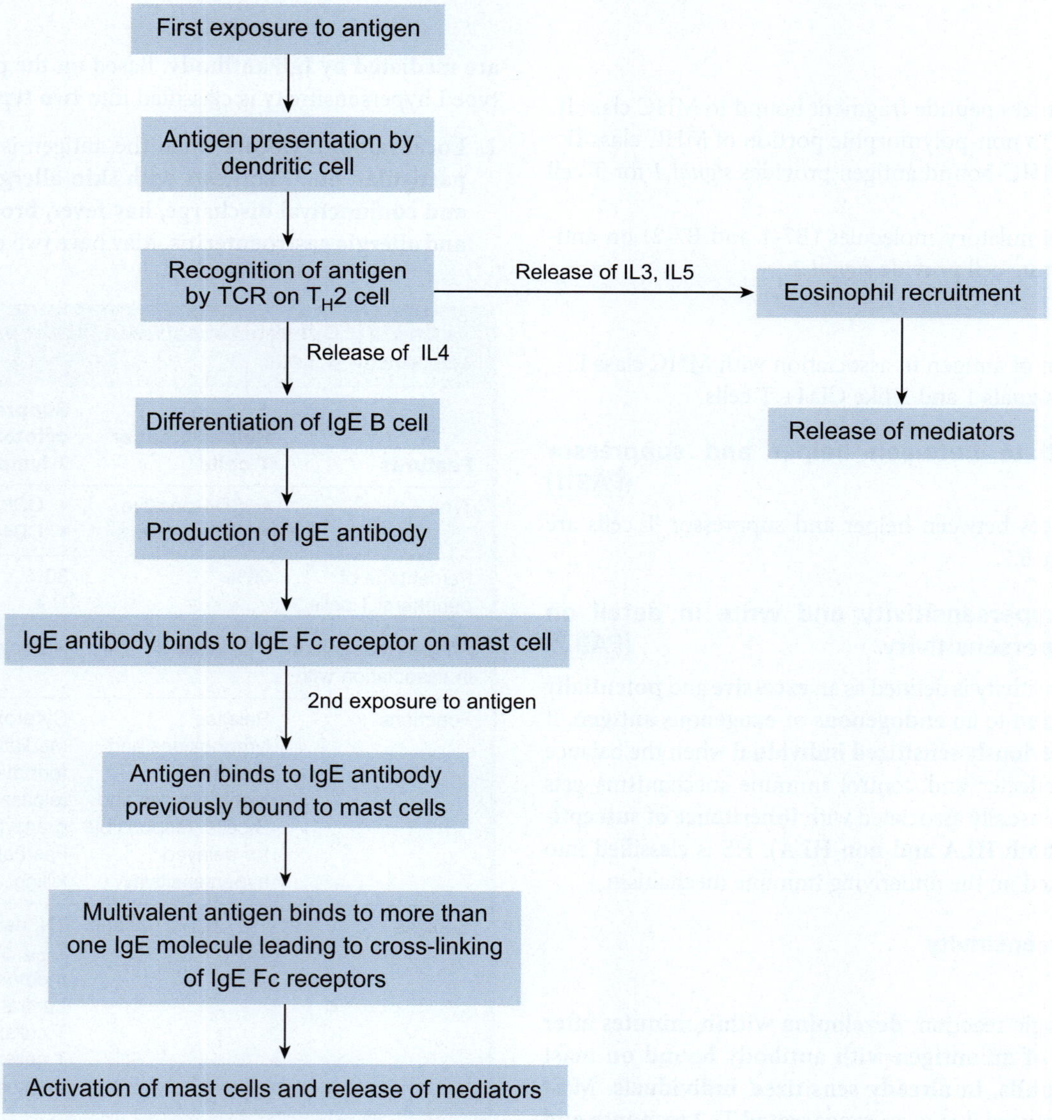

Flowchart 6.2 Mechanism underlying type I hypersensitivity.

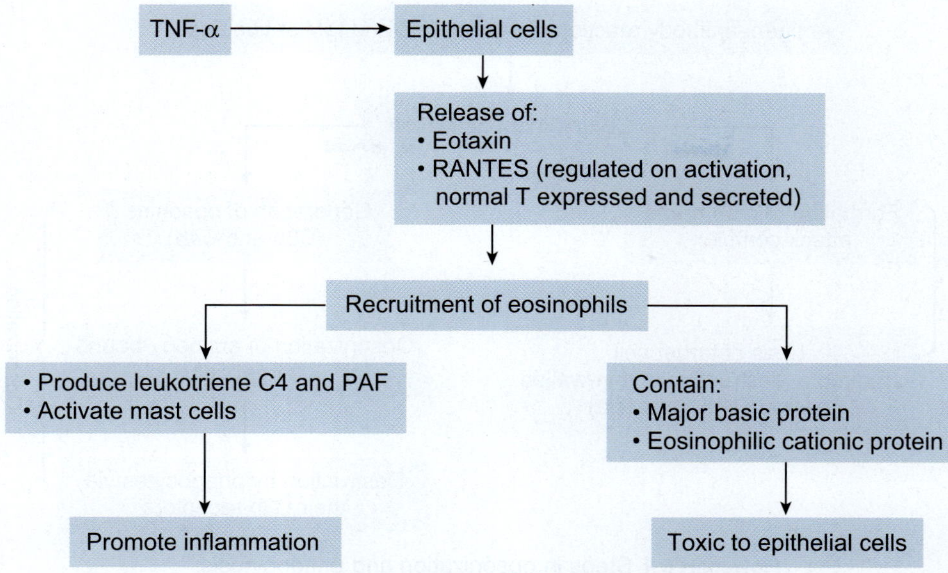

Flowchart 6.3 Role of eosinophils in type I hypersensitivity.

(b) **Chemotactic mediators**
 (i) Eosinophil chemotactic factor (ECF).
 (ii) Neutrophil chemotactic factor (NCF).

(c) **Enzymes**
Contained in granule matrix, for example proteases (tryptase, chymase) and acid hydrolases.

(d) **Proteoglycans**
Heparin and chondroitin sulphate (serve to package and store other mediators in the granules).

2. **Secondary mediators:** These are **synthesized de novo** and **released late**.
 (a) **Lipid mediators**
  (i) **Leukotrienes**
   - C_4, D_4 (vasoactive and spasmogenic—increase vascular permeability and induce bronchospasm).
   - B_4 (chemotactic for neutrophils, eosinophils and monocytes).
  (ii) **Prostaglandin D_2**
   - Generated by cyclooxygenase pathway.
   - Induces bronchospasm and increased mucous secretion.
  (iii) **Platelet-activating factor (PAF)**
   - Induces platelet activation and bronchospasm.
   - Releases histamine.
   - Increases vascular permeability.
   - Is chemotactic for neutrophils and eosinophils.
   - Activates inflammatory cells and causes their aggregation and degranulation.
 (b) **Cytokines** include TNF-α, ILs-1, -3, -4, -5, -6 {T_H2 response}, GMCSF, chemokines, and macrophage inhibitory protein (MIP-1α and β). Cytokines recruit and activate inflammatory cells and mast cells.

Q. What are mast cells? How do they contribute to type I hypersensitivity?

Ans. Mast cells are bone marrow-derived cells, widely distributed in tissues near blood vessels and nerves and in subepithelial sites. They contain membrane-bound granules that possess a variety of biological mediators including PAF, histamine, leukotrienes C_4, D_4, E_4, prostaglandins, cytokines, ECF and NCF.

Q. Write briefly on the role of eosinophils in type I hypersensitivity. (PA9.2)

Ans. Refer to Flowchart 6.3.

Q. Write in detail on type II hypersensitivity. (PA9.2)

Ans. Type II hypersensitivity is **mediated by antibodies directed towards antigens present on the surface of the cells or other tissue components**. These antigens may be **intrinsic to cell membrane** or **exogenous antigens absorbed on the cell surface** (e.g. a drug metabolite). Reaction occurs when antibodies bind to normal or altered cell surface antigens. A **sensitization phase** leads to production of antibodies against substances or metabolites that accumulate in cellular membrane structures. In the **effector phase**, target cells become coated with antibodies, a process termed opsonization, which leads to cellular destruction by: (1) phagocytosis, (2) antibody-dependent cellular cytotoxicity (ADCC) and (3) complement-dependent cytotoxicity (CDC).

Mechanisms Underlying Type II Hypersensitivity

I. Complement Dependant Mechanisms

1. **Opsonization and phagocytosis** (Flowchart 6.4)**:** Opsonization is the process by which a foreign particle like a microbe is coated with opsonins, e.g., immunoglobulins or complement proteins (particularly C3b) so as to facilitate the attachment and internalization of that particle by a phagocytic cell. IgG or IgM antibodies coating target cells can bind to Fc receptors present on cells such as macrophages and neutrophils and mediate phagocytosis and destruction.
2. **ADCC** (Flowchart 6.5) involves cell lysis without phagocytosis mediated by monocytes, neutrophils and NK cells. IgG antibodies can bind FcγRIII on NK cells and macrophages, mediating release of granzymes and perforin and resulting in cell death by apoptosis.

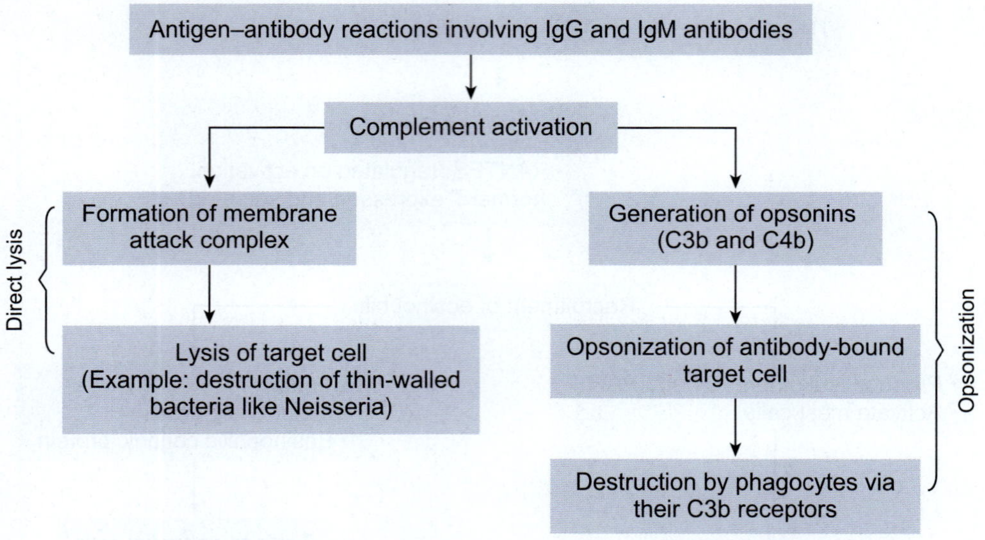

Flowchart 6.4 Steps in opsonization and phagocytosis.

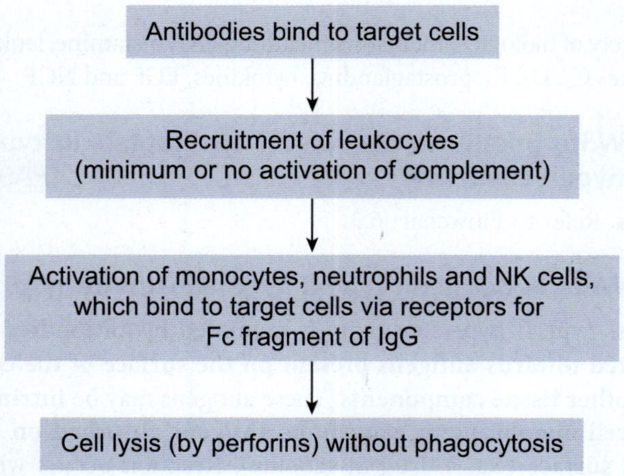

Flowchart 6.5 Antibody-dependent cellular cytotoxicity (ADCC).

Examples: Autoimmune haemolytic anaemia, agranulocytosis, thrombocytopenia and drug reactions.

3. **Complement and Fc receptor-mediated inflammation** (Flowchart 6.6)**:** Deposition of antibody in extracellular tissue initiates an antigen-antibody reaction leading to complement activation and release of C3a and C5a. Complement components activate inflammatory cells to cause the cell injury via ROS and lysosomal enzymes.
   Examples: Goodpasture syndrome (basement membrane containing collagen type IV in the lung and kidney is attacked by one's own antibodies).
4. **Lysis of target cells via MAC:** Complement activation also leads to production of the Membrane attack complex (MAC), which forms pores in the cellular membrane resulting in cytolysis.
   Examples: Incompatible transfusion reactions and haemolytic disease of newborn (erythroblastosis foetalis).

II. Complement Independant Mechanism

Antibody-mediated cellular dysfunction

Antibodies against cell surface receptors deregulate function without causing cell injury or inflammation.

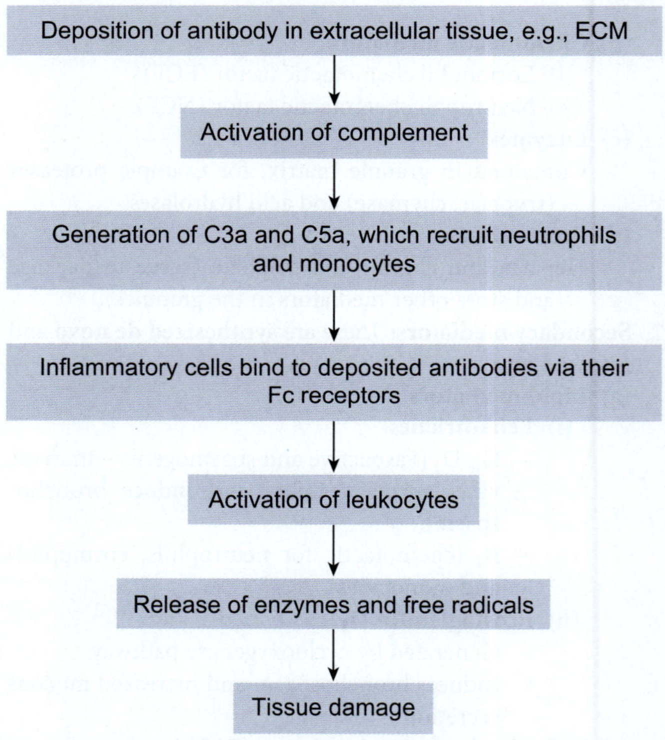

Flowchart 6.6 Complement and Fc receptor-mediated inflammation.

Examples:

- *Myasthenia gravis,* which is due to antibodies against acetylcholine receptors in the motor end plates of skeletal muscle. These antibodies impair neuromuscular transmission and cause muscle weakness.
- *Pemphigus vulgaris,* which is due to antibodies against desmosomes. These antibodies disrupt the intercellular junction and result in the formation of vesicles.

Q. Write in detail on type III hypersensitivity. (PA9.2)

Ans. Type III hypersensitivity is induced by antigen–antibody complexes that produce tissue damage as a result of their capacity to activate the complement system. It involves soluble antigens that are not bound to cell surfaces (contrary to those in type II hypersensitivity). When these antigens bind antibodies, immune complexes of different sizes form. Antigen–antibody complexes may be:

1. **Circulating** or **in situ.**
2. **Exogenous** (e.g. against infectious agents and drugs) or **endogenous** (e.g. against 'nuclear antigens' in SLE, 'immunoglobulins' in reactive arthritis, 'streptococcal cell wall antigens' in acute post-streptococcal glomerulonephritis and 'HBS antigen' in polyarteritis nodosa).
3. **Systemic** (acute serum sickness—prototype of a systemic immune complex disease) or **local** (Arthus reaction—local immune complex disease).

Pathogenesis

- Formation of antigen–antibody complexes (**first phase**).
- Deposition of immune complexes in various tissues (**second phase**).
- Initiation of an inflammatory reaction in dispersed sites throughout the body (**third phase**).

Factors Influencing Deposition of Immune Complexes in Various Tissues

1. Size of immune complexes:
   (a) Large complexes have antibody excess (complex with many free IgG Fc regions) and are readily removed by the mononuclear phagocytic system.
   (b) Small- and medium-sized complexes have antigen excess, are cleared less effectively and are the most pathogenic complexes.
2. Functional status of mononuclear phagocytic system (MPS): Intrinsic dysfunction or overload of MPS increases the probability of persistence of immune complexes in circulation and tissue deposition.
3. Charge of immune complex: Anionic versus cationic; charged cationic antigens are more likely to be deposited in the negatively charged glomerular basement membrane.
4. The three-dimensional structure of immune complex: Structural lattice is important in determining the deposition of immune complexes.
5. Valency of the antigen: The size of immune complexes depends on the valency of the antigen, and on the titre of the antibody.
6. Affinity of the antigen to tissue components and avidity of antibody: Certain complexes are deposited in specific organs in certain diseases. In SLE, the kidney is the prime target, whereas in rheumatoid arthritis, the joints are the principal target.
7. Haemodynamic factors: Immune-complex deposition is most likely where there is high blood pressure and turbulence.

Favoured Sites of Deposition of Immune Complexes

Renal glomeruli, joints, skin, heart, serosa and small blood vessels.

Morphology of Immune Complex-Mediated Tissue Injury

- Necrotizing vasculitis (fibrinoid necrosis and neutrophils in the vessel wall).
- Swelling and proliferation of endothelial and mesangial cells.
- Neutrophilic and monocytic infiltration into glomeruli
- Hypercellular glomeruli.
- *Immunofluorescence*: granular lumpy deposits of immunoglobulins and complement.
- *Electron microscopy*: electron-dense deposits.

Mechanism of Immune Complex-Mediated Tissue Injury (Flowchart 6.7)

- Type III hypersensitivity reactions are also termed **immune complex reactions.** Immune complex deposits in tissues activate complement and cause damage via the action of cleaved complement **anaphylotoxins** C3a and C5a, which, mediate the release of mediators from **mast cells.**
- This results in increased vascular permeability and recruitment of inflammatory cells into the tissue (mainly those with **lysosomal** action, leading to tissue damage through **phagocytosis** by **PMNs** and macrophages). **Platelet aggregation** occurs, resulting in microthrombus formation in the **vasculature.**
- **The reaction can take hours, days, or even weeks to develop,** depending on whether or not there is **immunological memory** of the precipitating antigen.
- Typically, clinical features emerge a week following initial antigen challenge and include **vasculitis, skin lesions, alveolar damage, glomerulonephritis and arthritis. Examples include SLE** (target-nuclear antigens)**, rheumatoid arthritis** ((target-antibody complexes specifically IgM to IgG), **post-streptococcal glomerulonephritis** (target-streptococcal cell wall antigens), etc.

Clinical Significance

- *Single large exposure of antigen* causes resolution of the disease due to catabolism of immune complexes (e.g. acute serum sickness, acute post-streptococcal glomerulonephritis).
- *Prolonged exposure to antigen* causes chronic disease (e.g. SLE).

Q. What is Arthus reaction? (PA9.2)

Ans. Arthus reaction (localized immune complex disease) typically manifests as a localized area of tissue necrosis resulting from **acute immune complex vasculitis involving complement fixing antibodies IgG and IgM.**

- It is usually elicited in the **skin.**
- Intracutaneous injection into an animal having circulating antibodies against the antigen result in formation of large immune complexes, which precipitate locally and trigger an inflammatory reaction.
- This leads to **fibrinoid necrosis** and **thrombosis** in the vessel wall.
- **Oedema, haemorrhage** and **ulceration** develop in a few hours and peak in 4–10 h after injection.

Q. Write in detail on type IV hypersensitivity. (PA9.2)

Ans. Type IV hypersensitivity is often called **delayed type hypersensitivity** as the reaction takes several days to develop. Unlike the other types, it is **not antibody-mediated** but rather

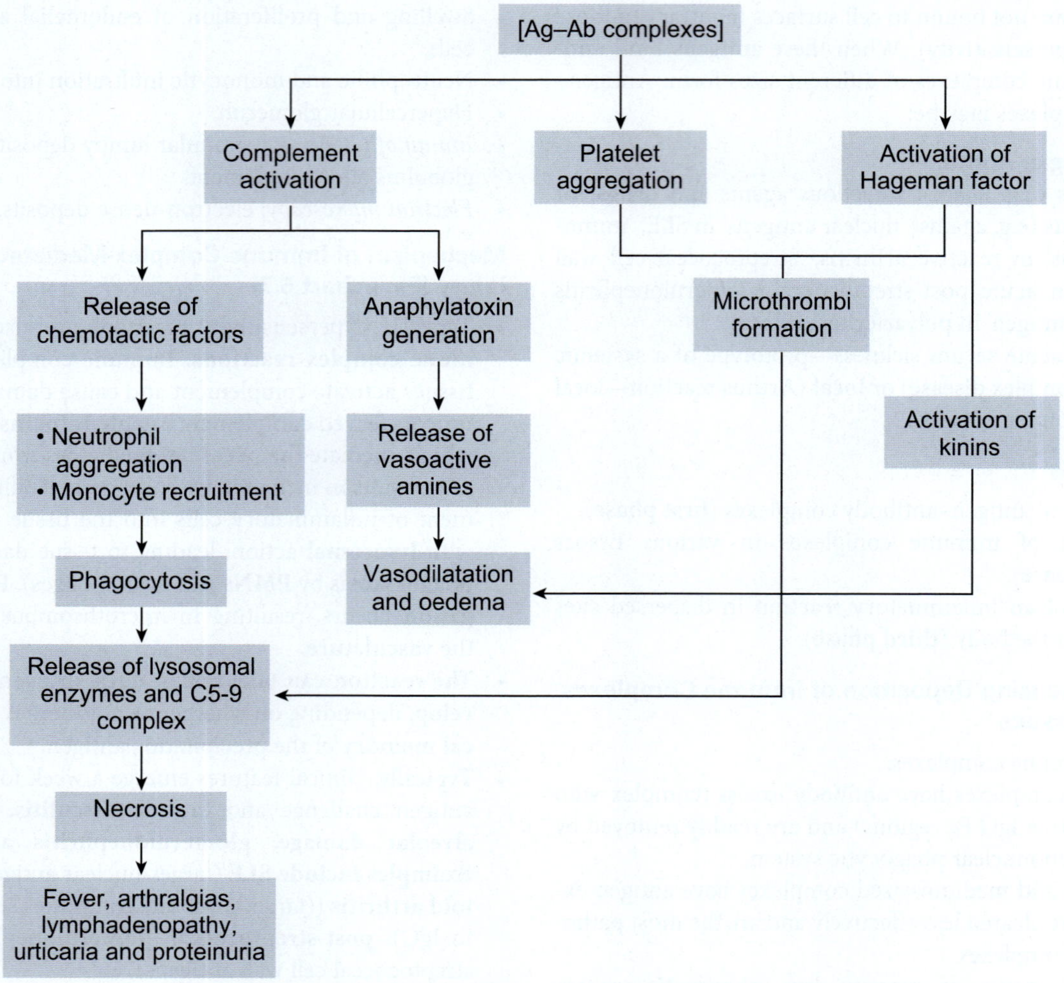

Flowchart 6.7 Mechanism of immune complex-mediated tissue injury.

is a type of **cell-mediated** response. Type IV hypersensitivity is initiated by specifically sensitized T cells and may be of two types:

1. ***Classic delayed hypersensitivity*** (DTH) mediated by CD4+ T cells.
2. ***Direct cell toxicity*** (cytolysis) mediated by CD8+ T cells.

Classic Delayed Hypersensitivity (DTH)

- It is the immunologic response to a variety of intracellular microbiologic agents, for example *M. tuberculosis, Mycobacterium bovis, Mycobacterium avium subsp.paratuberculosis,* viruses, fungi, protozoa, parasites, as well as conditions like contact dermatitis, type 1 diabetes mellitus, multiple sclerosis and graft rejection.
- The **classic prototype of DTH is tuberculin reaction** (intracutaneous injection of tuberculin (protein–liposaccharide component of tuberculous bacillus) in a previously sensitized individual resulting in reddening and induration, which starts after 8–12 h and peaks in 24–72 h.
- DTH like all other hypersensitivity reactions involve a **sensitization** phase and an **effector** phase (Flowchart 6.8).
- The **sensitization phase** starts with the **initial exposure to the antigen** and results in the development of **antigen-specific memory T cells**. This reaction is initiated by CD4 + T_H1 helper cells when they recognize a foreign antigen in a complex with the MHC class II on the surface of antigen-presenting cells (APCs; usually macrophages).
- The naïve CD4+ T lymphocytes develop into **activated T_H1 lymphocytes** (also designated **TDTH lymphocytes**).
- **A prolonged or repeat exposure** to the antigen results in the development of an **effector phase** which entails either a **T_H1 response** through the elaboration of cytokines by CD4+ lymphocytes or a cytotoxic response mediated by **CD8+ lymphocytes**.
- **T_H1 cytokines** (mainly, IL-2, IL-3, IFN-γ and TNF-β), as well as, **chemokines** (IL-8, macrophage chemotactic and activating factor, and macrophage-inhibition factor) enhance the function of cytokine-producing T lymphocytes (in an autocrine and paracrine fashion) and also activate macrophages.
- **IL-2** induces proliferation and increases survival of T lymphocytes. **IL-3** supports the growth and differentiation of T_H1 lymphocytes and NK cells. **IFN-γ, the master regulator**

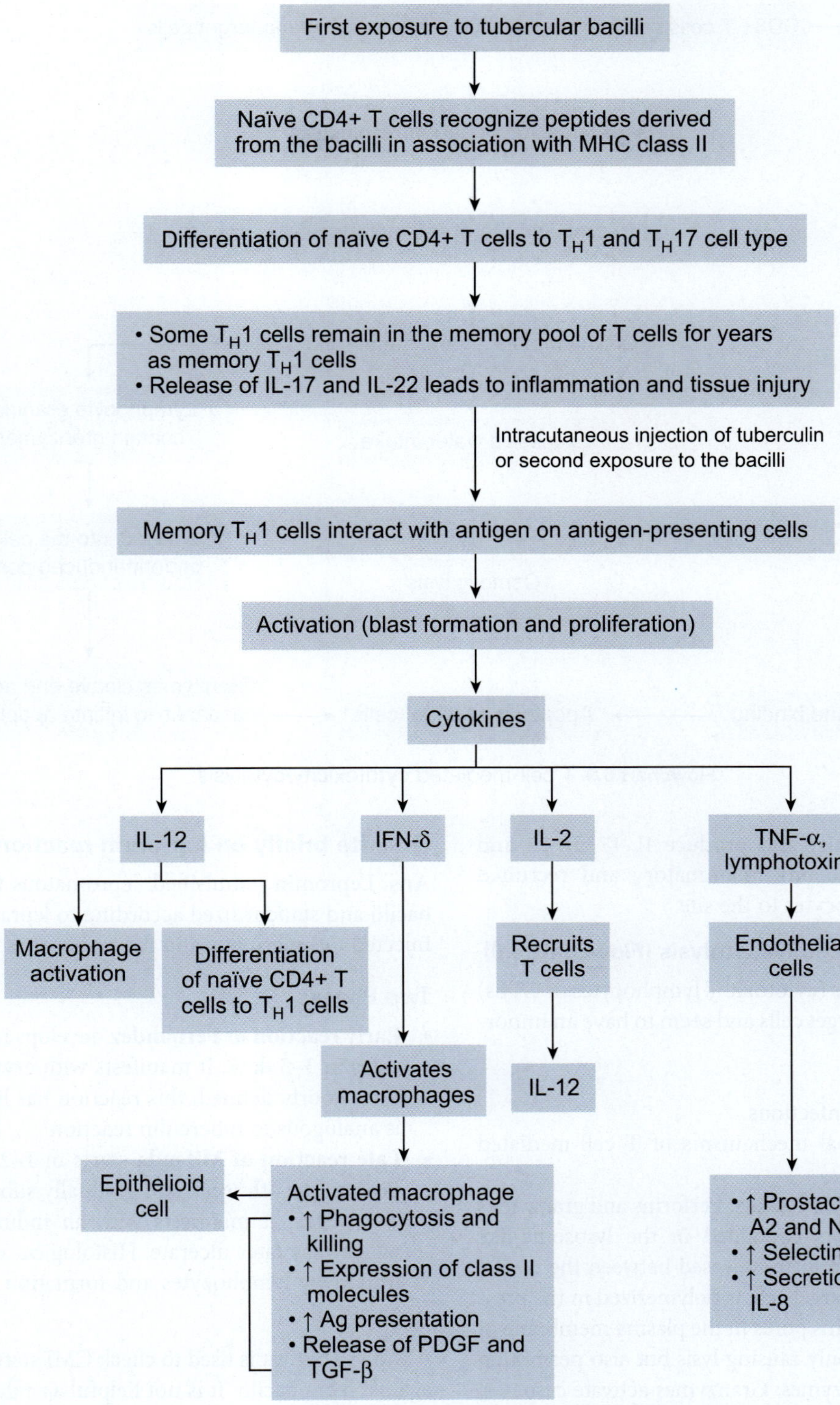

Flowchart 6.8 Sequence of events in development of DTH.

of type IV hypersensitivity, activates macrophages (enhances their phagocytic and killing potential, enhance their antigen presenting ability by increasing the expression of class II MHC molecules and mediate the production of cytokines that influence CD4+ lymphocytes, resulting in a harmful response that results in tissue damage (hypersensitivity) instead of a beneficial protective response (immunity).

- **Activated macrophages** and **dendritic cells** produce **IL-12**, which transforms the naive T cells into effector T cells of T_H1 type; **IL-1** and **TNF-α**, which increase the expression of adhesion molecules on endothelial cells, which facilitates the extravasation of additional inflammatory cells.
- The APCs may also release **IL-1, IL-6**, and **IL-23** which transform the naive T cells into effector T cells of T_H17 type. T_H17 type of T Cells are activated in some infections

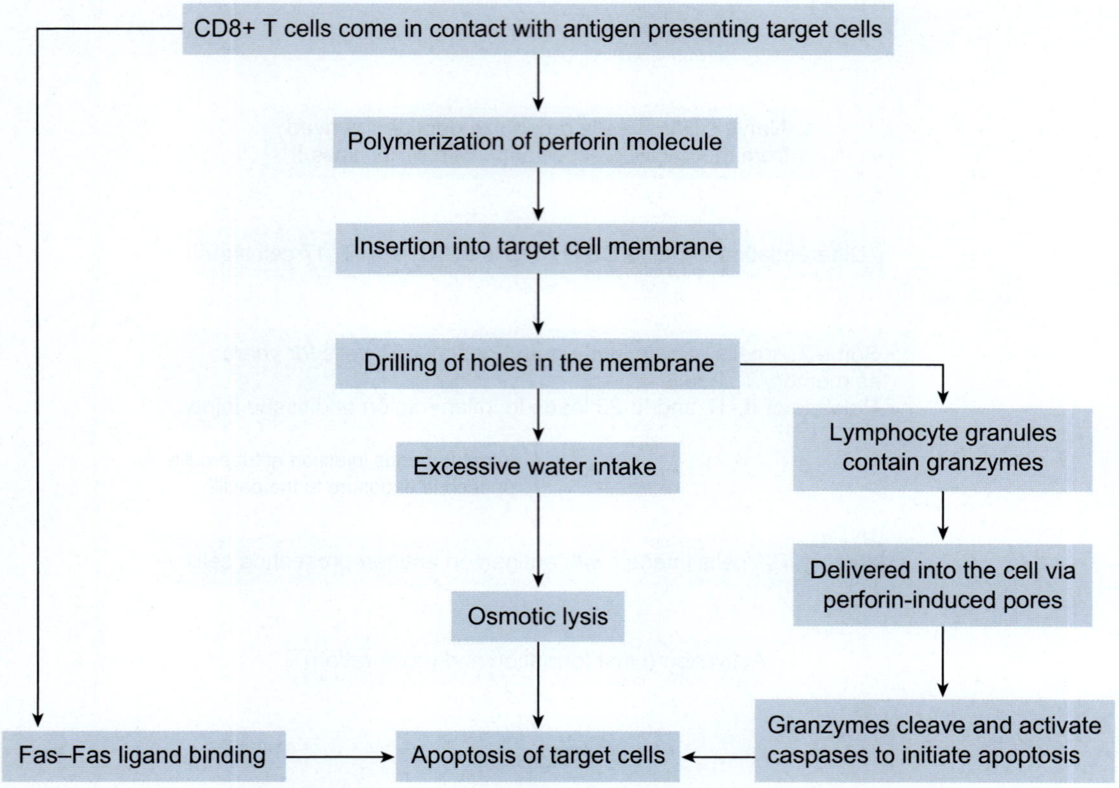

Flowchart 6.9 T cell-mediated cytotoxicity/cytolysis.

as well as autoimmunity and produce IL-17, IL-22 and chemokines which are pro-inflammatory and recruited polymorphs and monocytes to the site.

T Cell-Mediated Cytotoxicity/Cytolysis (Flowchart 6.9)

- Sensitized CD8+ T cells (cytotoxic T lymphocytes or CTLs) kill antigen-bearing target cells and seem to have an important role in:
  - Graft rejection.
  - Resistance to viral infections.
- There are two principal mechanisms of T cell-mediated damage:
  - **Delivery of cytotoxic proteins:** Perforins and granzymes are soluble mediators contained in the lysosome-like granules of CTLs. Perforin, released between the conjugated CTL and the target cell, is polymerized in the presence of Ca^{2+} and forms pores in the plasma membrane of the target cell, not only causing lysis but also permitting the delivery of granzymes. Granzymes activate caspases, normally present in an inactive proenzyme form that ultimately result in apoptotic death of the cell.
  - **Fas–Fas ligand-dependent killing:** The cross-linking of Fas receptor (on the target cells) by its ligand, membrane-bound FasL on the CTL, results in the activation of the extrinsic (death-receptor–initiated) pathway of apoptosisism.

Q. Tabulate differences between the different types of hypersensitivity. (PA9.2)

Ans. Differences between types I, II, III and IV hypersensitivity are summarized in Table 6.8.

Q. Write briefly on lepromin reaction. (PA9.2)

Ans. Lepromin (emulsified, lepromatous tissue rich in lepra bacilli and standardized according to lepra bacilli contents) is injected intradermally and the response is noted.

Two Phases

- **Early reaction of Fernandez** develops in 24–48 h and subsides in 3–5 days. It manifests with erythema and induration. Poorly defined, this reaction has little significance. It is analogous to tuberculin reaction.
- **Late reaction of Mitsuda** starts in 1–2 weeks, reaches its peak in the 4th week and gradually subsides over the next few weeks. It manifests with an indurated skin nodule, which may later ulcerate. Histological sections show infiltration by lymphocytes and formation of epithelioid and giant cells.

Note: This test is used to check CMI status of the individual against lepra bacilli. It is not helpful as a diagnostic test.

Q. Define immunologic tolerance. What are its different types? (PA9.1)

Ans. An individual is incapable of developing an immune response to a specific self-antigen and, hence, is capable of living in harmony with one's own cells and tissues. This is called immunologic tolerance. Tolerance is of two types—**central tolerance** and **peripheral tolerance**. **Central tolerance** develops very early in the life of an immune cell, which encounters the self-molecules in the body during development. This initiates a self-destruction pathway, which leads to the death of the auto-reactive cell before it attains maturity. This process, called

Table 6.8 Differences between types I, II, III and IV hypersensitivity

Features	Type I	Type II	Type III	Type IV
Reaction type	Anaphylactic	Cytotoxic	• Serum sickness • Arthus reaction	Delayed hypersensitivity
Cells involved	Mast cells, basophils, eosinophils, neutrophils, monocytes, CD4+ T cells, B cells	Non-sensitized macrophages, NK cells, neutrophils, eosinophils, B cells	Neutrophils, B cells	CD4+ T cells, macrophages, CD8+ T cells
Antibody type	IgE	IgG, IgM	IgG, IgM	None
Chemical mediators	IL-3, 4, 5; vasoactive amines	Complement system	Complement system	Lymphokines, IL-12, IL-2, INF-γ, TGF-β, TNF-α
Antigen presentation by APC	Required	Not required	Required	Required
Pre-sensitization	Required	Not required	Required	Required
Pathogenesis	Formation of IgE and immediate release of mediators to recruit inflammatory cells inducing inflammatory changes	Opsonization and phagocytosis, ADCC, antireceptor antibody type	Formation and deposition of Ag–Ab complexes → activates complement system → neutrophils recruited → release of lysosomal enzymes and other toxic agents	Sensitized T- lymphocytes mediate release of lymphokines T cell-mediated cytolysis
Time for onset	Minutes	Hours to days	Hours to days	Hours to days
Examples	Allergic bronchial asthma	Transfusion haemolytic reactions	Glomerulonephritis, rheumatoid arthritis	Transplant rejection

clonal deletion, helps ensure that 'self-reactive' T cells and B cells, that could develop the ability to destroy the body's own cells, do not mature and attack healthy tissues. Lymphocytes can only develop tolerance towards antigens that are present in the bone marrow (for B cells) and thymus (for T cells).

In **peripheral tolerance**, the body's immune cells might recognize a self-molecule but do not build up an immune response to it (switch off) because some of the chemical signals required to activate the T or B cell are absent. This is labelled clonal anergy. A special class of regulatory T cells that inhibits helper or cytotoxic T cell is involved in the development of peripheral tolerance.

1. **Mechanisms of development of central tolerance (clonal elimination or deletion)**
   (a) Central tolerance develops during lymphocyte development and operates in the thymus and bone marrow.
   (b) Here, T and B lymphocytes that recognize self-antigens are deleted before they mature into fully immunocompetent cells, preventing autoimmunity.
   (c) Self-antigens are present in both organs due to endogenous expression within the organ and importation of antigen due to circulation from peripheral sites.
   (d) In the case of **T cell central tolerance**, additional sources of antigen are made available in the thymus by the action of the transcription factors AIRE (**autoimmune regulator**) and Fezf2. A protein product of AIRE gene is crucial for deletion of immature self-reactive T cells.
   (e) **Positive selection** occurs first when näive T cells are exposed to antigens in the thymus. T cells, which have receptors with sufficient affinity for self-MHC molecules are selected. Other cells that do not show sufficient affinity to self-antigens will undergo a deletion process known as **death by neglect,** which involves apoptosis of the cells. This does not occur in B cells.
   (f) **Negative selection** of T cells with a very high affinity to self-MHC molecules is induced to anergy or lineage divergence to form T-regulatory cells.
   (g) Immature B cells in the bone marrow undergo negative selection when they bind self-peptides. B cell receptors recognize non-self antigen or pathogen associated molecular proteins (PAMPs). Auto-reactive B cells undergo apoptosis (clonal deletion), receptor editing (the self-reactive B cell changes specificity by rearranging genes and develops a new BCR that does not respond to self), go into a state of anergy (non-reactivity). Stimulation of CD40 on the B cell induces the expression of Fas on that cell and stimulation of B cell Fas by Fas ligand on the T cell causes the death of that anergic B cell.
2. **Mechanisms of development of peripheral tolerance**
   (a) **Clonal anergy**
      (i) Prolonged or irreversible inactivation of lymphocytes is labelled anergy.
      (ii) Activation of antigen-specific T cells requires two signals:
         – Recognition of peptide antigen in association with MHC molecule on the surface of antigen-presenting cell.
         – Second set of costimulatory signals provided by antigen-presenting cells.

(iii) Certain T cell-associated molecules such as CD28 must bind to their ligands B7-1 and B7-2.
(iv) If the antigen-presenting cell does not bear a CD28 ligand, a negative signal is generated to induce anergy.
(v) B cell anergy develops if B cells come across self-antigen in the absence of specific helper T cell.

(b) **Peripheral suppression by T cells**
(i) A population of T cells is called **'regulatory T cells'**. These cells have the ability to down regulate function of autoreactive T cells. This is mediated by secretion of cytokines.
(ii) CD4+ T cells of T_H2 type are the best-known 'regulatory cells' and are thought to mediate their action via cytokines like IL4, IL10 and TGF β.

(c) **Clonal deletion by activation-induced cell death**
(i) CD4+ T cells that recognize self-antigens may receive signals that promote their death by apoptosis.
(ii) Lymphocytes express Fas (CD95), a member of TNF receptor family.
(iii) Fas ligand (Fas L) is a member protein that is structurally homologous to the cytokine TNF, and is expressed mainly on activated T lymphocytes.
(iv) Engagement of Fas by Fas L induces apoptosis of activated T cells and may cause peripheral deletion of autoreactive T cells.
(v) Self-reactive B cells are also deleted by Fas L on T cells due to engaging of Fas on B cells.

(d) **Antigen sequestration:** Some antigens are hidden from the immune system because the tissues in which these antigens are located do not communicate with the blood and lymph, for example testis, eye and brain.

Q. Differentiate between central and peripheral tolerance. (PA9.1)

Ans. Differences between central and peripheral tolerance are enlisted in Table 6.9.

Table 6.9 Differences between central and peripheral tolerance

Features	Central tolerance	Peripheral tolerance
Origin	Thymus/bone marrow	Peripheral tissue
Mechanism	Clonal deletion of self-T/B cells	Clonal deletion, clonal anergy, peripheral suppression by T cells
Role in autoimmune diseases	Failure may not result in autoimmune diseases	Failure usually results in autoimmune diseases

Q. Write in detail on the mechanism of development of autoimmunity. (PA9.4)

Ans. Development of autoimmunity is related to:

- **Susceptibility genes** which influence the maintenance of self-tolerance.
- **Environmental triggers,** particularly **infections,** which promote the activation of self-reactive lymphocytes.

Mechanisms of Development of Autoimmunity

1. **Breakdown of T cell anergy**
   (a) Autoreactive T cells that escape clonal deletion are rendered anergic when they encounter self-antigens expressed on costimulator deficient antigen-presenting cells (APCs).
   (b) Anergy is broken if APCs are induced to express co-stimulatory molecules (induction may occur consequent to infections, tissue necrosis, inflammation, etc.).
2. **Failure of activation-induced cell death:** Defects (congenital or acquired) in the Fas–Fas ligand system (responsible for apoptosis) may lead to persistence and proliferation of autoreactive T cells in the peripheral tissues.
3. **Failure of T cell-mediated suppression:** Loss of regulatory/suppressor T cells that can limit the function of autoreactive T and B cells.
4. **Molecular mimicry**
   (a) Some infective agents share epitopes with self-antigens.
   (b) Immune response against such microbes produces a tissue damaging reaction, for example rheumatic heart disease: cross-reaction between antibodies to streptococcal M protein and cardiac glycoproteins.
5. **Polyclonal lymphocyte activation**
   (a) Several microorganisms and their products (e.g. bacterial lipopolysaccharides or endotoxins) are capable of inducing polyclonal B cell activation or CD4+ T cells activation in an antigen-independent manner. Because they stimulate all T cells that are associated with a set of V TCRS, they are called **super antigens** (SAgs).
   (b) They do so by binding to MHC class II on APC and β chains on TCR outside the antigen-binding groove.
   (c) This causes a massive immune response that is not specific to any particular epitope on the SAg.
   (d) Among T cells activated by super antigens, some may be reactive to self-antigens leading to autoimmunity.
   (e) SAgs produce an immune response that is effectively useless. Microbes produce SAgs as a defence mechanism to aid them in evading the immune system.
6. **Release of sequestered antigens (anatomic sequestration):** Any self-antigen that is completely sequestered during development is likely to be viewed as *foreign when introduced in the circulation*, for example spermatozoa {post-traumatic orchitis) and ocular antigens (uveitis).
7. **Exposure of cryptic self-antigens and epitope spreading (molecular sequestration):** A large number of self-determinants are not readily recognized by the immune system, and hence, T cells specific for such 'cryptic' self-epitopes are not deleted.

Evidence Implicating Genetic Factors in Development of Autoimmunity

- Familial clustering.
- Linkage of autoimmune diseases with HLA (Table 6.10).

Table 6.10 Linkage of autoimmune diseases with HLA

Disease	HLA allele
Rheumatoid arthritis anti-cyclic citrullinated peptides (CCP) antibody positive.	DR4
Type 1 diabetes	DR3, DR4, DQB1 position-β 57
Multiple sclerosis	DR15
Systemic lupus erythematosus	DR3, DR8, DR15
Ankylosing spondylitis	B27
Celiac disease	DQ2, DQ8

- Induction of autoimmune diseases in HLA-B27 transgenic rats.
- Linkage of autoimmune diseases with non-MHC genes, which may be either disease specific or associated with the multiple disorders, for example polymorphisms in **PTPN22**, polymorphisms in **NOD2** and the genes coding for **IL-2 receptor** and **IL-23 receptor** (Table 6.11).

Q. Classify autoimmune diseases. (PA9.4)

Ans. Autoimmune diseases can be organ specific or systemic. Classification of autoimmune diseases is given in Table 6.12.

Q. Describe the aetiopathogenesis and clinicopathological features of systemic lupus erythematosus (SLE). (PA9.5)

Ans. SLE is a classical prototype of a multisystem disease of autoimmune origin.

Table 6.11 Linkage of autoimmune diseases with non-MHC genes

Gene involved	Disease	Function
PTPN22	RA, IBD	Protein tyrosine phosphatase; affects signalling in lymphocytes
IL2RA	MS	α-chain of the receptor for IL-2; important in growth and survival of activated and regulatory T cells
IL23R	IBD, PS, AS	Receptor for T_H17 inducing cytokine IL-23; may affect differentiation of CD4+ cells into pathogenic T_H17 effector cells
CTLA4	RA	Terminates activation and promotion of regulatory T cells; inhibit T cell responses and interfere with self-tolerance
NOD2	IBD	May control resistance to gut commensals
ATG16	IBD	May be involved in autophagy of microbes

Table 6.12 Classification of autoimmune diseases

Organ specific	Systemic
• Autoimmune haemolytic anaemia • Atrophic gastritis (pernicious anaemia) • Multiple sclerosis (MS) • Good pasture syndrome • Insulin-dependent diabetes mellitus • Graves disease • Hashimoto thyroiditis	• Rheumatoid arthritis • Sjögren syndrome • Systemic lupus erythematosus (SLE)

Clinical Features

- **Chronic, remitting, relapsing, commonly febrile illness** characterized by **injury to skin, joints, kidneys and serosal membranes.**
- **Females** are more commonly affected than males.
- May be **acute or insidious** in onset; usually arises in the second or third decade (no age exempt).
- **Clinical manifestations of SLE include:**
  - Constitutional (fatigue, fever, arthralgia, weight changes).
  - Musculoskeletal (arthralgia, myalgia, arthritis, avascular necrosis).
  - Dermatologic (malar rash, photosensitivity, discoid lupus).
  - Renal (acute or chronic renal failure, nepritis).
  - Neuropsychiatric (seizure, psychosis).
  - Pulmonary (pleural effusion, pneumonitis, pulmonary hypertension, interstitial lung disease).
  - Gastrointestinal (nausea, dyspepsia, abdominal pain).
  - Cardiac (pericarditis, myocarditis).
  - Haematologic (leukopenia, lymphopenia, anaemia, or thrombocytopenia).
- Patients with the above clinical features usually give a positive family history of autoimmune disease.

Diagnosis of SLE

The classification of 1997 was replaced by SLICC (Systemic Lupus International Collaborating Clinics) classification in 2012. Further ACR and EULAR published new criteria for the classification of SLE in 2019 (Table 6.13).

Investigations

- Complete blood count (CBC) with differential count.
- Complement levels (low C3, C4 or CH50 levels).
- Kidney function tests
  - Serum creatinine.
  - Urinalysis with microscopy (an active urinary sediment defined as >5 RBCs per hpf; >5 WBCs/hpf in the absence of infection; or cellular casts limited to RBC or WBC casts).
  - Spot protein/spot creatinine ratio greater than 0.5 g/day can substitute for the 24-hour protein measurement.
- Liver function tests.
- Inflammatory markers (ESR and CRP).
- Direct Coombs test (assay for anti-red cell antibody in the absence of clinically evident haemolytic anaemia).
- Joint radiography (periarticular osteopaenia and soft-tissue swelling without erosions).
- Chest imaging studies (for interstitial lung disease, pneumonitis, pulmonary emboli, and alveolar haemorrhage).

Table 6.13 Single criteria in the four SLE classification criteria sets since 1982

ACR 1982	ACR 1997	SLICC 2012	EULAR/ACR 2019	
			Mucocutaneous	
1. Malar rash		1. Acute cutaneous LE*	Acute cutaneous LE	6
		or SCLE	SCLE	4
2. Discoid rash		2. Chronic cutaneous LE*	Discoid LE	4
3. Photosensitivity		3. Oral ulcers or nasal ulcers	Oral ulcers	2
4. Oral ulcers		4. Non-scarring alopecia	Non-scarring alopecia	2
5. Arthritis		5. Synovitis	Joint involvement	6
6. Serositis		6. Serositis	Serosal	
a) Pleuritis		Pleuritis	Effusion	5
b) Pericarditis		or pericarditis	Acute pericarditis	6
7. Renal disorder		7. Renal	Renal	
a) Persistent proteinuria		Proteinuria	Proteinuria	4
b) Cellular casts		or red cell casts		
		Histology compatible with lupus	ISN/RPS II/V	8
		nephritis	ISN/RPS III/IV	10
8. Neurologic disorder		8. Neurologic	Neuropsychiatric	
a) Seizures		Seizures	Seizure	5
b) Psychosis		Psychosis	Psychosis	3
		Mononeuritis multiplex		
		Myelitis		
		Peripheral or cranial neuropathy		
		Acute confusional state	Delirium	2
9. Hematologic disorder			Hematologic	
a) Hemolytic anemia		9. Hemolytic anemia	Coombs+ hemolytic anemia	4
b) Leukopenia			Leukopenia	3
c) Lymphopenia		10. Leukopenia		4
d) Thrombocytopenia		or lymphopenia		
10. Immunologic disorder		11. Thrombocytopenia	Thrombocytopenia	6
a) LE cell preparation			SLE-specific antibodies	6
b) Anti-DNA	a) Anti-DNA	12. Anti-dsDNA	Anti-dsDNA	2
c) Anti-Sm	b) Anti-Sm	13. Anti-Sm	Anti-Sm	
d) False-positive syphilis serology	c) Anti-phospholipid	14. Anti-phospholipid	Anti-phospholipid	3
		15. Low complements	Low complement	4
			C3 or C4 low	
			C3 and C4 low	
		16. Coombs test without hemolytic anemia		
11. ANA	11. ANA	17. ANA	Entry criterion ANA	

Note: Within each domain, only the highest-weighted criterion is counted toward the total score.
(*Source*: Martin Aringer et al, New Criteria for Lupus. *Curr Rheumatol Rep.* 2020; 22(6): 18. Published online 2020 May 13. doi: 10.1007/s11926-020-00896-6. Table 1.)

- Echocardiography (pericardial effusion, pulmonary hypertension, or verrucous Libman-Sacks endocarditis).
- Renal biopsy.

Antibody Tests

- Fundamental defect in regulatory mechanisms that sustain self-tolerance.
- Characterized by presence of antibodies to:
  - Nuclear antigens.
  - Cytoplasmic antigens.
  - Cell surface antigens.
  - Antigens of blood elements.
- **Antinuclear antibodies (ANAs)** include:
  - Antibodies to DNA.
  - Antibodies to histones.
  - Antibodies to non-histone proteins bound to RNA.
  - Antibodies to nucleolar antigens.
- Most reliable technique to demonstrate ANAs is indirect immunofluorescence (IF) which shows four basic patterns, namely:
  - Homogenous/diffuse nuclear staining: Antibodies to chromatin, histones and double stranded (ds) DNA.
  - Rim or peripheral staining patterns: Antibodies to ds DNA.
  - Speckled pattern: Most common and least specific pattern. IF shows uniform- and variable-sized specks, which indicate presence of antibodies to sm (Smith) antigen, RNP (ribonucleoprotein), SS-A and SS-B.
  - Nucleolar pattern: Most commonly seen in systemic sclerosis. IF shows discrete spots in the nucleus which indicate antibodies to nucleolar RNA.
- The fluorescence patterns are not absolutely specific for the type of antibody as there can be more than one antibody or a combination of patterns.
- ANA is the screening test with 95% sensitivity but is usually not diagnostic without clinical symptoms.
- **Antibodies to Sm antigen and ds DNA are however virtually diagnostic of SLE.**
- Correlation between presence of certain ANAs and clinical manifestations is noted, for example **high titers of ds DNA**

antibodies are found to be associated with active renal disease. Anti-ds-DNA is highly specific but sensitivity is variable depending on disease activity.

- Anti-SSA (Ro) /Anti-SSB (La) are present in 15% patients of SLE. More common in Sjogren syndrome.
- Antiphospholipid (AP) antibodies (antibodies against plasma proteins complexed to phospholipids, for example prothrombin, annexin V, β2 glycoprotein 1, proteins C and S as well as antibodies against RBCs, platelets and lymphocytes may also be seen in SLE).

Pathogenesis of SLE

Pathogenesis of SLE is thought to be multifactorial:

- **Genetic factors**
  - Increased risk in family members and concordance in monozygotic twins noted.
  - MHC genes are thought to regulate the production of autoantibodies (specific polymorphisms of HLA-DQ are linked to the production of anti-ds DNA, anti-Sm and AP antibodies).
  - Non-MHC genes may also contribute.
  - Lupus patients may have inherited deficiency of early complement components; for example, C4 or C1q C2 (lack of complement impairs removal of circulating immune complexes and defective phagocytic clearance of apoptotic cells).
  - The genome-wide association studies have indicated the involvement of more than sixty genetic loci. These loci encode proteins which are responsible for lymphocyte activation and cytokine (IFN) responses. Genes previously associated with other autoimmune diseases have been associated with SLE (e.g. *PTPN22* and diabetes; *STAT4* and rheumatoid arthritis).
  - Several genes associated with T-cell function and signalling have been found to be associated with SLE (*PTPN22, TNFSF4, PDCD1, IL10, BCL6, IL16, TYK2, PRL, STAT4,* and *RASGRP3*). Also, immune-complex processing and innate immunity genes, including several complement genes (*C2, C4A,* and *C4B*) have also been implicated.
- **Environmental factors**
  - Drugs such as hydralazine and procainamide are known to induce an SLE-like response.
  - Ultraviolet light may bring about changes in DNA such that it becomes immunogenic.
  - Sex hormones are thought to be involved in the pathogenesis (since females are affected more than males).
  - Silica dust and cigarette smoking may increase the risk of developing SLE.
  - Vitamin D deficiency has been implicated in autoimmunity and the development of rheumatic diseases, including SLE.
- **Immunologic factors**
  - Susceptibility genes interfere with normally existing self-tolerance. Defective elimination of self-reactive B cells in the bone marrow results in failure of self tolerance in B cells. Environmental insults induce apoptosis and defective clearance of the nuclei of the apoptotic bodies which in turn increases the burden of nuclear antigens (redistribution of cellular antigens during necrosis/apoptosis leads to a cell-surface display of plasma and nuclear antigens in the form of nucleosomes).
  - There is dysregulation of T cells which show abnormalities in effector activity such as CD8 cytotoxicity; T-regulatory, B-cell activity; migration; and adhesion.
  - Self-nucleic acids may mimic their microbial counterparts to activate TLRs which send signals to B cells specific for nuclear antigens as well as dendritic cells resulting in production of antinuclear antibodies. Dendritic cells produce type 1 IFN which stimulates B cells.
  - Tissue damaging antibodies are driven against self-antigens (results from an antigen-specific helper T cell-dependent B cell response). The lesions of SLE are mainly caused by immune complexes (type III HS).

Morphological Features of SLE

Most characteristic lesions result from deposition of immune complexes in the kidneys, connective tissues and skin.

Kidneys

- Light microscopic involvement is seen in 60%–70% cases; whereas, immunofluorescence (IF) and electron microscopic (EM) changes are seen in most cases.
- Six morphological patterns are recognized:
  1. Class I (Minimal mesangial): Rare; no changes seen on light microscopy; however, IF or EM can identify immune complex deposition in the mesangium.
  2. Class II (Mesangial proliferative): Also called mesangial lupus glomerulonephritis, this comprises 20% of all cases and manifests with minimal clinical symptoms. It is morphologically characterized by:
     (a) Increased intercapillary mesangial matrix and cells.
     (b) Granular mesangial deposits of immunoglobulins and complement on IF.
  3. Class III (focal proliferative): Manifests with mild to moderate haematuria and proteinuria. It is morphologically characterized by:
     (a) Involvement of less than 50% of all glomeruli.
     (b) Swelling and proliferation of endothelial and mesangial cells.
     (c) Neutrophilic infiltrate; fibrinoid deposits, and intercapillary thrombi. Extracapillary proliferation with crescent formation may also be seen.
     (d) Class III lupus nephritis is further subclassified as follows:
        (i) Class III (A), focal proliferative: Active lesions.
        (ii) Class III (A/C), focal proliferative and sclerosing: Active and chronic lesions.
        (iii) Class III (C) (focal sclerosing): Chronic lesions.
  4. Class IV (diffuse proliferative; Fig. 6.9: Overtly symptomatic and shows the following morphological features:
     (a) More than or equal to 50% glomeruli are affected.
     (b) Involvement of the entire glomerulus is labelled 'global' (IV-G) glomerulonephritis and part of the glomerulus is labelled 'segmental' (IV-S) glomerulonephritis.
     (c) There is proliferation of endothelial, mesangial and epithelial cells.
     (d) Epithelial crescents may be seen in Bowman's space.

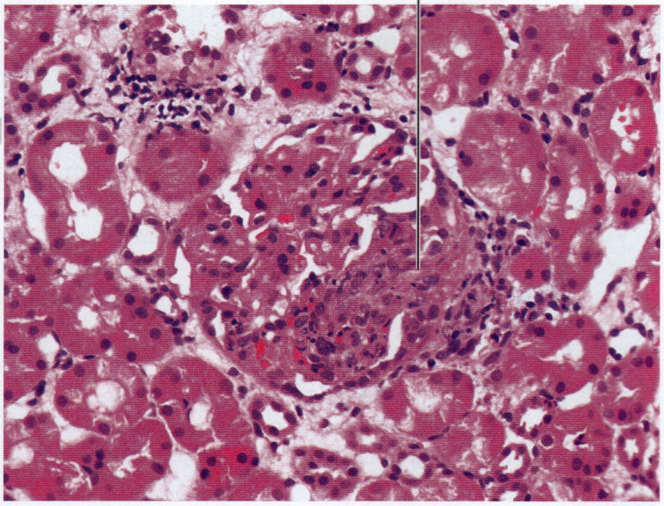

Fig. 6.9 Section from renal biopsy of a patient with lupus nephritis showing diffuse proliferative glomerulonephritis (H&E; 400×).

(e) Also present are fibrinoid necrosis and hyaline thrombi in glomeruli.

(f) Class IV lupus nephritis is also further subclassified, as follows:
   (i) Class IV-S: Diffuse segmental proliferative.
   (ii) Class IV-G: Diffuse global proliferative.
   (iii) Class IV-S or IV-G, active (A) or chronic (C).

5. Class V (Membranous): Comprises 15% of all cases and manifests with severe proteinuria with nephrotic syndrome. Main light microscopic change is widespread thickening of capillary walls.
6. Class VI (Advancing sclerosing): Represents end-stage renal disease wherein >90% glomeruli are sclerosed.

- The immune complexes may be deposited in the basement membrane, mesangium, subepithelial zone (between basement membrane and visceral epithelial cells, as in membranous glomerulonephritis) and subendothelial zone (between basement membrane and endothelium). When extensive, subendothelial deposits create a peculiar thickening of the capillary wall called '**wire loop lesions**'.
- Changes in interstitium and tubules may be seen in cases with diffuse involvement.
- **Prominent changes in other organs**
  (a) **Libman–Sacks endocarditis** (non-bacterial verrucous endocarditis) and pericarditis.
  (b) Capsular thickening, follicular hyperplasia, increased plasma cells and thickening of penicilliary arteries (onion skinning) in spleen.
  (c) Pleuritis, pleural effusion, alveolar injury in the form of oedema and haemorrhage and chronic interstitial fibrosis in lungs.
  (d) Acute necrotizing vasculitis of small vessels.
  (e) Cutaneous lesions (erythema on bridge of the nose and cheeks labelled butterfly rash, maculopapular lesions on the extremities, urticaria, bullae).
  (f) Non-erosive synovitis.
  (g) Endothelial damage by immune complexes results in intimal proliferation and occlusion of small vessels in CNS leading to neuropsychiatric manifestations.

Q. Write briefly on scleroderma. (PA9.7)

Ans. The term scleroderma is derived from the Greek words skleros (meaning hard or indurated) and derma (skin). It is characterized by skin hardening and induration, which is progressive in nature. Scleroderma is better termed systemic sclerosis (SS), as it is a systemic connective tissue disease that not only involves skin but also involves subcutaneous tissue, muscles, and internal organs (lungs, heart, digestive system, kidneys, muscles, joints, and nervous system).

Pathogenesis

Many factors have been implicated in the pathogenesis of SS including genetic, environmental (CMV infection, specific geographical locations), and immunological (ANA positivity) (Flowchart 6.10).

Accumulation of CD+ T cells in response to an unknown antigen as well as activation of humoral immunity

↓

Secretion of cytokines and their soluble receptors and enzymes and their inhibitors [profibrotic cytokins, include transforming growth factor-beta (TGF-beta), interleukin-4 (IL-4), platelet-derived growth factor (PDGF), and connective-tissue growth factor]

↓

Vascular changes (intimal proliferation, capillary dilatation and endothelial damage) and changes in the extracellular matrix compounds (Fibronectin; proteoglycans; and collagen types I, III, V and VII)

↓

Increased collagen deposition or disturbances in its degradation

Flowchart 6.10 Pathogenesis of scleroderma.

Clinical Spectrum and Diagnosis

SS has many clinical forms ranging from 'limited cutaneous SS' to 'diffuse skin sclerosis' and 'diffuse cutaneous SS with extensive internal organ involvement'. It may occasionally have a fulminant course (fulminant SS).

1. **Limited cutaneous SS**
   (a) **CREST syndrome** (calcinosis, Raynaud phenomenon, oesophageal hypomotility, sclerodactyly and telangiectasias) was the earlier term used to describe this condition.
   (b) Typically involves areas distal to the elbows and knees with the face and neck.
2. **Diffuse cutaneous SS**
   (a) Involves the trunk and the skin of the extremities proximal to the elbows and knees along with involvement of the face.
   (b) The GI, respiratory, renal, cardiovascular, musculoskeletal, endocrine and genitourinary systems are also frequently involved.

The main diagnostic features of SS are as follows:

Skin changes

- Morphea (localized scleroderma) manifests as solitary or multiple sclerotic dermal plaques.
- Early stages of SS show diffuse oedema of hands and feet followed by progressive skin tightening and sclerodactyly (claw hand).
- Other cutaneous changes associated with SS include calcinosis, telangiectasias, digital ulcers and pits, contractures, hyperpigmentation and hypopigmentation, characteristic mask like facies.

Vascular changes: Raynaud phenomenon, ischemic digital and leg ulcers.

Changes in lungs:

- Interstitial lung disease and pulmonary hypertension.
- Aspiration pneumonitis caused by oesophageal motility problems leading to reflux.
- Decreased thoracic compliance and respiratory muscle weakness.

Changes in the heart: Cardiomyopathy, congestive heart failure, arrhythmias.

Renal changes: Scleroderma renal crisis.

Changes in the joints: Arthralgia and arthritis, myopathy, myositis.

Gastrointestinal changes: Gastroesophageal reflux and abnormalities of motility and peristalsis of entire GIT leading to bloating, early satiety, stasis, and pseudoobstruction, oesophageal stricture.

Endocrine changes: Hypothyroidism.

Neurologic changes: Carpal tunnel syndrome and trigeminal neuralgia.

Immunological changes: SS-related autoantibodies (anticentromere, antitopoisomerase I, and anti-RNA polymerase III 3).

Morphology

- *Early stages* show oedema and collagen degeneration with perivascular mononuclear inflammation which at times becomes intense enough to obstruct the vascular lumina.
- *Late stages* of both localized and systemic scleroderma show collagenization/hyalinization of connective tissue of deep dermis, subcutaneous fat, fascia, and muscles with perivascular and interstitial lymphocytic and plasma cell infiltrate. Epidermis and adnexal structures show atrophy. There is thickening and luminal narrowing of small blood vessels. Diminished elastic tissue and dystrophic calcification of blood vessels may be seen.
- *Kidneys* are involved frequently and show thickening of the tunica intima of interlobular arteries owing to concentric proliferation of intimal cells and fibrinoid necrosis.
- *GIT* shows atrophy of the muscularis and replacement by fibrosis.
- *Skeletal muscle* shows interstitial fibrosis with degeneration.
- *Lungs* show interstitial fibrosis.

Q. Write briefly on Sjögren syndrome. (PA9.7)

Ans. Sjögren's syndrome is an autoimmune condition that can occur at any age, but is most common in older women.

Clinical Features

It presents with a triad of sicca symptoms—xerophthalmia (dry eyes or keratoconjunctivitis sicca), xerostomia (dry mouth), and parotid gland enlargement. Other less common manifestations include:

- Arthralgias and arthritis.
- Raynaud phenomenon and vasculitis.
- Pulmonary and gastrointestinal disease.
- Haematological abnormalities like anaemia and leukopenia.
- Lymphadenopathy.
- Neuropathy.
- Development of lymphoma.
- Cutaneous manifestations (dry skin or xeroderma, purpura, urticaria).

Primary Sjögren syndrome occurs in the absence of another underlying rheumatic disorder, whereas **secondary Sjögren syndrome** occurs secondary to another underlying collagen vascular disease, such as SLE, RA, or scleroderma. Inappropriate T cell and B cell activation are both implicated in the pathogenesis. In genetically susceptible individuals, a viral infection may trigger the disease. Autoimmunity to a cytoskeletal protein called alpha-fodrin is being investigated.

Diagnosis

Diagnosis of Sjögren syndrome requires at least two of the following three findings:

- Positive serum anti-SSA (Ro) and/or anti-SSB (La) antibodies or positive rheumatoid factor and ANA titer of at least 1:320.
- Ocular staining score of at least 3.
- Presence of focal lymphocytic sialadenitis.

Morphology

- Extensive lymphoid infiltrate at places forming germinal centres.
- Interstitial fibrosis and acinar atrophy.
- Epithelial-myoepithelial islands.

Q. Define transplant rejection. Describe the pathogenesis, clinical features and morphology of acute and chronic rejection. (PA9.3)

Ans. Transplant rejection is defined as recognition by the host of the grafted tissue as foreign. Rejection is a complex process in which both **CMI** and **circulating antibodies** play a role. The degree of immune response to a graft is determined by the degree of genetic disparity between the grafted organ and the host. **Xenografts,** which are grafts between members of different species, elicit the maximal immune response. **Autografts,** which are grafts taken from one part of the body to be put in another part (e.g. skin grafts), are not foreign and, therefore, do not undergo rejection. **Isografts,** which are grafts between genetically identical individuals (e.g. monozygotic twins), also undergo no rejection. **Allografts** are grafts between members of the same species that differ genetically. This is the most common form of transplantation. Their rejection depends on the degree of histocompatibility between the donor and the recipient.

A. T cell-Mediated Reactions (cellular rejection; Fig. 6.10):

Occurs due to cytotoxic CD8+ T lymphocytes-mediated killing of grafted cells or delayed hypersensitivity, triggered by activated CD4+ T helper cells, and is mediated by two main pathways:

1. **Direct pathway** (Flowchart 6.11)
   (a) Host CD8+ and CD4+ T cells directly recognize MHC molecules on the surface of the graft APC.
   (b) The transplanted organ carries passenger APCs in the form of interstitial dendritic cells. Such APCs have a high density of allo-MHC molecules, and are capable of directly stimulating the recipient's T cells.
   (c) The relative number of T cells that proliferate is therefore extraordinarily high as compared with the number of clones that target antigen presented by self-APC. Thus, this pathway is important in acute allo-rejection.
   (d) CD8+ T cells recognise class I MHC antigens in the graft, get activated and transform into cytotoxic T cells (CTLs). Graft cells are then killed by CTLs resulting in parenchymal and endothelial damage in the graft tissue. Host CD4+ helper T cells recognize class II MHC antigens in the graft, get activated and release cytokines which induce a DTH response.
2. **Indirect pathway**
   (a) Recipient T lymphocytes recognize antigens of the graft donor after they are presented by the recipient's own antigen-presenting cells.
   (b) Uptake and processing of MHC molecules shed from the grafted organ by host antigen-presenting cells.

B. Antibody-Mediated Reactions

These are due to preformed antibodies, (e.g. hyperacute rejection).

Clinicopathological Features of Rejection

1. **Hyperacute rejection**
   (a) Humoral rejection occurring immediately post-transplantation is called hyperacute rejection.
   (b) It occurs minutes or hours after transplantation and leads to a cyanotic, mottled and flaccid kidney excreting a few drops of bloody urine.
   (c) There is a rapid accumulation of neutrophils within arterioles, glomeruli and peritubular capillaries along with deposits of immunoglobulins and complement in the vessel wall. EM shows endothelial injury with fibrin-plated thrombi.

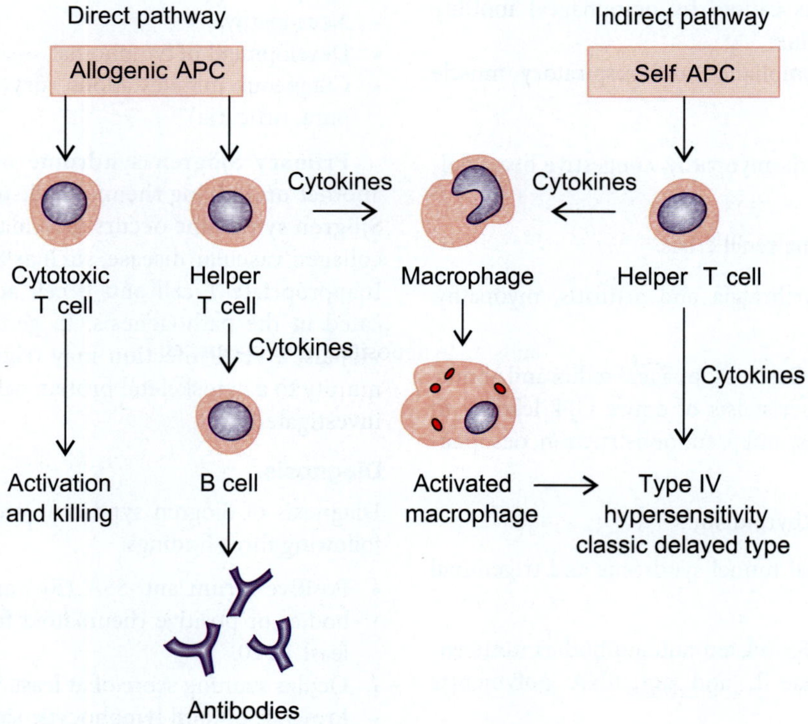

Fig. 6.10 T cell-mediated rejection.

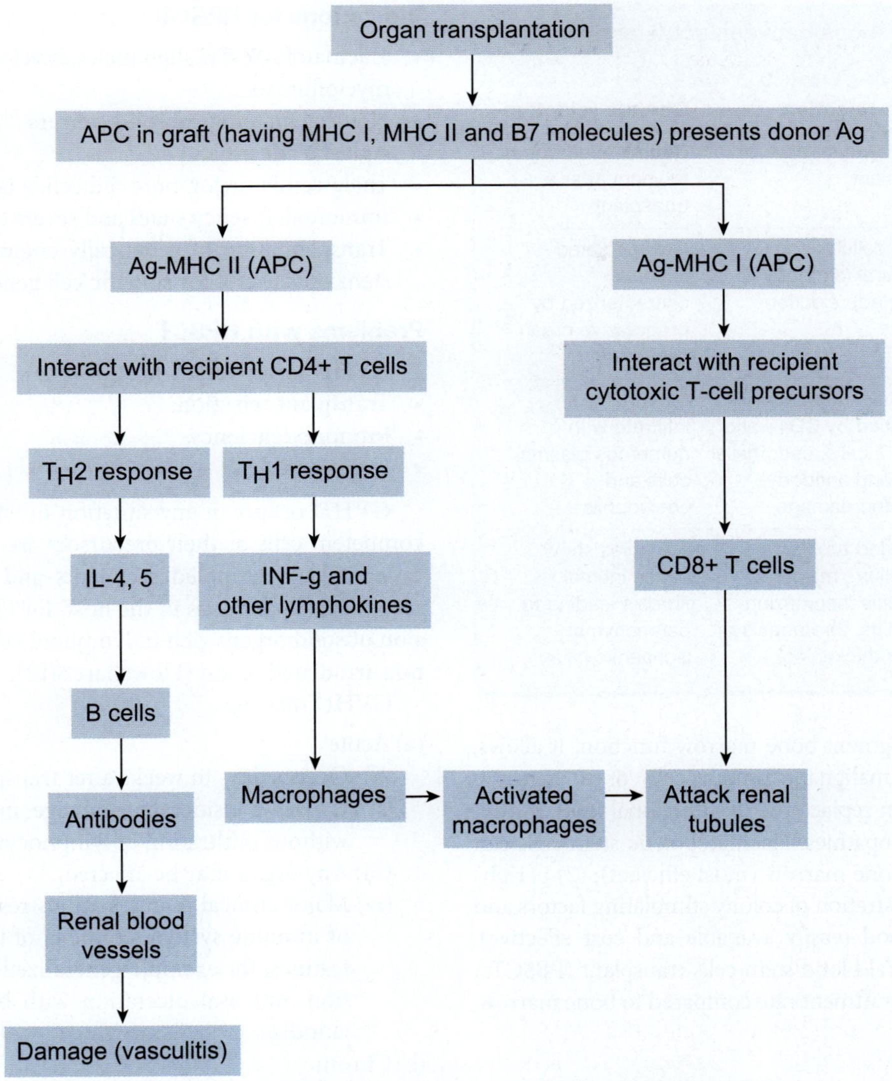

Flowchart 6.11 Direct pathway of cellular rejection.

2. **Acute rejection**
   (a) Occurs days, months or even years after transplant.
   (b) Both cellular and humoural responses involved.
   (c) **Acute cellular rejection** is mediated by T lymphocytes that have been activated against donor antigens. The donor dendritic cells (also called passenger leukocytes) enter the circulation and function as antigen-presenting cells (APCs).
   (d) **Humoral rejection** is primarily mediated by antibody and complement. It can occur immediately post-transplantation (**hyperacute**) or **during the first week**. The antibodies are either preformed antibodies or represent antidonor antibodies that develop after transplantation.

Features of acute cellular rejection:
- Increased serum creatinine with clinical signs of renal failure.
- Extensive interstitial mononuclear infiltrate, oedema and haemorrhage.
- Mononuclear cells in the glomerular and peritubular capillaries, which may invade tubules to induce tubular necrosis.
- Vascular endothelial injury mediated by CD8+ T cells.

Features of acute humoral rejection:
- Mediated primarily by the antidonor antibodies.
- Characterized by the necrotizing vasculitis, endothelial cell necrosis, neutrophilic infiltrate and deposition of immunoglobulins along with complement and fibrin.

3. **Chronic rejection**
   (a) Chronic rejection is both antibody- and cell-mediated and is characterized by progressive rise of serum creatinine over a period of 4–5 months.
   (b) It is dominated by vascular changes (dense intimal fibrosis), interstitial fibrosis, glomerular loss, tubular atrophy, shrinkage of renal parenchyma, interstitial infiltrate of plasma cells and eosinophils.

Q. Differentiate between acute and chronic transplant rejection. (PA9.3)

Ans. Differences between acute and chronic rejection are enlisted in Table 6.14.

Q. Write briefly on transplantation of haematopoietic cells. (PA9.3)

Ans. Bone marrow transplant (haematopoietic stem cell transplant or HPSCT) involves the administration of healthy haematopoietic stem cells in patients with dysfunctional/depleted bone

Table 6.14 Differences between acute and chronic rejection

Features	Acute rejection	Chronic rejection
Onset	Occurs within days of transplant	Occurs over months to years after a transplant
Components	Acute cellular and humoural (antibody-mediated) rejection	Cell-mediated rejection characterized by progressive organ dysfunction
Mechanism	Interstitial mononuclear infiltration by CD4+ and CD8+ T cells, endothelial injury and antibody-mediated damage	Mononuclear infiltrate with numerous plasma cells and eosinophils
Morphology	Damaged tubular epithelium, rejection vasculitis (necrotizing vasculitis, thrombosis or intimal thickening)	Arterioles show dense intimal fibrosis leading to parenchymal ischaemic injury

marrow in order to augment bone marrow function. It allows, either destruction of malignant/tumour cells or to generate functional cells that can replace the dysfunctional ones, for example in haemoglobinopathies. Haematopoietic stem cells can be collected from (1) bone marrow (most efficient); (2) peripheral blood after administration of colony stimulating factors and (3) umbilical cord blood (easily available and cost effective). Advantages of peripheral blood stem cells transplant (PBSCTs) include more rapid engraftment rate compared to bone marrow.

Types

1. ***Syngeneic Bone Marrow Transplantation***
   The donor and the recipient are identical twins therefore no graft versus host disease (GVHD) or graft failure ensues. However, it is difficult for most transplant patients to find an identical twin for transplantation.
2. ***Autologous Bone Marrow Transplantation***
   Haematopoietic stem cells are collected from the patient and are reinfused after purification methods. This prevents GVHD but the bone marrow products may contain abnormal cells that can cause relapse.
3. ***Allogenic Transplantation***
   The donor could be an HLA matched family member, unrelated matched donor or mismatched family donors (haploidentical).

Indications for HPSCT

- Haematological malignancies, myelodysplastic syndromes, myelofibrosis.
- Non-haematological solid cancers.
- Aplastic anaemia.
- Thalassemia major, pure red cell aplasia, sickle cell disease
- Immunodeficiency states and severe autoimmune disorders
- Transplantation of genetically engineered haematopoietic stem cells useful for somatic cell gene therapy.

Problems with HPSCT

- GVHD (graft-versus-host disease).
- Transplant rejection.
- Immunodeficiency.
- Infections.

GVHD occurs in any situation in which immunologically competent cells or their precursors are transplanted into immunologically crippled recipients and the transferred cells recognize alloantigens in the host, for example BMT, transfusion of solid organs rich in lymphoid cells, and transfusion of non-irradiated blood (Flowchart 6.12).

GVHD may be:

(a) Acute
   (i) Occurs days to weeks after transplant.
   (ii) Causes considerable damage mediated by cytokines without infiltration of lymphocytes.
   (iii) Any organ may be affected.
   (iv) Major clinical manifestations result from involvement of immune system, epithelia of the skin, liver and intestines, for example generalized rash with desquamation, mucosal ulceration with bloody diarrhoea and jaundice.

(b) Chronic
   (i) May follow acute GVHD or occur insidiously.
   (ii) Characterized by extensive cutaneous injury, destruction of skin appendages and fibrosis of dermis (differential systemic sclerosis).
   (iii) Manifests with chronic liver damage with cholestasis, oesophageal strictures and life-threatening infections (due to involution of thymus and depletion of lymphocytes in lymph nodes).

Q. Describe the physical and chemical nature of amyloid. (PA3.1)

Ans. Amyloid is an **amorphous, eosinophilic, pathologic, proteinaceous** substance deposited in **between cells** or **extracellularly**.

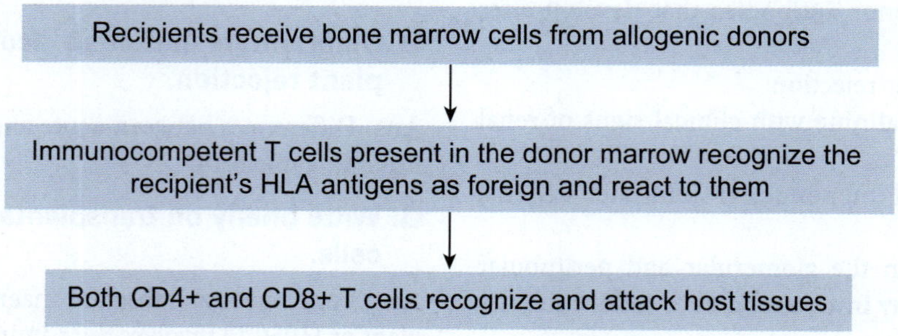

Flowchart 6.12 Mechanism of GVHD.

- First described by **Rokitansky** in 1842; it was named 'amyloid' by **Virchow**. It is not a distinct entity but a **group of diseases having in common deposition of similar appearing proteins** constituted by insoluble abnormal fibrils that injure tissue.
- The fibrils are formed by the **aggregation of misfolded, abnormally soluble proteins,** which bind to various **proteoglycans** and **glycosaminoglycans or GAGs (heparin and dermatan sulphate, apolipoprotein-E and serum amyloid P protein or SAP)**. Amyloid was so named because the charged sugar groups in the adsorbed proteins resulted in a staining pattern similar to amylase, it was however, later found to be unrelated to starch.

Physical Nature of Amyloid

The main physical constituents of amyloid are **non-branching fibrils of indefinite length and a diameter of 7.5–10 nm,** which on X-ray crystallography and infrared spectroscopy show a **cross-β-pleated sheet conformation (Fig. 6.11).**

Chemical Nature of Amyloid

- Amyloid is composed of **95% fibril proteins, 5% P (pentagonal) component** and other glycoproteins.
- There are 23 biochemically different fibril proteins, of which the most common ones are:

  AL (amyloid light chain) protein
  - The precursor protein is a clonal immunoglobulin light chain or light chain fragment, derived from plasma cells.

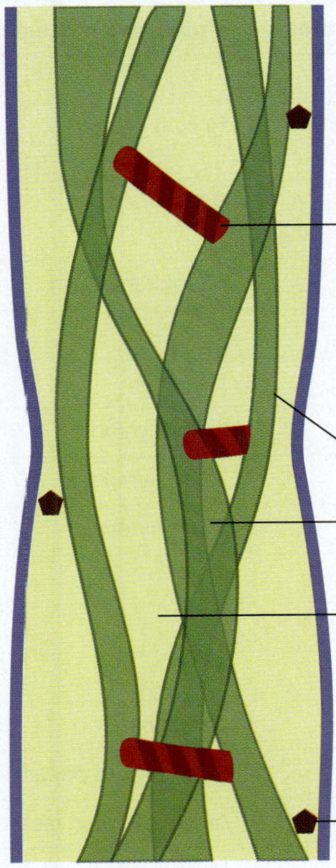

Fig. 6.11 Schematic representation of structure of amyloid fibril and P component. Each fibril is composed of β-pleated sheets of twin filaments arranged in a double helical pattern.

  - Most AL are composed of lambda light chains; some have kappa chains.
  - AL amyloidosis is associated with monoclonal B cell proliferations. It is labelled 'primary amyloidosis' because it is not associated with any primary disease and its clinical manifestations are due to effects of amyloid deposition. A large number of AL amyloidoses have marrow plasmacytosis.
  - Typical organs involved include the heart, kidney, peripheral nervous system, gastrointestinal tract, respiratory tract.

Heavy chain amyloidosis (AH): In a few cases, immunoglobulin chain amyloidosis fibrils contain only heavy-chain sequences rather than light-chain sequences, and the disease is termed AH rather than AL.

AA (amyloid-associated) protein
- It has a molecular weight of 8500 kDa and 76 amino acid residues.
- Derived from precursor SAA (serum amyloid-associated) protein; it is an acute phase reactant that circulates in the serum bound to high-density lipoprotein, HDL-3.
- AA protein deposits are associated with 'secondary amyloidosis', which occurs secondary to inflammatory conditions like tuberculosis, bronchiectasis, chronic osteomyelitis, autoimmune diseases and heroin abuse.

Transthyretin (TTR)
- TTR is a normal serum protein synthesized in the liver and choroid plexus that binds and transports thyroxine and retinal protein.
  Normal TTR usually deposits in the ventricles of elderly people (senile cardiac amyloidosis). This condition is mostly an incidental autopsy finding, but can sometimes present with heart failure and arrhythmias.
- A mutant form is deposited in familial amyloidotic polyneuropathies and in the hearts of aged individuals (senile systemic amyloidosis), gastrointestinal tract, and vitreous.
- The presentation of ATTR is fairly non-specific, but signs and symptoms typical of chronic heart failure, polyneuropathy, and carpal tunnel syndrome.

β2 microglobulin
- β2 microglobulin is a component of MHC Class I.
- It is a normal serum protein (light-chain component of the MHC) whose levels increase in patients on long-term haemodialysis.
- β_2 M is normally catabolized in the kidney after it is displaced from the MHC-I heavy chain in the proximal tubules, but in patients with decreased clearance the serum levels may mount.
- Aβ_2 M commonly deposits in the carpal ligaments, synovium, and bone, resulting in carpal tunnel syndrome, destructive arthropathy, bone cysts, and fractures. Other organs involved include the heart, gastrointestinal tract, liver, lungs, prostate, adrenals, and tongue

Aβ protein

- Aβ protein is a 4000 Da protein derived from amyloid
- It constitutes cerebral plaques in Alzheimer disease and is derived by proteolysis from a glycoprotein called amyloid precursor protein

Atrial natriuretic factor amyloidosis

- The precursor protein is atrial natriuretic factor (ANF), a hormone responsible for sodium and water homeostasis.
- As it is synthesized by the cardiac atria, the amyloid deposits are localized to the cardiac atria.
- It is highly prevalent in elderly people and is not clinically significant.
- ANF amyloidosis (AANF) is most common in patients with long-standing congestive heart failure, presumably because of persistent ANF production.

Calcitonin amyloid

- Patients with medullary carcinoma of the thyroid may develop localized amyloid deposition in the tumours, consisting of normal-sequence procalcitonin (ACal).
- The precursor protein is calcitonin, a calcium regulatory hormone synthesized by the thyroid.

Islet amyloid polypeptide amyloidosis

- In islet amyloid polypeptide amyloidosis (AIAPP), the precursor protein is an islet amyloid polypeptide (IAPP), also known as amylin, which modulates insulin activity, blood glucose levels, adiposity and body weight.
- IAPP is a protein secreted by the islet beta cells that are stored in the same granules as insulin.
- IAPP amyloid is found in insulinomas and in the pancreas of many patients with diabetes mellitus type 2.

Q. Classify amyloidosis. Describe the aetiology and clinicopathological features of the same. (PA3.1)

Ans. Classification of amyloidosis (Table 6.15): The classification of amyloidosis is based on the tissue distribution of amyloid deposits (**local or systemic amyloidosis**), the absence or presence of pre-existing disease (**primary or secondary amyloidosis**) and the **chemical type** of amyloid protein fibril (present day classification). The amyloidoses are named such that the name begins with a capital A (for amyloid) followed by an abbreviation for the fibril protein. For example, in myeloma-associated amyloidosis, the fibril protein is an immunoglobulin light chain (referred to as L) and the patients with these amyloidoses are said to have light-chain amyloidosis (AL).

Systemic Amyloidoses

Common types of systemic amyloidoses include:

1. **Reactive systemic amyloidosis or amyloidosis A (AA) or secondary amyloidosis**
   (a) AA is the most common systemic amyloidosis.
   (b) It occurs secondary to chronic inflammatory disorders, infections, and rarely neoplasms and typically involves the kidneys, liver and spleen.

Table 6.15 Classification of amyloidosis

Clinicopathological category	Associated conditions	Major fibril protein	Precursor protein
Systemic Amyloidosis			
Primary amyloidosis (Immunocyte dyscrasias associated amyloidosis)	Multiple myeloma and other monoclonal B cell proliferations	AL	Ig light chains
Secondary amyloidosis (Reactive systemic amyloidosis)	Chronic inflammatory conditions	AA	SAA
Haemodialysis-related amyloidosis	Chronic kidney disease	$A\beta_2m$	β2 microglobulin
Hereditary or Familial Amyloidosis			
Hereditary amyloidosis	—	AA	SAA
Familial Mediterranean fever	—	ATTR	Transthyretin
Familial amyloidotic neuropathies	—	ATTR	Transthyretin
Senile systemic amyloidosis	—	ATTR	Transthyretin
Localized Amyloidosis			
Senile cerebral	Alzheimer disease	Aβ	APP
Endocrine			
Thyroid	Medullary carcinoma	A Cal	Calcitonin
Islet of Langerhans	Type 2 Diabetes		Islet amyloid peptide
Isolated atrial amyloidosis	—	AANF	Arial natriuretic factor
Prion disease	Various prion diseases of the CNS	Misfolded prion proteins (PrP^{sc})	Normal prion protein

Source: Robbins & Cotran Pathologic Basis of Disease, Tenth Edition: Vinay Kumar, Abul K. Abbas, Jon C. Aster, Table 6.17, Page 261, Elsevier Inc., 2021.

(c) AA associated conditions include rheumatoid arthritis, ankylosing spondylitis, psoriasis, Crohn disease, ulcerative colitis, leprosy, tuberculosis, osteomyelitis, bronchiectasis, lymphomas, epithelial malignancies like renal cell carcinoma and heroin abuse, etc.

(d) Persistent inflammation, as seen in the aforementioned conditions, induces an increase in the synthesis of IL-6 and IL-1, both of which stimulate hepatocytes to synthesize more and more SAA, which in turn leads to amyloid deposition.

(e) Also, it has been postulated that monocyte-derived enzymes, that normally degrade SAA to soluble end products, which can be easily removed, may be defective leading to deposition of insoluble SAA aggregates. It is possible that a genetic abnormality leads to production of abnormally structured SAA molecules, which are resistant to the action of the monocyte-derived enzymes.

2. **Light-chain amyloidosis (AL) or primary amyloidosis**
   (a) AL is usually seen in association with plasma cell disorders (mostly just a monoclonal gammopathy in which abnormal protein is secreted without presence of an overt myeloma or a B cell lymphoma).
   (b) The precursor protein is a monoclonal immunoglobulin light-chain or light-chain fragment (free unpaired kappa or lambda chains, also called Bence–Jones proteins) synthesized by the neoplastic plasma cells.
   (c) These light chains and their fragments are amyloidogenic owing to their peculiar physical and chemical properties.
   (d) Organs mainly involved are the heart, kidneys, peripheral nervous system, gastrointestinal tract and respiratory tract.
3. **Heredofamilial amyloidosis**
   (a) This rare, familial amyloidosis that is location specific encompasses a variety of conditions.
   (b) Examples include:
      (i) Familial Mediterranean fever (autosomal recessive disorder characterized by excessive production of IL-1, fever, serositis and arthritis).
      (ii) Familial amyloidotic polyneuropathies (autosomal dominant disorders characterized by amyloid deposits in peripheral and autonomic nerves).

Localized Amyloidoses

Localized amyloidosis is usually seen in isolated organs, for example lungs, larynx, tongue, skin, urinary bladder where it presents as nodular masses.

Prion protein amyloidosis (APrP)

1. The precursor protein in APrP is a membrane glycoprotein called 'prion protein'.
2. APrP could be infectious (i.e. kuru and transmissible spongiform encephalitis) or genetic (i.e. Creutzfeldt–Jakob disease) in origin.
3. The infectious prion protein induces a conformational change in a native protease-sensitive protein, increasing the beta-pleated sheets. The accumulation of these beta-pleated sheets renders the protein protease-resistant and therefore amyloidogenic.
4. Autosomal dominant mutations in the prion protein gene increase its amyloidogenic potential.

Pathogenesis of Amyloidosis (Flowchart 6.13)

There are two types of amyloid proteins:

1. **Misfolded proteins** (*production of abnormal amounts of normal protein* which is unstable, self-associates to form oligomers and fibrils, called misfolded proteins). Misfolded amyloid proteins are thought to arise from infectious sources (prions), mutations, errors in transcription, translation, post-translational modification, or protein transport.
2. **Mutant proteins** (*production of normal amounts of abnormal/mutant protein* which is structurally unstable, prone to misfolding and subsequent aggregation). Abnormally folded

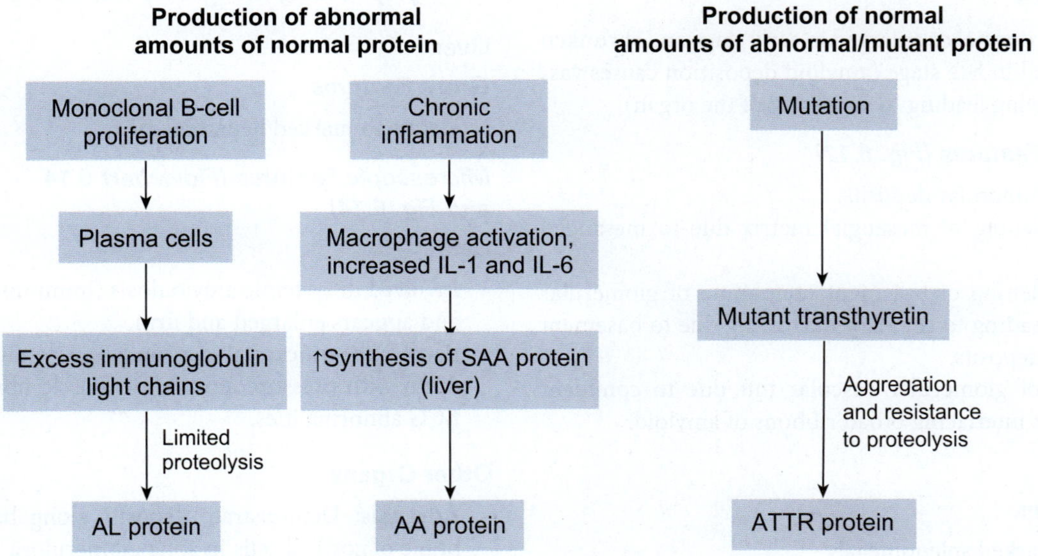

Flowchart 6.13 Pathogenesis of amyloidosis.

proteins get deposited in extracellular tissue as fibrils and disrupt normal tissue by causing pressure atrophy of adjacent cells and vascular narrowing; the latter leading to ischaemia.

Q. Write in detail on the morphological features amyloidosis. (PA3.2)

Ans. Amyloidosis is of two types:

- **Primary amyloidosis:** Affects kidneys, liver, spleen, lymph nodes, adrenal and thyroid.
- **Secondary amyloidosis:** Affects heart, kidneys, GIT, peripheral nerves, skin and tongue.

Gross Features

- Affected organs are enlarged, firm and waxy.
- Painting cut-surface with iodine imparts a yellow colour, which changes to bluish-violet after application of sulphuric acid.

Staining Characteristics

- **Congo red**
  - Ordinary light-pink or red colour.
  - Polarized light-apple green birefringence (due to cross-β-pleated configuration).
- **Metachromatic stains (Rosaniline dyes):** Examples are methyl violet and crystal violet. Amyloid takes up a rose pink colour with these dyes.
- **Fluorescent stains of Thioflavin T and S:** In ultraviolet light, amyloid fluoresces yellow.
- **Immunohistochemistry:** Anti-AA and anti-lambda, anti-kappa antibodies can be used to differentiate between different types of amyloid.
- **Toluidine blue:** Blue colour in ordinary light and dark red, birefringence under polarized microscopy.
- **Alcian blue:** Blue-green colour.
- **PAS (periodic acid-Schiff) and H&E stains:** Pink colour.

Histopathology

Kidneys (most common and most serious form of organ involvement).

Gross Features

- Kidneys are normal or enlarged in early stage and shrunken or contracted in late stage (amyloid deposition causes vascular narrowing leading to shrinking of the organ).

Microscopic Features (Fig. 6.12)

- Primarily glomerular deposits.
- Subtle thickening of mesangial matrix due to mesangial deposits.
- Uneven widening of basement membrane of glomerular capillaries leading to capillary narrowing due to basement membrane deposits.
- Distortion of glomerular vascular tuft due to confluent masses of or interlacing broad ribbons of amyloid.

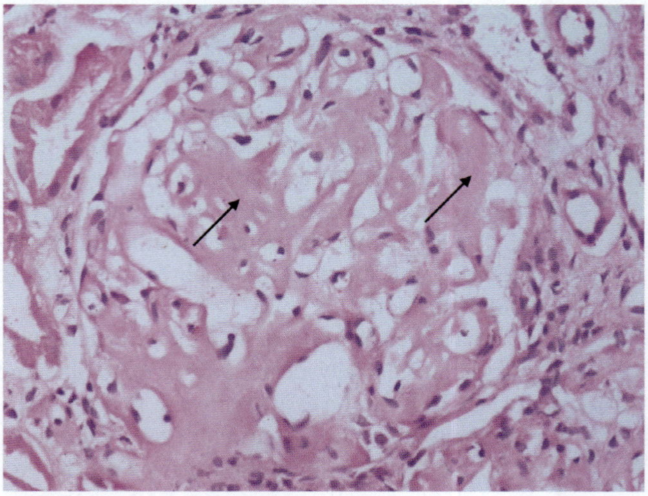

Fig. 6.12 Photomicrograph showing amyloid deposits in the glomerular vascular tuft resulting in its distortion *(arrows)*. The deposits are also seen in the arteriolar wall and peritubular connective tissue (H&E; 400×).

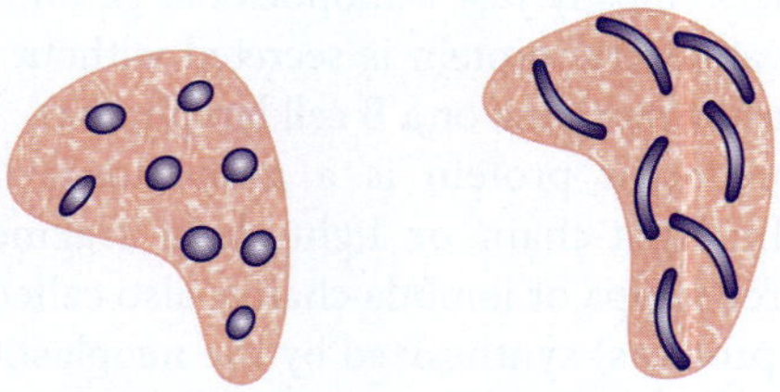

Fig. 6.13 Schematic diagram of spleen showing gross patterns of amyloid deposits.

Spleen

Gross Features

Moderate to marked splenomegaly.

Microscopic Features

There are two patterns of deposition (Fig. 6.13)

1. Sago spleen: Deposits largely limited to splenic follicles; entire follicle replaced by amyloid, leading to Tapioca-like granules.
2. Lardaceous spleen: Sparing of follicles; involvement of walls of splenic sinuses and connective tissue framework of red pulp, leading to large map like areas.

Liver

Gross Features

Moderate to marked hepatomegaly.

Microscopic Features (Flowchart 6.14 and Fig. 6.14)

Heart

- Involved in systemic amyloidosis (immunocyte dyscrasias) and appears enlarged and firm.
- Focal subendocardial accumulation within the myocardium with pressure atrophy of muscle fibres may induce ECG abnormalities.

Other Organs

- **Adrenals:** Demonstrate deposits along basement membrane of cortical cells in zona glomerulosa.

Deposition starts in space of Disse

↓

Amyloid deposits progressively encroached on adjacent parenchymal cells and sinusoids

↓

Deformity, pressure atrophy, replacement of hepatocytes

↓

Replacement of large areas of liver by amyloid

↓

Vascular involvement and deposits in Kupffer cells

Flowchart 6.14 Evolution of morphological changes in hepatic amyloidosis.

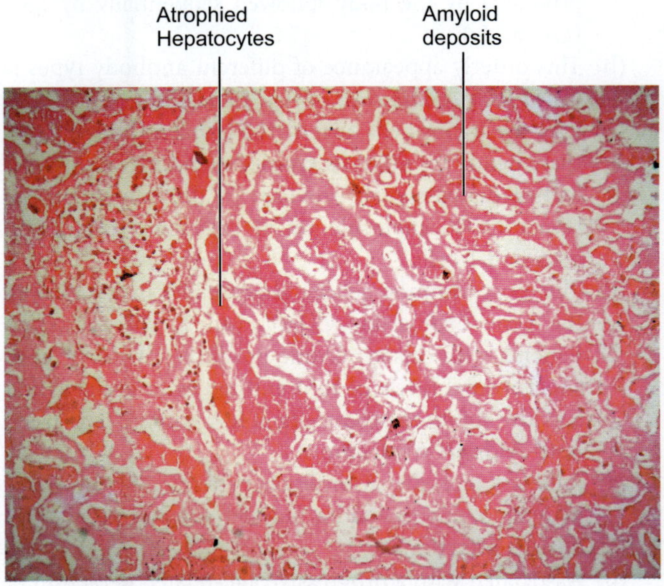

Fig. 6.14 Photomicrograph showing extensive amyloid deposits with distortion of the hepatic architecture (H&E; 400×).

- **GIT:** Early lesions affect blood vessels but later submucosa, muscularis and sub-serosa can be affected.
- **Tongue:** Undergoes enlargement (pseudo tumour formation or macroglossia).
- **Respiratory tract:** Shows diffuse involvement of large and small bronchioles.
- **Skin:** Primary amyloidosis shows masses of eosinophilic, amorphous material in dermis, and subcutaneous tissue. **Macular amyloidosis** shows focal eosinophilic deposits in papillary dermis with basal layer damage and pigment incontinence. **Lichenoid amyloidosis** shows hyperkeratosis, acanthosis, basal hydropic degeneration with small eosinophilic globules in papillary dermis and pigment incontinence.

Clinical Features

- **Early, non-specific:** Weakness, loss of weight and lightheadedness.
- **Skin and joints:** Mucocutaneous lesions (petechiae, purpura, waxy papules, nodules, or plaques), and carpal tunnel syndrome.
- **Renal involvement:** Nephrotic syndrome (proteinuria), renal failure and uraemia.
- **Cardiac involvement:** Conduction disturbances, arrhythmias, restrictive cardiomyopathy, congestive cardiac failure and constrictive pericarditis.
- **Tongue involvement:** Hampers speech and swallowing
- **GIT involvement:** Diarrhoea, malabsorption and digestive disturbances.

Diagnosis

Depends on demonstration of amyloid by:

- **FNAC** of abdominal fat (Smears and cell blocks are prepared and stained with Congo red).
- **Biopsy** of kidney (in case of renal involvement), rectum or gingiva.
- **Imaging** (cardiac amyloidosis can be visualized with gated MRI and technetium pyrophosphate).

Investigations for Primary Amyloidosis

- Serum/urine electrophoresis for M spike.
- Immunoelectrophoresis.
- Serum free light chain test (now commercially available for diagnosis and treatment monitoring; can also measure the ratio of kappa chains to lambda chains).
- Urine samples to demonstrate small quantities of monoclonal paraprotein or Bence–Jones protein.
- Bone marrow aspiration.
- Echocardiography for the evaluation of amyloid heart disease.
- Doppler studies for vascular involvement.

Q. Differentiate between primary and secondary amyloidosis. (PA3.1, 3.2)

Ans. Contrasting features of primary and secondary amyloidosis are enlisted in Table 6.16.

Table 6.16 Contrasting features of primary and secondary amyloidosis

Features	Primary amyloid	Secondary amyloid
Biochemical composition	AL (light chain proteins); lambda chains more than kappa	AA, derived from larger precursor SAA
Associated diseases	Plasma cell dyscrasias such as multiple myeloma, B cell lymphoma	Chronic inflammation, autoimmune diseases, cancers
Pathogenesis	Stimulus → monoclonal B cell-proliferation → excess of light chains → partial degradation → insoluble AL fibril	Stimulus → chronic inflammation → activation of macrophages → cytokines → partial degradation → insoluble AA
Incidence	More common in developed countries	Common worldwide
Distribution	Kidney, heart, bowel, nerves	Kidney, liver, spleen, adrenals
Stains	Specific immunoassays with anti-kappa antibodies	Immunoassays with anti-AA

Q. Write briefly on primary or congenital immune deficiency diseases.

Ans. Caused by mutations in genes involved in lymphocyte maturation or function.

Common Congenital Immune Deficiency Diseases

1. **XLA (X-linked agammaglobulinaemia or Bruton disease)**
   (a) Failure of B cell maturation and absence of antibodies (due to mutations in BTK gene, which encodes B cell tyrosine kinase, required for delivering maturation signals from pre-B cells and B cell receptors).
   (b) Absence of gammaglobulin in the blood.
   (c) Manifests by about 6 months of age, when there is depletion of maternal immunoglobulins.
   (d) Patients are susceptible to recurrent bacterial or viral infections and infections with *Giardia lamblia.*
2. **Common variable immunodeficiency**
   (a) Heterogeneous group of disorders characterized by hypogammaglobulinaemia, impaired immune response and increased susceptibility to infections.
   (b) Onset in second decade.
   (c) Defects in antibody production due to unknown cause.
   (d) Plasma cells are absent, perhaps due to a block in antigen-stimulated B cell differentiation.
   (e) These patients are also prone to develop autoimmune diseases as well as lymphoid tumours.
3. **Selective IgA deficiency:**
   (a) Most common of all primary immunodeficiencies.
   (b) Failure of IgA production due to unknown cause (seemingly caused by a block in the terminal differentiation of IgA-secreting B cells to plasma cells).
   (c) Since IgA is the most common immunoglobulin in mucosal surfaces, its deficiency leads to recurrent sinonasal and pulmonary infections as well as diarrhoea.
4. **X-linked SCID (severe combined immunodeficiency):** Failure of both T cell and B cell maturation due to the mutation in the common γ chain of the cytokine receptor, leading to failure of IL-7 signalling and defective haemopoiesis (IL-7 is the growth factor responsible for stimulating survival and expansion of B and T cell precursors).
5. **Autosomal SCID:** Failure of T cell development and a secondary defect in antibody responses, which are due to a defect in the gene coding for ADA (adenosine deaminase), leading to accumulation of toxic metabolites, which hamper lymphocyte maturation and proliferation. ADA is an enzyme involved in purine metabolism.
6. **X-linked hyper-IgM syndrome:**
   (a) In normal individuals, IgM is the first antibody to be produced by the body followed sequentially by IgG, IgA and IgE.
   (b) This orderly appearance of different antibody types is called *heavy chain class isotype switching.*
   (c) IgM-producing cells turn on the transcription of genes that encode for other isotypes, depending on the contact-mediated signals provided by the interaction between CD40 molecule on B cells and CD40L on activated T cells.
   (d) The most common genetic abnormality is mutation in the gene coding for CD40L (on X chromosome). Patients with this syndrome produce normal or even supernormal levels of IgM antibodies to antigens but lack the ability to produce IgG, IgA and IgE isotypes.
7. **Wiskott–Aldrich syndrome**
   (a) X-linked recessive disorder characterized by thrombocytopenia, eczema and a marked susceptibility to recurrent infections.
   (b) Associated with a progressive age-related depletion of T lymphocytes in the peripheral blood and lymph nodes.
   (c) Also, there is inability to synthesize antibodies to polysaccharide antigens and increased susceptibility to encapsulated pyogenic organisms.

Q. Write in detail on the aetiopathogenesis of acquired immunodeficiency syndrome (AIDS). (PA9.6)

Ans. Acquired immune deficiency syndrome (**AIDS**) is a spectrum of conditions caused by infection with the human immunodeficiency virus (HIV), which is a retrovirus (genus *Lentivirus* part of the family *Retroviridae*). Lentiviruses are single-stranded, enveloped RNA viruses, which enter the target cell, where the viral RNA genome is reverse transcribed into double-stranded DNA by a virally encoded reverse transcriptase that is transported along with the viral genome in the virus particle. The viral DNA is then integrated into the cellular DNA by a virally encoded integrase and host co-factors.

Two genetically different but related forms of HIV, namely HIV-1 and HIV-2, are implicated. HIV-1 was the first virus to

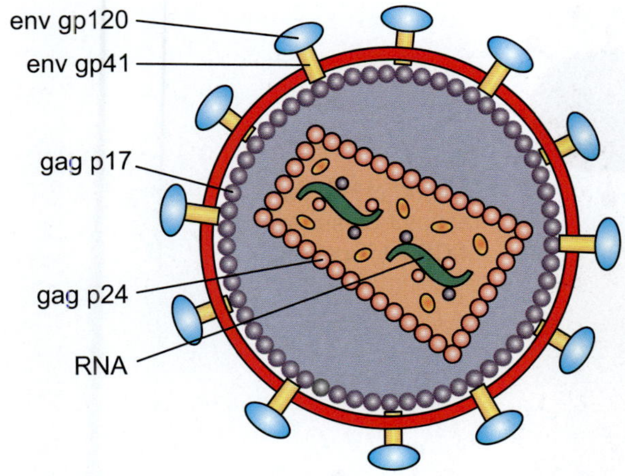

Fig. 6.15 Schematic representation of the structure of human immunodeficiency virus (HIV) virus.

be discovered (originally called LAV or HTLV-III). It is more virulent and infective and has been the cause for majority of HIV infections globally. Because of its relatively poor capacity for transmission, HIV-2 has largely remained confined to West Africa.

Structure of HIV Virus (Fig. 6.15)

- HIV virus is spherical in shape and contains an electron-dense, cone-shaped core which further contains:
  - Major capsid protein p24.
  - Nucleocapsid proteins p7/p9.
  - Two copies of genomic RNA.
  - Three viral enzymes (protease, reverse transcriptase and integrase).
- The viral core is surrounded by a matrix protein called p17.
- The viral envelope is studded with two glycoproteins, Gp120 and Gp 41, critical for infection.
- HIV proviral genome contains non-structural and regulatory genes like *LTR*, *vif*, *vpr*, *vpu*, *nef* and *rev*, which code for different viral proteins (Table 6.17).

Transmission Categories of HIV

- Male-to-male sexual contact.
- Heterosexual contact.
- Injection drug use.
- Male-to-male sexual contact and injection drug use.

Table 6.17 HIV genes coding for different viral proteins

Gag gene	Capsid protein p24, matrix protein p17, nucleocapsid protein p7/9
Poil gene	Reverse transcriptase, protease, integrase, ribonuclease
Env gene	Envelope glycoprotein gp160, cleaved in endoplasmic reticulum to gp120 (mediates CD4 and chemokine receptor binding), and gp41 (mediates fusion)

Routes of Transmission

- In 75%–80% cases HIV spreads by sexual contact (homosexual or bisexual population constituting the largest group) followed by blood and blood products, and needle or syringe use.
- It can also spread through other body fluids like rectal fluids, vaginal fluids, breast milk, sweat, urine, CSF, synovial, pleural, and pericardial fluid.
- These fluids must come in contact with damaged tissue or discontinuous mucous membrane or be directly injected into the bloodstream.
- Less commonly, HIV may spread from infected mother to child during pregnancy, birth, or breastfeeding (perinatal transmission). Health care workers can get HIV due to accidental inoculation with HIV-contaminated needle, or other sharp object (needle-stick injury).

Risk Factors

- Unprotected sexual intercourse, especially receptive anal intercourse.
- Multiple sexual partners.
- Previous or current sexually transmitted diseases (STDs).
- Sharing of intravenous (IV) drug paraphernalia.
- Receipt of blood products.
- Mucosal contact with infected blood or needle-stick injuries.
- Maternal HIV infection.

Infection of Cells with HIV (lifecycle of HIV/ Pathogenesis of HIV; Fig. 6.16)

The main targets of HIV infection are:

1. **Immune system:** HIV has selective tropism for host cells with CD4 molecular receptor like CD4+ T cells, macrophages/monocytes and dendritic cells/Langerhans cells.
   (a) ***CD4+ T lymphocyte*** (Flowchart 6.15).
   - HIV may be macrophage tropic (R5 virus strains) or CD4+ T cell tropic.
   - Its envelope has two glycoproteins, surface **Gp120** and **Gp41**.
   - Gp120 binds to CD4 molecule receptor on the host cell and undergoes conformational change that results in formation of a new recognition sites on Gp120 for the co-receptors **CCR5 or CXCR4** (T cell tropic-CXCR4 (α-chemokine) receptors are present on T cells, both freshly isolated and culture retained).
   - Gp120 then binds to the above chemokine receptors leading to a conformational change in Gp41. This second conformational change aids HIV in penetrating the cell membrane of the target cell to ultimately fuse with the host cell to form a syncytium.
   - This allows the viral core containing the HIV genome to enter the cytoplasm of the host cell.
   - The RNA genome of the virus then undergoes **reverse transcription** to synthesize a double stranded **complementary DNA (cDNA)**.

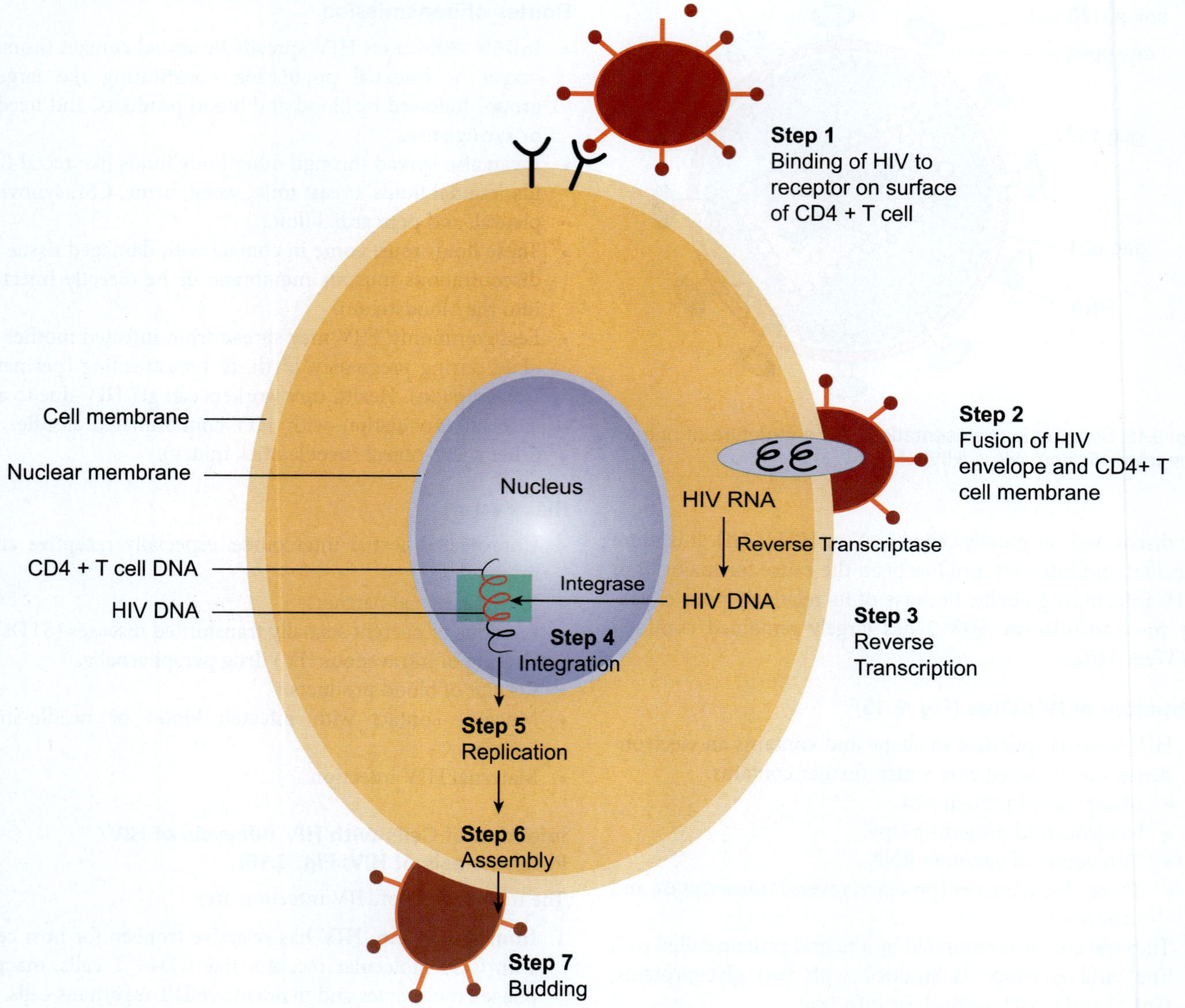

Fig. 6.16 Life cycle of HIV.

- In **quiescent CD4+ T cells** HIVcDNA remains in a linear episomal form in the cytoplasm. In dividing T cells HIV cDNA enters the nucleus and becomes integrated into the host genome using the protein **integrase**.
- Subsequent to integration, the provirus may remain silent (**latent infection**) or transcribe (**productive infection**) on exposure to antigen/cytokines.
- Transcription results in formation of a **complete viral particle,** which spreads between CD4^{+} T cells by two simultaneously ongoing routes: a) cell-free spread and b) cell-to-cell spread, also called **hybrid mechanisms**.
- In the cell-free spread, virus particles bud from an infected T cell, enter the blood/extracellular fluid and then infect another T cell following a chance encounter.
- HIV can also disseminate by direct transmission from one cell to another by a process of cell-to-cell spread.
- When there is extensive production of the new virus particles the infected host cell ruptures and dies (release of viral particles results in CD4+ T cell lysis).
- The virus can remain latent in the host lymphoid tissue for a long time. Active viral replication and dissemination however results in progression to AIDS.
- There is a specific decline in the CD4+ helper T cells, resulting in inversion of the normal CD4/CD8 T-cell ratio and dysregulation of B-cell antibody production.
- During the acute phase, HIV-induced cell lysis and killing of infected cells by CD8+ T cells accounts for CD4+ T cell depletion, although apoptosis may also be a factor. During the chronic phase, the consequences of generalized immune activation coupled with the gradual loss of the ability of the immune system to generate new T cells appear to account for the slow decline in CD4+ T cell numbers.

CD4+ molecule is a high-affinity receptor for HIV

↓

HIV gp120 binds with CD4 molecules

↓

Conformational changes in gp120 and formation of a new recognition site on it

↓

This new site binds to CCR5/CXCR4 (co-receptors) resulting in conformational change in gp41 with insertion of a fusion peptide present at the tip of gp41 into target cell membrane

↓

Viral core containing genome enters cytoplasm of cell

Flowchart 6.15 Steps in the binding of HIV virus to CD4+ T lymphocyte.

- Qualitative defects in T cells are observed in T cells even in asymptomatic patients (leading to clinical symptoms).

(b) ***Macrophages***

(i) Act as a factory and reservoir for the virus and a vehicle for HIV to be transported to other organs.

(ii) Provide a site for viral replication in late phase of the disease, when CD4+ T cell count is greatly decreased.

(iii) CCR5 (β-chemokine) receptors are present on monocytes/macrophage and freshly isolated peripheral blood T cells (not in vitro propagated T cell line).

(iv) T cell tropic-CXCR4 (α-chemokine) receptors are present on T cells, both freshly isolated and culture retained.

(v) M-tropic viruses are more efficient in transmitting AIDS but T-tropic HIV gradually accumulates and cause the final rapid phase of disease (being more virulent).

(c) ***Dendritic cells***

(i) Mucosal Langerhan cells capture the virus and transport it to regional lymph nodes.

(ii) Follicular dendritic cells in germinal centre of lymph nodes are reservoirs of HIV.

They have receptors for the Fc portion of immunoglobulins and can trap HIV virions coated with anti-HIV antibodies. They also have the capability of transmitting the virions to T lymphocytes.

2. **CNS**

(a) Viruses are carried to circulation by infected monocytes.

(b) Virus infects macrophages and microglia (HIV does not infect neurons).

(c) Neurological deficit is due to direct effect of Gp 120 or may be caused indirectly by viral products and soluble factors (IL-1, TNF-α, IL-6) produced by macrophages/microglia.

Progression of HIV Infection

- HIV infection has **two phases**. It starts as **acute infection** during which HIV infects CCR5 expressing memory T cells in the mucosal lymphoid tissue which is the largest reservoir of memory T cells.
- Host T cell lysis results in T cell depletion.
- Dendritic cells capture the virus and transport it to regional lymph nodes/peripheral lymphoid tissue.
- The virus replicates to cause viremia (acute retroviral/HIV syndrome). The rate of disease progression correlates directly with HIV RNA levels.
- This is followed by development of humoral and cellular immune response against viral antigens (cytotoxic T cell and anti HIV antibody) response.
- By about end of first week, the virus is detectable in blood using antigen tests such as polymerase chain reaction (PCR); however, antibody test findings are negative. During weeks 2–4, early antibodies to HIV may be detected.
- During weeks 10–24, the HIV viral load drops to its lowest point (**set point**) and antibodies develop higher affinity for viral antigens; therefore, antibody tests become positive for HIV. Seroconversion is now complete, and **chronic HIV infection** begins.

Q. Write briefly on the clinical presentation of HIV/AIDS.

Ans. HIV patients may present with signs and symptoms of any of the stages of HIV infection and their physical findings are usually those of the associated infection or malignancy. Manifestations include the following:

- **Acute seroconversion:** A self limited flu-like illness may be seen within 2–4 weeks of HIV infection when the patient manifests with fever, chills, rash, night sweats, muscle aches, sore throat, fatigue, lymph node enlargement and mouth ulcer.
- Later a stage called the **clinical latency stage (also called 'chronic HIV infection')** develops during which HIV is still

active but multiplies at very low levels. People with chronic HIV infection may not have any HIV-related symptoms, or only mild ones. This period can last a decade or longer.

- **Acquired immunodeficiency syndrome (AIDS)** is the condition that results from chronic HIV infection and is defined by an absolute CD4 cell count of less than 200 cells/μL and specific opportunistic infections or malignancies. The interval between acute HIV infection and AIDS is highly variable, with a median time of approximately 10 years.

Manifestations of AIDS include:

- Rapid weight loss or wasting.
- Recurring fever or profuse night sweats.
- Mucocutaneous exanthema.
- Persistent generalized lymphadenopathy (defined as lymph nodes enlarged to greater than 1 cm at two extrainguinal sites for at least 3 months without any obvious cause).
- Diarrhoea that lasts for more than a week.
- Sores/ulcers of the mouth, anus, or genitals.
- Oral and/or oropharyngeal and/or oesophageal candidiasis.
- Memory loss, depression, and other neurologic disorders. AIDS-associated dementia (HIV encephalopathy) manifests with loss of cognition.
- Manifestations resulting from opportunistic infections which occur when the immunity becomes very low.
- Manifestations resulting from anaemia, leucopenia, and thrombocytopenia.
- HIV-associated pneumonia, nephropathy, cardiomyopathy, septic arthritis, osteoporosis, osteomyelitis and myosotis.
- Dyslipidemia, hyperinsulinemia, hyperglycaemia, abnormal thyroid and gonadal function, inappropriate ADH secretion.

Sequelae include AIDS-associated dementia/encephalopathy and HIV wasting syndrome (chronic diarrhoea and weight loss with no identifiable cause).

Q. Enumerate the abnormalities of immune functions in AIDS.

Ans. HIV infection results in multiple abnormalities of immune functions, which include:

1. **Lymphopenia:** Selective loss of CD4+ T helper-inducer cells with reversal of CD4:CD8 ratio.
2. **Altered T cell functions in vitro**
   (a) Decreased lymphocyte proliferative response to mitogens and antigens.
   (b) Decreased cytotoxicity.
   (c) Decreased T helper cell function for B cells (decreased antibody production).
3. **Decreased T cell functions in vivo**
   (a) Loss of activated and memory T cells.
   (b) Defective type IV hypersensitivity.
   (c) Susceptibility to opportunistic infections and neoplasms.
4. **Altered monocyte/macrophage functions**
   (a) Decreased chemotaxis and phagocytosis.
   (b) Decreased HLA-II expression.
   (c) Decreased antigen presentation.
5. **Polyclonal B cell activation**
   (a) Hypergammaglobulinaemia and circulating immune complexes.
   (b) Decreased ability to mount an antibody response to a new antigen.
   (c) Loss of control/signals for B cell function in vitro.

Q. Enumerate the AIDS-defining opportunistic infections and neoplasms.

Ans. ***AIDS-defining opportunistic infections:***

Protozoal and Helminthic

- Cryptosporidiosis or isosporidiosis (enteritis).
- Toxoplasmosis (pneumonia or CNS infection).

Fungal

- Candidiasis (oesophageal, tracheal and pulmonary infections).
- Cryptococcosis (CNS infection).
- Coccidioidomycosis (disseminated infection).
- Histoplasmosis (disseminated infection).
- Pneumocystosis (pneumonia or disseminated infection).

Bacterial Infections

- Mycobacteriosis (*atypical* and *Mycobacterium tuberculosis*; pulmonary and extrapulmonary).
- Nocardiosis (pneumonia, meningitis and disseminated infections).
- *Salmonella* infections (disseminated).

Viral

- Cytomegalovirus (pulmonary, intestinal, retinal or CNS infections).
- Herpes simplex virus (localized or disseminated infection).
- Varicella zoster virus (localized or disseminated infection).
- Progressive multifocal leukoencephalopathy.

AIDS-Defining Neoplasms

- Kaposi sarcoma (Kaposi sarcoma herpes virus or KSHV).
- B cell non-Hodgkin lymphoma (EBV).
- Primary lymphoma of the brain (EBV).
- Invasive cancer of the uterine cervix (HPV).
- Anal carcinoma (HPV).

Q. Write briefly on Center for Disease Control (CDC) classification of categories of HIV infection.

Ans. The CDC classifies HIV infection into three categories, based on the presence of certain infections or diseases (Table 6.18).

Category A is asymptomatic HIV infection without a history of symptoms or AIDS-defining conditions.

Category B is HIV infection with symptoms that are directly attributable to HIV infection (or a defect in T-cell–mediated immunity) or that are complicated by HIV infection. These include bacillary angiomatosis, oropharyngeal candidiasis (thrush), vulvovaginal candidiasis, persistent or resistant pelvic inflammatory disease (PID), cervical dysplasia (moderate or severe)/cervical carcinoma in situ, oral hairy leukoplakia, idiopathic thrombocytopenic purpura, constitutional symptoms, such as fever (>38.5°C) or diarrhoea lasting more than 1 month, peripheral

Table 6.18 CDC classification of HIV infection

Clinical categories	CD4+ T cell categories		
	1 (≥500 cells/μL)	2 (200–499 cells/μL)	3 (<200 cells/μL)
A. Asymptomatic, acute primary HIV, or persistent generalized lymphadenopathy	A1	A2	A3
B. Symptomatic, not A or C conditions	B1	B2	B3
C. AIDS indicator conditions: including constitutional disease, neurologic disease or neoplasm			

Source: Data from Centers for Disease Control and Prevention: 1993 revised classification system and expanded surveillance definition for AIDS among adolescents and adults, MMWR 41(RR-17):1, 1992.

neuropathy, Herpes (shingles), involving two or more episodes or one or more dermatomes.

Category C is HIV infection with AIDS-defining opportunistic infections.

These three categories are further subdivided based on the CD4+ T-cell count. Categories A1, B1, and C1 are characterized by $CD4^+$ T-cell counts greater than 500/μL. Categories A2, B2, and C2 are characterized by CD4+ T-cell counts between 200/μL and 400/μL. HIV infections in patient with $CD4^+$ T-cell counts under 200/μL are designated as A3, B3, or C3.

Q. Write briefly on the laboratory diagnosis of AIDS.

Ans. Laboratory diagnosis of AIDS includes:

1. **Non-specific tests**
   (a) Decreased TLC.
   (b) Decreased lymphocyte count (<2000/mm^3).
   (c) Decreased CD4+ T cell count (<200 CD4+ T cells/μL) and reversal of T4:T8 ratio.
   (d) Thrombocytopenia.
   (e) Increased β2 microglobulin level.
   (f) Lymph node biopsy:
      (i) Early stage
      - Marked follicular hyperplasia.
      - Follicles extend to medulla and sometimes spread outside the capsule.
      - Mantle zone thinned out and germinal centres seem to merge with the interfollicular areas.
      - Presence of monocytoid B cells in and around sinusoids and in trabecular blood vessels.
      - Involvement of the B cell areas of the lymph node supports polyclonal B cell activation and hypergammaglobulinaemia.

      (ii) Disease progression
      - Severe follicular involution.
      - Follicles are depleted of cells.
      - Organized network of follicular dendritic cells disrupted.
      - Germinal centres become hyalinized.
      - Atrophic and small lymph nodes *(burnt out appearance)*.
      - In this stage, lymph nodes may harbour opportunistic infections.
      - The inflammatory response to infections in both nodal and extranodal sites may be atypical and sparse, for example granulomatous response to mycobacteria may not develop adequately because of deficient CD4+ T cells.
2. **Specific tests**
   (a) Antigen detection
      (i) Acute illness/seroconversion stage: p24 antigenaemia and viraemia, also appearance of IgM thereafter.
      (ii) Asymptomatic phase: decreased or absent free p24, but antibody-bound p24 antigen may be demonstrated.
      (iii) Clinical disease: increased free p24 antigen.

   Method: Antigen-capture ELISA
   In the first few weeks after infection and in terminal phase, the test is uniformly positive.

   (b) Antibody detection
      (i) Simplest and most widely used method.
      (ii) Negative in window period that follows infection (time taken for antibodies to appear); IgM appears first followed by IgG.

      Method: ELISA
      - Sensitive but not so specific.
      - *Types used*: 'Direct solid phase antiglobulin ELISA' and 'Capture ELISA specific for IgM antibody'.

      (iii) Western blot test: more specific than ELISA.
      (iv) PCR: Now 'new gold standard' test for diagnosis in all stages of HIV.

   (c) Direct virus isolation and culture in neoplastic T cell line.

As per CDC recommendations, diagnosis should start with a fourth-generation test that detects HIV in the blood earlier than antibody tests can; it identifies the viral protein HIV-1 p24 antigen, which appears in the blood before antibodies do. If this test is positive, an immunoassay that differentiates HIV-1 from HIV-2 antibodies should be performed. In patients with positive results on the initial antigen test but with negative or indeterminate results on the antibody differentiation assay, HIV-1 nucleic acid testing should be performed to determine whether infection is present.

7 Genetic and Paediatric Disorders

PART I: GENETIC DISORDERS

Q. Write briefly on the structure of a gene.

Ans. Human diseases that have a genetic basis arise from changes in the sequence or pattern of expression of genes. **A gene, which is the unit of heredity, is a piece of DNA that encodes a protein or RNA. It has a specific sequence of nucleotides that codes for a protein through a genetic code** (a sequence called **codon**) (Fig. 7.1).

- The boundaries of a gene are known as **start** and **stop codons.** The **start (initiator) codon** decides when to initiate the protein synthesis and the **stop (termination) codon** decides when to end it.
- The nucleotide sequence between the initiator and stop codon is the **exon** which is a region that contains the coding information that is both transcribed and translated into proteins and **introns** which are stretches between exons that do not code for a protein (**non-coding region**).
- On either side of a gene, there are non-coding regions called **flanking regions** that are responsible for the regulation of gene expression. They are called **regulatory regions**. These include **promoters** (regions which bind to transcription factors strongly or weakly), **enhancers** (regions that enhance the effects of a weak promoter) and **silencers** (regions that inhibit transcription).
- In the first stage of transcription, an enzyme called **RNA polymerase** binds to a **TATA** base sequence in the 5'-flanking region (at the 'front end' of the gene) adjacent to where transcription is initiated. There are other sequences in the region that serve as sites to which proteins that assist in transcription bind. This entire flanking region prior to the coding region of the gene is called the **promotor**.
- On the far end of the gene, past the coding region of introns and exons, is the **3'-flanking region** which largely remains untranslated.
- Once an mRNA is transcribed from the DNA coding region of a gene, it goes through several processing steps before it leaves the nucleus to be translated in the cytoplasm.
- Most of the human genome is located in the nucleus, with a small amount in the mitochondria.

Q. What are hereditary disorders?

Ans. These are disorders that are transmitted in the **germ line** through generations (therefore also called **familial**). The term congenital simply implies **'born with'**. Some congenital diseases are not genetic, for example, congenital syphilis. Not all genetic diseases are congenital; patients with Huntington disease, for example, begin to manifest their condition only after their twenties or thirties.

Q. What are alleles?

Ans. Alternative forms of same gene are called alleles. Genes with same alleles are called homozygous, while those with different alleles are called heterozygous. The most common functional allele at a locus is known as wild-type allele.

Q. Define gene polymorphism.

Ans. Gene polymorphism is an occurrence in a population of two or more genotypes in frequencies that cannot be accounted for by recurrent mutation. Genetic variations occurring in more than 1% of population would be considered useful polymorphisms for genetic linkage analysis. Such occurrences are generally long term. Genetic polymorphism may be balanced (such that allele frequencies are in equilibrium with one another at a given locus) or transient (such that a mutation is spreading through population in a constant direction).

Q. Define pleiotropy.

Ans. The phenomenon in which a single gene mutation leads to many phenotypic effects is called pleiotropism, for example **Marfan syndrome** is associated with widespread involvement

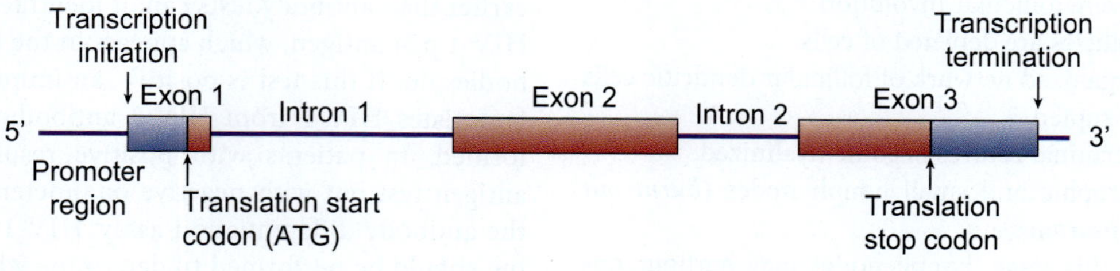

Fig. 7.1 Structure of a gene.

of the connective tissue component of skeleton, eye, cardiovascular system, etc. all of which result from a single mutation in the **gene fibrillin**.

Q. What are the different categories of genetic disorders? (PA11.1)

Ans. Different categories of genetic disorders are:

1. Those related to single-gene mutations of large effect **(Monogenic disorders):**
   (a) ***With classical Mendelian inheritance***
   (b) ***With non-classical inheritance***
   - ***Mitochondrial genes***
   - ***Trinucleotide repeats***
   - ***Genomic imprinting.***
2. Diseases with **multifactorial (polygenic) inheritance**, which involve both genetic and environmental influences **(complex multigenic disorders)**. They are caused by interaction between multiple variant forms of genes and environmental factors. These variations in genes are referred to as **'polymorphisms'**. Each variant gene causes a small increase or decrease in the risk of a disease. No single susceptibility gene is individually sufficient for inducing the disease. Several polymorphisms are required for the disease to occur.
3. Those arising from **structural** and **numeric aberrations** in autosomes and sex chromosomes **(chromosomal disorders).**
4. **Developmental defects**
   (a) *Agenesis* (complete absence of the organ, e.g. renal agenesis).
   (b) *Aplasia* (rudimentary organ with impaired development, e.g. aplasia of lung).
   (c) *Hypoplasia* (incomplete organ development so that the organ does not reach its normal size).
   (d) *Atresia* (incomplete development of the lumen in a luminal organ, e.g. oesophageal atresia).
   (e) *Dysplasia* (aberrant or defective tissue development, e.g. renal dysplasia).
   (f) *Deformation* (a condition arising from mechanical stress to normal tissue).
   (g) *Dysraphism* (results from failure of fusion like spina bifida).

Q. Define mutation. What are its types? (PA11.1)

Ans. Mutation refers to a permanent change in DNA. It can occur consequent to **errors in DNA replication, errors in DNA recombination, chemical or radiation damage to DNA.** DNA can be mutated either by **substitution, deletion** or **insertion of base pairs**. An **insertion** changes the number of DNA bases in a gene by adding a piece of DNA. A **deletion** changes the number of DNA bases by removing a piece of DNA. Small deletions may remove one or a few base pairs within a gene, while larger deletions can remove an entire gene or several neighbouring genes. **Duplication** consists of a piece of DNA that is abnormally copied one or more times.

Mutations can be classified based on:

1. **The cell type affected:** mutations which affect **germ cells** are transmitted to the progeny and may give rise to inherited diseases (**germ line mutations**). Mutations in the **somatic cells** are not transmitted to the progeny and may give rise to cancers and congenital malformations (**somatic mutations**).
2. **The effect of the mutation:** a type of mutation in which the altered gene product lacks the molecular function of the wild type gene is called a **loss of function, amorphic or null mutation**. This usually occurs due to deletion of the entire gene, nonsense mutation or a frameshift mutation. **Antimorphic mutation** is a type of mutation in which the altered gene product acquires function that is antagonistic to the wild type gene. When a mutation alters a gene product in such a way that it acquires a new molecular function it is labelled a **gain of function mutation**. These are generally due to missense mutation.
3. **The structural change in the chromosome:** rearrangement of genetic material results in structural change in chromosomes which could be subtle or prominent. Depending on the structural alterations mutations can be classified into -
   (a) **Genome mutations** involve loss or gain of whole chromosomes giving rise to monosomy or trisomy.
   (b) **Chromosome mutations** result from the rearrangement of genetic material to give rise to visible changes in the chromosome.
   (c) **Gene mutations** are the **most common mutations** associated with genetic diseases. They involve partial or complete deletion of a gene or often a single base.

Examples of Mutations

1. **Point mutations**
   - These can occur **within coding sequences** as well as **non-coding sequences.** The latter involve the regulatory sequences in the promoter/enhancer regions and not the exons.
   - Point mutations result from the substitution of a single nucleotide base by a different base, resulting in the replacement of one amino acid by the other in the protein, for example, sickle cell anaemia.
   - Such mutations alter the meaning of the genetic code and are thus called **missense mutations.**
   - Certain point mutations may change an amino acid codon to a **chain termination codon** or **stop codon**.
   - **Nonsense mutations** interrupt translation, leading to the formation of truncated proteins which are rapidly degraded.
   - If a base **substitution** occurs in the third position of the codon there is a good chance that a synonymous codon will be generated. Thus the amino acid sequence encoded by the gene is not changed and the mutation is said to be **silent.**
   - Point mutations are called **transition mutations** when a purine is substituted with another purine or when a pyrimidine is substituted with another pyrimidine and **transversion mutation** when a purine is substituted for a pyrimidine or a pyrimidine replaces a purine.
   - Point mutations or deletions involving regulatory sequences interfere with the binding of transcription factors leading to a gross reduction or complete absence of transcription (as seen in thalassaemias). Point mutations involving introns lead to defective splicing of intervening sequences.

2. **Frame shift mutations** occur when the insertion or deletion of one or two base pairs alter the reading frame of the DNA strand.
3. **Trinucleotide repeat mutations** are characterised by amplification of a sequence of three nucleotides; all affected sequences share guanine and cytosine, for example in fragile X syndrome, there are 200–400 tandem repeats of the sequence CGG within a gene called FMR1 (familial mental retardation-1), which prevents the normal expression of FMR1 gene leading to mental retardation.

Q. Write briefly on Mendelian inheritance disorders. (PA11.1)

Ans. Single gene defects (mutations) follow the Mendelian pattern of inheritance and are called Mendelian disorders. Mutations involving single genes usually follow one of the following three patterns of inheritance:

1. **Autosomal dominant (AD) disorders**
   (a) Only one abnormal allele is necessary to express the disease (manifests in the heterozygous state).
   (b) AD diseases are characterised by reduced penetrance, variable expressivity, and in some cases, late onset of the disease (e.g. familial polyposis, Huntington chorea). Each affected individual has an affected parent unless the condition has arisen from a new mutation in the germ cells forming that individual.
   (c) Phenotypic expression of an inherited mutant gene or percentage carriers of the gene who express the trait is called **penetrance.** When some individuals inherit the mutant gene but are phenotypically normal (i.e. a patient may have the abnormal gene but never expresses the disease), the trait is said to exhibit reduced penetrance.
   (d) If a trait is seen in all individuals carrying the mutant gene but they express the disease with different severity, it is called **variable expressivity** (e.g. neurofibromatosis).
   (e) The manifestations of these disorders depend on the nature of protein affected and the type of mutation. **'Loss of function mutations'** may affect proteins involved in control of complex metabolic pathways dependent on feedback regulation, such as mutation in gene responsible for synthesis of low density lipoprotein (LDL) receptor results in decrease in the number of the same leading to increased cholesterol levels; or structural proteins like collagen, a reduction of which leads to skeletal abnormalities. **'Gain of function mutations'** are less common and may lead to enhanced normal function of the protein, for example increased activity of enzymes; or may induce a new function in addition to the normal function of the protein, such as huntingtin in Huntington disease, which is neurotoxic to neurons.

   Examples: Von Willebrand disease, familial hypercholesterolaemia, adult polycystic kidney, Huntington chorea, congenital spherocytosis, familial polyposis, neurofibromatosis and Marfan syndrome.

   Neurofibromatosis is associated with neurofibromas, iris hamartomas (**Lisch nodules**), **café-au-lait spots,** skeletal lesions (**scoliosis**) and an increased incidence of other tumours (**acoustic neuromas, meningiomas, optic nerve gliomas and pheochromocytomas).**

   Marfan syndrome, due to a defect in fibrillin, primarily affects the skeleton (**eunuchoid habitus and arachnodactyly**), eyes (**dislocated lens**) and cardiovascular system (**mitral valve prolapse and dissecting aortic aneurysm**).
2. **Autosomal recessive (AR) disorders**
   (a) Largest group of Mendelian disorders.
   (b) Both abnormal alleles must be present (homozygous state) to express the disease.
   (c) Presence of a trait does not always affect the parents but siblings may be affected.
   (d) The chance of siblings getting affected is one in four.
   (e) May result from a consanguineous marriage.
   (f) Expression of the defect appears to be more uniform than in AD disorders.
   (g) Complete penetrance is common.
   (h) Onset is frequently early in life.
   (i) Because the affected individual may be an asymptomatic heterozygote, new mutations are rarely discovered clinically; several generations may pass before the descendants of such a person mates with other heterozygotes.

   Examples: Haemochromatosis, sickle cell anaemia, cystic fibrosis, Tay–Sachs disease, phenylketonuria, 21-hydroxylase deficiency, albinism, mucopolysaccharidoses (except Hunter syndrome), glycogenoses and galactosaemia.

   Lysosomal storage diseases are a group of diseases in which the absence of degrading enzymes leads to accumulation of complex substrates (e.g. sphingolipids and mucopolysaccharides) in the lysosome.

   Glycogenoses involve accumulation of glycogen in tissue due to increased synthesis or decreased degradation of glycogen.
3. **X-linked disorders**
   (a) All sex-linked disorders are X-linked; no Y-linked diseases are known.
   (b) Most X-linked disorders are recessive.
   (c) They are transmitted by heterozygous female carriers only to their sons.
   (d) Heterozygous females rarely express the complete phenotype of the disease as they have the paired normal allele. Due to inactivation of one of the X chromosomes in females (Lyon's hypothesis), it is possible for the normal allele to be inactivated resulting in full expression of the disease in heterozygote females.
   (e) An affected male does not transmit the disease to his sons, but all his daughters are carriers.

   Examples: Lesch–Nyhan syndrome (hyperuricaemia and self-mutilation due to deficiency of HGPRT), fragile X syndrome (mental retardation), haemophilia, glucose-6 phosphate dehydrogenase deficiency, testicular feminisation, chronic granulomatous disease of childhood and Wiskott–Aldrich syndrome.

Table 7.1 Differences between the various Mendelian disorders

Features	Autosomal dominant	Autosomal recessive	Sex-linked recessive
Transmission	Both males and females are affected and can transmit the disease. Only one parent of the index case has the disease. 50% of children are affected and 50% normal	Both parents must be carriers (heterozygotes or homozygotes). 25% of children are symptomatic, 50% carriers and 25% normal	Males express the disease. Affected male transmits abnormal gene to 100% of his daughters (asymptomatic carriers), who then transmit the disease to 50% of their sons
Penetrance/variable expressivity/ delayed onset of symptoms	Seen	Not seen	Not seen

Q. Differentiate between the various Mendelian disorders. (PA11.1)

Ans. Differences between the various Mendelian disorders are given in Table 7.1.

Q. What is multifactorial inheritance?

Ans. Multifactorial (polygenic) inheritance disorders occur consequent to multiple small mutations plus the effect of environment.

Examples: Cleft lip or palate, congenital heart disease, coronary artery disease, gout, type II diabetes mellitus, hypertension, open neural tube defects and congenital pyloric stenosis.

Q. Write briefly on chromosomal aberrations. (PA11.1)

Ans. Chromosomal aberrations can involve both the autosomes and the sex chromosomes and are classified into:

1. Numerical aberrations.
2. Structural aberrations.

Numerical Aberrations

- These are usually caused by a failure of chromosome division, which results in cells with an extra chromosome or a deficiency in chromosomes.
- Humans have 46 chromosomes consisting of 22 pairs of autosomes or somatic chromosomes and 2 sex chromosomes (XX = female and XY = male). The gametes contain a haploid number of chromosomes (n = 23).
- The union of two sex cells (egg and sperm), each with only haploid number of chromosomes, results in a diploid zygote (2n).
- **Hyperdiploidy** is a chromosomal number more than diploid and **hypodiploidy** is a chromosomal number less than diploid.
- **Aneuploidy** refers to the presence of an uneven multiple of 23 chromosomes. It is most frequently due to **non-disjunction**, in which one set of homologous chromosomes fails to separate during the first meiotic division (one gamete has 22 chromosomes and the other 24 chromosomes).
- **Polyploidy** is a condition in which a normally diploid cell or organism acquires one or more additional sets of chromosomes. In other words, the polyploid cell or organism has three or more times the haploid chromosome number (triploidy 69 chromosomes and tetraploidy 92 chromosomes). Polyploidy arises as the result of total non-disjunction of chromosomes during mitosis or meiosis.
- **Trisomy** is a numerical aberration with the presence of an extra chromosome (2n+1).
- **Monosomy** is a numerical aberration with the loss of one chromosome (2n–1).
- When non-disjunction occurs during mitosis of autosomal cells, the result is **mosaicism** (presence of two or more genetically different cell populations in the same patient; a common occurrence in Turner syndrome).

Structural Aberrations

- **Chromosomal translocation:** Chromosomal translocation (Fig. 7.2) is the transfer of a broken segment from one chromosome to another non-homologous chromosome. The process is usually **reciprocal** (fragments are exchanged between two chromosomes). Translocations are indicated by 't' followed by involved chromosome in numeric order. Structural rearrangements are defined as **balanced** if the complete chromosomal set is still present, though rearranged, and **unbalanced** if information is additional or missing. Unbalanced rearrangements include deletions, duplications or insertions of a chromosomal segment. Since there is no loss of genetic material and the full complement of DNA material is maintained, balanced chromosomal rearrangements may not result in disease. A disease can arise as a result of a balanced rearrangement if the breaks in the chromosomes occur in a gene, resulting in an absent or non-functional protein, or if the fusion of chromosomal segments results in a hybrid of two genes, producing a new protein product whose function is damaging to the cell.
  - A special pattern of translocation involving two acrocentric (centromere at the end; q very long, p very short) chromosomes is called **centric fusion type** or **Robertsonian translocation.** The break occurs close to the centromere and affects the short arm of both chromosomes. Transfer of the segment leads to a very large and a very small chromosome. The short fragment is lost and the carrier has 45 chromosomes.
  - **Isochromosomes** result when the centromeres divide horizontally and not vertically. One of the two arms of the chromosome is lost and the remaining is duplicated, resulting in a chromosome with two short arms or two long arms only (Fig. 7.3).
  - Three, or more breaks and more than two chromosomes can participate in exchange, leading to some very complicated rearrangements called **complex translocations**.

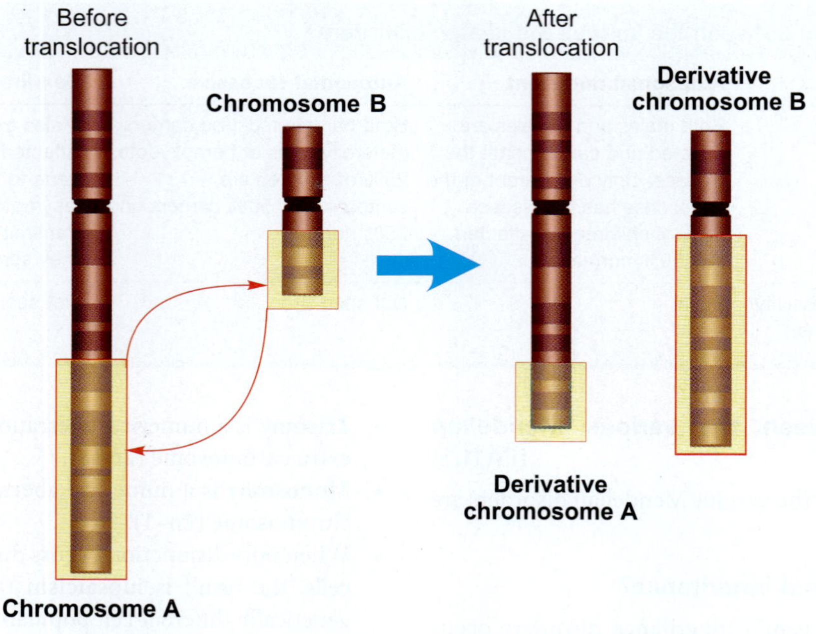

Fig. 7.2 Structural chromosomal abnormalities – reciprocal chromosomal translocation.

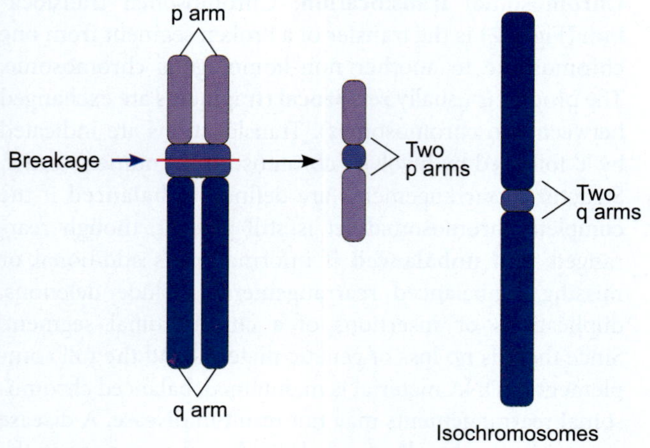

Fig. 7.3 Isochromosomes.

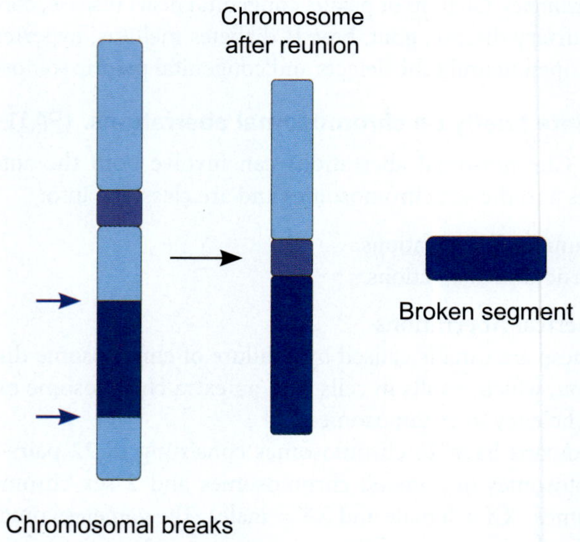

Fig. 7.4 Deletion.

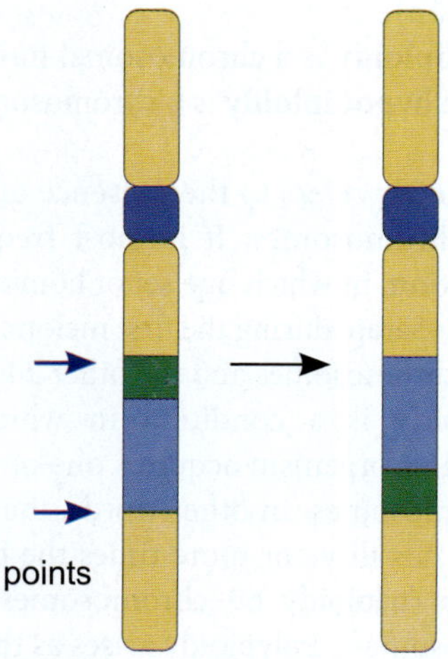

Fig. 7.5 Inversion.

- **Deletion:** Deletion is loss of a portion of a chromosome. A single break may delete a terminal segment (Fig. 7.4). Two breaks with loss of an intervening segment is called an interstitial deletion. Two interstitial breaks with reunion of the proximal and distal segments may result in formation of a **ring chromosome**. After loss of segments from each end of the chromosome, the arms unite to form a ring.
- **Inversion:** Inversions occur when there are two interstitial breaks in a chromosome and the segment reunites after rotation (Fig. 7.5). An inversion is termed **paracentric** when the segment involved lies wholly within one chromosome arm (either short or long arm) and **pericentric** when the two break-points are on the opposite sides of the centromere, and rejoining effectively inverts the central centromere-bearing segment.
- **Insertion:** A segment of a chromosome is deleted and transferred to a new position in some other chromosome, or into its homologue, or in a different location within the

same chromosome. The inserted segment may position itself with the same orientation to the centromere or may become inverted. This is usually a balanced rearrangement.

Q. What are mitochondrial DNA disorders? (PA11.1)

Ans. Mitochondrial DNA (mtDNA) disorders arise secondary to mutations in mitochondrial genes, which primarily code for enzymes involved in oxidative phosphorylation.

- The disorders are unique to females (mitochondrial genes are inherited by maternal inheritance, since ova have more mitochondria than sperms, which lose their mitochondria during fertilization).
- A female with an mtDNA defect transmits it to all her children.
- mtDNA in humans has 37 genes, of which 22 are transcribed into transfer RNAs and two into ribosomal RNAs. The remaining code for enzymes of oxidative phosphorylation pathway.
- Mitochondrial disorders, therefore, affect organs like CNS, skeletal and cardiac muscle, liver and kidney which are dependent on oxidative phosphorylation.
- Leber hereditary optic neuropathy, a neurodegenerative disease, is a prototype of mitochondrial disorders. It manifests with bilateral loss of central vision, cardiac conduction defects and neurological aberrations.

Q. Define genetic heterogeneity.

Ans. The phenomenon in which mutations at different genetic loci produce the same result is called genetic heterogeneity, for example retinitis pigmentosa, a disorder of abnormal retinal pigmentation and visual impairment can be caused by several different types of mutations.

Q. Write briefly on Lyon's hypothesis.

Ans. Components of Lyon's hypothesis:

1. Only one of the X chromosomes is genetically active; the other X chromosome of either maternal or paternal origin undergoes hyperpyknosis and is rendered inactive.
2. Inactivation of either the maternal or paternal X chromosome occurs at random among all the cells of the blastocyst, on or about the 16th day of embryonic life.
3. Inactivation of the same X chromosome persists in all the cells derived from one precursor cell.
   (a) The inactivated X chromosome is selectively reactivated in germ cells before first meiotic division, as both X chromosomes are required for normal oogenesis ('Modified Lyon's hypothesis'—modification is based on the observation that women continue to express many genes from their inactive X chromosome).
   (b) The inactive X chromosomes can be seen in the interphase nucleus as the darkly staining small mass in contact with the nuclear membrane known as **Barr body** or X chromatin.
   (c) It is present in all cells of a normal female. A buccal smear is made to demonstrate it.
   (d) Normal females have one Barr body and normal males none.
   (e) A male with Klinefelter syndrome and an XXY genotype has one Barr body.

Q. Enumerate the cytogenetic (karyotypic) disorders involving autosomes. (PA11.1)

Ans. Cytogenetic disorders involving autosomes include the following:

1. Autosomal trisomies affecting chromosomes 21 (**Down syndrome**), 18 (**Edwards syndrome**) and 13 (**Patau syndrome**).
2. One deletion (**cri du chat**) syndrome due to partial deletion of short arm of chromosome 5 (characterised by mental retardation, a cat-like cry, and ventricular septal defects).
3. Trisomies and deletions affecting 22q ('**DiGeorge syndrome**'—thymic hypoplasia, decreased T-cell immunity, parathyroid hypoplasia, hypocalcaemia; 'Velocardiofacial syndrome'—congenital heart disease, facial dysmorphism and delayed development).

Q. Write briefly on Down syndrome. (PA11.1)

Ans. Down syndrome is a cytogenetic disorder affecting chromosome 21.

Incidence

1 in 700 live births.

Genetic Abnormalities

- Trisomy of chromosome 21 (47, XX, + 21).
- Extra chromosome because of Robertsonian translocation of the long arm of chromosome 21 to another acrocentric chromosome like 22 or 14 [46, XX; der(14;21) (q10;q10); + 21].
- Least common mosaic pattern having some cells with 46 chromosomes and some with 47 chromosomes due to mitotic non-disjunction of chromosome 21 during early stage of embryogenesis (46, XX/47, XX, + 21).
- Trisomy of chromosome 21 is influenced by mother's age. Increased incidence is noted after 30 years of age.
- The extra chromosome is derived from non-disjunction of chromosome 21 during first meiotic division in ovum.

Clinical Features

- Mental retardation (IQ = 25–40).
- Flat facial profile and epicanthic folds, oblique palpebral fissure **(Mongolism/Mongolian idiocy).**
- Abundant neck skin.
- Congenital heart defects like atrial septal defects, endocardial cushion defects, atrioventricular valve malformations and ventricular septal defects (major cause of death during early life).
- Umbilical hernia.
- Intestinal stenosis.
- Hypotonia; gap between the first and second toe.
- Simian crease.
- Predisposition to acute leukaemia (lymphoblastic and myeloblastic).
- Neuropathological changes (like Alzheimer disease), seen after the age of 40 years.

Q. Write briefly on Edwards syndrome. (PA11.1)

Ans. Edwards syndrome is a cytogenetic disorder affecting chromosome 18.

Incidence

1 in 8000 live births.

Genetic Abnormalities

Trisomy of chromosome 18 (47, XX, + 18); mosaic type—46, XX/47, XX, + 18.

Clinical Features

- Mental retardation
- Micrognathia
- Prominent occiput
- Low-set ears
- Short neck
- Congenital heart defects
- Renal malformations
- Limited hip abduction
- Overlapping of fingers
- Rocker bottom feet.

Q. Write briefly on Patau syndrome. (PA11.1)

Ans. Patau syndrome is a cytogenetic disorder affecting chromosome 13.

Incidence

1 in 15,000 live births.

Genetic Abnormalities

Trisomy of chromosome 13 (47, XX, + 13); mosaic type—46, XX/47, XX, + 13; translocation type—46, XX, + 13, der(13;14)(q10;q10).

Clinical Features

- Microcephaly and mental retardation
- Microphthalmia
- Cleft lip and palate
- Polydactyly
- Congenital heart defects
- Renal malformations
- Umbilical hernia
- Rocker bottom feet.

Q. Enumerate the cytogenetic disorders involving sex chromosomes. (PA11.1)

Ans. Cytogenetic disorders involving sex chromosomes:

1. Klinefelter syndrome.
2. Turner syndrome.
3. Hermaphroditism and pseudohermaphroditism.

Q. Write briefly on Klinefelter syndrome. (PA11.1)

Ans. Klinefelter syndrome is characterised by male hypogonadism due to presence of two or more X chromosomes and one or more Y chromosome.

Incidence

1 in 850 live male births.

Genetic Abnormalities

- Classical type 47, XXY karyotype (82% cases).
- Maternal non-disjunction is slightly more common than paternal non-disjunction of sex chromosomes; increases with increase in age.
- Other variants: 46, XY/47, XXY; 47, XXY/48, XXXY; may have more number of X chromosomes.

Clinical Features

- Distinctive body pattern and other features emerge after puberty.
- Elongated body due to increased length between the soles and the pubic bone.
- 'Eunuchoid body habitus': long legs, small atrophied testes and small penis.
- Loss of secondary male characters like deep voice, male distribution of pubic hair, beard and moustache and body hair.
- Gynaecomastia.
- No mental retardation but mean IQ lower than normal.
- One of the most common causes of *male infertility.*

Hormone Levels

- Increased follicle stimulating hormone (FSH).
- Low testosterone.
- Increased estradiol.

Microscopic Findings

- Features of testicular atrophy may be seen.

Q. Write briefly on Turner syndrome. (PA11.1)

Ans. Complete or partial monosomy of X chromosome resulting in hypogonadism in the female phenotype.

Incidence

1 in 3000 female births.

Genetic Abnormalities

- Classic type: Entire X chromosome is missing (45, X).
- Structural abnormality of second X chromosome:
  - Deletion of small arm and formation of an isochromosome of the long arm—46, X, i(X) (q10).
  - Deletion of a portion of short and long arm, and formation of ring chromosome 46, X, r(X).
  - Deletion of a portion of short or long arm—46, X, del(Xq) or 46, X, del(Xp).
- *Mosaic pattern*: 45, X/46, XX; 45, X/46, XY; 45, X/47, XXX.

Pathogenesis

- During embryogenesis of ovaries, both X chromosomes are required.
- Normally foetal ovaries develop early in embryogenesis, but absence of second X chromosome leads to an accelerated loss of oocytes against a slow loss in normal female. By the age of 2 years, all the oocytes are destroyed.

- Ovaries are replaced by fibrous strands, with absence of ova and follicles (streak ovaries). Patients with Turner syndrome have been found to have deletions at the end of the short arm of X-chromosome (Xp-), including haploinsufficiency of the SHOX (short stature homeobox) gene, manifesting with short stature and orthopaedic abnormalities (e.g. cubitus valgus, Madelung deformity, micrognatia, and high-arched palate) and hearing impairment.

Clinical Features

- Infants present with peripheral oedema (lymph stasis) of the dorsae of hands and feet, and may have a swelling in the nape of neck (**cystic hygroma**) showing dilated lymphatic channels.
- With age, the swelling is replaced by bilateral neck webbing, loose skin on the back of neck and a low posterior hairline.
- Congenital heart diseases like coarctation of aorta and bicuspid aortic valve are the most common cause of death.
- Chest is broad and nipples are widely placed.
- Affected individuals may have streak ovaries (it is the single most important cause of primary amenorrhea), pigmented nevi, cubitus valgus and a short stature.
- Autoimmunity develops leading to hypothyroidism and glucose intolerance may also be seen.

Q. Describe disorders involving sex differentiation in both males and females.

Ans. An **XY karyotype** leads to differentiation of the primitive gonadal tissue into sex cords (seminiferous tubules) and Leydig cells, whereas an **XX karyotype** leads to preferential development of the germinal cortex into primordial follicles.

- A **true hermaphrodite** has both male and female gonads (ovary and testis).
- A **pseudohermaphrodite** is a person whose **phenotype** (appearance) is not in agreement with the **genotype** (true gonadal sex).
- A **male pseudohermaphrodite** is a genotypic male (XY with testes), who phenotypically resembles a female (e.g. testicular feminisation).
- A **female pseudohermaphrodite** is a genotypic female (XX with ovaries), who phenotypically resembles a male (e.g. virilization in congenital adrenal hyperplasia).
- **Testicular feminisation** is due to deficiency of androgen receptors (testosterone is unable to cause development of the seminal vesicles, epididymis) and vas deferens.

Q. Write briefly on testing for genetic diseases.

Ans. Genetic testing involves analysis of genetic material so as to establish diagnosis; decide on treatment; and aid in long term follow-up of a patient and family counselling. There are a wide variety of tests available for a large number of human disorders, including single gene diseases, polygenic diseases and chromosomal syndromes. Genetic testing can be of the following types:

- **Diagnostic testing in adults and adolescents:** Confirms a clinically suspected genetic disorder, for example Huntington's disease. It is indicated in patients with a family history of inherited cancer syndromes or suspected inherited predisposition to cancers and neurodegenerative diseases.
- **Presymptomatic or predictive genetic testing:** Used to assess the risk of development of a certain disease in a healthy person with our without a family history, for example cancer and heart disease.
- **Carrier testing:** can determine if a couple carries the risk of passing to their children a recessive allele for genetic diseases such as sickle cell anaemia or cystic fibrosis. It can also be done if one is in an ethnic group that has a high risk of a specific genetic disorder.
- **Preimplantation studies:** Done before conception (in invitro fertilisation) to diagnose a genetic disease in an embryo before it is implanted into the mother's uterus. It is undertaken when parents are known to be at risk of having a child with a genetic disorder.
- **Prenatal diagnosis:** Done after conception to diagnose a genetic disease or condition in the developing foetus. This type of testing is offered to couples with an increased risk of having a baby with a genetic or chromosomal disorder. Prenatal tests include screening blood, ultrasound (sonograms), amniocentesis, chorionic villus sampling (CVS) and percutaneous umbilical blood sampling (PUBS). Some important indications are the following:
  - Advanced maternal age (>34 years).
  - A parent who is a carrier of a balanced reciprocal translocation, Robertsonian translocation, or inversion (in these cases the gametes may be unbalanced, and hence the progeny would be at risk for chromosomal disorders).
  - A parent with a previous child with a chromosomal abnormality.
  - A parent who is a carrier of an X linked genetic disorder (to determine foetal sex).
- **Postnatal chromosome analysis:** It is usually performed on peripheral blood lymphocytes. Indications are as follows:
  a. Multiple congenital anomalies.
  b. Unexplained mental retardation or developmental delay.
  c. Suspected aneuploidy (e.g. features of Down syndrome) or sex chromosomal abnormality (e.g. Turner syndrome).
  d. Suspected fragile-X syndrome.
  e. Infertility and multiple spontaneous abortions.
- **Newborn screening:** is used to check for certain genetic disorders that can be diagnosed and treated early in life.

Genetic Testing Methods

Several different methods are currently used in genetic testing laboratories. The type of test depends on the type of abnormality being measured. The diagnosis of single gene disorders is mostly based on the identification of abnormal gene products or their clinical effects, such as anaemia (abnormal haemoglobin) or mental retardation (enzyme defects, e.g. Phenylketonuria). Subtle or submicroscopic changes in individual genes that cannot be detected by conventional karyotyping are now diagnosed by the use of recombinant DNA technology (PCR). There are two distinct approaches to the diagnosis of single-gene diseases: direct detection of mutations and indirect detection based on linkage of the disease gene with a harmless 'marker gene'. In general, three major types of genetic testing are available: cytogenetic, biochemical and molecular.

1. **Cytogenetic testing: Conventional cytogenetics** involves the examination of whole chromosomes for abnormalities whereas **molecular cytogenetics** is the study of genetic material at the level of nucleotide bases (e.g. FISH). T lymphocytes, are the most readily accessible cells for cytogenetic analysis because they are easily collected from blood and are capable of rapid division in cell culture. Amniotic fluid cells can be cultured for prenatal diagnosis. Cells can also be obtained directly from bone marrow and chronic villus biopsy. Following cell culture, chromosomes are fixed, spread and stained. The distinct bands of each chromosome revealed by staining allow for analysis of chromosome structure. Different banding techniques are available including G-banding (Giemsa) and Q-banding (Quinacrine fluorescent stain).
2. **Biochemical testing:** A mutation in any type of protein can result in impaired function or lack of function of the protein. Biochemical testing for genetic disease involves testing for the protein instead of the gene. Tests can be developed to measure the protein activity directly (enzymes), or measure the level of metabolites (indirect measurement of protein activity), or the size or quantity of protein as in case of structural proteins. These tests are typically performed on blood, urine, amniotic fluid, or cerebrospinal fluid. Proteins are not a stable as DNA. To prevent them from rapid degradation it is of utmost importance that the sample is properly collected and stored, and shipped promptly according to the laboratory's specifications.
3. **Molecular testing:** For small DNA mutations, direct DNA testing may be the most effective method, particularly if the function of the protein is unknown and a biochemical test cannot be developed. A DNA test can be performed on any tissue sample and requires very small amounts of sample. The quantity and quality of DNA preparation may vary, depending on the requirements of the assay. Majority of laboratories routinely purify DNA for the analysis, using some of the manual methods or commercial kits. The source of DNA could be any tissue with nuclear cells: usually, it is blood or buccal swab; in prenatal diagnosis these are CVS cells from amniotic fluid etc.

Q. Write briefly on karyotype analysis.

Ans. Photocapture of a stained preparation of chromosomes is referred to as the individual karyotype. Chromosomes can be studied in any cell of the body; however, they are best studied in lymphocytes. The cells to be studied are arrested in the metaphase by colchicine. They are then spread on to a slide and stained with a stain. When stained the chromosomal bands appear alternately dark and light. The staining technique using Giemsa staining is called G banding (Fig. 7.6). Other banding techniques include Q banding (quinacrine fluorescence stain), C banding (constitutive heterochromatin staining), and R banding (reverse Giemsa staining).

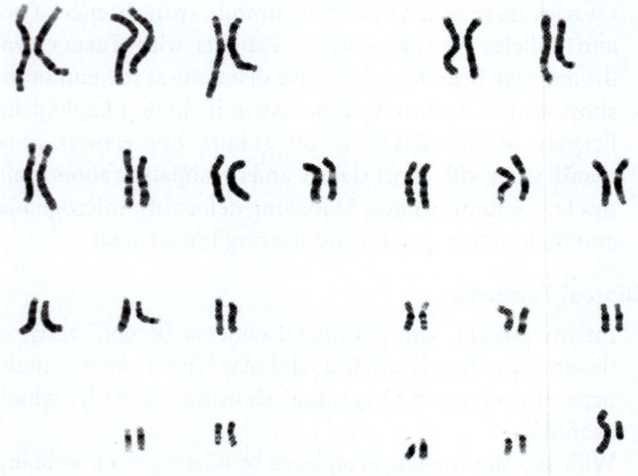

Fig. 7.6 Karyotype demonstration on G banding.

The following observations are made:

1. Differences in basic number of chromosomes.
2. Differences in the absolute sizes of chromosomes.
3. Differences in the position of centromeres (*metacentric chromosomes* are those in which the centromere is exactly in the middle, ***submetacentric*** *chromosomes* are those in which the chromosome is divided into a short (p) and a long (q) arm, and ***acrocentric*** *chromosomes* are those in which there is the centromere is very eccentrically placed and there is a very short and a very long arm).
4. Differences in the relative size of chromosomes (in case there is an interchange of segments of unequal lengths between two chromosomes).

Q. Write in detail on the methods for molecular testing of genetic diseases.

Ans. Hybridisation is defined as the process of double-stranded molecule formation that occurs between target DNA or RNA and their complementary nucleic acid probes.

Probes

Segments of DNA or RNA labelled with radioisotope or non-radioisotope reporter molecules, which may be:

1. Short single-stranded oligonucleotides.
2. Intermediate-sized complementary RNA probes.
3. Long double-stranded DNA probes.
   - Hybridisation can be accomplished in solution (polymerase chain reaction or PCR), on solid support such as nitrocellulose or nylon membranes (Southern blot), or at the cellular or subcellular level (in situ hybridisation).
   - Factors that affect the formation and stability of hybridisation are composition of sequences and temperature and salt concentration. Higher temperature and low salt level lead to stringent hybridisation, whereas low temperature and high-salt concentration lead to relaxed hybridisation with occasional

mismatched base pair. Guanine cytosine (GC)-rich sequence forms a more stable product than an adenine cytosine (AC)-rich sequence because the former contains more hydrogen bonds that require a higher temperature to dissociate the hybrid structure. A direct relationship exists between DNA stability and its melting temperature.

Southern Blotting

In this filter hybridisation method, denatured DNA is immobilised on an inert support that allows for the binding of a labelled nucleic acid probe.

Northern Hybridisation (Blotting)

- This is a sensitive and quantitative method for mRNA detection.
- RNA is denatured with a variety of reagents. To obtain a high-quality RNA yield, it is important to avoid contamination and to inhibit RNAases during processing of tissue.
- Although RNA is single stranded, denaturation is required for effective separation on agarose gel.
- Denaturation is typically performed by using formamide with subsequent separation by electrophoresis on a formaldehyde gel.
- Separated RNA on the gel will be transferred to filter paper by capillary action and hybridised in a similar way, as Southern method, to a complementary target molecule.
- These are hybridised with radiolabelled probes.

Dot Blot Hybridisation

This is a useful technique for quantitative measurement of target DNA sequences where the size of the target is known or is unnecessary. A membrane blotted with known DNA sequences will be hybridised with a test sample for the detection of a specific sequence.

Western Blotting

In this technique, electrophoretically separated components are transferred from a gel onto a solid support and probed with antibodies specific to certain epitopes on target protein.

In situ Hybridisation

- The technique is ideal for visualisation and localisation of specific nucleic acid sequences in cells. A tissue sample or cell preparation mounted on a slide can be used as a target for probe hybridisation.
- *In situ DNA*: The target for this technique is nuclear DNA and the probe sequences include centromeric, whole chromosome and specific gene.
- *In situ mRNA*: The target in this method is the mRNA transcript in the cytoplasm. The probes are manufactured in vitro by inserting a cloned DNA fragment of interest into a vector near a regulatory sequence (promoters) that direct RNA polymerase to transcribe sequence to RNA.
- A sense or antisense RNA probe can be generated depending on the orientation of inserted fragment. Each affected individual has an affected parent unless the condition has arisen from a new mutation in the germ cells forming that individual.
- The applications include gene localisation and determination of translocation, ploidy and gene amplification.

Q. Write briefly on polymerase chain reaction (PCR).

Ans. PCR is an in vitro technique of nucleic acid synthesis that allows for rapid, sensitive and specific replication of nucleic acid for the detection and isolation of a targeted sequence.

- The method involves exponential amplification of DNA, and is based on the function of DNA polymerase enzyme to create a new complementary DNA strand from a template strand.
- If RNA is used as a substrate, it is first reverse transcribed to obtain cDNA and then amplified by PCR.
- The technique requires a pair of oligonucleotide primers that complement the opposite ends of each strand of a target sequence and are aligned for DNA synthesis to proceed only in the region between the primers.
- A reaction mixture for PCR amplifications typically contains a DNA sample, a pair of primers, thermostable Taq DNA polymerase enzyme and 4-deoxynucleotide triphosphates (dNTPs) in a buffered solution.
- For the reaction to proceed, target DNA is first denatured by heating and the reaction mixture then cooled to a certain temperature to allow the primers to anneal to the DNA target and, lastly, extension by Taq DNA polymerase is brought about.
- Repeating these cycles leads to exponential production of the specific target.

Steps

The repeated cycles of DNA polymerase activity include the following:

1. **Denaturation:** Heat is typically used to break the hydrogen bonds between complementary bases of both strands.
2. **Annealing:** This entails the binding of the primers to the beginning sequence of one strand and to the end of the other strand.
3. **Extension:** DNA polymerase and triphosphorylated deoxynucleotides are added to the reaction including the primers to extend the complementary strand.

Types

1. **Simple PCR:** This entails the amplification of a single specific sequence by using a pair of primers complementary to the flanking sequences of the target and is routinely used for preparing more DNA targets for subsequent analyses.
2. **Multiplex PCR:** In this technique, a number of different primers are added to the same reaction mixture to screen for multiple abnormalities and to avoid unnecessary testing.

Q. Write briefly on fluorescence in situ hybridisation (FISH).

Ans. This is a method of identifying a chromosome or its parts by the use of specific probes that bind to specific DNA sequences (which are complementary).

- It is more useful than traditional karyotyping, as cells can be visualised even in interphase.
- It circumvents the need for dividing cells; even those cells that are not dividing or cannot be induced to divide can be mapped.
- The probes are attached with fluorescent dyes and are visualised under a fluorescent microscope.

Applications

- Karyotyping of cells/chromosomes in interphase.
- Using specific complementary DNA sequence, one can look for specific regions on a chromosome.
- Can be used for detection of numerical abnormalities, such as aneuploidy, microdeletions and complex translocations that are not readily visualised by karyotyping.
- Mapping/localisation of newly isolated genes of clinical importance.

Chromosome painting: It is visualisation of the entire chromosome using different fluorescent dyes.

Spectral karyotyping: Using computer-generated signals the entire human genome can be 'painted' and visualised simultaneously.

Q. Write briefly on array comparative genomic hybridisation.

Ans. Array comparative genomic hybridisation, also called **CMA (chromosomal microarray analysis)** or **CGH (microarray-based comparative genomic hybridisation),** is a technique to detect genomic variations, at a higher resolution level than chromosome-based CGH without prior knowledge of what these aberrations may be. DNA from a test sample and normal reference sample are labelled differentially, using different fluorescent dyes and hybridised to several thousand probes. The probes are derived from most of the known genes and non-coding regions of the genome, printed on a glass slide. The ratio of the fluorescence intensity of the test to that of the reference DNA is then calculated, to measure the copy number changes for a particular location in the genome.

Q. What are SNP genotyping arrays?

Ans. Single nucleotide polymorphism (SNP) genotyping arrays are newer genomic arrays based on identification of SNPs sites genome wide. SNPs are the most common DNA polymorphisms which occur after every thousand nucleotides throughout the genome. SNP arrays are used to find copy number abnormalities when the karyotype is normal but a structural abnormality is suspected.

Q. What is Multiplex ligation-dependent probe amplification (MLPA)?

Ans. MLPA is a variation of the multiplex PCR that allows amplification of multiple targets with a single primer pair. It is highly sensitive technique (because of it being a multiplex reaction) that allows quantification of nucleic acid sequences. It is applied to detect copy number changes (like deletions or duplications) of a gene, identify the methylation status of

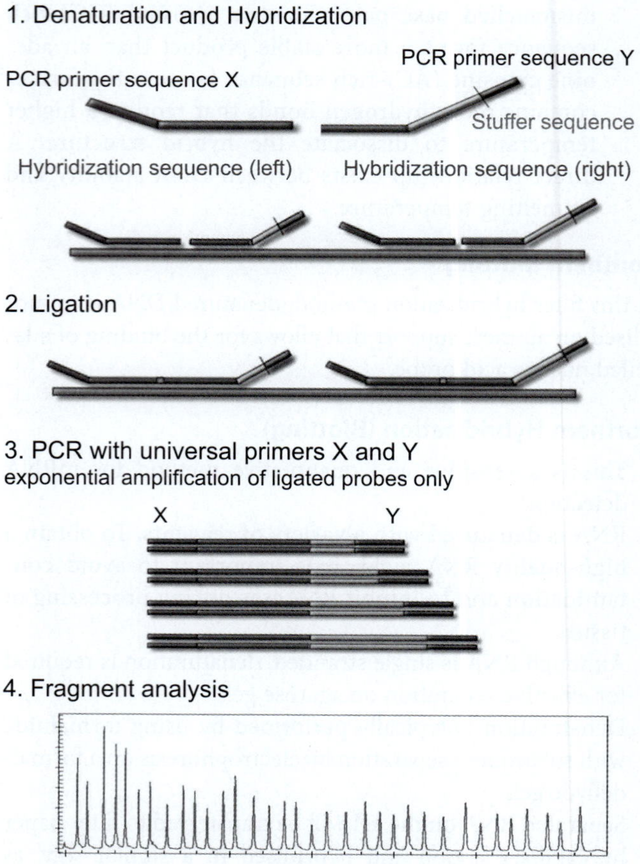

Fig. 7.7 MLPA technique. (*Source: Molecular Diagnostics,* 2nd Edition: George P. Patrinos, Wilhelm J. Ansorge, Figure 13.1: Eline M. Sepers, Jan P. Schouten, Elsevier Ltd., 2010.)

DNA, detect single nucleotide polymorphisms (SNPs) and point mutations and quantify mRNA. MLPA consists of the following steps (Fig. 7.7):

- Denaturation
- Hybridisation
- Ligation
- Amplification (by PCR)
- Fragment separation and data analysis.

Advantages of MLPA

- MLPA is a highly sensitive, rapid (results are available in 24 hours) and high-throughput technique.
- It can discern between point mutations, as well as duplication/deletion of genes. Other techniques, like sequencing are only capable of finding point mutations. Moreover, unlike FISH, MLPA can detect small gene alterations.
- MLPA can also be used to detect methylation patterns in DNA (Methylation specific-MLPA (MS-MLPA).

Limitations of MLPA

- MLPA is extremely sensitive to impurities. Therefore, there needs to be extreme caution when preparing samples and performing the technique.
- There can be a decrease in signal from a probe due to a rare polymorphism or mutation, and it might be necessary to test it by other techniques.

Q. Write briefly on the biochemical consequences of single gene Mendelian disorders.

Ans. The ability of a gene to be expressed depends upon the sex of the parent who passed on the gene. In some cases imprinted genes are expressed when they are inherited from the mother. In other cases they are expressed when inherited from the father. Genomic imprinting does not affect the DNA sequence itself, instead it affects gene expression by chemically modifying DNA and/or altering the chromatin structure. Often, genomic imprinting results in a gene being expressed only in the chromosome inherited from one or the other parent. While this is a normal process, when combined with genomic mutations, disease can result. For example, Prader–Willi syndrome and Angelman syndrome are two distinct diseases caused by a deletion in the same part of chromosome 15. When this deletion occurs on the chromosome 15 that came from the father, the child will have Prader-Willi syndrome. However, when the deletion occurs on the chromosome 15 that came from the mother, the child will develop Angelman syndrome.

Q. Write briefly on the biochemical consequences of single gene Mendelian disorders. (PA11.3)

Ans. The following mechanisms are involved in single-gene disorders:

1. Enzyme defects.
2. Defects in membrane receptors.
3. Abnormalities in the quantity, structure and function of non-enzymatic proteins.
4. Mutations leading to aberrant drug reactions.

Enzyme Defects

Mutations may result in the synthesis of a defective enzyme or synthesis of reduced quantity of a normal enzyme. The biochemical consequences of an enzyme defect in such a reaction may lead to three major consequences:

1. Defect in an enzyme in a major pathway may result in accumulation of the substrate or one or more intermediates. An increased level of one of the intermediates stimulates the minor pathway leading to an excess of other metabolites. Excess quantity of the substrate or the intermediates may lead to tissue injury, particularly if they are toxic in nature. For example, in galactosaemia, the deficiency of galactose-l-phosphate uridyltransferase leads to the accumulation of galactose and consequent tissue damage.
2. An enzyme defect can block a major pathway and lead to decreased amount of end product that may be necessary for normal function. For example, a deficiency of melanin may result from lack of tyrosinase, which is necessary for biosynthesis of melanin from its precursor, tyrosine leading to a clinical condition called albinism.
3. Failure to inactivate a tissue-damaging substrate, for example α1-antitrypsin (α1-AT) deficiency. Patients who have an inherited deficiency of serum α1-AT are unable to inactivate neutrophil elastase in their lungs. This leads to destruction of elastin in the alveolar walls, resulting eventually in pulmonary emphysema.

Defects in Membrane Receptors

Defective receptor mediated transport as seen in familial hypercholesterolaemia (decreased number or defective function of LDL receptors leads to impaired transport of LDL into cells and excessive cholesterol synthesis).

Abnormalities in the Quantity, Structure and Function of Non-enzymatic Proteins

Examples of genetic disorders with abnormalities in the quantity, structure and function of non-enzymatic proteins include haemoglobinopathies like sickle cell anaemia. Other proteins affected are collagen (osteogenesis imperfecta), dystrophin (muscular dystrophy), spectrin (spherocytosis), etc.

Mutations Leading to Aberrant Drug Reactions

Prototypical example is drug induced injury seen in glucose-6-phosphate deficiency. No haemolysis is seen in these patients under normal circumstances, however, administration of certain drugs like primaquine can result in severe haemolysis.

Q. Write briefly on enzyme defects and their consequences. (PA11.3)

Ans. Disorders associated with defects in enzymes include the following:

1. **Phenylketonuria (PKU)**
   - PKU is characterised by deficiency of **phenylalanine hydroxylase**, which converts **phenylalanine** to **tyrosine.**
   - Infants are normal at birth but they develop increased phenylalanine levels within a few weeks.
   - Rising phenylalanine levels impair development of the brain, leading to severe mental retardation.
   - Other clinical features are seizures, decreased pigmentation of the hair and skin, eczema and strong mousy or musty odour of sweat and urine (due to accumulation of minor pathway products).
2. **Galactosaemia**
   - Galactose comes from the metabolism of lactose (glucose + galactose). In the first step of galactose metabolism, galactose is converted to galactose-1-phosphate (Gal-1-P) by the enzyme galactokinase, which is then converted to uridine diphosphate galactose (UDP-galactose) by the enzyme galactose-1-phosphate uridylyltransferase, with UDP-glucose acting as the UDP donor. UDP-galactose can then be converted to lactose, by the enzyme lactose synthase or to UDP-glucose by UDP-galactose epimerase (GALE). In galactosemia, there is a total lack of *galactose-1-phosphate uridylyltransferase (GALT)* leading to accumulation of galactose-1-phosphate.
   - Galactose-1-phosphate is toxic and damages tissue resulting in neonatal cholestasis (may progress to cirrhosis), CNS damage (mental retardation), renal damage (aminoaciduria), and *Escherichia coli* sepsis. Excess galactose may be converted into polyol (alcohol sugar), which causes osmotic damage to the lens, nerve tissue, liver and CNS.

3. **Homocystinuria**: It is due to deficiency of **cystathionine synthetase**. It resembles Marfan syndrome (shares arachnodactyly and a dislocated lens). Differentiating features from Marfan syndrome include mental retardation, thromboembolic episodes (homocysteine damages endothelial cells) and osteoporosis.
4. **Alkaptonuria**
   (a) Alkaptonuria (ochronosis) is secondary to a lack of **homogentisic oxidase** required for the metabolism of phenylalanine.
   (b) There is an increase in homogentisic acid in urine, which is colourless at first but turns black after oxidation, upon exposure to light.
   (c) Homogentisic acid binds to collagen in connective tissue, tendons and cartilage (causing a crippling joint disease), and imparts a black colour to all these tissues.
5. **Lysosomal storage diseases** (See question on 'Lysosomal storage diseases').
6. **Glycogen storage diseases** (See question on 'Glycogen storage diseases').

Q. Write briefly on lysosomal storage diseases. (PA11.3)

Ans. Lysosomes contain a variety of hydrolytic enzymes that are involved in degradation of complex substrates, for example, sphingolipids and mucopolysaccharides, into soluble end products. Due to a lack of a lysosomal enzyme, catabolism of a substrate remains incomplete leading to accumulation of the partially degraded insoluble metabolites within the lysosomes.

- Approximately 40 lysosomal storage diseases have been identified.
- Lysosomal storage diseases have an AR transmission and commonly affect infants and children.
- Accumulation of insoluble intermediates may lead to the following:
  - Organ enlargement (hepatosplenomegaly or cardiomegaly).
  - CNS involvement (neuronal damage).
  - Macrophage activation and cytokine release aiding to widespread cellular dysfunction
- Traditionally, lysosomal storage diseases are classified based on the biochemical nature of the substrate or accumulated metabolite.

Examples

- **Tay–Sachs disease**: G_{M2} gangliosidosis
  - Enzyme deficiency: lysosomal hexosaminidase (α-subunit).
  - Metabolite accumulation: G_{M2} ganglioside.
  - It is primarily seen in Ashkenazi Jews.
  - Patients are normal at birth but develop signs of severe mental retardation within 6 months.
  - There is blindness, a cherry-red spot in the macula, muscle weakness, flaccidity and death by 2–3 years.
  - Histopathology shows ballooned neurons with cytoplasmic vacuoles which are actually distended lysosomes containing gangliosides which stain with fat stains like oil red O and Sudan black B. Retinal ganglion cells show the same changes. The normal colour of the macular choroid appears exaggerated due to the pallor of the adjacent swollen ganglion cells resulting in the 'cherry-red spot'.
- **Niemann–Pick disease**
  - Enzyme deficiency: sphingomyelinase.
  - Metabolite accumulation: sphingomyelin, primarily in macrophages (imparting a bubbly appearance) and in neurons.
  - Three variants: A, B and C; in the more severe type A, there is severe neuronal damage and mental retardation, massive hepatosplenomegaly and deterioration of psychomotor function (disease is fatal in early life).
  - In type B, neuronal damage is not present.
  - Type C was initially thought to be a variant of types A and B but is now considered a distinct clinicopathological and genetic entity. It is caused by mutations in two closely related genes—NPC1 and NPC2. Niemann–Pick type C is due to a primary defect in free cholesterol transport from the lysosomes to the cytoplasm and resultant accumulation in different organs especially in the nervous system. Patients have ataxia, dysarthria and psychomotor regression.
- **Gaucher disease**
  - AR disorder; most common lysosomal storage disease.
  - Enzyme deficiency: glucocerebrosidase or glucosylceramidase (primarily noted in Ashkenazi Jews).
  - Normally, the glycolipids derived from the breakdown of senescent blood cells are sequentially degraded (glucocerebrosidase cleaves glucose from ceramide). In Gaucher disease, the degradation stops at the level of glucocerebroside, which accumulates in the macrophages and CNS. Adverse results of Gaucher disease are caused not only by the accumulated glucocerebroside but also due to activation of macrophages which release various cytokines (IL 1, IL 2 and TNF).
  - The most common, type I (chronic non-neuronopathic form), accounts for 99% of cases of Gaucher disease. The glucocerebrosides accumulate in the mononuclear phagocytic system without affecting the CNS. Distended lysosomes give the macrophages a characteristic **fibrillary** or **wrinkled tissue paper appearance** (called **'Gaucher cells'**). There is massive hepatosplenomegaly, skeletal involvement (producing bone erosions and fractures), involvement of bone marrow (producing pancytopenia) and lymphadenopathy.
  - Types II (acute neuronopathic type) and III (intermediate between types I and II) have variable CNS involvement. Type II disease shows no preferential involvement of Jews and has an infantile acute cerebral pattern of presentation. Progressive CNS involvement leads to an early death. Type III disease shows systemic involvement with CNS disease which begins late in adolescence or adulthood.
- **Metachromatic leukodystrophy**
  - Enzyme deficiency: arylsulphatase A.
  - Metabolite accumulation: sulphatide.

- The myelin that is synthesised is abnormal, hence affecting the CNS and peripheral nerves.
- There is mental retardation, peripheral neuropathy and visceral organ abnormalities.

- **Krabbe disease**
  - Enzyme deficiency: galactosylceramidase.
  - Metabolite accumulation: galactocerebrosidase.
  - Similar to metachromatic leukodystrophy, there is synthesis of an abnormal myelin leading to progressive psychomotor retardation.
  - Sections from brain at autopsy reveal multinucleated globoid cells loaded with the galactocerebroside material.
- **Fabry disease**
  - Enzyme deficiency: α-galactocerebrosidase A.
  - Metabolite accumulation: ceramide trihexoside.
  - It is characterised by angiokeratomas on the skin, hypertension and renal failure (X linked recessive disease).
- **Mucopolysaccharidoses**
  - Mucopolysaccharides form a part of the ground substance synthesised by connective tissue fibroblasts, a certain fraction of which is degraded within lysosomes.
  - Mucopolysaccharidoses is characterised by accumulation of mucopolysaccharides due to lack of certain enzymes involved in their catabolic pathway.
  - Several clinical variants (MPS I to MPS VII) are known.
  - **Two well-recognised syndromes belonging to this category:**
    - ***Hurler syndrome*** (part of MPS I)
      - Enzyme deficiency: α-L-iduronidase.
      - Metabolite accumulation: dermatan sulphate and heparin sulphate.
      - Patients have severe mental retardation, coarse facial features, massive hepatosplenomegaly, clouding of the cornea, a high incidence of coronary disease owing to accumulation of the metabolites in the coronary vessels, joint stiffness and vacuoles in leukocytes in the peripheral blood.
    - ***Hunter syndrome*** (part of MPS II)
      - X linked inheritance.
      - Enzyme deficiency: L-iduronate sulphatase.
      - Metabolite accumulation: dermatan sulphate and heparin sulphate.
      - Absence of corneal clouding and a milder course differentiates it from Hurler syndrome.

Q. Write briefly on glycogen storage diseases or glycogenoses. (PA11.3)

Ans. Principal groups of glycogenoses are given in Table 7.2.

Q. Enumerate the different teratogens and write briefly on their effects.

Ans. Teratogens may be classified as follows:

1. **Non-infectious teratogens**
   (a) ***Alcohol***: Foetal alcohol syndrome occurs in the offspring of women who have more than 4–6 drinks per day. It results in intrauterine growth retardation, maxillary hypoplasia, mental retardation, microcephaly, atrial septal defects and hypoglycaemia at birth.
   (b) ***Smoking***: Associated with low birthweight and sudden infant death syndrome, smoking can lead to spontaneous abortions and placental abnormalities.
   (c) ***Cocaine***: Can cause abruptio placentae and premature labour in the mother and CNS infarcts, intraventricular haemorrhage, genitourinary and gastrointestinal abnormalities in the newborn.
   (d) ***Isotretinoin***: Used to treat acne; it may induce craniofacial abnormalities (small ears, micrognathia and cleft palate), cardiac defects and CNS malformations (microcephaly).
   (e) ***Diethylstilbestrol (DES)***: DES causes abnormalities in Mullerian structures, for example, vaginal adenosis and is a precursor of clear cell adenocarcinoma of cervix.
   (f) ***Thalidomide***: It is associated with limb abnormalities: amelia (absent limbs) and phocomelia (**seal-like limbs**).
   (g) ***Phenytoin***: If consumed during pregnancy, phenytoin is associated with hypoplasia of the distal phalanges, CNS abnormalities and cleft lip/palate.
   (h) ***Diabetes mellitus***: Children of diabetic mothers may manifest with increased birthweight (macrosomia), open neural tube defects, cleft lip/palate, respiratory distress syndrome and transposition of great vessels.

Table 7.2 Principal groups of glycogenoses

Clinicopathological category	Specific type	Enzyme deficiency	Morphological changes	Clinical features
Hepatic type	Hepatorenal (von Gierke disease)	Glucose-6-phosphatase	Hepato and renomegaly: intracytoplasmic accumulation of glycogen	Failure to thrive, stunted growth, hypoglycaemia, hyperuricaemia, hyperlipidaemia
Myopathic type	McArdle disease (type V)	Muscle phosphorylase	Skeletal muscle: accumulation of glycogen in the sarcolemmal location	• Painful cramps, myoglobinuria • No increase in lactic acid with exercise
Miscellaneous	• Generalized glycogenosis • Pompe disease (type II)	Lysosomal glucosidase (acid maltase)	Mild hepatomegaly, cardiomegaly, deposits in skeletal muscle	• Massive cardiomegaly, muscle hypotonia, cardiorespiratory failure within 2 years • Milder adult form with only skeletal muscle involvement, presents with chronic myopathy

2. **Infectious teratogens**
   (a) ***Cytomegalovirus (CMV)***
      (i) Most common in utero viral infection.
      (ii) Primarily transplacental transmission.
      (iii) May manifest with hearing loss, periventricular calcification, neonatal cholestasis, anaemia, thrombocytopenia, chorioretinitis (blindness) and microcephaly.
      (iv) Virus can be isolated from urine, saliva, blood and tissue. Histopathology reveals basophilic intranuclear inclusions labelled **'owl's eye appearance'**.
   (b) ***Rubella***
      (i) Primarily transplacental transmission.
      (ii) Manifests with nerve deafness (most common defect), congenital heart disease (patent ductus arteriosus), cataract and mental retardation.
      (iii) Positive serologic test (TORCH) indicates disease.
   (c) ***Toxoplasmosis***
      (i) Maternal infection secondary to exposure to cats.
      (ii) Primarily transplacental transmission.
      (iii) Manifests with chorioretinitis (blindness), periventricular calcifications, microcephaly, mental retardation and neonatal cholestasis.
      (iv) Positive serologic test (TORCH) indicates disease.
   (d) ***Herpes simplex***
      (i) Primarily perinatal transmission while passing through birth canal with active shedding of herpes genitalis (HSV-2 baby should be delivered by caesarean section, if viral shedding present).
      (ii) Permanent neurological sequelae common.
      (iii) Positive serologic test (TORCH) indicates disease.
   (e) ***Syphilis***
      (i) Primarily transplacental transmission.
      (ii) Symptoms and signs appear in first 1–2 months after birth and include mucocutaneous lesions, lobar pneumonia, persistent rhinitis (snuffles), osteochondritis and hepatomegaly.
      (iii) Prominent late manifestations are bone abnormalities **(saber shins)** and **Hutchinson's triad** (malformed, notched upper central incisors, interstitial keratitis leading to blindness and nerve deafness).
      (iv) Rising VDRL titer; positive FTA-ABS-IgM are diagnostic.

Q. Write briefly on the disorders associated with prematurity.

Ans. *Newborns may be classified as appropriate for gestational age (AGA), small for gestational age (SGA) or large for gestational age (LGA).*

- *Term newborns are those born between 37 and 42 weeks, preterm newborns are those born before 37 weeks and post-term newborns are those born after 42 weeks.*
- Infants born before completion of gestation usually weigh less than normal (2500 g).
- Prematurity is second only to congenital malformations as a cause of infant mortality.
- Preterm infants have immature organs, which predisposes them to various complications, such as immature lungs (that lack surfactant and are prone to develop respiratory distress syndrome), necrotising enterocolitis and intraventricular haemorrhage.

PART II: DISEASES OF INFANCY AND CHILDHOOD

Q. Write briefly on neonatal respiratory distress syndrome/hyaline membrane disease.

Ans. Characterised by formation of pulmonary hyaline membrane, neonatal respiratory distress syndrome is associated with the following conditions:

- Preterm infants.
- Infants born to diabetic mothers.
- Caesarean section delivery.
- Excessive sedation of mother during labour.
- Other birth-related asphyxias.

Aetiopathogenesis (Flowchart 7.1)

Clinical Features

- Dyspnoea, tachypnea, hypoxia and cyanosis.
- May be fatal in severe cases.

Decreased alveolar surfactant
↓
Increased alveolar surface tension and atelectasis
↓
Uneven perfusion and hypoventilation leading to hypoxaemia and CO_2 retention
↓
Acidosis and further reduction in surfactant synthesis
↓
Pulmonary vasoconstriction and hypoperfusion
↓
Endothelial and epithelial damage
↓
Leakage of plasma into alveoli
↓
Accumulation of fibrin and necrotic cells
↓
Hyaline membrane formation

Flowchart 7.1 Aetiopathogenesis of hyaline membrane disease.

Morphology

Gross: Lung or its part(s) are normal in size, solid, airless, reddish purple in colour and sink(s) in water.

Microscopic features: Collapsed alveoli, neutrophilic infiltration, eosinophilic hyaline membrane in the terminal bronchioles and alveolar ducts/alveoli.

Q. Define foetal hydrops. Enumerate and describe the two types of hydrops.

Ans. Foetal hydrops refers to accumulation of oedema fluid in the foetus during intrauterine growth. Fluid accumulation may vary from progressive generalised oedema of the foetus (hydrops) to a more localised isolated pleural/peritoneal collection. It may be *immune* or *non-immune* in origin.

1. **Immune hydrops (erythroblastosis foetalis; haemolytic disease of newborn):**
   (a) Haemolytic disease in the newborn is caused by blood group incompatibility between mother and child.
   (b) Occurs when the foetus inherits red cell antigenic determinants from the father that are foreign to the mother.
   (c) Immunisation of the mother by blood group antigens on foetal red cells and the free passage of antibodies from the mother through the placenta to the foetus is the basis of the disease.
   (d) Antigens may reach maternal circulation in the last trimester when the cytotrophoblast is no longer present as a barrier or during childbirth (foetomaternal bleed).
   (e) Most common incompatibility is Rh (D), followed by ABO blood group:
      (i) ***Rh incompatibility***:
      - When the mother is Rh-negative and the foetus is Rh-positive, the first child is usually unaffected; but all pregnancies in the future producing an Rh-positive foetus will be affected. Immunoglobulin containing anti-D antibodies should be administered within 72 h of delivery and/or at 28th week of pregnancy to Rh-negative mothers to prevent complications in the subsequent pregnancies.
      - If an Rh-negative mother has already been sensitised by Rh-positive blood due to prior transfusion, even the *first* Rh-positive child may be affected.
      - Such sensitised mothers form antibodies against Rh antigens.
      - Antibodies (Abs) cross placenta during the first pregnancy but usually in late third trimester; IgM isotype is the first antibody to be formed, which does not cross placenta, so the first child is mostly unaffected; but if there is heavy and early sensitisation of mother, then haemolytic symptoms are visible in the first child due to IgG formation (which is capable of crossing placenta).
      - Second Rh-positive foetus causes large amount of IgG antibody formation. These antibodies cross placenta and attach to Rh-positive foetal RBCs.
      - Destruction of such RBCs leads to anaemia and haemolytic jaundice. In severe cases, jaundice may lead to kernicterus and mental retardation; anaemia may cause extramedullary haematopoiesis and/or cardiac decompensation leading to *hydrops foetalis.*

      (ii) ***ABO incompatibility:***
      - This is less common compared to *Rh incompatibility* because anti-A and anti-B antibodies are IgM type, they do not cross the placenta.
      - Neonatal RBCs express blood group antigens A and B poorly, resulting in less sensitisation of the mother.
      - ABO haemolytic disease occurs exclusively in infants born to 'O' blood group mothers (IgG type anti-A and anti-B antibodies).
2. **Non-immune hydrops**
   (a) Major causes include cardiovascular defects, chromosomal anomalies (Turner syndrome, trisomies 18 and 21) and foetal anaemia (e.g. that associated with homozygous α-thalassaemia) resulting in intrauterine cardiac failure.
   (b) Transplacental infection with parvovirus B19 is emerging as an important cause of foetal hydrops.

Morphology of Hydrops

- Presence of dysmorphic features suggests underlying chromosomal abnormalities.
- Postmortem examination may reveal a cardiac anomaly.
- In hydrops associated with foetal anaemia, both the foetus and the placenta are characteristically pale.
- In most cases, there is hepatosplenomegaly.
- Compensatory erythroid hyperplasia may be seen in the marrow and extramedullary haematopoiesis may be seen in liver, spleen, kidneys and lungs.
- Haemolysis leads to increased unconjugated bilirubin.
- CNS is damaged when bilirubin levels are more than 20 mg/dL. Basal ganglia and brain stem are prone to deposition of bilirubin ***(Kernicterus).***

Q. Enumerate the common malignant tumours of infancy and childhood. (PA11.2)

Ans. Common malignant tumours of infancy and childhood are enlisted in Table 7.3.

Q. Enumerate the small round blue-cell tumours of childhood. (PA11.2)

Ans. Many childhood tumours are collectively termed 'small round blue-cell tumours of childhood' because they have a similar histological appearance, that is, presence of small round cells with a high N/C ratio. Subtle morphological clues may be present to distinguish between the tumours assisted by immunohistochemistry, electron microscopy and molecular analysis for chromosomal abnormalities. Following is a list of the most common tumours placed in this category:

- Ewing sarcoma and primitive neuroectodermal tumour
- Small cell osteosarcoma
- Leukaemia–lymphoma

Table 7.3 Common malignant tumours of infancy and childhood

0–4 years	5–9 years	10–14 years
Leukaemia	Leukaemia	Hepatocellular carcinoma
Retinoblastoma	Retinoblastoma	Soft-tissue sarcomas
Neuroblastoma	Neuroblastoma	Osteogenic sarcoma
Wilms tumour	Hepatocellular carcinoma	Thyroid carcinoma
Hepatoblastoma	Soft-tissue sarcomas	Hodgkin disease
Soft-tissue sarcomas	CNS tumours	
Teratomas	Ewing sarcoma	
CNS tumours	Lymphoma	

- Neuroblastoma
- Rhabdomyosarcoma
- Wilms tumour
- Retinoblastoma
- Medulloblastoma
- Desmoplastic small round blue-cell tumour.

Q. Describe the clinicopathological features of neuroblastoma. (PA11.2)

- **Ans.** Second most common solid malignancy of childhood after brain tumours; most common in infants (<1 year of age).
- **Mostly sporadic, rarely familial with AD transmission.**
- Familial cases are associated with germline mutations in the anaplastic lymphoma kinase (ALK) gene. Somatic gain of function mutations also seen in less than 10% cases (inhibitors of this kinase are being used as potential treatment for neuroblastoma). Germline mutations in the *PHOX2B* or *KIF1B* gene have been implicated in familial neuroblastoma. *MYCN* oncogene amplification within the tumour is a common finding in neuroblastoma.

Clinical Features

- Most common site is **adrenal medulla**; *other sites*—anywhere along sympathetic chain (paravertebral region of the posterior mediastinum and lower abdomen); 50%–60% of all neuroblastoma cases present with metastases.
- Usually present with a large abdominal mass, fever and weight loss.
- Watery diarrhoea syndrome may occur due to vasoactive intestinal peptide secretion.
- Rapid eye movements, ataxia, irregular muscle movements from paraneoplastic cause.
- Horner's syndrome due to damage to sympathetic trunk resulting in miosis, ptosis, enophthalmos, anhidrosis, in head, neck and thoracic tumours.
- Metastases may cause hepatomegaly, ascites and bone pain.
- In neonates, disseminated neuroblastomas may present with multiple cutaneous metastases and deep blue discolouration of the skin **(blueberry muffin baby)**.
- Also seen are paralysis in paraspinal tumours; skin bruising due to metastases to skin; raccoon eyes associated with metastases to orbit; pallor and anaemia due to infiltration of the bone marrow.
- About 90% tumours produce catecholamines and are associated with elevated levels of catecholamine metabolites like vanillylmandelic acid (VMA) and homovanillic acid (HVA) in the urine.

The important prognostic features of neuroblastoma are enlisted in Table 7.4.

Gross Morphology

- Neuroblastomas vary from being in situ lesions (small nodule) to large masses.

Table 7.4 Prognostic indicators of neuroblastoma

Features	Good prognosis	Bad prognosis
Age	<18 months	>18 months
Stage	1, 2a, 2b, 4s	III or IV
Ploidy	Hyperdiploid/near triploid	Near diploid
1p deletion and *N-myc* amplification	Absent	Present
Expression of TrkA (high-affinity growth receptor) indicating differentiation towards sympathetic ganglia lineage	Present	Absent
Expression of TrkB	Absent	Present
Mutations of neuritogenesis genes	Absent	Present
Morphology	Presence of Schwannian stroma and gangliocytic differentiation	Absence of Schwannian stroma and gangliocytic differentiation
Mitosis-karyorrhexis index	<200/5000 cells	>200/5000 cells

Source: *Robbins & Cotran Pathologic Basis of Disease,* Tenth Edition: Vinay Kumar, Abul K. Abbas, Jon C. Aster, Table 6.17, Page 261, Elsevier Inc., 2021.

- In situ lesions may regress to leave only small foci of fibrosis and calcification (spontaneous regression or therapy-induced maturation).
- Some tumours appear encapsulated and sharply demarcated, while others are highly infiltrative.
- Cut surface is soft, grey, brain-like with areas of necrosis and haemorrhage.

Microscopic Features

- Tumour is constituted by small, primitive-looking cells having dark nuclei, scant cytoplasm and poorly defined cell margins arranged in sheets.
- There is prominent mitotic activity, pleomorphism, and nuclear breakdown (karyorrhexis).
- Homer Wright pseudorosettes (tumour cells arranged around a central space filled with their fibrillar extensions) may be seen.

Staging

- Stage 1: Localised tumour that is completely surgically removed at diagnosis.
- Stage 2A: Unilateral tumour with incomplete gross resection; identifiable, ipsilateral and contralateral lymph nodes negative for tumour.
- Stage 2B: Localised tumour with or without complete gross resection; representative ipsilateral non-adherent lymph nodes positive for tumour; enlarged contralateral lymph nodes are negative for tumour microscopically.
- Stage 3: Unresectable unilateral tumour infiltrating across the midline with or without lymph nodes involvement or localised unilateral tumour with contralateral regional lymph nodes involvement.
- Stage 4: Any primary tumour with dissemination to distant lymph nodes, bone, bone marrow, liver, skin or other organs except defined for stage 4s.
- Stage 4s: Localised primary tumour (as defined for stages 1, 2A or 2B) with dissemination limited to skin, liver and/or bone marrow (less than 10% of nucleated cells are constituted by the neoplastic cells; more than 10% involvement of bone marrow is considered stage 4).

Q. Describe the clinicopathological features of retinoblastoma. (PA11.2)

Ans. Retinoblastoma is the most common malignant intraocular tumour of childhood.

- Develops in 80%–90% of those with mutant alleles in retinoblastoma (Rb) gene at 13q14.
- Need mutations in both alleles to inactivate Rb gene, which is a negative growth regulator.
- Patients with hereditary retinoblastoma have a germline mutation in one allele; develop tumours after somatic mutation in second allele ('second hit'); in sporadic cases, both alleles have somatic mutations.
- Familial forms may be multifocal and bilateral.
- Retinoblastomas are known to undergo spontaneous regression.
- These patients have a high incidence of secondary tumours (familial retinoblastoma predisposes to osteosarcoma and other soft-tissue sarcomas).
- Most cases are diagnosed before the age of 4 years (peak age 6 months to 2 years).

Clinical Features

- Poor vision, strabismus, a whitish hue to the pupil **(cat's eye reflex, leukokoria)**, pain in the eye and retinal detachment.
- Tendency to invade optic nerve; can invade uveal tract.
- Distant metastases to cranial vault, skeletal system.

Morphology

- Arises from neuroepithelial cells.
- Nodular, often with satellite lesions.
- Creamy white with chalky areas of calcification.
- May grow inward (endophytic) or outward toward choroid (exophytic) or in some cases are diffusely infiltrative.
- Composed of small round cells with hyperchromatic nuclei and scant cytoplasm (resembling retinoblasts).
- True rosettes called ***Flexner–Wintersteiner rosettes*** (clusters of cuboidal or short columnar cells arranged around a central lumen, which seems to have a limiting membrane resembling the external limiting membrane of the retina) are present and are unlike the pseudorosettes of neuroblastoma, which lack a true lumen.
- Tumour cells spread along the optic nerve or subarachnoid space.
- Distant metastases is seen in CNS, skull, distal bones and lymph nodes.

Prognosis

- **5 year survival:** Untreated the tumour is fatal, but with enucleation, chemotherapy and radiotherapy, survival rates are usually good (90% if unilateral, slightly less if bilateral).
- **Poor prognostic factors:** invasion of optic nerve, invasion of uveal tract or sclera, seeding of vitreous, involvement of anterior segment; extensive ocular tissue and tumour necrosis.

8 Neoplasia

Q. Define neoplasia. (PA7.1)

Ans. Neoplasia **(new growth)** is defined as excessive and unregulated proliferation that eventually becomes **autonomous** (independent of physiologic growth stimuli).

Q. Define oncology.

Ans. Oncology is the study of tumours and neoplasms (oncos in Greek means tumour). The term tumour was originally referred to any swelling, but is currently used most exclusively to refer to a neoplastic growth.

Q. Define cancer.

Ans. Cancer is the common term for malignant tumours (derived from the Latin word crab, indicating adherence to any part it seizes upon obstinately like a crab).

Q. What is clonality?

Ans. A tumour is said to be clonal when the entire population of cells within a tumour arises from a single cell that has incurred genetic change. A clonal neoplasm is therefore constituted by cells which carry the same genetic anomaly, for example in lymphoma and leukaemia, clonality is proven by the amplification of a single rearrangement of their immunoglobulin gene (for B cell lesions) or T cell receptor gene (for T cell lesions). The demonstration of clonality is now considered to be necessary to identify a lymphoid cell proliferation as neoplastic; however, as this is not always possible, clonality is not included in the definition of neoplasia.

Q. What are the two main components of all neoplasms? (PA7.1)

Ans. Histologically, almost all neoplasms are composed of two main components:

1. **Tumour cells that comprise the parenchyma** (also called specific component).
2. **Tumour stroma,** which is a supporting framework consisting of connective tissue and newly formed blood vessels elicited from adjacent tissues.

There is perpetual interaction between parenchyma and stroma, which directly influences the growth of the tumour.

Q. What is desmoplasia?

Ans. Hyperplasia of fibroblasts and formation of abundant collagen in the stroma as a reaction to infiltration by a cancer is labelled desmoplasia.

Q. Define a teratoma.

Ans. Teratoma is a tumour derived from a variety of cell types representing **more than one germ cell layer, usually all three.**

Characteristics:

- Derived from **totipotent cells (cells with an ability to differentiate into any cell type)**, teratomas are **usually encountered in gonads**. They sometimes develop in sequestered primitive cell rests elsewhere.
- Sacrococcygeal teratomas are the most common tumours in newborns, and mature cystic teratomas account for 10%–20% of all ovarian neoplasms.
- Teratomas are also frequently seen in the head and neck region, mediastinum and retroperitoneum.
- They range from benign, **well-differentiated mature cystic lesions** (Fig. 8.1), to those that are **solid** and **immature.** Additionally, teratomas may be **monodermal** and **highly specialised.**
- Rarely, within some mature teratomas certain elements (most commonly squamous components) undergo **malignant transformation.**

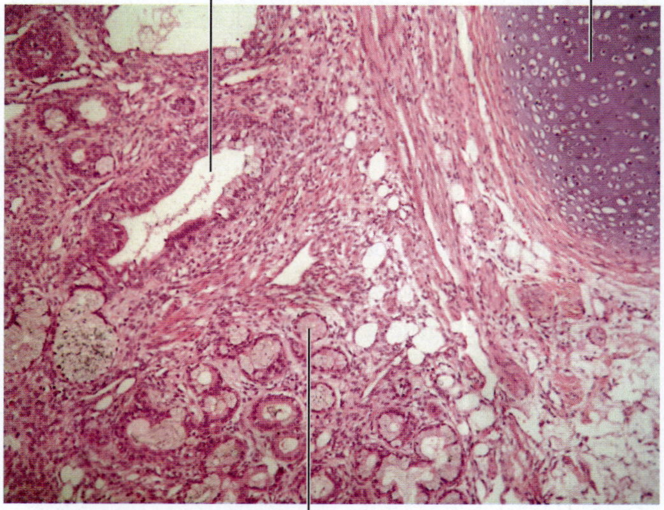

Fig. 8.1 Photomicrograph from a mature cystic teratoma showing glands lined by stratified columnar epithelium, mucinous glands and hyaline cartilage (H&E; 200×).

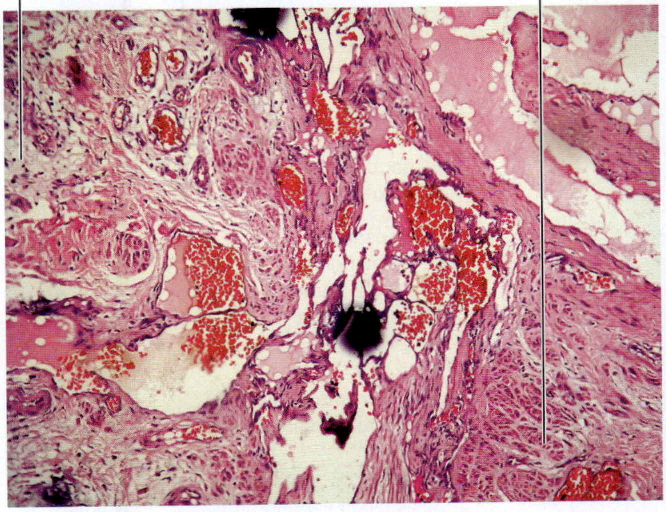

Fig. 8.2 Photomicrograph of a vascular hamartoma showing large caliber vessels, smooth muscle, and mature adipose tissue (H&E; 100×).

Q. Define a choristoma.

Ans. A choristoma is an **ectopic rest of normal tissue**, for example a rest of adrenal cells under the kidney capsule and pancreatic rest in the intestine.

Q. Define a hamartoma.

Ans. Aberrant differentiation may produce a mass of disorganised but mature, specialised cells/tissue indigenous to the particular site (thought to be either an anomalous development or a neoplasm in origin), for example hamartoma of the lung or a vascular hamartoma in soft tissue (Fig. 8.2). Although the underlying reasons for the aberrant differentiation are not fully understood, hamartomas are thought to be an anomalous development rather than neoplastic in origin). They are known to grow along with, and at the same rate as, the organ of origin and unlike neoplasms, only rarely invade or compress surrounding structures significantly.

Q. Define a blastoma.

Ans. Blastoma is a type of malignant tumour that arises in precursor cells and typically affects children and young adults. The nomenclature of the blastoma is based on its location in the body. For example, **retinoblastoma** is a blastoma of the eye, while **nephroblastoma** (Wilms' tumour) is a blastoma of the kidney.

Q. Differentiate between a hamartoma and a neoplasm.

Ans. Differences between a hamartoma and a neoplasm are summarised in (Table 8.1).

Table 8.1 Differences between a hamartoma and a neoplasm

Features	Hamartoma	Neoplasm
Definition	Disorganised focal overgrowth of mature tissue indigenous to a particular site	Abnormal, excessive, unregulated, autonomous proliferation of cells
Behaviour	Always benign	May be benign or malignant
Degree of differentiation	Well-differentiated cells, which completely resemble normal counterparts	Vary from well-differentiated to poorly differentiated anaplastic lesions
Clonality	Polyclonal	Monoclonal
Examples	Vascular hamartoma	Squamous cell carcinoma

Q. Classify neoplasms. (PA7.1)

Ans. Neoplasms can be classified into different types based on the following features:

1. **Gross or naked-eye appearance:**
   - **Benign lesions** are usually encapsulated and circumscribed and grow along broad fonds (have pushing margins).
   - **Malignant lesions** are usually unencapsulated, ill-defined and infiltrating. They can have several different gross appearances, that is, annular (endophytic), ulcerative, fungating (exophytic or cauliflower-like), scirrhous (showing excessive fibrosis) or mucoid (containing abundant mucin).
2. **Histological appearance and histogenetic/embryological considerations:**
   - **Cell of origin**, that is, epithelial or connective tissue, undifferentiated stem cells or highly specialised cells/tissue.
   - **Vascular/lymphatic invasion.**
   - **Capsular invasion.**
   - **Histopathological margins** (infiltrating or expansile).
3. **Behavioural characteristics** (indolent, borderline aggressive or frankly aggressive).
4. **Aetiological characteristics** (tumour induced by radiation, chemical or viral carcinogens; tumour of primary or secondary origin).
5. **Functional characteristics** (some tumours secrete hormones or proteins with characteristic effects on the body, for example adrenocorticotropic hormone (ACTH), parathormone (PTH) and antidiuretic hormone (ADH) secreted by lung carcinoma and keratin produced by well-differentiated squamous cell carcinoma).

Presently, tissue of origin and behavioural pattern is the basis of classification of most neoplasms.

Q. Define and classify benign tumours. (PA7.1)

Ans. Benign tumours are neoplasms, that grow as cohesive expansile masses, and do not invade, **infiltrate** or **metastasize.** They are usually encapsulated (the capsule is made of a rim of compressed connective tissue derived largely from the native stroma).

Table 8.2 Classification and nomenclature of tumours

Tissue of origin	Benign	Malignant
1. *Tumours of one parenchymal cell type*		
a. Mesenchymal origin		
i. Connective tissue and its derivatives	Fibroma Lipoma Chondroma Osteoma	Fibrosarcoma Liposarcoma Chondrosarcoma Osteosarcoma
ii. Endothelial and related tissues		
A. Blood vessels	Haemangioma	Angiosarcoma
B. Lymph vessels	Lymphangioma	Lymphangiosarcoma
C. Synovium	—	Synovial sarcoma
D. Mesothelium	—	Mesothelioma
E. Haematopoetic tissue	—	Leukaemia, lymphoma
iii. Muscle		
A. Smooth	Leiomyoma	Leiomyosarcoma
B. Skeletal	Rhabdomyoma	Rhabdomyosarcoma
b. Epithelial origin		
i. Squamous cells	Squamous papilloma	Squamous cell carcinoma
ii. Basal cells	—	Basal cell carcinoma
iii. Lining of glands and ducts	Adenoma	Adenocarcinoma
A. Respiratory epithelium	Bronchial adenoma	Bronchogenic carcinoma
B. Transitional epithelium	Transitional papilloma	Transitional cell carcinoma
C. Germ cells	—	Malignant germ cell tumours (embryonal carcinoma, seminoma)
c. Tumour of melanocytes	Nevus	Malignant melanoma
2. *Tumours of more than one cell type (mixed tumours derived from a single germ cell layer)*		
a. Salivary glands	Pleomorphic adenoma	Carcinoma in pleomorphic adenoma
b. Renal anlage	—	Wilms tumour
3. *Tumours of more than one cell type (mixed tumours derived from more than one germ cell layer)*	Teratoma	Teratocarcinoma

Nomenclature and Classification (Table 8.2)

1. **Tumours of mesenchymal origin:** Designated by adding suffix 'oma' to the cell of origin, for example fibroma, lipoma, osteoma and chondroma (Fig. 8.3).

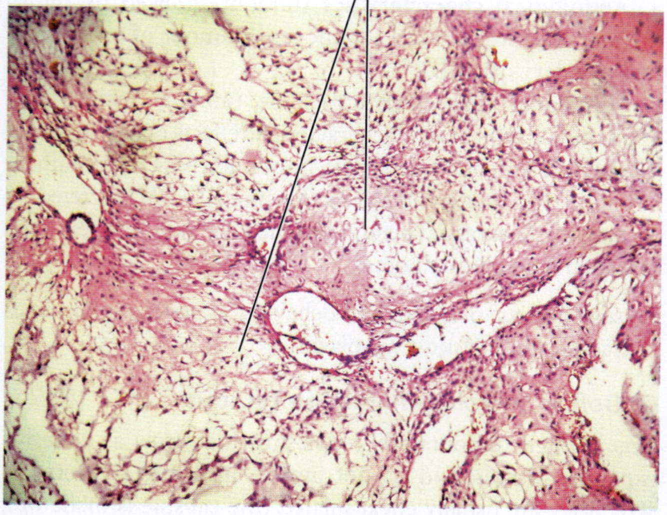

Fig. 8.3 Photomicrograph of a chondroma showing lobules of benign appearing cartilage separated by fibrous septae (H&E; 100×).

2. **Tumours of epithelial origin are variously classified:**
   (a) Some based on the cell of origin, such as squamous cell papilloma (Fig. 8.4).
   (b) Others based on the microscopic architecture, eg, adenoma (glandular pattern; Fig. 8.5), papilloma (finger-like

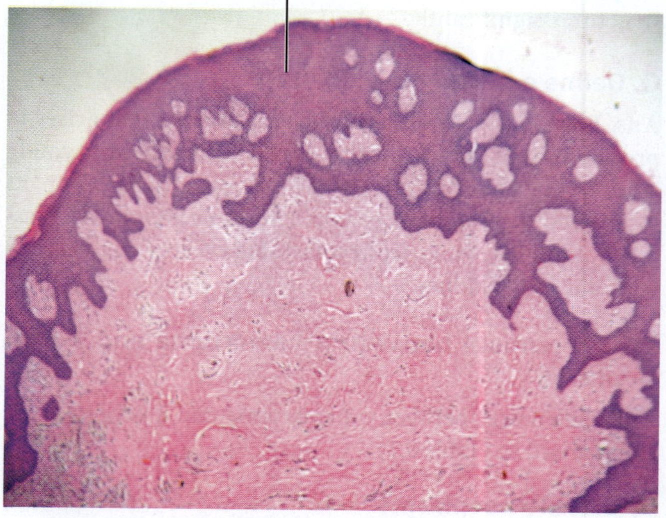

Fig. 8.4 Photomicrograph of a squamous papilloma showing hyperplastic squamous lining covering fibrovascular tissue (H&E; 100×).

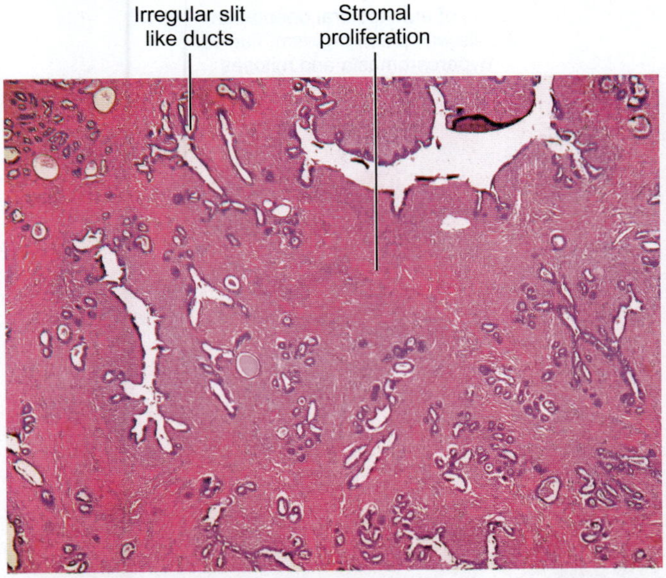

Fig. 8.5 Photomicrograph of fibroadenoma breast showing stromal proliferation with compression of ducts, which appear irregular and slit like (H&E; 100×).

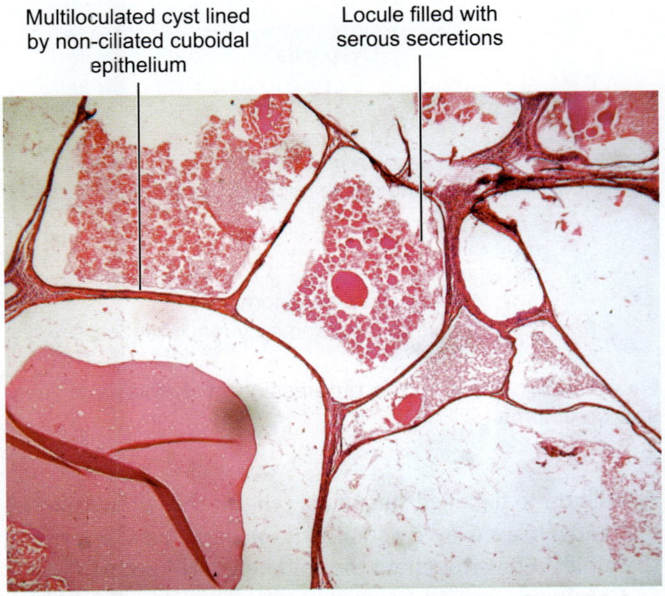

Fig. 8.6 Photomicrograph of a serous cystadenoma ovary showing a multiloculated cyst lined by serous epithelium (non-ciliated epithelium resembling ovarian surface epithelium H&E; 100×).

or warty projections), cystadenoma (cystic masses; Fig. 8.6) and papillary cyst adenoma (papillary cystic masses).

3. **Mixed tumours:** Divergent differentiation of a single line of parenchymal cells resulting in tumours comprising more than one cell type; usually derived from one germ cell layer, for example pleomorphic adenoma of the salivary gland (Fig. 8.7).

Q. Define differentiation. (PA7.1)

Ans. Differentiation is the extent to which neoplastic cells resemble comparable normal cells, both morphologically and functionally. The cells in benign tumours are almost always well differentiated and resemble their normal cells of origin.

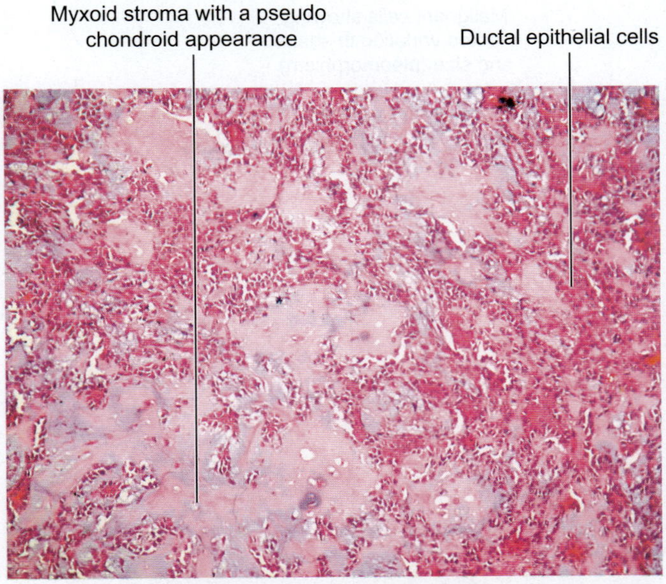

Fig. 8.7 Photomicrograph of pleomorphic adenoma of salivary gland showing a biphasic pattern resulting from the admixture of two components—epithelial (comprised of ducts and cords lined by epithelial and myoepithelial cells) and stromal (comprised of fibromyxoid elements) (H&E; 100×).

Cancers, however, vary from being well differentiated to poorly differentiated.

- **Well-differentiated cancers** show progressive maturation or specialization of undifferentiated cells as they proliferate. **Poorly differentiated or undifferentiated cancers** show proliferation without differentiation or maturation.
- Well-differentiated squamous cell carcinomas of the epidermis elaborate keratin, just as well-differentiated hepatocellular carcinomas elaborate bile. Highly anaplastic undifferentiated cells, whatever is their tissue of origin, loose their resemblance to the normal cells from which they have arisen.

Q. Define anaplasia. Enumerate the morphological features indicative of anaplasia. (PA7.1)

Ans. Anaplasia is defined as lack of differentiation; literal meaning is 'reverse differentiation'. It is usually a hallmark of malignant transformation.

Morphological Features Indicative of Anaplasia.

- Pleomorphism (variation in size and shape of cells; Fig. 8.8.
- Anisonucleosis (variation in size of nuclei).
- Abnormal nuclear morphology:
  - Abundant and darkly staining (hyperchromatic) DNA.
  - Coarsely clumped chromatin or clumping of nuclear chromatin along the nuclear membrane resulting in prominent appearing nucleoli.
  - Increased nucleocytoplasmic ratio (normal from 1:4 to 1:6; may approach 1:1).
- Numerous mitoses with abnormal, atypical, bizarre, tri, quadri and multipolar spindles (abnormal mitoses are seen in malignant tumours only; Fig. 8.9).
- Loss of polarity (orientation of cells) resulting in sheets or large masses of tumour cells that grow in disorganised fashion.
- Presence of the tumour giant cells which have pleomorphic, sometimes bizarre, hyperchromatic nuclei.

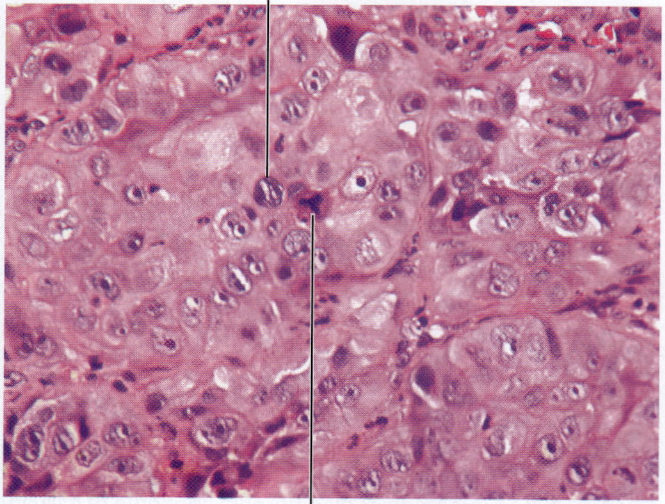

Fig. 8.8 Photomicrograph of a squamous cell carcinoma showing marked cellular pleomorphism with presence of atypical mitosis (H&E; 200×).

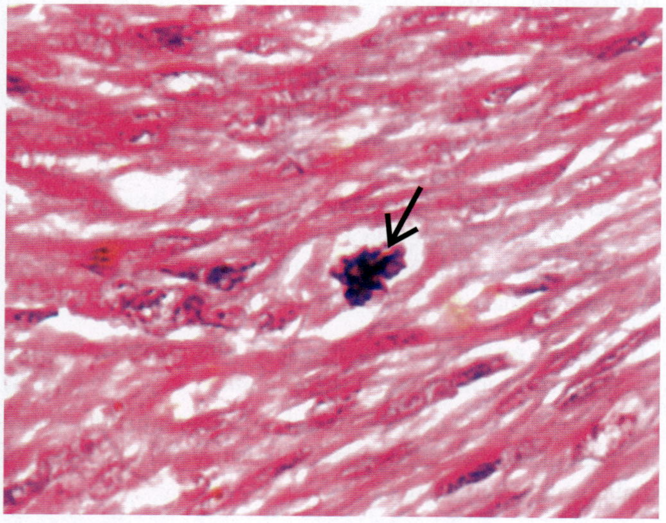

Fig. 8.9 Photomicrograph of a high-grade sarcoma showing an abnormal multipolar mitosis (arrow) (H&E; 400×).

Q. Define dysplasia. Enumerate the steps in the course of progression of dysplasia to invasive cancer. (PA7.1)

Ans. Dysplasia (disordered growth) is defined as the loss of architectural orientation of cells with respect to one another along with presence of pleomorphism, nuclear hyperchromatism and mitoses (Fig. 8.10). Dysplasia can be low grade or high grade (see 'carcinoma in situ' in next paragraph). The risk of low grade dysplasia transforming into high-grade dysplasia and eventually cancer is low. High-grade dysplasia, however, represents an advanced progression toward malignant transformation. For example, the usual progressive maturation of tall cells in the basal layer of stratified squamous epithelium to flattened squamous cells on the surface may be lost and replaced by a scrambling of dark, basal-appearing (basaloid) cells throughout the epithelium. (Flowchart 8.1).

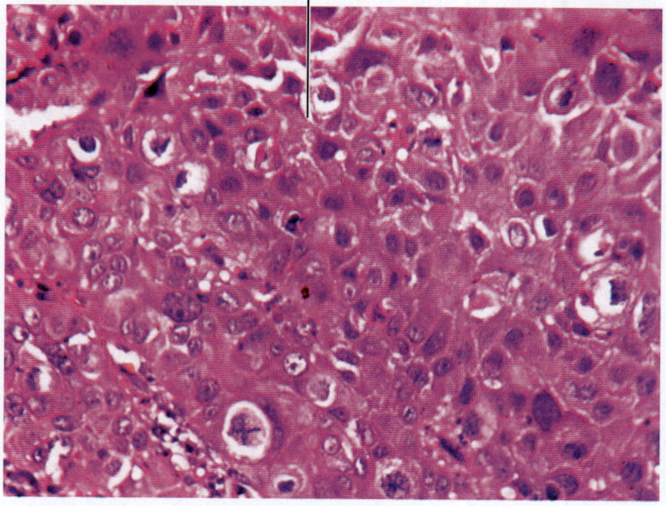

Fig. 8.10 Section from dysplastic epithelium showing anisonucleosis and loss of nuclear polarity (H&E; 200×).

Dysplasia
↓
Carcinoma in situ
(Dysplasia involving the entire thickness of the epithelium)
↓
Invasive carcinoma
(Frank invasion into the stroma by malignant cells)

Flowchart 8.1 Steps in the progression of dysplasia to invasive carcinoma.

Carcinoma in situ ('cancer in place') is a lesion in which the dysplastic cells show essentially no maturation and grow rapidly without regulation; however, they remain localised, and do not invade past the basement membrane into the subepithelial tissue or stroma.

Invasive carcinoma is the final step in this sequence of events. It is the stage in which the malignant cells have invaded beyond the basement membrane and have acquired the potential to metastasize. Invasive carcinoma, if left untreated, is almost always fatal.

Differences between metaplasia and dysplasia are shown in Table 8.3.

Q. Differentiate between dysplasia and anaplasia. (PA7.1)

Ans. Differences between dysplasia and anaplasia are shown in Table 8.4.

Table 8.3 Differences between metaplasia and dysplasia

Features	Metaplasia	Dysplasia
Definition	Reversible change in which one adult cell type (epithelial or mesenchymal) is replaced by another adult cell type	Loss of uniformity of the individual cells (mainly epithelial) as well as lack of architectural orientation with respect to one another
Cellular pleomorphism	Usually not seen	Present
Nuclear atypia	Usually not seen	Hyperchromatic and abnormally large atypical nuclei may be seen
Mitotic figures	Few	Many
Orientation with respect to one another (tissue architecture)	Maintained	Loss of ordered maturation as in dysplastic stratified squamous epithelium
Reversibility	Reversible, if triggering factors are removed	May become irreversible if it involves whole thickness of the epithelium
Example	Columnar to squamous epithelium in respiratory tract of chronic smokers	Cervical intraepithelial neoplasia (CIN)

Table 8.4 Differences between dysplasia and anaplasia

Features	Dysplasia	Anaplasia
Definition	Lack of uniformity of individual cells with architectural distortion	Lack of morphological and functional differentiation of cells
Behaviour	A potentially precancerous condition, which may or may not progress to cancer	Anaplasia is usually a hallmark of malignant transformation
Tissue involved	Mainly epithelium	Both epithelium and mesenchyme
Cellular pleomorphism and nuclear atypia	Present, but usually low grade	High grade
Mitotic figures	Present, usually not atypical	Abnormal and atypical figures may be seen (tripolar, quadripolar and multipolar spindles)
Tumour giant cells	Absent	Present

Q. Define and classify malignant tumours (refer to Table 8.2). (PA7.1)

Ans. Malignant tumours are neoplasms that **infiltrate**, **invade** and **metastasize.** They may be:

- **Epithelial in origin (ecarcinomas),** usually named after (1) their parent organ or tissue of origin, for example adenocarcinoma of intestine and squamous cell carcinoma of the cervix or oral mucosa, or (2) their architectural pattern—a carcinoma with a glandular growth pattern termed an adenocarcinoma (Fig. 8.11). One producing recognisable squamous cells (arising from any of the stratified squamous epithelia of the body) is termed a squamous cell carcinoma (Fig. 8.12). Also, it is a common practice to specify, whenever possible, the organ of origin of the malignancy (e.g. renal adenocarcinoma, bronchogenic squamous cell carcinoma, etc.).

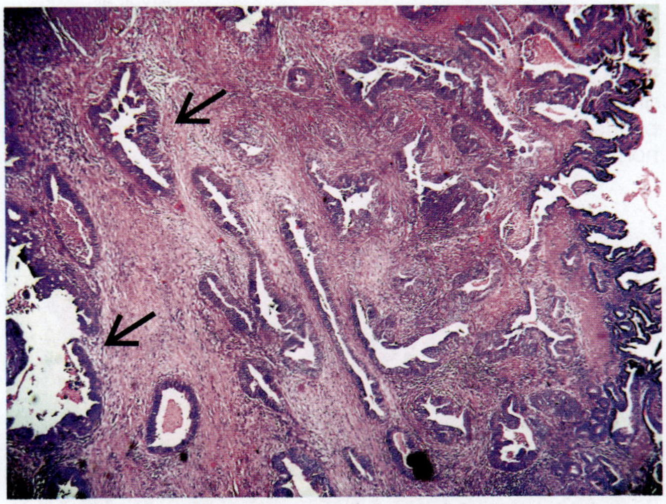

Fig. 8.11 Section from adenocarcinoma gall bladder showing malignant glands invading its wall (arrows) (H&E; 100×).

- **Mesenchymal** or **connective tissue in origin (sarcomas),** for example, malignant neoplasm of fibroblasts is labelled fibrosarcoma and one composed of fat cells is called liposarcoma. Malignant tumour derived from osteoblasts is called an osteogenic sarcoma (Fig. 8.13).
- A malignant neoplasm may be composed of very primitive, undifferentiated cells, in which case it is designated merely as an **undifferentiated malignant tumour** or when possible, **undifferentiated carcinoma or undifferentiated sarcoma.**

Q. Differentiate between benign and malignant tumours.

Ans. Differences between benign and malignant tumours are shown in Table 8.5.

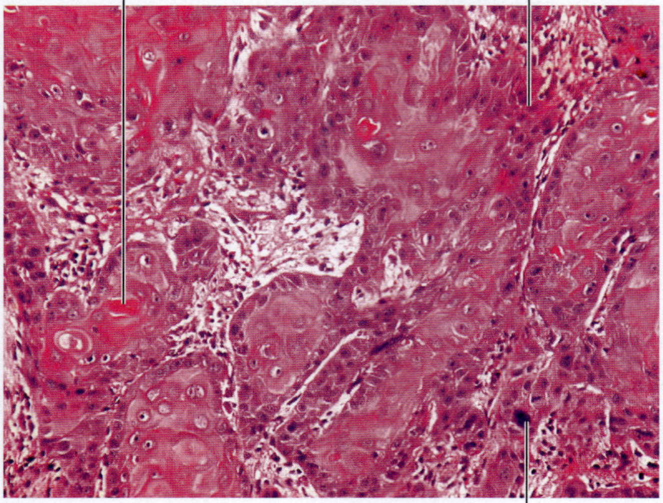

Fig. 8.12 Photomicrograph from oral mucosa showing a well-differentiated squamous cell carcinoma with numerous keratin pearls. The tumour cells show a striking resemblance to normal squamous cells (H&E; 100×).

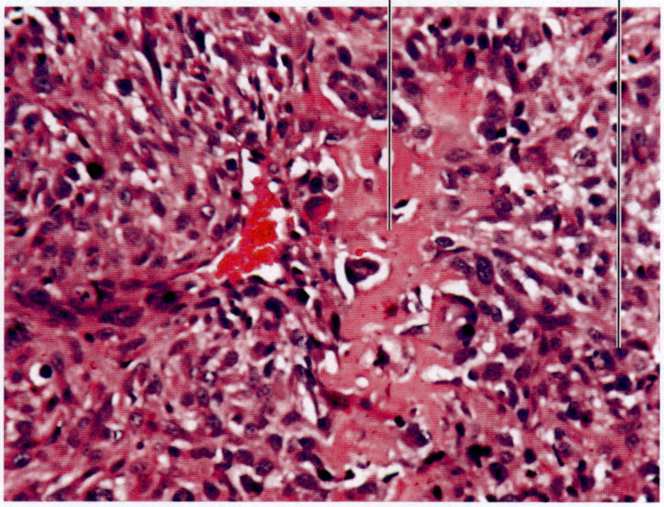

Fig. 8.13 Section from an osteosarcoma showing highly pleomorphic stromal cells laying down pink tumour osteoid (H&E; 200×).

Q. Define local invasion.

Ans. Most cancers are accompanied by progressive infiltration and destruction of the surrounding tissue, referred to as local invasion or direct spread.

Q. Define metastasis. Write briefly on the various pathways of spread of the tumours.

Ans. Tumour implants discontinuous with the primary tumour, confirm the malignant nature of a tumour and are labelled metastases. All cancers metastasize with a few exceptions, for example, basal cell carcinoma (rodent ulcer) and gliomas of the central nervous system, which are locally invasive and rarely metastasize. Metastases can occur **via lymphatics, blood vessels, across body cavities (transcoelomic spread), body fluids (e.g. cerebrospinal fluid), tumour implantation**, etc.

Table 8.5 Contrasting features of benign and malignant tumours

Features	Benign	Malignant
Gross features		
Boundaries	Encapsulated/well circumscribed	Ill circumscribed/ unencapsulated
Size	Usually small	Usually large
Secondary changes	Less frequent	More frequent
Surrounding tissue	Compressed	Invaded
Microscopic features		
Pattern	Resembles tissue of origin	Poor resemblance to tissue of origin
Polarity	Retained	Lost
Anaplasia	Absent	Present
Mitoses	Present, few, typical	Present, many, atypical as well as typical
Tumour giant cells	Rare, without atypia	Common, with atypia
Cytogenetic changes	Rare	Common
Physiology of cells/function	Maintained	Lost
Growth rate	Low	High
Local invasion	Rare	Common
Metastasis	Absent	Present

Pathways of Spread of the Tumours

1. **Direct seeding of body cavities and surfaces:** Penetration of a tumour into a natural open field/space, for example pleural, pericardial, subarachnoid and synovial. Sometimes mucinous tumours of appendix and ovary (both benign and malignant) fill the peritoneal cavity with a gelatinous neoplastic mass called **'pseudomyxoma peritonei'.**
2. **Lymphatic spread**
   (a) Functional lymphatics are absent in tumours and lymphatic vessels located at the surface are sufficient for lymphatic spread.
   (b) Tumour cells invade the wall of the lymphatics and may grow within it in a continuous manner or detached groups of malignant cells may embolize into lymphatics to reach the draining lymph nodes. The tumour emboli reach the subcapsular sinus where they grow to later replace the entire lymph node. Lymphatic spread tends

to follow natural routes of lymphatic drainage and is the usual route for dissemination of **epithelial malignancies**; sarcomas may also use this route.

(c) Since **carcinoma of the breast** usually arises in the upper outer quadrant, it generally disseminates first to the axillary lymph nodes. Cancers of the inner quadrant may drain through lymphatics to the nodes within the chest along the internal mammary artery. Thereafter the infraclavicular and supraclavicular nodes may become involved. **Carcinoma of the lung** arising in the major respiratory passages metastasizes first to the perihilar, tracheobronchial and mediastinal nodes. Local lymph nodes, however, may sometimes be bypassed—**skip metastasis**—because of venous–lymphatic anastomoses, or because inflammation or radiation has obliterated channels. An example of local lymph nodes getting bypassed and metastasis developing in a distant group of lymph nodes is **'Virchow's lymph node'** (cancers of abdominal organs metastasising in the supraclavicular lymph node). A tumour spreading against the normal flow of lymphatics is called **'reterograde metastasis'** (carcinoma prostate metastasising to supraclavicular lymph node).

(d) Drainage of tumour cell debris and antigens may induce reactive hyperplasia and lymphadenopathy **(sinus histiocytosis and dermatopathic lymphadenopathy)**. Therefore nodal enlargement in proximity to a cancer does not necessarily mean dissemination of the primary lesion.

(e) A **'sentinel' lymph node** is defined as the first node in the regional lymphatic chain to receive lymph flow from the primary tumour. Sentinel node mapping can be done by injection of radiolabelled tracers or blue dyes.

3. **Haematogenous spread**
   (a) Typical of **sarcomas** but also seen in carcinomas
   (b) Arteries have thick walls, are less penetrable than veins. **Capillaries and venues are generally invaded.** After venous invasion, blood-borne cells follow venous flow to reach the draining sites of the organ of origin (Fig. 8.14).
   (c) All portal blood flows to liver and all caval blood flows to lungs; therefore, **liver and lungs are the most frequently involved organs in haematogenous dissemination. Brain is the most common site for metastasis from lungs, kidneys and adrenals.**
   (d) Cancers in the vicinity of vertebral column, for example **thyroid and prostate, metastasize to the vertebrae via paravertebral plexus.**

Q. Write briefly about the biology of the tumour growth.

Ans. Rate of growth of the tumour depends on:

1. **Doubling time** of tumour cells (time taken by the tumour cells to double their volume or number of cells).
2. **Growth fraction** (fraction of the tumour cells that are in the replicative pool).

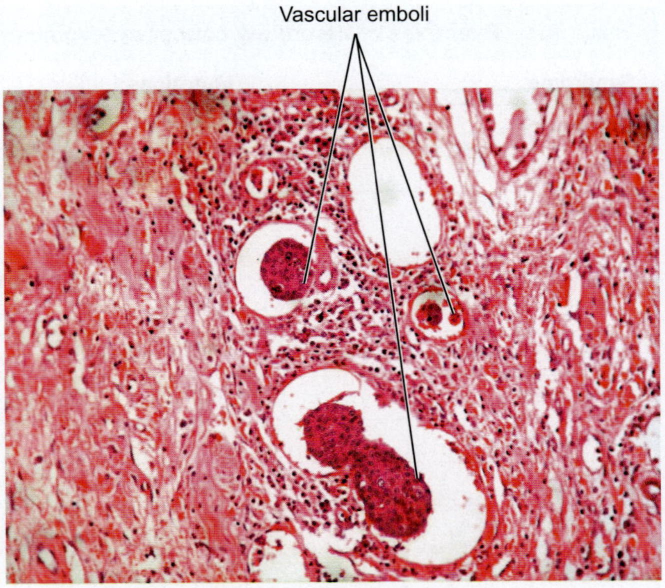

Fig. 8.14 Section showing vascular tumour emboli (H&E; 100×).

3. Rate at which cells are shed and lost in the growing lesion.
4. **Fast-growing tumours have a high-cell turnover** (high rate of, both proliferation and apoptosis); the tumour growth is possible only if rate of proliferation is greater than rate of apoptosis.
5. Most anticancer drugs act on cells, which are in the growth cycle.
6. Tumours with high growth fraction are more susceptible to radio and chemotherapy.
7. Debulking with surgery and radiation shifts tumour cells from G_0 to G_1 phase.
8. Rate of growth is proportional to the level of differentiation of cells.

Q. Write briefly about the epidemiology of malignant tumours.

Ans. Cancer is a leading cause of death worldwide, accounting for a large number of deaths. Lung, stomach, liver, colon and breast cancer cause most cancer deaths each year. The frequency of different cancers differs between men and women. Most cancers can be attributed to five leading behavioural and dietary risks: high body mass index, low fruit and vegetable intake, lack of physical activity, tobacco and alcohol use. In India, breast cancer is the most common, and stomach cancer is the leading cause of death by cancer for the population as a whole. Breast cancer and lung cancer kill the most women and men, respectively. The following are the most common malignant tumours encountered worldwide:

Men: lung, prostate, colon or rectum, stomach, leukaemia and lymphoma, liver.

Women: breast, colorectal, lung, cervical, thyroid, leukaemia and lymphoma, ovary.

Children: acute leukaemia, CNS tumours, lymphomas, neuroblastoma, bone sarcomas.

Table 8.6 Examples of hereditary cancer syndromes

Syndrome	Mutations	Associated cancers
Cowden	PTEN	Breast, thyroid, endometrial
FAP	APC	Colorectal, GI, CNS, Gastric, Bone, Skin
Lynch	MSH2, MLH1, MSH6, PMS2, EPCAM	Coloreactal
Turcot	MSH2, MLH1, MSH6, PMS2 (biallelic)	Large intestine, CNS
Hereditary breast-ovarian cancer	BRCA1 and BRCA 2	Breast, ovarian, prostate, pancreatic
Li Fraumeni	TP53	Sarcomas, breast, lung, brain, adrenal gland
Von Hippel Lindau	VHL	Renal cell carcinoma
MEN 1	MEN	Pancreatic islet cell, adenomas of parathyroid and pituitary
MEN 2A	RET	Thyroid, pheochromocytoma, parathyroid adenoma
RB	RB1	Retinal, pineal, osteosarcoma, melanoma, sarcoma

Q. Write briefly on the epidemiological factors influencing neoplasia. (PA7.2)

Ans. The following factors influence the development of neoplasia:

I. Familial and Genetic Factors (Inherited Predisposition to Cancer)

1. **Autosomal dominant-inherited cancer syndromes (Table 8.6)**
   (a) The autosomal dominant inheritance of a single mutant gene greatly increases risk of developing a tumour. The inherited mutation is generally a point mutation occurring in a single allele of a tumour suppressor gene. Defect in the second allele occurs in the somatic cell, as a consequence of deletion or recombination. As in other autosomal dominant conditions, both incomplete penetrance and variable expressivity occur.
   (b) *Examples are as follows:*
      (i) **Retinoblastoma (RB):** Approximately 40% of RBs are inherited. Carriers of a mutant RB tumour suppressor gene have a 10,000-fold increased risk of developing RB, usually bilateral. They also have a greatly increased risk of developing a second cancer, usually osteogenic sarcoma.
      (ii) **Familial polyposis coli (FAP):**
      - Presents with polypoid adenomas at birth and shows 100% conversion to familial polyposis coli by age of 50 years.
      - The genetic defect in FAP is a germline mutation in the adenomatous polyposis coli (APC) gene. Syndromes once thought to be distinct from FAP are now recognised to be a part of the phenotypic spectrum of FAP.
      - Syndromes with a germline mutation in the APC gene include FAP, Gardner syndrome, some families with Turcot syndrome and attenuated adenomatous polyposis coli (AAPC).
      - **Gardner syndrome** is characterized by colonic polyposis typical of FAP, along with osteomas (skull and mandible), dental abnormalities and soft tissue tumours. **Turcot syndrome** is characterized by colonic polyposis typical of FAP, along with CNS tumours (medulloblastoma). **AAPC** is characterised by fewer colonic polyps as compared to classic FAP, which tend to develop late (average age 36 years), and involve proximal colonic area.

      (iii) **Multiple endocrine neoplasia (MEN) syndromes:**
      - The term **MEN** encompasses several distinct autosomal dominant syndromes featuring both benign and malignant tumours derived from endocrine and non-endocrine tissue.
      - There are two major forms of MEN—type 1 and type 2—which are distinguished based on the genes involved and hormones secreted (**MEN 1**—adenomas of pituitary, parathyroid and pancreas; **MEN 2**—medullary carcinoma thyroid, pheochromocytoma and parathyroid tumours).
      - Other component neoplasms include adrenocortical tumours; visceral and cutaneous lipomas; meningiomas; facial angiofibromas and thymic, gastric and bronchial carcinoids.
      - MEN 1 follows Knudson's 'two-hit' model for tumour suppressor gene carcinogenesis. First hit is a heterozygous MEN 1 germline mutation, inherited from one parent (familial cases) or developed in an early embryonic stage (sporadic cases) and present in all cells at birth. Second hit is a MEN 1 somatic mutation, usually a large deletion, which occurs in predisposed endocrine

cells. MEN 2 is caused by a mutation of RET proto-oncogene.

(iv) **Neurofibromatosis (NF) or von Recklinghausen disease:**
- NF is an autosomal dominant disorder that affects bones, nervous system, soft tissue and skin.
- At least eight different clinical phenotypes of NF have been identified, and they are linked to at least two genetic disorders. Commonly abbreviated **NF1** (neurofibromatosis type 1), the first is also known as **von Recklinghausen disease.** It occurs following mutation of neurofibromin 1 on chromosome 17q11.2.
- Neurofibromin is a tumour suppressor gene whose function is to inhibit p21 RAS oncoprotein. In absence of the inhibitory control of RAS oncoprotein by this gene, there is uncontrolled cellular proliferation and manifestation mainly as neurofibromas and Café au lait spots.
- **Neurofibromatosis type 2** (also called **'central neurofibromatosis'**) is a result of mutation of protein merlin (also known as 'Neurofibromin 2' or 'schwannomin') on chromosome 22q12. It accounts for only 10% of all cases of NF. Normal function of merlin is not well understood.

(v) **Li-Fraumeni syndrome:** Results from germline mutation of P53 (see P53).

2. **Defective DNA repair syndromes**
   (a) Human syndromes with DNA repair deficiencies cause genomic instability which is the driving force behind cancer development. There are four categories of DNA repair genes:
      (i) Mismatch repair genes.
      (ii) Base excision repair genes.
      (iii) Nucleotide excision repair genes.
      (iv) Double strand break repair genes.
   (b) Mostly autosomal recessive in inheritance, common examples of DNA repair defects include **xeroderma pigmentosa, ataxia telangiectasia** and **Bloom syndrome**. Xeroderma pigmentosa manifests with extreme sensitivity to UV radiation and predisposition to basal cell carcinoma, squamous cell carcinoma and malignant melanoma. Rarely defective DNA repair syndromes may be autosomal dominant in inheritance, as in HNPCC (hereditary non-polypoid colonic cancer caused by inactivation of a DNA mismatch repair gene).
3. **Familial cancers**
   Cancers with a high frequency of occurrence within a family are called familial cancers, for example carcinomas of breast, colon, uterus, ovary, stomach and some sarcomas. Familial cancers have the following features:
      (i) Early age of onset
      (ii) Multiple primary cancers in a single individual (such as bilateral breast cancer)
      (iii) No clearly identifiable pattern of transmission.

Table 8.7 Racial and geographic variations in various cancers

Race	Commonly seen cancers
White Europeans	Carcinoma skin, lung, breast, prostate and colorectal region
Black Africans	Carcinoma of penis, cervix, and liver
Japanese	Carcinoma stomach
South East Asians	Nasopharyngeal carcinoma (more common in Chinese)
Indians	Oral and gastrointestinal cancers, carcinoma cervix, and breast

II. Racial and Geographic Factors

Disparities in cancer incidence, mortality and survival in relation to race and ethnicity, and geographical location have been observed indicating that racial and geographical factors have a role to play in cancer incidence and characteristics (Table 8.7).

III. Environmental and Cultural Factors

1. **Cigarette smoking** is known to be associated with oral cancer, carcinoma of larynx, pharynx, oesophagus, lungs, pancreas and urinary bladder.
2. **Alcohol abuse** causes cancers of oropharynx, larynx, oesophagus and liver. Alcohol and smoking together increase the incidence of cancer of the upper airways and digestive tract.
3. **Industrial and environmental carcinogens** include UV rays, smog, arsenic, asbestos, benzene, vinyl chloride and β-naphthylamine.
4. **Infectious agents** like Human Papilloma Virus (HPV) implicated in carcinoma cervix and head and neck cancers.
5. **Diet:** Following factors predispose to malignancies:
   (a) Obesity
   (b) Deficiency of vitamin A, tocopherols, selenium and zinc
   (c) Diet rich in animal fats; low in fibre content.
6. **Age:** Most cancers are seen after fifth decade; some cancers may be seen in childhood.
7. **Sex:** Males are more commonly affected, except in carcinoma breast, gall bladder, thyroid and hypopharynx.

IV. Predisposing Factors for Specific Malignancies

1. **Carcinoma of cervix:** Young age at first coitus, high frequency of sexual intercourse, multiplicity of partners and multiparity contribute to increasing probability of carcinoma cervix.
2. **Penile carcinoma:** Rare in Jews and Muslims (because they are customarily circumcised); common in other communities.
3. **Cancer of cheek and tongue:** Associated with betel nut and tobacco chewing.

V. Interactions Between Genetic and Non-genetic Factors

Inherited variations (polymorphisms) in enzymes that metabolise procarcinogens to carcinogens can determine the susceptibility to cancer, for example polymorphisms in gene coding for *P-450* confers inherited susceptibility to lung cancer in smokers.

VI. Non-hereditary Predisposing Conditions

1. **Chronic inflammation and cancer:**
   (a) An increased risk of cancer has been noted in chronic inflammatory conditions, such as chronic irritation and oral cancers, **Marjolin's ulcer** and squamous cell carcinoma, ulcerative colitis and adenocarcinoma colon, *Helicobacter pylori* gastritis and carcinoma stomach and viral hepatitis/cirrhosis and hepatocellular carcinoma.
   (b) Inflammation increases expression of cyclooxygenase-2 (COX-2), which induces conversion of arachidonic acid into prostaglandins, which in turn are found to be increased in cancers, for example colonic cancer. The role of COX-2 inhibitors in cancer treatment and the potential association between cancer and chronic inflammation is being explored.
   (c) Chronic inflammation is associated with repair and proliferation, thus increasing the tissue stem cell pool, which is vulnerable and susceptible to transformation.
2. **Precancerous conditions:** Certain non-neoplastic and benign disorders have a well-defined association with cancer. Increased incidence of cancer in precancerous lesions is mostly attributed to continuous regenerative cell replication. These lesions include:
   (a) Actinic or solar keratosis.
   (b) Barrett oesophagus.
   (c) Leukoplakia of oral cavity, vulva and penis.
   (d) Chronic atrophic gastritis.
   (e) Paget disease of bone.
   (f) Multiple villous adenomas of colon.
   (g) Neurofibromatosis.
   (h) Long-standing ulcerative colitis.
   (i) Cirrhosis of liver.
   (j) Chronic bronchitis (heavy smokers).
   (k) Chronic irritation of the oral cavity.
   (l) Old burn scar **(Marjolin ulcer)**.
3. **Immunodeficiency states:** Individuals with deficient T cell immunity are predisposed to cancers particularly those caused by oncogenic viruses.

VII. Role of Hormones in Cancer

Hormone-related cancers include carcinoma of the breast, endometrium, ovary, prostate, testis, and thyroid as well as osteosarcoma. Hormone-mediated carcinogenesis is unique and involves both endogenous and exogenous hormones which stimulate cell proliferation, and thus increase the possibility of accumulation of random genetic errors. Excessive estrogen (estrogen therapy or estrogen secreting granulosa cell tumour of the ovary) can induce breast cancer and carcinoma of the endometrium. Daughters of mothers who receive estrogen therapy during pregnancy can sometimes present with adenocarcinoma of the vagina. Cancers which can be experimentally induced in mice include SCC of cervix, benign and malignant hepatic tumours, testicular Leydig cell tumours, and renal tumours. Anabolic steroids have been implicated in the pathogenesis of benign and malignant hepatic tumours. Oral contraceptives (OCs), which include an estrogen and high-dose progesterone, reduce the risk of ovarian and endometrial cancers. A modest increase in risk of breast cancer has been found to be associated with OC use. The risk is thought to be greatest for those who began to use OCs before the age of 20 years, and tended to decline with increasing age at diagnosis. Hormone replacement therapy (HRT) is thought to increase the risk of breast cancer proportionate to duration of usage.

Q. Write briefly on the molecular basis of cancer/carcinogenesis. (PA7.2)

Ans. Carcinogenesis is initiated by non-lethal genetic damage to a cell (**mutation**), which could be: (1) inherited in germ line or (2) acquired (due to chemicals, radiation and viruses). Occurrence of a mutation is followed by clonal expansion of the mutated cell (Fig. 8.15). Mutations that are directly responsible for neoplastic transformation are called **'driver mutations'**. The first driver mutation is called an **'initiating mutation'**. Tumour cells can acquire driver mutations through point mutations, deletions, amplifications and gene re-arrangements. Besides the 'driver mutations' that cause the disease, cells also accumulate a number of other mutations with seemingly no direct role in this evolutionary process. They are called **'passenger mutations'**. There is increasing evidence that shows that passenger mutations also play a major role in tumourigenesis because they have a bearing on areas such as epigenetics, in mitochondrial DNA, immunogenicity and even response to chemotherapy. In addition to frank mutations, there are **'epigenetic aberrations'** which also contribute to malignancy, for example DNA methylation and histone modifications. The word 'epigenetics' refers to the study of mitotically and/or meiotically heritable changes in gene expression that occur without changes in the DNA sequence. Such changes (epigenetic aberration) underlie a wide variety of pathologies. Unlike mutations, epigenetic aberrations are considered reversible with drugs that reduce the influence of DNA or histone modifying factors, making them potential therapeutic targets.

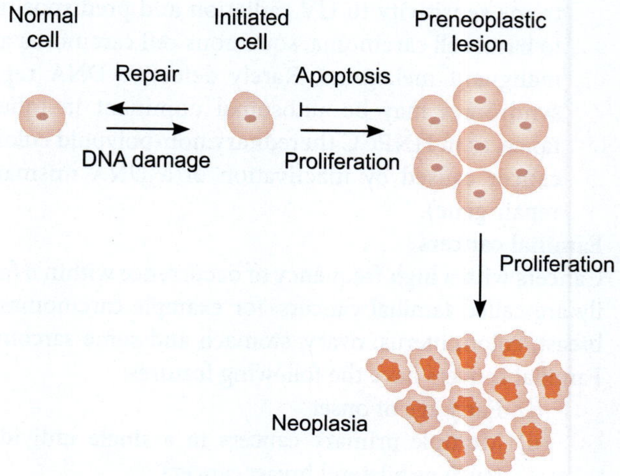

Fig. 8.15 Molecular basis of carcinogenesis.

Q. Write briefly on the role of non-coding RNAs in cancer. (PA7.2)

Ans. Genomic studies have revealed that only 2% of the entire human genome represents protein coding genes and the vast portion of the genome comprises of non-coding RNAs (ncRNAs). These ncRNAs do not transcribe into proteins but they have a significant role in regulating the transcription of protein coding transcripts into RNA and translation into functional proteins. They are classified into small non-coding RNAs called **micro RNAs (miRNAs)** and **long non-coding RNAs (lncRNAs)**. lncRNAs are a class of RNA transcripts with a length greater than 200 nucleotides. IncRNAs regulate gene expressions and functions at transcriptional, translational, and post-translational levels. In the past decade, it has been demonstrated that the dysregulated lncRNA and mRNA profile is widely involved in the pathogenesis of many diseases, including cancer, metabolic disorders and cardiovascular diseases. Many lncRNAs have been shown to be potential biomarkers and targets for the diagnosis and treatment of cancers, including lung (MALAT-1), breast (HOTAIR), liver (HULC) and colorectal cancers (XLOC), as well as haematological malignancies (NEAT1 in multiple myeloma). MicroRNAs (miRNAs) that play a crucial role in cancer development are also termed as **oncomirs** and have been identified in the peripheral blood circulation and mononuclear cells of cancer patients, such as breast cancer (miRNA-195 and let-7a), lung carcinoma (miR-21, miR-210 and miR-486-5p) and prostate cancer (miR-141). miRNAs are endogenous, short non-coding, single stranded RNAs that function in post-translational regulation of gene expression. Aberrant miRNA expression has been associated with amplification or deletion of miRNA genes, abnormal transcriptional control of miRNAs, as well as dysregulated epigenetic changes. miRNAs may function as either oncogenes or tumour suppressors under certain conditions. The dysregulated miRNAs induce sustained proliferative signalling, suppression of growth suppressors, evasion of cell death, activation of invasion and metastasis and induction of angiogenesis.

Q. Write briefly on cancer regulatory genes. (PA7.2)

Ans. There are four main classes of **cancer regulatory genes**:

1. **Proto-oncogenes**
   (a) Dominant.
   (b) Cause 'gain of function' (excessively increase one or more of the normal functions of the encoded gene product).
   (c) Can transform cells despite the presence of a normal counterpart.
2. **Tumour suppressor genes**
   (a) Recessive.
   (b) Mutations in these genes cause a 'loss of function'.
   (c) Both normal alleles of tumour suppressor genes must be damaged to transform cell.
3. **Genes regulating apoptosis and cancer**
   (a) Apoptosis in a normal cell is guided by cell death receptor CD95.
   (b) *BAD*, *BID*, *BAX* and TP58 are proapoptotic.
   (c) *Bcl*-2 and *Bcl*-X are antiapoptotic.
   (d) Mutant form of *Bcl*-2 gene is seen in B cell lymphomas, carcinoma breast, thyroid and prostate.
   (e) CD95 has been found to be depleted in hepatocellular carcinoma.
4. **DNA repair genes**
   (a) Defects in DNA repair genes predispose to mutations (mutator phenotype).
   (b) Both alleles of DNA repair genes must be inactivated to induce genomic instability (recessive inheritance).

Table 8.8 Differences between anti-oncogenes and proto-oncogenes

Features	Anti-oncogenes	Proto-oncogenes
Other name	Tumour suppressor genes	Precursor genes for oncogene
Function	They suppress cell proliferation, and promote differentiation and maturation of cells	They promote normal cell growth and differentiation
Inheritance	Recessive. Homozygous inactivation, that is loss of both normal copies of gene is required for carcinogenesis	Dominant. Mutation in a single copy may lead to oncogenic conversion
Action	Act passively, that is cancer-promoting genes dominate and lead to tumour formation due to loss of normal function of anti-oncogenes	Act actively, ie, gene products of oncogenes directly lead to tumour formation
Examples	*P53*, *RB* gene, *BRCA*-1 and 2, *TGF*-β, *APC*, *WT-1* and *NF*	*myc*, *N-myc*, *erb*B1/2/3

APC, *Adenomatous polyposis coli* gene; NF, neurofibroma; RB, retinoblastoma; TGF-β, transforming growth factor-β; WT, Wilms tumour.

Q. Differentiate between anti-oncogenes and proto-oncogenes. (PA7.2)

Ans. Differences between anti-oncogenes and proto-oncogenes are enlisted in Table 8.8.

Q. Enumerate the steps involved in carcinogenesis. (PA7.2)

Ans. Carcinogenesis is a multistep process. The steps involved in carcinogenesis are depicted in Flowchart 8.2.

Q. Write briefly on role of cyclins, CDK (cyclin-dependent kinases) and CDK inhibitors in regulating G_1/S cell cycle transition/pathogenesis of neoplasia. (PA7.2)

Ans. Cyclin D, the first cyclin to increase in the cell cycle, appears in mid-G phase, but is no longer detectable in the S phase. There are three forms of cyclin D, named Dl, D2 and D3; but to simplify matters, the general term 'cyclin D' is used. Cyclin D, like other cyclins, is unstable and is

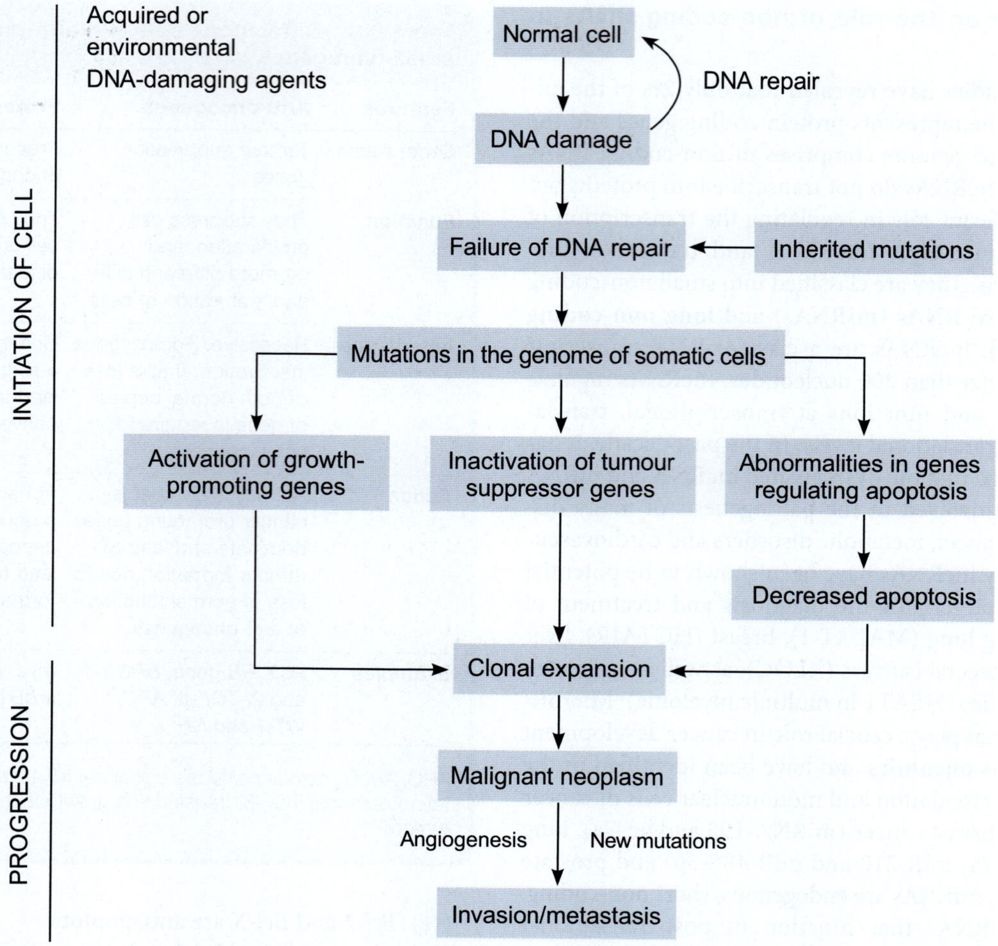

Flowchart 8.2 Steps involved in carcinogenesis.

degraded through **ubiquitin—proteasome pathway**. During the G phase of the cell cycle, cyclin D binds to and activates CDK4, forming a *cyclin D–CDK4 complex.* This complex plays a critical role in the cell cycle by phosphorylating the retinoblastoma susceptibility protein (pRB). '**The phosphorylation of RB is a molecular ON–OFF switch for the cell cycle**'. In its hypophosphorylated state, RB prevents cells from replicating by forming a tight, inactive complex with the transcription factor E2F. Phosphorylation of RB dissociates the complex and releases the inhibition on E2F transcriptional activity (see Fig. 8.16 and Flowchart 8.3).

Q. Write in detail on cancer-related genes and their effect on cell growth. (PA7.2)

Ans. Alterations in the controlling genes, typically by mutation, are major genetic hallmarks of cancer (Fig. 8.17) and include:

Excessive and Autonomous Growth

- Genes that promote autonomous cell growth in cancer cells are called **oncogenes** and their normal cellular counterparts are called **proto-oncogenes.**
- Proto-oncogenes are physiological regulators of cell proliferation and differentiation, and are often involved in signal transduction and execution of mitogenic signals, usually through their protein products.
- Oncogenes are mutated forms of normal proto-oncogenes, different from the latter in the following ways:
  - Presence of mutation/s in the structure of the gene.
  - Ability to promote autonomous and excessive cellular proliferation in the event of overexpression, even in the absence of normal mitogenic signals.
- Activation of oncogenes can be induced by:
  - *Point mutation* and *deletion* (as in *RAS* oncogene implicated in carcinoma of colon and pancreas).
  - *Chromosomal translocation*, as in Philadelphia chromosome (translocation of C-ABL proto-oncogene from chromosome 9 to chromosome 22) and translocation of *c-MYC* proto-oncogene from chromosome 8 to chromosome 14 (seen in 75% cases of Burkitt lymphoma).
  - *Gene amplification* (chromosomal alterations that result in increased number of copies of a gene) as in the case of *n-MYC* implicated in neuroblastoma, and ERB-B2 in breast and ovarian cancer. The expression of oncogenes can be regulated by **microRNAs** that control gene expression by downregulating them. Mutations in such miRNAs can lead to the activation of oncogenes.

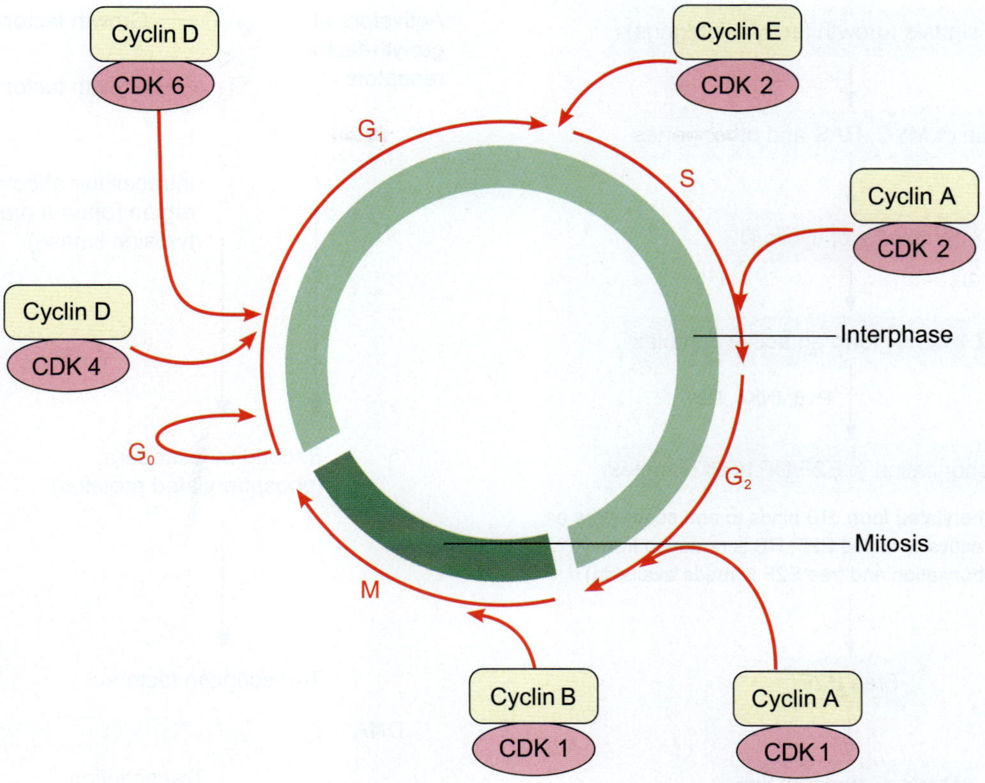

Fig. 8.16 Cyclins and cell cycle.

- **Oncoproteins** are products of oncogenes, which resemble products of proto-oncogenes, but are devoid of important regulatory mechanisms (Table 8.9). They include:
  - *Growth factors (GFs):*
    - These are polypeptides elaborated by many cells that normally act on another cell to stimulate its proliferation (paracrine action), for example PDGF in glioblastomas, TGF-α in sarcomas and FGF in carcinoma of bowel and breast.
    - Many cancer cells are capable of synthesizing the same growth factors that stimulate their growth. An oncogene may cause a cell to secrete growth factors, even though it does not normally do so, thus inducing its own uncontrolled proliferation (autocrine loop) and proliferation of neighbouring cells, for example osteosarcomas encode β-chain of PDGF and the same tumours also express receptors for PDGF.
    - A group of related oncogenes that encode homologues of fibroblast growth factors (FGFs), for example HSTF-1 (heparin-binding secretory transforming factor-1) and INT-2 (also known as fibroblast growth factor-3) are activated in several gastrointestinal and breast tumours; β FGF, a member of the fibroblast growth factor family, is expressed in human melanomas but not in normal melanocytes. Hepatocyte growth factor and its receptor c-MET are overexpressed in follicular carcinoma of thyroid.
  - *Growth factor receptors*: Receptors can be divided into two categories: **intracellular receptors**, found inside of the cell (in the cytoplasm or nucleus), and **cell surface receptors**, which are found in the plasma membrane. The ligands of intracellular receptors are hydrophobic molecules, since they have to traverse the plasma membrane in order to reach their receptors, for example, receptors for steroid hormones, such as the sex hormones. Binding of the hormone to its receptor induces conformational changes in the receptor, allowing the receptor–hormone complex to enter the nucleus and exposing regions of the receptor that have DNA-binding activity, which in turn enhances the transcription of certain genes. In the case of cell-surface receptors the ligands can be large and hydrophilic as it does not have to traverse the cell membrane. Cell-surface receptors have three different domains: an extracellular ligand-binding domain, hydrophobic domain extending through the membrane, and an intracellular domain, which transmits the signal. There are three common types of cell surface receptors: ligand-gated ion channels, G protein-coupled receptors, and receptor tyrosine kinases. Receptor kinases add phosphate groups to receptor proteins at the surface of the cell (which receive protein signals from outside the cell and transmit them to the inside of the cell). Tyrosine kinases add phosphate groups to the amino acid tyrosine in the target protein. They can cause cancer by turning the receptor on permanently (constitutively), even without signals from outside the cell (Flowchart 8.4).

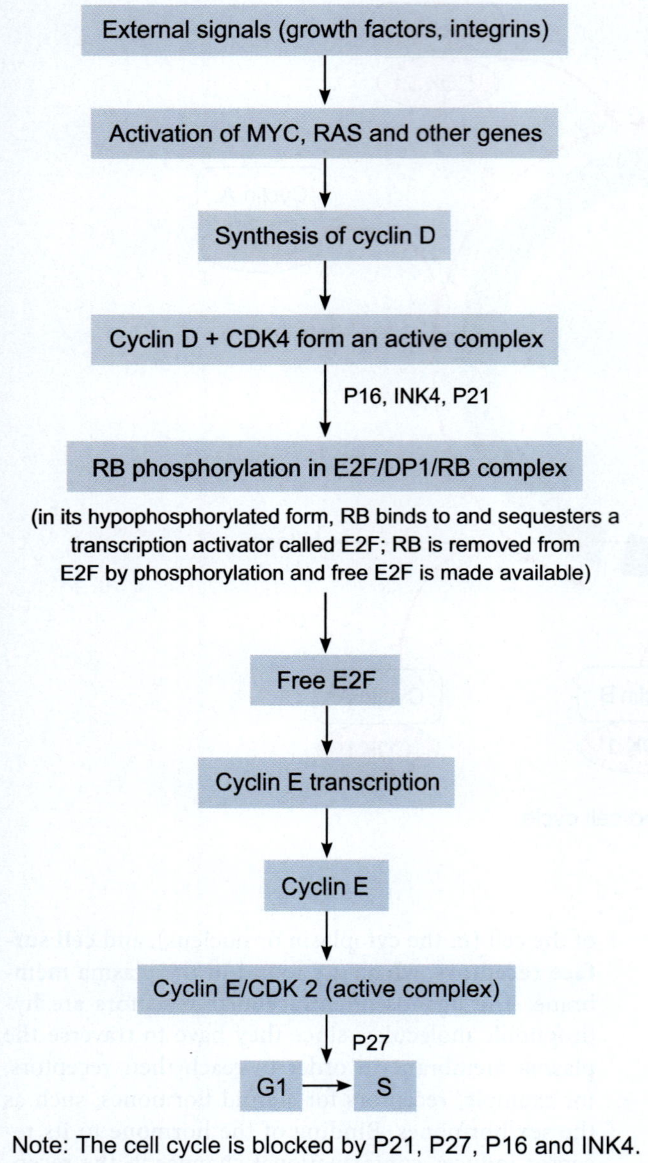

Flowchart 8.3 Role of cyclins, CDKs and CDK inhibitors in regulating G1/S cell cycle transition.

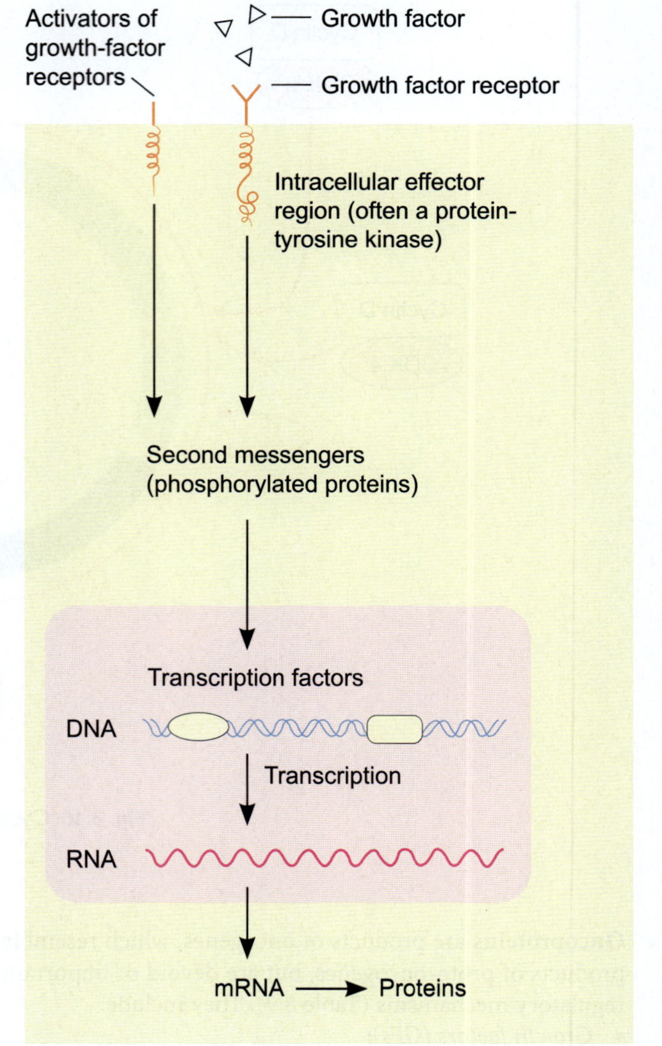

Fig. 8.17 Mechanisms involved in excessive unregulated growth.

Examples

- Point mutations in ERB-B1 (EGF receptor) found in a subset of lung adenocarcinomas and squamous cell carcinoma result in constitutive activation of EGFR tyrosine kinase.
- Amplification of ERB-B2 results in overexpression of HER2 receptor and its constitutive tyrosine kinase activity leading to carcinomas of breast, lung, ovary and stomach.
- Gene rearrangements may activate other receptor tyrosine kinases, for example ALK.tyrosine kinase.

▪ *Signal transduction proteins*

- Normal signal transduction proteins, which transduce signals from the growth factor receptors on the cell surface to the nucleus, may get mutated, for example, **mutated RAS (rat sarcoma) gene.**
- Point mutations involving **RAS family genes** - HRAS (bladder and kidney tumours), KRAS (adenocarcinoma colon, lung and pancreas) and NRAS (melanoma and haematology maignancies); HRAS and KRAS were named after their discoverers, namely Jennifer Harvey and Werner Kirsten and NRAS was named so as it was initially identified in neuroblastoma cells); are the most common form of abnormality affecting a proto-oncogene in human tumours. As a member of the family of small G proteins, it is mainly implicated in the pathogenesis of carcinoma of colon, lungs and pancreas.
- In the inactive state, RAS proteins bind guanosine diphosphate (GDP); when cells are stimulated by growth factors or other receptor–ligand interactions, RAS becomes activated by exchanging GDP for GTP (guanosine triphosphate; see Fig. 8.18; Flowchart 8.5).
- Activated RAS, in turn, acts on MAP (mitogen-activated protein) kinase pathway by recruiting cytosolic protein RAF-1 (RAF proto-oncogene serine/threonine-protein kinase also known as proto-oncogene c-RAF or simply c-Raf). In addition to MAP path-

Table 8.9 Important oncogenes and associated cancers

Category	Proto-oncogene	Associated cancers	Mechanism	Gene functions
Growth factors (mitogens) 1. PDGF-β 2. TGF-α 3. FGF 4. c-MET	 SIS RAS HST-1, INT-2 HGF	Glioblastomas, fibrosarcomas, osteosarcomas, breast and bowel carcinomas, melanomas, and follicular carcinoma thyroid	Overexpression and amplification	Induces cell proliferation.
Receptors for growth factors 1. EGF receptors 2. c-Kit receptors 3. RET receptor 4. FMS like tyrosine kinase receptor	 ERB-1 (HER-1), ERB-2 (HER2/neu) c-Kit RET FLT-3 gene	Breast cancer, gastrointestinal stromal tumours, non-small cell lung cancer, and pancreatic cancer	Overexpression, amplification, and point mutation	Transduce signals for cell growth and differentiation.
Cytoplasmic tyrosine kinases 1. Regulatory GTPases 2. Non-GF receptor tyrosine kinases	 RAS ABL-BCR gene in CML-Philadelphia chromosome	Colorectal, breast, ovarian, gastric, head and neck, pancreatic, lung and brain cancers, CML and acute leukaemias	Point mutation and translocation	Cell proliferation, migration, and differentiation
Cytoplasmic serine/threonine kinases and their regulatory subunits	Raf kinase, and cyclin-dependent kinases	Adenocarcinomas of the pancreas, colon, thyroid and myeloid leukemia	Overexpression	Involved in cell cycle regulation, cell proliferation, differentiation, and apoptosis
Nuclear transcription factors	Myc gene (C-MYC, N-MYC, and L-MYC)	Burkitt lymphoma, neuroblastoma, and small cell carcinoma lung	Translocation and amplification	Regulate transcription of genes

FGF, Fibroblast growth factor; PDGF, platelet-derived growth factor; TGF, transforming growth factor; EGF, epidermal growth factor; c-MET, tyrosine-protein kinase Met or hepatocyte growth factor receptor (HGFR); c-Kit, mast/stem cell growth factor receptor (SCFR), also known as protooncogene c-Kit or tyrosine-protein kinase Kit or CD117; RET, rearranged during transfection.

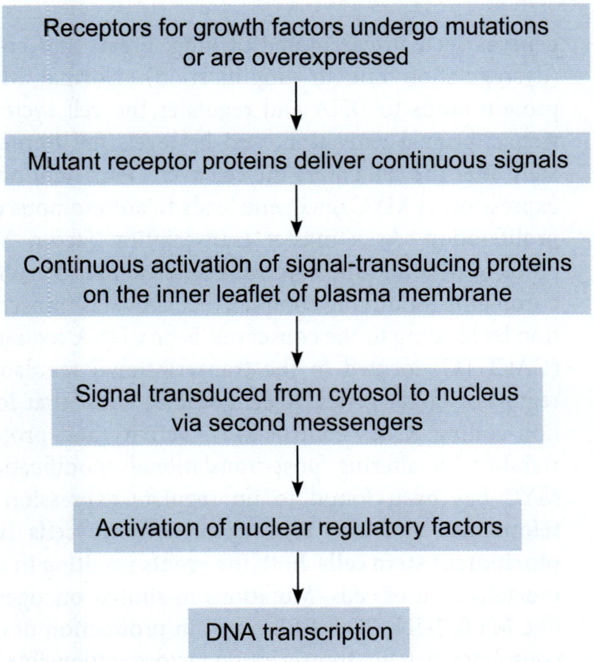

Flowchart 8.4 Role of growth factor receptors in evolution of carcinogenesis.

way, there is activation of the P13K/AKT pathway as well.

- The MAP kinases so activated target nuclear transcription factors, and thus promote mitogenesis.
- In normal cells, the activated signal-transmitting stage of the RAS protein is transient because its intrinsic GTPase activity hydrolyses GTP to GDP, thereby returning RAS to its quiescent ground state.
- Mutations that reduce the GTPase activity of the RAS protein result in an activated GTP-bound form that receives continuous signals.
- **BRAF** is a human gene that encodes a protein called B-Raf (**proto-oncogene B-Raf**). It is also known as **serine/threonine-protein kinase B-Raf** and is part of a signalling pathway known as the RAS/MAPK pathway, which controls several important cell functions (growth and division/proliferation, differentiation, cell movement, and apoptosis). Activating point mutations in the BRAF gene makes a protein that is involved in sending signals in cells and in cell growth and may be found in some types of cancer, including melanoma and colorectal cancer.

▪ ***Nuclear regulatory molecules*: Myc** is a family of proto-oncogenes that code for transcription factors. The Myc

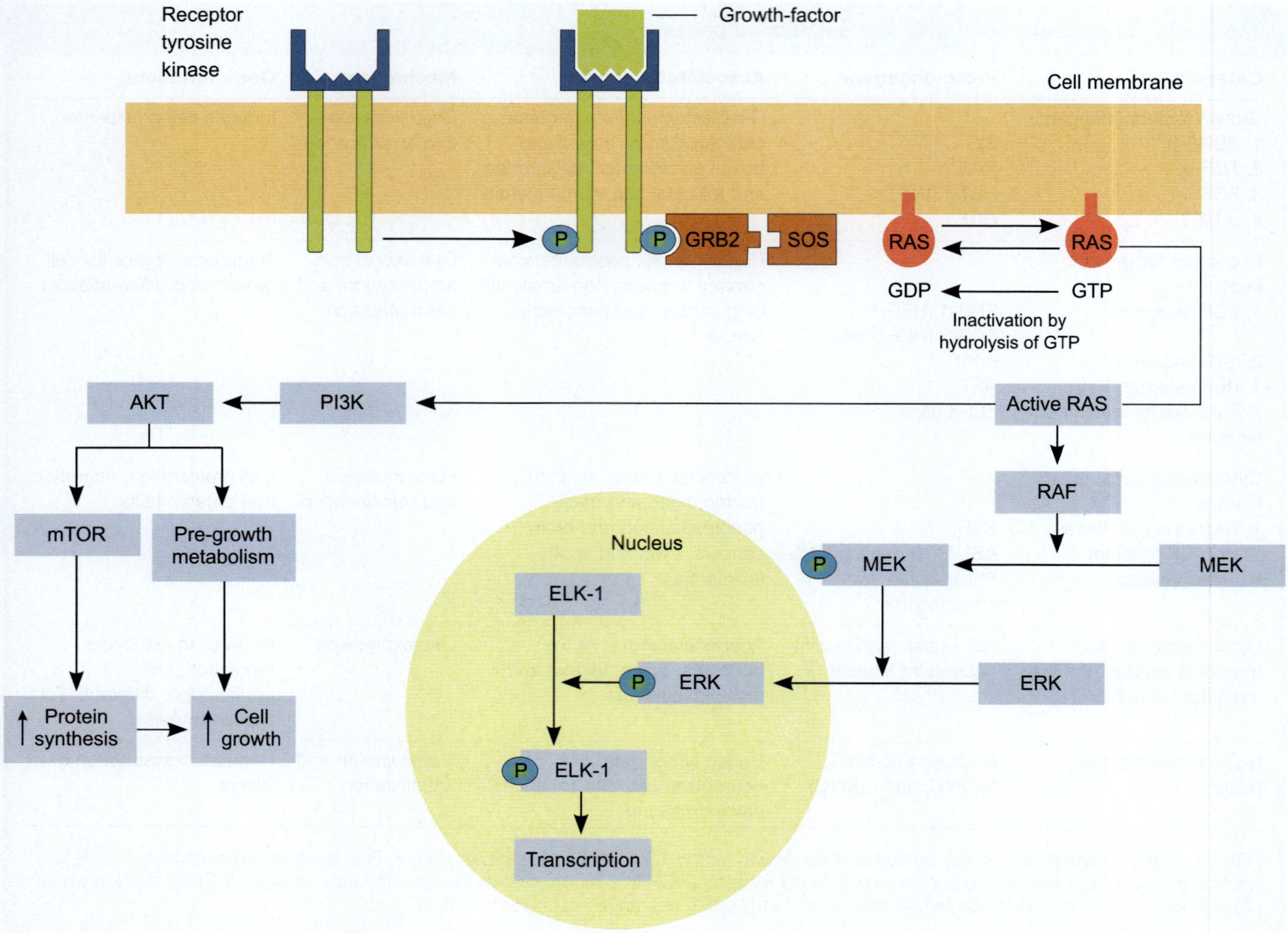

Fig. 8.18 Role of RAS oncogene in cellular growth and neoplasia. (GRB2 – Growth factor receptor-bound protein 2; SOS – Son of sevenless group of genes encoding guanine nucleotide exchange factors; RAS – Rat sarcoma gene; RAF – Rapidly accelerated fibrosarcoma; MEK – Mitogen-activated protein kinase kinase, also known as MAP2K; ERK – Extracellular regulated kinases; ELK1 – ETS Like-1 protein; AKT – A serine/threonine-specific protein kinase).

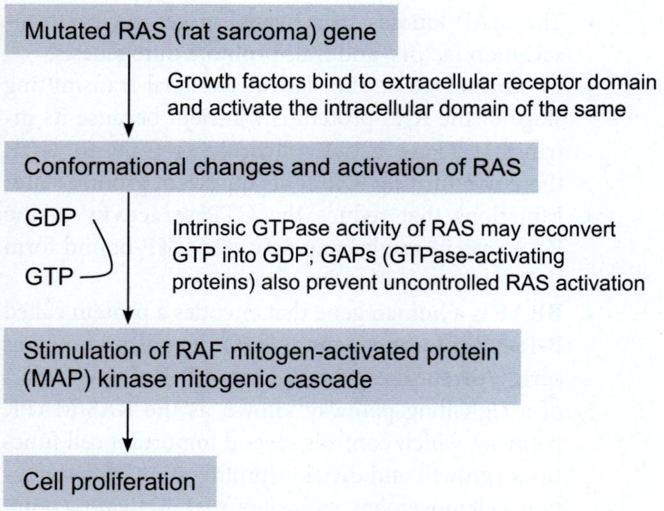

Flowchart 8.5 Role of RAS-signalling pathway in cancer.

family consists of three related human genes: c-myc (MYC), l-myc (MYCL), and n-myc (MYCN). Overexpression of **MYC gene** occurs with **t(8;14) in Burkitt lymphoma** or may be a result of **amplification** of the gene as seen in carcinoma of lung, breast and colon (dysregulation due to amplification). Normal MYC protein binds to DNA and regulates the cell cycle by transcriptional activation, and its levels fall immediately after the cell enters the cell cycle. Persistent overexpression of MYC oncogene leads to autonomous cell proliferation. As a master transcription factor, Myc binds to Max and the Myc/Max heterodimer recruits a chromatin-modifying complex that activates transcription by binding to the conserved E-box DNA sequence (CACGTG) located in the transcriptional regulatory region of target genes. Recent studies show that long non-coding RNAs control MYC activity and protein stability by altering post-translational modification. MYC has been found to up regulate expression of **telomerase** and also **reprogram somatic cells into pluripotent stem cells,** both the events resulting in immortalisation of cells, Mutations in similar oncogenes like MYB, JUN, FOS, REL result in production of oncoproteins that are transcription factors responsible for regulating the expression of Cyclins which are growth promoters.

- ***Cell-cycle regulatory proteins:*** Normal cell cycle is under control of cyclins and CDK A, B, E and D. Checkpoint is $G_1 \rightarrow S$ phase. Mutations in cyclins (particularly cyclin D) and CDKs (in particular CDK4) may aid in induction of cancer, for example 'overexpression of cyclin D' is implicated in carcinoma of breast, liver and mantle cell lymphoma, and 'amplification of CDK4' in multiple myeloma, glioblastomas and sarcomas.

Refractoriness to Growth Inhibition (Loss of Growth-Suppressing Anti-Oncogenes)

Anti-oncogenes or tumour suppressor genes prevent entry of cells in mitotic pool and push cells into the G_0 phase. Mutated anti-oncogenes behave like growth-promoting genes. The following are the important tumour suppressor genes involved in growth inhibition:

1. ***RB gene***
   (a) Approximately 60% of retinoblastomas are sporadic, and the remaining 40% are inherited. To explain the inherited and sporadic occurrence of this seemingly identical tumour, **Knudson proposed his now famous *'two-hit' hypothesis of oncogenesis.***
   (b) He suggested that in **hereditary cases** one genetic change ('first hit') is inherited from an affected parent, and is therefore present in all somatic cells of the body; whereas, the second mutation ('second hit') occurs in one of the many retinal cells (which already carry the first mutation).
   (c) In **sporadic cases**, however, the two mutations (hits) occur somatically within a single retinal cell whose progeny then form the tumour.
   (d) The mutations required to produce retinoblastoma involve the ***RB* gene**, located on **chromosome 13ql4**.
   (e) **Both normal alleles of the *RB* locus must be inactivated (two hits) for the development of retinoblastoma.**
   (f) In **familial cases**, children are born with one normal and one defective copy of the *RB* gene. They lose the intact copy in the retinoblasts through some form of somatic mutation (point mutation, deletion of 13q 14 or even complete loss of the normal chromosome 13).
   (g) In **sporadic cases**, both normal *RB* alleles are lost by somatic mutation in one of the retinoblasts.
   (h) Patients with familial retinoblastoma are also at a greatly increased risk of developing **osteosarcoma** and **some other soft-tissue sarcomas.**
   (i) Inactivation of the *RB* locus has been noted in several other tumours, including **adenocarcinoma of the breast, small cell carcinoma of the lung and bladder carcinoma.**
   (j) Most importantly, alterations in the key regulators of the cell cycle or RB pathway (involving **INK4a proteins, cyclin D-dependent kinases and RB family proteins**) are present in most cancer cells. The RB gene can loose its normal suppressor action and go into the proliferative mode by various mechanisms (loss of function mutations affecting RB; gene amplification of CDK4 and cyclin D; loss of cyclin-dependant kinase inhibitors like p16/INK4 and inhibition of RB by binding of viral oncoproteins to it).

RB pathway:

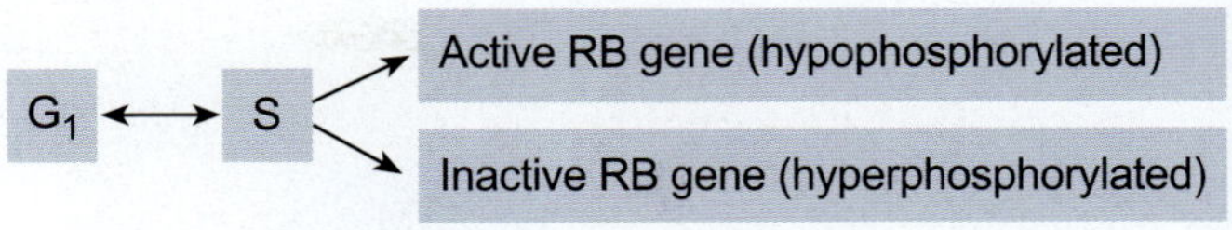

- The **retinoblastoma gene** encodes a 110-kDa **phosphoprotein (pRB)** that is expressed in almost every cell of the human body and contributes to growth regulation in these cells.
- The most important target of the retinoblastoma protein is cellular transcription factor **E2F**. E2F is a potent stimulator of cell cycle entry into S phase.
- E2F activity consists of an E2F polypeptide and a DP protein (E2F/DP heterodimeric complex).
- In the hypophosphorylated form (which occurs early in G_1), *RB* binds to E2F, inactivates E2F as a transcription factor and shuts the expression of E2F target genes off (Fig. 8.19).
- Phosphorylation of pRB by Cyclin/CDK complexes in mid-to-late G_1 causes pRB to lose its affinity for E2F.
- The free E2F/DP transcription factor can now activate transcription of E2F target genes.
- In a normal cell during mitosis, **phosphatase 1-like protein (PP1)** removes all phosphates from pRB.

2. ***Tp53 gene (p53)*:** Situated on short arm of **chromosome 17**, it is also called '**protector of the genome**' as *P53* mutation is present in more than half of all human cancers. It is a transcriptional activator, regulates the expression of **MDM2** and the genes involved in growth arrest, DNA repair and apoptosis. Some important examples are listed below.
   (a) Growth arrest: p21, Gadd45, and 14-3-3s.
   (b) DNA repair: p53R2.
   (c) Apoptosis: Bax, Apaf-1, PUMA and NoxA.

Regulation of p53 (Fig. 8.20)

Expression of MDM2 is activated by p53. Binding of p53 by MDM2 triggers the degradation of p53 via the ubiquitin system. Phosphorylation of p53 will disrupt its binding with MDM2. DNA damage may activate protein kinase (such as ATM, DNA-PK, or CHK2) to phosphorylate p53, thereby increasing p53 level. Since MDM2 expression is

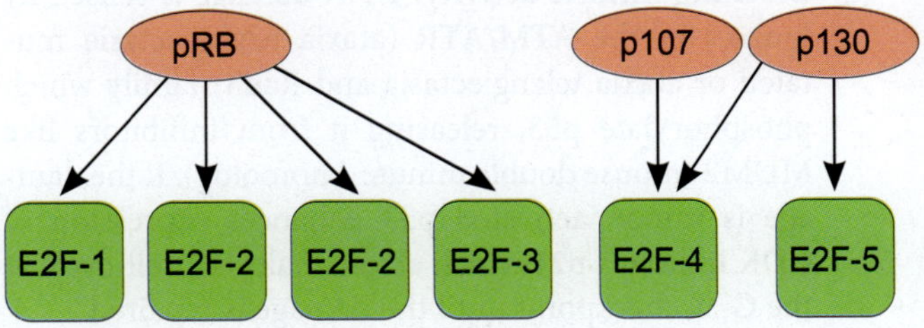

Fig. 8.19 E2F and RB interaction. E2F-1 to E2F-5 induce cell-cycle transition from G1 to S phase and are under regulation by pRB, p107, and p130.

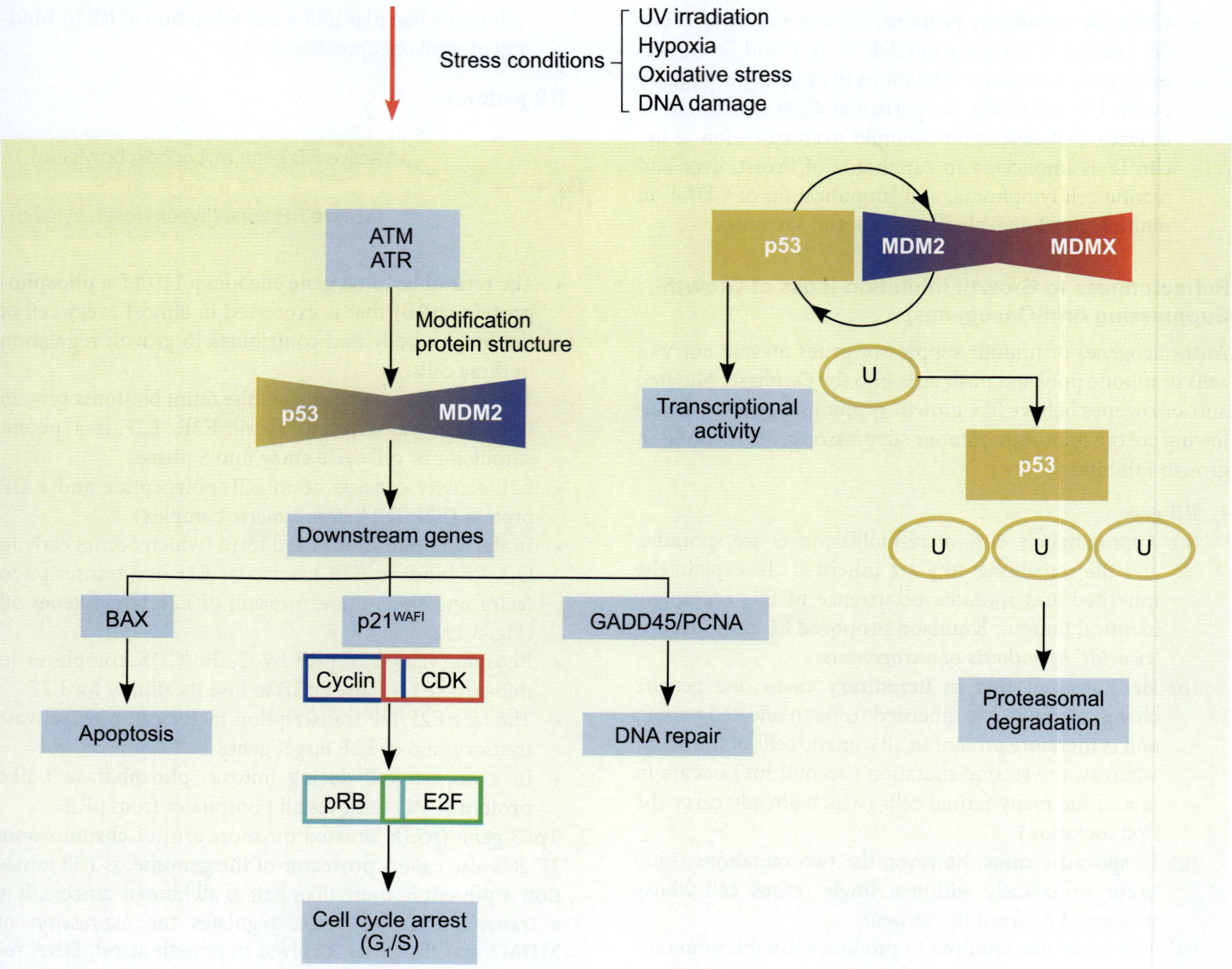

Fig. 8.20 Regulation of p53 (MDM2 – Mouse double minute 2 homolog; MDMX – Murine double minute X; ATM/ATR pathway – serine/threonine protein kinases that are recruited and activated by DNA double-strand breaks. It phosphorylates p53 which initiates activation of the DNA damage checkpoint, leading to cell cycle arrest, DNA repair or apoptosis).

activated by p53, the increase of p53 also increases MDM2, but it has no effect while p53 is phosphorylated. After the DNA damage is repaired, the ATM kinase is no longer active, p53 will be quickly dephosphorylated and destroyed by the accumulated MDM2.

Functions of P53 (Fig. 8.21)

(a) **Blocking mitotic activity:** DNA damage is sensed by kinases of the ATM/ATR (ataxia telangiectasia mutated or ataxia telangiectasia and Rad3) family which phosphorylate p53, releasing it from inhibitors like MDM2 (mouse double minute 2 homolog). If the damage is minor, activated p53 enhances expression of CDK inhibitor p21 which arrests/halts the cell-cycle at the G_1/S checkpoint until the damage is repaired.

(b) **Role in promoting apoptosis:** If the damage is major and cannot be repaired, *p53* triggers the cell to commit suicide by apoptosis (activates apoptosis, inducing *BAX* gene to bring the defective cell to an end). Apoptosis can be induced by the binding of Caspase 9 to cytochrome c and Apaf1. p53 may activate the expression of Apaf1 and Bax. The latter can then stimulate the release of cytochrome c from mitochondria.

(c) **Role in senescence:** P53 is essential for the senescence response to short telomeres.

(d) **Inhibition of angiogenesis:** As tumours grow they need to recruit new blood vessels to supply them, and p53 inhibits that by (1) interfering with regulators of tumour hypoxia that also affect angiogenesis, such as HIF1 and HIF2 (hypoxia-inducible factor 1 alpha and 2 alpha), (2) inhibiting the production of angiogenic promoting factors, and (3) directly increasing the production of angiogenesis inhibitors, such as arresten.

(e) **Effect on adult stem cells:** Mechanical signals such as hypoxia affect levels of p53 in these niche cells through

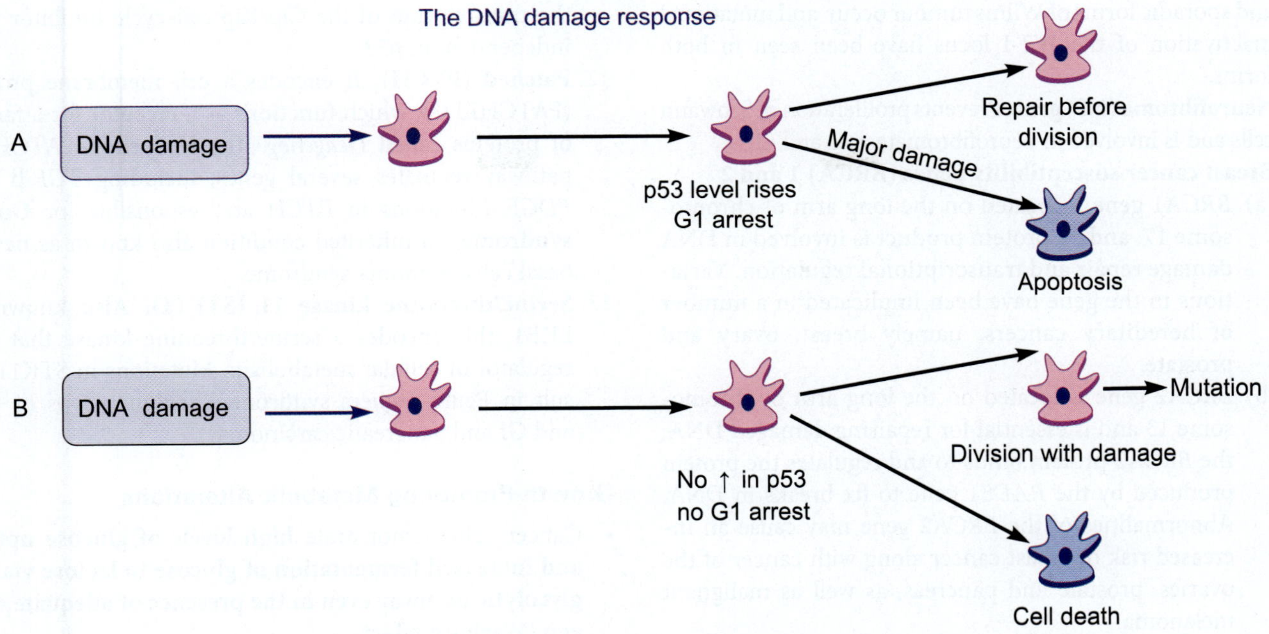

Fig. 8.21 DNA damage response of p53.

the hypoxia inducible factors, HIF-1α and HIF-2α. While HIF-1α stabilizes p53, HIF-2α suppresses it. Suppression of p53 has been found to reprogram differentiated cells into stem cells.

(f) **Role in disease:** *TP53* is the most frequently inactivated gene in human cancers. Its inactivation leads to the production of mutant p53 proteins that loose wild-type p53 tumour suppression functions and simultaneously acquire new oncogenic properties like deregulated cellular proliferation, increased chemoresistance, and unregulated invasion and metastasis. Mutated form of *p53* is associated with a variety of cancers, chiefly, carcinomas of lung, head, neck, colon and breast. It also contributes to sequential development of carcinoma in situ in invasive carcinoma. Cancers of multiple organs (breast, lung, brain, adrenals, and bone and soft tissue sarcomas) are caused by damage to both alleles of p53 (**Li-Fraumeni syndrome**). p53 family has other members like p63 (required for squamous differentiation) and p73 (a potent pro-apoptotic factor after chemotherapy induced DNA damage), both of which show relative tissue specificity unlike p53, which is ubiquitously present.

(g) **Therapeutic use:** P53 deficiency cripples the normal functioning of the cell. Restoring its function therefore would be a major step in curing many cancers. This can be achieved by altering the mutant conformation of p53 back to an active form. Other promising targets for cancer therapeutics are the proteins and molecules associated with p53 function, for example the molecular chaperone Hsp90, which interacts with p53 in vivo. Thus, pharmacological reactivation of p53 presents itself as a viable cancer treatment option. The first commercial gene therapy, Gendicine, was approved in China in 2003 for the treatment of head and neck squamous cell carcinoma. It delivers a functional copy of the p53 gene using an engineered adenovirus.

3. ***Transforming growth factor*** (TGF-β): Inhibitor of cell proliferation, TGF-β acts on G_1 phase. Its mutant form has impaired-growth-inhibiting effect, leading to uncontrolled cell proliferation and cancer as in carcinoma of pancreas, colon and stomach.
4. ***Adenomatous polyposis gene (APC)***
   (a) APC is a component of WNT-signalling pathways which controls cell adhesion and polarity during embryogenesis. An important function of the APC protein is to downregulate β-catenin.
   (b) In the absence of WNT-signalling, APC causes proteasomal degradation of β-catenin by forming a 'destruction complex', thus preventing its accumulation in the cytoplasm. In the event of *APC* gene inactivation, there is disruption of this complex, thereby increasing cellular levels of β-catenin, which, in turn, translocates to the nucleus.
   (c) In the nucleus, β-catenin forms a complex with TCF-α transcription factor which upregulates cellular proliferation by promoting the transcription of *c-MYC, CYCLIN Dl* and other genes.
   (d) APC is mutated in familial adenomatous polyposis and sporadic colonic carcinomas. Also, colonic tumours in some cases have normal APC genes but mutated β-catenin, which is not inhibited by APC.
   (e) Dysregulation of the APC–β-catenin pathway is also present in more than 50% of hepatoblastomas and in approximately 20% of hepatocellular carcinomas.
5. **Wilms tumour (WT)-1 gene:** The *WT-1* gene, located on chromosome l 1p13, is associated with the development of Wilms tumour. It is a transcriptional activator of genes involved in renal and gonadal differentiation. Both inherited

and sporadic forms of Wilms tumour occur, and mutational inactivation of the *WT*-I locus have been seen in both forms.

6. **Neurofibroma (NF) gene:** Prevents proliferation of Schwann cells and is involved in neurofibromatosis-1 and -2.
7. **Breast cancer susceptibility genes (BRCA) 1 and 2**
   (a) *BRCA*1 gene is located on the long arm of chromosome 17, and its protein product is involved in DNA damage repair and transcriptional regulation. Variations in the gene have been implicated in a number of hereditary cancers, namely breast, ovary and prostate.
   (b) *BRCA*2 gene is located on the long arm of chromosome 13 and is essential for repairing damaged DNA; the *BRCA*2 protein binds to and regulates the protein produced by the *RAD*51 gene to fix breaks in DNA. Abnormalities of the *BRCA*2 gene may cause an increased risk of breast cancer along with cancer of the ovaries, prostate and pancreas, as well as malignant melanoma.
8. **von Hippel–Lindau (VHL) gene:** Germline mutation of *VHL* gene on chromosome 3p is associated with hereditary renal cell carcinoma, pheochromocytoma, haemangioblastoma of the central nervous system, retinal angiomas and renal cysts. Mutations in *VHL* gene are sometimes also noted in sporadic renal cell cancers. VHL covalently binds ubiquitin chains to protein substrates promoting their degradation by proteasomes, the most important substrate being HIF1 alpha. HIF1 alpha is hydroxylated in the presence of oxygen and binds to ubiquitin ligase to undergo degradation.This alters gene expression in response to hypoxia.
9. **Phosphatase and tensin homologue (PTEN) gene:** This is located on chromosome 10 and is frequently deleted in endometrial cancer and glioblastoma. *PTEN* activity causes cell cycle arrest and apoptosis as well as inhibition of cell motility. It has been proposed that *PTEN* blocks the cell cycle by increasing the transcription of the p27 Cip/Kip cell-cycle inhibitor and stabilising the protein. With loss of *PTEN*, the cells continuously replicate.
10. **Cadherins**
    (a) Cadherins are a family of transmembrane proteins that play an important role in cell adhesion. They are dependent on calcium ions to function, hence their name. Loss of Cadherins induces loss of cohesion of cells, which then invade locally as well as metastasize.
    (b) Different members of the cadherin family are found in different locations. E-Cadherins are found in epithelial tissue, N-Cadherins are found in neurons and P-Cadherins are found in the placenta.
    (c) Reduced cell-surface expression of E-Cadherins is noted in many cancers, for example oesophagus, colon, breast and ovary. Germline mutations of E-cadherin gene predisposes to familial gastric carcinomas.
11. **Kruppel-like factor 6 (KLF6):** This encodes a transcription factor that has many target genes, including *TGF*-α and *TGF*-β receptors, and is found to be mutated in more than 70% of primary prostate cancers. It has been proposed that *KLF*6 inhibits cell proliferation by increasing the transcription of the Cip/Kip cell-cycle inhibitor *p21*, independent of *p53*.
12. **Patched (PTCH):** It encodes a cell membrane protein (PATCHED1), which functions as a receptor for a family of proteins called *Hedgehog*. The Hedgehog–PATCHED pathway regulates several genes, including *TGF*-β and *PDGF*. Mutations in *PTCH* are responsible for **Gorlin syndrome**, an inherited condition also known as nevoid basal cell carcinoma syndrome.
13. **Serine/threonine kinase 11 (STK11):** Also known as LKB1, this encodes a serine/threonine kinase that is a regulator of cellular metabolism. Mutations in STK11 result in Peutz–Jeghers syndrome (benign polyps of GIT and GI and pancreatic carcinomas).

Growth-Promoting Metabolic Alterations

- Cancer cells demonstrate **high levels of glucose uptake and increased fermentation of glucose to lactose via the glycolytic pathway even in the presence of adequate oxygen (Warburg effect)**.
- Positron emission tomography (PET scan) uses this glucose hunger of cancer cells to visualise tumour cells. This procedure involves injecting patients with F-fluorodeoxyglucose, which is a non-metabolisable derivative of glucose and is preferentially taken up by rapidly proliferating tumour cells.
- This preference exhibited for aerobic glycolysis by rapidly proliferating tumour cells over mitochondrial oxidative phosphorylation is because the former provides the tumour cells with metabolic intermediates necessary for synthesis of cellular components not provided by the latter.
- Also, while in the rapidly growing normal cells, aerobic glycolysis stops when the cells are no more proliferating, in cancer cells aerobic glycolysis continues due to enhanced action of oncogenes and decreased action of tumour suppressor genes (owing to pro-growth signalling factors like P13K/AKT signalling, upregulated transcription factor MYC and receptor tyrosine kinase activity).

Evasion of Apoptosis and Cellular Ageing

Cancer cells demonstrate abnormalities of both the intrinsic and extrinsic pathways but the former are more commonly encountered, for example overexpression of anti-apoptotic gene BCL2 in follicular lymphomas.

Stem Cell-Like Replicative Potential

- It has been found that some of the cancer cells behave like stem cells. 'Cancer stem cells' can arise either through transformation of normal stem cells or through genetic aberrations in mature cells which make de-differentiate to push them into a stem cell-like state.
- The ability of 'cancer stem cells' to continuously replicate is attributed to inactivation of senescence signals and reactivation of telomerase.

The characteristics of a malignant cell are depicted in Fig. 8.22.

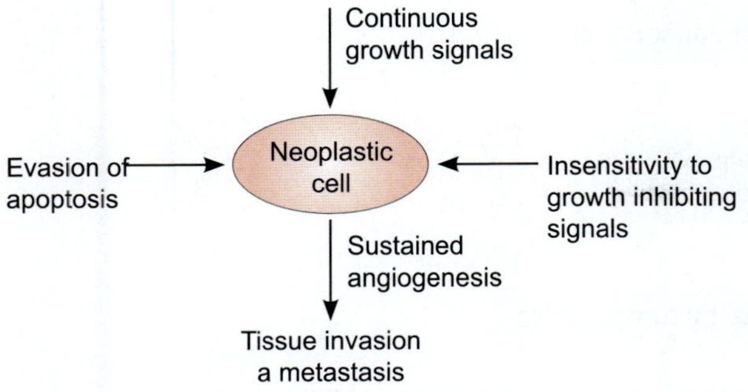

Fig. 8.22 Characteristics of a malignant cell.

Q. Write briefly on angiogenesis. (PA7.1)

Ans. Neoplasms cannot enlarge beyond 2 mm in diameter unless they undergo neovascularisation as the maximal distance across which oxygen and nutrients can diffuse from surrounding blood vessels is 1–2 mm.

- Neovascularisation perfuses the tumour and newly formed endothelial cells stimulate the growth of adjacent tumour cells by secreting polypeptide growth factors such as insulin-like growth factors (IGFs) and PDGF.
- Angiogenesis is required not only for tumour growth, but also for metastasis. Without access to the vasculature, the tumour cells cannot spread to distant sites.
- Sprouting of new vessels from already-existing ones is called neoangiogenesis; whereas, vasculogenesis occurs by recruitment of endothelial cell precursors. Tumour blood vessels differ from the normal vasculature by being leaky and unorganised.
- The pro-angiogenic factors are produced by tumour cells or derived from inflammatory cells (e.g. macrophages) that infiltrate tumours. Hypoxia activates transcription factor Hypoxia-inducible factor (HIF)-1α which in turn activates proangiogenic factors like VEGF and bFGF. Other promoters of angiogenesis include angiopoietins 1 and 2. Inhibitors of VEGF are being used for the treatment of advanced cancers. These are not curative but can prolong survival.
- Under normal circumstances, p53 increases expression of anti-angiogenic factors like thrombospondin-1, angiostatin, tumstatin and endostatin. Loss of p53, therefore, allows angiogenesis. Gain of function mutations in RAS and MYC enhance the production of VEGF.
- Stromal and tumour cells both release proteases which induce release of antiangiogenic factors like angiostatin and endostatin and proangiogenic factors like bFGF. Angiogenic inhibitors are being used for cancer therapy.

Q. Describe the mechanism and biology of invasion and metastasis. (PA7.1)

Ans. In the early stage of tumourigenesis, the cells are not invasive and metastatic. Progressive genetic aberrations are associated with the appearance of new clones with invasiveness and metastatic ability. Highly metastatic cells often acquire alterations in more genes than non-metastatic cells. Potentially important genes associated with epithelial metastasis include twist-related protein (TWIST) and the zinc-finger group gene SNAIL; these genes encode transcription factors which increase epithelial-mesenchymal interactions. The following are the steps involved in invasion and metastasis (Flowchart 8.6; Fig. 8.23):

1. **Invasion:** The loss of cell-cell adhesion capacity due to **loss of E-cadherin** function allows malignant cells to dissociate from the primary tumour mass (normally cells are attached to each other by adhesion molecules, namely, E-cadherins). **Changes in cell-matrix interaction** enable the cells to invade the surrounding stroma; the process of invasion. This involves the secretion of **degrading enzymes like matrix metalloproteinases or MMPs, cathepsin and urokinase plasminogen activator**. These aid in degradation of the basement membrane and extracellular matrix and also increase the expression/suppression of proteins involved in the control of motility and migration. Because invasive cells are capable of dramatically changing their cell shape to a nonpolarised, motile, spindle-shaped cell resembling a fibroblast, some hypothesise that neoplastic cells dedifferentiate to a more motile mesenchymal cell phenotype. This is referred to as **Epithelial-Mesenchymal transition (EMT)**. The tumour must also initialise angiogenesis, without which the tumour would fail to develop.
2. **Intrvasation:** The blood vessels in the vanity of the tumour facilitate the detached tumour cells in entering the circulation to metastasize to distant sites; the process called intravasation. Blood is normally not a conducive environment for **circulating tumour cells** (CTCs) to survive due to the physical shear forces in the blood stream and the surveillance by immune cells, particularly natural killer cells. Tumour cells protect themselves from these by secreting substances like thrombin, cathepsin B, and MMPs with the consequence of platelets aggregating around the tumour cells, a process known as **tumour cell-induced platelet aggregation**. This helps in extravasation and the subsequent arrest at distant organ sites.
3. **Extravasation:** CTCs have to leave the circulation, a step described as extravasation, which is made possible by secretion of factors that induce vascular hyperpermeability like protein **angiopoietin-like-4 and MMP-1 and 2**. Tumour cells seem to have an affinity for certain organs by virtue of release of chemokines specific for each organ and the expression of appropriate chemokine receptors on the surface of the tumour, for example expression of chemokine receptor 4 (CXCR4) in breast cancer. Tumours with CXCR4 expression migrate to organs that express high levels of its ligand CXCL12. CXCL12 is expressed in the common sites of metastasis for breast cancer: lung, liver, bone marrow and brain.
4. **Micrometastases formation:** After extravasation, CTCs arrive at the target organ and release growth factors into the circulation which upregulate VEGF-A, placental growth factor (PlGF), transforming growth factor-β (TGFβ), and other inflammatory proteins. Consequently, VEGF receptor (VEGFR) 1-positive bone marrow-derived haematopoietic progenitor cells are recruited and the ECM

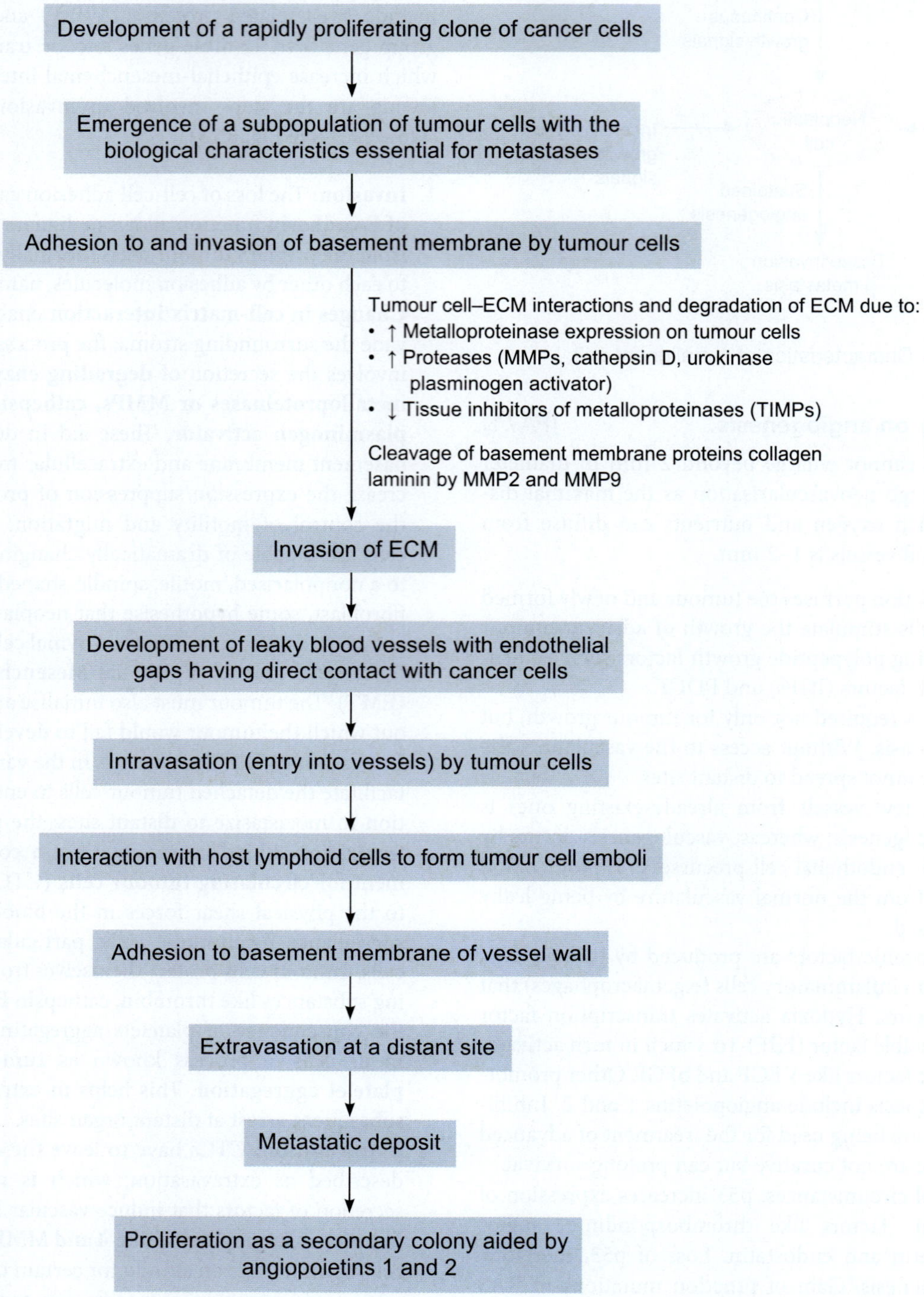

Flowchart 8.6 Sequence of events in invasion and metastasis.

is modulated at these sites. This already 'primed' tissue, which does not yet harbor tumour cells, provides the 'soil' for future metastasis. The activation of cMet and its downstream molecules has several effects on the cascade of metastasis. EMT, invasion and proliferation is promoted by activation of PI3K/Akt/mTOR or FAK. Intravasation is promoted by increasing neoangiogenesis. Involved pathways are STAT3, PI3K/Akt, and RAS. Additionally, cMet is a key regulator of the transcription factor HIF-1α. HIF-1α also promotes neoangiogenesis in hypoxic tissue.

Q. Write briefly on chemical carcinogenesis. (PA7.3)

Ans. ***Induction of cancer by chemicals depends on:***

- Dose, duration and mode of administration of the chemical.
- Individual susceptibility.
- Associated predisposing factors.

Chemical carcinogens covalently attach to cellular proteins and DNA. Only sufficiently reactive 'electrophiles' are capable of directly interacting with these macromolecules. Nucleophilic or chemically inert compounds, such as

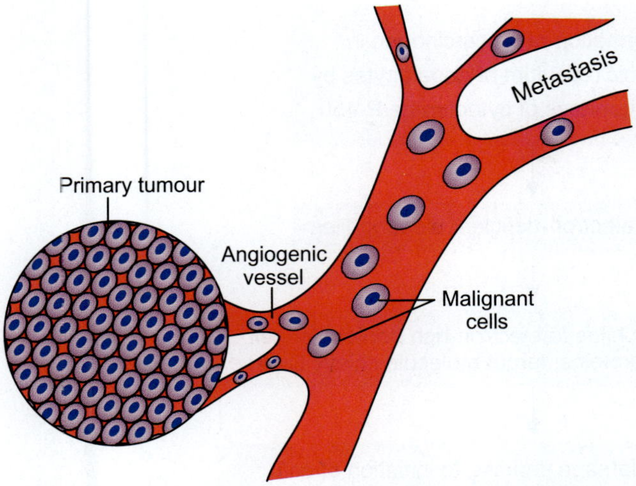

Fig. 8.23 Steps in invasion and metastasis.

aromatic and heterocyclic amines do not react directly with cellular constituents—they require enzymatic conversion into their ultimate carcinogenic forms—they are termed 'procarcinogens'. Cytochrome P450 (CYP) enzymes are central to the metabolic activation of these procarcinogens [polycyclic aromatic hydrocarbons (PAHs)] to active intermediates, which are then converted to the ultimate carcinogens. Historically, CYP1A1 was believed to be the main enzyme that catalyses activation of PAHs. However, recent studies have established that CYP1B1, a newly identified member of the CYP1 family, plays a very important role in the metabolic activation of PAHs. Differences in the susceptibility of individuals to the adverse action of procarcinogens may, in part, be due to differences in the levels of expression of CYP1A1 and 1B1 and to genetic variations in the CYP1A1 and 1B1 genes.

Stages of Chemical Carcinogenesis

- **Initiation:** results from exposure of cells to sufficient dose of the carcinogen. The change induced is sudden and irreversible, and has memory. Initiation alone, however, is not sufficient for tumour formation.
- **Promotion:** is an epigenetic event (change in gene expression without change in DNA) which entails proliferation and clonal expansion of the altered and initiated cell. It has the following characteristics:
  - It is mitogenic (not mutagenic) and causes both mutated and normal cells to proliferate. Long delay is possible between administration of initiating agent and promoting agent.
  - The cellular changes resulting from the application of promoters do not affect DNA directly, and are reversible.
  - Promoters include phorbol esters, phenols, hormones, artificial sweeteners and phenobarbital. TPA (tetradecanoylphorbol acetate) and other phorbol esters activate protein kinase C, which leads to activation of signal transduction pathways that increase DNA replication and cell division.
  - Endocrine disruptors are involved in breast, ovarian, colon and prostate cancers and include estrogen and androgen receptors.
- **Progression :** Results from further mutations arising due to genetic instability during promotion and adds to the ability of invasiveness and metastasis of the malignant cell. Examples of agents aiding in progression include inflammation, asbestos, benzene, benzoyl peroxide, other peroxides, oxidative stress, etc.

Initiators

1. **Direct-acting carcinogens**—Do not require metabolic activation and include:
   (a) **Alkylating agents** (associated with lymphomas, AML, bladder cancer). Examples include:
      (i) Anticancer drugs, such as cyclophosphamide, chlorambucil, busulfan, melphalan and nitrosoureas.
      (ii) β-propiolactone.
      (iii) Dimethyl sulphate.
      (iv) Diepoxybutane.
   (b) **Acylating agents**
      (i) 1-acetyl imidazole.
      (ii) Dimethyl carbamyl chloride.
2. **Indirect-acting procarcinogens**—Require metabolic activation and include:
   (a) **Polycyclic aromatic hydrocarbons** (found in tobacco, smoke, fossil, fuel, soot, tar, mineral oils and smoked animal foods)
      (i) Anthracenes (associated with lung and skin cancer).
      (ii) Benzopyrene (associated with cancer of oral cavity).
      (iii) Methylcholanthrene (associated with sarcomas).
   (b) **Aromatic amines and azo dyes**
      (i) β naphthylamine (associated with carcinoma of urinary bladder).
      (ii) Benzidine (role in pathogenesis of hepatocellular carcinoma).
      (iii) Azo dyes like butter yellow, scarlet red (role in pathogenesis of hepatocellular carcinoma).
   (c) **Naturally occurring products**
      (i) Aflatoxin B_1 (role in pathogenesis of hepatocellular carcinoma).
      (ii) Cycasin (role in hepatobiliary tumours).
      (iii) Safrole (carcinogenic and genotoxic).
      (iv) Betel nuts (oral cancer).
   (d) **Miscellaneous**
      (i) Nitrosamines and amides (role in pathogenesis of gastric carcinoma).
      (ii) Vinyl chloride monomer (implicated in the pathogenesis of angiosarcoma of liver).
      (iii) Asbestosis (may lead to bronchogenic carcinoma and mesothelioma).
      (iv) Nickel, lead, cobalt and chromium (cause epidermal hyperplasia and basal cell carcinoma).

Stages of chemical carcinogenesis are shown in Flowchart 8.7.

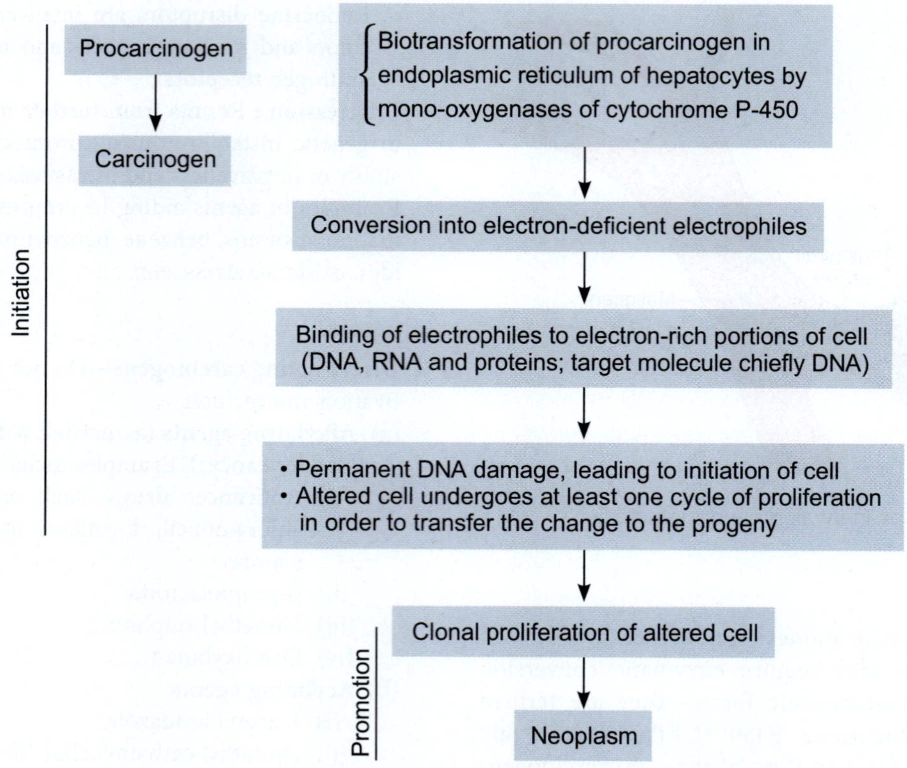

Flowchart 8.7 Stages of chemical carcinogenesis.

Table 8.10 Contrasting features of initiators and promoters

Features	Initiators	Promoters
Sequence of application	Applied first	Applied after initiator
Mechanism	Induction of mutation	• Not mutagenic; instead are mitogenic • Induce cell cycling and reinforce the action of initiators rather than inducing a mutation
Dose	Single for a short time	Repeated over a long time
Response	Sudden	Delayed
Molecular change	Permanent/ irreversible	Reversible
Examples	Most chemical carcinogens, radiation	Hormones, phorbol esters

The contrasting features of initiators and promoters are listed in Table 8.10.

Q. Write briefly on microbial carcinogenesis. (PA7.3)

Ans. Carcinogenic microbiological agents mainly include oncogenic DNA and RNA viruses as well as bacteria like *Helicobacter pylori*.

1. **Oncogenic DNA viruses:** Genomes of oncogenic DNA viruses integrate into and forms stable associations with host genome, for example E6 proteins of high-risk HPV types complex with *p53* to enhance its degradation. Oncogenic DNA viruses include:
   (a) **Human papilloma virus (HPV):** HPV has more than 100 distinct subtypes of which types 1, 2, 4 and 7 cause benign squamous papillomas or warts. Squamous cell carcinomas (SCCs) of cervix and anogenital region, as well as, oral and laryngeal cancers are associated with HPV 16, 18, 31, 33, 35 and 51 and their precursor lesions; whereas, HPV 6 and 11 cause genital lesions with low-malignant potential. HPV genome is present in **episomal (non-integrated)** form in benign warts and preneoplastic lesions. In cancers, the viral genome appears to be **integrated** into the host DNA. HPV proteins have the following effects on the cell cycle:
      (i) E6 and E7 block p53 and RB cell-cycle suppression pathways, respectively.
      (ii) E6 proteins of high-risk HPV type complex with p53 to enhance its degradation. It also stimulates the expression of telomerase reverse transcriptase (TERT) which immortalizes cells. E6 proteins of low-risk HPV types have low affinity for p53 and do not affect its stability.
      (iii) Increased p53 degradation causes a block in apoptosis (p53 increases activity of BAX, which is proapoptotic).
      (iv) E7 from high-risk types binds to RB protein, releasing sequestered E2F from the RB–E2F complex, triggering entry of cells in the S phase. E7 also inactivates CDK inhibitors like p21 and p27.
      (v) E7 from low-risk types has a lower affinity for RB protein, and is slow in transforming cells.

(b) **Epstein–Barr virus (EBV):** EBV is implicated in the pathogenesis of
  (i) African form of Burkitt lymphoma.
  (ii) B-cell lymphoma in immunosuppressed individuals.
  (iii) Hodgkin lymphoma.
  (iv) Nasopharyngeal carcinoma.
  (v) Gastric carcinoma.
  (vi) NK cell lymphoma.

  Mechanism of EBV-induced oncogenesis is shown in Flowchart 8.8.

(c) **Hepatitis viruses:** 70%–80% hepatocellular carcinoma is due to HBV and HCV. Effects of HBV are mainly indirect; it causes chronic liver cell injury, and regenerative hyperplasia (increased pool of cycling cells are at risk for genetic changes). HBV also encodes a regulatory element called **HBX protein,** which disrupts normal growth control of infected liver cells by transcriptional activation of an insulin-like growth factor II and receptors for insulin-like growth factor I. Overexpression of the foetal growth factor IGF-II, IGF-I receptor (IGF-IR) and cytoplasmic downstream effectors, such as insulin-receptor substrates (IRS) contribute to proliferation, antiapoptosis and invasive behaviour. HBX protein also binds to p53 and interferes with its growth-suppressing activities.

(d) **Human herpes simplex virus (HHV) 8:** HHV 8 has an established role in **Kaposi sarcoma, B cell lymphomas and multicentric variant of Castleman disease.** HHV-8 infects host macrophages and primitive mesenchymal cells, which differentiate into endothelial cells under the influence of several cytokines like IL6, IL8 and MIP. It also interferes with the tumour suppressor pathways, mainly those of p53 and RB gene.

2. **Oncogenic RNA viruses**
  (a) Retroviruses are the only RNA viruses that seem to have oncogenic potential in humans. They contain 'reverse transcriptase', which induces reverse transcription of viral RNA to synthesise viral DNA. The viral DNA moves to host cell nucleus and gets incorporated in it. The prototypic example of an oncogenic RNA virus is human T cell leukaemia virus (HTLV)-1.
  (b) HTLV-1 causes adult T cell leukaemia–lymphoma (ATLL) endemic in Japan and Caribbean basin.
  (c) It has tropism for CD4 + T cells and is transmitted by passage of infected T cells during sexual intercourse, blood product transfusion and breast feeding.

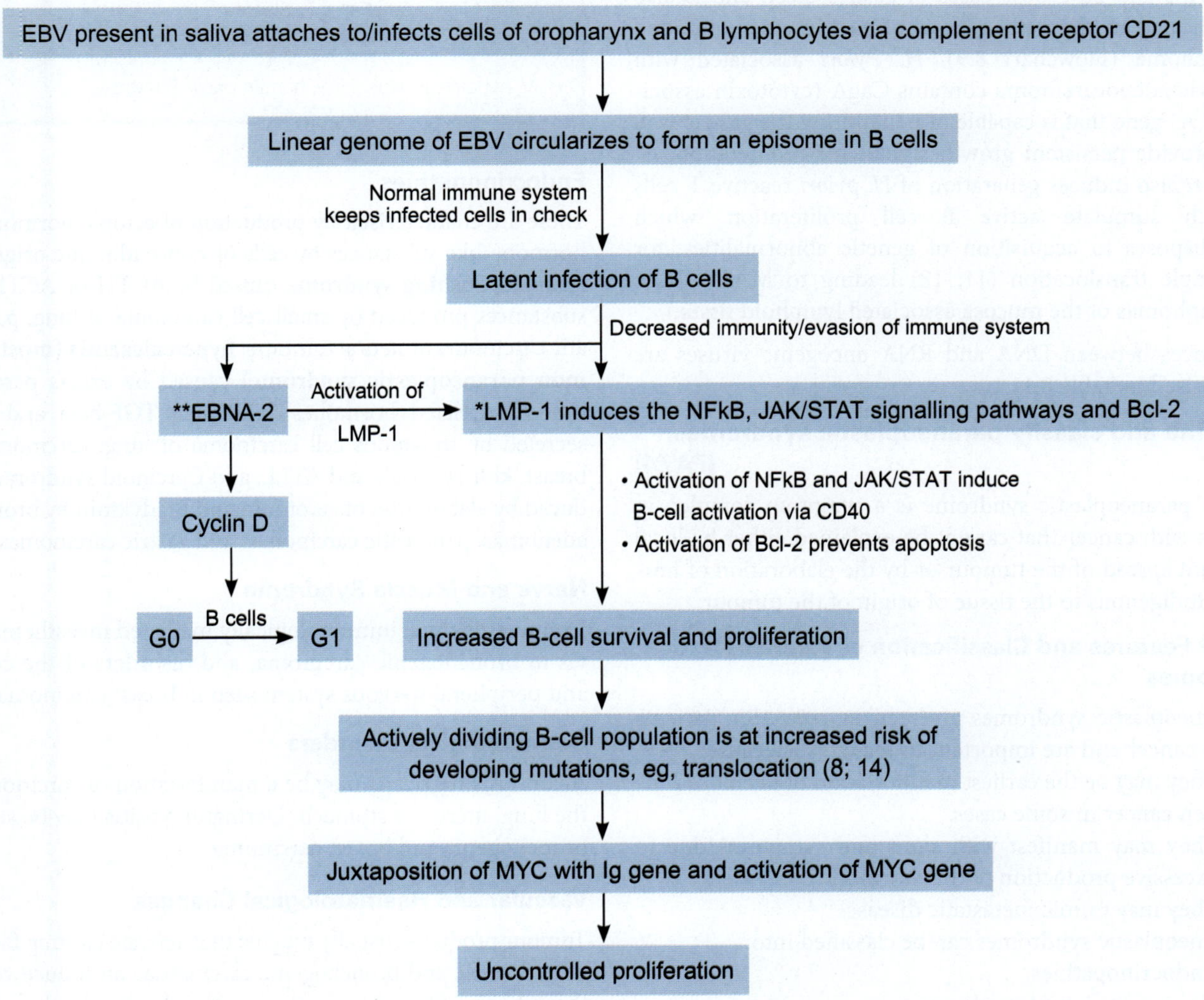

***LMP-1 – Latent membrane protein-1. **EBNA-2 – Epstein–Barr nuclear antigen 2.**

Flowchart 8.8 Mechanism of EBV-induced oncogenesis.

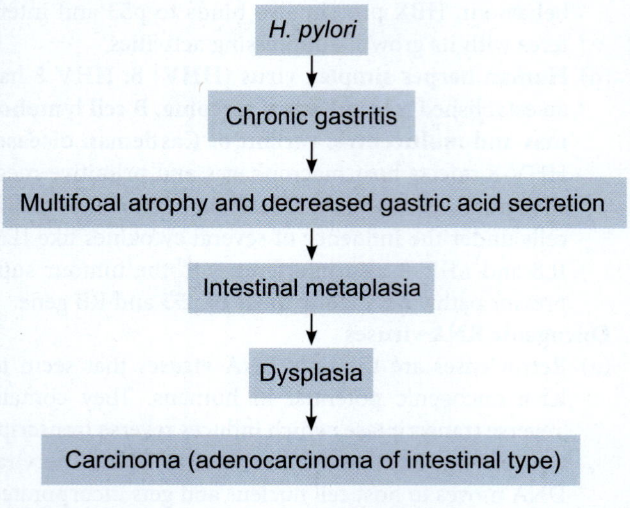

Flowchart 8.9 Mechanism of ***Helicobacter pylori***-induced oncogenesis.

(d) It contains *gag*, *pol* and *env* genes typical of other retroviruses. It also contains '*TAX*' gene, which activates several host cell genes involved in proliferation and differentiation of T cells and interferes with DNA repair functions.

3. **Helicobacter pylori:** Can be demonstrated in 90% cases of gastritis and 20%–30% cases of gastric ulcer, and is also implicated in the pathogenesis of gastric carcinoma and lymphoma (Flowchart 8.9). *H. Pylori* associated with gastric adenocarcinoma contains CagA (cytotoxin associated A) gene that is capable of penetrating the gastric wall to provide persistent growth signals for proliferation. *H. Pylori* also induces generation of *H. pylori* reactive T cells which stimulate active B cell proliferation, which predisposes to acquisition of genetic abnormalities, for example translocation (11; 18) leading to MALTOMAs (lymphomas of the mucosa associated lymphoid tissue).

Differences between DNA and RNA oncogenic viruses are summarised in Table 8.11.

Table 8.11 Differences between DNA and RNA oncogenic viruses

Features	DNA oncogenic virus	rna oncogenic virus
Viruses	HPV, EBV, HBV, KSHV	HTLV-1
Genome	Double-stranded DNA	Single-stranded RNA
Reverse transcriptase	Absent	Present
Interaction with host genome	Linear DNA genome forms a double-stranded circle within infected cell and then covalently integrates into host genome	First RNA is transcribed into DNA, which then integrates into host genome
Name of gene	*Early region A* gene	*src* gene
Name of protein	T antigen	*src* protein
Function of protein	Protein kinase, ATPase activity, binding to DNA, and stimulation of DNA	Protein kinase that phosphorylates tyrosine and disturbs the growth control process
Location of protein	Primarily nuclear, but sometimes in plasma membrane	Plasma membrane

HBV, hepatitis B virus; HPV, human papilloma virus.

Q. Define and classify paraneoplastic syndromes. (PA7.4)

Ans. A paraneoplastic syndrome is a symptom complex in patients with cancer that cannot be explained either by local or distant spread of the tumour or by the elaboration of hormones indigenous to the tissue of origin of the tumour.

Salient Features and Classification of Paraneoplastic Syndromes

- Paraneoplastic syndromes are seen in 10%–15% patients with cancer and are important to recognise because:
  - They may be the earliest manifestation of occult or hidden cancer in some cases.
  - They may manifest with signs and symptoms due to excessive production of that hormone.
  - They may mimic metastatic disease.
- Paraneoplastic syndromes can be classified into:
  - Endocrinopathies.
  - Nerve and muscle syndrome.
  - Dermatological disorders.
  - Vascular and haematological changes.
  - Bone and soft-tissue changes.

Endocrinopathies

These are characterised by production of ectopic hormones or hormone-like substances by cells of non-endocrine origin, for example **Cushing syndrome** caused by ACTH or ACTH-like substances produced by small-cell carcinoma of lung, pancreatic carcinoma or neural tumours; **hypercalcaemia (most common paraneoplastic syndrome)** caused by excess parathormone or related hormones (TNF-alfa, TGF-beta and IL-1) secreted by squamous cell carcinoma of lung, carcinomas of breast, kidney, ovary and ATLL; and Carcinoid syndrome produced by elaboration of serotonin and bradykinin by bronchial adenomas, pancreatic carcinomas and gastric carcinomas.

Nerve and Muscle Syndrome

Examples include immunologically mediated myasthenia gravis in bronchogenic carcinoma, and disorders of the central and peripheral nervous system seen in breast carcinoma.

Dermatological Disorders

Acanthosis nigricans may be a manifestation of carcinoma of the lung, uterus or stomach. Dermatomyositis may be seen in bronchogenic and breast carcinoma.

Vascular and Haematological Changes

Tumour products (usually mucins that activate clotting factors) of pancreatic and bronchogenic carcinoma can induce venous thrombosis **(Trousseau sign).** Non-bacterial thrombotic endocarditis (due to hypercoagulability) is seen in many advanced cancers; and anaemia may develop in association with thymic neoplasms (cause is unknown).

Bone and Soft-Tissue Changes

Hypertrophic osteoarthropathy and clubbing are common presenting symptoms of bronchogenic carcinoma (cause is unknown).

Q. Write briefly on laboratory diagnosis of cancer.

Ans. The modalities for laboratory diagnosis of cancer include:

1. **Cytological methods**
   The main techniques used for cytological diagnosis are:
   (a) FNAC: FNAC of tumours involves aspirating constituent cells of the tumour followed by cytological examination of the stained smear. This method is used most commonly for the assessment of palpable lesions in accessible sites (salivary glands, breast, thyroid, skin, sift tissue and lymph nodes). FNAC under imaging guidance enables one to aspirate the deeper relatively inaccessible lesions. FNAC is an extremely reliable, rapid and useful technique. Both 'air-dried May–Grünwald–Giemsa (MGG)-stained smears' and 'wet (95% ethanol)-fixed Haematoxylin-and-Eosin stained smears' are prepared from the FNAC material and examined.

   Fine needle aspiration cytology (FNAC) → Direct
   Fine needle aspiration cytology (FNAC) → Image guided

   (b) Exfoliative cytology: Due to loss of cohesiveness, neoplastic cells are continuously shed from tumours into the surrounding space. These are called exfoliated cells and can be examined in the following preparations:
      (i) Papanicolaou smears (for carcinoma cervix).
      (ii) Sputum and bronchial washings (for bronchogenic carcinoma).
      (iii) Pleural, pericardial and peritoneal fluid (for local cancers).
      (iv) Urine (for urothelial malignancies).
      (v) Cerebrospinal fluid (for CNS tumours).
      (vi) Gastric secretions (for gastric carcinoma).
   Diagnostic reliability of exfoliative cytology varies between 80% and 97%.
2. **Histopathology:** Histopathological diagnosis entails microscopy supported by clinical and investigative data. Formalin fixation is required for routine histopathology and glutaraldehyde fixation is required for electron microscopy. Frozen sectioning aids in rapid/intraoperative diagnosis.
3. **Histochemistry/cytochemistry (special stains):** These are diagnostic tools for identifying **chemical composition of cells for the purpose of tumour diagnosis and classification** (Table 8.12).

Table 8.12 Special stains in tumour diagnosis

Substances	Stain
Basement membrane/ collagen	PAS, reticulin, Van Gieson, Masson trichrome
Glycogen	PAS with diastase loss
Glycoproteins	PAS with diastase persistence
Mucins of epithelial origin	Mucicarmine
Acid mucins (of mesenchymal origin)	Alcian blue
Argyrophilic/argentaffin granules/fungi	Silver stains
Fat	Oil red-O, Sudan black B
Enzymes	Acid phosphatase (prostatic malignancy) and alkaline phosphatase (chronic m yeloid leukaemia), myeloperoxidse (acute myeloid leukaemia), NASD chloroacetate esterase (myeloid series, mast cells)
Calcium	von Kossa, Alizarin red

PAS, Periodic acid–Schiff.

4. **Immunohistochemistry/immunocytochemistry:** Immunohistocytochemistry (IHC) is an immunological method of recognising a cell based on recognition of specific components called 'antigens'. 'Specific antibodies' against antigens are raised by hybridoma technique and labelled monoclonal antibodies. Antigen–antibody complexes on the slides (histological sections or cytology smears) are made visible for microscopic identification by labels (fluorochromes or enzyme systems). Most tumour markers are proteins but some oncogenes, tumour suppressor genes, tumour proliferation markers, DNA alterations and patterns of gene expression are also considered to be tumour markers. IHC enables us to differentiate between a benign or malignant neoplasm, and aids in specific typing of a cancer (Table 8.13).

   Uses
   - Categorisation of undifferentiated neoplasms.
   - Specific typing of leukaemias/lymphomas.
   - Determination of site of origin of a metastatic tumour.
   - Detection of molecules that have *prognostic* or *therapeutic* significance, such as ER–PR receptors in carcinoma breast.
   - Expression of protein products of oncogenes.
   - Differentiating benign from malignant lesions.
   - Demonstration of infectious agents using specific antibodies against microbial DNA and RNA.
5. **Intermediate filaments (IFs):** IFs are a family of related proteins that share common structural features. They have an average diameter of 10 nanometers, which is between that of microfilaments (which are smaller) and microtubules (which are larger). Most types of intermediate filaments are cytoplasmic except lamins, which are nuclear. The most important function of intermediate filaments is to provide mechanical support to the plasma membrane, where they come in contact with other cells or with the extracellular matrix. Unlike microfilaments and microtubules, intermediate filaments do not participate in cell motility. In higher vertebrates, the subunits composing intermediate filaments constitute a superfamily of α-helical proteins that is divided into subtypes on the basis of similarities in sequence (Table 8.14).
6. **Electron microscopy (EM):** EM is used for confirming or substantiating tumour diagnosis based on:
   (a) Presence and type of cell junctions.
   (b) Presence of microvilli.
   (c) Shape of nucleus, features of nuclear membrane and nucleoli.

Table 8.13 Common immunohistochemical markers used for tumour diagnosis

Tumour	IHC marker
Epithelial tumours (carcinomas)	• EMA • CEA • Low molecular weight keratins (CAM 5.2, AE1-AE3) • Cytokeratin cocktail, CK7, CK20, CEA, and EMA • Alternative epithelial markers—p63, MOC-31, and TTF1
Mesenchymal tumours (sarcomas)	• Vimentin (general mesenchymal marker) • Desmin, myogenin, muscle specific actin, myoglobin, Myo D1 (muscle markers) • CD31, CD34, factor VIII antigen (vascular markers for vascular tumours and endothelial cells) • D2-40 (marker for lymphatic origin) • α-1-Chymotrypsin (for fibrohistiocytic origin)
Melanoma	Vimentin, S 100, HMB 45, Melan A, Mart 1
Histiocytic neoplasms	CD68, lysozyme, CD1a (Langerhans cells)
Lymphomas	Leukocyte common antigen (LCA or CD45), pan B markers—CD19, CD20, immunoglobulins, pan T marker—CD3, Markers for Hodgkin (RS cells)—CD15, 30
Neuroendocrine tumours	Neuron specific enolase, chromogranin, synaptophysin, CD56, and CD57
Trophoblastic tumours	HCG
Papillary carcinoma thyroid	CK 19, HBME1, Thyroglobulin
Medullary carcinoma of thyroid	Calcitonin
Follicular carcinoma of thyroid	Thyroglobulin, low molecular weight keratin, EMA, TTF1
Carcinoma of ovary	CA 125
Cancer of bowel, pancreas, and breast	CEA
Carcinoma of breast	CA-15.3
Cell proliferation/ apoptosis markers	Ki-67, bcl2

CEA, Carcinoembryonic antigen; EMA, epithelial membrane antigen; HCG, human chorionic gonadotropin; IHC; immunohistocytochemistry.

(d) Cytoplasmic organelles.
(e) Presence of dense bodies in the cytoplasm.

7. **Tumour markers:** These are substances found in blood, urine, body fluids or tissue, the levels of which might be elevated in association with a cancer. Tumour markers may be used to help diagnose cancer, predict a patient's response to cancer therapy, check a patient's response to treatment or determine cancer recurrence. More than 20 tumour markers are currently in use (Table 8.15).

Table 8.14 'Intermediate filaments' and their significance in the tumour diagnosis

Keratins	Carcinomas, mesotheliomas, and germ-cell tumours
Vimentin	Sarcomas, melanomas, and lymphomas (mesenchymal tumours)
Desmin	Myogenic tumours
Neurofilaments	Neural tumours
GFAP	Glial tumours

GFAP, Glial fibrillary acidic proteins.

Table 8.15 Role of Tumour Markers in the Diagnosis of Neoplasia

Tumour marker	Associated neoplasm
AFP	Hepatocellular carcinoma, non-seminomatous germ cell tumours
PSA	Prostatic carcinoma
HCG	Trophoblastic tumours
Calcitonin	Medullary carcinoma of thyroid
VMA	Pheochromocytoma
CA-125	Carcinoma of ovary
CEA	Cancer of bowel, pancreas, and breast
CA-15-3	Carcinoma of breast
CA 19-9	Carcinoma of breast, pancreas, colon
NSE	Neuroblastoma, oat cell carcinoma lung and other neuroendocrine tumours
Catecholamines	Pheochromocytoma and neuroblastoma
CD30	Hodgkin disease, ALCL
Monoclonal immunoglobulins	Multiple myeloma and other monoclonal gammopathies

AFP, α-Fetoprotein; ALCL, anaplastic large cell lymphoma; CEA, carcinoembryonic antigen; HCG, human chorionic gonadotropin; NSE, neuron specific enolase; PSA, prostate-specific antigen; VMA, vanillylmandelic acid.

Modern Aids in the Tumour Diagnosis

1. **Flow cytometry:** Recognition and quantification of several parameters simultaneously by making single-cell suspensions of cells, which are made to pass through a chamber in a single file. Fluids, blood and bone marrow can be processed directly; whereas, homogenisation is necessary for solid tissue. Each cell is struck by a focused laser beam, and the properties of scattered and fluorescent light is measured to characterise the cell.

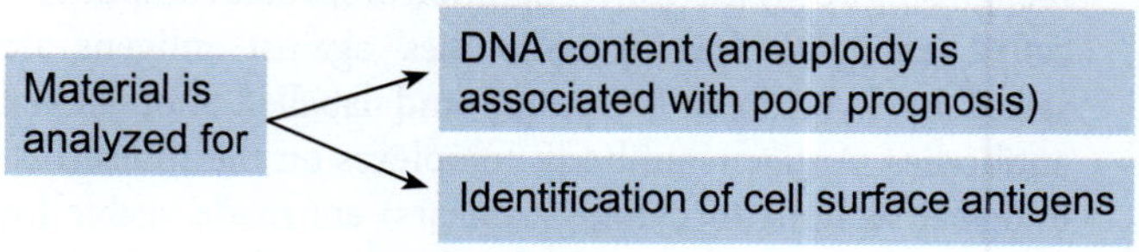

2. **In situ hybridisation:** Molecular technique by which nucleic acid sequences (cellular/viral DNA and RNA) are

localised by specifically labelled nucleic acid probes *directly in the cell* rather than after DNA extraction, for example, localisation of oncogenes.

3. A variety of DNA-/RNA-based techniques in which DNA/RNA are extracted and analysed, for example **DNA analysis by Southern blot and RNA analysis by Northern blot** are also available.
4. A molecular cytogenetic technique called **spectral karyotyping** is a highly sensitive method that allows the examination of all chromosomes in a single experiment. This technique, which is based on 24-colour chromosomal painting with a mixture of fluorochromes, can detect all types of chromosomal rearrangements in tumours including very small translocations and insertions.
5. Another available technique, **comparative genomic hybridisation,** is more frequently used in research laboratories as it requires a lot of time and effort. This technique allows the analysis of genome amplification and chromosomal gains and losses in tumour cells. It has been used to differentiate primary from metastatic carcinomas, and to identify primary tumours of uncertain origin.
6. **DNA microarray analysis and proteomics:** These methods are used to obtain gene expression signatures (molecular profiles) of cancer cells. DNA microarray techniques reveal the RNA expression from as many as 30,000 different genes using gene–chip technology. Conventional DNA probes are substituted by silicon chips that contain the entire range of genes, and high-resolution scanners are used for measurement. *Proteomics* determines the protein profiles of tumours. With the methods currently in use, protein profiles from about 3,000 genes can be obtained.
7. Validation of new markers for cancer diagnosis can be done on multiple tissue samples, using **tissue arrays.** In this technique, core samples are obtained from tissues embedded in a paraffin block and used to prepare a new block that may contain hundreds of tissue fragments. These multiple samples are then used to test the expression of potential tumour markers by immunohistochemical or in situ hybridisation techniques.

The above molecular methods can be used for:

- **Analysis of molecular cytogenetic abnormalities and mutational analysis:** Certain genetic alterations are associated with poor prognosis, and hence their detection allows stratification of patients for therapy. As an example, amplification of the *N-MYC* gene and deletions of 1p bode poorly for patients with neuroblastoma. These can be detected by routine cytogenetics, and also by fluorescent in situ hybridisation (FISH) or polymerase chain reaction (PCR) assays.
- **Study of oncogenic viruses at molecular level:** Oncogenic viruses can contribute to different steps of the carcinogenic process. In addition to elucidate the aetiology of several human cancers, the study of oncogenic viruses has been invaluable to the discovery and analysis of key cellular pathways that are commonly rendered dysfunctional during carcinogenesis, in general.
- **Detection of minimal residual disease:** After treatment of patients with leukaemia or lymphoma, the presence of minimal disease or the onset of relapse can be monitored by PCR-based amplification of unique nucleic acid sequences generated by the translocation. For example, detection of *BCR-ABL* transcripts by PCR gives a measure of the residual leukaemia cells in treated patients with chronic myeloid leukaemia.
- **Diagnosis of hereditary predisposition to cancer:** As was discussed earlier, germline mutations in several tumour suppressor genes, including *BRCA*1, *BRCA*2 and the *RET* proto-oncogene are associated with a high risk of developing specific cancers. Thus, detection of carriers of these mutations in family members of affected patients or in those at high risk of carrying the mutation can be achieved by molecular methods.

Q. Write briefly on immune response to cancer.

(PA7.5)

Ans. T cell is the most important cell responsible for direct recognition and killing of tumour cells. T cells carry out immunologic surveillance, then proliferate and destroy newly transformed tumour cells after recognizing tumour-associated antigens or TAAs. T cells may in some instances require the presence of humoral antibodies directed against the tumour cells (antibody-dependent cellular cytotoxicity) to initiate the interactions that lead to the death of tumour cells. In contrast, suppressor T cells inhibit the immune response against tumours.

Cytotoxic T lymphocytes (CTLs) recognize antigens on target cells and lyse these cells. These antigens may be cell surface proteins or may be intracellular proteins that are expressed on the surface in combination with class I MHC molecules. Natural killer (NK) cells too are effector cells with tumoricidal activity. In contrast to CTLs, NK cells lack the receptor for antigen detection but can still recognize normal cells from tumour cells. The underlying mechanism for this ability to discriminate is not clear. Evidence suggests that class I MHC molecules on the surface of normal cells inhibit NK cells and prevent lysis. Thus, the decreased level of class I molecule expression characteristic of many tumour cells may allow activation of NK cells and subsequent tumour lysis.

Macrophages can kill specific tumour cells when activated via lymphokines (soluble factors produced by T cells) and interferons. Under certain circumstances, macrophages may present TAAs to T cells and stimulate tumour-specific immune response. There are two classes of tumour-associated macrophages (TAM): (a) TAM-1 (M1) cells facilitate T cell killing of tumours and (b) TAM-2 (M2) cells which promote tumour tolerance. Dendritic cells are dedicated antigen-presenting cells present in barrier tissues. They take up tumour-associated proteins, process them, and present TAAs to T cells to stimulate the CTL response against tumour.

Lymphokines induce growth and activation of other immune cells (interleukin-2, also known as T-cell growth factor, and the interferons. IL-12 is produced by dendritic cells and specifically induces CTLs, thereby enhancing antitumour immune responses.

Humoral antibodies do not appear to confer significant protection against tumour growth. Most antibodies cannot recognize TAAs. Cytotoxic antibodies are directed against surface antigens of tumour cells. These antibodies can exert anti-tumour effects through complement fixation or destroy tumour cells with T cells (ADCC).

9 Infectious Diseases

Infectious diseases are caused by pathogenic microorganisms, such as bacteria, viruses, parasites, or fungi, and can spread, directly or indirectly, from one person to another. They are also known as ***transmissible diseases* or *communicable diseases***, and are typically characterized by ***clinically evident symptoms*** and ***signs*** of disease resulting from the infection and 'presence and growth of pathogenic biological agents in the host'. In certain cases, infectious diseases may be asymptomatic for much or even their entire course. An ***infection*** is not synonymous with an *infectious disease*, as some infections do not cause visible illness in the host but lie dormant.

The term ***infectivity*** describes the ability of an organism to enter, survive and multiply in the host, while ***infectiousness*** of a disease indicates comparative ease with which the disease is transmitted to other hosts. Transmission of a pathogen can occur in various ways including physical contact, contaminated food, body fluids, objects, airborne inhalation, or through vector organisms. ***Virulence*** is defined as the likelihood of an organism causing severe or aggressive disease (degree of pathogenicity).

A ***contagious disease*** is a subset of infectious disease that is infective or easily transmitted. Other types of infectious diseases with more specialized routes of infection, such as vector transmission or sexual transmission, are usually not regarded as 'contagious,' and often do not require medical isolation (sometimes loosely called quarantine) of victims. ***Zoonotic diseases*** are infectious diseases of animals that can cause disease when transmitted to humans.

Some of the major historical events in infectious disease pathology are briefly summarized as following:

- **Leeuwenhoek**, in the 17th century reported the microscopic observation of 'other heretofore unseen creatures', but they were regarded as incidental findings.
- When **Agostino Bassi** in the late 18th century linked a disease in the silkworm with a fungal parasite (*Botrytis paradoxa*), he extended his views to suggest that many contagious diseases, such as smallpox, typhus, plague and cholera were also due to live organisms—as yet undiscovered.
- **Louis Pasteur**, one of the founders of microbiology, put forward the 'germ theory of disease' (establishing that microorganisms can cause disease). Pasteur extended this theory to explain the causes of many diseases—including anthrax, cholera, tuberculosis and smallpox—and their prevention by vaccination. He is best known for creating the first live attenuated vaccines, including rabies vaccine for humans.
- In 1882, **Koch**, a German physician, became famous for isolating *Bacillus anthracis*, the tuberculosis bacillus *(Mycobacterium tuberculosis)* and *Vibrio cholerae*, and for his development of *Koch postulates*. Koch postulated that a specific microorganism can be linked to a disease provided:
  - The organism is found in lesions caused by the disease; the organism can be isolated on culture.
  - Inoculation of the organism causes lesions in experimental animals.
  - The organism can be recovered from experimental animals.
- **Ronald Ross**, an English military physician posted in India, demonstrated in 1897 that mosquitoes carry malaria.
- **Oswald Avery** demonstrated that an avirulent *Streptococcus pneumoniae* could be transformed into a virulent phenotype by the transfer of DNA. This pioneered further research in molecular epidemiology of infectious diseases.

Epidemiology is an important tool used to study disease in a population. For infectious diseases, it helps to determine if a disease outbreak is sporadic (occasional occurrence), endemic (regular cases often occurring in a region), epidemic (an unusually high number of cases in a region), or pandemic (a global epidemic).

Q. Write in detail on classification of infectious diseases.

Ans. Infectious diseases are classified based on the type of causative microbes and host immune status. Causative microbes can be ***primary pathogens*** or ***opportunistic pathogens***:

- ***Primary pathogens*** are those, which cause disease in a normal, healthy host, due to their intrinsic virulence.
- Organisms that cause disease in a host who is immunosuppressed are termed as ***opportunistic pathogens***. These may be a part of normal host flora (*Candida*) or may be acquired from the environment (e.g. introduction via surgical or traumatic wound infections). Impairment of host defenses may have a genetic basis (chronic granulomatous disease) or may be acquired (in intake of broad-spectrum antibiotics, immunosuppressive chemicals, exposure to chemotherapeutic agents and ionizing radiation, or infections such as HIV).

Infectious agents belong to a wide range of classes, namely, bacteria, viruses, fungi, protozoa, chlamydiae, rickettsiae, mycoplasma and helminths.

Table 9.1 Organ system approach of classification of bacterial diseases

Organ system	Causative organisms
Meningitis	Pneumococci, meningococci, *Haemophilus influenzae*, *Listeria*
Sinusitis	Pneumococci, *H. influenzae*, *Moraxella*
Acute otitis media	Pneumococci, *H. influenzae*, *Moraxella*
Pharyngitis	Group A streptococci
Chest cavity	
1. Pneumonias	
(a) Community accuired	Pneumococcus, *Staphylococcus aureus* and *H. influenzae*
(b) Atypical	*Mycoplasma pneumoniae*, *Chlamydiae pneumonia* and *Legionella pneumophila*
(c) Tuberculous	*M. tuberculosis*
2. Pleuritis and lung abscess	Anaerobic bacteria (*Peptostreptococcus*, *Bacteroides*, *Fusobacterium* species), *Staphylococcus*, *Klebsiella*, *Haemophilus*, *Pseudomonas*, *Nocardia*, *Escherichia coli*, *Streptococcus*, and mycobacteria
3. Endocarditis	*Streptococcus viridans*, *S. aureus*, and Enterococci
Abdomen	
1. Gastritis	*Helicobacter pylori*
2. Enteric infections	*Campylobacter jejuni*, *Salmonella*, *Shigella*, *Clostridium*
3. Peritonitis	*E. coli* and *S. aureus*
4. Liver abscesses and biliary tract infections	*Bacteroides*, *Enterococcus*, *E. coli*, *Klebsiella*, *Staphylococcus* and *Streptococcus*
Skin infections	Gram-positive cocci (*S. aureus* and *Streptococcus pyogenes*)
Urinary tract infection	*E. coli*, other Enterobacteriaceae, *Staphylococcus saprophyticus*, and *Pseudomonas aeruginosa*

Table 9.2 Classification of bacterial diseases based on causative organisms

Disease	Causative agent
Anthrax	*B. anthracis*
Brucellosis	*Bacillus melitensis, Bacillus abortus, Bacillus suis and Bacillus canis*
Bronchopneumonia	*S. aureus, S. pneumoniae, H. influenzae and Klebsiella pneumoniae*
Bubonic plague	*Yersinia pestis*
Cholera	*V. cholerae*
Chancroid	*Haemophilus ducreyi*
Clostridial diseases:	
1. Gas gangrene	*Clostridium perfringens*
2. Tetanus	*C. tetani*
3. Botulism	*C. botulinum*
4. Clostridial food poisoning	*C. perfringens*
Cat scratch diseases	*Bartonella henselae*
Diphtheria	*Corynebacterium diphtheriae*
Gonorrhea	*Neisseria gonorrhoeae*
Leprosy	*Mycobacterium leprae*
Leptospirosis	Genus *Leptospira*
Lyme disease	*Borrelia burgdorferi*
Lobar pneumonia	*S. aureus, S. pneumoniae, H. influenzae and K. pneumoniae*
Meningitis	*E. coli, H. influenzae, Neisseria meningitides, S. pneumoniae*
Pertussis	*Bordetella pertussis*
Primary atypical pneumonia	*M. pneumoniae*, *C. pneumonia* and *L. pneumophila*
Tuberculosis	*M. tuberculosis*
Tularemia	*Francisella tularensis*
Typhoid	*Salmonella typhi*
Urinary tract infection	*E. coli*, other Enterobacteriaceae, *S. saprophyticus* and *P. aeruginosa*

Q. Write in detail on diseases caused by bacteria. (PA10.4)

Ans. Bacterial cells are prokaryotes (group of organisms whose cells lack a nucleus or any other membrane-bound organelle). Bacterial cell wall usually consists of peptidoglycan which is a polymer composed of mixed sugars and amino acids. Peptidoglycans are the structural elements of all bacterial cell walls. They constitute almost 95% of the cell wall in some Gram-positive bacteria and as little as 5% of the cell wall in Gram-negative bacteria. Most commonly used classifications reflect major differences in bacterial cell wall structure and to some extent mechanisms involved in disease caused by them.

Bacterial diseases can be classified based on the organ systems involved or the nature of the aetiological agent that causes the disease (Tables 9.1 and 9.2):

Classification of Bacteria

Bacteria can be classified based on the following characteristics:

1. **Gram staining** (Figs. 9.1 and 9.2):
   (a) Gram-positive (purple/violet) organisms have a single, thick, cell wall surrounding the cell membrane that retains crystal violet stain. It consists of a peptidoglycan layer without any lipopolysaccharide (LPS). Gram-negative (pink) organisms have inner and outer membranes, with the outer membrane having LPS molecules. The cell wall is sandwiched between the bilayer. Examples of Gram-positive and Gram-negative cocci include *S. pyogenes* and *S. aureus*, and *N. gonorrhoeae* and *N. meningitides*, respectively.
   (b) Some organisms, however, require stains other than the Gram stain for their demonstration, for example, mycobacteria or *Nocardia*, which show acid fastness on Ziehl–Neelsen or similar stains.
   (c) Still other organisms may need to be demonstrated by culture in special media, serology, or molecular techniques.

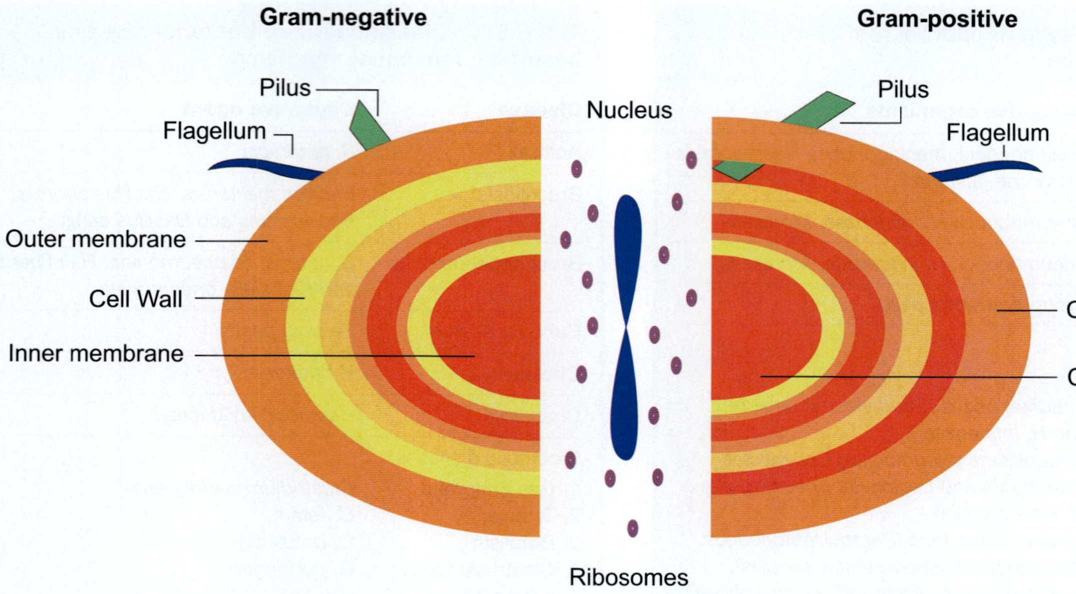

Fig. 9.1 Cell wall structure in Gram-positive and Gram-negative organisms.

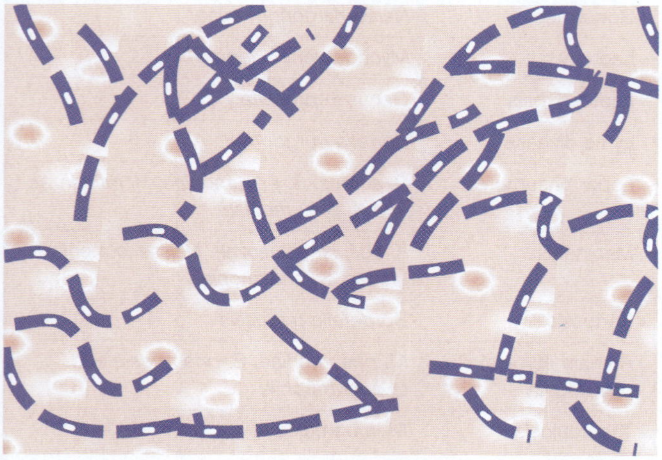

Fig. 9.2 Gram-positive bacilli.

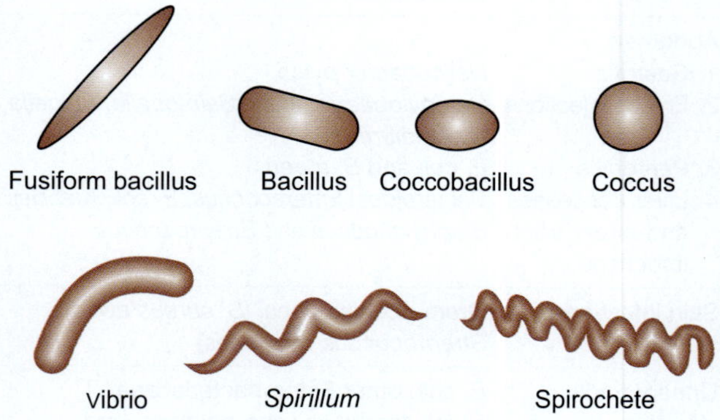

Fig. 9.3 Bacterial morphology shapes.

2. **Shape** (Fig. 9.3): Following binary fission, the newly formed bacteria spontaneously assume a characteristic shape. This shape varies significantly among species of bacteria and may be employed in course of isolate identification, for example:
   (a) *Spherical bacteria or cocci*: Examples include *Streptococcus* and *Staphylococcus*.
   (b) *Rod-shaped bacteria or bacilli*: Can be subdivided based on their ability to form spores. The non-spore formers are *Corynebacterium* and *Listeria* (a coccobacillus), whereas *Bacillus* and *Clostridium* produce spores.
   (c) *Curved or spiral bacteria*: Include treponemes, borrelias, leptospiras, *Spirillum*.
   (d) *Filamentous bacteria*: Include *Actinomyces*, *Nocardia*, mycobacteria.
3. **Metabolic behavior (aerobic or anaerobic):** The spore-forming bacteria can again be divided based on their mode of respiration: *Bacillus* is a facultative anaerobe, while *Clostridium* is an obligate anaerobe. Aerobic and anaerobic bacteria in the mouth, particularly *Streptococcus mutans*, contribute to dental plaque, a major cause of tooth decay. In the colon, majority of bacteria are anaerobic, including *Bacteroides* species.
4. **Location (intracellular vs. extracellular):** Many bacteria remain extracellular when they invade the body, while others can survive and replicate either outside or inside of host cells (*facultative intracellular* bacteria), and some grow only inside host cells *(obligate intracellular* bacteria).
5. **Antigenic composition and DNA sequence**: Identification of bacteria and classification is increasingly using molecular methods. Diagnostics using such DNA-based tools, such as polymerase chain reaction, are becoming increasingly popular due to their specificity and speed, compared to culture-based methods.

Mechanism of Bacterial Injury

1. **Bacterial adhesion:** Bacterial adhesions bind bacteria to host cells. Examples of adhesions include lipoteichoic acids, M protein, and protein F, which are expressed on the surface of *S. pyogenes*. Lipoteichoic acid and protein F bind to

fibronectin, and M protein prevents phagocytosis by host macrophages. Protein F may also help *S. pyogenes* to evade immune response by aiding the entry of the organism into epithelial cells. *Fimbriae* or *pilli* are filamentous proteins on surface of Gram-negative bacteria. Strains of *E. coli* that cause urinary tract infections uniquely express a specific P pilus, which binds to a specific moiety expressed on urothelial cells.

2. **Intracellular growth of bacteria**
   (a) Intracellular location of the bacterium protects it from the immune response of the body (e.g., antibodies), and also aids in its spread to other sites (migration of macrophages carries *M. tuberculosis* from lung to lymphatics). *M. tuberculosis* is among many bacteria which are capable of activating alternative complement pathway. This results in opsonization with C3b. The C3b-coated organisms bind to CR3 complement receptor on macrophages and are taken into the cell. Once within macrophages, they prevent the fusion of phagosome with a lysosome to form a phagolysosome and escape destruction.
   (b) Gram-negative bacteria have projections on their surface, which bind to host cells to form pores in host cell membrane, and then inject proteins that mediate rearrangement of cell cytoskeleton, facilitating bacterial entry. Organisms like *Shigella* inhibit host protein synthesis and cause rapid lysis of the host cell.
3. **Bacterial toxins**
   (a) The cell-associated toxins are referred to as endotoxins and the extracellular diffusible toxins are referred to as exotoxins. In bacteriology, an **endotoxin** is synonymous with LPS complex associated with the outer membrane of Gram-negative pathogens, such as *E. coli, Salmonella, Shigella, Pseudomonas, Neisseria, H. influenzae, B. pertussis,* and *V. cholerae*. LPS is composed of a long-chain fatty acid (lipid A) connected to a sugar chain. Attached to the sugar is a variable carbohydrate chain (0 antigen), which is used to serotype and discriminate between different strains of bacteria. Toxicity is associated with the lipid component (lipid A) and immunogenicity is associated with the polysaccharide components.
   (b) Low levels of LPS induce natural immunity, whereas high levels of LPS release cytokines, activate coagulation cascade and also the complement pathway to induce septic shock, disseminated intravascular coagulation (DIC), and adult respiratory distress syndrome; LPS also acts as a B cell mitogen and stimulates the multiplication of B cells and the secretion of immunoglobulins, especially immunoglobulin G (IgG) and immunoglobulin M (IgM).
   (c) Bacteria also secrete a variety of **enzymes,** such as proteases, hyaluronidases, coagulases, fibrinolysins and lipases.
   (d) **Exotoxins** are usually proteins that act enzymatically. The production of the toxin is generally specific to a particular bacterial species that produces the disease associated with the toxin (e.g. only *C. tetani* produces tetanus toxin; only *C. diphtheriae* produces the diphtheria toxin). Usually, virulent strains of the bacterium produce the toxin while non-virulent strains do not, and the toxin is the major determinant of virulence. Both Gram-positive and Gram-negative bacteria produce soluble protein exotoxins. Neurotoxins produced by *C. botulinum*, and *C. tetani* inhibit release of neurotransmitters, resulting in paralysis. Toxins associated with *B. anthracis, V. cholerae* and *E. coli* are involved in alteration of the intracellular signaling mechanisms. RTX toxins of Gram-negative bacteria, streptolysin O produced by *S. pyogenes*, and *S. aureus* alpha toxin are called pore forming toxins as they are capable of forming pores on the eukaryotic membrane disrupting the selective influx and efflux of ions.
   (e) **Superantigens** are bacterial toxins that stimulate a very large number of T lymphocytes by binding to distinct regions outside the peptide-binding cleft of the major histocompatibility class II molecules (MHC II), expressed on the surface of antigen-presenting cells, and to specific Vβ elements on the T-cell receptor of T lymphocytes. This leads to massive T-lymphocyte proliferation and cytokine release, which induce capillary leakage and shock.

Bacterial Infections

Staphylococcal Infections

Rosenbach described the two pigmented colony types of staphylococci and proposed the nomenclature: ***S. aureus*** (yellow) and ***Staphylococcus albus*** (white) way back in 1884. The latter is now named ***Staphylococcus epidermidis***. More than 20 species of *Staphylococcus* are described in the literature, of which, *S. aureus* and *S. epidermidis* are considered most significant in terms of human pathogenicity. *S. aureus* colonizes mainly the nasal passages, but it may also be found in the skin, oral cavity, and gastrointestinal tract. ***S. epidermidis*** is an inhabitant of the skin and causes opportunistic infections. *S. saprophyticus* is a common cause of urinary tract infections in young women.

S. aureus organisms are pyogenic, non-motile, Gram-positive *cocci* that form grape-like clusters (Fig. 9.4).

Pathogenesis

Staphylococci possess numerous virulence factors, which include:

1. ***Surface proteins***: These are involved in adherence to host cells and promote colonization.
2. ***Enzymes that degrade proteins***: Include invasins that promote bacterial spread in tissues (leukocidin, kinases, hyaluronidase); and lipases and proteinases that degrade lipids and proteins on skin surface leading to abscesses.
3. ***Surface factors that inhibit phagocytic engulfment (capsule and Protein A)***: Staphylococci have a 'polysaccharide capsule' that allows them to attach to constituent materials of prosthetic valves and catheters and to resist host cell phagocytosis. Immunoglobulin-binding 'Protein A' binds to Fc portion of immunoglobulins and protects it from antibody-mediated killing.

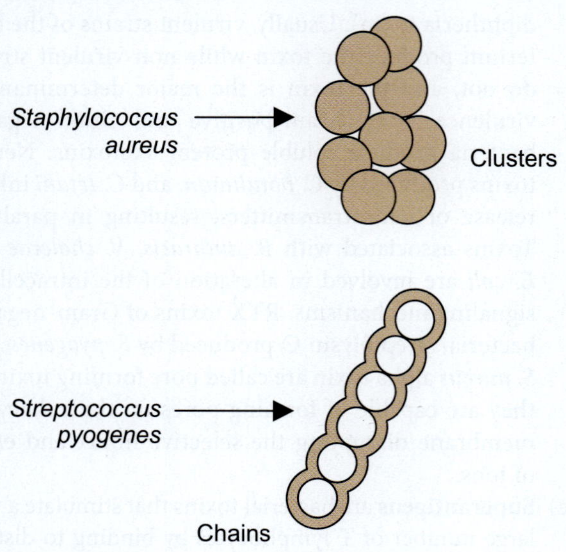

Fig. 9.4 Bacterial arrangements.

4. **Toxins**
   (a) Membrane-damaging toxins that lyse eukaryotic cell membranes, for example haemolysins, leukotoxin, leukocidin.
   (b) Systemic release of α-toxin causes septic shock (α-toxin inserts itself into the plasma membrane and forms pores to dramatically increase intracellular calcium levels).
   (c) Enterotoxins and toxic shock syndrome toxin (TSST-1) are superantigens that may cause toxic shock.
   (d) Staphylococcal enterotoxins cause vomiting when ingested, and the bacterium is a leading cause of food poisoning.
   (e) Exfoliative toxins (serine proteases) split skin by cleaving protein desmoglein 1, which holds epidermal cells together. This can cause superficial epidermis to split away from deeper skin, making patient vulnerable to secondary infections.

Clinical Manifestations (Fig. 9.5)

- *S. aureus* can lead to infections in any of major organs of the body **(osteomyelitis, endocarditis, pericarditis, respiratory tract infections and bacteremia).**
- Ocular infections include **conjunctivitis** and **endophthalmitis.**
- It is a common cause of **burns and wound infections.**
- It is also responsible for many serious **community- and nosocomially acquired infections,** being the most frequently isolated bacterial pathogen from patients with hospital-acquired infections, especially patients with implants or prosthetic devices.
- **Asymptomatic *S. aureus* colonization** occurs intermittently in children and adults, most commonly in anterior nasal vestibule, and occasionally on skin, hair, nails, axillae, perineum and vagina.
- **Invasive infections of the skin** can occur in previously healthy individuals, ranging from **impetigo to abscess formation, cellulitis and lymphadenitis.**
- Infection of nail bed by *S. aureus* is called **paronychia.**
- *S. aureus* is also a cause of a number of toxinoses, including **toxic shock syndrome (TSS), food poisoning, staphylococcal scalded skin syndrome (SSSS), and necrotizing pneumonia.** TSS is due to a toxin-producing strain of *S. aureus*. It is usually associated with tampon-wearing menstruating women. There is a 1- to 4-day prodrome of high fever, mental confusion, diarrhea, hypotension, pharyngitis, and an erythematous rash that occurs during or soon after menses. The rash occurs predominantly on the hands and feet, and resolves with desquamation in 7–10 days.
- SSSS also called **Ritter disease,** is caused by the exfoliative B toxins. It is an exfoliative dermatitis that most frequently

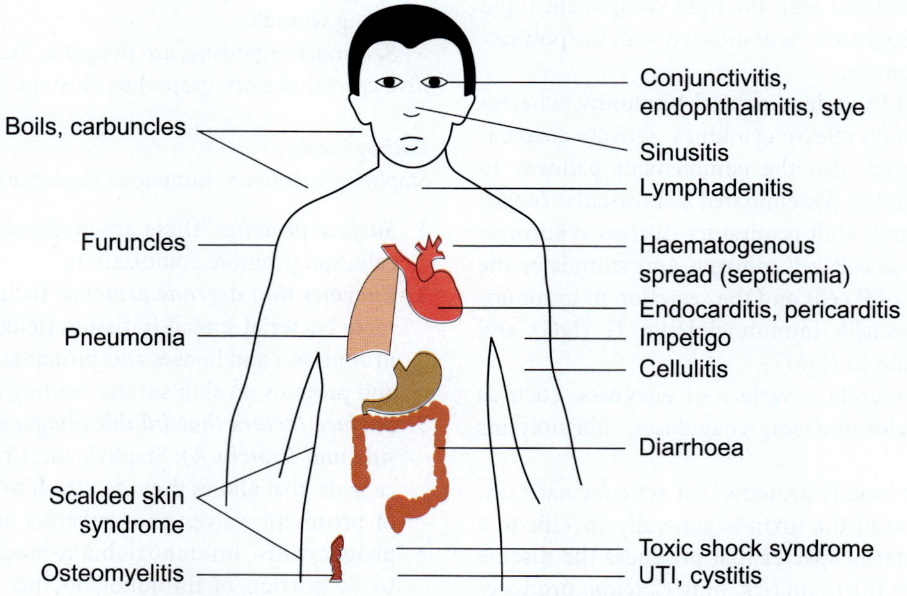

Fig. 9.5 Clinical manifestations of staphylococcal infection.

occurs in children with staphylococcal infections of nasopharynx or skin.
- **Chronic abscess formation of apocrine gland regions**, most frequently of axilla, is known as **hidradenitis suppurativa**.

Morphology

S. aureus causes pyogenic inflammation with a tendency for local destructiveness as in a furuncle or boil. A carbuncle is associated with deep suppuration that spreads laterally beneath deep subcutaneous fascia and then erupts in multiple adjacent skin sinuses.

Streptococcal Infections

S. pyogenes (group A streptococcus) is an important species of Gram-positive extracellular bacterial pathogen that colonizes throat or skin. It is covered with an outer hyaluronic acid capsule and a layer of group A carbohydrate, a polymer of rhamnose with *N*-acetylglucosamine side chains. In addition, molecules of M protein attached to bacterial membrane extend from cell surface as coiled fibers that appear as fibrils on the surface of the bacterium. Streptococci divide in one plane and thus occur in pairs or chains of varying lengths (Fig. 9.4). *S. pneumoniae,* the most important α-haemolytic *Streptococcus*, is a common cause of community-acquired pneumonia and meningitis in adults. *S. viridans* group includes several species of α-haemolytic streptococci that are not only part of normal oral flora but are also a common cause of endocarditis. Finally, *S. mutans* is major cause of dental caries.

Pathogenesis

- Many streptococci have **hyaluronic acid capsules** that resist phagocytosis.
- *S. pyogenes* expresses **M protein**—a surface protein that prevents bacteria from being phagocytosed. Poststreptococcal acute rheumatic fever is an autoimmune disease caused by antistreptococcal M protein antibodies that cross-react with cardiac myosin.
- M protein, **fibronectin-binding protein (Protein F),** and **lipoteichoic acid** also aid in adherence of the bacteria to the host cells.
- Streptococci release invasins, such as **streptokinase, streptodornase (DNase B), hyaluronidase, and streptolysins and exotoxins, such as pyrogenic (erythrogenic) toxin,** which causes the rash of scarlet fever and systemic TSS.
- **Pneumolysin** is a cytosolic bacterial protein released on disruption of *S. pneumoniae.* Pneumolysin inserts into target cell membranes and lyses them. This toxin also activates the classical pathway of complement, reducing the complement available for opsonization of bacteria.
- *S. mutans* produces caries by converting sucrose to lactic acid (which causes demineralization of tooth enamel) and by secreting high-molecular-weight glucans that promote bacterial colonization and plaque formation.

Clinical Manifestations (Fig. 9.6)

- *S. pyogenes* is one of the most frequent pathogens of humans. It is estimated that between 5% and 15% of normal individuals harbor the bacterium, usually in respiratory tract, without signs of the disease. As normal flora, *S. pyogenes* can cause a variety of suppurative infections when defenses are compromised.
- *S. pyogenes* is a leading cause of **puerperal sepsis.**
- Acute *S. pyogenes* infections may be present as **pharyngitis, scarlet fever (streptococcal pharyngitis with rash), impetigo (infection of superficial layers of skin), or cellulitis (infection of deep layers of the skin).** Scarlet fever is caused by a strain of *S. pyogenes* that generates an erythrogenic toxin. It produces an erythematous rash (having a sandpaper consistency) that begins on trunk and limbs, and then resolves with desquamation. Also seen are circumoral pallor and changes in tongue, which initially has a '**white-strawberry**' followed by a 'red-strawberry' appearance.
- Invasive, toxigenic infections can result in **necrotizing fasciitis, myositis and streptococcal TSS.**

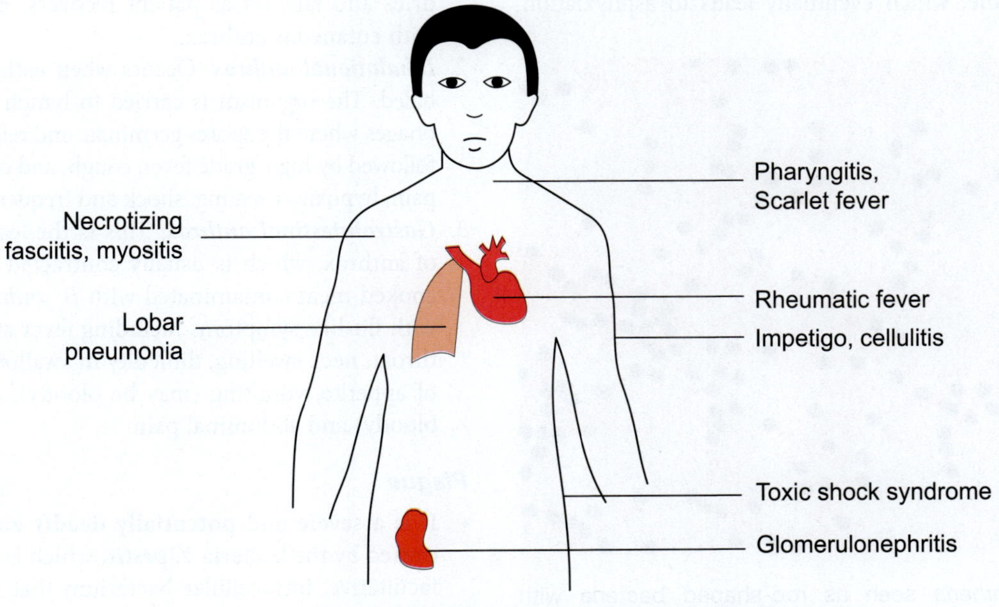

Fig. 9.6 Clinical manifestations of streptococcal infection.

- *S. pneumoniae* is an important cause of lobar pneumonia.
- Patients may **develop immune-mediated poststreptococcal sequelae, such as acute rheumatic fever and acute glomerulonephritis**, following acute infections caused by *S. pyogenes*.

Morphology

- Although *Streptococcus* causes lesions that are similar to those caused by *Staphylococcus* (furuncles, carbuncles, and impetigo), there is less tendency for inducing destruction of host tissues. Streptococcal lesions are typically characterized by diffuse interstitial neutrophilic infiltrate.
- **Erysipelas** is characterized by rapidly spreading erythematous cutaneous swelling that may begin on face or, less frequently, body, or an extremity. On histologic examination, there is a diffuse neutrophilic inflammatory reaction in dermis and epidermis extending into subcutaneous tissues with extensive oedema. Leukocytic infiltration is more intense around vessels and skin adnexa.
- Streptococcal pharyngitis is marked by oedema, epiglottic swelling and punctate abscesses of tonsillar crypts.

Diphtheria

Diphtheria is caused by a Gram-positive, aerobic, non-motile, rod-shaped bacteria with clubbed ends classified as actinobacteria, which undergo snapping movements just after cell division resulting in characteristic Chinese letter like forms (Fig. 9.7), ***C. diphtheriae*** is transmitted from person-to-person through aerosols or skin shedding.

Clinical Manifestations

- *C. diphtheriae* may demonstrate **asymptomatic carriage** or manifest as **clinical diphtheria**, which may be **nasopharyngeal** and **cutaneous**.
- **Pharyngeal diphtheria** varies from **mild pharyngitis** to **airway obstruction** due to the **formation of a pseudomembrane**. The bacteria induce an intense fibrinosuppurative exudate, the coagulation of which creates a tough, dirty, gray membrane, which eventually leads to asphyxiation. Involvement of cervical lymph nodes may cause profound swelling of the neck **(bull neck diphtheria)**.
- **Toxin-mediated damage** causes life-threatening systemic complications, principally **loss of motor function** (e.g. difficulty in swallowing) and **congestive heart failure** due to the action of diphtheria toxin on peripheral motor neurons and the myocardium.
- **Infection of chronic wounds** is common. The skin lesions in cutaneous diphtheria are also usually covered by a grey-brown pseudomembrane.

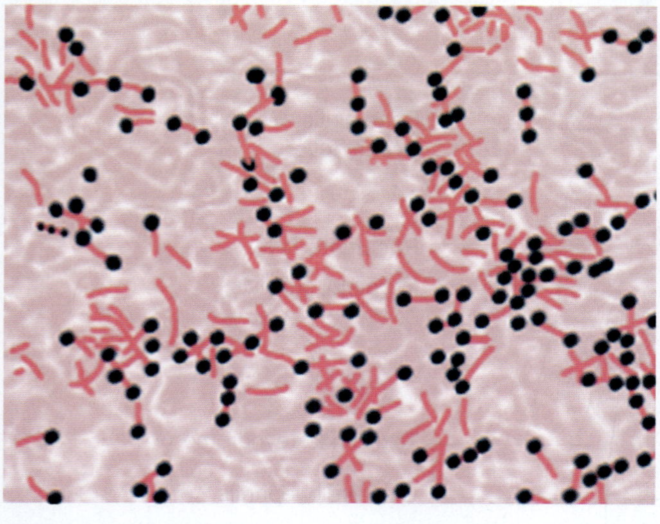

Fig. 9.7 *C. diphtheria* seen as rod-shaped bacteria with clubbed ends arranged in a Chinese letter pattern.

Morphology

Histological sections typically show marked neutrophilic infiltration, vascular congestion, interstitial oedema and fibrin exudation. The release of exotoxins induces generalized hyperplasia of the reticuloendothelial system and may cause degeneration of myelin sheaths of nerves, and fatty change and necroses of the myocardium liver, kidneys and adrenals.

Anthrax

Anthrax is a **zoonotic infection** caused by ***B. anthracis***, which is a large, spore-forming, Gram-positive, rod-shaped bacterium. It is a common pathogen in animals that have contact with soil contaminated with *B. anthracis* spores. Anthrax spores can be ground to a fine powder, making them a potential weapon for bioterrorism. *B. anthracis* produces potent toxins and a polyglutamyl capsule, which is antiphagocytic. The tissue damage in anthrax is by virtue of anthrax toxins, which have A and B subunits. Of these, the B subunit is the carrier molecule, which delivers the toxic A subunit. *B. anthracis* also possesses a polyglutamyl capsule which prevents its phagocytosis.

There are **three major anthrax syndromes**:

1. ***Cutaneous anthrax***: Comprises the bulk of anthrax; begins as a painless pruritic papule, which eventually develops into a vesicle. This is accompanied by regional lymphadenopathy. After the vesicle ruptures, the remaining ulcer becomes covered with a characteristic black eschar, which dries and falls off as patient recovers. Bacteremia is rare with cutaneous anthrax.
2. ***Inhalational anthrax***: Occurs when anthrax spores are inhaled. The organism is carried to lymph nodes by macrophages where the spores germinate and release toxins. This is followed by high-grade fever, cough, and chest or abdominal pain, hypoxia, sweating, shock and frequently death.
3. ***Gastrointestinal anthrax***: This is the least common form of anthrax, which is usually contracted by eating undercooked meat contaminated with *B. anthracis*. It manifests with flu-like symptoms including fever and tiredness, sore throat, neck swelling, difficulty in swallowing, nausea, loss of appetite, vomiting (may be bloody), diarrhea (may be bloody) and abdominal pain.

Plague

- It is a severe and **potentially deadly zoonotic infection** caused by the bacteria ***Y. pestis***, which is a Gram-negative, facultative, intracellular bacterium that is transmitted by fleabites or aerosols.

- It causes a highly invasive, frequently fatal systemic infection (also named '**Black Death**').
- The three most common forms of plague include:
  - **Bubonic plague (infection of lymph nodes).**
  - **Pneumonic plague (infection of lungs).**
  - **Septicaemic plague (infection of blood).**
- Rodents, such as rats, carry the disease and plague affects humans when they are bitten by a flea that carries the plague bacteria from an infected rodent. In rare cases, one may get the disease while handling an infected animal. Pneumonic plague can spread from human-to-human via respiratory droplets.
- The incubation period (time between being infected and developing symptoms) is typically 2–7 days.

Clinical Manifestations

- The major manifestations of bubonic plague include **malaise, fever with chills, headache, myalgias (muscle pain), painful lymphadenopathy (gland swelling called a bubo is not only commonly found in groin, but may also occur in armpits or neck, or site of the infection).**
- Symptoms of pneumonic plague include **cough, difficulty in breathing, fever, and frothy, bloody sputum.**
- Septicaemic plague may cause death even before the onset of symptoms. Symptoms include **abdominal pain, bleeding, diarrhea, fever, nausea, and vomiting.**

Morphology

- The distinctive histologic features of plague include appearance of **protein and polysaccharide-rich effusions, marked tissue swelling, necrosis of tissues with haemorrhage and thrombosis, and massive neutrophilic infiltrates.**
- **Bubonic plague** usually affects legs and is marked by a **small pustule or ulcer**. This is followed by **enlargement of the draining lymph nodes, which become soft and pulpy, and may rupture through skin.**
- In **pneumonic plague, there is a severe, confluent, haemorrhagic, and necrotizing bronchopneumonia, often with fibrinous pleuritis.**
- In **septicaemic plague, lymph nodes** throughout the body develop **foci of necrosis**. The bacteremia may induce **DIC** with widespread haemorrhages and thrombi.

Diagnosis

- Blood culture
- Culture of lymph node aspirate (bubo aspirates)
- Sputum culture (in pneumonic plague).

Typhoid Fever

Typhoid fever (also known as '**enteric' or 'bilious fever**') is caused by the Gram-negative bacillus, ***Salmonella typhi.*** Extent of infection by *Salmonella* species depends on the bacterial type and its strain. *Salmonella* possesses **antigens to protect itself and cause destruction**; these include **heat-stable cell wall LPS known as somatic or 'O' antigen**, and **flagellar or H antigens** derived from structural proteins, which form the hair-like filaments for movement of the bacterium and, in addition, its **PS capsular Vi (for virulence) antigen** found at surface of freshly isolated strains.

Table 9.3 Clinical manifestations of typhoid

Disease period	Signs and symptoms	Pathology
1st week	Fever, chills, headache, abdominal tenderness	Bacteremia
2nd week	Rash, diarrhoea or constipation, hepatosplenomegaly	Hyperplasia of ileal Peyer's patches, and typhoid nodules in spleen and liver
3rd week	Complications of intestinal bleeding and perforation, shock, melena, ileus, coma	Ulceration over Peyer's patches, perforation with peritonitis, septicaemia
4th week	Resolution of symptoms/relapse, cholecystitis, chronic faecal carriage of bacteria	—

Pathogenesis

Common worldwide, typhoid is transmitted by **ingestion of food or water contaminated with faeces from an infected person.** Inside **lumen of intestine,** the bacterium multiplies by **attaching to microvilli** of the intestinal surface. **Bacteria perforate through the intestinal wall and are phagocytosed by macrophages.** *S. typhi* alters its structure to resist destruction and allow it to exist within the macrophage. **Preferential colonization** is seen in Peyer's patches in ileum, followed by **hyperplasia of Peyer's patches and eventual ulceration of overlying mucosa.** The organism may spread via lymphatics to get access to the mononuclear phagocytic system and then disseminate throughout the body.

Clinical Manifestations (Table 9.3)

Typhoid is characterized by a **sustained, slowly rising fever accompanied by profuse sweating, diarrhoea, a rash of flat rose-coloured spots, tender hepatosplenomegaly, and elevation of liver transaminases.** Less commonly, there is **relative bradycardia, malaise, headache, cough, rarely epistaxis, abdominal pain and delirium.** The illness classically lasts for 3–4 weeks. By the end of 3rd week recovery commences.

Complications

- **Bleeding** from congested Peyer's patches or eroded vessels in ulcer base
- **Perforation** in distal ileum (which is frequently fatal). May be followed by septicaemia and peritonitis
- **Metastatic abscesses** in other organs
- **Osteomyelitis, endocarditis, glomerulonephritis, and infection of genitourinary tract or meningitis**
- *S. typhi* shows a **predilection for gallbladder, where infection tends to become chronic,** especially in individuals with a pathologic gallbladder condition **(Typhoid Mary).**

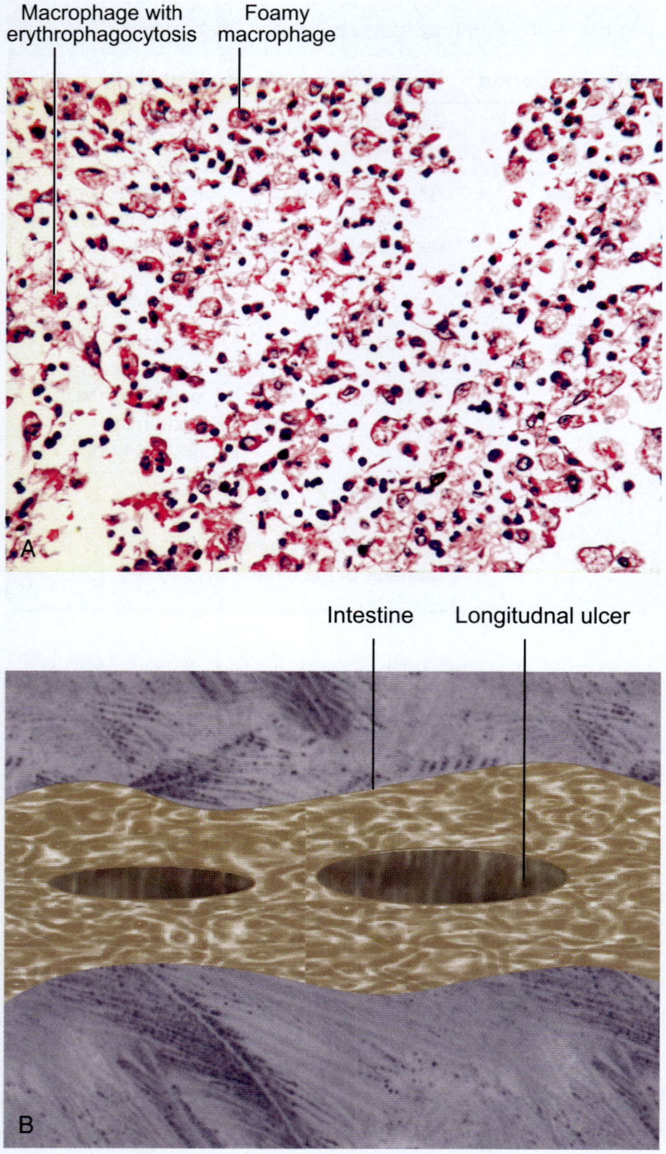

Fig. 9.8 (A) Section from typhoid intestine showing numerous macrophages, some with prominent erythrophagocytosis *(arrow)*. (B) Typhoid ulcer oriented along the longitudinal axis of small bowel.

Morphology (Fig. 9.8)

- Ileum shows **superficial mucosal ulcers aligned along Peyer's patches**, in the background of chronic non-specific inflammation with **numerous macrophages and prominent erythrophagocytosis.**
- Lamina propria may show neutrophilic infiltration.
- Draining lymph nodes show reactive hyperplasia.
- Liver may show focal hepatocytic necrosis with replacement of the parenchyma by macrophage aggregates called '**typhoid nodules**'.

Diagnosis

- **Peripheral blood** shows **leukopenia** with **relative lymphocytosis** and rarely **thrombocytopenia.**
- Isolation of *Salmonella* species from **blood (culture positive during 1st week of fever).**
- **Isolation of *Salmonella* species from stool or urine** (culture positive in 2nd or 3rd week).
- '**Widal test**' is a serological test for enteric fever. It demonstrates agglutinating antibodies against O-somatic and H-flagellar antigens in the blood. Since patients are often exposed to other bacteria that induce cross-reactivity, many people have antibodies against other pathogens, which react with antigens in the Widal test, causing a false-positive result. Test results need to be interpreted carefully in light of past history of enteric fever, typhoid vaccination, and general level of antibodies in endemic areas (rising titer is more important; >1:160 is convincing).
- **'Typhidot'** is a dot ELISA kit that detects IgM and IgG antibodies against the outer membrane protein (OMP) of the *S. typhi*. The test becomes positive within 2–3 days of infection and identifies both IgM and IgG antibodies.
- Indirect haemagglutination test, indirect fluorescent antibody test, and indirect enzyme-linked immunosorbent assay (ELISA) for IgM and IgG antibodies to *S. typhi* polysaccharide, as well as monoclonal antibodies against *S. typhi* flagella are promising, but the success rates of these assays vary greatly in the literature.

Nocardia

Nocardia are aerobic Gram-positive bacteria that grow as aerial structures with terminal spores, which appear like hyphae on culture. The majority of cases are caused by **the *Nocardia asteroides* complex (at least 50% of invasive infections).** The *N. asteroides* complex is comprised of *Nocardia abscessus*, *Nocardia cyriacigeorgica*, *Nocardia farcinica*, and *N. nova*. Other known pathogenic species of *Nocardia* include *Nocardia transvalensis* complex, *Nippostrongylus brasiliensis*, and *Nocardia pseudobrasiliensis*.

Clinical Manifestations

Nocardia are soil inhabitants and usually cause **opportunistic infections** in **immunocompromised individuals.** *N. asteroides* causes respiratory infections (**pneumonia** and **lung abscess**) and may extend to involve **central nervous system (CNS) or cause disseminated infection**, while other species, mainly ***Nocardia brasiliensis***, infect **skin. Respiratory infection with *N. asteroides* causes an indolent illness with fever, weight loss, and cough, which may be mistaken for tuberculosis or malignancy. CNS symptoms include headache, lethargy, confusion, seizures, or sudden onset of neurological deficit.**

Morphology

The diagnosis of nocardiosis depends on identification of **beaded and branched thin Gram-positive organisms** in a suppurative background. ***Nocardia* stain with modified acid-fast stains (Fite–Faraco stain),** unlike *Actinomyces,* which may appear similar on Gram stain of tissue. Chronic lesions may be surrounded by granulation tissue and fibrosis. Granulomatous inflammation is generally not seen.

Neisserial Infections

- *Neisseria* are **Gram-negative diplococci**; their adjacent sides are flattened giving the pair the shape of a **coffee bean** (Fig. 9.9).

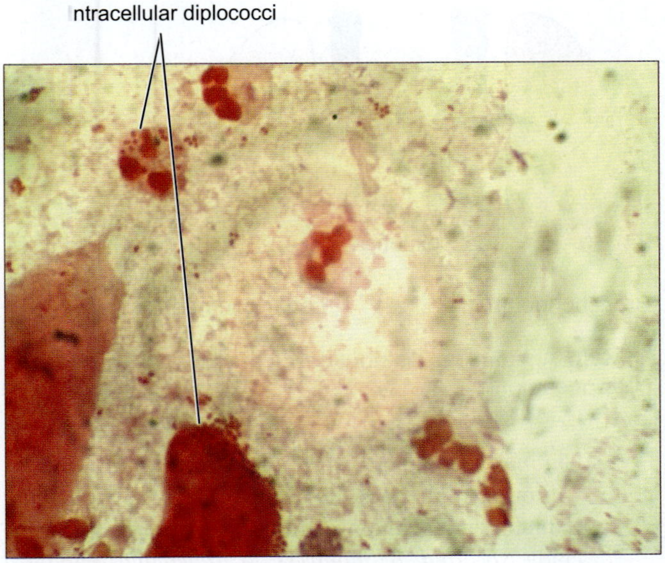

Fig. 9.9 *N. gonorrhoeae* diplococci demonstrated in urethral discharge of a patient of gonococcal urethritis.

- They are aerobic (grow best on enriched media, such as lysed sheep's blood agar or 'chocolate' agar).
- *Neisseria* inhabit mucosal surfaces. There are two clinically significant species:
- ***N. gonorrhoeae:*** Also referred to as the gonococcus; *N. gonorrhoeae* is responsible for the disease gonorrhea.
- ***N. meningitidis:*** Also referred to as the meningococcus; *N. meningitidis* is responsible for meningitis.
- There are four types of *N. gonorrhoeae* based on the presence of fimbriae; T1, T2, T3, and T4. *N. meningitidis* is serotyped by the antigenic character of its capsular polysaccharide; several groups including A, B, C, 29E, W-135, and Y are recognized.
- Humans are the only host of *N. gonorrhoeae* and **transmission is via sexual contact** (gonorrhea is a sexually transmitted disease). Fimbriae (pili) are very important for the gonococcus to attach to host cells. *N. gonorrhoeae* lacking fimbriae are avirulent.
- *N. meningitidis* inhabits the **human nasopharynx**. The virulence of *N. meningitidis* is associated with its antiphagocytic capsule and meningococcal LPS.

Clinical Manifestations

- *N. gonorrhoeae* causes **symptomatic urethritis** in men. **In women, the infection is often asymptomatic and so might go untreated**. Untreated infection can lead to pelvic inflammatory disease, which, in turn, can cause infertility or ectopic pregnancy.
- **Disseminated infection** can cause **septic arthritis** accompanied by a **haemorrhagic rash**.
- Neonatal *N. gonorrhoeae* infection can cause blindness and, rarely, sepsis.

Chancroid (Soft Chancre)

- Chancroid is a **sexually transmitted, ulcerative infection caused by *H. ducreyi*, a small, Gram-negative, facultative anaerobic bacillus**, which is highly infective.
- Chancroid is one of the **most common causes of genital ulcers in Southeast Asia**, where it probably serves as an important cofactor in the transmission of HIV-1 infection.
- It is known to spread to other anatomical sites by autoinoculation.

Clinical Manifestations

- The organism has an incubation period of 5–7 days. The disease typically begins as a **small inflammatory papule** at the site of inoculation; within days, the papule **may erode to form an extremely painful deep irregular ulceration.**
- In males, the primary lesion is usually on the penis; in females, most lesions occur in the vagina or the periurethral area. Unlike the primary chancre of syphilis, the ulcer of chancroid is not indurated, and multiple lesions may be present.
- **Regional lymphadenopathy** is very common. In untreated cases, inflamed nodes may erode overlying skin to produce chronic, draining ulcers.

Morphology

- Microscopically, the ulcer of chancroid contains **three zones**, a superficial zone of neutrophilic debris and fibrin; a middle zone of granulation tissue and oedema; and a deep zone of lymphoplasmacytic inflammation. Coccobacilli can sometimes be demonstrated by Gram or silver stains.
- *H. ducreyi* is a fastidious bacterium requiring a relatively expensive nutritive base to grow on and is an extremely difficult organism to culture from clinical specimens. DNA amplification techniques have shown a somewhat improved diagnostic sensitivity but are only performed in a few laboratories.

Granuloma Inguinale

Granuloma inguinale (donovanosis) is a sexually transmitted chronic inflammatory disease caused by ***Klebsiella granulomatis***, formerly *Calymmatobacterium granulomatis*, a Gram-negative rod. It is endemic in tropical and subtropical climates.

Clinical Manifestations

- The average incubation period varies between 2 and 4 weeks.
- The initial lesion may be a **papule, a subcutaneous nodule or an ulcer**, which after few weeks converts into a **raised, soft, painless, beefy-red, superficial ulcer with characteristic rolled edges.**
- The **lesion spreads by peripheral extension** and may have **satellite lesions (pseudobuboes).** This is generally **not accompanied by inguinal lymphadenopathy**.
- Untreated cases are characterized by development of **extensive scarring, often associated with lymphatic obstruction and lymphedema (elephantiasis) of external genitalia.**

Morphology

- Main pathology is an ulcerative lesion accompanied by abundant granulation tissue, which on gross examination appears as a soft, fleshy, painless mass.

- Active lesions are marked by epithelial hyperplasia (pseudoepitheliomatous/pseudocarcinomatous reaction). A mixture of neutrophils and mononuclear inflammatory cells is usually present at the base of the ulcer.
- Culture of the organism is difficult, so morphologic examination of smears or biopsy is the mainstay of the diagnosis.

Pneumonia

Pneumonia may be defined as a **collection of inflammatory exudate in lung parenchyma distal to terminal bronchioles, mostly resulting in consolidation (solidification) of lung part(s).**

Classification

1. **Aetiological**:
   (a) *Community-acquired or acute bacterial pneumonia:*
      (i) *Streptococcus pneumoniae* (most common causative organism; typically has lobar distribution).
      (ii) *Hemophilus influenzae and Moraxella catarrhalis* (complicate COPD).
      (iii) *Staphylococcus aureus* (occurs secondary to viral infections).
      (iv) *Legionella pneumophilia (seen in organ transplant patients).*
      (v) *Enterobacteriaceae* (infect chronic alcoholics).
      (vi) *Pseudomonas* (seen in cystic fibrosis and burn patients).
      (vii) *Atypical organisms* (include *Mycoplasma pneumoniae, Chlamydophilia pneumoniae, Coxiella burnetii* and viruses-respiratory syncytial virus, parainfluenza virus, human metapneumovirus, influenza A and B, and adenovirus). They are labelled 'atypical' as they are not demonstrable with Gram-stain and do not grow on routine culture media.

   (b) *Healthcare-associated pneumonia*: Distinct clinical entity defined by the following criteria: hospitalization of at least two days within recent past; attending a long-term care facility, a hospital or a haemodialysis clinic; recent intravenous antibiotic therapy, wound care or chemotherapy. Causative organisms include:
      (i) *Staphylococcus aureus* (methicillin sensitive).
      (ii) *Staphylococcus aureus* (methicillin resistant).
      (iii) *Pseudomonas* species.
      (iv) *Streptococcus pneumoniae.*

   (c) *Hospital-acquired pneumonia*: Defined as pulmonary infections acquired during course of hospital stay. Causative organisms include:
      (i) Gram-negative rods.
      (ii) *Enterobacteriaceae.*
      (iii) *Pseudomonas, Staphylococcus aureus* (methicillin resistant).

   (d) *Aspiration (inhalation) pneumonia*: Usually seen in debilitated, comatose or unconscious patients. Aspiration of gastric contents results in chemical irritation (due to gastric acid) and also bacterial infection. It is typically associated with anaerobic infection (oral flora) mixed with aerobic organisms.

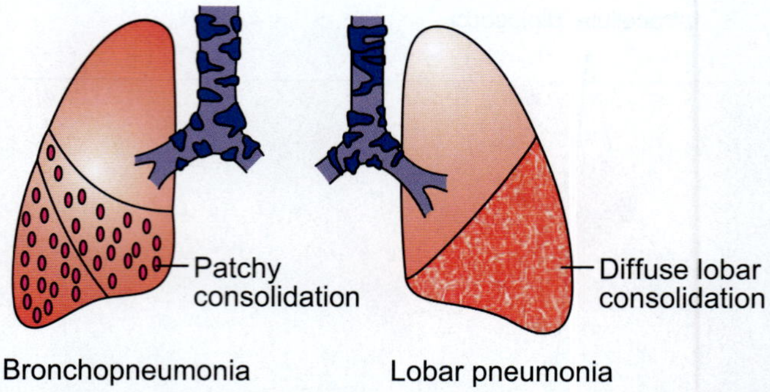

Fig. 9.10 Anatomical distribution of bronchopneumonia and lobar pneumonia.

   (e) *Chronic pneumonia*: It is a localized lesion with or without lymph node involvement, typically showing granulomatous inflammation. Causative organisms include *Nocardia, Actinomyces, M. tuberculosis*, atypical mycobacteria, histoplasmosis, *Coccidioides immitis* and *Blastomyces dermatitidis.*

   (f) *Necrotizing pneumonia* and *lung abscess*: It is caused by anaerobic oral flora mixed with or without aerobic organisms, for example *Staphylococcus aureus, Klebsiella pneumoniae, Streptococcus pyogenes, Pneumococcus* (type III).

   (g) *Pneumonia in an immunocompromised host*: Caused by opportunistic agents, which rarely infect normal hosts, namely, Cytomegalovirus, *Pneumocystis jiroveci, Mycobacterium avium-intracellulare,* invasive aspergillosis and invasive candidiasis. This presents with pulmonary infiltrates with or without other signs.

2. **Based on Anatomical Distribution** (Fig. 9.10):
   (a) *Lobular/bronchopneumonia*: Type of pneumonia that begins with acute bronchitis with later extension to the surrounding alveoli. Lower lobes and right middle lobe are most commonly involved and show a patchy area of consolidation.
   (b) *Lobar pneumonia*: Complete or near complete consolidation of a lobe of the lung.

Pathogenesis

Pneumonia may result whenever defense mechanisms of respiratory system are impaired or immunity of host is low. The normal respiratory defense mechanisms include:

- Nasal clearance (sneezing, blowing).
- Tracheobronchial clearance (mucociliary action).
- Alveolar clearance (alveolar macrophages).

Predisposing Factors

- Loss or suppression of cough reflex as in coma, anesthesia and drugs (most common cause of lobar pneumonia is microaspiration of oropharyngeal secretions during sleep followed by inhalation of aerosol drops).
- Injury to mucociliary apparatus/impaired ciliary function, as in cigarette smoking, inhalation of hot or corrosive gases.
- Impaired phagocytic or bactericidal action of alveolar macrophages.
- Pulmonary congestion and oedema.
- Accumulation of secretions, as in bronchial obstruction.

of less cross-reactivity due to BCG vaccination and sensitization by non-tuberculous mycobacteria. IGRAs also appear to be at least as sensitive as the TST for active tuberculosis.

The differences between primary and secondary tuberculosis are listed in Table 9.5.

Leprosy (PA10.3)

Leprosy or **Hansen disease** is a chronic infectious disease caused by the bacterium ***Mycobacterium leprae***. Transmission occurs by **close and prolonged contact with an infected individual or through nasal droplets**. Leprosy may be seen in animals like armadillo and chimpanzee, besides humans. The bacterium can also be grown in laboratory by injection into footpads of mice.

Pathogenesis

- Genetic factors are thought to play a role in the pathogenesis of leprosy (based on the observation of clustering of leprosy in certain families).
- In addition, malnutrition and prolonged exposure to infected persons may aid in development of the overt disease.
- The incubation period can vary from 2 to 10 years.

Classification

- The older system of classification included six categories: indeterminate leprosy, tuberculoid leprosy, borderline tuberculoid leprosy, mid-borderline leprosy, borderline lepromatous leprosy, and lepromatous leprosy (Table 9.6).
- ***World Health Organization (WHO)*** has replaced the older, more complicated classification system with a simpler system that identifies two main types of leprosy—*paucibacillary* and *multibacillary.* Paucibacillary leprosy is defined as five or fewer skin lesions with the absence of bacilli in skin smears, and multibacillary leprosy is defined as six or more skin lesions and positive skin smears.
- ***Paucibacillary leprosy*** (Fig. 9.14) encompasses indeterminate, tuberculoid, and borderline tuberculoid leprosy. It is characterized by one or more hypopigmented skin macules, which show sensory loss (due to damaged peripheral nerves caused by the host's immune cells).
- ***Multibacillary leprosy*** (Fig. 9.15) includes mid-borderline, borderline lepromatous and lepromatous leprosy. It is associated with symmetric skin lesions, nodules, plaques and

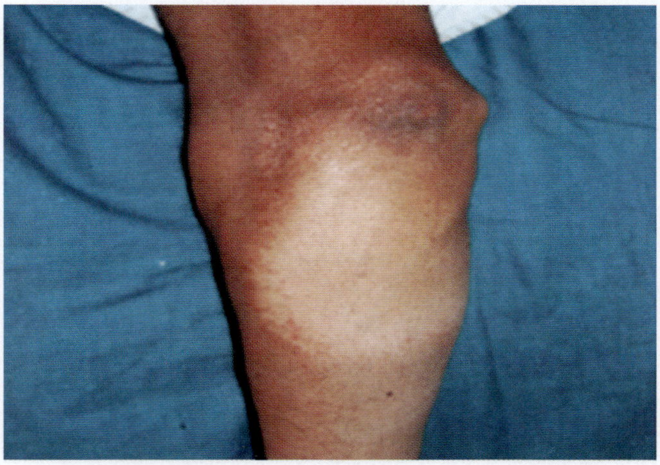

Fig. 9.14 Large, well-defined, hypopigmented plaque of paucibacillary leprosy showing irregular borders.

Table 9.6 Differences between tuberculoid and lepromatous leprosy

Features	Tuberculoid leprosy	Lepromatous leprosy
T cell-mediated immunity	Well developed	Absent/very weak
Lepromin test	Strongly positive	Negative
Skin lesions	Asymmetrical, single or few, well-defined, hypopigmented patches/plaques or erythematous macular lesions; all with sensory loss	Symmetrical multiple, ill-defined, hypopigmented or erythematous, maculopapular or nodular lesions; sensory loss late and less prominent
Histopathology	Well-formed epithelioid cell granulomas eroding basal layer of epidermis as well as dermal nerves, no clear grenz zone, paucibacillary	Foamy macrophages laden with lepra bacilli (lepra cells/ Virchow cells) in dermis separated from epidermis by a clear grenz zone. The lepra cells are usually dispersed around neuromuscular structures and appendages, multibacillary
CD4+ T cells	Present in abundance at periphery of granuloma	Almost absent
CD8+ T cells	Very few; at center of lesion	Present (more in number) in a diffuse manner
Infectivity	Low	High
Involvement	Mostly nerve (severely affected, may be destroyed), skin	Skin, peripheral nerves, anterior eye, upper airways, testes, feet, hands
Complications	Related to nerve damage like paralysis, distinct sensory disturbances	Type II immune complex-mediated reaction or ENL causing vasculitis, glomerulonephritis, nerve-related damage
Prognosis	Milder disease; better prognosis	Extensive, progressive disease; bad prognosis

ENL, Erythema nodosum leprosum.

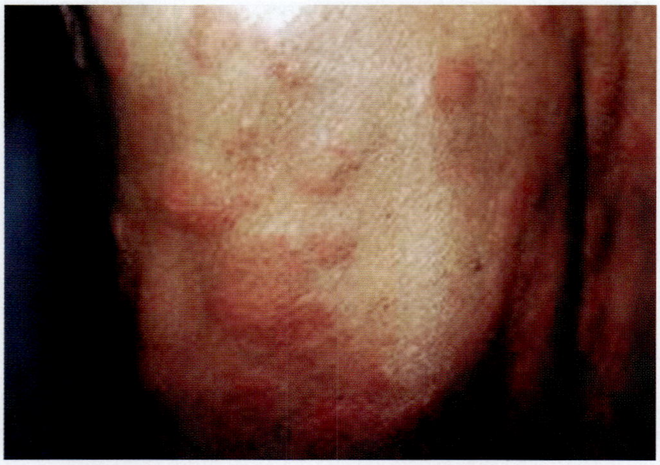

Fig. 9.15 Multiple, large, variable-sized plaques of lepromatous leprosy.

frequent involvement of nasal mucosa. However, detectable nerve damage is a late occurrence.

- ***Borderline leprosy*** is of intermediate severity, and is the most common form. Skin lesions resemble tuberculoid leprosy, but are larger, more numerous, and irregular; peripheral nerve involvement with loss of sensation is common. This type is unstable and may convert into lepromatous leprosy or may undergo a reversal reaction. Borderline tuberculoid leprosy shows epithelioid cells and fair number of lymphocytes. Borderline lepromatous leprosy shows mainly histiocytes and a few scattered lymphocytes. Mid-borderline leprosy shows sheets of epithelioid cells with very few giant cells. Lymphocytes are few and located in the perineurial zone.

Clinical Features

- Involvement of nasal passages can result in a **chronically stuffy nose** and **epistaxis** may occur due to mucosal erosion.
- Eye damage may lead to **blindness**.
- Men with lepromatous leprosy may experience **erectile dysfunction (impotence)** and become **infertile (testicular involvement)**.
- **Deformities** may result from muscle weakness.

Reactions in Leprosy

- During the course of treatment (or even in untreated leprosy), a sudden change in the status of host immune response may produce leprosy reactions—an acute inflammatory state. These reactions manifest with fever and inflammation of the skin as well as peripheral nerves, and may affect the lymph nodes, bone marrow, liver, spleen, joints, testes, kidneys, and anterior chamber of eye.
- ***Type I reaction:*** This is a cell-mediated immune reaction (delayed or type IV hypersensitivity) to mycobacterial antigens in skin and nerves. It may be upgrading or downgrading depending on the predominantly activated cell type, that is, CD4+ T cells or CD8+ T cells, respectively. Patients with borderline disease are usually affected. A downgrading reaction represents a shift toward lepromatous pole, and a reversal reaction represents a shift toward tuberculoid pole.

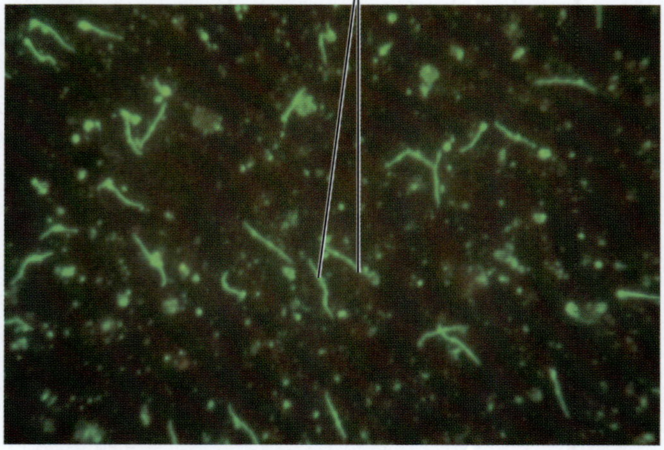

Fig. 9.16 Demonstration of *Treponema pallidum* on FTA-ABS test.

- ***Type II reaction:*** Also called erythema nodosum leprosum, it is a type III (immune complex mediated) reaction to mycobacterial antigens, usually seen in lepromatous and borderline lepromatous subtypes (which are clinical variants with antigen excess).

Diagnosis

Microscopic examination of a sample of infected skin tissue (slit smear examination) confirms diagnosis.

Syphilis

Syphilis is a **venereal disease** with **multisystem involvement**. It is often called '**the great imitator**' because many of its signs and symptoms are indistinguishable from those of other diseases.

Causative Organism

Treponema pallidum (Fig. 9.16), a spirochaete bacterium, is the causative organism of syphilis. It has the following salient features:

- An axial protoplasmic flagella wound around slender, helical protoplasm.
- Its presence is confirmed by dark field examination, silver stains and immunofluorescence examination.
- It is sexually transmitted (through bacteria laden secretions/intimate contact).
- Transplacental transmission (congenital syphilis) is well known.

Pathogenesis

Endarteritis is secondary to binding of spirochetes to endothelial cells through host fibronectin molecules, and is mediated by delayed hypersensitivity.

Clinical Features

1. ***Primary stage***
   (a) Starts with a single, firm, non-tender raised red lesion (*chancre;* Fig. 9.17) on penis, cervix, vagina, arms, or as multiple sores *(chancres).*

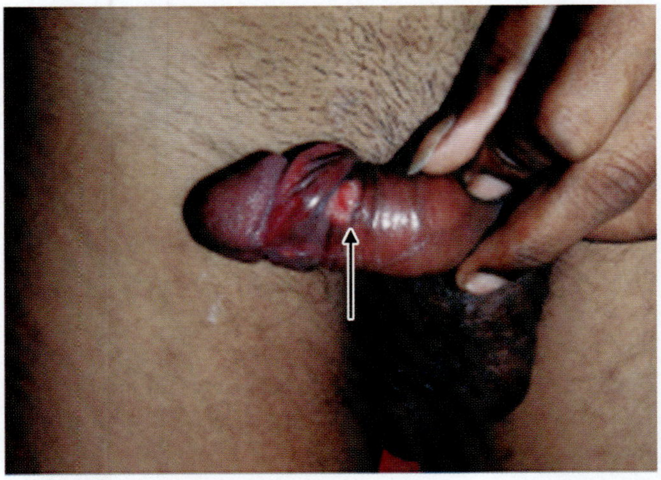

Fig. 9.17 Primary chancre showing typical clean, well-defined, indurated, non-tender ulcer.

(b) The time between infection with syphilis and start of the first symptom can range from 10 to 90 days (average 21 days).

(c) Chancre heals in a few days (even without therapy).

2. ***Secondary stage***
   (a) Skin rash and mucous membrane lesions characterize secondary stage.
   (b) This stage typically starts with development of a rash on one or more areas of the body.
   (c) Characteristic rash of secondary syphilis appears as rough, red, or reddish-brown spots, both on palms of hands and soles (Fig. 9.18A–B).
   (d) In addition to the rash, symptoms of secondary syphilis may include fever, lymphadenopathy, sore throat, patchy hair loss, headache, weight loss, muscle aches and fatigue.
   (e) Moist areas of the skin, for example anogenital region, axillae and inner thighs may develop broad-based, elevated plaques (condyloma lata; Fig. 9.19).
   (f) The signs and symptoms of secondary syphilis may resolve with or without treatment. Without treatment, the infection progresses to latent and tertiary stages of the disease.
3. ***Latent stage***
   (a) The latent (hidden) stage of syphilis begins when primary and secondary symptoms disappear.
   (b) The infected person will continue to have syphilis even though there are no signs or symptoms.
   (c) The latent stage can last for years.
4. ***Tertiary stage***
   (a) About 15% of people who have not been treated for syphilis go into late tertiary stage of syphilis (which can appear even 10–20 years after infection was first acquired).
   (b) Manifestations include neurosyphilis (meningovascular, tabes dorsalis, general paresis), aortitis (aneurysms, aortic regurgitation), gumma formation (hepar lobatum, involvement of skin, bone, etc.) and others.

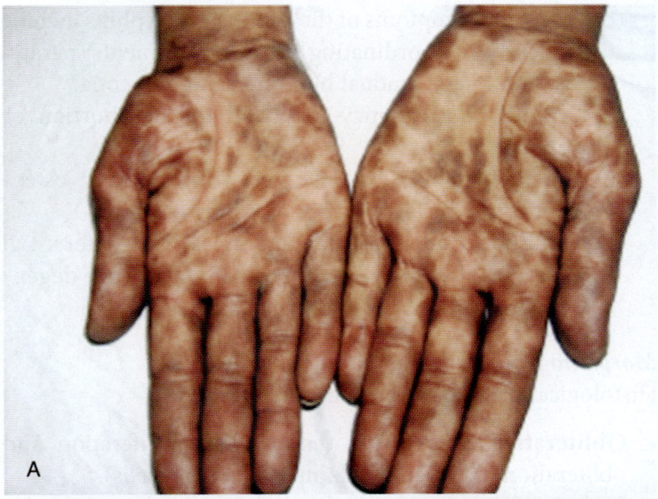

A

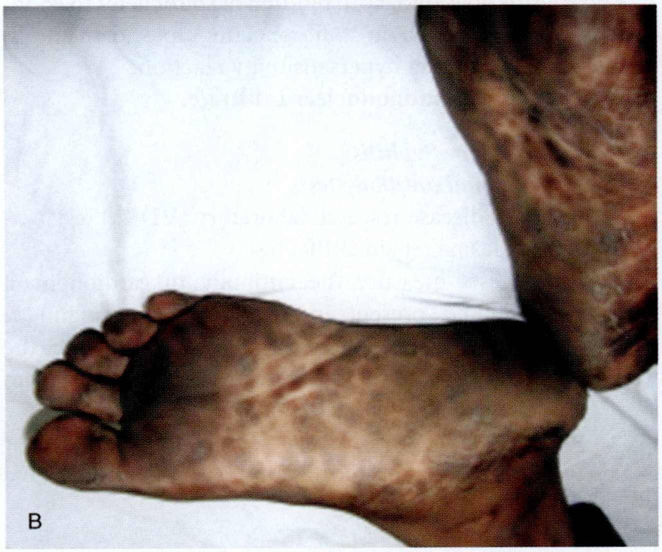

B

Fig. 9.18 (A and B) Palmoplantar involvement by secondary syphilis showing coppery-red annular eruption on which central tenderness may be elicited with a match head or pin head.

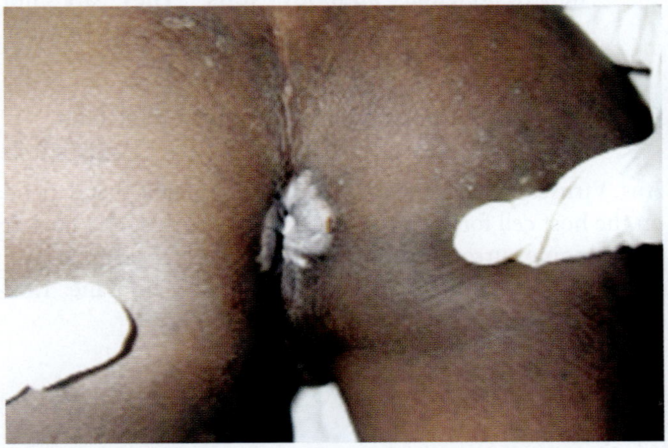

Fig. 9.19 Typical perianal greyish-white moist plaque (condyloma lata) in secondary syphilis.

(c) Signs and symptoms of the late stage of syphilis include difficulty in coordinating muscle movements, paralysis, numbness, gradual blindness and dementia.
(d) Syphilis in pregnancy may lead to late abortion or stillbirth.
(e) Infantile syphilis may manifest with the rash, osteochondritis, periostitis, liver and lung fibrosis.
(f) Childhood syphilis may manifest with interstitial keratitis, Hutchinson teeth and eighth nerve degeneration.

Morphology

Histological hallmarks of syphilis include:

- **Obliterative endarteritis** (endothelial proliferation and obliteration of lumen by plump endothelial cells).
- Endarteritis is secondary to binding of spirochetes to endothelial cells through host fibronectin molecules, and is mediated by delayed hypersensitivity reaction.
- **Plasma cell-rich mononuclear infiltrate.**

Diagnostic Tests for Syphilis

1. ***Non-treponemal antibody tests***
   (a) Venereal disease research laboratory (VDRL) test
   (b) Rapid plasma regain (RPR) test
   These tests measure the antibody to cardiolipin, a phospholipid present in both host tissues and *T. pallidum*, and become positive 4–6 weeks after the infection (so immunofluorescence of exudates from the chancre is important for diagnosis early in the infection). They are used as screening tests and for monitoring response to therapy because they become negative after therapy.
2. ***Treponemal antibody tests***
   (a) FTA-ABS (fluorescent treponemal antibody absorption) test
   (b) Microhaemagglutination assay for *T. pallidum* antibodies
   These tests measure antibodies that specifically react with *T. pallidum*, become positive 4–6 weeks after the infection, and remain positive even after successful treatment. They are more specific than non-treponemal antibody tests. They are not recommended as primary screening tests because they are expensive.

Q. Write in detail on diseases caused by viruses. (PA10.4)

Ans. Viruses are very tiny intracellular organisms that depend on the host cell for their replication. They consist of a nucleic acid genome surrounded by a protein coat (capsid) that may in some cases be further encased in a lipid membrane. Thus the three basic components of a virus are:

- Nucleic acid
- Protein coat
- Lipid membrane.

The nucleic acid core of the virus may either be deoxyribonucleic acid or ribonucleic acid (DNA or RNA, respectively) in nature. A complete virus particle (also called 'virion') delivers its DNA or RNA genome into the host cell. The virion may then insert its genetic material into its host and take control of the host's functions. Some viruses may remain dormant inside host cells for long periods (the lysogenic phase). But when a dormant virus is stimulated, it enters the active (lytic) phase: new viruses are formed, which self-assemble, and burst out of the host cell, killing the cell and going on to infect other cells. Viruses are classified on the basis of size and shape, chemical composition and structure of the genome, and mode of replication.

Mechanisms of Viral Injury

The affinity of viruses towards certain cells and not others is called tissue tropism, and is determined by several factors, including:

- ***Host cell receptors for the virus***: HIV gp120 binds to CD4+ T cells, and to chemokine receptors CXCR4 (mainly on T cells) and CCR5 (mainly on macrophages).
- ***Inhibition of cellular transcription and translation***: Viruses may inhibit host cell DNA, RNA, or protein synthesis (poliovirus inactivates cap-binding protein, which is essential for translation of host cell mRNAs, but leaves translation of the virus mRNAs unaffected).
- ***Local host factors***: Enteroviruses replicate in the intestine, in part, because they can resist inactivation by acids, bile, and digestive enzymes. Rhinoviruses replicate only within the upper respiratory tract because they survive optimally at lower temperature of upper respiratory tract.

Once viruses are inside host cells, they can kill the cells and/or cause tissue damage in a number of ways:

- Viral proteins may insert into the host cell's plasma membrane and directly damage it or promote cell fusion (HIV, measles virus and herpes viruses).
- Viruses may lyse host cells (respiratory epithelial cells are killed by influenza virus replication, liver cells by yellow fever virus and neurons by poliovirus and rabies virus).
- Viruses may interfere with apoptosis or accelerate it. Some virus proteins (including TAT and gp120 of HIV, and E1A protein of adenovirus) can induce cell death. In contrast, some viruses encode one or more genes that inhibit apoptosis (e.g. homologs of cellular *Bcl-2* gene). Apoptotic cell death is thought to be a protective host response to remove virus-infected cells.
- Cytotoxic T lymphocytes may play a role in injuring host lymphocytes as they recognize the viral proteins within them.
- Viruses may damage cells involved in host antimicrobial defense, leading to secondary infections. For example, viral damage to respiratory epithelium predisposes to subsequent development of pneumonia by *S. pneumoniae* and *H. influenzae. HIV* depletes CD4+ helper lymphocytes, and thereby causes opportunistic infections.
- Some viruses can cause *persistent cell proliferation and transformation* [e.g. EBV (Epstein Barr virus), HBV, human papillomavirus, or HTLV-1], resulting in cancer.

Measles

Aetiopathogenesis

- Measles is usually seen in unvaccinated individuals or in case of vaccination failure. It is caused by **ssRNA virus of the paramyxovirus family (rubeola virus)** and **spreads by respiratory droplets.**
- The virus initially multiplies within **upper respiratory epithelial cells,** and then spreads to **lymphoid tissues,** where it can **replicate in mononuclear cells, including T lymphocytes, macrophages, and dendritic cells.**
- Attachment to respiratory epithelial cells is via receptors, mainly, **CD46** (a complement regulatory protein) and **signalling lymphocyte activation molecule** (SLAM). The virus then spreads by the blood throughout the body.

Clinical Manifestations

- The **incubation period** of measles (from exposure to onset of rash) is generally 14 days (range 7–18 days). Patients are usually contagious from 4 days before until 4 days after onset of the rash.
- Patient presents with **fever, cough, coryza (running nose), conjunctivitis, and an erythematous maculopapular rash** (a hypersensitivity reaction to viral antigens in the skin).
- **Koplik spots**—a rash (enanthem) present on mucous membranes—is considered pathognomonic of measles. This is typically seen as clustered, white lesions on the buccal mucosa near each Stenson duct (opposite the maxillary second molars). On microscopy Koplik spots appear as ulcerated mucosal lesions with neutrophilic exudate.

Complications

- Diarrhoea
- Middle-ear infection
- Keratitis
- Pneumonia
- Encephalitis, frequently resulting in permanent brain damage [subacute sclerosing panencephalitis (SSPE)].

Histopathology

- Skin vessels are dilated and surrounded by a mononuclear perivascular infiltrate.
- Lymphoid organs show follicular hyperplasia.
- Random giant cells called ***Warthin–Finkeldey cells*** may be observed.
- **Eosinophilic intranuclear and intracytoplasmic inclusions** may be seen in the mononuclear epithelial and giant cells.

Investigations

- Measles serology
- Viral culture (rarely done)

Mumps

Aetiopathogenesis

It is a transient inflammation of **salivary glands** caused by an **RNA virus** that usually **also involves testes, pancreas, and CNS** (causes aseptic meningitis and encephalitis).

Clinical Manifestations

- It spreads by **respiratory droplets** to **enter respiratory epithelium, salivary gland tissue**, and **T cells** in lymph nodes.
- It can then **spread to other sites, including CNS, testis and ovary and pancreas. Aseptic meningitis** is the most common extrasalivary complication of mumps infection.
- Others include **orchitis** leading to sterility, **pancreatitis** and **encephalitis.**

Histopathology

1. ***Mumps parotitis***
   (a) Involvement is bilateral in 70% cases; affected glands are enlarged, congested and inflamed.
   (b) Interstitium is oedematous and shows infiltration by histiocytes and lymphocytes, which may damage the acini.
   (c) Ductal lumina may show necrotic debris.
2. ***Mumps orchitis***
   (a) Haemorrhage and infarction is common.
   (b) Scarring may follow and lead to sterility.
   (c) Microscopy shows mononuclear cell infiltration.
3. ***Mumps pancreatitis***
   (a) Lesions may be destructive and result in parenchymal and fat necrosis.
   (b) Neutrophil-rich inflammation is invariably present.
4. ***CNS***: Demyelination and perivascular cuffing may be seen.

Infectious Mononucleosis

Aetiopathogenesis

- It is a **benign and self-limiting lymphoproliferative disease caused by EBV**. Also known as **'kissing disease' or 'Pfeiffer disease' or 'glandular fever'**.
- EBV infects **B lymphocytes** to induce reactive lymphocytosis with presence of atypical lymphocytes known as ***Downey bodies.***
- It is typically transmitted from asymptomatic individuals through **close contact and oropharyngeal secretions** (earning it the name 'the kissing disease') or by **sharing utensils**. It may also be transmitted through **blood.**
- The virus binds to **CD21 on the surface of B cells** in oropharynx.
- Circulating B cells then spread the infection throughout **mononuclear phagocytic system,** that is, **liver, spleen** and **peripheral lymph nodes.**
- EBV infection of B lymphocytes results in a humoural and cellular response to the virus. (The **humoural immune response directed against EBV structural proteins is the basis for the test used to diagnose infectious mononucleosis.**) The T lymphocyte response is essential for the control of EBV infection; natural killer cells and CD8+ cytotoxic T cells control proliferating B lymphocytes infected with EBV.

Clinical Features

Mononucleosis is seen most commonly in adolescents and young adults, and is characterized by **lymphadenopathy,**

fever, sore throat, muscle soreness and fatigue. Other less common manifestations include:

- Massive splenomegaly and/or hepatomegaly.
- Petechial haemorrhages and skin rash.
- Headache and loss of appetite.
- Dizziness or disorientation.

Complications

- Hepatitis
- Meningitis and encephalitis
- Pneumonitis
- Rupture of spleen
- EBV is also implicated in the genesis of malignancies like nasopharyngeal carcinoma, Burkitt lymphoma, and B cell variety of non-Hodgkin lymphoma.

Histopathology

- ***Lymph nodes***
  - Atypical lymphocytes in paracortical region.
  - Enlarged lymphoid follicles with infiltration by atypical lymphocytes.
- ***Liver***
  - Atypical lymphocytes in portal areas and sinusoids.
  - Scattered isolated/individual cell necrosis or foci of parenchymal necrosis common.
- ***CNS***: Congestion, oedema, perivascular mononuclear cells and leptomeningeal infiltrate.

Diagnosis

- **Peripheral blood examination**
  - Absolute lymphocytosis.
  - Numerous large atypical lymphocytes with abundant basophilic cytoplasm showing vacuolation with an oval, indented, folded nucleus.
- **Mononucleosis test**
  - Includes the **monospot test** and EBV antibody test.
  - Monospot test is a heterophile antibody test for rapid diagnosis of EBV.
  - The test may be falsely negative early in course of the infection.

Poliomyelitis

Aetiopathogenesis

- It is caused by **poliovirus**, which is a spherical, unencapsulated **RNA virus of the enterovirus genus.**
- There are **three major strains of poliovirus, types I, II and III**. Polio is an acute infection of both the meninges and motor neurons of spinal cord and brainstem. The latter may produce permanent paralysis.
- Poliovirus, like other enteroviruses, is transmitted by the **fecal–oral route**. It first infects tissues in the **oropharynx**, is secreted into **saliva** and swallowed, and then multiplies in **intestinal mucosa** and **lymph nodes**, causing a transient viremia and fever.
- Virus spread to the **nervous system** may be secondary to viremia or by retrograde transport of the virus along axons of motor neurons.

Circulating viruses cross the blood–brain barrier and cause **inflammation (itis) of the grey matter (polio) of the spinal cord (myelin)**. Motor neurons are involved. In fatal cases, destruction is found in cerebral ganglia, reticular formation, cerebellar nuclei, hypothalamus, thalamus and cerebral cortex.

Clinical Features

- Non-specific symptoms, for example moderate fever, headache, vomiting, constipation, coryza and sore throat occur 6–20 days after exposure.
- The illness may subside entirely (minor or abortive poliomyelitis), abate temporarily, or progress directly to involve the CNS (major poliomyelitis) 2–6 days after onset, which may be paralytic or non-paralytic).
- Early in paralytic poliomyelitis the patient exhibits.
- Signs of meningeal irritation.
- Weakness.
- Hyperesthesia (increased sensitivity to stimuli).
- Severe muscle pain.
- Spasm of involved muscles or accentuated tendon reflexes.

Histopathology

Gross

Swelling, softening, congestion and petechial haemorrhages in the organ affected.

Microscopy

Affected tissue shows congestion, interstitial oedema and infiltration by lymphocytes.

German Measles (Rubella)

- Also called '**3-day measles**', it is transmitted by **close personal contact and usually presents with fever, headache, arthralgia and painful postauricular lymphadenopathy**.
- This is followed by the onset of a maculopapular rash, which begins on head and spreads downward.
- In **pregnant women**, it can affect the foetus to cause.
- Cardiac anomalies, such as, ventricular septal defect and patent ductus arteriosus.
- Cataract
- Deafness
- Mental retardation and delayed milestones
- Seizures
- Microcephaly
- Intrauterine death.

Parvovirus B19

Produces erythema infectiosum (fifth disease), which typically manifests with a confluent maculopapular rash, usually beginning on the cheeks (giving a **'slapped-face' appearance**) and extending centripetally to involve trunk.

Viral Haemorrhagic Fevers

Viral haemorrhagic fevers are systemic infections characterized by fever and haemorrhages. They are caused by **enveloped RNA viruses belonging to four different families: *arena virus, filo virus, bunya virus* and *flavivirus***. The viruses survive in animals and are transmitted by insects.

Virus enters bloodstream by bite of an insect/ mucous membrane exposure

↓

Endothelial cell dysfunction

↓

Increased vascular permeability

↓

Widespread haemorrhage and necrosis

↓

Disseminated intravascular coagulation

Flowchart 9.2 Pathogenesis of manifestations of viral haemorrhagic fevers.

Humans are infected when they come in contact with infected hosts and vectors. Manifestations vary from a ***mild illness*** **(fever, myalgias, headache, rash, neutropenia and thrombocytopenia) to** ***life-threatening disease*** (haemodynamic disturbances and shock; Flowchart 9.2).

Herpes Virus

Herpes viruses are large encapsulated viruses having a **double stranded DNA genome**. They cause acute infection followed by latent infection in which the viruses persist in a non-infectious form with periodic reactivation. There are nine types of human herpes viruses (HHVs), belonging to three subgroups defined by the type of cell most frequently infected and site of latency (Table 9.7):

- **α-Group viruses**: Herpes simplex virus (HSV)-1, HSV-2 and varicella zoster virus (VZV).
- **β-Lymphotropic viruses**: CMV, Human Herpes Virus-6 or HHV-6 (which causes exanthem subitum, also known as roseola infantum and sixth disease—a benign rash of infants), and HHV-7 (which is not yet associated with a specific disease).
- **γ-Group viruses**: EBV and Kaposi sarcoma-associated herpes virus (KSHV)/HHV-8—the cause of Kaposi sarcoma.

Herpes Simplex Infection

- **Causative organisms are HSV-1 and HSV-2**, both of which cause **primary and secondary** as well as **acute and latent infections**.
- Both viruses replicate in the skin and mucous membranes at the ***site of entry (oropharynx*** **and** ***genitals)*** and produce infective virions, which induce vesicular lesions. The virions then spread to sensory neurons that innervate the primary sites.
- Virus is transported along axons to neuronal cell bodies where the virus establishes latent infection and is not immunologically recognized. In an immunocompetent individual, infection resolves in a few days, but the virus remains dormant in nerve cells. Reactivation occurs repeatedly when the virus travels from neurons to skin and mucous membranes.

Clinical Manifestations

- **Oral herpes** can be caused by HSV-1 or HSV-2 infection. In primary herpetic gingivostomatitis, the typical clear lesions are the first to develop followed by ulcers. The infection, often initially on the lips, spreads to all parts of the mouth and pharynx.
- Reactivation from the trigeminal ganglia can result in what are known as **cold sores.** Intraepithelial vesicles (due to intracellular oedema and ballooning of cells) are formed, which burst and crust, and can lead to superficial ulceration.

Table 9.7 Types of herpes viruses

Herpes type	Name	Target cell	Site of latency	Transmission
1	HSV-1	Epithelial cells	Neurons	Close contact
2	HSV-2	Epithelial cells	Neurons	Close contact usually sexual
3	VSV	Epithelial cells	Neurons	Contact or respiratory route
4	EBV	B lymphocytes, epithelial cells	B lymphocytes	Saliva
5	CMV	Epithelial cells, monocytes, and lymphocytes	Monocytes and lymphocytes	Contact, blood transfusions, transplantation, congenital
6	Herpes lymphotropic virus	T lymphocytes	T lymphocytes	Contact, respiratory route
7	HHV-7	T lymphocytes	T lymphocytes	Unknown
8	HHV-8 KSHV	Endothelial cells	Unknown	Possibly exchange of body fluids

CMV, Cytomegalovirus; EBV, Epstein–Barr virus; HHV-7, human herpes virus-7; KSHV, Kaposi sarcoma-associated herpes virus; VSV, varicella zoster virus.

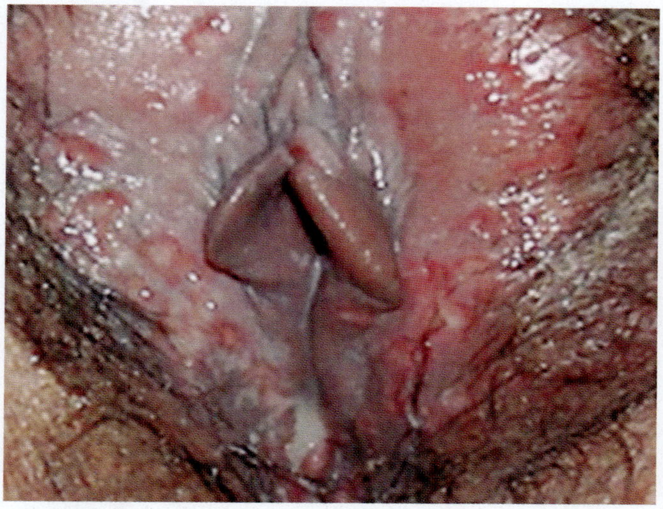

Fig. 9.20 Genital herpes erosions involving inner labia majora.

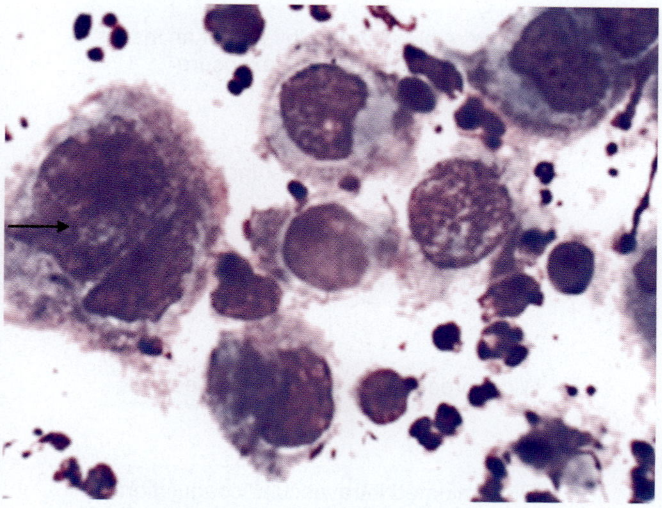

Fig. 9.21 Herpes infected enlarged keratinocytes with multinucleated syncytial cells *(arrow)*.

- **Gingivostomatitis** encountered in children is usually caused by HSV-1. It is a vesicular eruption extending from tongue to retropharynx causing cervical lymphadenopathy.
- Swollen, erythematous HSV lesions of fingers or palm (**herpetic whitlow**) occur in infants and occasionally, in healthcare workers.
- **Herpes keratitis** is an infection of the eye primarily caused by HSV-1. It can be recurrent and may lead to blindness.
- **Herpes gladiatorum** is contracted by wrestlers. It spreads by direct contact from skin lesions on one wrestler to his/her opponent, and usually appears in the head and neck region (which are frequent sites of contact in wrestling holds).
- **Genital herpes** (Fig. 9.20) is usually the result of HSV-2 with about 10% of cases being the result of HSV-1. Primary infection is often asymptomatic, but sometimes, painful lesions can develop on glans or shaft of the penis in men and on vulva, vagina, cervix, and perianal region of women. HSV-2 can be transmitted to neonates during passage through birth canal of infected mothers. HSV-2 disease in the neonate can vary from being mild to severe with generalized lymphadenopathy, splenomegaly, and necrotic foci throughout the lungs, liver, adrenals and central nervous system.
- **Eczema herpeticum** is characterized by confluent, pustular, or haemorrhagic blisters, often with bacterial superinfection and viral dissemination to internal viscera.
- **Herpes bronchopneumonia** can result from insertion of an airway through oral herpes lesions.
- **Herpes hepatitis** can cause liver failure.
- HSV can be a cause of inflammation of rectum and anus (**proctitis**).
- **HSV encephalitis** due to HSV-1 infection is the most common sporadic viral encephalitis.
- **HSV meningitis** is the result of HSV-2 infection and usually resolves spontaneously.

Morphology

- Morphologic hallmark of HSV infection is ***large pink-to-purple intranuclear (Cowdry type A)*** *inclusions,* which push nuclear chromatin to periphery.
- There is ***mild increase in cellular size*** along with formation of ***multinucleated syncytial cells*** *that also have inclusions* (Fig. 9.21).

Cytomegalovirus

Aetiopathogenesis

- CMV can produce a variety of disease manifestations, depending on age of the host, and, more importantly, on the host's immune status.
- The **major glycoprotein envelope of CMV binds to epidermal growth factor receptor (EGFR) to gain entry into different cells.**
- CMV infects and **remains latent in white blood cells, and can be reactivated in the event of depressed cell-mediated immunity (CMI).** In immunocompromised patients, CMV can cause life-threatening illness.

Morphology

CMV produces cellular and nuclear enlargement true to its name. **A large intranuclear inclusion surrounded by a clear halo (owl's eye appearance)** is its morphological hallmark (Fig. 9.22).

Dengue Fever

Aetiopathogenesis

- Dengue (**break-bone**) **fever** is an infectious disease common in tropics. It occurs in epidemic form from time-to-time.
- Dengue is transmitted by several species of mosquitoes within the genus *Aedes*, principally ***Aedes aegypti.***
- **Dengue fever virus (DENV) is an RNA virus of family Flaviviridae; genus *Flavivirus*.** Other members of the same genus include yellow fever virus, West Nile virus, St. Louis encephalitis virus, Japanese encephalitis virus, tick-borne encephalitis virus, Kyasanur forest disease virus, and Omsk haemorrhagic fever virus.
- The virus has **four different types**; infection with one type usually gives lifelong immunity to that type, but only

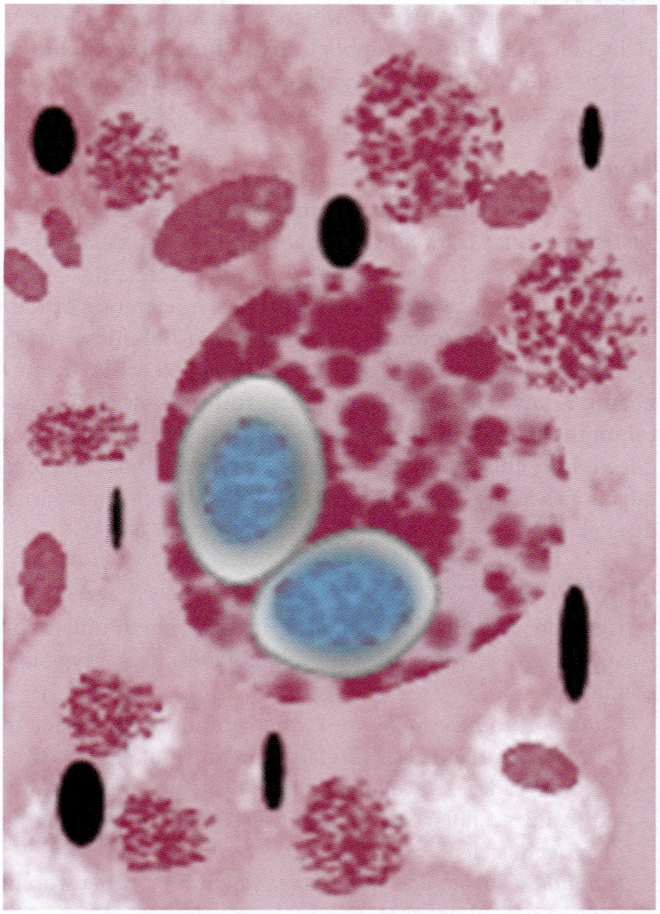

Fig. 9.22 A typical owl's eye intranuclear inclusion in CMV-infected cells.

short-term immunity to others. Subsequent infection with a different type increases the risk of severe complications.

Clinical Features

- The **WHO's 2009 classification** divides dengue fever into **two groups: uncomplicated and severe.**
- **Most people** infected with dengue virus are **asymptomatic** or only have **mild symptoms**, such as an **uncomplicated fever.** Others present with a more severe illness, which in a small proportion of cases may be life threatening.
- The incubation period ranges from 3 to 14 days, but most often is about 4–7 days.
- The characteristic symptoms of dengue are **sudden-onset fever, headache (typically located behind the eyes), muscle and joint pains and rash**. The course of infection is divided into **three phases: febrile, critical and recovery**. The febrile phase involves high fever, often over 40°C (104°F), and severe generalized aches and pains; this usually lasts 2–7 days. This is followed by a maculopapular rash, after which the disease proceeds to the critical phase, which is marked by resolution of the high fever. During this phase, there may be significant fluid accumulation in the chest and abdominal cavity due to increased capillary permeability and leakage. The recovery phase occurs next, with resorption of the leaked fluid into the bloodstream. This is characterized by severe itching and bradycardia, and leads to depletion of fluid from the circulation and decreased blood supply to vital organs. Another rash may occur with either a maculopapular or vasculitic appearance, which is followed by peeling of the skin.
- In a **small proportion of cases**, the disease develops into a **life-threatening dengue haemorrhagic fever, resulting in bleeding, low circulating levels of platelets and blood plasma leakage, or into dengue shock syndrome, where dangerously low blood pressure occurs.** Polymorphisms in particular genes have been linked with increased risk of severe dengue complications.

Q. Write briefly about chlamydial, rickettsial and mycoplasma infections. (PA 10.4)

Ans. These microbes are grouped together because, like other bacteria, they divide by binary fission and are sensitive to antibiotics, but they lack certain structures (e.g. *Mycoplasma* lacks a cell wall) or metabolic capabilities (e.g. *Chlamydia* cannot synthesize adenosine triphosphate). *Chlamydia* and rickettsiae are obligate intracellular organisms that replicate in membrane-bound vacuoles in epithelial cells and cytoplasm of endothelial cells, respectively.

Chlamydiae

- *Chlamydia trachomatis* is a small Gram-negative, aerobic, intracellular bacterium. ***C. pneumoniae*** is one of the main causative agents of **pneumonia and bronchitis**. It has also been linked with artherosclerosis and multiple sclerosis.
- ***C. trachomatis*** infection causes **urogenital infections *(non-gonococcal urethritis)*, inclusion conjunctivitis, lymphogranuloma venereum, epididymitis, prostatitis, pelvic inflammatory disease, pharyngitis, conjunctivitis and trachoma.**
- *C. trachomatis* exists in two forms during its unique life cycle. The infectious form— the '**elementary body**'—is a metabolically inactive, spore-like structure, which is taken up by host cells, primarily by receptor-mediated endocytosis. The bacteria prevent fusion of endosome and lysosome. Inside the endosome, the elementary body differentiates into a metabolically active form called the '**reticulate body**' that is capable of infecting additional cells.
- *C. trachomatis* urethritis is characterized by a mucopurulent discharge which on microscopy shows mainly neutrophils. The lesions of lymphogranuloma venereum show a suppurative (neutrophilic inflammatory) response with an occasional granuloma. Intracytoplasmic chlamydial inclusions can be demonstrated in epithelial or inflammatory cells.
- Regional lymphadenopathy is common. Affected nodes show a granulomatous inflammatory reaction associated with irregularly necrosis (stellate abscesses), which may lead to extensive fibrosis, which, in turn, may cause lymphatic obstruction with lymphedema.
- Chlamydiae cannot be demonstrated by Gram staining. While culturing of the organism can confirm the diagnosis, this method is limited to research laboratories. For routine diagnostic use, newer and inexpensive diagnostic tests that depend upon identification and amplification of the genetic

material of the organism have replaced the older, time-consuming culture methods.

Rickettsial Infections

- *Rickettsial organisms* are **vector-borne, Gram-negative, obligate intracellular bacteria** that are divided into **two antigenically defined groups: spotted fever group and typhus group**. *Rickettsia* cause Rocky Mountain spotted fever (*Rickettsia rickettsia*), rickettsial pox (*Rickettsia akari*), epidemic typhus (*Rickettsia prowazekii*), and murine or endemic typhus (*Rickettsia typhi*). *Orientia* (formerly *Rickettsia*) *tsutsugamushi* causes scrub typhus.
- Patients present with **fever and exanthem**; eventually there is **visceral involvement**; symptoms include **nausea, vomiting, abdominal pain, encephalitis, hypotension, acute renal failure, respiratory distress and coma.**
- The organisms proliferate in the endothelial cell cytoplasm and then either burst the cell (typhus group) or spread from cell-to-cell (spotted fever group).

Mycoplasma

- The causative agent of mycoplasmal pneumonia is ***M. pneumoniae*, a short rod-shaped bacterium, lacking a cell wall (unlike bacteria).** Unlike viruses, it does not need a host cell for replication.
- It belongs to the **class Mollicutes**, the smallest known free-living microorganisms.
- The organism can be **excreted from the respiratory tract** for several weeks after onset of the acute infection and is difficult to grow in the laboratory.
- It inhibits ciliary movement thereby causing **prolonged paroxysmal cough** and has two peculiar features: **first, an affinity for respiratory epithelial cells; and second, the ability to produce hydrogen peroxide, which is responsible for cellular damage.**

Q. Write briefly about fungal infections.

Ans. Fungi are **eukaryotes with thick chitinous cell walls**. Their cell membranes contain ergosterol. Fungi grow either as **budding yeast cells or as filamentous hyphae**. Hyphae may be **thick or thin septate** (with cell walls separating individual cells) or **aseptate**, and show **branching at various different angles**. Fungi may cause **superficial or deep infections**.

- **Superficial fungal infections involve the skin, hair and nails**. Fungal species that remain limited to superficial layers of the human skin are known as **dermatophytes**. The common term for dermatophytic infections is 'tinea'. **Dermatophytic infections are referred to as 'tinea' followed by part of the body affected (e.g. tinea pedis: 'athlete's foot'; tinea capitis: 'ringworm of the scalp').** Certain other fungal species are capable of invading the **subcutaneous tissue to cause subcutaneous mycoses (abscesses or granulomas, e.g. sporotrichosis).**
- **Deep fungal infections** can spread systemically to involve deeper/visceral organs. Vital organs are invaded and destroyed in immunocompromised hosts, but the lesions usually heal or remain latent in immunologically competent hosts. Examples of fungi which can cause deep mycoses include ***Histoplasma*, opportunistic fungi like *Candida, Aspergillus, Mucor, Cryptococcus* and *Pneumocystis jiroveci (carinii).***

Candida

It is a part of **normal flora (commensal) of the skin, mouth, gastrointestinal tract and vagina,** and does not usually produce any disease. However, some *Candida* species, most often *Candida albicans,* can cause human fungal infections, particularly in **immunocompromised persons (diabetics, AIDS patients, burn patients, patients receiving steroids, immunosuppressive therapy, transplants, and those with haematolymphoid malignancies).** *Candida* can be directly introduced into the blood by intravenous lines and catheters, during peritoneal dialysis, cardiac surgery, or intravenous drug abuse.

Pathogenesis

- *Candida* can adapt to changes in host environment by switching between different phenotypes in a reversible manner.
- *Candida* produces *adhesins* (which aid in its adherence to host cells) and *enzymes* (*proteinases* contribute to invasiveness, degrade extracellular matrix proteins, and *catalases* aid in intracellular survival and resist oxidative killing by phagocytic cells).
- *Candida* also secretes *adenosine*, which blocks neutrophil oxygen radical production and degranulation.

Clinical Manifestations

- *Candida* can cause superficial to disseminated deep mycosis **(vaginitis; oral thrush; diaper rash; endocarditis; meningitis; osteomyelitis; and renal, intracerebral and hepatic abscesses).**
- In immunocompetent persons, candidiasis is usually a very localized infection of the skin or mucosal membranes. Most common type of superficial candidiasis is infection of oral mucosa (thrush), which is characterized by formation of a dirty-looking pseudomembrane, composed of colonies of organisms and inflammatory debris. Other forms of oropharyngeal candidiasis include **glossitis, stomatitis and angular cheilitis (perleche). Candidal oesophagitis** presents with dysphagia, and endoscopy demonstrates white pseudomembranes on oesophageal mucosa.
- Mucocutaneous candidiasis includes **intertrigo, diaper candidiasis, paronychia and onychomycosis**. Intertriginous candidiasis is most commonly seen in the skin folds including axillae, groin, inter- and submammary folds, intergluteal folds, interdigital spaces and umbilicus. Main predisposing factors include moisture, heat, and friction; obesity, diabetes mellitus, warm water immersion or occlusion of the skin, and the use of broad-spectrum antibiotics are additional factors.
- *Candida* vaginitis is a common form of vaginal infection in women, especially those who are diabetic or pregnant, or on oral contraceptive pills. It is usually associated with intense itching and a thick, curd-like discharge.

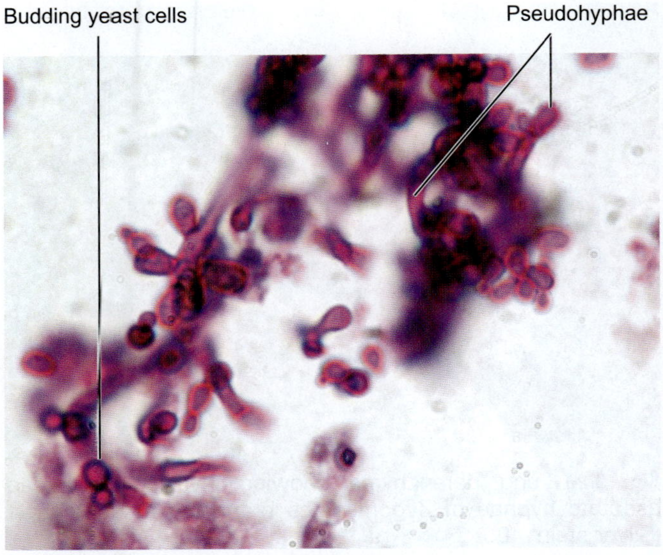

Fig. 9.23 Yeast forms of *Candida* (small, thin-walled ovoid cells of 4–6 μm that reproduce by budding), and pseudohyphae (PAS stain; 400×).

- **Severe disseminated candidiasis or candidal sepsis** usually occurs in a setting of severe immunosuppression and can eventually cause death due to shock and DIC.

Morphology

Candida exists as a **yeast form (small, thin-walled ovoid cells of 4–6 μm that reproduce by budding) as well as pseudohyphae**. These are best demonstrated by **silver methenamine** and **periodic acid–Schiff (PAS) stains** (Fig. 9.23). *Candida* grows well on routine blood agar and fungal media. Biphasic blood cultures and lysis centrifugation may facilitate recovery. In tissue sections, *C. albicans* can appear as yeast-like forms (blastoconidia), pseudohyphae, and, less commonly, true hyphae. Pseudohyphae are important diagnostic clue for *C. albicans* and represent budding yeast cells joined end-to-end at constrictions, thus simulating true fungal hyphae. **Three types of histopathological reactions may be seen depending on the host immunity**:

- No cellular response
- Suppurative response
- Granulomatous response.

Cryptococcosis

Cryptococcosis is a rare fungal infection caused by inhalation of ***Cryptococcus neoformans*, an encapsulated fungus** that is ordinarily found in soil. Cryptococcosis mostly occurs in **immunocompromised individuals** (such as those who are HIV infected; on corticosteroids or cancer chemotherapy; or suffering from Hodgkin disease, SLE and sarcoidosis). **Once inhaled, the infection may heal on its own, remain localized in the lungs, or spread throughout the body (dissemination).** In people with normal immune system, the infection may have no symptoms. However, in people with impaired immune systems, *Cryptococcus* may even spread to the brain (causing meningoencephalitis).

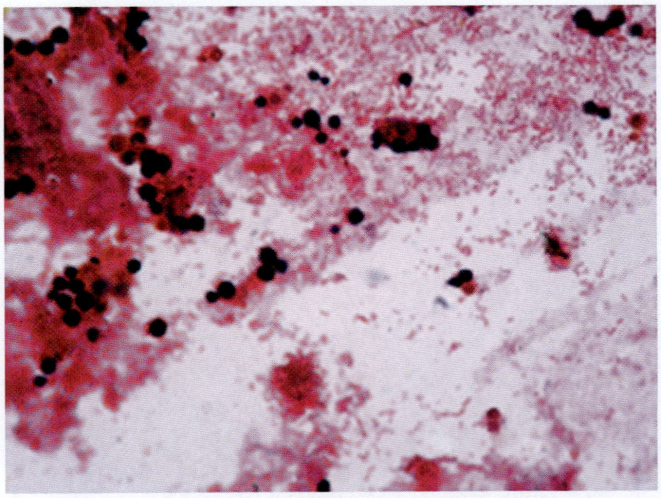

Fig. 9.24 Yeast forms of *C. neoformans* (Silver stain).

Disseminated cryptococcosis usually involves the skin, liver, spleen, adrenals and bones.

Pathogenesis

Virulence is due to capsular polysaccharides and enzymes, which prevents phagocytosis by alveolar macrophages and inhibits leukocyte recruitment and migration.

Morphology

- *Cryptococcus* has yeast but no pseudohyphal or hyphal forms.
- Its yeast form is 5–10 μm in size (extremely variable in size) and has a thick gelatinous capsule that is valuable for diagnosis (Fig. 9.24).
- **Capsular polysaccharide stains intense pink/red with PAS and mucicarmine** in tissues, and can be detected with antibody-coated beads in an agglutination assay.
- **India ink preparation gives a negative image, visualizing thick capsule as a clear halo**, but do not stain the yeast.
- In immunosuppressed patients, organisms may evoke virtually no inflammatory reaction, so gelatinous masses of fungi are seen in the tissue (gelatinous reaction).
- In non-immunosuppressed patients, the fungi induce a chronic granulomatous reaction composed of macrophages, lymphocytes, and foreign-body-type giant cells. Rarely, suppuration can be seen.

Molds

Aspergillosis

This **saprophytic fungus sporulates** and **produces conidia (asexual spores)** that are **readily aerosolized.** Molecular studies of *Aspergillus* isolated from opportunistic infections show many different strains of *Aspergillus,* suggesting that **immune status of the host is more important than fungal pathogenicity** as far as the nature of infection is concerned. ***Aspergillus fumigatus*** is the most common species to cause disease, and it produces severe invasive infections in immunocompromised individuals.

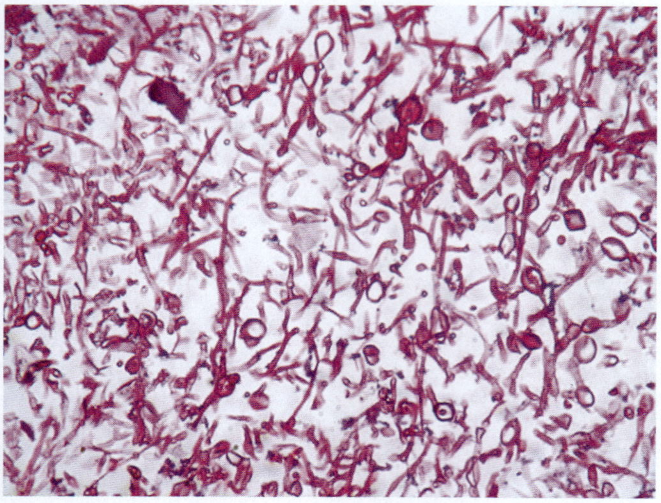

Fig. 9.25 Septate filaments of *Aspergillus* showing branching at acute angles (PAS stain; 200×).

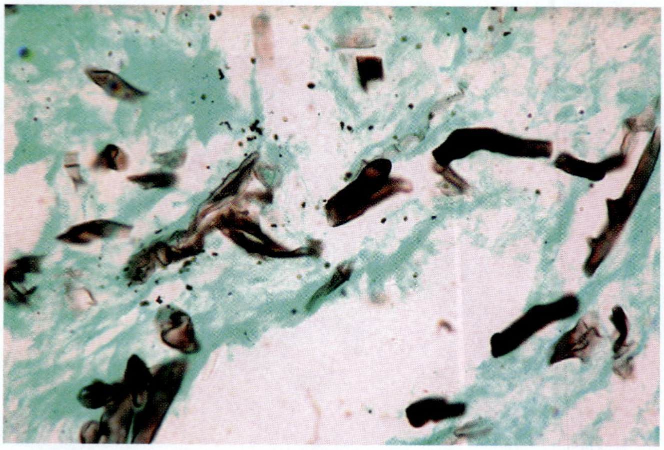

Fig. 9.26 Lung parenchyma showing invasion by broad aseptate hyphae of Zygomycetes branching at right angle (Silver stain' 400×).

Pathogenesis

- The small size of *Aspergillus* spores enables them to reach alveoli where they are taken up by alveolar macrophages, which secrete cytokines and chemokines to elicit adaptive immune responses.
- *Aspergillus* also produces several virulence factors, including *adhesins, antioxidants, enzymes* and *toxins*.
- *Aspergillus* species is a source of *aflatoxin*, which is a major cause of liver cancer in Africa. Sensitization to *Aspergillus* spores can produce an allergic alveolitis.
- ***Allergic bronchopulmonary aspergillosis*** results from hypersensitivity arising from superficial colonization of bronchial mucosa and may eventually result in chronic obstructive lung disease.
- ***Colonizing aspergillosis (aspergilloma)*** occurs when there is growth of the fungus in pulmonary cavities with minimal or no invasion of the tissues. Cavities usually result from pre-existing tuberculosis, bronchiectasis, old infarcts, or abscesses. Masses of fungal hyphae called fungus balls are seen lying free within the cavities. They may be surrounded by minimal inflammatory reaction to marked chronic inflammation and fibrosis.
- ***Invasive aspergillosis*** is an opportunistic infection that is confined to immunosuppressed and debilitated hosts.

Morphology

- ***Aspergillus*** **forms fruiting bodies (particularly in cavities) and septate filaments, which are 5–10-μm thick and branch at acute angles** (Fig. 9.25).
- ***Aspergillus*** **has a tendency to invade blood vessels**; therefore, areas of haemorrhage and infarction are usually superimposed on necrotizing, inflammatory tissue reactions.
- In **invasive aspergillosis, the primary lesions are usually in the lung, but widespread haematogenous dissemination is common**. The pulmonary lesions take form of necrotizing pneumonia with sharply delineated, rounded, grey foci with haemorrhagic borders, often referred to as ***target lesions.***

Zygomycosis (Mucormycosis)

- Zygomycetes form **non-septate, broad (6–50 μm) fungal hyphae with frequent right-angle branching**, which are readily demonstrated in the necrotic tissues by haematoxylin and eosin, or special fungal stains.
- Also called **mucormycosis** or **phycomycosis, zygomycosis** is an **opportunistic infection** caused by 'bread mould fungi', including *Rhizopus, Absidia, Cumunghanrella* and *Mucor,* which belong to the class Zygomycetes.
- The **three primary sites of invasion are nasal sinuses, lungs and gastrointestinal tract,** depending on whether spores (which are widespread in dust and air) are inhaled or ingested.
- Most commonly in diabetics, the fungus may spread from nasal sinuses to orbit and brain, giving rise to **rhinocerebral mucormycosis**. The Zygomycetes cause local tissue necrosis, invade arterial walls, and penetrate periorbital tissues and cranial vault. **Meningoencephalitis** follows, sometimes complicated by cerebral infarctions when fungi invade arteries and induce thrombosis.
- Lung involvement with Zygomycetes (Fig. 9.26) may be secondary to rhinocerebral disease, or it may be primary in patients with haematologic neoplasms. Lung lesions combine areas of haemorrhagic pneumonia with vascular thrombi and distal infarctions.

Q. Write briefly on the aetiopathogenesis and diagnosis of mycetoma.

Ans. Mycetoma can be classified as a **eumycetoma**—a fungal disease, or **actinomycetoma**—an old name for actinomycosis.

Eumycetoma

- This is a **chronic, specific, granulomatous, fungal disease, which mainly affects the foot**. *Mycetoma pedis* is also known as **Madura foot.** This infection is endemic in Africa, India, and Central and South America and is usually acquired while performing agricultural work.

- It generally afflicts men between 20 and 40 years old. The disease is acquired by contacting grains of fungal spores that have been discharged onto soil.
- Infection usually manifests as an open area or break in the skin. It is clinically characterized by draining sinuses, granules and tumefaction.
- The disease usually involves **cutaneous and subcutaneous tissue**, and may also spread to **underlying fascia and bone. Sinuses discharge serosanguinous fluid containing granules that vary in size, colour and degree of hardness, depending on aetiologic species, and are hallmark of *Mycetoma*.**
- Eumycetoma may be of several varieties, depending upon colour of granulous discharge:
  - Red—*Actinomadura pelletieri.*
  - White or yellow—*Acremonium* species, *Aspergillus nidulans, Pseudallescheria boydii.*
  - Black—*Curvularia lunata, Exophiala jeanselmei, Madurella grisea, Madurella mycetomatis.*

Actinomycetoma

- Actinomycosis is a rare, chronic, and slowly progressive granulomatous disease **caused by filamentous Gram-positive anaerobic bacteria from the Actinomycetaceae family (genus *Actinomyces*)**, such as *Actinomyces israelii* or *Actinomyces gerencseriae*. It can also be caused by *Propionibacterium propionicus*.
- *Actinomyces* are commensals of the human oropharynx, gastrointestinal tract, and urogenital tract. When tissue integrity is breached through a mucosal lesion they can invade local structures and organs and become pathogenic.
- The condition tends to affect certain areas of the body and can be classified into **four main types:**
  - Oral cervicofacial actinomycosis
  - Thoracic actinomycosis
  - Abdominal actinomycosis
  - Pelvic actinomycosis.

Clinical Manifestations of Mycetoma

- Mycetoma is a chronic, suppurative infection of subcutaneous tissue and contiguous bone. The feet are most common site for infection and account for at least two-thirds of cases (Fig. 9.27).
- Other sites include lower legs, hands, head, neck, chest, shoulder and arms. Most cases start out as a small hard painless nodule, which over time begins to soften on the surface and ulcerate to discharge fluid containing grains.
- The infection slowly spreads to adjacent tissue, including bone, often causing considerable deformity.

Laboratory Diagnosis of Mycetoma

- *Direct microscopy*: Microscopic examination of crushed granules can be done using either 10% KOH and Parker ink, or calcofluor white mounts.
- *Tissue sections*: Tissue sections show **grains,** which are interwoven mycelia lined by intensely eosinophilic material **(Splendor Hoeppli phenomenon). Eumycotic mycetoma** shows septate hyphae, 2–6 μm in dm, staining positive with H&E (Fig. 9.28), GMS (Grocott methenamine silver), and PAS. **Actinomycotic mycetoma** shows delicate, branched, Gram-positive filaments sometimes showing beading and measuring less than 1 μm.
- *Culture*: Clinical specimens should be inoculated onto primary isolation media, like Sabouraud dextrose agar.

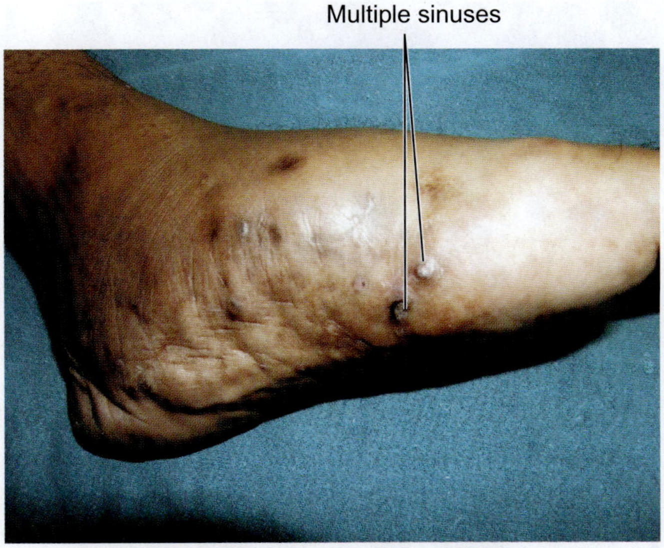

Fig. 9.27 Mycetoma foot showing numerous draining sinuses.

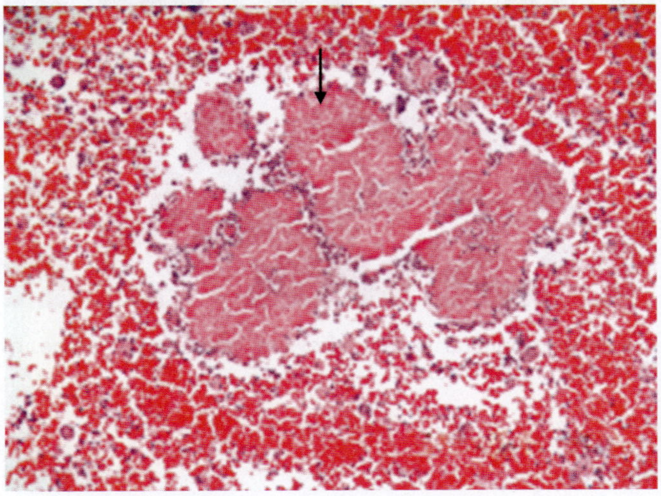

Fig. 9.28 H&E stained section showing a eumycetoma with intensely eosinophilic material (Splendor–Hoeppli phenomenon) surrounded by septate hyphae, 2–6 μm in diameter.

Q. Write briefly on protozoan infections.

(PA10.1, 10.4)

Ans. Parasitic protozoa are single-celled eukaryotes that are major causes of morbidity and mortality in developing countries. They can replicate intracellularly within a variety of cells (e.g. *Plasmodium* in red blood cells, Leishmania in macrophages) or extracellularly in urogenital system, intestine or blood. Common protozoal infections are discussed below.

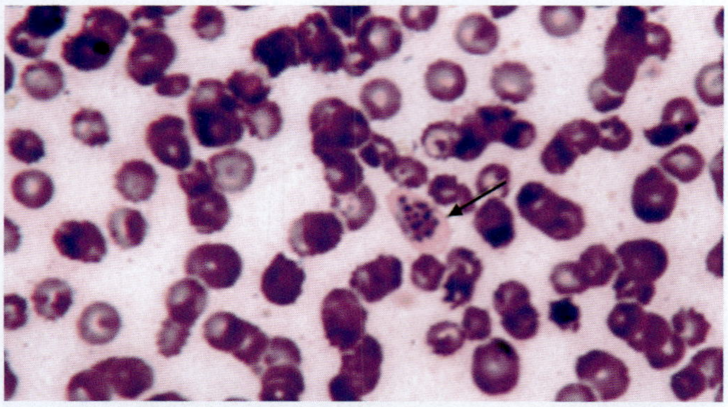

Fig. 9.29 Schizont form of malarial parasite *(arrow)*.

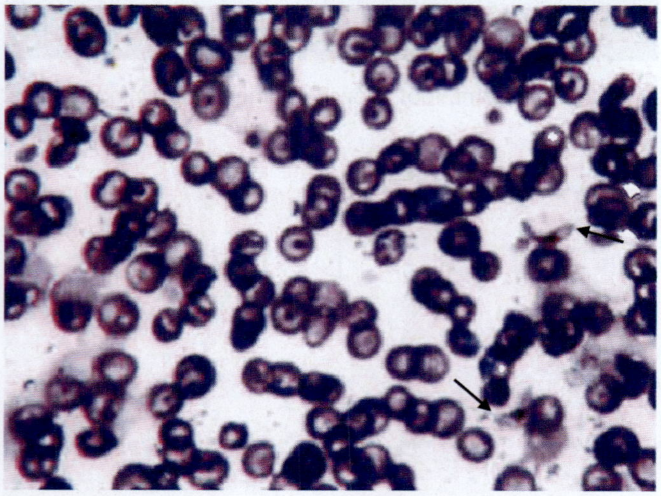

Fig. 9.30 Peripheral smear showing gametocyte stage of *P. falciparum (arrows)*.

Malaria (PA10.1)

Malaria is transmitted by female ***Anopheles* mosquito**. It is caused by parasites of the species ***Plasmodium*** that spread from person-to-person through bites of infected mosquitoes. The common first symptoms are **fever, headache, chills and vomiting, and these appear 10–15 days after a person is infected**. If not treated promptly with effective medicines, malaria can cause severe illness that is often fatal. There are four types of human malaria caused by *Plasmodium falciparum, Plasmodium vivax* (Fig. 9.29), *Plasmodium malariae,* and *Plasmodium ovale,* respectively. *P. falciparum* (Fig. 9.30) and *P. vivax* are the most common. *P. falciparum* is by far the most deadly type of malaria. Unique features of *P. falciparum* are:

- High parasitemia.
- Severe anaemia.
- Frequent occurrence of renal failure, pulmonary oedema and death.
- *P. falciparum* causes RBCs to clump together (rosetting) and also sticks to endothelial lining.
- Several proteins including *P. falciparum erythrocyte membrane protein (PfEMP1)* form knobs on surface of the RBCs. PfEMP1 binds to ligands on endothelial cells including CD36, thrombospondin, VCAM1, ICAM1, and E selectin. This binding causes ischaemia, which is responsible for manifestations of cerebral malaria.

Features common to *P. vivax* and *P. malariae* include:

- Mild anaemia
- Splenic rupture
- Nephrotic syndrome.

Life Cycle

The life cycle of malarial parasite is depicted in Flowchart 9.3.

Causes of Resistance to Malaria

- Inherited alterations in RBCs (presence of HbS, HbC, and absence of Duffy antigen).
- Repeated and prolonged exposure to *Plasmodium* species (stimulates an immune response that reduces severity of malaria).

Histopathology

Spleen

- Congested and enlarged (may exceed 1000 g in weight).
- Parenchyma is gray-black because of granular, brown-black, birefringent haemozoin pigment.
- May become extremely fibrotic and brittle with a thickened capsule (fibrocongestive splenomegaly).
- Phagocytic activity of reticuloendothelial cells is increased.

Liver

- Liver is enlarged.
- Sections show pigmented Kupffer cells, which are heavily laden with malarial parasite.

Kidneys. May be enlarged with presence of pigment in glomeruli and haemoglobin casts in tubules.

Nervous System

- Brain vessels are plugged with parasitized RBCs, each with a dot of haemozoin.
- Perivascular ring haemorrhages due to local hypoxia and vascular stasis, as well as, small focal inflammatory aggregates **(malarial or Durck granulomas)** may be seen.
- Also seen sometimes are degeneration of neurons and focal ischaemic softening.

Leishmaniasis

Leishmaniasis is a **chronic inflammatory disease of the skin, mucous membranes and viscera caused by an obligate intracellular protozoan transmitted through bites of infected sand fly.**

- It is endemic throughout Middle East, South Asia, Africa and Latin America.
- Life cycle involves two forms: ***promastigotes,*** which develop and live extracellularly in the sand fly vector and the ***amastigote*** form that multiplies intracellularly in the host macrophages.

Sporozoites reach blood by bite of an infected mosquito (female Anopheles)

↓

They invade and attach to liver cells (binding to hepatocytic receptors for proteins thrombospondin and properdin)

↓

Multiply asexually in the liver cells

Hepatic phase

↓

Merozoites (asexual haploid forms) released into circulation when hepatocytes rupture

↓

Bind to RBCs via lectin on glycophorin molecules of RBC membrane (*P. vivax* binds to Duffy Ag)

↓

Merozoites release proteases from a special organelle called Rhoptry

Erythrocytic phase

↓

Multiply in RBCs, within which parasites grow in membrane-bound digestive vacuoles and hydrolyse haemoglobin via serotonin enzymes, converting haem to haemozoin

Note: First stage of parasite in RBCs is ring stage, followed by trophozoite and schizont form (Figure 7.15).

Some merozoites develop into sexual forms called gametocytes that infect mosquito when it takes a blood meal

↓

Once ingested, the parasite gametocytes taken up in the blood will further differentiate into male or female gametes (Fig. 7.16) and then fuse in the mosquito gut

↓

This produces an ookinete that penetrates the gut lining and produces an oocyst in gut wall

↓

When the oocyst ruptures, it releases sporozoites that migrate through the mosquito's body to its salivary glands, where they are then ready to infect a new human host

Flowchart 9.3 Life cycle of malarial parasite.

- Mammals including rodents, dogs and foxes are reservoirs of *Leishmania*.
- Parasite specific CMI is the main host immune response.

The clinical types of leishmaniasis are listed in Table 9.8.

Table 9.8 Types of leishmaniasis

Type of disease	Causative species
Cutaneous disease	*Leishmania major*, *L. mexicana*, *L. aethiopica*, *L. braziliensis*
Visceral pathology (Kala azar)	*L. donovani*, *L. chagasi*

Life Cycle

The life cycle of Leishmania is depicted in Flowchart 9.4.

Pathogenesis

- *Promastigotes* produce two surface glycoconjugates, important for their virulence, namely, *lipophosphoglycan* and *Gp63*. *Lipophosphoglycan* forms a dense glycocalyx, which:
  - Activates complement to deposit C3b on the parasite surface, and
  - Inhibits complement by preventing membrane complex attack insertion into the parasite membrane.

Sand fly bites infected humans and animals

↓

Macrophages with amastigotes are ingested

↓

Amastigotes differentiate into *promastigotes,* which multiply in the digestive tract of sand fly and migrate to its pharynx ready for transmission to host during a bite by sand fly

↓

Promastigotes (flagellate forms) are released into host dermis with sand fly saliva

↓

Phagocytosed by macrophages and transformed into round *amastigotes (aflagellate forms)*

↓

Multiply within macrophages

↓

Macrophages rupture and amastigotes are released

Flowchart 9.4 Life cycle of *Leishmania*.

  - C3b coated on the parasite binds to Mac1 and CR1 on macrophages initiating promastigote phagocytosis by macrophages.
- *Lipophosphoglycan* neutralizes oxygen radicals and inhibits lysosomal enzymes, protecting the parasite in the phagolysosome.
- *Gp63,* a zinc-dependent proteinase that cleaves complement and some lysosomal antimicrobial enzymes; also promotes promastigote adhesion to macrophages.

Histopathology

- Invasion by parasite-laden macrophages throughout reticuloendothelial cells leads to systemic disease (hepatosplenomegaly, lymphadenopathy, pancytopenia, fever and weight loss).
- Phagocytic cells crowd the bone marrow, lymph nodes, liver, lungs, GIT, kidneys, pancreas and testes.
- Hyperpigmentation of the skin (***black fever***) may be seen.
- Liver becomes fibrotic in the later stages.
- Normal architecture of the spleen may be replaced by sheets of histiocytes, which are parasite laden.
- Plasma cells are increased in number.
- Kidney biopsy may show mesangioproliferative glomerulonephritis and/or amyloidosis.

Cutaneous Leishmaniasis

Cutaneous leishmaniasis usually manifests with a single ulcer on exposed skin (***tropical sore***). It starts as a papule surrounded by induration, progresses to a shallow expanding ulcer with irregular borders, which usually heals by involution without treatment. Histopathology shows well-formed granulomatous reaction or ill-defined histiocytic aggregates with intracellular parasite.

Mucocutaneous Leishmaniasis

Moist, ulcerating and non-ulcerating lesions arise in larynx, nasal septum and vulva after the skin lesion has healed. Histopathology usually shows sheets of histiocytes, lymphocytes, and plasma cells. Occasionally a well-formed granulomatous reaction may be seen.

Diffuse Cutaneous Leishmaniasis in Anergic Patients

Starts as a single nodule and spreads to the whole body as bizarre nodular lesions (resemble keloids and verrucae; they may sometimes be mistaken for the nodules of lepromatous leprosy).

Amoebiasis

- Amoebiasis is caused by ***E. histolytica* (*Entamoeba histolytica*), a protozoan parasite, which spreads by faecal–oral transmission.**
- Amoeba proteins involved in tissue invasion include:
  - *Cysteine proteases,* which lyse proteins of extracellular matrix.
  - *Lectins* on parasite surface that bind to carbohydrates on colonic epithelium and RBCs.
  - *Channel forming proteins* that contain an *amoeba pore* that makes pores in plasma membrane and lyses it.
- It is important to distinguish the *E. histolytica* cyst from the cysts of non-pathogenic intestinal protozoa, such as *Entamoeba coli. E. histolytica* cysts have a maximum of four nuclei, while the commensal *E. coli* cyst has up to eight nuclei. Additionally, in *E. histolytica,* the endosome is

Ingestion of cysts
(Infectious forms of *E. histolytica* which have a chitinous wall and 4 nuclei and are resistant to gastric acids)

↓

Cysts colonize the mucin-secreting epithelial cells of colon

↓

In the colonic lumen, cysts release trophozoites or amoeboid forms
(lack of mitochondria and Krebs cycle enzymes makes them obligate fermenters of glucose to ethanol;
Metronidazole targets pyruvate–oxido-reductase, an enzyme critical in this fermentation)

↓

Dysentery, intestinal pain and fever

Flowchart 9.5 Life cycle of *Entamoeba histolytica*.

centrally located in the nucleus, while it is usually eccentric in *E. coli.* Chromatoidal bodies in *E. histolytica* cysts are rounded, while they are jagged in *E. coli. Virulent strains* of *E. histolytica* show ingested RBCs, whereas *non-virulent* strains do not.

Life Cycle

The life cycle of *E. histolytica* is depicted in Flowchart 9.5.

Pathology

- **Caecum, ascending colon, sigmoid, rectum and appendix are involved in that order.** In severe full-blown cases, entire colon may be involved.
- *Amoebae* invade crypts of colonic glands and burrow through the wall up to muscularis mucosae (which acts as a barrier to the infection). Thereafter they fan out laterally forming a ***flask-shaped*** **ulcer** (Fig. 9.31).

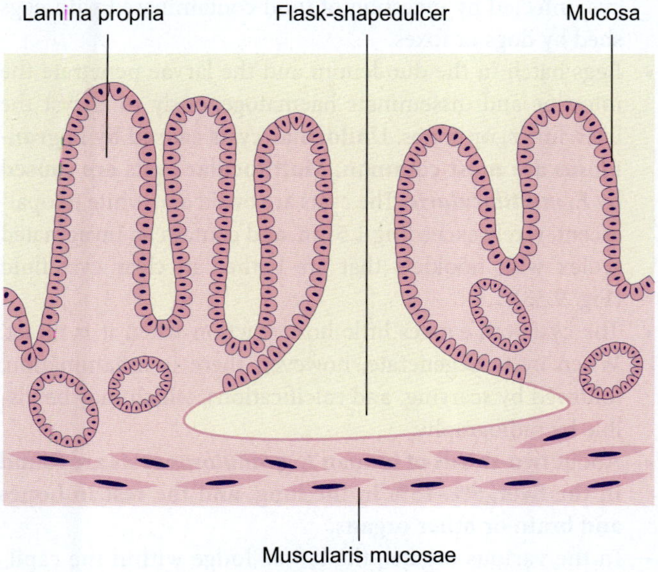

Fig. 9.31 A flask-shaped amoebic ulcer.

- The ulcer contains large areas of liquefactive necrosis and very few inflammatory cells. A sharp line divides the necrotic and viable mucosa. Trophozoites are found on the surface of the ulcers, in the exudate and in the crater. They are also frequently found in the submucosa, muscularis propria, serosa and small veins of the submucosa.
- ***Ameboma* is a napkin-like constrictive lesion** (comprised of granulation tissue), which may be confused with carcinoma colon.
- In 40% patients, parasites penetrate portal vessels leading to **solitary and multiple abscesses in the liver (*amoebic liver abscesses*) filled with chocolate coloured, odourless, pasty (*anchovy sauce-like*) material.** These may undergo secondary bacterial infection causing suppuration.

Diagnosis

- Asymptomatic human infections are usually diagnosed by finding **cysts shed in the stool.** Various sedimentation procedures have been developed to recover the cysts from faecal matter.
- In symptomatic infections, the **motile form (trophozoite) can often be seen in fresh faeces.** Amoebic trophozoites can also be demonstrated in **histopathology sections,** where they appear as spherical or oval-shaped bodies (15–20 µm in diameter) with a thin cell membrane and single nucleus with prominent nuclear border and central karyosome. Trophozoites resemble macrophages because of a comparable size and presence of multiple vacuoles; the parasite, however, has a smaller nucleus with a large karyosome. The PAS procedure stains the cytoplasm of the trophozoite red. The organism appears black when stained with Heidenhain iron haematoxylin method. Presence of trophozoites containing RBCs is indicative of tissue invasion.
- ***Serological tests:*** Serology becomes positive about 2 weeks after infection. The levels of antibody are much higher in individuals with liver abscesses.

Q. Write briefly on helminthic infections. (PA10.2, 10.4)

Ans. The helminths are **worm-like, multicellular parasites. They undergo sexual reproduction in the definitive host and asexual multiplication in an intermediary host.** The clinically important helminths are classified according to their physical characteristics, internal morphology (appearance of their egg, larval and adult stages), and the host/vector they inhabit. Flukes (Trematodes) are leaf-shaped flatworms with prominent oral and ventral suckers. Tapeworms (Cestodes) are elongated, segmented, hermaphroditic flatworms that inhabit the intestinal lumen. Larval forms, which are cystic or solid, inhabit extraintestinal tissues. Roundworms (Nematodes) are bisexual, cylindrical worms. They inhabit intestinal and extraintestinal sites.

Tapeworms (Cestodes): Cysticercosis and Hydatid Disease

Taenia solium **and** ***Echinococcus granulosus*** are cestodes (tapeworms) that cause cysticercosis and hydatid infections, respectively. Both diseases are caused by larvae that develop following ingestion of tapeworm eggs:

Cysticercosis

- ***T. solium*** **tapeworms** consist of a **head (scolex) that has suckers and hooklets that attach to the intestinal wall, a neck, and many flat segments called proglottids that contain male and female reproductive organs.**
- When pigs ingest the proglottids or eggs, the eggs hatch, penetrate their intestinal wall, and spread to skeletal muscle, especially the neck, tongue and trunk. There, the larvae mature into encysted cysticerci over 2–3 months.
- The cysticerci suppress the host inflammatory response and survive in tissues for months to years. The life cycle is completed when humans ingest inadequately cooked pork that contains viable cysticerci or eggs.
- The larvae hatch, penetrate the gut wall, disseminate haematogenously, and encyst in many organs. The egg-containing faeces usually contaminate water supplies in endemic areas. If this water is used to irrigate fruits and vegetables, eggs are ingested with the contaminated food. Thus, people who have never visited endemic countries can also develop infection.
- Autoinfection involves the retrograde transmission of proglottids from the intestines into the stomach with subsequent release of *T. solium* eggs into the gut.
- The clinical syndromes caused by *T. solium* are categorized as **neurocysticercosis or extraneural cysticercosis** [intestinal infection, subcutaneous nodules (Fig. 9.32), and ocular cysts]. Neurocysticercosis can manifest with convulsions and other neurological signs of increased intracranial pressure.
- Neurocysticercosis is further divided into parenchymal and extraparenchymal disease. Parenchymal disease is characterized by infection within the brain parenchyma. Extraparenchymal disease develops when cysticerci migrate to the CSF of the ventricles, cisterns and subarachnoid space or within the eyes or spinal cord.

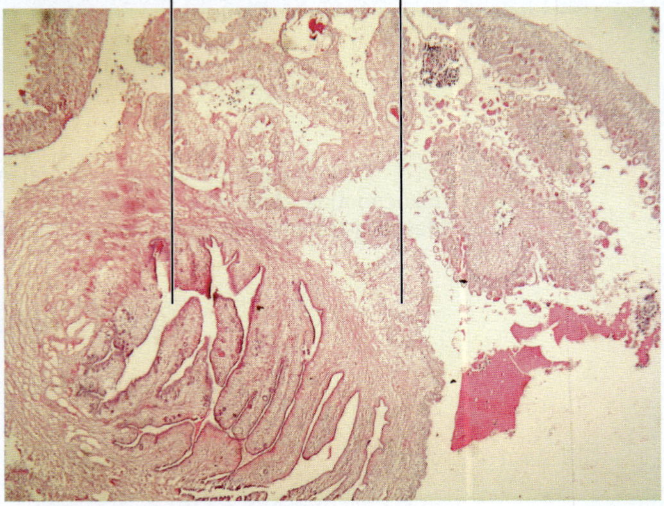

Fig. 9.32 Cysticercosis (H&E; 100×).

Hydatid Disease

- It is caused by ingestion of eggs of echinoccal species. Of the four known species of ***Echinococcus,*** **three are of medical importance in humans. These are** ***E. granulosus,*** **causing cystic echinococcosis;** ***Echinococcus multilocularis,*** **causing alveolar echinococcosis (AE); and** ***Echinococcus vogeli. E. granulosus*** **is the most common of the three.** *E. multilocularis* is rare but is the most virulent, and *E. vogeli* is the rarest.
- Humans are accidental intermediate hosts for echinicoccus, infected by ingestion of food contaminated with eggs shed by dogs or foxes.
- Eggs hatch in the duodenum and the larvae penetrate the intestine and disseminate haematogenously to encyst the liver, lungs, or bones. **Unilocular cysts caused by** ***E. granulosus*** **are most common. Multilocular cysts are caused by** ***E. multilocularis.*** The cysts are ovoid and white to opalescent, rarely exceeding 1.5 cm, and contain an invaginated scolex with hooklets that are bathed in clear cyst fluid (Fig. 9.33).
- The cyst wall evokes little host reaction when it is intact. When cysts degenerate, however, there is inflammation, followed by scarring, and calcifications, which may be visible by radiography.
- About **two-thirds of human** ***E. granulosus*** **cysts are found in the liver, 5%–15% in the lung, and the rest in bones and brain or other organs.**
- In the various organs, the larvae lodge within the capillaries and incite an inflammatory reaction composed

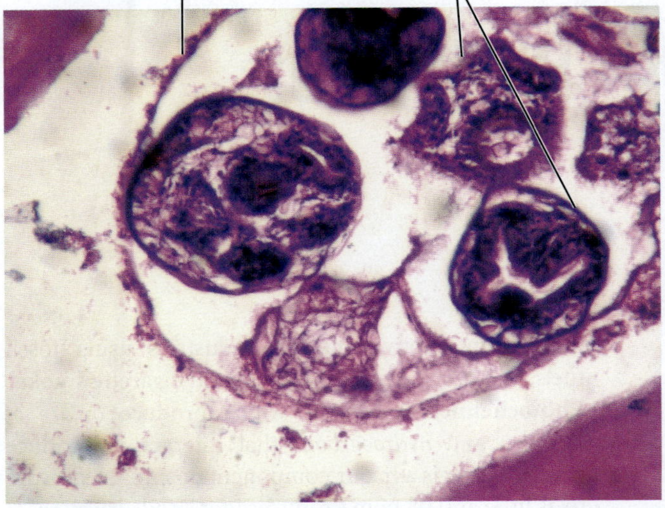

Fig. 9.33 Echinococcosis liver showing invaginated scolices embedded in the cyst wall (H&E; 200×).

principally of mononuclear leukocytes and eosinophils. Many such larvae undergo encystation.

- The cysts (Fig. 9.34) have an inner, nucleated, germinative layer and an outer, opaque, non-nucleated layer. The outer non-nucleated layer is distinctive and has innumerable delicate laminations as though made up of many layers of gelatin. Outside this opaque layer, there is a host inflammatory reaction that produces a zone of fibroblasts, giant cells, and mononuclear and eosinophilic cells. In time, daughter cysts develop within them.

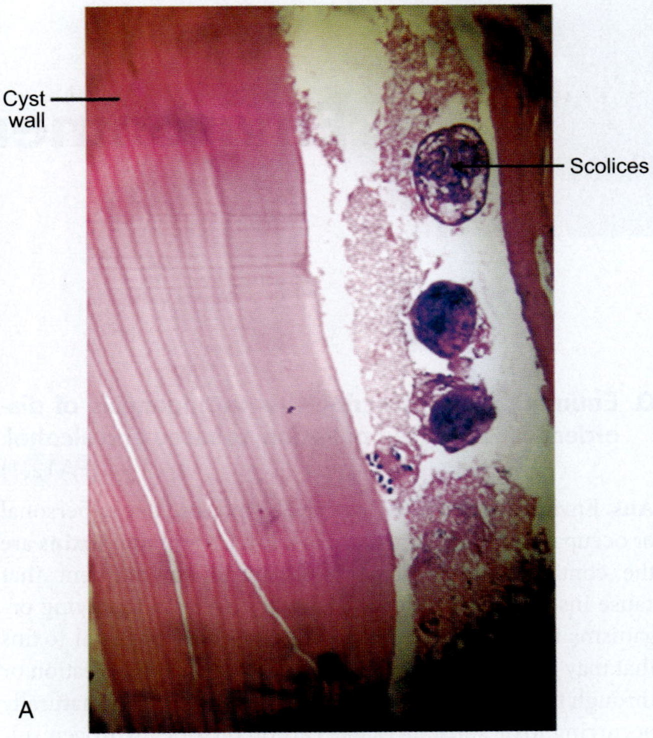

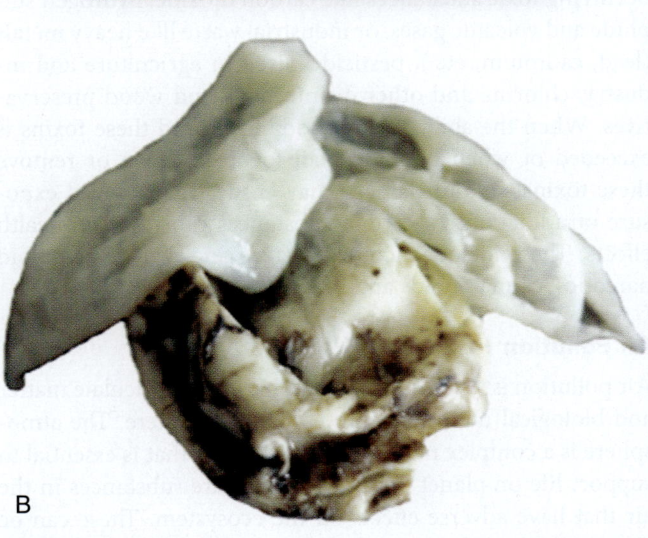

Fig. 9.34 (A) Photomicrograph of Echinococcosis liver showing the cyst wall with scolices (H&E; 100×). (B) Gross picture of an infected (thickened) echinococcal cyst.

10 Environmental Pathology

Q. Enumerate and describe the pathogenesis of disorders caused by air pollution, tobacco and alcohol. (PA12.1)

Ans. Environmental pathology can be induced due to personal or occupational exposure to toxins. **Environmental toxins** are the contaminants released into natural environment that cause instability in the ecosystem and harm to the living organisms inhabiting it. **Xenobiotics** are environmental toxins that may be absorbed into the body by inhalation, ingestion or through the skin and mucosal surfaces. They include naturally occurring toxic substances like carbon dioxide, hydrogen sulphide and volcanic gases, or industrial waste like heavy metals (lead, cadmium, etc.), pesticides used in agriculture and industry, chlorine and other disinfectants and wood preservatives. When the ability of our body to defend these toxins is exceeded or when our body fail to break down or remove these toxins, serious damage may ensue. Self-induced exposure or addictions to certain substances can result in health effects. These include alcohol, tobacco and drugs like opioid narcotics, cannabinoids and sedative-hypnotics.

Air Pollution

Air pollution is the introduction of harmful particulate matter and biological molecules into earth's atmosphere. The atmosphere is a complex natural gaseous system that is essential to support life on planet Earth. Pollutants are substances in the air that have adverse effects on the ecosystem. These can be chemical, physical or microbiological substances; may be solid particles, liquid droplets, or gases; may be of natural origin or man-made; could be primary or secondary. Primary pollutants include ash from a volcanic eruption, CO gas from vehicular emission, and sulphur dioxide released from industrial emissions. Secondary pollutants form in the air when primary pollutants react with the atmospheric contents (e.g. ground level ozone). There could be outdoor or indoor hazards.

1. **Outdoor:** This is mainly a problem of industrialized countries. Major sources of outdoor pollution include:
   (a) **Combustion of fossil fuels** originating from vehicles, power plants, and factories, which release emissions that are a complex mixture of *CO, oxides of nitrogen, hydrocarbons, diesel exhaust particles,* and *other particulates including lead oxide* from tetraethyl lead contained in leaded gasoline. CO is a non-irritant, colourless, and odourless gas produced by imperfect combustion of carbonaceous material. Its sources include automotive engines, industries using fossil fuels, and home heating with oil, and cigarette smoke.
   (b) **Photochemical reactions** which produce *oxides of nitrogen* and *hydrocarbons* that interact to produce ozone, which is a major component of smog. Exposure to as little as 0.08 ppm produces increased airway reactivity and inflammation in lungs leading to cough, chest discomfort and decreased lung function.
   (c) **Power plant emissions** that have *sulphur dioxide,* which is absorbed in the upper and lower airways, where it releases (bisulphite) and SO (sulphite), which cause local irritation. Sources of sulphur dioxide include volcanoes, industries, coal and petroleum combustion, etc. Further oxidation of SO_2, usually in the presence of a catalyst, such as NO_2, forms H_2SO_4 (acid rain).
   (d) **Waste from incinerators/industry/smelters** that contains *acid aerosols, organic compounds,* and *particles,* which alter mucociliary reflexes and increase the incidence of respiratory infections.
   (e) **Volatile organic compounds (VOCs)** that are basically organic solvents and vapours, which cause outdoor air pollution. They could be methane (CH_4) derived or non-methane (NMVOCs) in nature. *Methane* is a hydrocarbon and a greenhouse gas. It gives rise to ozone. The aromatic NMVOCs include benzene, toluene and xylene, which have been implicated in carcinogenesis. VOCs are used in manufacturing, dry cleaning and as components of paint removers and aerosol sprays.
   (f) **Chlorofluorocarbons (CFCs)** which are released into the atmosphere from air conditioners, refrigerators, aerosol sprays, etc. The air containing CFCs rises to stratosphere where they come in contact with other gases and damage the ozone layer. This allows harmful ultraviolet rays to reach the earth's surface leading to skin cancer, diseases of the eye, etc.
2. **Indoor pollutants:** Sources of indoor air pollutants are cooking stoves (gas and wood), furnaces, radon, construction materials, furniture, allergens derived from pets, dust mites, fungal spores and bacteria. The effects of major indoor air pollutants are summarized as follows:
   (a) **CO:** CO pollution of indoor air can reduce exercise capacity and aggravate myocardial ischemia. It is an important cause of accidental death due to oxygen deprivation (haemoglobin has 200 times higher affinity for CO than for O_2; besides carboxyhaemoglobin interferes with release of oxygen from oxyhaemoglobin

causing further tissue hypoxia). Diagnosis of CO poisoning is confirmed by measuring carboxyhaemoglobin levels. CO poisoning presents in two ways:

(i) ***Acute CO poisoning:***
- Cherry red skin and mucus membrane.
- Petechial haemorrhages.
- Hypoxic injury to brain, liver and renal tubules.

(ii) ***Chronic CO poisoning:***
- Diffuse neuronal loss and focal cerebral demyelination (CNS disturbances, hearing loss, blindness, and paralysis).
- May cause glomerulopathy and acute tubular necrosis.

(b) **Nitrogen dioxide (NO_2):** Predisposes to respiratory infections.

(c) **Wood smoke:** Contains oxides of nitrogen and carbon particulates, is an irritant, and predisposes to lung infections.

(d) **Formaldehyde:** Causes eye and nose irritation, and asthma.

(e) **Radon:** Radioactive gas derived from uranium widely present in soil and homes; can cause lung cancer in uranium miners.

(f) **Asbestos fibres:** Occupational exposure can produce lung cancer and mesotheliomas.

(g) **Mineral fibres:** Used in maintenance and construction; may cause skin and airway irritation.

(h) **Bioaerosols:** Include microbiologic agents that cause infections, such as Legionnaire disease, viral agents, common cold, as well as allergens derived from pet dander, dust mites, fungi, and moulds that cause allergic rhinitis/asthma.

Alcohol

- *Ethanol* is mainly absorbed in the stomach and small intestine; depending on the blood levels, it is then distributed to all tissues and fluids of the body.
- Drunk driving in most states is defined as a concentration of 80 mg/dL in the blood; inebriation generally results at a blood alcohol level of 200 mg/dL and coma, death and respiratory arrest usually occur at levels of 300–400 mg/dL.
- Habitual drinkers can tolerate blood alcohol levels up to 700 mg/dL. This metabolic tolerance is attributed to an increased induction of the cytochrome P-450 xenobiotic-metabolizing enzyme CYP2E1, which accelerates the metabolism of ethanol as well as that of other drugs and chemicals like cocaine and acetaminophen.
- *Methanol* is metabolized to formaldehyde and formic acid, resulting in metabolic acidosis, dizziness, vomiting, blurred vision or blindness and respiratory depression.
- Ethanol in blood is transformed to acetaldehyde in the liver by three enzyme systems.

Adverse Effects of Alcohol

1. **Acute effects:** Acute alcohol intake exerts its effects mainly on CNS, but can also induce hepatic and gastric damage. The following are chief manifestations of acute alcoholic toxicity:
   (a) CNS: Disordered cortical, motor and intellectual behaviour followed by CNS depression.
   (b) Liver: Acute alcoholic hepatitis (manifests with fever, right hypochondrial tenderness, jaundice and histology of the liver shows focal hepatocyte necrosis, Mallory hyaline, neutrophilic infiltrate and fat accumulation).
   (c) Stomach: Acute gastritis or ulceration.
2. **Chronic effects:** Chronic alcohol intake has deleterious effects on specific organs as described:
   (a) **Liver:** Fatty change, hepatitis, cirrhosis, portal hypertension or hepatocellular carcinoma are possible effects (alcohol oxidation by ADH causes reduction in nicotinamide adenine dinucleotide or NAD levels as ADH reduces NAD to NADH. NAD is required for fatty acid oxidation in liver and conversion of lactate into pyruvate. Its deficiency, therefore, causes accumulation of fat in the liver of alcoholics). Metabolism of ethanol by MEOS (CYP2E1) produces reactive oxygen species that causes lipid peroxidation of cell membranes leading to injury. Formation of adducts with tubulin results in impaired function of microtubules and transport of lipoproteins. Alcohol may also induce release of endotoxin, a product of Gram-negative bacteria from the intestinal flora, which stimulates release of tumour necrosis factor (TNF) and other cytokines, causing cell injury.
   (b) **Nervous system:** Thiamine deficiency is common in alcoholics and is known to induce degeneration of nerve cells, reactive gliosis and atrophy of cerebellum and peripheral nerves. Two syndromes are closely associated with chronic alcohol intake, namely, **Wernicke syndrome**, which presents with ataxia, disturbed cognition, ophthalmoplegia, nystagmus and **Korsakoff syndrome**, which is believed to result from a combination of alcohol toxicity, poor nutrition and thiamine deficiency, and manifests with severe memory loss.
   (c) **CVS:** Chronic alcohol intake causes injury to myocardium leading to *dilated congestive cardiomyopathy*, which is thought to be due to direct toxicity rather than thiamine deficiency. High blood alcohol levels have a vasopressor effect due to release of catecholamines, which may induce hypertension. Heavy consumption of alcohol also leads to decreased levels of high-density lipoproteins (HDL) and contributes to *coronary artery disease.*
   (d) **GIT:** Alcohol can cause massive bleeding from gastritis/gastric ulcer or oesophageal varices and acute or chronic

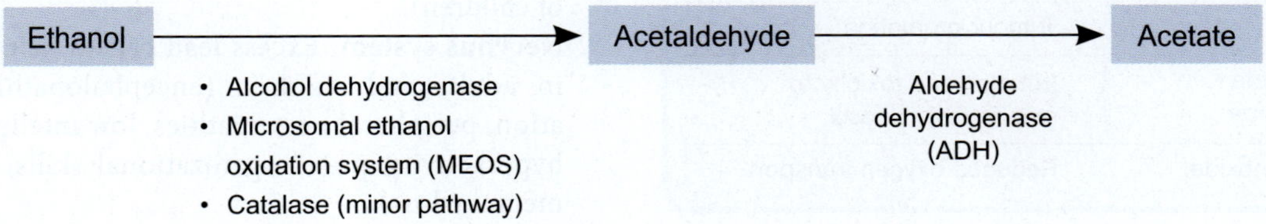

pancreatitis. It is also associated with increased risk of cancer *of the oral cavity,* and *oesophagus.* Ethanol is not a direct-acting carcinogen; but one of its metabolites, acetaldehyde, may act as a tumour promoter. Ethanol inhibits detoxification of chemical carcinogens such as nitrosamines, which have been associated with tumours of the upper gastrointestinal tract.

(e) **Reproductive system:** Heavy long-term consumption of alcohol is known to cause testicular atrophy in men and reduced fertility and spontaneous abortions in women.

(f) **Skeletal muscle:** Alcohol causes rhabdomyolysis, which, in turn, leads to muscle weakness and pain.

(g) Ethanol is a substantial source of energy; therefore, chronic alcoholism commonly leads to **malnutrition and deficiencies.**

(h) Alcohol intake during pregnancy can induce **foetal alcohol syndrome**, which manifests in infants as microcephaly, growth retardation and facial abnormalities; older children may show a reduction in mental functions.

Smoking

Tobacco is the most frequent exogenous cause of human cancer. Main contributor is cigarette smoking, but pipes, snuff, bidis and tobacco chewing are also harmful. Cigarette smoke inhaled by the smoker is constituted by a particulate phase (tar) and a gas phase. There are more than 40 established carcinogens in cigarette smoke. In addition to these, cigarette smoke contains carcinogenic metals, such as arsenic, nickel, cadmium, and chromium; promoters, such as acetaldehyde and phenol; toxins and irritants, such as nitrogen dioxide, formaldehyde, and hydrogen cyanide; and carbon monoxide (CO). Nicotine, another very important constituent of cigarette smoke, is the reason behind tobacco addiction. It can induce increased heart rate, blood pressure, cardiac output, and coronary flow by increasing circulating catecholamines. The important toxic chemicals present in tobacco smoke are enlisted in Table 10.1. ***Smoking associated cancers*** *include cancer of the larynx, lung, oesophagus, pancreas, urinary bladder* and *oral cavity.*

Table 10.1 Toxic chemicals in cigarette smoke and their effects

Chemicals	Effects
• Tar • Polycyclic aromatic hydrocarbons • Nitrosamines	Carcinogenesis
• Nicotine	Ganglionic stimulation, depression and tumour promotion
• Phenol	Tumour promotion
• Formaldehyde • Nitrogen oxide	Irritation and toxicity to respiratory mucosa
• Carbon monoxide	Reduced oxygen transport

Other Effects of Smoking:

- Ischaemic heart disease (due to accelerated atherosclerosis, increased platelet aggregation and impaired lung function, which causes reduced myocardial oxygen supply).
- Peptic ulcer disease.
- Cerebrovascular accident (CVA).
- Chronic respiratory disease (exacerbates bronchitis, asthma and pneumoconiosis).
- Increased incidence of low birthweight, prematurity and spontaneous abortion as a consequence of maternal smoking.

Other Toxic Agents

Mercury

- *Source*: Industrial contamination of ocean (from bacteria to fish to humans) and paints.
- *Effects*: CNS disturbances, hearing loss, blindness, spasticity, paralysis and glomerulopathy.

Cyanide

- *Sources*: Combustion of wool, silk and plastic upholstery
- *Effects*: Hypoxic injury to brain, liver and kidney.

Mushroom Poisoning

- *Sources*: *Amanita phalloides* and *Amanita muscaria.*
- *Effects*: Vomiting, abdominal cramps, CNS changes, renal and hepatic necrosis.

Insecticides

- *Sources*: Chlorinated hydrocarbons, DDT, chlordane and organophosphates.
- *Effects*: Hyperexcitability, muscle twitching to paralysis, cardiac arrhythmias, delirium, convulsions and coma.

Methanol

- *Source*: Organic solvents.
- *Effects*: Toxic necrosis of retinal ganglion cells with blindness.

Q. Write briefly about lead toxicity.

Ans. Lead exposure occurs through contaminated air, water and food.

Sources: House paints, gasoline, mines, foundries, batteries, automatic exhaust, urban soil and spray paints. Most of the absorbed lead is taken up by bone and teeth.

Effects:

1. **Bones:** Radiodense deposits in epiphyses (excess lead interferes with vitamin D metabolism and calcium homoeostasis thereby interfering with normal remodelling of calcified cartilage and primary bone trabeculae in the epiphyses of children).
2. **Nervous system:** Excess lead causes *neurological effects* in adults and children (encephalopathies, demyelination, peripheral neuropathies, low intellectual capacity, hyperactivity, poor organizational skills, headache and memory loss).

3. **Gingiva:** Lead line (lead stimulates hyperpigmentation of the gums).
4. **Blood:** Lead has high affinity for sulfhydryl groups and interferes with enzymes involved in haeme synthesis; iron incorporation into haeme is impaired leading to microcytic hypochromic anaemia, and basophilic stippling. The levels of erythrocyte protoporphyrin are increased.
5. **Kidney:** Chronic tubulointerstitial disease (excretion of lead occurs via the kidney).
6. **GIT:** Abdominal pain or colic.

Q. Write briefly about the effects of climate change on human health.

Ans. During the preceding 1000 years, maximum warming of earth has taken place in the last 50 years. Rising levels of CO_2, methane and ozone (greenhouse gases) along with water vapour lead to increased absorption and re-emission of infrared energy, which radiates from the surface of the earth and is normally lost into space. This event raises the global temperature (greenhouse effect).

- Increase in global temperature increases the surface heat absorption leading to:
  - Loss of ice and snow.
  - Increased content of atmospheric water vapour due to increased evaporation from water bodies.
  - Increased release of CO_2 and methane from organic matter in thawing ice (such as arctic).
  - Decreased removal of CO_2 by diatoms due to their reduced growth; increased CO_2 increases the acidity of oceans which in turn disrupts the marine ecosystem.
  - Increased heat energy in oceans induces variability in the weather events casing floods, droughts and storms.
- Climate change brings about **cardiovascular, cerebrovascular** and **respiratory diseases** (owing to increased temperature and air pollution); **increased incidence of food- and water-borne diseases** (contamination due to floods and disruption of clean water supply); **increased incidence of vector-borne infections** (due to increased temperature) and **malnutrition** (weather changes harm the crop production).

Q. Write briefly about the biological effects and mechanism of action of ionizing radiation.

Ans. Radiation describes a process in which high-energy particles or waves travel through a medium or space. There are two distinct types of radiation:

- **Ionizing radiation:** The word *radiation* is commonly used in reference to ionizing radiation only (i.e. having sufficient energy to ionize an atom). This occurs when an electron is stripped (or 'knocked out') from an electron shell, and leaves the atom with a net positive charge, for example alpha particles (consist of two neutrons and two protons), beta particles (consist of energized electrons), gamma rays (consist of photons with a frequency of greater than 10^{19} Hz) and X-rays (electromagnetic waves with a wavelength smaller than about 10 nm).
- **Non-ionizing radiation:** Energy radiating (i.e. travelling outward in straight lines in all directions) from its source. The energy of non-ionizing radiation is less and instead of producing charged ions when passing through matter, there is only sufficient energy to change the rotational, vibrational or electronic valence configurations of molecules and atoms, for example UV rays, infrared waves, microwaves and sound waves.

Radiation Units

1. **Curie (Ci):** The amount of radiation emitted by a source (one Ci = 3.7×10^{10} disintegrations per second of a radionuclide/radioisotope).
2. **Gray (Gy):** The energy absorbed by the target tissue per unit mass; corresponds to the absorption of 10^4 erg/g of tissue and is equivalent to exposure of tissues to 100 RAD (radiation absorbed dose). The unit 'cGy' (centigray) terminology has replaced 'R' (rads).
3. **Sievert (Sv):** Has replaced a term called 'rem'. Sv quantifies a unit of equivalent dose that depends on the biological rather than the physical effects of radiation (measures the relative biological effectiveness of the radiation).

Morphological Effects of Radiation

- Deletions, breaks, translocations and fragmentation of chromosomes.
- Disorderly mitotic spindles, polyploidy and aneuploidy.
- Nuclear swelling/condensation/clumping of chromatin.
- Breakdown of nuclear membrane.
- Apoptosis.
- Formation of giant cells, pleomorphic nuclei, cytoplasmic swelling, degeneration of mitochondria and endoplasmic reticulum and defects in plasma membrane.
- Vascular changes, for example endothelial swelling and proliferation with hyalinization of vessel wall.

Hazards of Radiation

These are caused by the whole body irradiation having short wavelength and high frequency. It may be electromagnetic waves like X-rays or particulate materials like α particles, β particles, electrons, protons, neutrons, mesons and deuterons. The clinical manifestations depend on the dose and duration of exposure to such radiation (Table 10.2).

Chronic Effects of Radiation

Result from damage to the genetic material in dividing cells, causing abnormalities of cell growth, such as cancer. Damage to reproductive cells has been shown to lead to birth defects. External radiation therapy for cancer may cause nausea, vomiting and loss of appetite, skin changes including hair loss, redness, peeling, sores, thinning of the skin, dilated blood vessels just beneath the skin's surface (spider veins) and skin cancer. Radiation to the lungs can cause radiation pneumonitis and fibrosis. Radiation to GIT may cause ulcers, fibrosis, strictures and cancer. Testes and ovaries show tubular atrophy and stromal fibrosis, respectively, and CNS may show necrosis, gliosis and cancer.

Q. Write briefly on common drug induced reactions.

Ans. Therapeutic drugs can induce a variety of adverse drug reactions. Common drug induced reactions are enlisted in the Table 10.3.

Table 10.2 Hazards of radiation

0–1 Sv	1–2 Sv	2–10 Sv	10–20 Sv	>50 Sv	
Main site of injury	None	Lymphocytes	Bone marrow	Small bowel	Brain
Main signs and symptoms	None	Moderate granulocytopenia and lymphopenia	Leukopenia, haemorrhage, hair loss, and vomiting	Nausea, vomiting, diarrhoea, and electrolyte imbalance	Ataxia, coma, convulsions, and vomiting
Time of development	—	1 Day to 1 week	2–6 Weeks	5–14 Days	1–4 h
Lethality	None	None	Variable	100%	100%

Table 10.3 Common drug-induced reactions

Organ system	Adverse effects	Drugs implicated
Bone marrow and blood	Granulocytopenia, pancytopenia, aplastic anaemia, thrombocytopenia, haemolytic anaemia	Antineoplastic agents, chloramphenicol, immunosuppressants, penicillin, methyldopa, heparin, quinidine
GIT	Gastritis, peptic ulcer, pancreatitis	Aspirin, NSAIDs, thiazide diuretics
Liver	Fatty change, hepatitis, cholestatic jaundice	Tetracycline, oestrogens (including contraceptive agents), acetominaphen, chlorpromazine, halothane isoniazid
CVS	Arrhythmias, cardiomyopathy	Theophylline, hydantoins, digoxin, doxorubicin and daunorubicin
CNS	Tinnitus, dizzy spells, acute dystonic reactions, Parkinson like reaction, respiratory depression	Salicylates, sedatives, antipsychotics
Respiratory system	Asthma, pneumonitis, interstitial fibrosis	Salicylates, nitofurantoin, bleomycin, busulphan
Urinary system	Glomerulonephritis, acute tubular necrosis, tublointerstitial disease	Salicylates, phenacetin, aminoglycosides, amphotericin B, cyclosporin, penicillamine
Skin	Urticaria, papulovesicular eruptions, petechiae, exfoliative dermatitis, fixed drug eruptions, pigmentation or skin discolouration	Antibiotics, minocycline, sulphonamides, hydantoins, antineoplastic agents

Q. Write briefly about exogenous oestrogens and their effects.

Ans. Oestrogen is extensively used in:

1. **Menopausal hormone therapy (MHT)**
   (a) Given to postmenopausal women to prevent progression of osteoporosis, distressing menopausal symptoms like hot flushes and reduce the likelihood of myocardial infarction (protective role of MHT in myocardial infarction has been demonstrated only in women under the age of 60 years; no protection in women who start MHT after 60 years is seen).
   (b) Unopposed oestrogen therapy increases the risk of **endometrial cancer;** risk is reduced or eliminated when progestins are added.
   (c) MHT may cause an increase in risk of **breast carcinoma** after a median time of 5–6 years (risk of breast carcinoma is marginally reduced with oestrogen-only therapy in females who have undergone hysterectomy).
   (d) MHT increases the risk of **venous thromboembolism (deep vein thrombosis, pulmonary embolism and stroke)** by about twofold.
2. **Oral contraceptives (OCs)**
   (a) Usually contain a synthetic oestradiol and a variable amount of progestin; few preparations contain progesterone only. OCs inhibit ovulation and prevent implantation.
   (b) Current prevailing opinion is that OCs do not cause an increase in breast cancer risk.
   (c) OCs have a protective role in endometrial and ovarian cancer.
   (d) May increase risk of cervical carcinoma in women infected with HPV virus (increased risk may be due to increased sexual activity).
   (e) Increase risk of thromboembolism. OCs induce a hypercoagulable state as they increase hepatic synthesis of coagulation factors.
   (f) Risk of cardiovascular disease increases in women over 35 years who are smokers.
   (g) Well-defined association between the use of OCs and hepatic adenoma.

Nutritional Disorders

11

Q. Define protein-energy malnutrition (PEM). (PA12.2)

Ans. The seven major classes of nutrients include carbohydrates, fats, proteins, vitamins, dietary fibre, minerals and water. Based on the requirement, these may be classified as *macronutrients* (needed in relatively large amounts) or *micronutrients* (needed in smaller quantities). The macronutrients include carbohydrates, fats, fibre, proteins and water, while the micronutrients include minerals and vitamins. Non-infectious diseases (cardiovascular diseases, cancers, diabetes and chronic respiratory problems) contribute majorly to the global morbidity and mortality and are all linked to poor nutrition. Infectious diseases on the other hand can result in malnutrition.

Protein-energy malnutrition (PEM) is defined as inadequate consumption of protein and/or energy resulting in a range of clinical syndromes, namely **kwashiorkor** (protein deficiency) and **marasmus** (overall lack of calories). There are two protein compartments in the body: the somatic protein compartment (skeletal muscle mass) and the visceral protein compartment, represented by the visceral organs (mainly the liver). The former is affected more in marasmus (calorie deficiency), while the latter is depleted severely in kwashiorkor (protein deficiency). The most common victims of PEM worldwide are children. A child whose weight falls to less than 80% of normal is considered malnourished. The diagnosis of PEM is usually more obvious in its severe form. In the milder form of disease one can compare the body weight for a given height with standard tables and arrive at a diagnosis. Other parameters that are helpful include evaluation of fat stores, muscle mass and serum proteins. With loss of fat, major storage form of energy, thickness of skin folds (which includes skin and subcutaneous tissue) is reduced. If somatic protein compartment is catabolized, the resultant reduction in muscle mass is reflected by reduced circumference of mid arm. Measurement of the serum proteins (albumin, transferrin and others) provides a measure of adequacy of visceral protein compartment.

Q. Differentiate between kwashiorkor and marasmus. (PA12.2)

Ans. Differences between kwashiorkor and marasmus are enlisted in Table 11.1.

Q. Write briefly about the metabolism of vitamin A.

Ans. Vitamin A (fat-soluble vitamin) is the generic term used for a group of related compounds namely, **retinal, retinol and retinoic acid.**

- **Retinol (an alcohol):** Retinol is preformed vitamin A, usually found in animal sources. It is stored in the liver as a 'retinol ester'. On being released from the liver it binds to 'retinol binding protein' (RBP) to be transported to the peripheral tissues. It is thus also called the *transport form* of vitamin A.
- **Retinal (an aldehyde):** It is the form found in visual pigment and can be easily converted by the body to retinoic acid.
- **Retinoids:** Refers to both natural and synthetic chemicals that are structurally related to vitamin A but may not have similar activity.

Sources

- **Animal sources:** Liver, fish, eggs, milk and butter are important dietary sources of preformed vitamin A.
- **Yellow and green leafy vegetables (spinach, carrots and squash)** supply large amounts of **beta-carotene and other carotenoids** that can be converted by the body into retinol and are referred to as **provitamin A carotenoids** (Flowchart 11.1**)**. The uptake of retinol in the peripheral tissue is dependent on cell surface receptors that are specific for RBP rather than retinol.

Functions

1. **Visual process:** The retina is located at back of the eye. When light passes through the lens, it is sensed by the retina and converted to a nerve impulse for interpretation by the brain.
   (a) *Retinol* is transported to the retina via circulation and accumulates in retinal pigment epithelial cells; retinol is esterified to form a *retinyl* ester, which can be stored.
   (b) When needed, retinyl esters are broken apart (hydrolysed) and isomerized to form 11-*cis-retinol,* which can be oxidized to form 11-*cis-retinal.*
   (c) 11-*cis*-retinal can be shuttled across to rod cells, where it binds to a protein called opsin to form the visual pigment, *rhodopsin (also known as visual purple).*
   (d) Rod cells with rhodopsin can detect very small amounts of light, making them important for night vision. Absorption of a photon of light catalyses isomerization of 11-*cis-retinal* to *all-trans-retinal,* and results in its release. This isomerization triggers a cascade of events, leading to generation of an electrical signal to optic nerve.
   (e) Once released, *all-trans-retinal is converted to all-trans-retinol,* which can be transported across retinal epithelial cell, thereby completing the visual cycle.
   (f) Inadequate retinol available to the retina results in impaired dark adaptation, known as **'night blindness'.**

Table 11.1 Differences between kwashiorkor and marasmus

Features	Kwashiorkor	Marasmus
Definition	Protein deficiency with adequate calorie intake	Starvation with a lack of overall calories
Age	<3 years	0–2 years
Clinical features		
Skeletal muscle	Relatively spared as visceral protein is decreased and somatic protein remains unchanged	Muscle protein catabolized for gluconeogenesis, loss of muscle mass **(broomstick extremities)**
Subcutaneous fat	Spared	Mobilized for energy (decreased adipose tissue leptin stores leading to lipolysis)
Liver protein stores	Markedly deprived/reduced—sometimes life-threatening	Depleted only marginally
Serum protein levels	Markedly decreased	Normal/slightly decreased
Oedema	Pitting oedema (which may be generalized or dependent) and ascites often present due to loss of plasma oncotic pressure as a result of hypoalbuminemia	Absent
Extremities	Oedematous	Patient looks emaciated; head appears too large as compared to body
Growth/mental retardation	Present but much less	Present; more severe
Weight loss	60%–80% of normal weight for the age and sex	Falls below the 60% of normal range
Skin lesions	**'Flaky paint'** appearance (alternating zone of hyperpigmentation, desquamation and hypo pigmentation)	Not generally seen
Hair changes	Loss of colour, alternating bands of pale and darker hair (flag sign), excessive hair fall	Not generally seen
Hepatomegaly	Presents with fatty change (decreased synthesis of ApoB-100 required for assembly of VLDL)	Not seen
Appetite	Lost; patient is apathetic, listless	Hungry and alert
Small bowel	Decrease in mitotic index in crypts, associated with mucosal atrophy and loss of villi and concurrent loss of brush border disaccaharides leading to diarrhoea	Rarely seen
Thymic and lymphoid atrophy	More marked	Less marked
Immune deficiency/recurrent infections	Present, lesser	Immune deficiency (mostly T cell) present, prone to recurrent infection

2. **Role in orderly differentiation of epithelium:** Retinoic acid is involved in switching on genes responsible for differentiating keratinocytes (immature skin cells) into mature epidermal cells. Retinoids also play a role in orderly maturation of mucus epithelial cells and deficiency of vitamin A results in metaplasia of mucus cells to keratin producing cells (squamous metaplasia).
3. **Role in gene transcription:** The production of retinoic acid is tightly regulated, as it acts a ligand for nuclear receptors. All-trans-retinoic acid (ATRA) regulates gene transcription by binding to nuclear receptors known as retinoic acid receptors (RARs), which are bound to DNA as heterodimers with retinoid 'X' receptors (RXRs). RAR and RXR must dimerize before they can bind to the DNA. The RAR-RXR heterodimer recognizes retinoic acid response elements (RAREs) on the DNA whereas the RXR-RXR homodimer recognizes retinoid 'X' response elements (RXREs) on the DNA; several RAREs near target genes have been shown to control physiological processes.
   (a) *All-trans-retinoic acid (ATRA)* exerts its effect by binding to retinoic acid receptor (*RAR*), which in turn is associated with nuclear receptors for 9-*cis*-retinoic acid (*RXR*) *forming RAR/RXR heterodimers*. These bind to promoter regions of multiple genes encoding for growth factors and tumour suppressor genes.
   (b) *ATRA* induces temporary remission of acute promyelocytic leukaemia and the *retinoic acid isomer,* 13-*cis retinoic acid,* has been used in the treatment of neuroblastoma.
4. **Role in host resistance to infections:**
   (a) Promotes the proliferation and differentiation of T cells (into regulatory T cells) through an indirect mechanism involving an increase in IL-2.
   (b) Important for T cell homing to the intestine, influences dendritic cell function and contributes to increased

Sources

Meats (preformed vitamin A) ↓ Vegetables (carotenes, provitamin A)

Absorbed as retinol ester and beta carotene by intestinal cells

↓

Transported to the liver as retinol in chylomicrons

↓

Taken up by liver cells through apolipoprotein receptors

↓

Undergoes esterification

↓

More than 90% stored in the liver in the Ito cells

↓

Rest transported to the tissues bound to retinol-binding protein (RBP)

↓ Oxidation

Retinoic acid

Note: The uptake of retinol in the peripheral tissue is dependent on cell surface receptors that are specific for RBP rather than retinol.

Flowchart 11.1 Sources and metabolism of vitamin A.

IgA secretion, which is important for the immune response in mucosal tissues.

(c) Maintains and restores integrity of mucosa.

Q. Enlist the manifestations of vitamin A deficiency.

Ans. Manifestations of vitamin A deficiency:

- First symptom of vitamin A deficiency is **decreased night vision** (vision in dim light).
- Ocular changes due to vitamin A deficiency are collectively known as **xerophthalmia (dry eye)**.
- First change is dryness of the conjunctivae, wherein; normal lacrimal and mucous-secreting epithelium is replaced by keratinized epithelium.
- This is followed by accumulation of keratin debris as small opaque plaques called **Bitot spots** (Fig. 11.1). There is erosion of surface of cornea, inducing formation of *corneal ulcers*, which may later lead to **softening and destruction of cornea (keratomalacia) and blindness.**
- The epithelium lining upper respiratory passage and urinary tract is replaced by keratinized squamous epithelium **(squamous metaplasia;** Fig. 11.2).
- Loss of mucociliary apparatus predisposes to secondary bacterial infections.

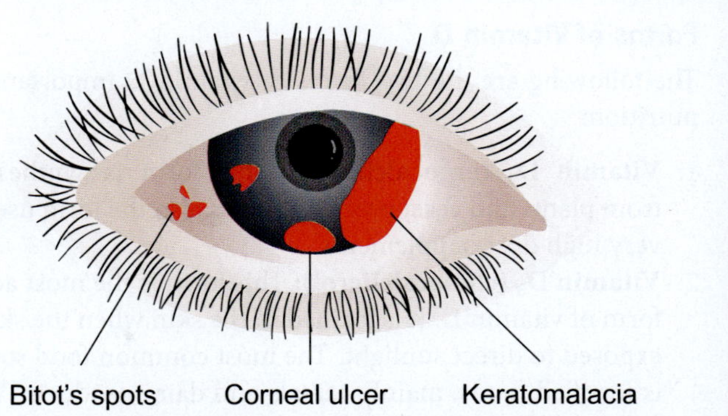

Fig. 11.1 Eye changes in vitamin A deficiency.

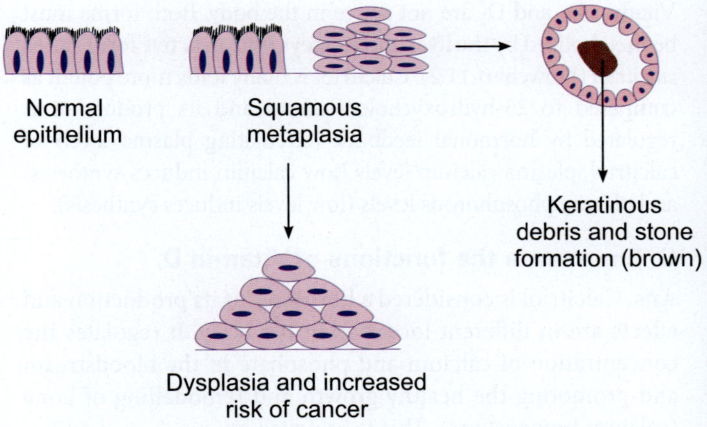

Fig. 11.2 Effects of vitamin A deficiency on skin and mucosa.

- Desquamation of keratinous debris in the urinary tract leads to renal and urinary bladder stones.
- Hyperplasia and hyperkeratinization of epidermis results in plugging of ducts of adnexal glands producing **follicular or papular dermatosis.**

Q. Write briefly on hypervitaminosis A.

Ans. Acute vitamin A toxicity manifests with symptoms similar to a space-occupying lesion in the brain. Chronic toxicity has the following manifestations:

- Nausea, vomiting, stomach discomfort
- Dry, scaly, peeling, and itchy skin, yellowish discolouration of the skin, cracks at the corners of the mouth, seborrhoea
- Hair loss and coarseness of hair
- Bone pain
- Poor appetite, fatigue
- Liver injury
- Headache, nervousness, irritability, dizziness, vision disturbances, cerebral oedema, papilledema (due to increased intracranial pressure)
- Hypercalcaemia, gastric mucosal calcinosis, heart valve calcification.

Q. Write briefly about the metabolism of vitamin D.

Ans. Vitamin D is necessary for the formation, growth and repair of bones. It also enhances immune function and improves muscle strength. Requirement for vitamin D increases as people age. It is stored mainly in the liver.

Forms of Vitamin D

The following are the two forms of vitamin D important for nutrition:

1. **Vitamin D_2 (ergocalciferol):** This form is synthesized from plants and yeast precursors. It is also the form used in very high dose supplements.
2. **Vitamin D_3 (cholecalciferol):** This form is the most active form of vitamin D. It is formed in the skin when the skin is exposed to direct sunlight. The most common food source is fortified foods, mainly cereals and dairy products. Vitamin D_3 is also present in fish liver oils. Human breast milk contains only small amounts of vitamin D_3.

Vitamin D_2 and D_3 are not active in the body. Both forms must be metabolized by the liver and kidneys into an active form called *calcitriol* (Flowchart 11.2). Calcitriol is many folds more potent as compared to 25-hydroxycholecalciferol and its production is regulated by hormonal feedback (circulating plasma levels of calcitriol, plasma calcium levels (low calcium induces synthesis) and plasma phosphorous levels (low levels induces synthesis).

Q. Enumerate the functions of Vitamin D.

Ans. Calcitriol is considered a hormone, as its production and effects are in different locations in the body. It regulates the concentration of calcium and phosphate in the bloodstream and promoting the healthy growth and remodelling of bone (calcium homeostasis). This is achieved by:

- Increasing intestinal absorption of calcium and phosphorus.
- Mobilizing calcium from bone to blood by causing osteoclastic reabsorption in collaboration with parathormone in the scenario of hypocalcaemia.
- Increasing distal tubular reabsorption of calcium, again, in collaboration with parathormone.

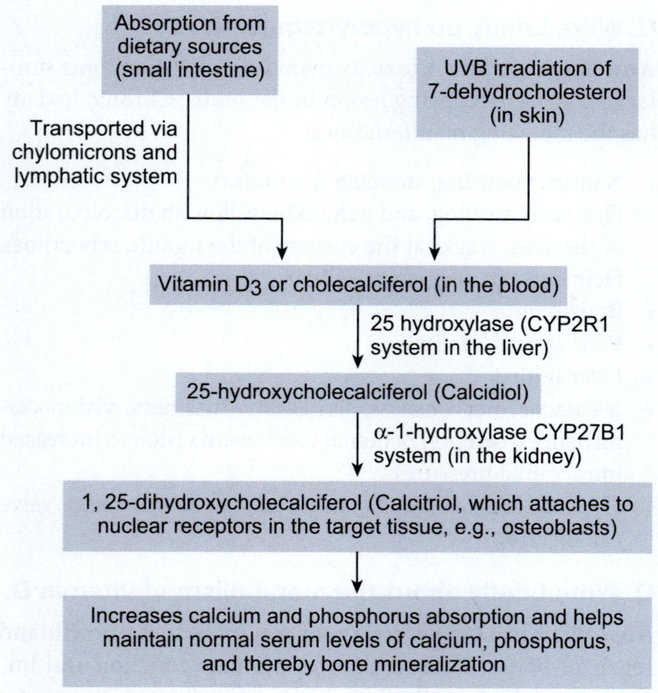

Flowchart 11.2 Sources and metabolism of vitamin D.

- Calcitriol also affects neuromuscular and immune function and has antiproliferative effects.

Q. Write briefly on the salient features of vitamin D deficiency.

Ans. Vitamin D deficiency can be caused by:

- The most common cause is inadequate exposure to sunlight. Thus, vitamin D deficiency occurs mainly among people who do not spend much time outdoors.
- Since breast milk contains only small amounts of vitamin D, breastfed infants are at risk of rickets.
- In malabsorption disorders, patients cannot absorb vitamin D because it is a fat-soluble vitamin, which is normally absorbed with fats in the small intestine.
- The body may not be able to convert vitamin D to an active form. Certain kidney and liver disorders and several rare hereditary disorders interfere with this conversion, as do certain drugs, such as some anticonvulsants and rifampin.

Bone Changes in Vitamin D Deficiency

- Vitamin D deficiency leads to overgrowth of epiphyseal cartilage. Unlike normal bone where cartilage resorption occurs and it is orderly replaced by osteoid matrix, there is persistence of overgrowth of cartilage with formation of irregular and distorted masses, which may project into marrow cavity. This results in enlarged costochondral junctions.
- Osteoid matrix is deposited on inadequately mineralized cartilaginous remnants.
- Also, there is abnormal overgrowth of capillaries and fibroblasts in the disorganized zone.
- Deformed bones are structurally weak.

Manifestations of Vitamin D Deficiency (Fig. 11.3)

- Manifests with **rickets** in children and **osteomalacia** in adults.
- In young infants who have rickets, the entire skull may be soft. Older infants may be slow to sit and crawl, and the spaces between the skull bones (fontanelles) may be slow to close.
- In children aged 1–4 years, bone growth may be abnormal, causing an abnormal curve in the spine and **bow legs or knock-knees**. These children may be slow to walk.
- For older children and adolescents, walking is painful. The pelvic bones may flatten, narrowing the birth canal in adolescent girls.
- Deformities of skeleton like **craniotabes** (parietal bones buckle inwards by pressure; with the release of pressure, elastic recoil snaps the bone back into its original position), **frontal bossing, squared appearance of frontal head** (due to excess of osteoid), **rachitic rosary** (overgrowth of cartilage or osteoid tissue at the costochondral junction), **pigeon chest deformity** (weakened metaphyseal areas of the ribs are subject to the pull of respiratory muscles and thus bend inward, creating anterior protrusion of the sternum) and **Harrison groove** (created by the inward pull at the margin of the diaphragm) are also seen.
- In adults, the spine is affected (**lumbar lordosis**), pelvis and leg bones weaken. Affected areas may be painful to touch,

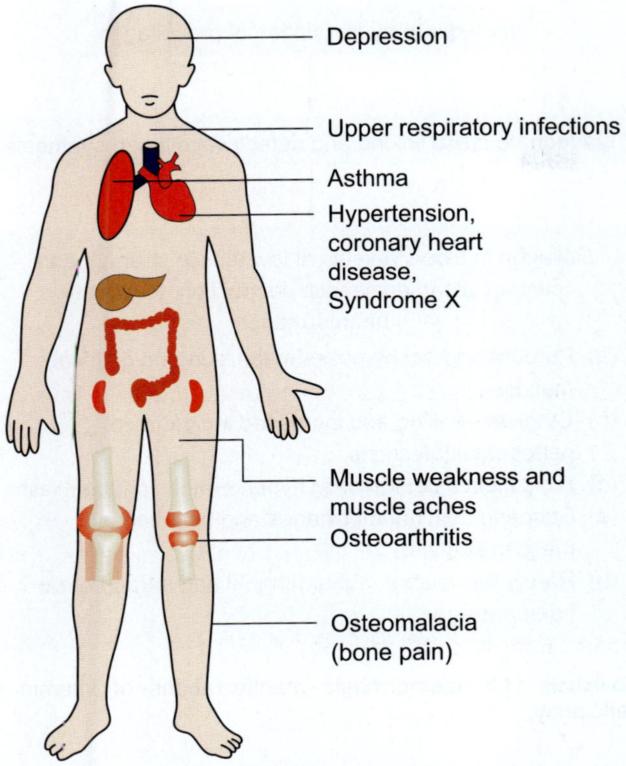

Fig. 11.3 Manifestations of vitamin D deficiency.

and fractures may occur. X-ray shows reduced bone density and radiolucent transverse defects in the neck of femur, ribs, scapula and pubic rami **(Milkman-Looser syndrome).**

- Biochemical changes in vitamin D deficiency include low levels of 25-hydroxy vitamin D, 1,25-dihydroxy vitamin D; calcium; phosphate and increased levels of alkaline phosphatase (owing to increased osteoclastic activity).

Factors Predisposing to Rickets and Osteomalacia

- Inadequate synthesis or dietary deficiency of vitamin D.
  - Inadequate exposure to sunlight.
  - Limited dietary intake of fortified foods.
  - Poor maternal nutrition during pregnancy and breast-feeding.
- Decreased absorption of vitamin D (fat-soluble vitamin)
  - Cholestatic liver disease.
  - Biliary tract obstruction.
  - Pancreatic insufficiency.
  - Diseases of small intestine.
- Deranged vitamin D metabolism.
  - Impaired synthesis of 25-hydroxy vitamin D.
  - Increased degradation of vitamin D and 25-hydroxy vitamin D.
  - Decreased synthesis of 1,25-dihydroxy vitamin D.
  - Resistance to action of 1,25-dihydroxy vitamin D.

Q. Write briefly about vitamin E deficiency.

Ans. Vitamin E belongs to a group of eight closely related fat-soluble compounds (four tocopherols and four tocotrienols) of which α-tocopherol is the most active.

- **Sources** include vegetables, nuts, grains and their oils, dairy products, fish and meat.
- **Absorption** requires normal biliary and pancreatic function.
- **Transported** in the blood in chylomicrons.
- **Stored** mainly in the fat depots; also in minor amounts in the liver and muscle.
- **Functions** as an antioxidant (terminates free radical generated lipid peroxidation reactions and prevents damage to the cellular and subcellular membranes). Vitamin E deficiency is common in individuals suffering from fat malabsorption, patients on total parenteral nutrition, and in premature infants (as the liver and gastrointestinal tract have not matured in them).
- **Pathologic changes** due to vitamin E deficiency are characteristically seen in the **nervous system (degeneration of axons in the posterior columns of the spinal cord and loss of neurons in the dorsal root ganglia). Vitamin E-deficient RBCs are more susceptible to oxidative damage and have a shorter half-life.**
- **Manifestations** include depressed tendon reflexes, ataxia, dysarthria, loss of position and vibration sense, muscle weakness, impaired vision and disorders of eye movement.

Q. Write briefly about vitamin K deficiency.

Ans. Vitamin K is a cofactor for a liver microsomal carboxylase, which carboxylates the glutamyl residues in certain proteins to carboxyglutamates, for example clotting factors like prothrombin, factors VII, IX and X. Carboxylation provides a calcium-binding site to allow calcium-dependent interactions of the clotting factors.

- Activation of **proteins** C and S also requires vitamin K-dependent carboxylation.
- Vitamin K–dependent carboxylation of **osteocalcin** (a protein secreted by osteoblasts) increases calcium and osteocalcin interaction and thereby favours bone calcification.
- Endogenous intestinal bacteria synthesize the vitamin, therefore, it is required in very small amounts in the diet.
- Active reduced form is converted to an epoxide after vitamin K reacts with its substrate; the epoxide reduced back by a liver epoxide reductase.
- Deficiency is seen in
  - Malabsorption syndromes (vitamin K is a fat-soluble vitamin).
  - Ingestion of broad spectrum antibiotics (which destroy the gut flora).
  - Neonatal period when the intestinal flora is not well developed, liver reserves are small and breast milk is low on vitamin K.
- **Deficiency** manifests as **bleeding diathesis (haematomas, haematuria, melena, ecchymoses and bleeding from the gums).**

Q. Write briefly about the sources, functions and deficiency of vitamin C.

Ans. The **sources** of vitamin C includes milk, fish, liver, fruits and vegetables; cannot be synthesized endogenously, thus humans are dependent on dietary intake. It is **absorbed** in the small intestine and stored in a variety of tissues particularly in the adrenal cortex.

Functions of Vitamin C

- **Role in collagen synthesis**
  - Accelerates hydroxylation and amidation reactions (hydroxylation of dopamine to norepinephrine).
  - Activates prolyl and lysyl hydroxylases for hydroxylation of procollagen (hydroxylation is important for a stable helical structure and cross linking).
  - Prevents oxidation of tetrahydrofolate to maintain folic acid levels.
  - Keeps iron in the reduced state to aid in its absorption.
- **Antioxidant action**
  - Scavenges free radicals and regenerates the antioxidant form of vitamin E; vitamins C and E act in concert to reduce atherosclerosis by reducing the oxidation of LDL.

Manifestations of Vitamin C Deficiency (Scurvy; Flowchart 11.3; Fig. 11.4)

- **Haemorrhagic diathesis.**
- **Skeletal changes** (Flowchart 11.4): Defect in osteoid formation (unlike rickets, in which the defect is in mineralization or calcification).
- **Delayed wound healing** (abnormal collagen synthesis and impaired fibroblast maturation).
- **Anaemia due to blood loss** (due to folic acid deficiency, hemorrhagic diathesis, deranged iron metabolism).
- **Dental lesions** (impaired dentine development, swollen bleeding gums, and gingivitis).

Inadequate hydroxylation of procollagen

↓

Inadequate cross linking and defective collagen synthesis

↓

Collagen in blood vessels of low tensile strength and susceptible to enzymatic destruction, leading to haemorrhages

(a) Purpura and ecchymoses in the skin and gingival mucosa.
(b) Gingival swelling and increased incidence of periodontal infections.
(c) A distinctive perifollicular hyperkeratotic papular rash.
(d) Subperiosteal haemorrhages and bleeding into the joint spaces.
(e) Rarely retrobulbar, subarachnoid and intracerebral haemorrhages.

Flowchart 11.3 Haemorrhagic manifestations of vitamin C deficiency.

Q. Write briefly about thiamine deficiency.

Ans. Vitamin B Complex is a group of substances, which are essential for the normal working of the body and, although not biochemically similar, are generally found together in the same foods. They include thiamine (vitamin B_1), riboflavin (vitamin B_2), pyridoxine (vitamin B_6) and cyanocobalamin (vitamin B_{12}).

- Thiamine plays an important role in helping the body metabolize carbohydrates and fats to produce energy. Absorption of thiamine in the gut is followed by its phosphorylation resulting in formation of thiamine pyrophosphate, which has three important functions:

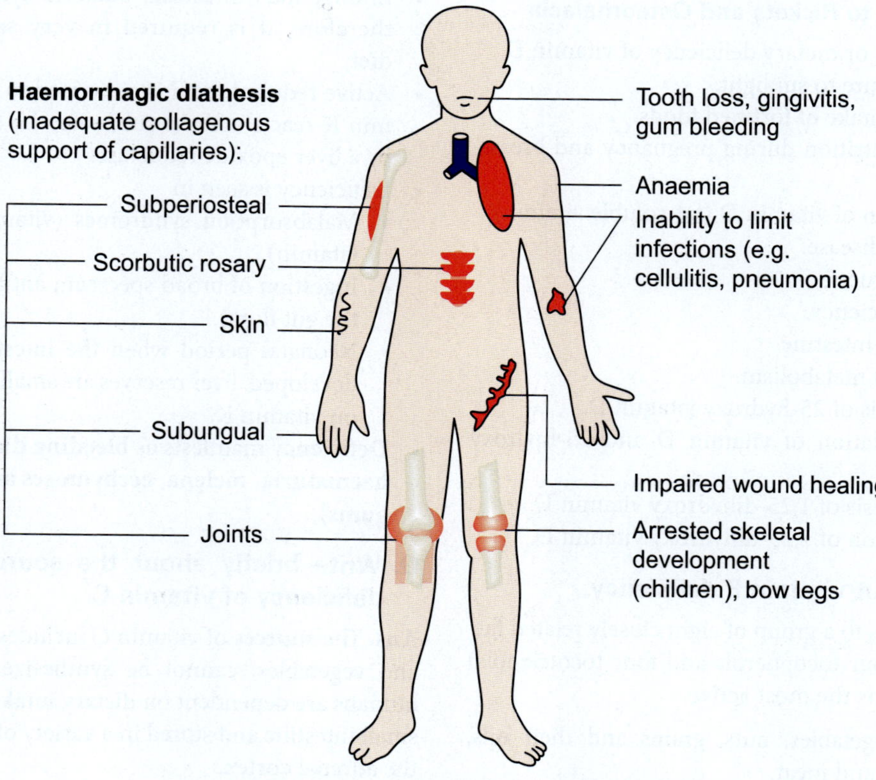

Fig. 11.4 Manifestations of vitamin C deficiency.

Normal cartilaginous matrix

↓ Vitamin C deficiency

Inadequate or defective osteoid formation (unlike rickets, in which the defect is in mineralization or calcification)

↓

Cartilaginous overgrowth
(a) Weak scorbutic bone.
(b) Bow legs.
(c) Abnormal depression of sternum and outward projection of the ends of ribs.

Flowchart 11.4 Skeletal changes in vitamin C deficiency.

- It regulates the oxidative decarboxylation of α-keto acids, responsible for synthesis of adenosine triphosphate.
- It is a cofactor for transketolase in pentose phosphate pathway.
- It maintains the integrity of neural membrane and ensures normal nerve conduction.

- Thiamine is essential for normal growth and development, and helps to maintain proper functioning of the heart, nervous and digestive systems.
- It is water-soluble and cannot be stored in the body; however, once absorbed, the vitamin concentrates in muscle tissue.
- **Sources** include green peas, spinach, liver, beef, pork, beans, nuts, bananas, whole grains, unpolished rice and legumes.
- **Deficiency** manifests as **Wernicke–Korsakoff syndromes** or **dry** and **wet beriberi**, and usually results from malnutrition, alcoholism, diets high in thiaminase-rich foods (raw freshwater fish, raw shellfish and ferns) and antithiamine factors (tea and coffee), debilitating illness, consumption of polished rice and protracted diarrhoea.
- **Dry beriberi** (Fig. 11.5) causes wasting and partial paralysis resulting from damaged peripheral nerves. It is also associated with tingling or loss of feeling (sensation) in hands and feet, mental confusion, speech difficulties and involuntary eye movements (nystagmus). It is thought to result from degeneration of myelin.
- **Wet beriberi** (Fig. 11.6) mainly affects the heart; it causes vasodilation, peripheral oedema, paroxysmal nocturnal dyspnoea, increased heart rate and eventually heart failure. The chronic form of wet beriberi consists of three stages. In the first stage, peripheral vasodilatation occurs, leading to a high-cardiac-output state. This leads to salt and water retention mediated through renin–angiotensin–aldosterone system in the kidneys. As the vasodilation progresses, the kidneys detect a relative loss of volume and respond by conserving salt. With salt retention, fluid is also absorbed into the circulatory system. The resulting fluid overload leads to oedema of dependent extremities. By the time significant oedema occurs, the heart has been exposed to a severely high workload in order to pump required cardiac output needed to satisfy end-organ requirements. This causes parts of the heart muscle to undergo overuse injury.

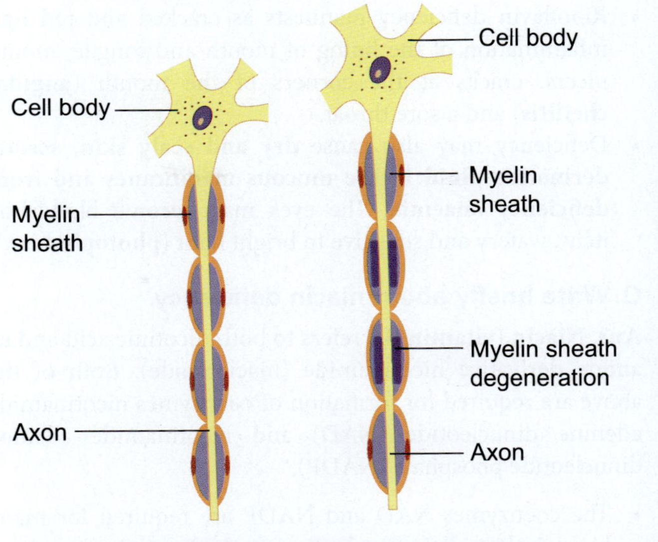

Fig. 11.5 Myelin degeneration in dry beriberi.

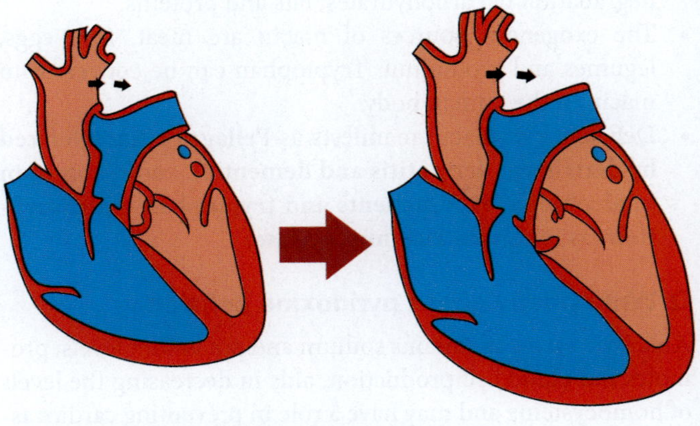

Fig. 11.6 Dilated heart showing flabby chambers in wet beriberi.

- A more rapid form of wet beriberi is termed **acute fulminant cardiovascular beriberi** or **Shoshin beriberi**. In this form, oedema may not be present. Instead, cyanosis of hands and feet, tachycardia, distended neck veins, restlessness and anxiety occur. It is because of damage to the heart muscle and its inability to cope with the demands of the body. Treatment with thiamine causes low-output cardiac failure because systemic vasoconstriction is reinstated before the heart muscle recovers.

Q. Write briefly about riboflavin deficiency.

Ans. Riboflavin is a yellow or yellow-orange coloured vitamin, which can be used as a food colouring. Large quantities of riboflavin are often included in multivitamins. The excess is excreted in the urine, causing the urine to be coloured bright yellow.

- **Deficiency** of riboflavin can be **primary**, which is diet related, or **secondary**, which may be a result of conditions that affect absorption in the intestine, the body not being able to use the vitamin, or an increase in the excretion of the vitamin from the body.

- Riboflavin deficiency manifests as cracked and red lips, inflammation of the lining of mouth and tongue, mouth ulcers, cracks at the corners of the mouth (**angular cheilitis**) and a sore throat.
- Deficiency may also cause **dry and scaly skin, scrotal dermatitis, fluid in the mucous membranes and iron-deficiency anaemia**. The eyes may become bloodshot, itchy, watery and sensitive to bright light (**photophobia**).

Q. Write briefly about niacin deficiency.

Ans. Niacin (vitamin B_4) refers to both nicotinic acid and its amide derivative nicotinamide (niacinamide). Both of the above are required for formation of coenzymes nicotinamide adenine dinucleotide (NAD) and nicotinamide adenine dinucleotide phosphate (NADP).

- The coenzymes NAD and NADP are required for many biological oxidation–reduction (redox) reactions responsible for energy generation in tissues by the biochemical degradation of carbohydrates, fats and proteins.
- The exogenous sources of niacin are meat, fish, eggs, legumes and groundnut. Tryptophan can be converted to niacin in the human body.
- Deficiency of niacin manifests as **Pellagra (characterized by diarrhoea, dermatitis and dementia)**, and is **common in alcoholics, HIV patients and tryptophan malabsorption (as is seen in Hartnup disease)**.

Q. Write briefly about pyridoxine deficiency.

Ans. Pyridoxine maintains sodium and potassium levels, promotes red blood cell production, aids in decreasing the levels of homocysteine and may have a role in preventing cardiovascular problems. Pyridoxine is precursor to pyridoxal phosphate, cofactor for enzyme aromatic amino acid decarboxylase, which is involved in the following reactions:

(a) 5-Hydroxytryptophan → Serotonin.
(b) Levodopa → Dopamine.

- **Sources** of pyridoxine include milk, meat, egg yolk, fish, legumes and vegetables.
- The following predispose to pyridoxine deficiency:
  - Pregnancy and infancy (due to increased demand).
  - Alcoholism (acetaldehyde, an alcohol metabolite, induces rapid degeneration of pyridoxine).
  - Drug intake (isoniazid and oestrogen).
- Manifestations of pyridoxine deficiency include anaemia, nerve damage, seizures, skin problems and oral ulcers.

Note: ***Folic acid and vitamin B_{12} are discussed in Chapter 23.***

Q. What are trace elements.

Ans. The human body needs a number of minerals in trace (milligram) or ultra trace (microgram) quantities. These are listed in Table 11.2. Of the 18 microminerals thought to be essential only four have been studied in detail.

Table 11.2 Functions and deficiency manifestations of trace elements

Mineral	Functions	Deficiency
Iron	Component of haemoglobin and other iron containing metalloenzymes (cytochromes)	Microcytic hypochromic anaemia
Zinc	Component of various enzymes specially oxidase	Anaemia, impaired growth and sexual maturation, hepatosplenomegaly, skin rash, alopecia
Copper	Involved in collagen synthesis and suppression of free radicals	Anaemia, impaired collagen synthesis and wound healing, lethargy, neurological deficits and muscle weakness
Manganese	Component of metalloenzymes	Abnormalities of connective tissue and bone
Molybdenum	Agent for electron transfer; component of xanthine oxidase	Clinical features not well defined; however, neurological abnormalities have been noted
Selenium	Component of glutathione peroxidase	Haemolytic anaemia and degeneration of skeletal and cardiac muscle (myopathy and cardiomyopathy)
Fluoride	Unknown	Tooth decay
Iodine	Component of thyroid hormone	Goitre
Cobalt	Required for biosynthesis of vitamin B_{12} family of coenzymes	B_{12} deficiency
Magnesium	Intracellular ion which acts as a cofactor in oxidative phosphorylation in the synthesis or utilization of ATP	Interference with oxidative phosphorylation

Q. Write briefly on the role of diet in carcinogenesis.

Ans. The human diet is a highly complex and variable mixture of naturally occurring and synthetic chemicals. The naturally occurring chemicals include macronutrients (fat, carbohydrate and protein), micronutrients (vitamins and trace metals) and non-nutrient constituents. Several carcinogens and anticarcinogens have been identified in the human diet.

Dietary Carcinogens

These are broadly classified into four categories:

1. **Naturally present carcinogens:** 'Aflatoxin', is an example of a naturally occurring dietary carcinogen. It is a mycotoxin produced by *Aspergillus flavus,* and is implicated in the pathogenesis of hepatocellular carcinoma. Aflatoxicosis is caused by intake of grains and nuts contaminated by the fungus.
2. **Carcinogens forming during food preparation:** Burnt or barbecued foods contain a group of carcinogenic substances

called polycyclic aromatic hydrocarbons, which are produced if food is overheated. High intake of fried and broiled food, such as meats, can increase the risk of breast, colon, prostate and pancreatic cancers.

3. **Preservatives and colouring agents added to food:** Artificial sweeteners (like saccharine and cyclamates) are known to cause bladder cancer. Cured, pickled or salty foods contain nitrates, which have been implicated in gastric cancer.
4. **Substances that are converted into carcinogens in the body:** Sodium nitrite which may be present in drinking water and vegetables gets converted to nitrosamine, which is a carcinogen.

Cancer-Preventing Diets

- Fruits and vegetables in the diet are thought to lower the risk of cancer.
- Retinoic acid promotes differentiation of mucous-secreting epithelial cells; therefore, diets containing β-carotene and retinoic acid can reverse metaplastic and precancerous lesions of the respiratory tract.
- High fibre content with low animal fat content in the diet prevents colonic carcinoma (high fat and low fibre content means high level of bile salts and acids in intestine, leading to increased levels of free radicals and carcinogenic by-products of bile acid metabolism).
- Folic acid, selenium, β-carotene, vitamin C and vitamin E are thought to prevent free radical damage to cell and its DNA; thus, preventing 'cancer initiation'. Vitamin A enhances immunity and may control free radical production by modulating inflammatory reactions.

Q. Write briefly on the definition, etiopathogenesis and pathologic consequences of obesity. (PA12.3)

Ans. Obesity is defined as abnormal or excessive fat accumulation that presents a risk to health. A crude population measure of obesity is the **body mass index (BMI)**—a person's weight (in kilograms) divided by the square of his or her height (in meters). The BMI, also known as the **Quetelet index**, is used more commonly than **body fat percentage** to define obesity. A person with a BMI of 30 or more is generally considered obese. A person with a BMI equal to or more than 25 is considered overweight. The most commonly used definitions, established by the World Health Organization provide values listed below (Table 11.3).

Table 11.3 Definitions of obesity (established by World Health Organization)

BMI (kg/m²)	Classification
<18.5	Underweight
18.5–24.9	Normal weight
25.0–29.9	Overweight
30.0–34.9	Class I obesity
35.0–39.9	Class II obesity
≥40.0	Class III obesity

Any BMI ≥35 or 40 is **severe obesity** which is further classified into:

- Severe obesity—BMI greater than 40 kg/m².
- Morbid obesity—BMI of 40–50 kg/m².
- Super obese—BMI greater than 50 kg/m².

In children, a BMI above the 85th percentile (for age-matched and sex-matched control subjects) is commonly used to define overweight, and a BMI above the 95th percentile is commonly used to define obesity.

Adiposity (percent fat) increases as a curvilinear function of BMI. **Fat-free mass** (mass of skeletal muscles and visceral organs) also increases in relation to BMI.

Aetiolopathogenesis of Obesity (Fig 11.7)

1. **Energy expenditure**
   (a) Energy expenditure (EE) of the human body has three main components: resting metabolic rate (RMR), activity-related energy expenditure (AEE), and diet-induced thermogenesis (DIT). RMR is defined as the metabolism of an individual at rest (energy requirements for maintenance of vital body functions). In sedentary adults, RMR accounts for 60%–75% of total daily EE. A low RMR is a predisposing factor for weight gain.
   (b) AEE is further categorized into exercise activity thermogenesis (EAT) and non-exercise activity thermogenesis (NEAT). NEAT is the predominant contributor to EE and comprises all physical activities other than sports/exercises. DIT is the increase in metabolic rate associated with the ingestion of food. DIT accounts for 5%–15% of total EE (energy is spent on digestion, absorption and metabolism).
   (c) Most studies do not support hypotheses of altered RMR and/or DIT in obesity, but lower NEAT and EAT are thought to contribute to body weight gain. When an individual ingests more energy than it expends, a positive energy balance develops and excess energy is stored as high-energy molecules. 60%–80% of excess energy is converted into fat.
   (d) Low metabolic efficiency implies an increase in heat production at the expense of ATP production (and conversion into triglycerides). Enhanced metabolic efficiency has been reported to contribute to obesity.
2. **Genetic contribution to obesity**
   (a) A widely held view is that obesity results from an interaction between environment/lifestyle and genetic susceptibility.
   (b) Obesity is polygenic in inheritance with contribution from several genes. Genome-wide association study-based data suggest a genetic predisposition for obesity with identification of more than 140 genetic chromosomal regions related to obesity. A few genes with a large effect on BMI have been identified including genes encoding components of **leptin** and **melanocortin signalling,** as well as genes along a specific region of chromosome 15 responsible for **Prader-Willi syndrome**. In contrast to such monogenetic cases,

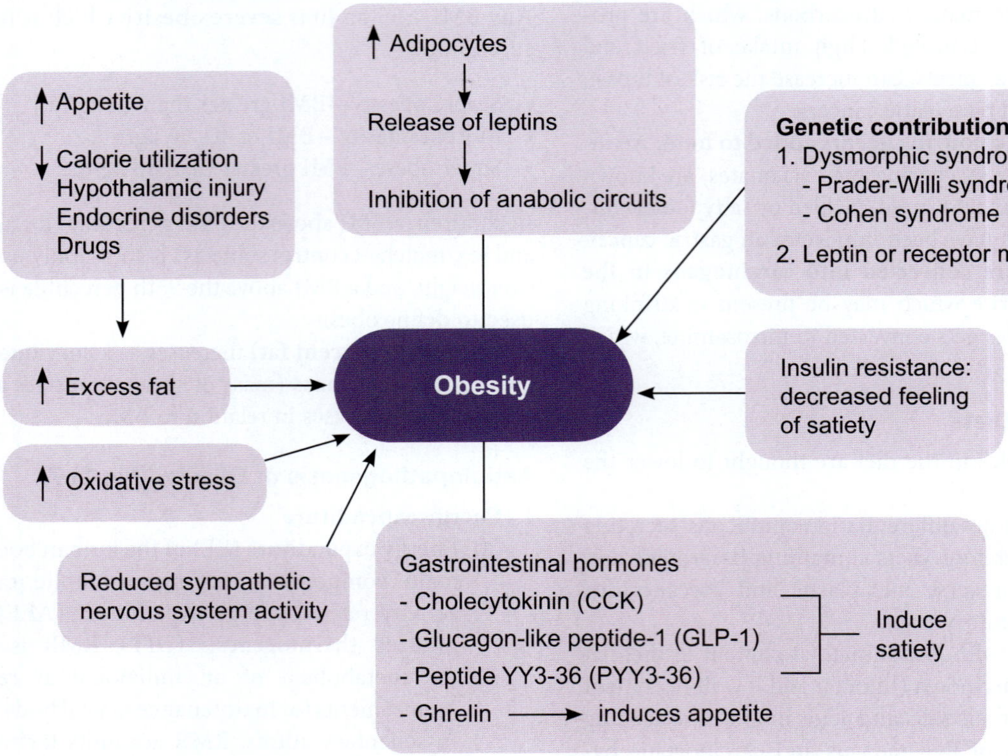

Fig. 11.7 Etiopathogenesis of obesity.

common obesity is thought to be associated with a large number of genes with small effect sizes.

3. **Sympathetic nervous system (SNS):** Feeding, especially carbohydrate overfeeding is associated with increased SNS activity. Fasting on the other hand reduces SNS activity. Leptin and insulin are the most likely mediators of SNS activity. The SNS promotes pancreatic insulin release, adipolysis, skeletal muscle glucose uptake and hepatic glucose mobilization. Reduced SNS-mediated adipose tissue lipolysis is thought to contribute to increased lipid accumulation and obesity. Altered regulation of core temperature by the SNS also predisposes to weight gain (lower core temperature, lower RMR).
4. **Homeostatic and hedonic pathways**
   (a) Of the two major systems that control food intake, the **homeostatic pathway** stimulates eating behaviour when energy stores are low. The **hypothalamus and brainstem** have been identified as its central processing units, which coordinate with the peripheral signals (circulating concentrations of nutrients, gastrointestinal hormones, insulin, leptin and vagal afferents), to determine the hunger versus satiety responses in order to adjust food intake. The **hedonic**, or reward-based, pathway can override the homeostatic system.
   (b) The neurohumoral mechanisms that regulate the body weight have three components:
      (i) The **afferent system,** which generates humoural signals. It is mainly constituted by **appetite suppressing signals** from (1) **leptin and adiponectin** produced by adipocytes, (2) **insulin** produced by pancreas, (3) **resistine** produced by macrophages and (4) **ghrelin** produced by the endocrine cells of the stomach and (5) peptide YY (PYY) and glucagon-like peptide (GLP-1) from the ileum and colon.
      (ii) The **central processing unit**, located primarily in hypothalamus. Integrates afferent signals.
      (iii) The **effector system** carries out 'orders' from hypothalamic nuclei in the form of feeding behaviour and energy expenditure.

Adipocytes communicate with the hypothalamic centres by secreting **leptin**—a member of the cytokine family. **Leptin seems to have a more important role than insulin in the CNS control of calorie balance**. When there is an abundance of stored energy in form of adipose tissue, resultant high levels of leptin cross blood–brain barrier, binding to leptin receptors. Leptin receptor signalling has two effects: it inhibits anabolic circuits that normally promote food intake and inhibit energy expenditure. Hence, over a period of time, energy stores (adipocytes) are reduced and weight is lost. This, in turn, reduces circulating levels of leptin, and a new equilibrium is reached. This cycle is reversed when adipose tissue is lost and leptin levels are reduced below a threshold. In obese people with elevated leptin levels, impaired leptin signalling, that is, leptin resistance, is implicated. The **leptin-melanocortin pathway** plays a major role in energy balance. Leptin stimulates **POMC (pro-opiomelanocortin) neurons** in the arcuate nucleus to produce a series of **melanocortin peptides**. The melanocortin α-MSH binds with high affinity to melanocortin 3 receptor (MC3R) and MC4R in the paraventricular nucleus. Mutations in genes involved in the leptin-melanocortin tract have been found to be associated with (childhood-onset) obesity.

Decreased serotonin signalling in the hypothalamus is hypothesized to contribute to obesity by impairing negative feedback from ingested energy on food intake, thus promoting over consumption. Serotonin activates the anorexigenic α-melanocyte-stimulating hormone (α-MSH), a product of pro-opiomelanocortin (POMC) neurons, and inhibits the orexigenic neuropeptide Y (NPY) and Agouti-related peptide (AgRP) neurons located in the arcuate nucleus of the hypothalamus.

Insulin contributes to post-prandial metabolism, is involved in nutritional feedback: and its effects on the hypothalamus promote satiety, whereas it enhances dopamine release in the striatum. Obesity is characterized by insulin resistance, and insulin-mediated nutritional feedback may be impaired in obesity.

Gut hormones and peptides are important modulators of metabolism and food intake, thereby contributing to the control of energy balance. Hypoglycaemia induces release of **ghrelin**, which acts on **neuropeptide Y (NPY) and agouti-related peptide (AgRP) neurons in the arcuate nucleus of the hypothalamus**. The neurotransmitters thus released act on **melanin-concentrating hormone (MCH) and orexin** to **increase appetite and induce adipose tissue deposition**. Also known as **orexigenic or hunger hormone**, it is primarily produced in the gastric fundus. Its levels go up during fasting and its secretion is suppressed postprandially. Ghrelin stimulates appetite and human obesity is associated with reduced postprandial ghrelin suppression. **Anorexigenic intestinal hormones**, include glucagon-like peptide 1 (GLP1), peptide YY (PYY), and cholecystokinin (CCK) (Fig. 11.7).

5. **Gut microbiota:** This facilitates the digestion of dietary components and it has been hypothesized that gut microbiota contribute to weight gain through this mechanism.

Co-morbidities of Obesity

Overweight and obesity are major risk factors for a number of chronic diseases, including diabetes, metabolic syndrome, cardiovascular diseases and cancer. Once considered a problem only in high-income countries, overweight and obesity are now dramatically on the rise in low- and middle-income countries; particularly, in the urban settings. Obesity is most commonly caused by a combination of excessive food intake, lack of physical activity and genetic susceptibility, although a few cases are caused due to endocrine disorders, medications or psychiatric illness. Other obesity-associated conditions include gallstones, pancreatitis, abdominal hernia, non-alcoholic steatohepatitis (NASH), gastroesophageal reflux disease (GERD), polycystic ovarian disease, abnormal pulmonary function, sleep apnoea, deep vein thrombosis, osteoarthritis and gout.

SECTION II

HAEMATOLOGY

Normal Haematopoiesis and Disorders of Red Cells

12

Q. Write briefly on the normal sequence of development of cells of haematopoietic system. (PA13.1)

Ans. Haematopoiesis is the formation of formed elements of blood from stem cells. There are **three main types of mature cells in the circulation, namely, red blood cells (erythrocytes), white blood cells (leukocytes) and platelets (thrombocytes).** Red blood cells (RBCs) are responsible for oxygen transport, white blood cells (WBCs) for body defense and platelets for coagulation and maintenance of the homeostasis (blood vessel integrity and prevention of blood loss). **Haematopoietic stem cells (HSCs)** in the bone marrow reside in a specialized microenvironment known as the HSCs niche, composed of osteoblasts, mesenchymal cells and sinusoidal vessels. Cytokines control the differentiation of HSCs. External factors like hypoxia also contribute to control of haematopoiesis, for example hypoxia results in a compensatory increase in the number of erythrocytes.

Haematopoiesis begins in the yolk sac during the third week of foetal embryonic development. HSCs that give rise to lymphoid and myeloid cells are thought to take origin from the mesoderm of the intraembryonic aorta/gonad/mesonephros (AGM) region, with some evidence pointing to an origin within a small subset of yolk sac-derived cells. In the third month of embryogenesis, stem cells derived from the AGM and/or yolk sac migrate to the liver. In the fourth month of development, stem cells migrate to the bone marrow to initiate haematopoiesis at this site. Bone marrow throughout the skeleton is haematopoietically active at birth and remains active up to puberty (Table 12.1). By the age of 18 years, only the vertebrae, ribs, sternum, skull, pelvis and proximal epiphyseal regions of the humerus and femur retain red marrow, the remaining marrow becoming yellow, fatty and inactive. Thus, in adults, only about half of the marrow space is active in haematopoiesis. With an increased demand for blood cells in the adult, the fatty marrow can transform to red, active marrow and haematopoiesis can start in other organs besides bone marrow (the latter is called **extramedullary haematopoiesis**).

Table 12.1 Sites of haematopoiesis

Foetus	• 0–2 Months	Yolk sac
	• 2 months of gestation to 2 weeks after birth	Liver, spleen
	• 5–9 months	Bone marrow
Infants		Bone marrow (all bones)
Adults		Vertebrae, ribs, sternum, skull, sacrum and pelvis, proximal ends of femur

HSCs are rare, nucleated cells in the bone marrow which show immunological positivity for CD34 (a cell surface protein responsible for their homing into the marrow after infusion) and negativity for CD38. These cells resemble a small or medium-sized lymphocytes and give rise to the committed haemopoietic progenitors, which are restricted in their developmental potential (demonstrated by in vitro culture techniques). Colony-forming unit (CFU)-GEMM is an example of an earliest detectable mixed myeloid precursor which gives rise to granulocytes, erythrocytes, monocytes and megakaryocytes. Lymphocytes also differentiate from a common lymphoid precursor.

The stem cells can self-renew to maintain the marrow cellularity. Bone marrow functions as an environment for stem cell survival, growth, and development. It is composed of stromal cells (adipocytes, fibroblasts, endothelial cells and macrophages) and a microvascular network. The stromal cells lay down the extracellular matrix and secrete growth factors (cytokines), which aid in haematopoiesis. Cytokines including interleukin-3 and GM-CSF induce cell proliferation, while other cytokines including flt-3 ligand and kit ligand protect cells from apoptosis and sensitize them to the effects of growth promoting cytokines. Cytokines also facilitate the interactions between stem cells and elements in the microenvironment including extracellular matrix components. Regulators of HSCs include transforming growth factor-beta (TGF-β) and tumour necrosis factor-alpha (TNF-α). These modulate cell cycle activity and engraftment. Newly discovered cytokines including Wnt and the notch ligand family may also have important effects on stem cell biology. The homing of stem cells, which involves surface adhesion molecules, makes it possible to perform bone marrow transplantation by infusing donor stem cells into the peripheral blood. Circulating marrow derived stem cells have the peculiar property of being able to seed other tissues and develop into non-haematopoietic cells as well.

Haematopoietic Growth Factors

The various haematopoietic growth factors are tabulated in Table 12.2.

Table 12.2 Haematopoietic growth factors and their effects

Haematopoietic growth factors	Main effects
IL-1, -2, -3, -6	• Exert their primary effects early in stem cell differentiation, and are therefore, important for the differentiation of multiple blood lineages. • IL-1 and -2 are B and T cell regulators. • IL-3 stimulates granulocytes, macrophages, eosinophils, and megakaryocyte colonies. • IL-6 converts lymphocytes into cytotoxic lymphocytes, increases the expression of IL-2R receptor, and converts B cells into plasma cells.
IF-γ	Increases NK cell activity and decreases apoptosis.
IF-α	Increases NK cell activity and promotes class II antigen expression on B and T cells.
EPO	• It is a heat-stable glycoprotein having a molecular weight of 36 kD, which acts on BFU-E and CFU-E. • EPO gene is present on human chromosome 7q21. It is the prime regulator of erythropoiesis and is responsible for differentiation and proliferation of erythropoietic cells. • Hypoxia induces the release of 'renal erythropoietic factor' from juxtaglomerular cells of kidney. • Renal erythropoietic factor acts on a plasma α globulin to form erythropoietin.
G-CSF	Promotes the differentiation of granulocytes as well as development of fully mature neutrophils from stem cells.
GM-CSF	Induces an increase in neutrophils, eosinophils, macrophages, and sometimes lymphocyte counts.
TPO	Most potent cytokine promoting proliferation and maturation of megakaryocytes.

EPO, Erythropoietin; G-CSF, granulocyte colony-stimulating factor; GM-CSF, granulocyte macrophage colony-stimulating factor; IF-α, interferon-α; IF-γ, interferon-γ; IL, interleukin; TPO, thrombopoietin.
Note: G-CSF, GM-CSF, and TPO exert their effects later in the differentiation cascade, and their effects are more lineage specific.

Sequence of Development of Cells of Haematopoietic System

The formed elements of blood (RBCs, granulocytes, monocytes, platelets, and lymphocytes) have a common origin from **pluripotent HSCs**. The pluripotent stem cell gives rise to two main types of multipotent progenitors: the **common lymphoid** and the **common myeloid stem cell**. The **common lymphoid stem cell** in turn gives rise to **precursors of T cells (pro-T cells), B cells (pro-B cells) and natural killer cells** (Flowchart 12.1; Fig. 12.1).

From the **common myeloid stem cell** arises at least three types of **committed stem cells** capable of differentiating along the **erythroid/megakaryocytic, eosinophilic and granulocyte macrophage** pathways. The committed stem cells are called *CFUs*, because each can give rise to colonies of differentiated progeny. The various committed stem cells give rise to the morphologically recognizable precursors of the differentiated cells, such as proerythroblasts, myeloblasts, megakaryoblasts, monoblasts and eosinophiloblasts, which in turn give rise to mature progeny.

Erythropoiesis

Proerythroblast (Pronormoblast)

- This earliest precursor of the erythrocyte-forming series measures about 14–20 µm in size.
- It has a fine, uniform, intensely staining nuclear chromatin (as opposed to a myeloblast), and one or two prominent nucleoli. The nucleus of a proerythroblast is large, occupies almost 80% of the cell.
- The cytoplasm is mild to moderate in amount, more basophilic than that of a myeloblast and agranular.
- Proerythroblasts are seen in the circulating blood only under pathological conditions like extramedullary haematopoiesis, breakdown of the blood–bone marrow barrier by tumour metastases, or erythroleukaemia.
- Erythroblasts undergo mitosis to give rise to *normoblasts*.

Erythroblast (Normoblast)

- An ***early (basophilic) normoblast*** is 12–16 µm in size; has a more basophilic cytoplasm (due to abundant ribonucleic acid) than a proerythroblast; and has a deeply staining, large nucleus with clumped chromatin (wheel with broad spokes pattern) and inconspicuous nucleoli. A blue, a perinuclear halo and a small pale area (Golgi apparatus) may be seen due to active RNA synthesis.
- An ***intermediate (polychromatic) normoblast*** is 12–16 µm in size. It is labelled 'polychromatic' because it has a cytoplasm that is essentially basophilic but is taking on a pink hue due to initiation of haemoglobinization. The nuclear size is smaller than an early normoblast and stains intensely.
- ***Late (orthochromatic) normoblast*** is a cell that is no longer able to divide. Its size varies between 8 and 12 µm and its cytoplasm is more abundant and pink than an intermediate normoblast. The nuclei of these cells gradually condense and are eventually expelled from the cells. Polychromatic and orthochromatic normoblasts may be released into the bloodstream whenever haematopoiesis is activated or when the turnover of blood cells is increased (haemolysis), such as in myeloproliferative diseases and bone marrow malignancy, which destroy the blood–bone marrow barrier.
- The orthochromatic normoblasts give rise to enucleated young erythrocytes containing abundant ribosomes that precipitate into reticular (net-like) structures after special

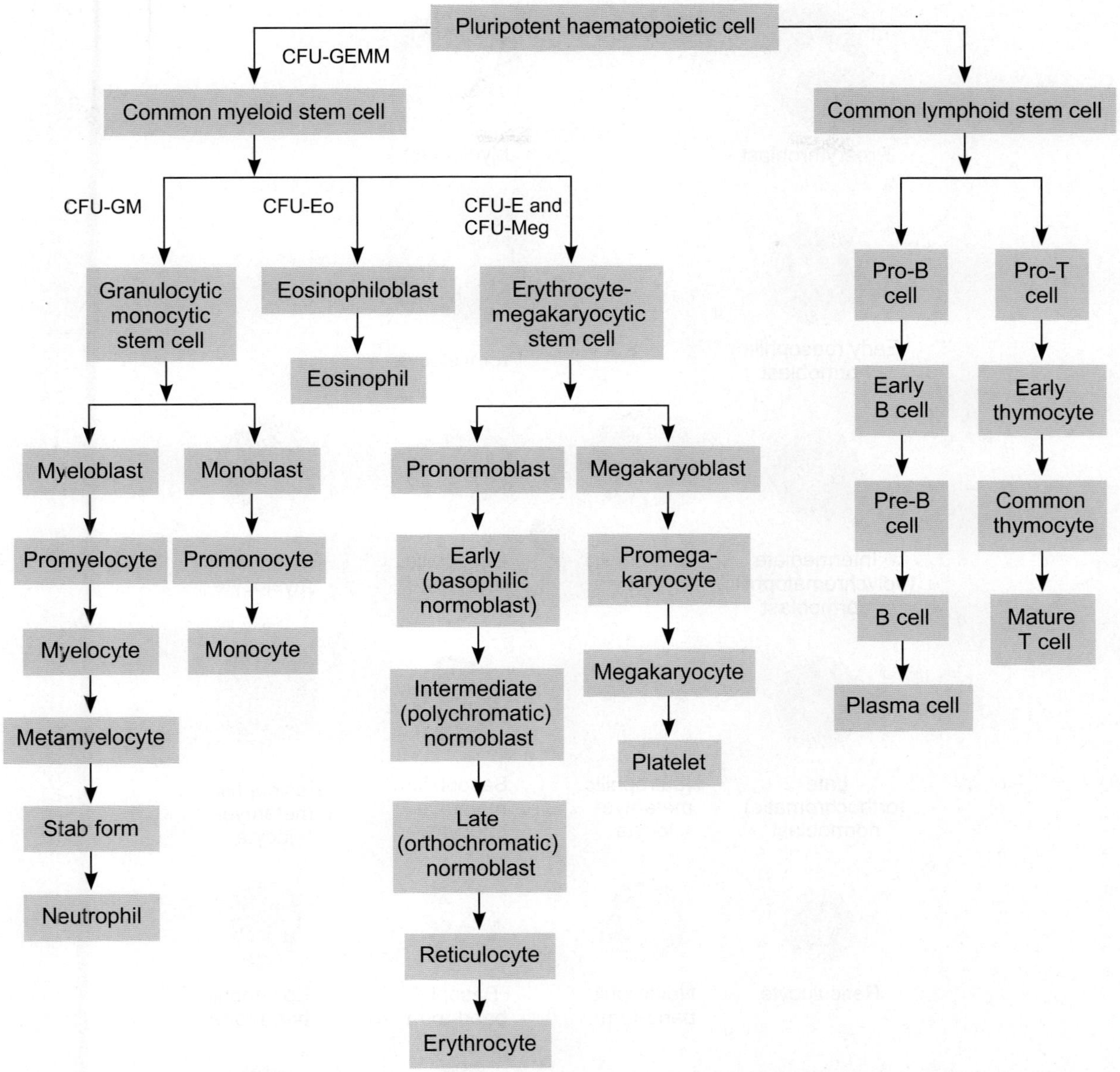

Flowchart 12.1 Normal sequence of development of cells of haematopoietic system. CFU-GEMM, Colony-forming unit granulocytes, erythrocytes, monocytes, and megakaryocytes; CFU-GM, colony-forming unit granulocytes and monocytes; CFU-E0, colony-forming unit eosinophils; CFU-E, colony-forming unit erythrocytes; CFU-Meg, colony-forming unit megakaryocytes.

staining and are labelled ***reticulocytes***. *Reticulocyte count* can be done by supra vital staining with dyes like new methylene blue or brilliant cresyl blue. Reticulocytes are normally found in the peripheral blood in the range of 0.5%–2.5% in adults and 2%–6% in infants. Their number increases in conditions of rapid erythropoiesis (post-haemorrhage, haemolysis, or in patients of anaemia on therapy).

- Reticulocytes give rise to ***mature erythrocytes***—biconcave cells with a diameter of 6.7–7.7 μm and a thickness of 1.7–2.4 μm. They lack a cell nucleus and most organelles, in order to provide maximum space for haemoglobin. They have a central pale area that occupies less than one-third of the total area of the cell. The cytoplasm of erythrocytes is rich in haemoglobin, an iron-containing molecule that transports oxygen and is responsible for the red colour of the cells. The red cell membrane is a highly deformable, non-expansile, trilaminar structure composed of a lipid layer which is traversed by several transmembrane proteins like glycophorin A (GPA) and anion exchanger 1 (AE1, formerly called band 3 protein). The cytoplasmic side of the cell membrane has a network of several cytoskeletal proteins, for example, spectrin, actin, protein 4.1 and ankyrin. The spectrin network is largely responsible for the shear elastic properties of the red cells. Integral and peripheral proteins connect the lipid bilayer and spectrin network. Important lipids include phospholipids and unesterified cholesterol. Their ability to undergo changes in their shape allow them to negotiate the circulatory system, specially the capillaries that have a diameter of only 3.5 μm. Besides the flexible membrane, the biconcave and discoid RBC has a high surface-to-volume ratio that also facilitates reversible deformation of the RBC as it repeatedly passes through microcirculation. Pathological conditions affecting red cell shape can interfere with its elasticity. Approximately

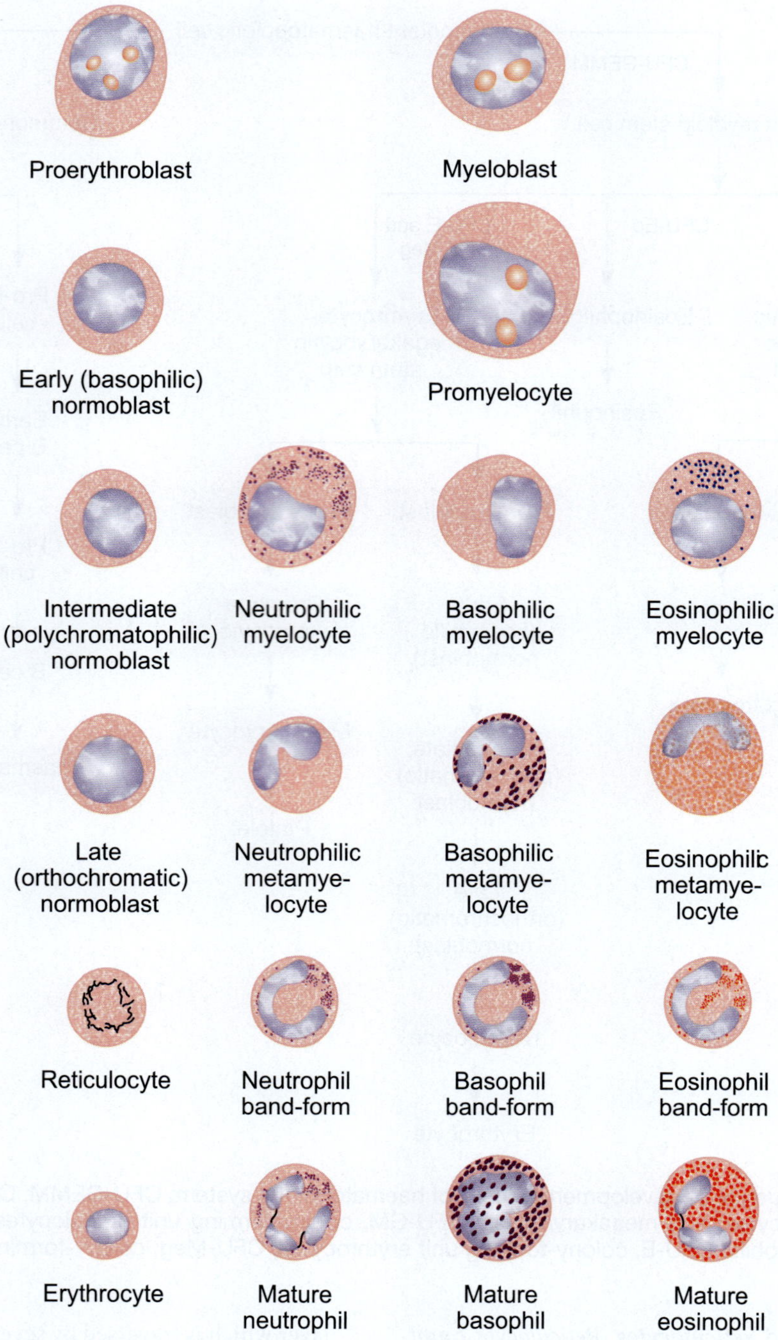

Fig. 12.1 Sequence of maturation of the erythrocytic and granulocytic series.

2.4 million new erythrocytes are produced every second in human adults. The cells develop in the bone marrow and circulate for about 100–120 days in the blood before their components are recycled by macrophages.

Leukopoiesis

Myeloblast

- Least mature cell in the granulocyte lineage.
- Round-to-ovoid in shape and about 15–20 μm in size.
- Has a high nuclear/cytoplasmic (N/C) ratio; fine, 'grainy' nuclear chromatin; delicate nuclear membrane; and 2–5 nucleoli.
- Cytoplasm is moderately blue and agranular.

Promyelocyte

- Is the product of myeloblast division, and usually grows larger than the progenitor cells (20–25 μm).
- Nucleus shows an increasingly coarse chromatin structure, is eccentrically located; the lighter zone over its indentation corresponds to the Golgi zone.
- The cytoplasm is basophilic, moderate to abundant, and contains large *azurophilic* or *primary granules* containing peroxidases, hydrolases and other enzymes.
- Promyelocytes may be released into the bloodstream in conditions associated with increased granulocyte production (shift to left).

Myelocyte

- Promyelocyte mitosis gives rise to a *myelocyte*, which is smaller (18–20 µm) in size.
- Nucleus is ovoid and has clumped chromatin.
- The cytoplasm becomes paler with maturation and shows *special* or *secondary granules,* which begin to appear at this stage. With successive mitoses, the number of azurophilic granules decreases.

Metamyelocyte

- Is the product of the final myelocyte division, and further maturation of the nucleus occurs with contraction and condensation.
- Metamyelocytes are incapable of cell division.
- The nuclei slowly take on the shape of a kidney bean.
- Cytoplasmic granules are fine and pinkish-blue.
- Myelocytes and metamyelocytes normally appear in the peripheral blood only during increased cell production in response to stress or infections.

Band Cell

The term *band cell* is used when the beginning of segmentation is visible, but the indentations do not cut more than two-thirds of the way across the nucleus.

Segmented Neutrophil

- This is 12–14 µm in size and represents the final stage in the myeloid lineage.
- Shows segmentation of nuclei such that the nuclear segments are connected only by narrow chromatin bridges, which should be no thicker than one-third of the average diameter of the nucleus.
- The chromatin is denser than the chromatin in band neutrophils. Upon staining, the cytoplasm of segmented neutrophilic granulocytes appears nearly colourless to pink or violet and is granular.
- A left shift to smaller numbers of segments is a discreet symptom of reactive activation of this cell series. A right shift or hypersegmentation usually accompanies vitamin B_{12} and folic acid deficiencies.

Eosinophilic Granulocytes

- Eosinophils arise from the same stem cell population as neutrophils and mature in parallel with them.
- The cell that is the precursor for the earliest recognizable eosinophil, the *eosinophilic myelocyte*, is morphologically indistinguishable from that which gives rise to neutrophils and monocytes or to basophils.
- In the early eosinophilic myelocyte, the granules are large and take the basophilic stain. As the cell matures, the granules appear olive-green and finally the characteristic red-orange.
- Nuclear maturation is similar to that of the neutrophil. Mature eosinophils are slightly larger than neutrophils [average diameter of 16 µm, have a bilobed nucleus, and provide immunity against parasites and foreign proteins (allergies)]. The different types of leukocytes in the peripheral blood are shown in Fig. 12.2.

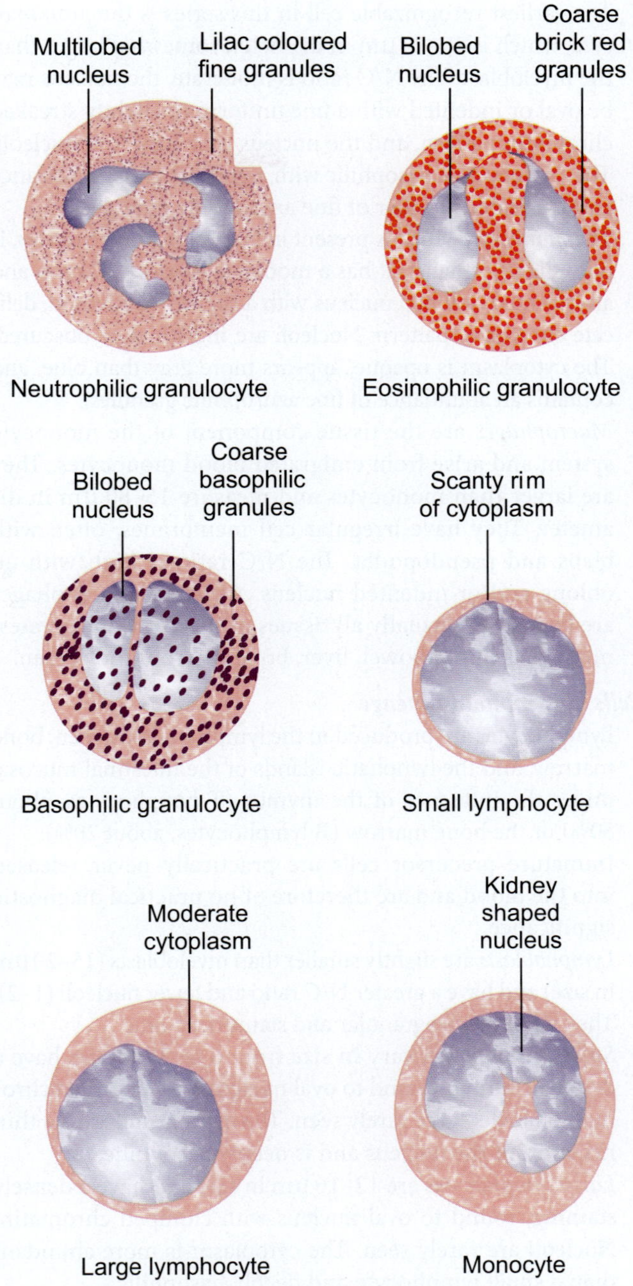

Fig. 12.2 Types of leukocytes in the peripheral blood.

Basophilic Granulocytes

- Similar to eosinophils, basophils (basophilic granulocytes) mature in parallel with cells of the neutrophil lineage.
- Basophilic precursors have large, black-violet stained granules.
- The first recognizable stage is a basophilic myelocyte, with the appearance of the specific basophil granules.
- In mature basophils, which are relatively small, these granules often overlie the two compact nuclear segments.
- Elevated basophil counts are seen mainly in hypersensitivity reactions and chronic myeloproliferative diseases, especially chronic myeloid leukaemia.

Cells of Monocytic Lineage

- In normal marrow, it is not possible morphologically to distinguish the *monoblast* from the *myeloblast*.

- The earliest recognizable cell in this series is the *promonocyte*, which is 15–20 μm in diameter, somewhat larger than the myeloblast. The N/C ratio is moderate, the nucleus may be oval or indented with a fine uniform or slightly streaked chromatin pattern, and the nucleus may have 2–5 nucleoli. The cytoplasm is basophilic with a ground-glass appearance and a variable number of fine azurophilic granules.
- The *monocyte*, which is present in both blood and marrow, is only slightly smaller; it has a moderate to low N/C ratio and an indented or lobed nucleus with a slightly condensed, delicate chromatin pattern. Nucleoli are indistinct or obscured. The cytoplasm is opaque, appears more gray than blue, and contains an abundance of fine azurophilic granules.
- *Macrophages* are the tissue component of the monocyte system and arise from emigrated blood monocytes. They are larger than monocytes and measure 15–80 μm in diameter. They have irregular cell membranes, often with blebs and pseudopodia. The N/C ratio is high with an oblong and/or indented nucleus. Although macrophages are located in virtually all tissues of the body, the greatest number is in the bowel, liver, bone marrow and spleen.

Cells of Lymphoid Lineage

- Lymphocytes are produced in the lymph nodes, spleen, bone marrow, and the lymphatic islands of the intestinal mucosa, under the influence of the thymus (T lymphocytes, about 80%) or the bone marrow (B lymphocytes, about 20%).
- Immature precursor cells are practically never released into the blood and are therefore of no practical diagnostic significance.
- *Lymphoblasts* are slightly smaller than myeloblasts (15–20 μm in size) and have a greater N/C ratio and fewer nucleoli (1–2). The cytoplasm is agranular and stains deep blue.
- *Small lymphocytes* vary in size from 6 to 9 μm and have a densely staining, round to oval nucleus with clumped chromatin. Nucleoli are rarely seen. The cytoplasm forms a thin rim around the nucleus and is deeply basophilic.
- *Large lymphocytes* are 12–16 μm in size and have a densely staining, round to oval nucleus with clumped chromatin. Nucleoli are rarely seen. The cytoplasm is more abundant than a small lymphocyte and deeply basophilic.
- Only about 5% of small lymphocytes and about 3% of large ones show *granules*. The family of large lymphocytes with granules consists mostly of *natural killer cells*.
- *T or B lymphocytes* are morphologically indistinguishable and undergo transformation in response to specific immunological stimuli.
- The final stage of B lymphocyte maturation (in bone marrow and lymph nodes) is *plasma cells*. *Plasma cells* vary in size from 14 to 20 μm. The cytoplasm is amphophilic and agranular with a well-defined, clear Golgi zone adjacent to the nucleus. The nucleus is eccentric in location and contains coarsely clumped chromatin arranged as radial bars (*cartwheel-like appearance*).

Megakaryopoiesis (Thrombopoiesis)

- Platelets originate from *megakaryocytes*, the largest of all haematopoietic cells, whose number is less than 1% of the total nucleated marrow cells.
- Megakaryocytes arise from the *multipotential HSCs* and then from a *committed progenitor cell, the colony-forming unit–megakaryocyte (CFU–Meg)*.
- Megakaryocyte proliferation is largely regulated by *thrombopoietin*. Endomitosis (nuclear division without cytoplasmic division) is typical of megakaryocytic development.
- The committed progenitor cells are morphologically identical to lymphocytes.
- The earliest recognizable precursor, the *megakaryoblast*, is 25–30 μm and has a large 2–4 lobed nucleus and a small amount of basophilic cytoplasm. During the course of maturation, nuclear lobes increase and spread out, and red-pink granules become visible.
- *Promegakaryocytes* are larger than megakaryoblasts and originate from the latter by endoduplication (nuclear chromatin replicates repeatedly in multiples of two without actual division of the cell). The cytoplasm of promegakaryocytes is deeply basophilic and granular. The nucleus is large and indented.
- In the *mature megakaryocyte*, basophilia has disappeared, and the granules are clustered into small aggregates. It is about 100 μm in size and contains 4–16 nuclear lobes, and coarsely clumped chromatin. Budding megakaryocytes develop invaginated surface membranes that provide a membrane reserve for proplatelet formation.
- *Proplatelets* are pseudopodial extensions of megakaryocytes that progressively branch and thin out. They are formed at the ends of proplatelets and released by microtubular action.
- *Platelets* are 1–4 mm in size; disc shaped; anucleate structures with a normal count of 150,000–400,000/μL. They have a lifespan of 7–10 days and about 70% of the total number circulates in the blood.

Q. Discuss the aetiology, classification and clinical features of anaemia. (PA13.3, 13.4, 13.5)

Ans. 'Anaemia' is derived from the Greek word (ναιμια) (an-haîma) meaning 'without blood', indicating a deficiency of red blood cells (RBCs) and/or haemoglobin. It is defined as a state in which the blood haemoglobin level is below the normal reference range for the patient's age and sex (Table 12.3) and anaemia is graded into mild, moderate and severe based on the haemoglobin value and clinical presentation (Table 12.4).

Table 12.3 Anaemic ranges of haemoglobin

Age/sex (years)	Hb (g/dL)
Children (0.5–4)	<11.0
Children (5–12)	<11.5
Children (12–15)	<12.0
Adult men	<13.0
Non-pregnant women	<12.0
Pregnant women	<11.0 (the lower limit is reduced in pregnancy)

Source: WHO grading.

Table 12.4 Grading of anaemia based on its severity and clinical features

Mild	9.5–13.0 g/dL (often no signs or symptoms, commonly remains untreated)
Moderate	8.0–9.5 g/dL (may present with symptoms, requires management to prevent development of complications)
Severe	<8.0 g/dL (symptoms usually present, may be life-threatening and require prompt management)

Classification of Anaemia

Anaemia can be due to a decrease in the quantity of circulating RBCs, represented by a reduction in haemoglobin concentration (Hb), haematocrit (Hct), or RBC count. Anaemias are classified based on:

1. The cause of anaemia **(aetiological classification).**
2. The morphology of red cells **(morphological classification).**

1. **Aetiological classification of anaemia**
   (a) **Anaemia of blood loss (may be acute or chronic):**
      (i) **Acute:** Trauma, major surgical procedures and postpartum bleeding.
      (ii) **Chronic:** Hookworm infestation, bleeding peptic ulcer, carcinoma colon, IBD, haemorrhoids and excessive menstrual loss.
   (b) **Impaired production of red cells:**
      (i) **Nutritional deficiency:** Iron (affects haemoglobin synthesis), vitamin B_{12} and folate (affect DNA synthesis), vitamin C deficiency.
      (ii) **Inherited genetic defects:**
         - Defects leading to stem cell depletion (Fanconi anaemia).
         - Defects affecting erythroblast maturation (Thalassaemia syndromes, Congenital dyserythropoietic anaemias).
      (iii) **Erythropoietin deficiency:** Renal failure and anaemia of chronic disease.
      (iv) **Immune-mediated disturbance of proliferation and differentiation of stem cells:** Hypoplastic or aplastic anaemia and pure red cell aplasia.
      (v) **Marrow invasion** (Myelophthisic anaemia): Leukaemia, lymphoma, secondary carcinoma, fibrosis and granulomatous disease.
      (vi) **Inflammatory iron sequestration:** Anaemia of chronic disease.
      (vii) **Unknown mechanisms:** Endocrine disorders (hypothyroidism, hypoadrenalism and hypopituitarism) and hepatic disease.
   (c) **Due to excessive destruction of red cells (haemolytic anaemias)**
      (i) **Genetic disorders:** Red cell membrane, enzyme abnormalities, haemoglobinopathies, such as sickle cell disease and thalassaemias.
      (ii) **Acquired disorders:** Immune, toxic, mechanical and infectious causes.

2. **Morphological classification of anaemia (Table 12.5)**
   These days, complete blood counts (CBC) and RBC cellular indices are calculated on automated counters and placed on laboratory reports. The morphological classification of anaemia is based on red cell indices, which include:
   (a) ***Mean corpuscular volume (MCV):*** It defines the size of the red blood cells and is expressed as femtolitres (fL) or as cubic microns. The mean volume of the red cell may be calculated from the formula:
   MCV = PCV (%) × 10/RBC count in millions/mm^3 expressed in fL.
   Note:
      (i) '10' is introduced to convert the haematocrit reading from PCV in 100 mL to PCV per litre.
      (ii) $1 fL = 1 \times 10^{-15}$ L.
   Normal range of MCV: 80–100 fL
   (b) ***MCH (mean corpuscular haemoglobin):*** It is the average amount of haemoglobin per red blood cell and is calculated by dividing the haemoglobin value by the red blood cell count.
   MCH (pg) = Hb (g/dL) × 10/RBC count in millions/mm^3.
   Note: $1 pg = 1 \times 10^{-12}$ g.
   Normal range: 29.5 ± 2.5 pg (27–32 pg)
   (c) ***MCHC (mean corpuscular haemoglobin concentration):*** It is the average concentration of haemoglobin per red blood cell and is calculated by dividing the haemoglobin by the haematocrit.
   MCHC (% or g/dL) = Hb (g/dL) × 100/PCV (%).
   ***Normal range*: 32.5 ± 2.5 (30%–35% or g/dL).**
   Note: MCHC has an upper physiological limit as red cells cannot possess haemoglobin beyond a certain limit; anaemia can therefore never be 'hyperchromic'.
   (d) ***Red cell distribution width (RDW):*** It represents the coefficient of variation of the red blood cell volume distribution (size) and is expressed as a percentage.
   Normal value for RDW is 13 ± 1.5%.
   Based on the red cell indices and morphology of red cells, anaemia is classified as follows:
      (i) ***Macrocytic anaemia*** (MCV >100 fL; MCH within normal range), which may further be of two types:
         - *Megaloblastic*: Due to vitamin B_{12} or folate deficiency.
         - *Non-megaloblastic*: Usually seen in association with haemolytic and post-haemorrhagic anaemia, as well as conditions associated with excessive red cell lipid content (thin macrocytosis due to hepatic disease and post-splenectomy).
      (ii) ***Normocytic normochromic anaemia*** (MCV 80–100 fL; MCH within normal range): This is associated with most haemolytic anaemias, anaemia from chronic illness, anaemia due to acute blood loss, marrow hypoplasia or aplasia, hypersplenism, chronic renal and liver disease, sideroblastic anaemia, hypothyroidism, adrenal insufficiency, and PNH.

Table 12.5 Morphological abnormalities of red cells in different types of anaemias

Abnormalities	Description	Morphology
Polychromatophilia or polychromasia	Red cells staining bluish-grey; they represent young reticulocytes and are seen in the conditions associated with accelerated erythropoiesis	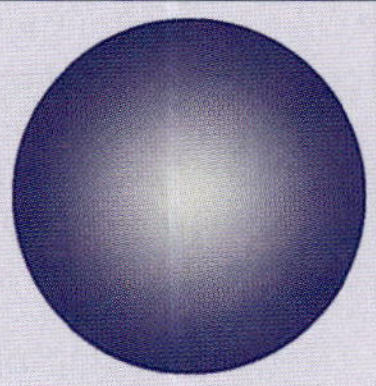
Punctate basophilia or basophilic stippling	Presence of fine or coarse purple-blue granules in the cytoplasm of red cells, representing ribosomal aggregates *Causes:* β-thalassaemia, haemoglobinopathies, lead and arsenic poisoning	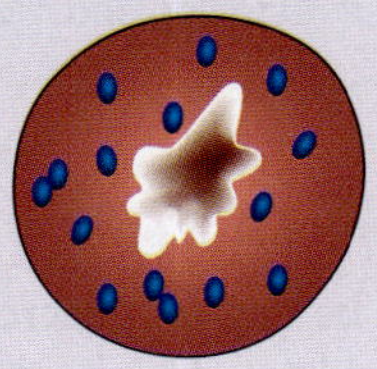
Anisocytosis	Variation in size of the cell as seen in iron deficiency	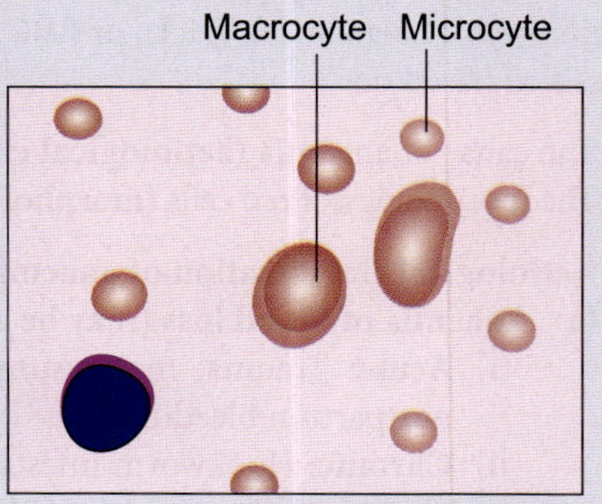
Microcytes	Small red cells (MCV < 80 fL) with decreased amount of haemoglobin *Causes:* Iron deficiency anaemia, thalassaemia, anaemia of chronic disease, lead poisoning and sideroblastic anaemia	
Macrocytes	Large red cells (MCV > 100 fL; size > 8.5 microns, normal MCH). May be round or oval *Causes:* Impaired DNA synthesis (B_{12} and folate deficiency), accelerated erythropoiesis, excessive surface membrane (liver disease or splenectomy)	
Poikilocytosis	Variation in shape of the cell as seen in thalassaemia	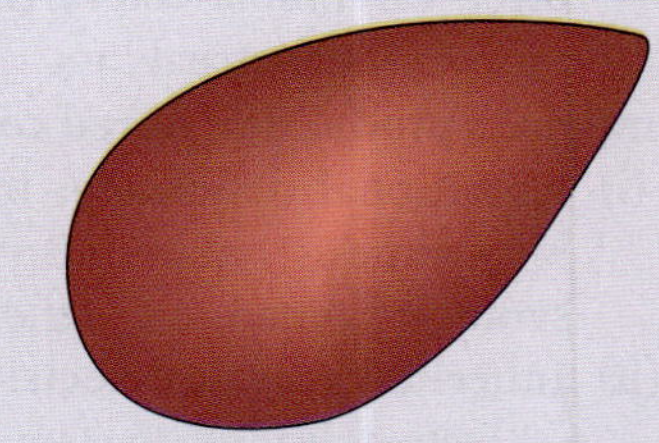
Target cells (codocytes)	Flat red cells with a central mass of haemoglobin (dense area), surrounded by a ring of pallor (pale area) and an outer ring of haemoglobin (dense area) *Causes:* Iron deficiency, chronic liver disease, hyposplenism and haemoglobinopathies	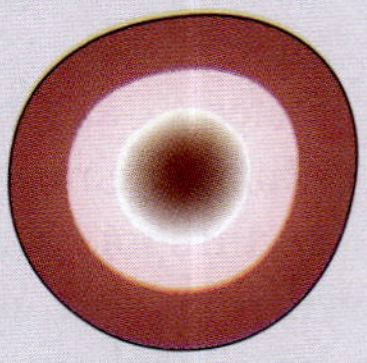
Howell–Jolly bodies	Remnants of nuclear material left after the nucleus is extruded, these are normally removed by spleen *Causes:* Non-functioning or absent spleen and megaloblastic anaemia	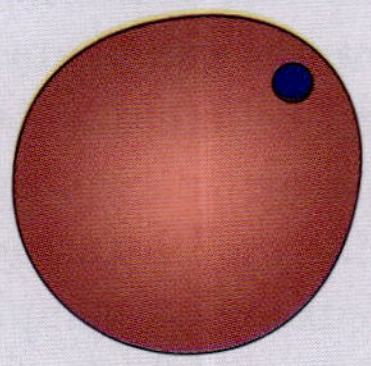
Heinz bodies	These are formed from denatured aggregated haemoglobin. Cells containing Heinz bodies are normally removed by spleen. They do not stain with Romanowski stains but can be demonstrated by Supravital stains like new methylene blue *Causes:* Thalassaemia, asplenia and chronic liver disease	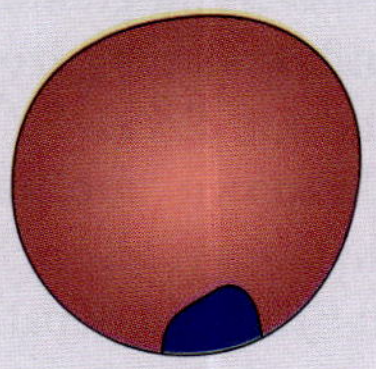
Spherocytes	Dark appearing (densely haemoglobinized) red cells with no central pallor (normal or decreased MCV and increased MCHC) *Causes:* Immune haemolytic anaemia, haemolytic disease of newborn, burns and hereditary spherocytosis	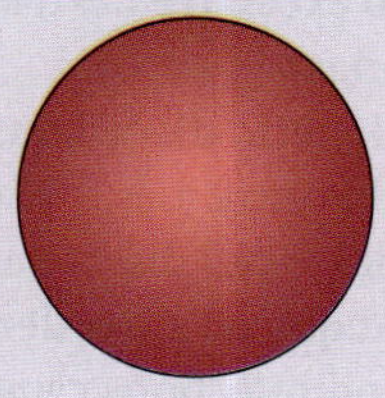

Table 12.5 Morphological abnormalities of red cells in different types of anaemias (*cont.*)

Abnormalities	Description	Morphology
Sickle cells (drepanocytes)	Curved red cells with pointed ends *Causes:* Sickle-cell anaemia, HbS-β thalassaemia	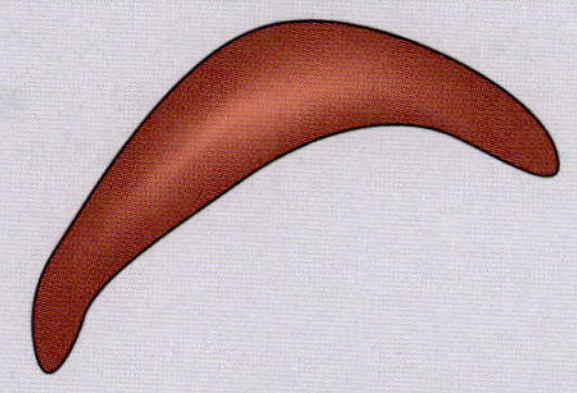
Teardrop cells (dacrocytes)	Red cells in the shape of teardrops; they are pathological and should be followed up *Causes:* Infiltrative disorders of bone marrow (e.g. myelofibrosis); may be seen in megaloblastic anaemia, β-thalassaemia, renal failure and tuberculosis	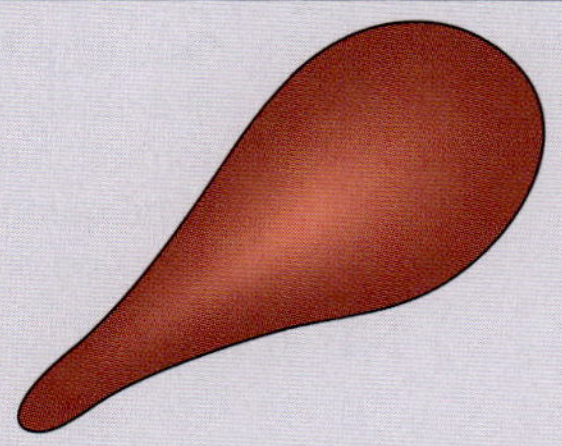
Schistocytes	Fragmented red cells *Causes:* Mechanical stress, for example microangiopathic haemolytic anaemia, thermal injury and severe burns	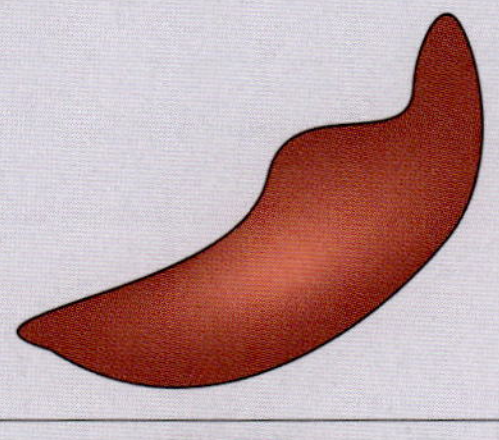
Bite cells	Red cells with peripheral single or multiple arcuate defects (bites) *Causes:* Red cells enzyme defects (G-6-PD deficiency and Pyruvate kinase deficiency)	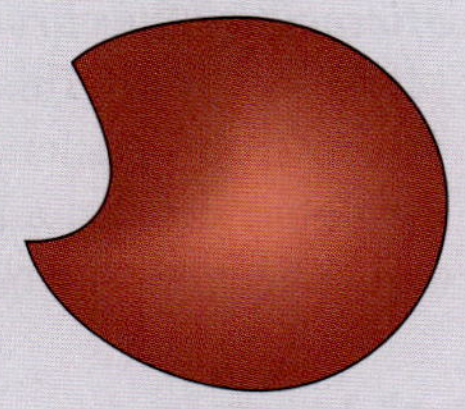
Acanthocytes (spur or spicule cells)	Spheroidal red cells with a few spiny/thorny projections (5–10 in number with irregular thickness and spacing) *Causes:* Post-splenectomy, alcoholic cirrhosis, pyruvate kinase deficiency, autoimmune haemolytic anaemia (AIHA), severe burns and renal disease	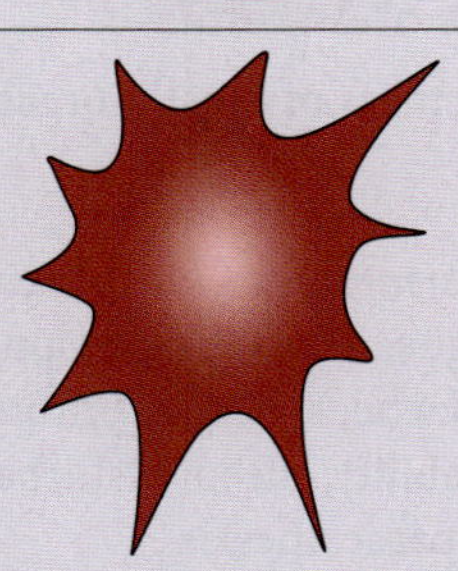
Echinocytes (Burr or sea urchin cells)	Small cells or cell fragments bearing shorter, more regular spines 10–30 in number, evenly spaced *Causes:* Uraemia, pyruvate kinase deficiency, blood storage, ATP depletion, calcium accumulation and contact with glass	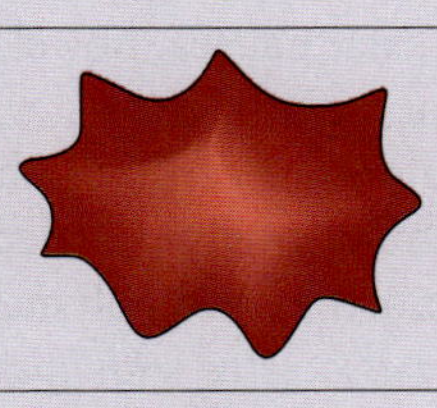
Elliptocytes	Elliptical cells *Causes:* Hereditary elliptocytosis, thalassaemia, sickle cell trait, iron deficiency, megaloblastic and myelophthisic anaemia	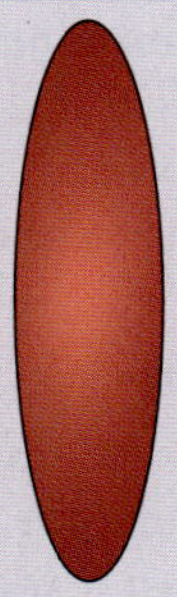

(Continued)

Table 12.5 Morphological abnormalities of red cells in different types of anaemias (*cont.*)

Abnormalities	Description	Morphology
Stomatocytes	Uniconcave red cells with a slit-like area of central pallor *Causes:* Hereditary stomatocytosis, alcoholism, cirrhosis, obstructive liver disease	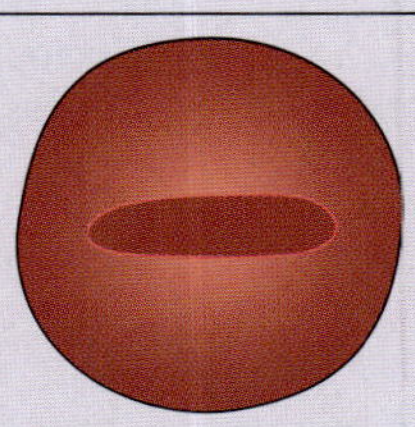
Agglutination	True agglutination is irregular clumping of red cells into grape like clusters (in contrast with pseudoagglutination or rouleaux formation which is observed in paraproteinemias, hypergammaglobulinemia and fibrinogenemia which causes stacking of red cells like coins)	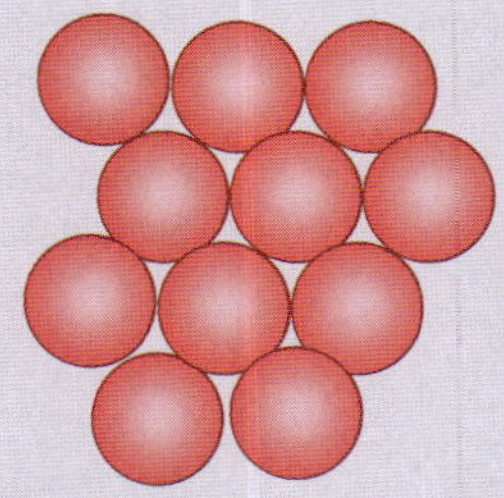

MCV, Mean corpuscular volume.

(iii) ***Microcytic hypochromic anaemia*** (MCV <80 fL; MCH <27 pg): This category includes anaemia due to iron deficiency, thalassaemia, other haemoglobin defects, anaemia of chronic disorders, and congenital sideroblastic anaemia.

Symptoms of Anaemia

Acute: Shortness of breath, organ failure and shock.

Chronic

1. *General symptoms (due to tissue hypoxia)*
   (a) Fatigue, lassitude, dyspnoea, palpitations, dizziness, headache, syncope, tinnitus and vertigo.
   (b) Irritability, sleep disturbances, lack of concentration and paraesthesias.
   (c) Anorexia, nausea, bowel disturbances and pica (craving for ice or dirt).
   (d) Symptoms of cardiac failure (palpitations, difficulty in breathing, swelling in dependent parts).
   (e) Amenorrhea and polymenorrhea.
2. *Symptoms associated with haemolysis*: Skeletal abnormalities (due to expansion of marrow), growth retardation, jaundice and gallstones.
3. *Symptoms associated with defective erythropoiesis*: Iron overload leading to heart and endocrine failure.

Signs of Anaemia

- Pallor of skin and mucous membranes, nail beds and palpebral conjunctivae.
- Tachycardia with a wide pulse pressure, ejection systolic murmur; best heard over the pulmonary area.
- Cardiac dilatation and later, signs of cardiac failure including oedema.
- Pulmonary findings—tachypnea and rales.
- In some cases hepato-splenomegaly.
- Proteinuria and impaired tubular concentrating capacity.

Q. Outline the laboratory approach to evaluation of anaemia.

Ans. The first step in the diagnosis of anaemia is the **confirmation of its existence.** Next one needs to investigate for the **type** and **the underlying cause and pathogenesis**. An **adequate history** and **a thorough physical examination** are imperative for determining the aetiology. **Confirmatory tests** are then undertaken to type the anaemia in order to institute appropriate therapy. A rational approach in determining aetiology of anaemia is to start with **CBC** followed by **peripheral blood smear (PBS) examination.** Often, the aetiology of a patient's anaemia can be determined based on the red blood cells showing specific changes in shape and size (anaemia may be microcytic, MCV <84 fL or macrocytic, MCV >96 fL) or the red cells may show certain morphological abnormalities which give an indication towards the diagnosis (Table 12.5).

The laboratory approach to evaluation of anaemia is outlined in the Flowchart 12.2.

Q. Enumerate the causes of microcytic hypochromic anaemia and enlist their salient features.

(PA14.2, 14.3)

Ans. Microcytic hypochromic anaemia is classified under the following broad headings:

- **Defect in Haem synthesis**
  - Iron deficiency anaemia.
  - Anaemia of chronic disease.
- **Defect in globin chain synthesis**
  - Alpha-, and beta-thalassaemia.
  - HbE syndrome.
  - HbC syndrome.
  - Unstable haemoglobinopathies.

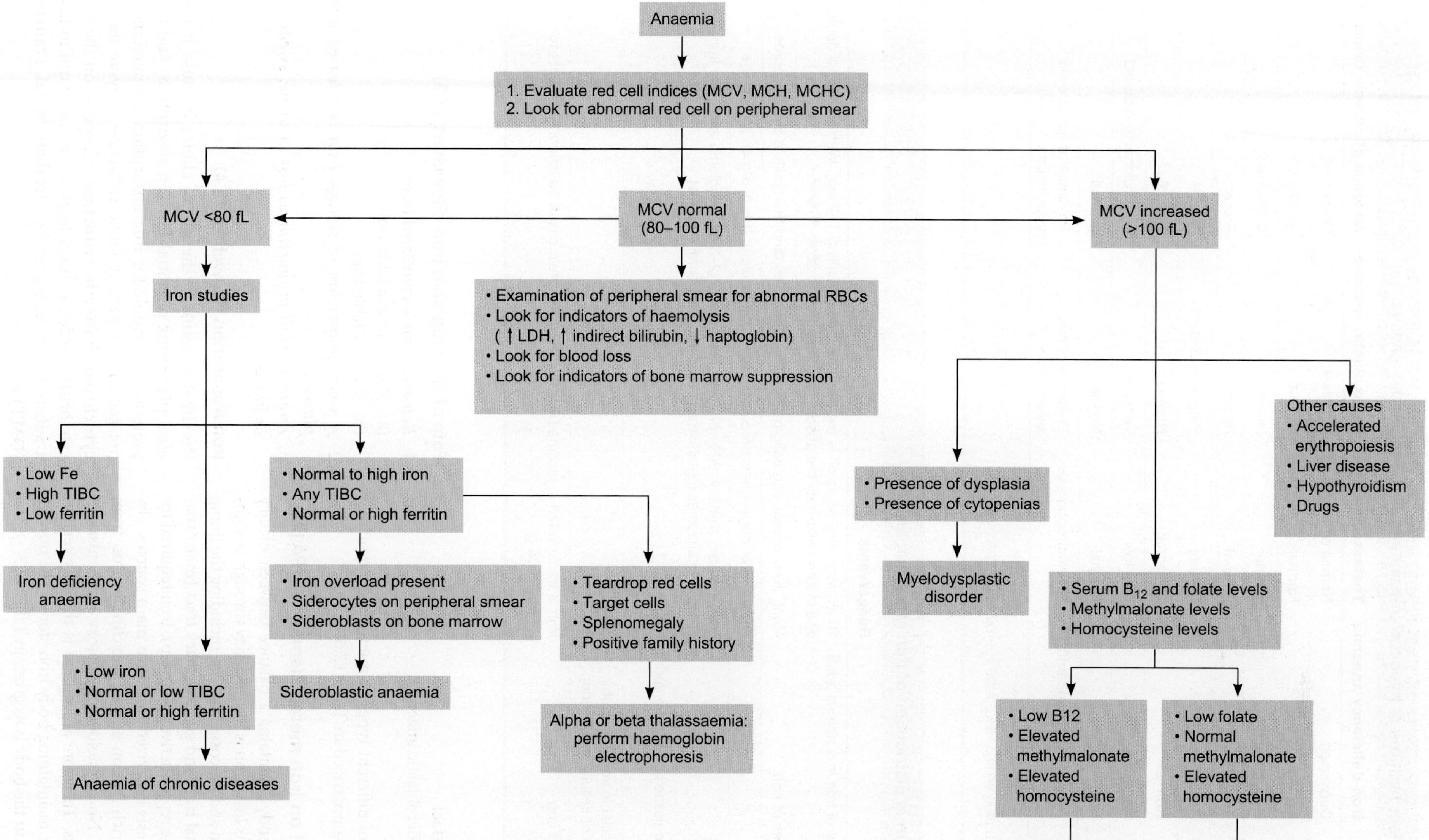

Note: CBC: complete blood count, MCV: mean corpuscular volume, RBC: red blood cell
Fe: Iron, TIBC: total iron-binding capacity (transferrin), LDH: lactate dehydrogenase

Flowchart 12.2 Laboratory approach to evaluation of anaemia.

Table 12.6 Salient features of hypochromic anaemias due to various causes

Features	Iron-deficiency anaemia	Thalassaemia	Sideroblastic anaemia	Anaemia of chronic disorders
Serum iron	Decreased	Normal or increased	Increased	Decreased
TIBC	Raised	Normal	Normal	Decreased
Serum ferritin	Decreased	Normal	Increased	Decreased
Marrow iron stores	Absent	Present	Present	Present
Iron in normoblasts	Absent	Present	Ring sideroblasts	Absent
Hb electrophoresis	Normal	Abnormal	Normal	Normal
Red cell indices	Reduced	Very low	Very low	Low, normal to reduced
RDW	High	Normal	Normal	Normal
Diagnostic feature/ investigation	Decreased serum ferritin	Hb electrophoresis	Presence of ring sideroblasts	Presence of normocytic population

RDW, Red cell distribution width; TIBC, total iron-binding capacity.

Table 12.7 Normal distribution of iron in the human body

Parameter	Range/value
Average daily intake of iron in a normal adult	10–20 mg; 10% of which is usually absorbed (equalling 1–2 mg). With increased demand and in iron deficiency the absorption can go up to 20%–30%
Chief dietary sources of iron	Meat, liver, kidney, egg yolk, green leafy vegetables, and fruit; milk is a poor source
Total body iron	The value of body iron is proportionate to body weight. It is 3–5 g on an average
Functional iron	Haemoglobin contains 80% of the functional iron (2–3 g), myoglobin and other iron-containing enzymes (catalase and cytochrome) contain the rest
Storage or available tissue iron (ferritin and haemosiderin)	1 g
Essential or non-available iron (myoglobin and other enzymes of cellular respiration)	0.5 g
Plasma or transport iron	Iron is transported in plasma bound to a glycoprotein called *transferrin*; amounts to 0.003–0.004 g

- **Sideroblastic defect**
  - Hereditary sideroblastic anaemia.
  - Lead toxicity.

Salient features of different types of microcytic hypochromic anaemias are summarized in Table 12.6.

Q. Write in detail on iron metabolism. (PA14.1)

Ans. The human body maintains a balance between dietary uptake of iron and its loss. Iron is lost each day through sloughing of cells from skin and mucosal surfaces, including the lining of the gastrointestinal tract and genitourinary tract (menstruation in women in the reproductive age group). Iron required for haemoglobin synthesis is derived from two main sources—by ingestion of foods rich in iron and by recycling of iron from senescent red cells. No physiologic regulatory mechanism of iron excretion exists. Therefore absorption is the only regulatory mechanism for maintaining body iron stores. The normal distribution of iron in the body is as given in Table 12.7.

Fate of Haemoglobin Iron (Flowchart 12.3)

1. ***Released iron is converted into:***
   (a) Storage or available iron.
   (b) Non-available iron.
2. ***A small proportion of storage iron is released into the plasma.***
3. ***Another small proportion is lost in urine, sweat, faeces or blood.***

Iron Absorption (Flowchart 12.4)

Proximal intestine is the site of choice because it has the ideal pH (redox potential for iron absorption) and the key proteins responsible for iron absorption are maximally expressed in this part. A ferric reductase enzyme **duodenal cytochrome b (dcytb) reductase**, expressed on the enterocyte brush border, reduces ferric to ferrous form to make it a substrate for transport by **Divalent Metal Transporter (DMT) 1.**

Aged or senescent RBCs

↓

Phagocytosis by reticuloendothelial system

↓

Breakdown of haemoglobin

↓

Release of iron into circulation

↓

Binding of released iron to '**Transferrin**'

↓

Reutilization of iron by marrow erythroblasts for haemoglobin synthesis

Flowchart 12.3 Fate of haemoglobin iron.

Iron released from food as ferric or ferrous form

↓ Ascorbic acid increases absorption | Tannins, phosphorus and phytic acid reduce absorption

Ferrous form is absorbed in duodenum and upper jejunum (as ferric ions polymerize and become less soluble with increase in the duodenal pH)

Flowchart 12.4 Iron absorption.

Types of Dietary Iron

- *Non-haem iron* (found as inorganic iron in vegetables, less readily absorbed).
- *Haem iron* (found in animal products and more readily absorbed).

Mucosal Uptake of Haem and Non-Haem Iron: Absorption of Iron Occurs Through Two Distinct Pathways

1. **Non-haem iron:** Enters the apical and basolateral portions of villus enterocytes by the action of transporter protein **DMT1.** Inside the cell, most of the iron is stored as mucosal ferritin and not absorbed. These ferritin-containing cells are later exfoliated from the mucosal surface into the intestine at the end of their 3–4-day lifespan. The remaining iron is transported to plasma by **ferroportin (IREG-1 transporter)** and **hephaestin (an iron oxidase)**.
2. **Haem iron:** Mechanism not well understood but it is thought that haem enters the mucosal surface unchanged to release iron within the cells by the action of the enzyme **haem oxygenase**. Iron from this source follows the same pathway as non-haem iron except that a small portion of the haem iron passes into the plasma intact to bind to haemopexin, a haem-binding protein.

Regulators of Iron Absorption

1. **Dietary regulator:** An increase in dietary iron reduces absorption, as the mucosal cells have accumulated iron and 'block' additional uptake.
2. **Stores regulator:** Increased iron stores in the liver induce release of the hepatic peptide **hepcidin** that decreases intestinal mucosal iron ferroportin release. The enterocytes retain any absorbed iron and are sloughed off in a few days. As body iron stores fall, there is a decrease in hepcidin, which induces intestinal mucosa to release the absorbed iron into circulation.

Storage and Transport of Iron

- Iron is transported in the plasma bound to a beta globulin named '**transferrin**' that is synthesized in the liver.
- Transferrin bound iron is utilized by the erythroid cells of the marrow for haemoglobin synthesis. Iron uptake occurs via '**transferrin receptors**' present on erythroid precursors.
- Percentage of total iron-binding protein to which iron is attached is called '**percentage saturation**' **(percentage saturation = serum iron/total iron-binding capacity (TIBC); normal value 33%).**
- Iron derived from the phagocytosis of senescent red cells is stored in bone marrow, liver, spleen and skeletal muscle as **ferritin** and **haemosiderin.**
- Ferritin is relatively unstable and has a spherical outer shell of protein called apoferritin and an inner core of trivalent iron.
- Haemosiderin is more stable, therefore less readily mobilized to haemoglobin formation.
- Ferritin levels are raised in acute leukaemias, inflammation and Hodgkin disease.
- Ferritin levels are decreased in liver disease.

Iron Excretion

Normal average excretion of iron in urine, faeces and sweat per day is about 0.5–1 mg. Another 0.5–1.0 mg is lost in menses.

Q. Outline the aetiopathogenesis, clinical features and blood picture of iron-deficiency anaemia (IDA).

Ans. IDA is the most common type of anaemia met with in clinical practice.

Causes

- **Pathological blood loss:** Peptic ulcer, haemorrhoids, hiatus hernia, carcinoma stomach and colon, chronic aspirin ingestion, oesophageal varices, ulcerative colitis, hookworm infestation, haematuria, repeated epistaxis, haemoptysis and pathological uterine bleeding.
- **Increased physiological demand:** Growing children and women in reproductive age group.
- **Inadequate intake**
  - **Nutritional deficiency:** Poverty, dietary fads, anorexia and poor bioavailability of non-haem iron.
  - **Impaired absorption:** Gastroenterostomy, tropical sprue, celiac disease, atransferrinaemia, abnormal transferring function or antibodies to transferring receptors.

- **Plummer–Vinson (Paterson–Kelly) syndrome:** Syndrome complex of chronic iron deficiency, dysphagia due to post-cricoid web and glossitis.

Stages of Iron Deficiency

1. Storage iron depletion.
2. Iron-deficient erythropoiesis.
3. Frank iron-deficiency anaemia.

Clinical Features

Signs and symptoms of iron deficiency are due to:

- **Anaemia:** Lassitude, weakness, fatigue, dyspnoea, palpitations, angina, CCF and pallor.
- **Epithelial tissue changes**
  - Nails: Thin, lusterless, brittle, show ridging and flattening; presence of koilonychia (spoon-shaped nails).
  - Tongue: Atrophy of papillae, shiny or glazed tongue, glossitis and angular stomatitis.
  - **Plummer–Vinson (Paterson–Kelly) syndrome:** Characterized by chronic iron deficiency, dysphagia and glossitis; seen in middle-aged to elderly women who have chronic iron deficiency and a fine web or band composed of desquamating epithelial cells at the oesophageal entrance (postcricoid web). These patients present with dysphagia to solids.
- **Pica:** This is defined as a craving to eat substances like dirt, clay, salt, hair and is a typical manifestation of iron deficiency.
- **Recurrent infections:** Iron deficiency induces defective lymphocyte-mediated immunity and impairs bacterial killing by phagocytes leading to impaired immunity and recurrent infections.

Laboratory Diagnosis

The first and most sensitive parameters to indicate iron deficiency are serum ferritin and stainable iron in tissue stores. These are very useful in differentiating iron deficiency from the anaemia of chronic disorders. The percentage saturation of transferrin with iron and free erythrocyte protoporphyrin values become abnormal only after the tissue stores are depleted of iron. A decrease in the haemoglobin concentration follows because iron is unavailable for haem synthesis. Red blood cell indices become abnormal after several months of depletion of tissue stores of iron.

1. **General blood parameters**
   (a) **Hb:** Decreased
   (b) **Haematocrit:** Reduced
   (c) **RBC count:** Decreased
   (d) **RBC indices:** Reduced/low (MCV < 80fL; MCH < 25pg; MCHC <27g/dL)
2. **Peripheral smear** (Fig. 12.3)
   (a) **Microcytic hypochromic cells** (red cells are smaller than normal and have increased central pallor). Microcytosis appears in the smear much before MCV decreases.
   (b) **Anisocytosis or variation in cell size** (anisocytosis is indicated by increased **red cell distribution width (RDW; >15% in IDA; normal 11.5%–14.5%)** and is more marked in IDA than in thalassaemia for the same haemoglobin value).

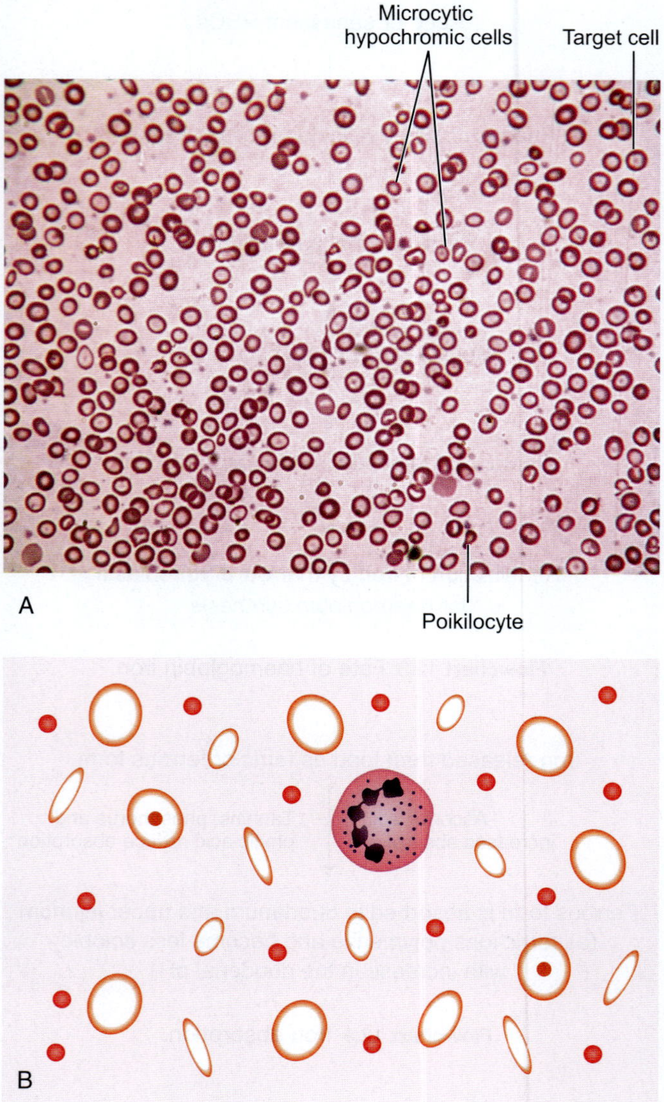

Fig. 12.3 (A) Leishman-stained peripheral blood smear (PBS) and (B) schematic diagram of iron-deficiency anaemia showing marked hypochromia and anisocytosis with presence of a fair number of microcytes, target cells and poikilocytes.

   (c) **Poikilocytosis or variation in cell shape** (less marked in IDA than in thalassaemia for the same haemoglobin value).
   (d) **Normoblasts, elliptocytes, pencil-shaped cells, ring/pessary cells** and **target cells** (usually seen in severe anaemia).
   (e) Normal, increased or decreased **platelet count (reactive thrombocytosis)** and unremarkable **WBCs.**
3. **Reticulocyte count:** Normal or decreased (in post-haemorrhagic anaemia reticulocyte count may be mildly raised).
4. **Iron studies**
   (a) Decreased serum iron (<50 μg/dL; normal range 40–140 μg/dL).
   (b) Reduced percentage saturation (<16%; normal range 30%–40%).
   (c) Reduced serum ferritin (most useful; <15 μg/L; normal range 15–300 μg/dL).

(d) High TIBC (350–450 µg/dL; normal range 310–340 µg/dL).
(e) Raised serum transferrin receptor fragments assay (sTFR) by immunological methods (3.5–7.1 µg/dL; normal range 0.57–2.8 µg/dL).
(f) Erythrocyte ferritin is decreased in iron deficiency and free erythrocyte zinc protoporphyrin (FEP) levels are increased in disorders of haem synthesis including iron deficiency (>200 µg/dL; normal range 30–50 µg/dL). Normally protoporphyrin binds iron to form haem in erythroid precursors. In IDA, protoporphyrin fails to bind iron and its levels increase. In thalassaemia FEP levels are normal.

5. **Bone marrow**
(a) Presence of erythroid hyperplasia; increase mainly in mature cells.
(b) Predominant cell is a polychromatic normoblast, which is smaller than normal (micronormoblastic maturation).
(c) Cytoplasm shows ragged borders.
(d) Cytoplasmic maturation lags behind that of the nucleus (due to delayed haemoglobinization).
(e) Prussian blue stain shows decreased iron stores.

Differential Diagnosis

- **Heterozygous form of** β-thalassaemia/β-thalassaemia trait
  - RBC count normal to increased (decreased in iron-deficiency anaemia).
  - MCV and MCH disproportionately lower than degree of anaemia.
  - RDW normal in thalassaemia (increased in iron-deficiency anaemia).
  - Target cells abundant (few in iron-deficiency anaemia).
  - Basophilic stippling and nucleated RBCs commonly seen (not seen or rare in iron deficiency).
  - Normal iron studies (deranged values in iron deficiency)
  - Increased HbF (normal in iron deficiency).
- **Anaemia of chronic disorders**
  - Serum iron decreased.
  - Serum ferritin normal or increased (decreased in iron deficiency).
  - TIBC normal or decreased (increased in iron deficiency).
  - Percentage saturation decreased to normal (decreased in iron deficiency).
- **Sideroblastic anaemia**
  - Serum iron normal or increased (decreased in iron deficiency).
  - Serum ferritin normal or increased (decreased in iron deficiency).
  - TIBC normal (increased in iron deficiency).
  - Percentage saturation normal or increased (decreased in iron deficiency).

Q. Write briefly on sideroblastic anaemia.

Ans. The sideroblastic anaemias are inherited or acquired disorders characterized by:

- Refractory anaemia with a variable number of hypochromic red cells in peripheral smear.
- Excess of iron and ring sideroblasts in the marrow.

Siderocytes and sideroblasts are erythrocytes and erythroblasts, respectively, containing cytoplasmic iron granules. Sideroblasts can be normal or abnormal. Normal sideroblasts contain a few scattered cytoplasmic granules, which are basically due to presence of unutilized iron remaining during haemoglobin synthesis. Abnormal sideroblasts may either contain numerous coarse diffusely present cytoplasmic granules as seen in dyserythropoiesis or show rings on Prussian blue staining (ringed sideroblasts).

Classification

1. Hereditary sideroblastic anaemia	2. Acquired sideroblastic anaemia
X-linked disorder associated with deficient activity of the enzyme aminolevulinic acid synthetase (ALA synthetase) involved in haeme synthesis. Females are generally carriers and do not manifest with the disease whereas affected males manifest with frank anaemia.	(a) Idiopathic or primary (a type of myelodysplasia): Occurs in middle aged or elderly individuals who show defective maturation of erythroid cells owing to a defect at the level of the haematopoietic stem cell. It may be associated with chromosomal, WBC and platelet abnormalities and can be of the following types: (i) Refractory anaemia with ring sideroblasts. (ii) Refractory anaemia with ring sideroblasts and thrombocytosis. (iii) Refractory anaemia with multilineage dysplasia and ring sideroblasts. (b) Secondary, which may be due to: (i) *Drugs*, for example isoniazid (pyridoxine antagonist), alcohol abuse and lead toxicity. (ii) *Haematological disorders*, for example acute leukaemia, lymphoma, haemolytic anaemia, myelofibrosis and polycythaemia vera. (iii) *Others*, for example hypothermia, rheumatoid arthritis and carcinoma.

Characteristic Features

- Affects middle-aged to elderly individuals who present with insidious onset moderate to severe anaemia.
- The peripheral smear shows a **dimorphic picture** with **microcytic, hypochromic** and **normocytic cells.**
- Iron overload with characteristic **ringed sideroblasts** are seen in the bone marrow (iron enters mitochondria surrounding the nucleus, cannot exit and appears as **'rings'** with Prussian blue staining).
- Siderocytes called **Pappenheimer bodies** (containing non-haem iron granules) are seen in the RBCs.

- Bone marrow shows erythroid hyperplasia and ineffective erythropoiesis. Dyserythropoiesis is common.
- There is marked increase in serum iron and transferrin saturation.

Q. Describe the aetiopathogenesis, clinical features and haematological picture of macrocytic anaemia. (PA15.1, 15.2, 15.3, 15.4)

Ans. A **macrocyte** is defined as a large red cell with increased volume (**MCV** >100 fL), diameter (>8.5 μL) and thickness. Increased thickness is perceived as a loss of central pallor. **MCH** is >31.5 pg; and **MCHC** is normal.

A **megaloblast** is so labelled when a large erythroid cell shows nuclear-cytoplasmic asynchrony (maturation of nucleus lags behind maturation of cytoplasm due to impaired DNA synthesis caused by the deficiency of vitamin B_{12} and folate).

Macrocytosis may be:

- **Megaloblastic** (with impaired DNA synthesis).
- **Non-megaloblastic** (with normal DNA synthesis).

Megaloblastic macrocytosis can result from:

1. Deficiency of vitamin B_{12} and/or folate.
2. Resistance to B_{12} or folic acid therapy due to metabolic inhibitors of DNA synthesis or folate metabolism.

To understand the genesis of megaloblastic anaemia, it is essential to understand the metabolism of vitamin B_{12} and folate. The salient features pertaining to metabolism of vitamin B_{12} and folate are listed in Table 12.8.

Metabolism of Vitamin B_{12}

1. ***Dietary sources***: B_{12} is predominantly present in animal products (meat, muscle, fish, eggs, cheese and milk); therefore, pure vegetarians may suffer from its deficiency. B_{12} is synthesized by bacteria in nature. In humans, these bacteria are normal inhabitants of large bowel but B_{12} cannot be absorbed from this site and thus humans are entirely dependent on dietary sources.

Table 12.8 Salient features of vitamin B_{12} and folate metabolism

Features	B_{12}	Folate
Content in food	• Vegetables: Poor source • Meat: Rich source • Milk: Good source	• Vegetables: Rich source • Meat: Moderate source • Milk: Poor source
Effect of cooking	10%–30% Loss	60%–90% Loss
Adult: Daily requirement	2–4 μg	200 μg
Adult: Daily intake	5–30 μg	100–500 μg
Site of absorption	Ileum	Duodenum and jejunum
Body stores	• 2–5 mg • Adequate for 3 years	• 5–20 mg • Adequate for 4 months

2. ***Absorption***: May be of two types:
   (a) Active (Flowchart 12.5)
   (i) Carrier molecules are involved.
   (ii) Responsible for absorption of physiological amounts of vitamin B_{12}.
   (iii) Highly efficient but slow (takes 8–12 h from ingestion to attainment of peak levels in blood).
   (b) Passive mechanism
   (i) No carrier molecule involved.
   (ii) Seen with supraphysiological doses of vitamin B_{12}.
   (iii) Absorption occurs through the buccal, gastric and jejuna mucosa.
3. ***Transportation***: **Cobalamin** is a general term for compounds with biologic vitamin B_{12} activity. These compounds are involved in nucleic acid metabolism, methyl transfer, myelin synthesis and repair. They are necessary for the formation of normal RBCs. Cobalmin has a **transport form (methylcobalamin)** and a **storage form (adenosylcobalamin)**. There are three major **vitamin B_{12}-binding proteins in plasma** namely **transcobalamins I, II** and **III**.
   Transcobalamin I (Haptocorrin)
   - α-1 Globulin synthesized by granulocytes.
   - 70%–80% of endogenous B_{12} is bound to TC I.
   - Required for storage and not essential for transport; therefore, its absence does not lead to clinical signs of B_{12} deficiency.

   Transcobalamin II
   - β-Globulin synthesized in liver.
   - Essential for transport of B_{12} from organ to organ and from cell to cell (B_{12} bound to TC II is known as holo-transcobalmin or holo-TC).
   - Deficiency leads to severe megaloblastic anaemia.

   Transcobalamin III
   - Binds a small amount of B_{12}.
4. ***Storage***
   (a) The liver stores large amounts of vitamin B_{12} followed by the kidneys, heart and brain.
   (b) B_{12} is excreted through bile and shedding of intestinal epithelial cells (enterohepatic reabsorption helps to retain vitamin B_{12}).
5. ***Functions***
   It is very important for normal haematopoiesis and plays a key role in the normal functioning of the brain and nervous system. It acts as a coenzyme for the following biochemical reactions (Flowchart 12.6).
   (a) Lack of adenosylcobalamin leads to accumulation of methylmalonyl CoA and its precursor propionyl CoA, which induce synthesis of fatty acids which get incorporated in the neuronal lipids to cause the neurological manifestations of B_{12} deficiency.
   (b) Absorbed N5-methyl tetrahydrofolate (FH4) gives away a methyl group to synthesize methionine from homocysteine in a step requiring cobalamin and generates FH4, which is reconjugated to N5,10-methylene FH4 for use in thymidylate and purine synthesis. Lack of B_{12} impairs this reaction, which in turn interferes with normal DNA synthesis to cause megaloblastic maturation.

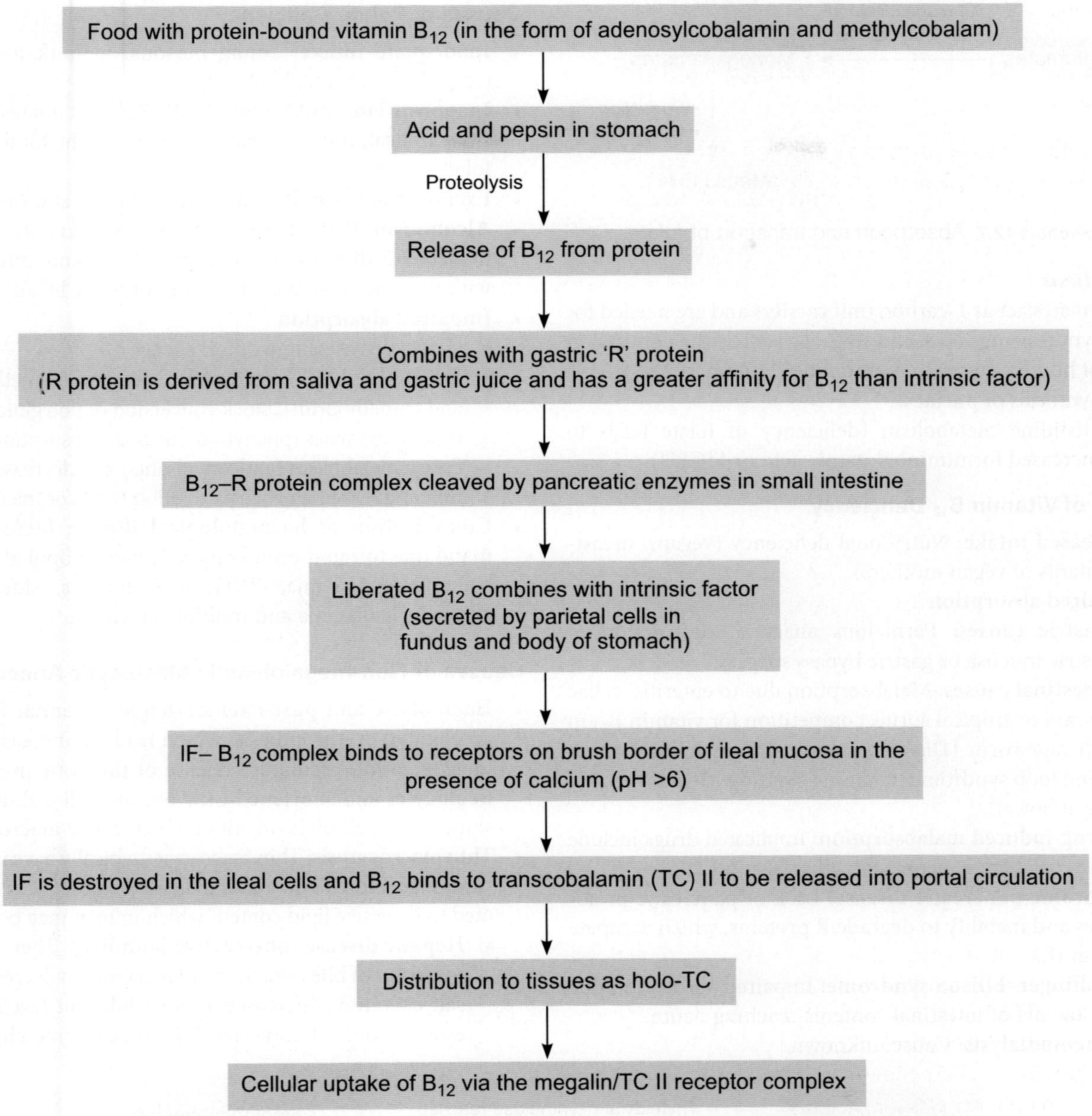

Flowchart 12.5 Absorption of vitamin B_{12} by active mechanism.

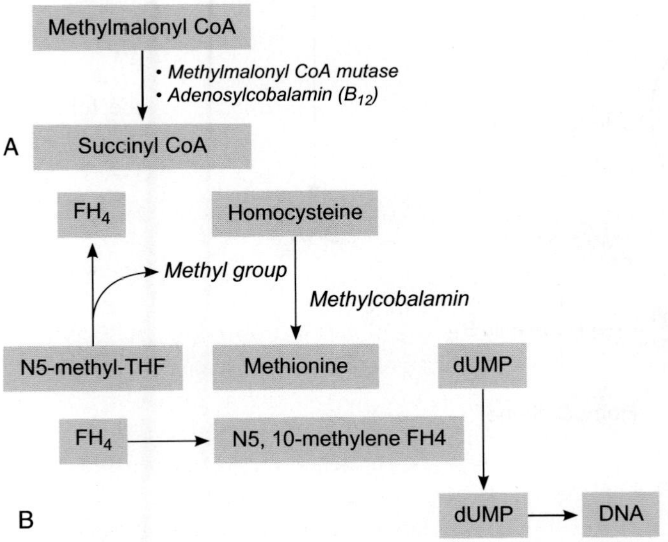

Flowchart 12.6 (A) and (B) Biochemical reactions involving vitamin B_{12}.

Metabolism of Folate

1. ***Dietary sources***: Green leafy vegetables are a rich source of folate. Moderate amounts are present in meat, and milk is a poor source.
2. ***Absorption, transport and storage***
   (a) Folate is a yellow compound with a chemical name pteroylglutamic acid (PGA).
   (b) It exists in nature as a polyglutamate (conjugated folate).
   (c) For its action as a coenzyme, it must be converted to dihydro or tetrahydro form.
   (d) Folate is absorbed in the proximal jejunum and ileum; the mechanism of absorption, however, is unclear.
   (e) Folate circulates free or bound to albumin in the plasma as N5-methyl FH4 (Flowchart 12.7).
   (f) Storage in liver is in polyglutamate form.

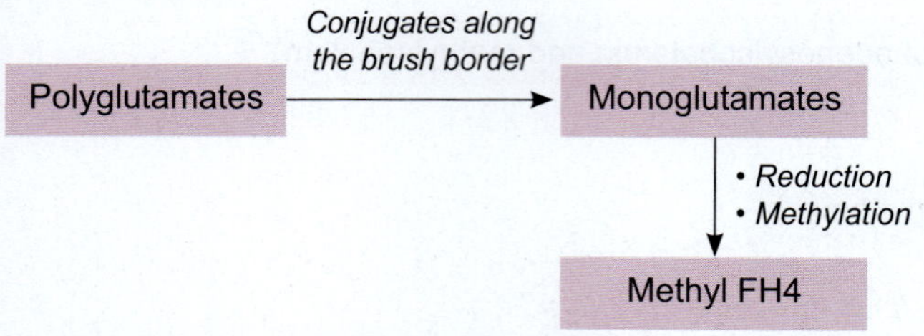

Flowchart 12.7 Absorption and transport of folate.

3. *Functions*
   (a) Folates act as 1-carbon unit carriers and are needed for synthesizing DNA and RNA, as well as the conversion of homocysteine to methionine (Flowchart 12.8).
   (b) Synthesis of purines.
   (c) Histidine metabolism (deficiency of folate leads to increased formiminoglutamic acid or FIGLU).

Causes of Vitamin B_{12} Deficiency

- **Decreased intake:** Nutritional deficiency (vegans, breast-fed infants of vegan mothers).
- **Impaired absorption**
  - **Gastric causes:** Pernicious anaemia, destruction of gastric mucosa or gastric bypass surgery.
  - **Intestinal causes:** Malabsorption due to enteritis, celiac disease or tropical sprue, competition for vitamin B_{12} in fish tapeworm (*Diphyllobothriumlatum*) infestation or blind loop syndrome (bacterial overgrowth in diverticulae of bowel).
  - **Drug-induced malabsorption:** Implicated drugs include PAS, colchicine, neomycin, ethanol and KCL.
  - **Chronic pancreatic disease:** Lack of pancreatic proteases and inability to degrade R proteins, which compete with IF.
  - **Zollinger–Ellison syndrome:** Impaired absorption due to low pH of intestinal contents reaching ileum.
  - **Haemodialysis:** Cause unknown.

Causes of Folate Deficiency

- **Inadequate intake:** Young persons on junk food diets, elderly and terminally ill people.
- **Inappropriate cooking methods:** Polyglutamates are sensitive to heat; boiling, steaming or frying the food destroys folate content.
- **Excess utilization**: Pregnancy, haemolysis and tumours.
- **Alcoholism:** Reduces serum folate levels are attributed to inadequate diet, excessive urinary loss and interference with the enterohepatic circulation of folate by alcohol.
- **Impaired absorption**
  - Celiac disease and tropical sprue.
  - Drugs that block dihydrofolate reductase (methotrexate and trimethoprim), block conversion of polyglutamates to monoglutamates (phenytoin), decrease absorption and increase metabolism (anticonvulsants) and decrease absorption and increase urinary excretion (oral contraceptives).
- **Complication of haematological illness:** Increased demand due to rapid proliferation of haematopoietic cells in haemolytic anaemia, PNH, myelofibrosis, sideroblastic anaemia, leukaemia and multiple myeloma.

Causes of Non-megaloblastic Macrocytic Anaemia

- **Haemolytic and post-haemorrhagic anaemia:** Result in accelerated erythropoiesis, which leads to increased reticulocyte count, premature release of the bone marrow reticulocytes and shortened time between all cell divisions/ skipping of cell division, all of which cause macrocytosis.
- **Thin macrocytosis:** Thin macrocytes typically have increased surface area to volume ratio. Increased surface area is attributed to excessive lipid content which in turn may be seen in:
  - **Hepatic disease (obstructive jaundice):** There is accumulation of bile salts in the plasma due to decreased bile salt excretion. Increased plasma bile salt levels reduce esterification of cholesterol, increasing free cholesterol

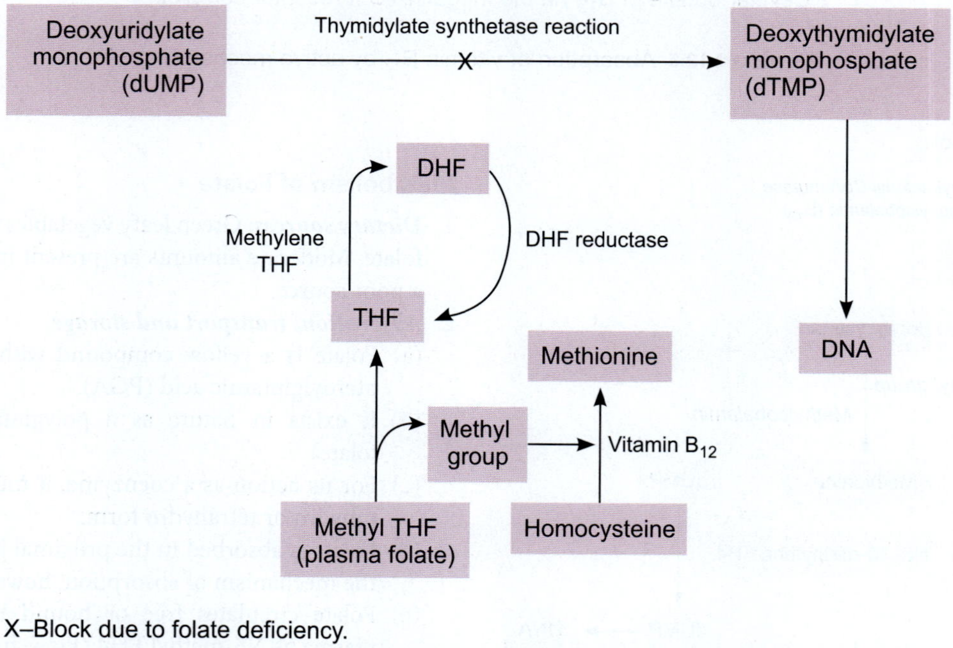

Flowchart 12.8 Role of B_{12} and folate in DNA synthesis.

levels, which in turn increases uptake of cholesterol by red cells, ultimately increasing the membrane surface area.
  - **Post-splenectomy state:** During maturation of reticulocytes in spleen, there is loss of lipids; in the absence of spleen, there is decreased loss and excessive accumulation of lipids in the RBC membrane resulting in increased surface area.
- **Myelodysplastic syndrome (MDS)**
  - Aplastic anaemia.
  - 5q-refractory anaemia syndrome.
  - Acquired sideroblastic anaemia.
  - Hereditary dyserythropoietic anaemia.
- **Miscellaneous**
  - Alcoholism.
  - Hypothyroidism.
  - Myelophthisic anaemia.

Clinical Features of Vitamin B_{12} Deficiency

- **General signs and symptoms of anaemia:** Weight loss, angular cheilosis, dermatitis, osteomalacia, pallor, icterus (lemon tint), low-grade fever (in severe anaemia), mucocutaneous bleeding (with thrombocytopenia).
- **Neurological manifestations:** Vitamin B_{12} deficiency causes **sensorimotor demyelinating peripheral neuropathy** (leading to paraesthesias and numbness) and **cerebral changes** (leading to dementia, psychosis or personality changes). This can be accompanied by involvement of **pyramidal tracts** (causing spastic paraparesis, cerebellar dysfunction and optic neuropathy). Vitamin B_{12} is required for transmethylation reactions, which are essential for myelin synthesis. B_{12} deficiency therefore affects white matter of dorsal/posterior and lateral columns of spinal cord leading to sensory ataxia and loss of position and vibration sense. Involvement of multiple pathways is labelled as **'subacute combined degeneration of the spinal cord'**.
- **Splenomegaly and hepatomegaly:** Mild and non-tender.
- **Gastrointestinal symptoms:** Weight loss and poorly localized abdominal pain.
- **Glossitis:** Loss of papillae leading to a smooth beefy red tongue.
- **Skin and hair changes:** Premature greying of hair and melanin pigmentation of skin with sparing of mucosa.
- **Infertility:** Reversible with correction of deficiency.

Clinical Features of Folate Deficiency

Folate deficiency mainly manifests with **megaloblastic anaemia** and **glossitis**. **Subacute combined degeneration is not seen** and **peripheral neuropathy is rare**.

Laboratory Diagnosis of Megaloblastic Anaemia

- **General blood parameters**
  - RBC count and haemoglobin levels are decreased.
  - MCV is increased (>100 fL) and MCH is decreased (less than 33 pg).
  - Reticulocyte count is normal.
- **Peripheral smear** (Fig. 12.4A and B)
  - Red cells show anisopoikilocytosis with the presence of **macrocytes** and **macroovalocytes** (large oval RBCs).

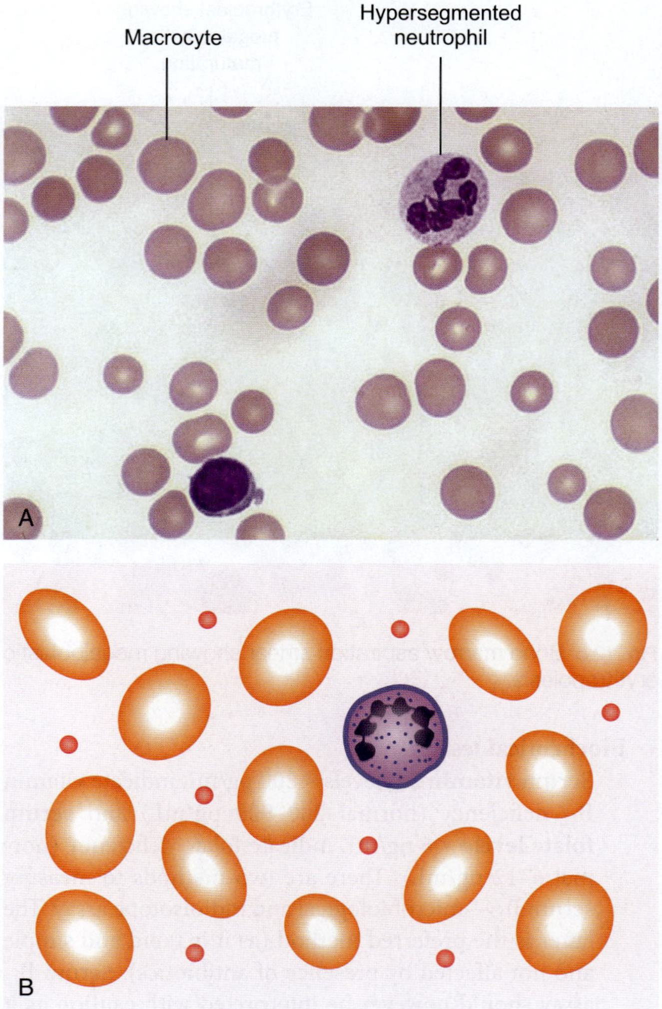

Fig. 12.4 (A) A Leishman-stained PBS of macrocytic anaemia and (B) schematic diagram of the same showing numerous macrocytes macro-ovalocytes and a hypersegmented neutrophil *(arrow)*.

  - Also present are **Howell–Jolly bodies** (nuclear remnants left after the nucleus is extruded) and **Cabot rings** (arginine-rich histones that are formed due to abnormal histone synthesis, accumulate as rings in red cells).
  - **Neutrophil hypersegmentation** is seen which is defined as greater than 5% neutrophils having more than five lobes or presence of at least one six-lobed cell. This is the first haematological abnormality to be seen in megaloblastic anaemia and is thought to be due to decreased production and a compensatory prolonged lifespan of circulating neutrophils (senile neutrophils).
- **Bone marrow**
  - Shows megaloblastic hyperplasia. Nuclei of erythroblasts are large with fine and open sieve-like chromatin. Haemoglobinization of the cytoplasm proceeds at a normal rate; whereas, nuclear maturation lags behind that of the cytoplasm (compared with iron deficiency anaemia in which the cytoplasmic maturation lags behind that of the nucleus). This is called nuclear-cytoplasmic asynchrony (Fig. 12.5).
  - Giant metamyelocytes and stab forms are seen.
  - Megakaryocytes may be large and abnormal.

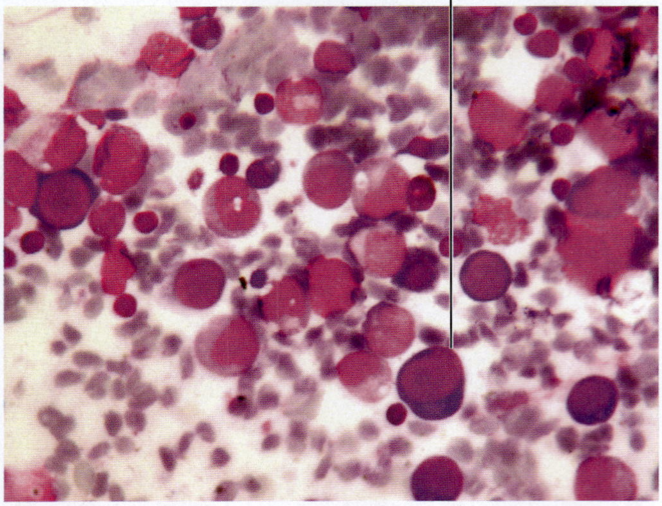

Fig. 12.5 Bone marrow aspiration smear showing megaloblastic erythropoiesis.

- **Biochemical tests**
  - **Serum vitamin B_{12}** levels <200 pg/mL indicate vitamin B_{12} deficiency (normal 200–900 pg/mL) and **serum folate levels** <6 ng/mL indicate folate deficiency (normal 6–12 ng/mL). There are two methods to measure serum B_{12}—microbiological and radioisotope assay. The latter is the preferred method (as it is rapid and simple and not affected by presence of antibiotics). Serum B_{12} assay should however be interpreted with caution as it represents the total and not metabolically active B_{12}.
  - **Holotranscobalamin (holo-TC)** is considered active B_{12} and is the earliest biomarker for B_{12} deficiency.
  - **Elevated methylmalonic acid (MMA) level indicates depletion of B_{12} stores.**
  - **Isolated decreased levels of holo TC** supports vitamin B_{12} deficiency and **a combination of decreased holoTc** and **increased MMA** (reference range: 0.08–0.28) and **homocysteine** indicate a metabolically manifest B_{12} deficiency. Increased MMA levels may also seen in renal failure. MMA levels can be used to monitor the response to treatment. MMA levels remain normal in folate deficiency. **Homocysteine levels** may be elevated with both vitamin B_{12} and folate deficiency. Hyperhomocystinaemia has been linked with increased risk of thrombosis as well as cardiovascular risk.
  - Red cells normally contain 20–50 times more folate than serum and **red cell folate assay is more reliable than serum folate assay.**
  - Measurement of urinary excretion of **formiminoglutamic acid (FIGLU)** after giving histidine load was used earlier to assess the folate levels; it is less specific and sensitive than the serum and RBC assays.
  - It is necessary to measure folate levels because vitamin B_{12} deficiency must be differentiated from folate deficiency as a cause of megaloblastic anaemia. Folate supplementation can mask vitamin B_{12} deficiency and may improve the anaemia but the neurological deficit continues to progress.
  - **Schilling test:** Schilling test is useful for diagnosing intrinsic factor deficiency, as in classic pernicious anaemia. It measures absorption of free radiolabelled vitamin B_{12}. Radiolabelled vitamin B_{12} is given orally, followed in 1–6 h by 1000 mcg (1 mg) of parenteral vitamin B_{12}, which reduces uptake of radiolabelled vitamin B_{12} by the liver. Absorbed radiolabelled vitamin B_{12} is excreted in urine, which is collected for 24 h. The amount excreted is measured and the percentage of radiolabelled vitamin B_{12} is determined. If absorption is normal, $\geq$ 9% of the dose given appears in the urine. Reduced urinary excretion (if kidney function is normal) indicates inadequate vitamin B_{12} absorption. Improved absorption with the subsequent addition of intrinsic factor to radiolabelled vitamin B_{12} confirms the diagnosis of pernicious anaemia.

    The test is often difficult to do or interpret because of incomplete urine collection or renal insufficiency. In addition, because the Schilling test does not measure absorption of protein-bound vitamin B_{12}, the test does not detect defective liberation of vitamin B_{12} from foods, which is common among the elderly.

    If the malabsorption is identified, the Schilling test can be repeated after a 2-week trial of an oral antibiotic. If antibiotic therapy corrects malabsorption, the likely cause is intestinal overgrowth of bacteria (e.g. blind-loop syndrome).

Q. Write briefly on anaemia due to blood loss.

Ans. Anaemia due to excessive bleeding results when loss of red blood cells exceeds production of new red blood cells.

Anaemia Due to Acute Blood Loss

- A healthy adult tolerates a loss of about 500 mL of whole blood without any ill effects.
- When more is lost, compensatory mechanisms come into play (the blood flow to skin and skeletal muscle is reduced, conserving the blood flow to vital organs like brain, kidney and heart.) If bleeding continues, compensatory mechanisms fail and hypovolaemic shock develops.
- Most expansion of plasma volume is seen in the first 24 h of blood loss.

Anaemia Due to Chronic Blood Loss

Compensatory mechanisms replenish the plasma volume and red cell loss. However, if the blood loss continues, body iron stores are depleted and anaemia due to iron deficiency appears.

Q. Define normocytic normochromic anaemia and enumerate its causes.

Ans. Normocytic normochromic anaemia is characterized by normal size of RBCs (normal MCV) and normal haemoglobinization (MCH).

Causes of normocytic normochromic anaemia are listed in Table 12.9.

Table 12.9 Causes of normocytic normochromic anaemia

Decreased red cell production	Increased red cell loss
• Anaemia of chronic illness	• Acute blood loss
• Marrow hypoplasia or aplasia	• Hypersplenism
• Myeloproliferative diseases	• Haemolytic disorders
• Myelofibrosis	• Haemoglobinopathies (sickle cell disease)
• Chronic renal failure	• Hereditary spherocytosis
• Chronic liver disease	• Glucose-6-phosphate dehydrogenase deficiency
• Sideroblastic anaemia	• Microangiopathic anaemias
• Hypothyroidism	• Autoimmune haemolytic anaemia
• Adrenal insufficiency	• PNH

PNH, Paroxysmal nocturnal haemoglobinuria.

Q. Outline the pathogenesis and laboratory findings of anaemia of chronic disease.

Ans. Anaemia of chronic disease is the most common cause of normocytic anaemia and the second most common form of anaemia worldwide (after iron-deficiency anaemia). Microcytosis and hypochromia usually occur later as the disease progresses. It occurs in a wide variety of chronic diseases including infective or inflammatory conditions, neoplasms and collagen vascular disorders, for example rheumatoid arthritis. The diagnosis of anaemia of chronic disease is not usually applied to anaemias associated with renal, hepatic or endocrine disorders.

Pathogenesis (Flowchart 12.9)

The major concern in this type of anaemia is that the marrow erythroid cells do not show increased expansion in response to anaemia. There are three main underlying mechanisms:

1. Mildly shortened red cell survival (cause unknown)
2. Impaired erythropoiesis due to decrease in both erythropoietin (EPO) production and marrow responsiveness to EPO
3. Impaired intracellular iron metabolism and restricted movement of iron from reticuloendothelial system (RES) to erythroid cells, which is due to:
   - Production of lactoferrin by inflammatory cells (which avidly binds iron; iron bound to lactoferrin is shunted to macrophages as there are no receptors for lactoferrin on erythroid cells).
   - Increased synthesis of apoferritin in inflammation (apoferritin binds to increased amounts of iron and diverts circulating iron to storage pool).

Laboratory Investigations

- Peripheral smear shows normocytic normochromic anaemia.
- Serum iron, transferrin levels and total iron-binding capacity are reduced.
- Ferritin levels are elevated and reticuloendothelial iron is increased.

Q. Define haemolysis. Classify haemolytic anaemia. (PA16.1)

Ans. Haemolysis is defined as premature destruction of red cells such that they have a shortened life span (<120 days). In the initial stages of haemolysis, increased bone marrow activity can compensate for the ongoing destruction of red cells; a stage called **compensated haemolysis.** There can be a six- to eightfold increase in red cell number due to compensatory bone marrow hyperplasia. Haemolytic anaemia results when the bone marrow activity can no more compensate for the shortened RBC survival. The three main characteristics of haemolytic anaemia are:

- Premature destruction of red cells.
- Accumulation of products of haemoglobin breakdown.
- Accelerated erythropoiesis in bone marrow.

The abnormal breakdown of RBCs may occur either within the blood vessels (intravascular haemolysis) or outside (extravascular haemolysis).

Classification of haemolytic anaemia is given in Table 12.10.

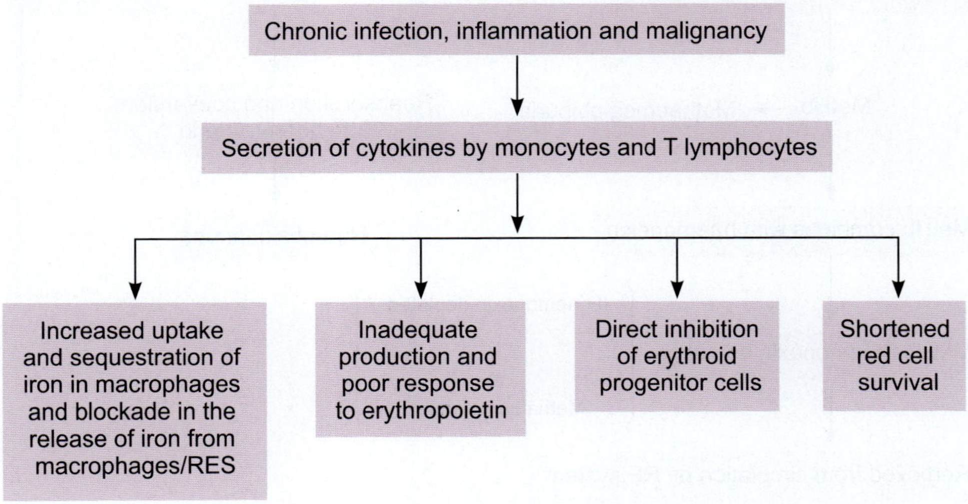

Flowchart 12.9 Pathogenesis of anaemia of chronic disease.

Table 12.10 Classification of haemolytic anaemias

Intrinsic/intracorpuscular abnormalities	Extrinsic/extracorpuscular abnormalities
Hereditary • Membrane cytoskeleton disorders: Spherocytosis and elliptocytosis • Red cell enzyme deficiency: Pyruvate kinase, G6PD • Disorders of haemoglobin synthesis: ▪ Deficient globin synthesis, for example thalassaemia syndrome ▪ Structural abnormality of globin chain (haemoglobinopathies), for example, sickle cell anaemia **Acquired** • Membrane defect: Paroxysmal nocturnal haemoglobinuria (PNH)	**Immune haemolytic anaemia** • Autoimmune (idiopathic, SLE, malignant neoplasms) • Alloimmune • Drug induced **Mechanical trauma to red cells (microangiopathic haemolytic anaemia)** Thrombotic thrombocytopenic purpura (TTP), DIC and prosthetic heart valves **Infections** Malaria and bacterial diseases **Chemical injury** Lead poisoning **Sequestration in mononuclear phagocyte system** Hypersplenism

Q. Enumerate the causes of intravascular haemolysis. (PA16.2)

Ans. Intravascular haemolysis entails lysis of red cells within the circulation to release their contents into plasma. Causes of intravascular haemolysis include:

- Microangiopathic haemolytic anaemia or mechanical trauma to red cells [Haemolytic-uraemic syndrome (HUS), DIC, and thrombotic thrombocytopenic purpura (TTP)].
- Physical injury (mechanical trauma and thermal injury).
- Paroxysmal Nocturnal Haemoglobinuria (PNH).
- G6PD (glucose-6-phosphate dehydrogenase) deficiency.
- Autoimmune haemolytic anaemia.
- Mechanical heart valves.
- March haemoglobinuria (seen in vigorous exercise).
- Pregnancy-induced hypertension.
- Infections—*P. falciparum* and *Clostridium perfringens.*
- Disseminated malignancy.
- Haemolytic uraemic syndrome.

The sequence of events occurring in intravascular haemolysis has been depicted in Flowchart 12.10.

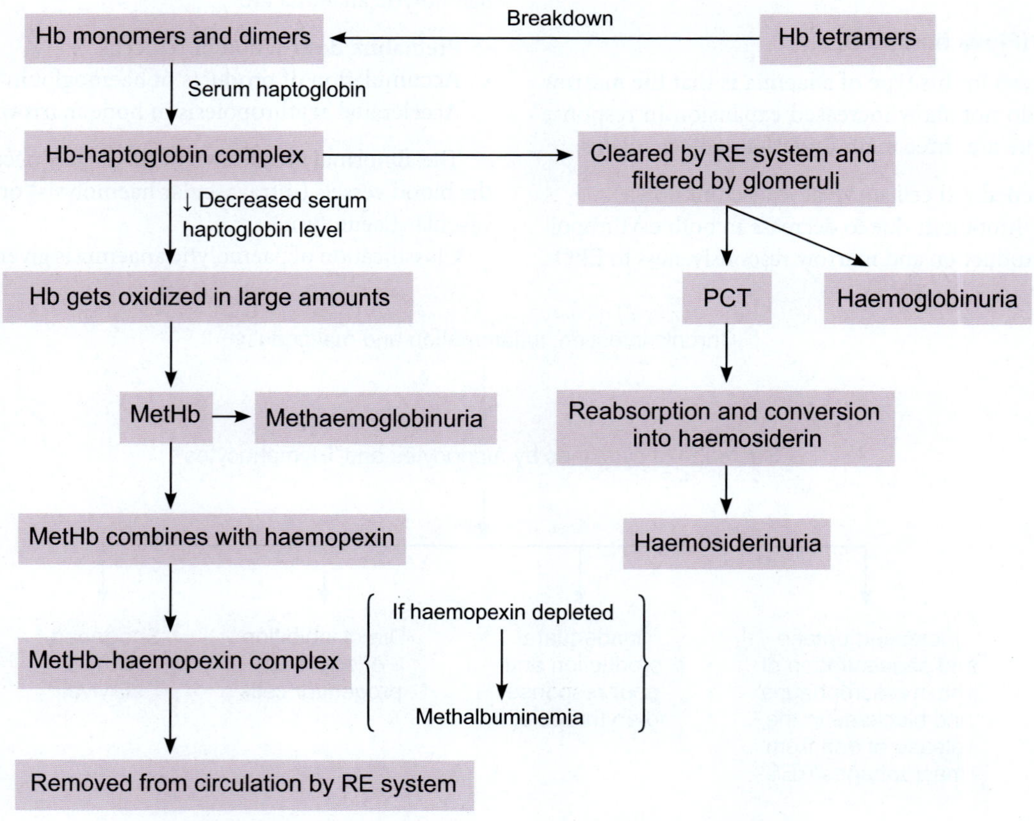

Flowchart 12.10 Sequence of events in intravascular haemolysis.

Table 12.11 Differences between intra- and extravascular haemolysis

Feature	Intravascular haemolysis	Extravascular haemolysis
Incidence	Less common	More common
Site	In peripheral blood	In RE organs (spleen, bone marrow, etc.)
Plasma haemoglobin	Present	Absent
Methaemoglobin	Present	Absent
Haemoglobinuria	Present	Absent
Haemosiderinuria	Present	Absent
Unconjugated bilirubin	Mild increase	Marked increase
Serum haptoglobin	Decreased	Normal
Serum LDH	Markedly increased	Mildly increased
Serum ferritin	Low	Normal-high
Iron stores	Decreased	Increased

Q. Enumerate the causes of extravascular haemolysis. (PA16.2)

Ans. Red cells are taken up by the RES where destruction takes place extravascularly. Causes of extravascular haemolysis include:

- All red cell membrane defects, for example hereditary spherocytosis.
- Sickle cell anaemia.
- Premature destruction of RBCs, for example thalassaemia or other haemoglobin synthesis disorders.
- Splenomegaly (hypersplenism).

Q. Differentiate between extravascular and intravascular haemolysis. (PA16.2)

Ans. Differences between intra- and extravascular haemolysis are tabulated in Table 12.11.

Q. Enumerate the steps in the laboratory diagnosis of haemolytic anaemia. (PA16.2, 16.5)

Ans. Diagnosis of haemolytic anaemia entails performing tests, which identify evidence for increased red cell breakdown, compensatory erythroid hyperplasia and damage to red cells, which are all important features of haemolysis.

Laboratory Evidence of Increased RBC Breakdown

- Increased serum bilirubin (mainly unconjugated).
- Increased faecal stercobilinogen.
- Increased urinary urobilinogen.
- Increased plasma LDH (LDH2 > LDH1).
- Shortened red cell lifespan (decreased from normal 120 days to 30–40 days) demonstrated by 51chromium labelled method.

Laboratory Evidence of Intravascular Haemolysis

- Decreased or absent serum haptoglobin and haemopexin (haemoglobin-binding proteins).
- Haemoglobinaemia, haemoglobinuria and methaemalbuminaemia.
- Haemosiderinuria.
- Jaundice.

Laboratory Evidence of Compensatory Erythroid Hyperplasia

- Increased reticulocyte count.
- Macrocytosis, polychromasia and stippling.
- Erythroid hyperplasia with increased iron stores (in most cases).

Laboratory Evidence of Damage to RBCs

- Presence of fragments of red cells (schistocytes) and spherocytes in the peripheral smear.
- Positive direct Coombs test, if haemolysis is immunological in origin.

Q. Enumerate the hereditary abnormalities of red cell membrane. Write briefly on the molecular pathology, laboratory diagnosis and clinical features of hereditary spherocytosis (HS).

Ans. Membrane disorders include **HS, elliptocytosis, and stomatocytosis. HS**, the commonest of these, is an inherited disease characterized by an intrinsic **defect in red cell membrane that results in less deformable, spheroidal RBCs, which are vulnerable to splenic sequestration and destruction.** It is **autosomal dominant** in 75% cases; remaining being recessive.

Molecular Pathology

- Spectrin, ankyrin, protein 4.1 and band 3 are main cytoskeletal proteins that are responsible for maintenance of normal shape, strength and flexibility of red cell membrane. The most common abnormality is a quantitative reduction in spectrin. In some patients, spectrin is unable to attach to protein 4.1.
- Any defect in these cytoskeleton proteins is associated with reduced membrane stability and loss of membrane fragments as the cells are exposed to shear stress in the circulation.
- Reduction in cell surface to volume ratio forces cells to assume shape of least surface area for a given volume that is a sphere.

Pathophysiology (See Flowchart 12.11)

Clinical Features

- Presents in childhood with anaemia, splenomegaly, jaundice and gallstones.
- Aplastic crisis (triggered by parvovirus B19) and haemolytic crisis are common occurrences. The former is characterized by aplasia, worsening of anaemia, and reticulocytopenia. The latter is characterized by sudden massive haemolysis, fever, abdominal pain and rarely shock.

Laboratory Diagnosis

- **General haematological parameters:**
  - Reduced values of Hb and MCV.

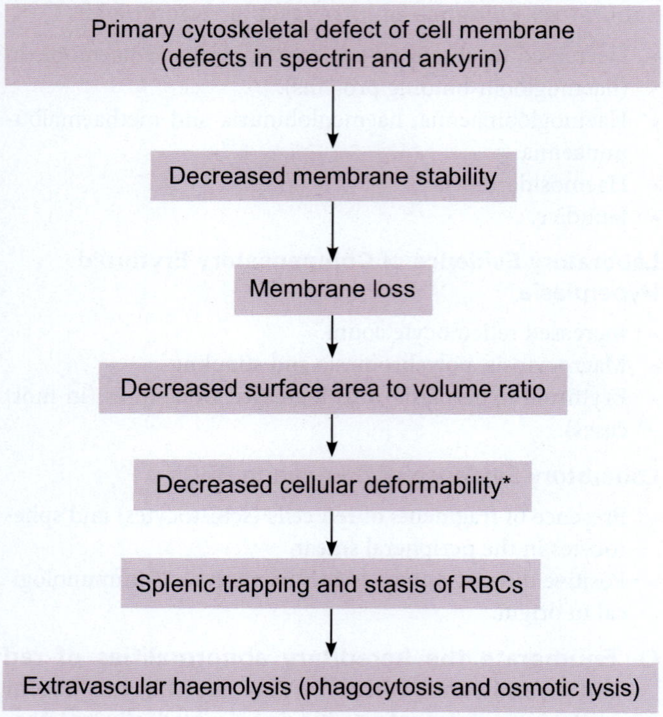

*The discoid shape of the normal RBCs allows extreme degrees of deformation required to leave cords of Billroth and enter the splenic sinusoids. Due to their spherical shape and limited deformability, spherocytes are sequestered in the splenic cords.

Flowchart 12.11 Pathophysiology of haemolysis in hereditary spherocytosis.

- Increased MCHC.
- Increased reticulocyte count.

- **Peripheral smear (Fig. 12.6):** Anisocytosis with presence of microspherocytes and spherocytes (dark appearing red cells with no central pallor). Unlike the spherocytes seen in other conditions, spherocytes in HS are uniform in size and density.
- **Bone marrow:** Erythroid hyperplasia (haemolytic picture).
- **Osmotic fragility test:** Determines the susceptibility of RBCs to haemolysis when they are subjected to osmotic stress; osmotic fragility is increased in HS.

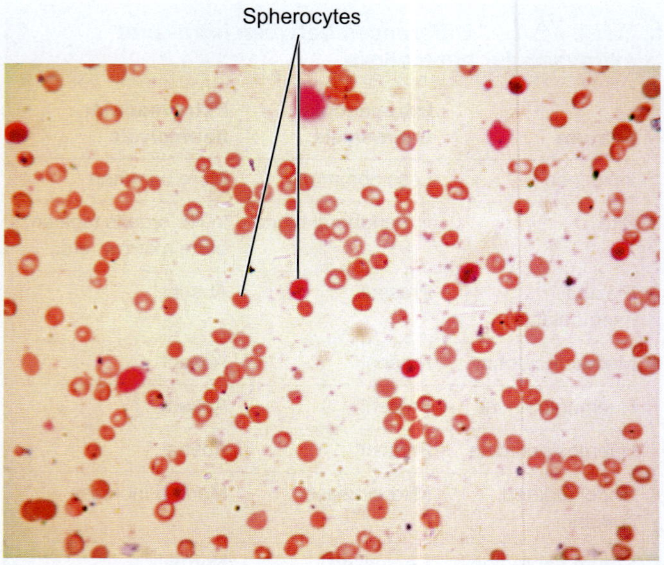

Fig. 12.6 Leishman-stained peripheral blood smear showing spherocytes and microspherocytes.

- **Autohaemolysis:** Spontaneous haemolysis when blood is incubated at 37°C for 48 h. Increased in HS; lysis of 10%–15% RBCs as compared to <4% in normal red cells.
- **Direct Coombs test:** Negative (differentiates it from acquired spherocytosis of AIHA in which Combs test is positive).
- **Increased serum bilirubin.**
- **Electrophoretic analysis of spectrin and other cytoskeleton protein levels (confirmatory test).**

Treatment

Splenectomy (after splenectomy, spherocytes persist but anaemia is corrected).

Q. Write briefly on G6PD deficiency anaemia.

Ans. Red cell enzyme defects mainly include **pyruvate kinase deficiency** (defect in glycolytic pathway) and **G6PD deficiency** (defect in hexose monophosphate shunt).

Role of G6PD (Glucose-6-Phosphate Dehydrogenase) Enzyme in HMP Pathway (Flowchart 12.12)

- Red cells are vulnerable to injury by endogenous and exogenous oxidants, which are normally inactivated by reduced glutathione (GSH).

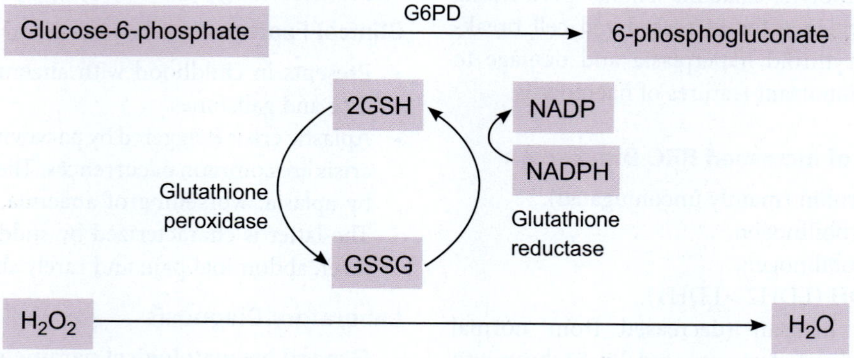

Flowchart 12.12 Role of glucose-6-phosphate dehydrogenase *(G6PD)* enzyme in HMP pathway.

- Abnormalities that affect enzymes required for GSH production reduce the ability of the cells to protect themselves from oxidative injury, leading to haemolysis.
- Prototype is the haemolytic anaemia associated with deficiency of G6PD.

Genetic Variation of G6PD Enzymes

More than 400 variants are identified. The inheritance of the mutant gene is an X-linked recessive trait. Induction of haemolysis is never spontaneous and always occurs in the presence of an environmental agent. Haemolysis develops after a lag period of 2–3 days and may be:

- Drug induced: Primaquine, chloroquine, sulfonamides, phenacetin, and aspirin in large doses.
- Infection induced: Viral hepatitis, pneumonia, and typhoid fever.
- Food induced: Fava beans.

Mechanism of Haemolysis

- Haemolysis is produced by action of free radicals as a response to oxidative stress, for example, H_2O_2, which is normally neutralized by GSH. Free radicals induce oxidation of sulfhydryl group of globin chain.
- Denaturation of haemoglobin chains results in precipitation as **Heinz bodies** (appear as dark inclusions within cells). Attachment of Heinz bodies to membrane aids to deformity of RBCs and intravascular haemolysis.
- When these cells pass through the splenic cords, macrophages pluck out Heinz bodies along with cytoplasm, giving appearance of '**bite cells**'. Loss of membrane results in formation of spherocytes and extravascular haemolysis.

Laboratory Diagnosis of G6PD Deficiency Anaemia

During Normal Phase

No anaemia is evident but red cell survival is decreased. Defective variant enzymes can be detected by molecular techniques.

During Haemolytic Phase

- Features of intravascular haemolysis (during active phase).
- Rapid fall of haematocrit with reticulocytosis (during recovery phase).
- *PBS*: Heinz bodies (demonstrated by supravital stains like crystal violet) and bite cells.
- *G6PD assay*:
  - Indirect assays, based on decreased ability to reduce dye. Methods used are met haemoglobin reduction test (MRT), fluorescent screening test and ascorbate cyanide screening test.
  - Direct enzyme assay in RBC.

Q. Write briefly on the pathophysiology, clinical features and laboratory diagnosis of sickle cell disease. (PA16.3)

Ans. Disorders of haemoglobin synthesis include disorders associated with deficient globin synthesis, for example, thalassaemia syndrome and structural abnormalities of globin chain synthesis, for example, haemoglobinopathies. **Sickle cell disease** is a hereditary haemoglobinopathy, which is **characterized by point mutation-substitution of glutamic acid (CTG) by valine (CAG) at 6th position in β-globin chain.**

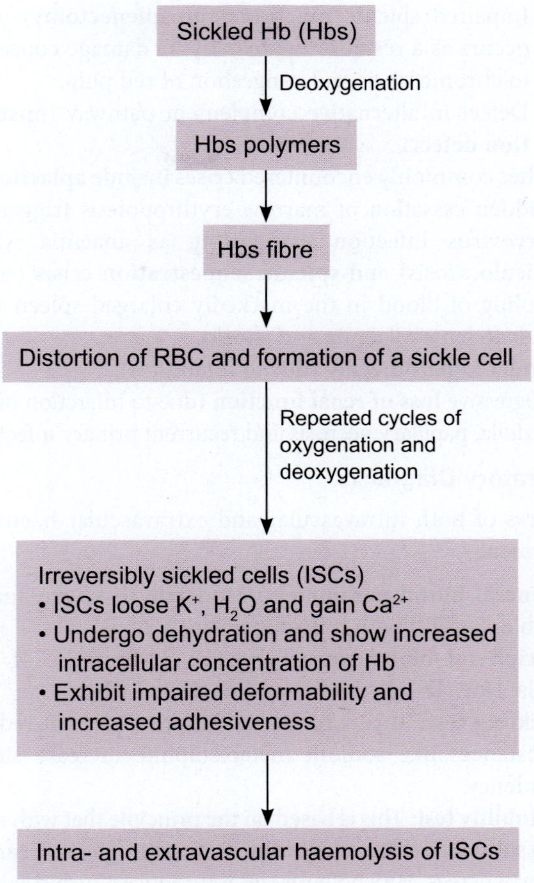

Flowchart 12.13 Pathogenesis of haemolysis in sickle cell anaemia.

Pathophysiology (See Flowchart 12.13)

Factors Affecting Sickling

- **Amount of HbS:** Heterozygotes do not show sickling except under severe hypoxia.
- **Interaction with other type of Hb:** HbF inhibits polymerization of HbS and hence, sickling (so, the disease manifests 5–6 months after birth). HbC and HbD promote sickling (HbSC is the more severe form of disease).
- **MCHC value:** Any condition (like dehydration) that increases MCHC increases sickling.
- **pH:** Fall in pH increases sickling.
- **Oxygen concentration:** Increased oxygen concentration increases sickling.

Clinical Features

- **Severe anaemia and generalized impairment of growth** and development due to hypoxia.
- **Vasoocclusive complications,** which include acute chest syndrome, dactylitis (hand-foot syndrome) and stroke.
- **Chronic hyperbilirubinaemia** and **cholelithiasis.**
- **Septicaemia** and **meningitis** caused by **Pneumococci** and ***H. influenzae*** are common. Patients are also predisposed to ***Salmonella* osteomyelitis.** Increased susceptibility to infection is attributed to the following:

- Impaired splenic function (**autosplenectomy**), which occurs as a result of hypoxic tissue damage consequent to chronic stasis and congestion of red pulp.
- Defect in alternative complement pathway (**opsonization defect**).

- Other commonly encountered crises include **aplastic crisis** (sudden cessation of marrow erythropoiesis triggered by parvovirus infection manifesting as anaemia without reticulocytosis) and **splenic sequestration crisis** (sudden pooling of blood in the markedly enlarged spleen which leads to hypovolaemia and shock).
- Tender **hepatomegaly** (due to infarction).
- Progressive **loss of renal function** (due to infarction of renal medulla, papillary necrosis and recurrent urinary infections).

Laboratory Diagnosis

Features of both intravascular and extravascular haemolysis are present.

- **General blood parameters:** Moderate to severe anaemia (Hb 6–8 g/dL) with reticulocytosis.
- **Peripheral blood smear** (Fig. 12.7): Presence of sickle cells; Howell–Jolly bodies and nucleated RBCs.
- **Sickling test:** This is based on the principle that reducing substances like sodium metabisulphite increase sickling tendency.
- **Solubility test:** This is based on the principle that with reducing substances like sodium dithionite, HbA gives a clear solution; whereas, HbS polymerizes to produce a turbid solution.
- **Hb electrophoresis:**
  - Decreased/absent HbA (normal adult Hb).
  - Increased HbS (abnormal Hb).
  - Increased HbF (2%–20%, compensatory increase).
- **Osmotic fragility test:** Osmotic fragility is decreased due to the sickle shape, which has large scope for expansion of volume without rupture of the red cell.

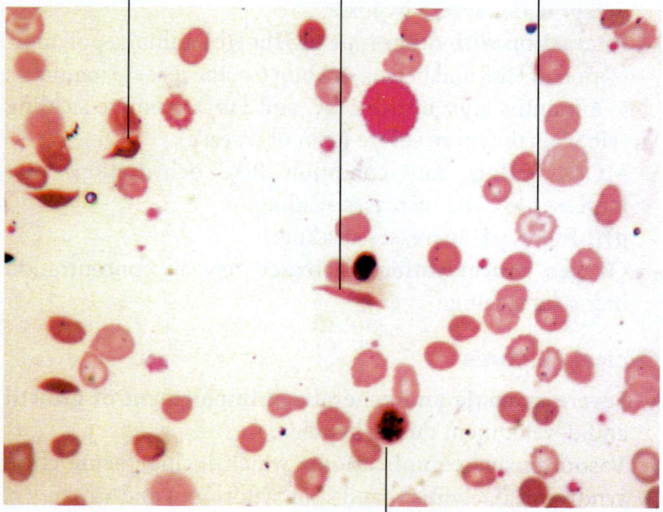

Fig. 12.7 Leishman-stained peripheral blood smear from sickle cell anaemia showing sickle cells, poikilocytes, target cells and nucleated RBCs.

Q. Describe the molecular pathology, clinical features and laboratory diagnosis of thalassaemias. (PA16.3)

Ans. Normally, HbA is the predominant type of haemoglobin found in adults. It comprises two α chains and two β chains; β chains are coded by two globin genes, each located on one of the two chromosome 11; whereas, α chains are coded by two pairs of genes, one pair located on each chromosome 16. Thalassaemias are a heterogenous group of genetic disorders characterized by a reduction in the synthesis of one or more haemoglobin polypeptide chains.

Common Types of Thalassaemias

1. **α-Thalassaemia:** Affects the synthesis of α chains and its severity depends on the number of α genes deleted. Based on the number of dysfunctional α genes, α-thalassaemia is classified into:
   (a) **α-thalassaemia trait:** One or two α genes are deleted or dysfunctional. Majority of the patients are asymptomatic; some show reduced MCV and MCH and a microcytic hypochromic anaemia.
   (b) **Haemoglobin H disease:** This is caused by functional inactivation of 3–4 α genes. There is microcytic hypochromic anaemia (Hb-7–11 g/dL); hepatosplenomegaly, jaundice, gall stones and leg ulcers. Haemoglobin electrophoresis shows 4%–10% HbH (β4 haemoglobin). No bony deformities or features of iron overload are evident.
   (c) **Haemoglobin Bart (hydrops fetalis):** All four α genes are inactive. There is inability to make either HbA or HbF. The excess β chains form Hb Bart's. There is intrauterine death at 25–40 weeks or the foetus dies immediately after birth.
2. **β-Thalassaemia:** Also called *Cooley anaemia or Mediterranean anaemia,* β-thalassaemia is characterized by a total lack or reduction in the synthesis of structurally normal β-globin chains with normal synthesis of α chains resulting in reduced levels of HbA. β-thalassaemia is a common blood disorder, which occurs most frequently in Mediterranean countries, North Africa, the Middle East, India, Central and Southeast Asia. Depending on the severity it is classified into:
   (a) β-Thalassaemia minor (trait).
   (b) β-Thalassaemia intermedia.
   (c) β-Thalassaemia major.

Molecular Pathology of β-Thalassaemia

- β-Thalassaemia is mainly due to point mutations (in contrast to gene deletion in α-thalassaemia).
- Two major groups of mutations are recognized:
  - Non-deletion forms: These defects involve a single base substitution or small insertions near or upstream of the β-globin gene: most often, mutations occur in the promoter regions, and less often, abnormal splice variants are believed to contribute to the disease.
  - Deletion forms: Deletions of different sizes involving the β-globin gene produce different syndromes such as (β^0) or hereditary persistence of fetal haemoglobin syndrome (a benign condition in which which increased fetal haemoglobin (HbF) production continues well into adulthood.

- Alleles without a mutation that reduces function are characterized as (β). Mutations are characterized as (β^0) if they prevent any formation of β chains, and as (β^+) if they allow some β chain formation to occur.
- **Promoter region mutations** lead to β^+-thalassaemia.
- **Chain terminator mutations** lead to β^0-thalassaemia. These result from either of the two following mechanisms:
  - Frame shift mutation (introduction of stop codon).
  - Point mutation (introduction of stop codon).
- **Splicing mutations** (most common cause of thalassaemia) may occur:
  - *At the junction of exon and intron:* β^0-thalassaemia.
  - *In intron:* β^+-thalassaemia.
- **Translation defect of exon** leads to β^0-thalassaemia.
- ***β-Thalassaemia major may be:***
  - Homozygous β^0-thalassaemia (β^0/β^0).
  - Homozygous β^+-thalassaemia (β^+/β^+).
  - Double heterozygous (β^+/β^0) thalassaemia.
- ***β-Thalassaemia minor/trait is:***
  - Heterozygous (β^0/β, β^+/β).

Pathogenesis (See Flowchart 12.14)

Clinical Features of β-Thalassaemia

- **β-Thalassaemia major**
  - Manifests 6–9 months after birth (as HbF decreases).
  - Presents with severe anaemia, requiring regular blood transfusions.
  - Untransfused patients show **failure to thrive; growth retardation** and **early death.**
  - **Mongoloid** or **thalassaemia facies** is typical (marrow expands due to erythroid hyperplasia leading to bossing of skull, hypertrophied maxillae and hair on end appearance on X-ray).
  - **Extramedullary haematopoiesis** may lead **to hepatosplenomegaly.** Other manifestations include **recurrent infections, spontaneous fractures, hypersplenism and leg ulcers.**
  - Transfused patients may end up with **secondary haemochromatosis** (iron chelators are given for treatment of the same). Iron deposition in the pancreas, liver and heart leads to diabetes, cirrhosis and arrhythmias, heart block or cardiac failure, respectively.
  - **Definite prevention and treatment of β-thalassaemia major:**
    - Prenatal diagnosis by DNA analysis and abortion.
    - Bone marrow transplantation from HLA-identical sibling.
- **β-Thalassaemia minor (trait).**

Patient is asymptomatic with mild or no anaemia and is commonly is diagnosed accidentally on peripheral smear examination.

Laboratory Diagnosis of β-Thalassaemia Major

General Blood Parameters

- Hb varies between 2 and 6 g/dL.
- Haematocrit, MCV, MCH and MCHC are severely decreased.
- RBC count is decreased.
- WBC count is increased with a shift to left of neutrophil series (presence of myelocytes and metamyelocytes).
- Platelet count may be normal or decreased (decrease is due to massive splenomegaly).

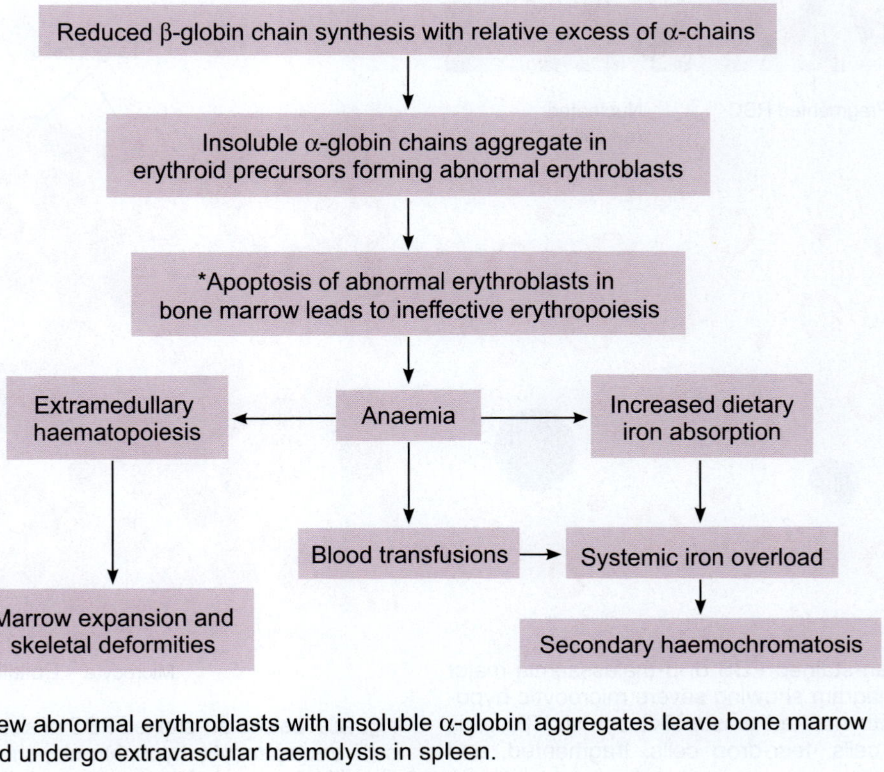

Flowchart 12.14 Pathophysiology of β-thalassaemia.

Peripheral Blood Smear (Fig. 12.8)

- Severe microcytic hypochromic anaemia with marked anisopoikilocytosis.
- Basophilic stippling, target cells, poikilocytes, fragmented red cells, pencil cells, cells with Cabot rings and numerous nucleated red cells.

Bone Marrow

- Normoblastic erythroid hyperplasia.
- Ineffective erythropoiesis.
- Predominance of intermediate and late normoblasts (smaller in size than normal).
- Increased reticuloendothelial iron with siderotic granules in the cytoplasm of normoblasts.

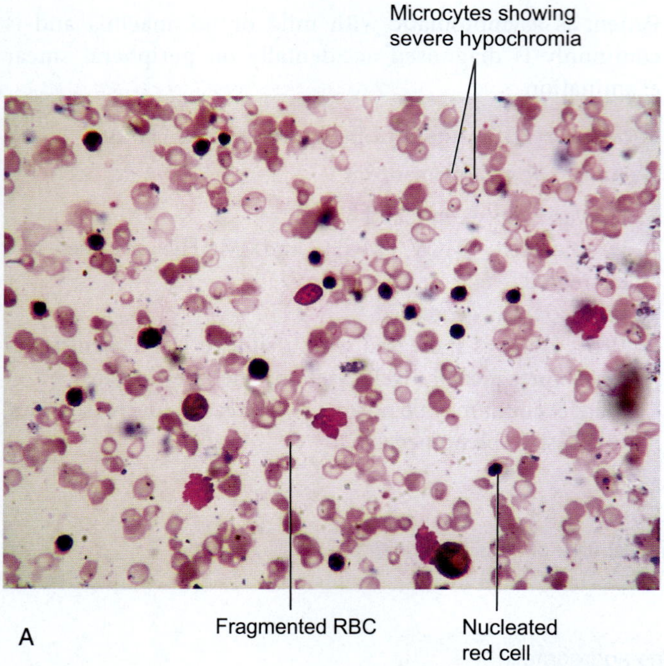

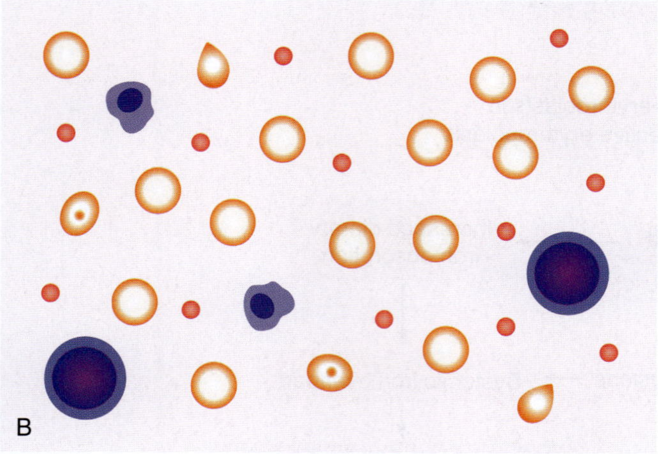

Fig. 12.8 (A) Leishman-stained PBS of β-thalassaemia major and (B) schematic diagram showing severe microcytic hypochromic anaemia with marked anisopoikilocytosis. There is presence of target cells, tear-drop cells, fragmented, and nucleated red cells.

Hb Electrophoresis

- HbA: Absent/markedly decreased.
- HbA_2: Normal/decreased/increased.
- HbF: Markedly increased (10%–98%).

Other Findings

- Increased unconjugated bilirubin and urinary urobilinogen.
- Markedly increased serum iron.
- Increased percentage transferrin saturation (>70%).
- Markedly increased serum ferritin (300–3000 mg/dL).
- Decreased osmotic fragility.

Laboratory Diagnosis of β-Thalassaemia Trait

General Blood Parameters

- Hb and haematocrit mildly decreased with increase in the reticulocyte count.
- MCV, MCH and MCHC decreased out of proportion to degree of anaemia.
- RBC count higher as compared to iron deficiency anaemia for the same haemoglobin value.

Peripheral Blood Smear (Fig. 12.9)

- Hypochromic microcytic RBCs with mild anisopoikilocytosis
- Target cells, basophilic stippling, poikilocytes, pencil cells, cells with Cabot rings and nucleated red cells may be present but are fewer as compared to β-thalassaemia major.

Bone Marrow

Mild erythroid hyperplasia.

Haemoglobin Electrophoresis

Increased HbA_2 (3.6%–9%; normal 1%–3.5%).

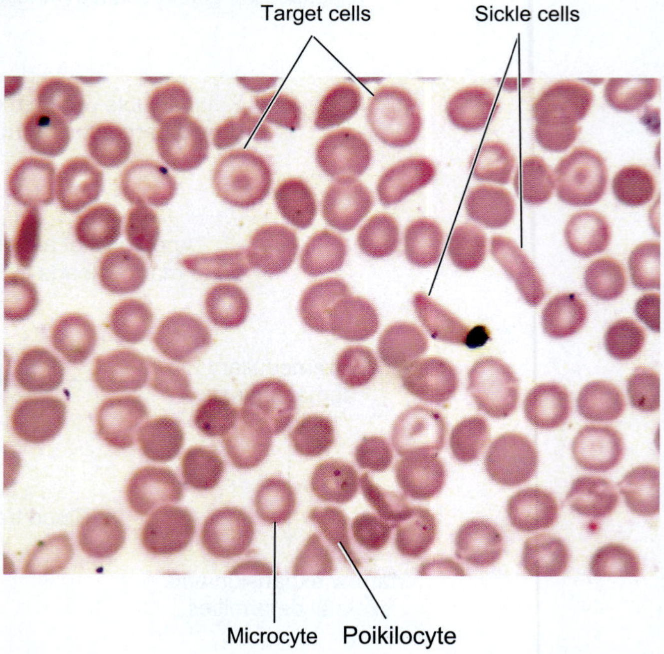

Fig. 12.9 Leishman-stained PBS of sickle-thalassaemia trait; red cells are microcytic hypochromic, show mild anisopoikilocytosis with presence of target cells, poikilocytes and sickle cells.

Osmotic Fragility Test

Shows decreased osmotic fragility.

Q. Write briefly on paroxysmal nocturnal haemoglobinuria (PNH).

Ans. PNH is the only example of an acquired defect in red cell membrane. It is characterized by chronic haemolytic anaemia with intermittent haemoglobinuria. It may be associated with aplastic anaemia, myelodysplastic syndrome and rarely acute leukaemia.

Pathology

- Mutation in phosphatidylinositol glycan A (PIGA) gene that codes for glycosyl-phosphatidylinositol (GPI) protein, which acts as an anchor of GPI-linked proteins to the cell membrane.
- The following GPI-linked membrane proteins regulate complement factors and are absent in PNH.
  - CD55 or decay-accelerating factor.
  - CD59 or membrane inhibitor of reactive lysis.
  - C8-binding protein (homologous restriction factor).

GPI-linked proteins interact with C3b and C4b to dissociate the convertase complexes of both classic and alternative complement pathways thus stopping amplification of activation by complement. RBCs, platelets and granulocytes are more sensitive to complement lysis when these proteins are absent.

Laboratory Diagnosis

General Blood Parameters

- **Evidence** of intravascular haemolysis.
- **Decreased** Hb, RBC, WBC and platelet counts (pancytopenia).
- **Increased** reticulocyte count and occasionally raised HbF.

Peripheral Blood Smear

Anaemia with macrocytosis and polychromasia.

Bone Marrow

- Hypercellular marrow with normoblastic erythroid hyperplasia.
- Some dyserythropoiesis is seen.
- Iron stores are decreased.
- Intermittent clinical haemoglobinuria (acute haemolytic episodes which occur mostly at night and are identified by passage of brown coloured urine in the morning).
- Haemosiderinuria and venous thrombosis are common.

Sucrose Haemolysis Test

A screening test for PNH, it is more sensitive than Hams test given below, though lacks specificity. Sucrose enhances complement binding to RBCs and haemolysis is by classic pathway of complement. Sucrose lysis test is done to find out degree of haemolysis (>10% haemolysis is diagnostic of PNH).

Hams Test (for Definitive Diagnosis of PNH)

The patient's cells undergo haemolysis (by alternative complement pathway) in compatible acidified serum at 37°C. The serum may be the patient's own or from another normal subject. 10%–50% lysis indicates a positive test.

Q. Write briefly on autoimmune acquired haemolytic anaemia (AIHA). (PA16.4)

Ans. AIHAs are a group of acquired disorders in which antibodies develop against red cell antigens and cause destruction of red cells.

Classification

1. **Based on antibody type**
   (a) Warm antibody AIHA
      (i) Primary or idiopathic.
      (ii) Secondary
         – Drugs (methyldopa, penicillin and quinidine).
         – Autoimmune disorders (SLE, others).
         – Haematologic malignancies like chronic lymphocytic leukaemia and lymphomas.
   (b) Cold antibody AIHA
      (i) Cold haemagglutinin disease.
      (ii) Paroxysmal cold haemoglobinuria.
      (iii) Cold AIHA associated with mycoplasma infection.
2. **Based on aetiology**
   (a) Idiopathic autoimmune acquired haemolytic anaemia (50%).
   (b) Secondary autoimmune acquired haemolytic anaemia (50%).
      (i) Drugs, for example methyldopa, penicillins, procainamide and phenothiazine.
      (ii) Chronic lymphocytic leukaemia.
      (iii) Malignant disorders like lymphomas.
      (iv) Infections like ***M. pneumoniae***, infectious mononucleosis, cytomegalovirus and rubella.
      (v) SLE and other connective tissue disorders.
      (vi) Immune deficiency states (common variable immunodeficiency).
      (vii) Miscellaneous: Carcinoma, sarcoidosis, ovarian teratoma post-transplant.

Warm Antibody AIHA

- Most common form of immune haemolytic anaemia.
- Caused by warm antibodies, which react with RBCs at 37°C.
- Majority of warm antibodies are of the IgG class.
- Most RBC destruction is extravascular. IgG-coated RBCs bind to Fc receptors on macrophages resulting in loss of RBC membrane during passage through spleen. This converts the RBCs to spherocytes, which are removed by the spleen.
- Clinical features include anaemia, jaundice, hepatosplenomegaly and manifestations of underlying disease.
- Diagnosis is based on presence of anaemia with reticulocytosis, evidence of haemolysis, spherocytes in peripheral blood and positive direct (antibodies on the red cell surface) and indirect Coombs tests (antibodies in the serum).

Cold Antibody AIHA

- Caused by cold agglutinins, which are IgM antibodies that bind and agglutinate RBCs at low temperatures (0–4°C).
- It is of two types, cold haemagglutinin disease (CHAD) and paroxysmal cold haemoglobinuria (PCH). CHAD is characterized by a haemolytic anaemia due to autoantibodies that act as RBC agglutinins at low temperatures; whereas, PCH is

characterized by episodes of acute haemolysis due to autoantibodies that act as red cell lysins at low temperatures.

- Most cells with bound IgM pick up C3b but are not lysed in the periphery.
- When they travel to warmer areas, the weakly bound IgM is released, but the coated C3b remains.
- C3b being an opsonin, the cells are phagocytosed by the mononuclear phagocytic system (haemolysis is extravascular).
- The typical blood picture is of anaemia with reticulocytosis, red cell agglutination and a positive direct antiglobulin test.

Q. Write briefly on Coombs test. (PA16.4)

Ans. Antiglobulin testing, also known as the Coombs test, is an immunology laboratory procedure used to detect the presence of antibodies against circulating RBCs. The destruction of these red blood cells by antibodies directed against them is described diagnostically as autoimmune haemolytic anaemia. Antiglobulin testing can be either direct antiglobulin testing (DAT) or indirect antiglobulin testing (IAT).

1. Direct Coombs Test

In this test, patient's red cells are washed and suspended in saline. Rabbit anti-human globulin is added. Agglutination of red cells indicates the presence of antibodies on the surface of red cells.

Indications:

- Haemolytic disease of newborn.
- Autoimmune haemolytic anaemia.

2. Indirect Coombs Test (ICT)

(a) In this test, normal red cells and rabbit anti-human globulin are added to the patient's serum. This produces agglutination of red cells if antibodies are present in the serum.

(b) ICT detects the incomplete antibodies present in a person's serum.

(c) The serum from the patient is taken and added to a suspension of O^+ RBCs. If the serum contains incomplete antibodies against Rh antigen, it will coat the O^+ RBCs. The suspension is washed many times to remove excess unbound antibodies in the serum.

(d) Thereafter, Coombs serum is added. If agglutination occurs, the test is said to be positive.

Indications:

- In crossmatching of blood to detect incomplete antibodies in donor's serum.
- In case of Rh-negative mother, whose first child is Rh-positive, and wants second conception.

Q. Define pancytopenia. Enumerate its causes. (PA17.1)

Ans. Pancytopenia is defined as simultaneous presence of anaemia (Hb <13.5 g/dL), leucopenia (TLC<4×10^9/L) and thrombocytopenia (150×10^9/L).

Causes

- **Hypocellular bone marrow:** Aplastic anaemia, hypoplastic MDS, cytotoxic drugs and radiotherapy.
- **Cellular marrow with systemic disease:** Megaloblastic anaemia, hypersplenism, tuberculosis, Kala-azar, brucellosis, severe infection, alcohol and autoimmune diseases.
- **Cellular marrow with primary marrow disease:** Bone marrow infiltration as seen in lymphoma, acute leukaemia, myeloma, carcinoma, paroxysmal nocturnal haemoglobinuria, disseminated tuberculosis, myelofibrosis and marrow metastasis.

Q. Write briefly on aplastic anaemia. (PA17.1, 17.2)

Ans. Aplastic anaemia is a condition in which bone marrow failure results in pancytopenia (anaemia, granulocytopenia and thrombocytopenia) in the absence of any abnormal cells in marrow or blood.

Classification of Aplastic Anaemia

1. **Congenital:** Fanconi's anaemia and Schwachman–Diamond syndrome.
2. **Acquired:** Primary or idiopathic (no definite cause) and secondary (definite or likely agent can be identified).

Causes of Secondary or Acquired Aplastic Anaemia

- **Infections:** Hepatitis viruses, EBV, human immunodeficiency virus (HIV), parvovirus and mycobacteria.
- **Radiation and chemicals:** Benzene, lindane (gamma benzene hexachloride) and DDT.
- **Drugs:** Drugs can produce aplastic anaemia either due to direct toxic effect (dose-dependent and predictable response) or idiosyncratic reactions (dose-independent and unpredictable response). The following drugs are implicated in aplastic anaemia:
  - Cytotoxic (alkylating agents and antimetabolites).
  - Antibacterial (chloramphenicol, sulfonamides, isoniazid and arsenicals).
  - Antirheumatic (oxyphenbutazone, phenylbutazone, indomethacin, gold salts and D-penicillamine).
  - Antidiabetic (tolbutamide and chlorpropamide).
  - Miscellaneous (chlorothiazide, mepacrine, hydralazine, acetazolamide, potassium perchlorate, carbamazepine and carbimazole).
- **Other causes:** Pancreatitis, PNH and eosinophilic fasciitis.

Pathogenesis

Haematopoietic failure due to various mechanisms, for example decreased number of stem cells in the marrow (primary stem cell abnormality), defective stem cells or a defective microenvironment that fails to sustain normal haematopoiesis. Immune-mediated destruction is also implicated.

Clinical Features

- Petechiae, ecchymoses, nasal and GIT bleeding due to thrombocytopenia.
- Infections due to neutropenia.
- Weakness, easy fatigability, pallor and breathlessness due to anaemia.

Laboratory Diagnosis

Aplastic anaemia is diagnosed if any two of the following are present:

- Hb ≤ 10 g/dL.
- Neutrophil count ≤1500/mm^3.
- Platelet count ≤50,000/mm^3.

Peripheral Smear

- Shows a normocytic-normochromic anaemia, leucopenia (neutropenia with relative lymphocytosis) and thrombocytopenia.
- Mild macrocytosis is occasionally seen.
- Corrected reticulocyte count is low.
- May be differentiated from **infiltrative causes of pancytopenia** based on the absence of teardrop poikilocytes and a leukoerythroblastic picture, both of which suggest an infiltrative process. The presence of dyserythropoietic cells and hypogranulated neutrophils indicates **myelodysplasia** and differentiates aplastic anaemia from dysplastic causes of pancytopenia.

Bone Marrow

Dry tap; markedly hypocellular or acellular marrow with increased iron stores.

Grading of Aplastic Anaemia

Aplasia is said to be 'severe' if any two of the following are present:

1. Neutrophil count is less than 500/mm^3.
2. Platelet count is less than 20,000/mm^3.
3. Anaemia with a corrected reticulocyte count* <1%
4. Marrow biopsy showing <25% of normal cellularity, or 25%–50% marrow cellularity with <30% haematopoietic cells.

Criteria for 'very severe' aplasia are similar, except granulocyte count ≤ 200/mm^3.

13 Disorders of Leukocytes and Lymphoreticular System

Q. Enumerate the disorders of WBCs. (PA18.1)

Ans. The disorders of leukocytes are broadly classified as follows:

Leukocytosis: Increase in the number of circulating leukocytes beyond the upper limit of normal (>11,000/mm^3; normal range 4000–11,000/mm^3). Leukocytosis is traditionally classified into various types depending on the type of leukocyte, which shows an increase in number, for example neutrophilic leukocytosis (Table 13.1). Neutrophils exit the marrow and enter the blood where they exist as two compartments, the **marginal compartment** and the **circulating compartment**. The neutrophils in the marginal compartment do not circulate freely, but are adherent to the vascular surface, and constitute almost half of the total neutrophils in the blood compartment. Neutrophilia may result from a shift of cells from the marginal to the circulating pool (shift neutrophilia) without an increase in the total blood granulocyte pool (TBGP) or from a true increase in TBGP size (true neutrophilia).

- **Leucopenia:** Total leukocyte count below the lower limit of normal (<4000/mm^3). Granulocytopenia is defined as a reduced number of blood granulocytes, namely neutrophils, eosinophils, and basophils. However, the term granulocytopenia is often used synonymously with neutropenia.
- **Leukoerythroblastic reaction:** Presence of immature WBCs as well as nucleated red cells in the peripheral blood. It may be due to **(1) Myelophthisis**—invasion of the bone marrow by tumour, fibrosis, granulomatous processes, storage disorders, etc. It is associated with 'teardrop" RBCs; **(2) myelofibrosis**—same pathophysiology as myelophthisis, but fibrosis is the primary marrow pathology; **(3) haemorrhage or haemolysis** (rarely, in severe cases).
- **Leukaemoid reaction:** Markedly increased leukocyte count with the presence of immature white cells in the peripheral blood but non-leukaemic in origin.

Q. Write briefly on the quantitative disorders of neutrophils. (PA18.1)

Ans. Neutrophilia (Fig. 13.1) is defined as absolute peripheral neutrophil count more than 7500/μL.

Causes of neutrophilia are given in Table 13.1.

Neutrophilia may be accompanied by a shift to the left and the presence of **toxic granules** and **Döhle bodies.**

(a) **Toxic granules:** Dark blue/purple granules in the cytoplasm of neutrophils. They represent azurophilic granules and result from impaired cytoplasmic maturation during accelerated generation of neutrophils.

(b) **Döhle bodies:** Pale inclusion bodies in the periphery of cytoplasm of neutrophils, which represent rough endoplasmic reticulum.

Neutropenia is defined as a reduction in the number of neutrophils to less than 1500/mm^3. It is classified as **mild, moderate or severe,** based on the absolute neutrophil count (ANC). Mild neutropenia is present when the ANC is 1000–1500 cells/μL, moderate neutropenia is present with an ANC of 500–1000/μL, and severe neutropenia refers to an ANC lower than 500 cells/μL. The risk of bacterial infection is increases with the severity and duration of the neutropenia. **Agranulocytosis** is a more severe type of neutropenia, which indicates virtual absence of neutrophils in peripheral blood (ANC is lower than 100/μL).

Neutropenia may be due to abnormality in any of the three compartments or their subcomponents: bone marrow (mitotic or mature storage pools); blood (circulating and marginal pools); or tissues (sequestration). Neutropenia can be caused by any of the following, alone or in combination:

1. **Insufficient or damaged bone marrow stem cells**
   (a) **Disorders of the pluripotent myeloid stem cells and committed myeloid progenitor cells**—congenital forms of neutropaenia, aplastic anaemia, drugs (antimicrobials, arsenicals, analgesics and cytotoxic drugs), bone marrow replacement or infiltration (granulomatous disorders, leukaemias, myeloproliferative disorders, MDS, myeloma, lymphoma and metastasis), ionising radiation, and bone marrow fibrosis.

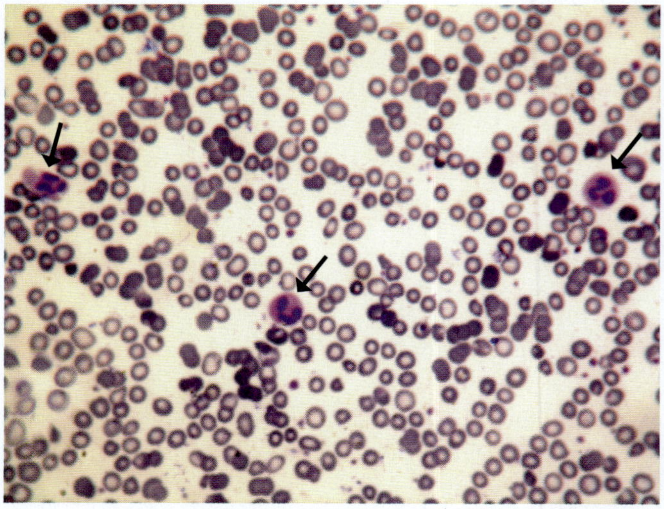

Fig. 13.1 PBS showing neutrophilia.

Table 13.1 Causes of leukocytosis

Neutrophilic leukocytosis (neutrophilia)	Absolute peripheral neutrophil count more than 7500/μL	• **Physiological:** Exercise (shift neutrophilia), newborns, pregnancy, labor, extreme temperatures, and emotional stress. • **Pathological:** May be due to: *Acute infections (true increase):* Furuncles, abscesses, tonsillitis, appendicitis, otitis media, osteomyelitis, cholecystitis, salpingitis, meningitis and peritonitis caused by Gram-positive cocci, (e.g. staphylococci, streptococci, pneumococci, meningococci and gonococci), *Escherichia coli, Pseudomonas aeruginosa, Actinomycosis,* certain fungi (e.g. *Coccidioides immitis*), spirochetes and viruses (rabies, poliomyelitis, herpes zoster and varicella), rickettsiae and parasites *Non-infectious causes:* Burns, postoperative state, acute myocardial infarction, acute attacks of gout, acute glomerulonephritis, rheumatic fever, collagen vascular diseases, Hodgkin lymphoma and solid tumours, drugs (e.g. glucocorticoids, epinephrine, lithium), cytokines (G-CSF and GM-CSF), myeloproliferative disorders, metabolic causes (ketoacidosis, uraemia), acute haemorrhage or haemolysis, after splenectomy
Eosinophilic leukocytosis (eosinophilia)	Defined as the absolute eosinophil count exceeding 600/μL	• **Parasitic infestations:** Ascariasis, toxocara, filariasis, strongyloidosis and trichinosis • **Pulmonary disorders:** *Loeffler syndrome*: Transient lung infiltrates on X-ray chest, eosinophilia and cough caused due to migration of helminthic larva through the lungs. *Tropical pulmonary eosinophilia*: Seen in filaria endemic regions; characterized by cough with wheezing, lung infiltrates and eosinophilia • **Type I hypersensitivity reactions:** Hay fever, asthma, urticaria and rhinitis • **Malignancies:** Hodgkin disease, chronic myeloid leukaemia and eosinophilic leukaemia • **Drugs:** Penicillin and iodides • **Idiopathic hypereosinophilic syndrome** (persistent high eosinophilia >1500/μL for more than 6 months without any identifiable cause and with the evidence of organ involvement and dysfunction due to cytokines released from eosinophilic granules) • **Collagen vascular diseases:** Rheumatoid arthritis and Churg–Strauss syndrome • **Skin diseases:** Atopic dermatitis, Bullous pemphigoid and eczema
Basophilic leukocytosis (basophilia)	Defined as increase in basophil count to more than 100/μL	• **Inflammatory conditions:** Inflammatory bowel disease, chronic airway inflammation, chronic dermatitis, viral infections and chronic sinusitis • **Myeloproliferative disorders:** Chronic myelogenous leukaemia, polycythaemia vera and myelofibrosis • **Endocrinological causes:** Hypothyroidism, ovulation and oestrogens • **Others:** Chronic haemolytic anaemia, Hodgkin disease and splenectomy
Monocytosis	Defined as a peripheral monocyte count more than 1000/μL	• **Infections:** Tuberculosis, brucellosis, listeriosis, bacterial endocarditis, syphilis, infectious mononucleosis and other viral infections, protozoal and rickettsial infections (e.g. kala-azar, malaria and Rocky Mountain spotted fever) • **Autoimmune diseases:** Systemic lupus erythaematosus, rheumatoid arthritis and inflammatory bowel disease • **Malignancies:** Hodgkin disease, MDS and certain leukaemias, such as chronic myelomonocytic leukaemia (CMML) and AML-M4 and AML-M5 • **Miscellaneous:** Sarcoidosis and carcinomas
Lymphocytosis	Defined as increase in the absolute count of lymphocytes beyond 4000/μL in adults	• **Infections** like pertussis, infectious mononucleosis, brucellosis, tuberculosis, secondary syphilis, cytomegalovirus, EBV, mumps, measles, varicella, toxoplasmosis and infective hepatitis • **Malignancies** like ALL, CLL and NHL • **Autoimmune disorders** like SLE • **Drugs** like phenytoin

(b) **Ineffective erythropoiesis**—megaloblastic anaemia, MDS, severe infections like typhoid, paratyphoid, septicaemia, military tuberculosis, HIV, influenza, infectious mononucleosis scrub typhus, malaria and kala azar.

2. **Increased destruction**
   (a) **Immune neutropaenia**
      (i) Idiopathic
      (ii) Secondary—Felty syndrome, SLE and neonatal isoimmune neutropenia, drugs
   (b) **Hypersplenism**
3. **Shift from circulating to marginal pool**
   Haemodialysis and cardiopulmonary bypass.

Q. Write briefly on the morphological/qualitative disorders of neutrophils. (PA18.1)

Ans. The following are the common morphological or qualitative disorders of neutrophils:

1. **Drumstick appendage** (Fig. 13.2): Neutrophils from women exhibit a small additional X chromosome structure, known as a 'drumstick'. A drumstick appears as a nuclear appendage about 1–1.5 μm in diameter attached to the nucleus by a filament. Drumsticks are not seen in individuals having only one X chromosome [males (XY), Turner's syndrome (XO) and testicular feminization

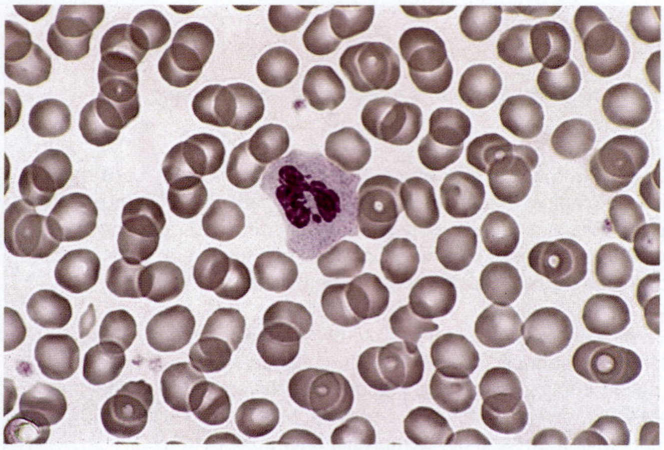

Fig. 13.2 Drumstick appendage. (*Source*: Gillian Rozenberg, *Microscopic Haematology: A Practical Guide for the Laboratory*, Figure B1-7, Pages 46–91, Elsevier, Churchill Livingstone, 2011.)

(XY)]. Their presence in >20% neutrophils (or at least six drumsticks per 500 neutrophils) is indicative of female sex chromosomes.

2. **Hypersegmentation or right shift of neutrophil nuclei** (Fig. 13.3): Average lobe count is increased such that greater than 3% neutrophils show more than 5 lobes; may be seen in megaloblastic anaemia, uraemia, and leukaemias.
3. **Ring-shaped nuclei:** Nucleus is ring or doughnut shaped; can be seen in acute myeloid leukaemia, chronic granulocytic leukaemia and megaloblastic anaemia.
4. **Detached nuclear fragments:** Nuclear fragments in the neutrophilic cytoplasm can be seen in dysgranulopoiesis, cancer chemotherapy and HIV.
5. **MPO deficiency:** Neutrophils appear normal on Romanowsky stain but are not counted as neutrophils by the cell counters employing a myeloperoxidase stain. This condition can be inherited and may be seen in refractory anaemia or blast crisis of chronic myeloid leukaemia (CML).
6. **Toxic granulation** (Fig. 13.4): Increased granulation wherein the neutrophilic azurophilic granules appear more basophilic (darkly staining) and larger than normal. This results from impaired cytoplasmic maturation during accelerated generation of neutrophils. Causes include severe bacterial infections, normal pregnancy and therapy with cytokines.
7. **Hypogranulation:** Reduced granulation in neutrophil cytoplasm usually seen in MDSs.
8. **Vacuoles in the cytoplasm of granulocytes:** Found in infections, ethanol toxicity and **Jordan anomaly** (cytoplasmic vacuoles seen in association with neutral lipid storage diseases).
9. **Döhle bodies** (Fig. 13.5): These are small pale blue cytoplasmic inclusions, often located in the periphery of the cell. They represent rough endoplasmic reticulum; and are usually seen in infective states, severe burns, postchemotherapy, pregnancy, etc.
10. **Auer rods** (Fig. 13.6): Needle- or rod-shaped eosinophilic structures, which occur in the cytoplasm of immature leukocytes (blasts) in patients with acute myelogenous

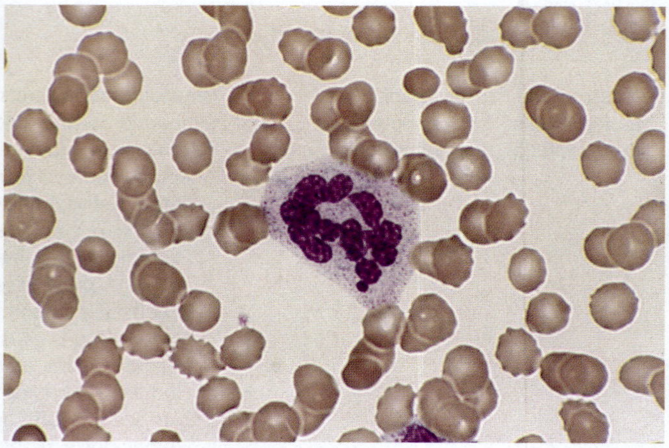

Fig. 13.3 Hypersegmented neutrophil. (*Source*: Gillian Rozenberg, *Microscopic Haematology: A Practical Guide for the Laboratory*, Figure B1-14, Pages 46–91, Elsevier, Churchill Livingstone, 2011.)

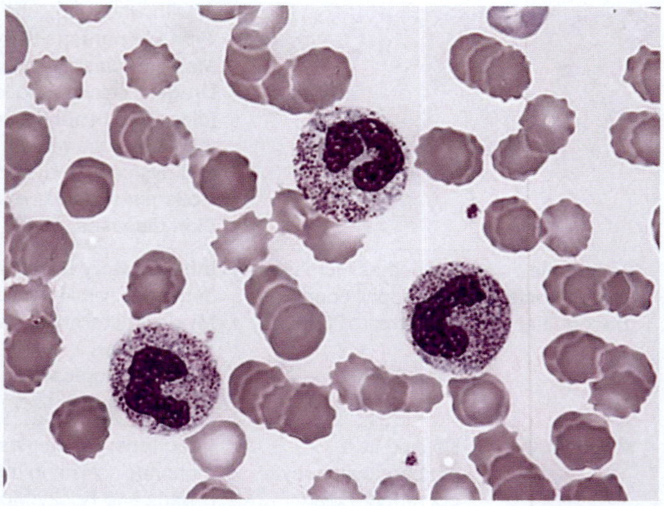

Fig. 13.4 Toxic granulation. (*Source*: Richard A. McPherson and Matthew R. Pincus, *Henry's Clinical Diagnosis and Management by Laboratory Methods,* Figure 33-1, Pages 601–655, Elsevier, Saunders, 2011.)

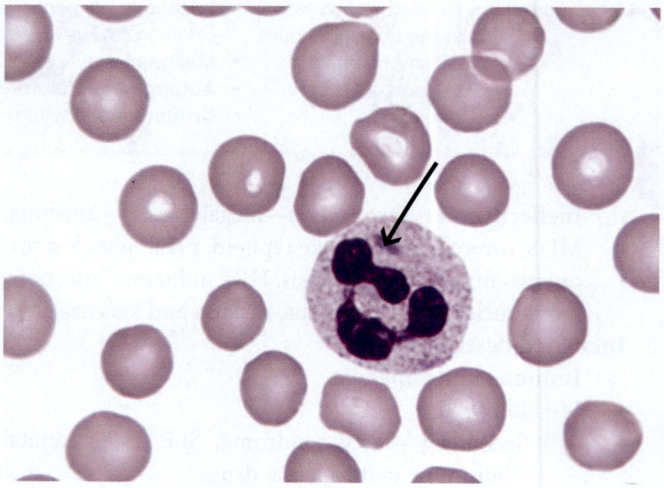

Fig. 13.5 Döhle bodies. (*Source*: Bernadette Rodak George Fritsma Elaine Keohane, *Hematology: Clinical Principles and Applications*: Non-malignant Leukocyte Disorders, Figure 28-13, Pages 408–426, Elsevier, Saunders, 2012.)

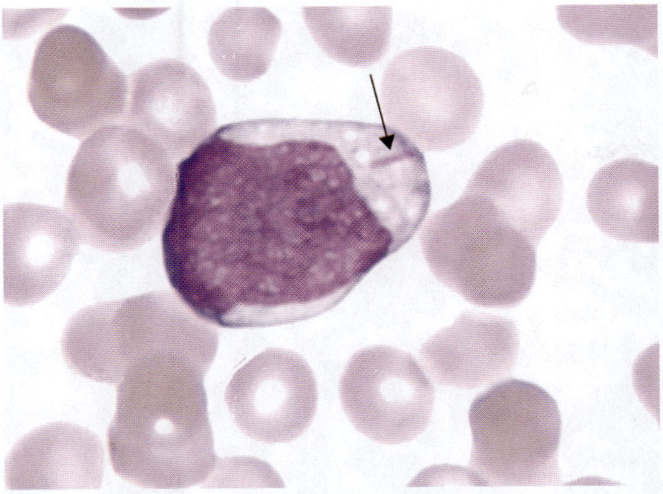

Fig. 13.6 Auer rods. (*Source*: *Mosby's Dictionary of Medicine,* Nursing & Health Professions, Figure: Auer rod (Carr and Rodak, 2009), Elsevier, 2010.

leukaemia (AML). These structures are formed from coalescing primary (azurophilic) granules. Auer rods occur singly in AML FAB subtypes M1, M2 and M4. Cells with numerous Auer rods are common in the hypergranular form of AML FAB M3 and are called **'faggot' cells.**

11. **Macroneutrophils:** Neutrophils twice the size of a normal neutrophil with tetraploid DNA content; occasionally seen in the blood of healthy subjects; could be inherited or may be seen in association with administration of G-CSF and megaloblastic anaemia.
12. **Necrobiotic/apoptotic neutrophils:** Dense homogenous pyknotic nuclei; found occasionally in healthy subjects and in patients with AML.
13. **Shift to the left:** Presence of precursors of granulocytes like stab forms, metamyelocytes and myelocytes in the peripheral blood (decrease in the number of neutrophil lobes); may be seen in normal individuals, in pregnancy or neonates, severe infections and bone marrow infiltrative disorders (leukoerythroblastic picture).
14. **Neutrophilic hyposegmentation:** Single- or bilobed neutrophils (Pelger–Huët cells) can be inherited (**Pelger–Huët anomaly;** Fig. 13.7) or acquired (pseudo-Pelger–Huët cells). Pseudo-Pelger–Huët cells can be seen in patients with acute leukaemia, MDS, idiopathic myelofibrosis (MF), chronic granulocytic leukaemia, therapy with colchicine, ibuprofen, infectious mononucleosis, malaria, myxedema and CLL.
15. **Alder–Reilly granules:** Alder–Reilly granules are large, coarse, dark purple, azurophilic granules that may be found in the cytoplasm of granulocytes, lymphocytes, and monocytes (Fig. 13.8). These are characteristically found in the Alder–Reilly anomaly and mucopolysaccharidoses.
16. **Chédiak–Higashi granules:** Chédiak–Higashi granules are large, red or blue granules that appear in the cytoplasm of granulocytes, lymphocytes or monocytes in patients with the Chédiak–Steinbrinck–Higashi syndrome (Fig. 13.9).
17. **May–Hegglin anomaly:** Small, basophilic, cytoplasmic granules, which represent aggregated ribosomes; usually seen in neutrophils (Fig. 13.10). Inherited as an autosomal

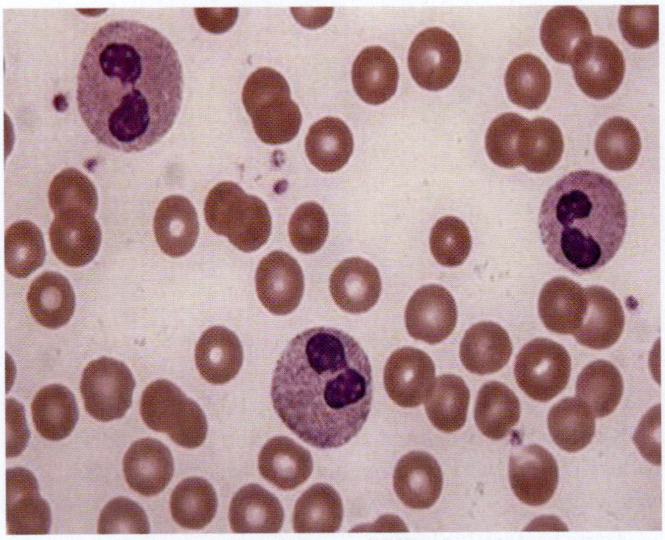

Fig. 13.7 Pelger–Huët anomaly. (*Source*: Enid Gilbert-Barness, Raj Kapur, Luc Laurier Oligny, et al., *Potter's Pathology of the Fetus, Infant and Child: Hematopoietic System,* Figure 29.1.20, Elsevier, Mosby, 2007.)

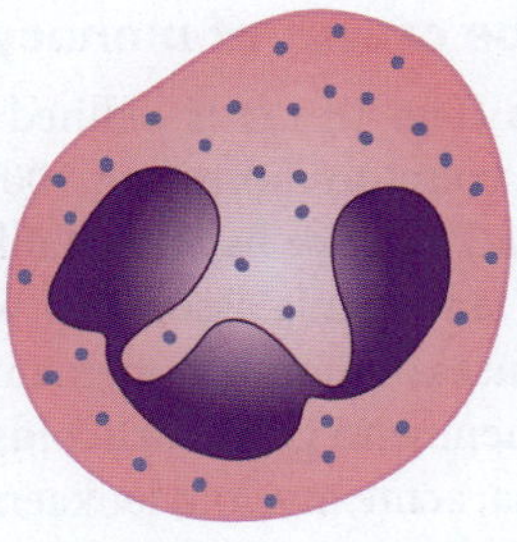

Fig. 13.8 Alder–Reilly granules.

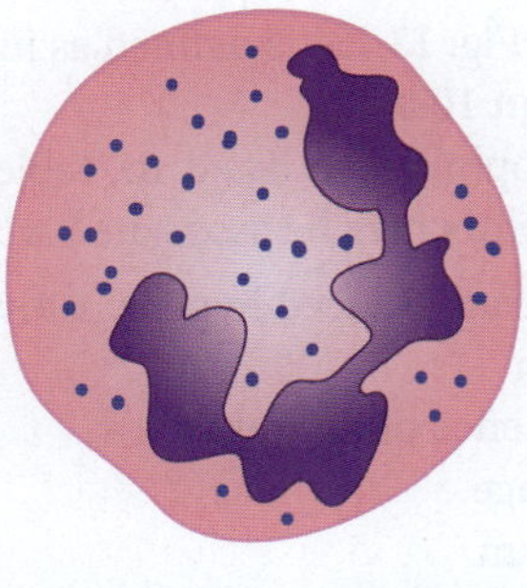

Fig. 13.9 Chédiak–Higashi granules.

dominant trait, this anomaly is associated with leukopaenia and abnormally large platelets (causing mild bleeding).

18. **Defective neutrophilic function can manifest in the form of (1) defective chemotaxis** (lazy leukocyte syndrome, corticosteroid therapy, aspirin intake and alcohol toxicity); **(2) defective phagocytosis** (deficient opsonization as in hypogammaglobulinemia or hypocomplementemia, postsplenectomy, and in sickle cell disease); or **(3) defective killing** (chronic granulomatous disease, Chédiak–Higashi syndrome, and AML).

Q. Write briefly on quantitative disorders of eosinophils. (PA18.1)

Ans. Eosinophilia (Fig. 13.11) is defined as the absolute eosinophil count exceeding 600/μL.

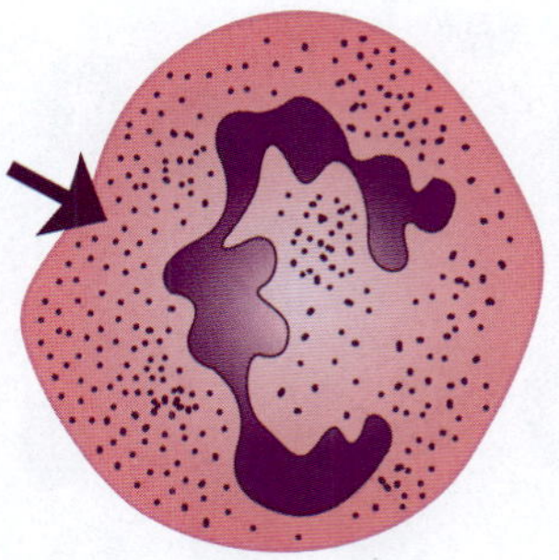

Fig. 13.10 May–Hegglin granules.

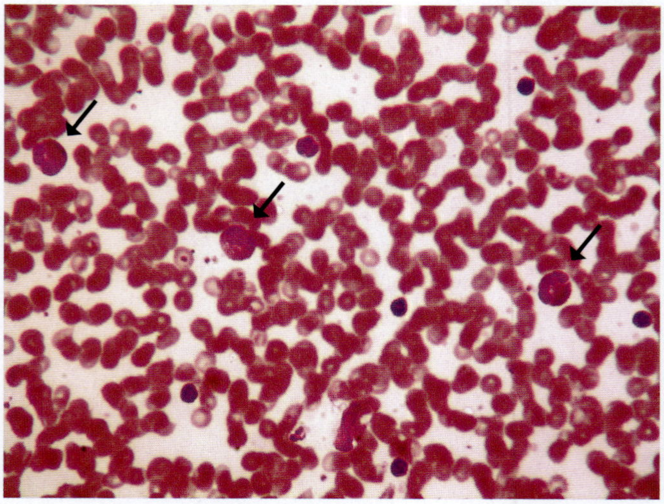

Fig. 13.11 PBS showing eosinophilia.

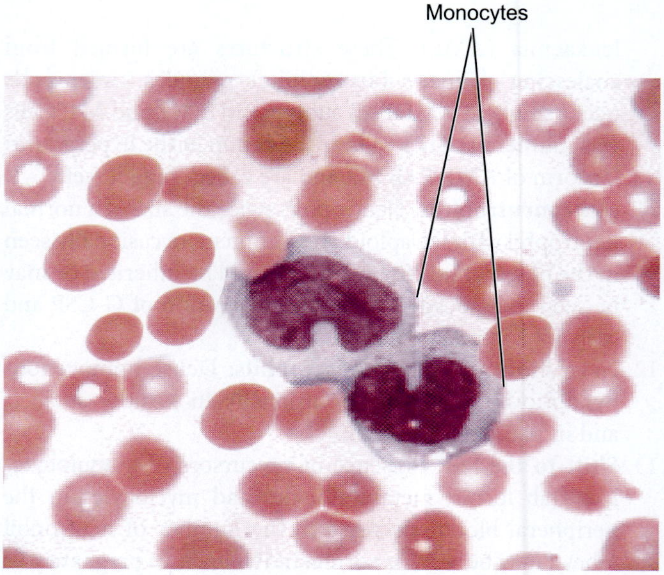

Fig. 13.12 PBS showing monocytosis.

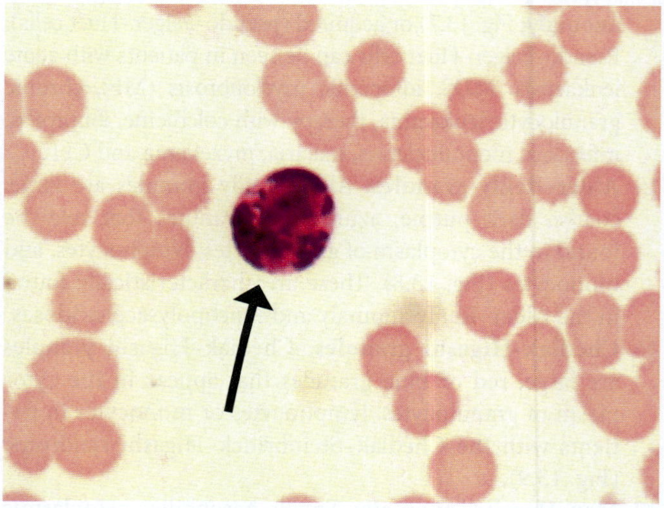

Fig. 13.13 PBS showing a basophil.

Causes of eosinophilia are listed in Table 13.1.

Eosinopenia is defined as a reduction in eosinophil count to less than 40/μL Eosinopenia may be associated with the following:

- Acute bacterial infection
- Glucocorticoid administration
- Hypogammaglobulinemia
- Physical stress
- Thymoma

Q. Enumerate the causes of monocytosis.

Ans. Monocytosis (Fig. 13.12) is defined as increase in peripheral monocyte count to more than 1000/μL.

Causes of monocytosis are listed in Table 13.1. **Monocytopenia** is a form of leukopenia associated with a deficiency of monocytes. The causes of monocytopenia include acute infections, stress, treatment with glucocorticoids, aplastic anaemia, hairy cell leukaemia, acute myeloid leukaemia, treatment with myelotoxic drugs and genetic syndromes.

Q. Enumerate the causes of basophilia.

Ans. Basophilia (Fig. 13.13) is defined as increase in basophil count to more than 100/μL

Causes of basophilia are listed in Table 13.1. **Decreased circulating basophils** may be associated with the following:

- Anaphylaxis, drug induced hypersensitivity and urticaria
- Acute infection
- Congenital absence of basophils
- Posthaemorrhage
- Hyperthyroidism
- Ionizing radiation
- Neoplasia
- Ovulation
- Drugs (e.g. corticosteroid, adrenocorticotropic hormone [ACTH] therapy, chemotherapeutic agents, thyroid hormones)

Q. Write briefly on quantitative disorders of lymphocytes. (PA18.1)

Ans. Absolute lymphocytosis (Fig. 13.14) is defined as increase in the absolute count of lymphocytes beyond 4000/μL in adults.

Causes of lymphocytosis are listed in Table 13.1.

Lymphopaenia is defined as the decrease in lymphocyte count to less than 1500/μL. It can be associated with aplastic anaemia, high dose steroids, AIDS, Hodgkin lymphoma and irradiation.

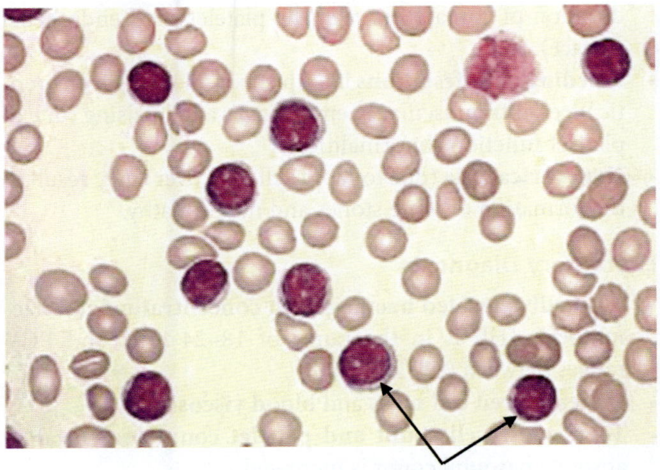

Fig. 13.14 PBS showing lymphocytosis.

Q. What are leukaemoid reactions? (PA18.1)

Ans. Leukaemoid reactions are characterized by an increase in the total leukocyte count beyond 25,000/µL. They are seen in response to infections, haematological and non-haematological malignancies and various toxic states. The bone marrow shows proliferation without presence of any abnormal cells. Leukaemoid reactions can be of two types:

1. **Myeloid leukaemoid reactions:** Total WBC count is markedly increased with a predominance of cells of myeloid series including an occasional immature cell (myelocytes, promyelocytes and myeloblasts).
   Causes
   - Infections like pneumonia, septicaemia and meningococcal meningitis
   - Secondary to non-haematological malignancies
   - Acute haemolysis
   - Eclampsia
   - Severe burns
2. **Lymphoid leukaemoid reactions:** Total WBC count is markedly increased with a predominance of cells of lymphoid series.
   Causes
   - Infectious mononucleosis
   - Cytomegalovirus, mumps, measles, rubella
   - Pertussis, tuberculosis, syphilis, brucellosis and infective hepatitis
   - CLL
   - Carcinoma

Q. Differentiate between leukaemoid reactions and chronic myeloid leukaemia (CML). (PA18.2)

Ans. Comparative features of leukaemoid reactions and CML are tabulated in Table 13.2.

Table 13.2 Contrasting features of leukaemoid reactions and chronic myeloid leukaemia (CML)

Features	Leukaemoid reactions	CML
Clinical features	Clinical features of the causative disorder	Splenomegaly, lymph node enlargement, and anaemia
Blood examination		
• TLC	Moderate increase; rarely exceeds 100 ×/L	Usual range 20–500 × 10^9/L
• Immature cells	Usually few	Usually numerous
• WBC morphology	*Toxic granules* (increased number of intensely staining primary granules) and *Döhle bodies* (discrete round to oval cytoplasmic bodies, 1–2 mm, stain blue-grey with Romanowsky stains) are seen in infective cases	Uncommon
• Eosinophilia and basophilia	Absolute eosinophilia or basophilia not seen	Absolute eosinophilia or basophilia is usually seen
• Anaemia	Slight or absent	Present and progressive
• Platelets	Normal or increased	Increased; may decrease in accelerated phase and blast crisis
• LAP score	High	Low
Autopsy	No infiltration of organs and tissues	Leukaemic infiltration of organs and tissues is present

LAP, Leukocyte alkaline phosphatase; TLC, total leukocyte count; WBC, white blood cell.

Q. Define and enumerate the myeloproliferative disorders?

Ans. Myeloproliferative disorders occur due to clonal expansion of a multipotent haematopoietic progenitor cells with the overproduction of one or more of the formed elements of blood. These conditions may evolve into acute leukaemia. The following conditions are included under this category of diseases:

- CML t(9;22)(q34;q11), BCR/ABL positive.
- Chronic neutrophilic leukaemia.
- Chronic eosinophilic leukaemia NOS.
- Primary myelofibrosis (MF) JAK2 or MPL mutation.
- Polycythemia vera JAK2V617F or exon 12 mutation.
- Essential thrombocythemia (ET) JAK2 mutation.
- Chronic myeloproliferative disease, unclassifiable.

Q. Define and classify polycythaemia?

Ans. It is defined as neoplastic proliferation of erythroid, granulocytic and megakaryocytic elements. Polycythaemia can be classified as:

1. **Relative:** Relative polycythaemia results from haemoconcentration due to reduced plasma volume (seen in

dehydration—low fluid intake, vomiting, diaorrhea and excessive sweating). The red cell mass remains within the normal range in relative polycythaemia.

2. **Absolute:** Absolute polycythaemia is associated with an actual increase in the red cell mass and is further classified into the following subtypes:
   (a) **Primary (polycythaemia vera):** Denotes absolute polycythaemia of unknown aetiology, which is associated with decreased erythropoietin levels.
   (b) **Secondary (erythrocytosis):** Erythrocytosis secondary to increase in production of erythropoietin as a consequence of hypoxia. It is seen in association with the following conditions:
      (i) High altitude.
      (ii) Cyanotic congenital heart diseases (TOF—Tetralogy of Fallot and Eisenmenger complex).
      (iii) Pulmonary diseases (e.g. COPD).
      (iv) Chronic carbon monoxide poisoning and smoking.
      (v) Abnormal haemoglobin with high oxygen affinity.
      (vi) Increased production of erythropoietin or erythropoietin-like substance by tumours and other conditions, as in, cerebellar haemangioblastoma, renal tumours (carcinoma, adenoma and sarcoma), polycystic kidney disease, uterine leiomyoma, hepatocellular carcinoma and pheochromocytoma.

Q. Outline the clinical features and laboratory diagnosis of polycythaemia vera.

Ans. Polycythaemia vera is a clonal stem cell disorder characterized by an increased production of formed elements of blood by a hyperplastic marrow; however, the disease is generally dominated by an elevated haemoglobin concentration (haematocrit >52% in an adult male and >48% in an adult female).

Aetiology

Mutation in Janus 2 kinase gene (JAK2V617F) is thought to render the erythropoietin receptor hypersensitive to erythropoietin. JAK2 is a tyrosine kinase involved in signalling pathway of the erythropoietin receptor, and causes not only erythrocytic but also granulocytic and megakaryocytic proliferation.

Clinical Features

Seen in middle-aged males who present with dusky red colour of the face (ruddy cyanosis). Complaints are related to the increased viscosity and stasis of blood and include:

- **Headache, dizziness, vertigo, visual disturbances, tinnitus and syncope** (due to decreased cerebral perfusion).
- **Pruritus** (due to histamine release from neoplastic basophils and mast cells).
- **Peptic ulceration** (due to excessive histamine).
- **Splenomegaly** and **hepatomegaly.**
- Symptoms of **peripheral vascular insufficiency** and **thrombotic complications** usually affecting the brain and heart; hepatic vein thrombosis resulting in Budd–Chiari syndrome (thrombosis occurs due to stasis and increased duration of contact between the platelets and endothelial surface).
- **Bleeding manifestations** like epistaxis, bleeding from peptic ulcer, intramuscular haemorrhages and bruising (due to platelet function abnormalities).
- **Hyperuricaemia** (due to rapid cell turn over) may result in the formation of urate stones and nephropathy.

Laboratory Diagnosis

- **Markedly elevated haemoglobin concentration** and **haematocrit** (Hb is in the range of 18–24 g/dL and PCV ranges between 0.60 and 0.70).
- **Increased red cell mass** and **blood viscosity.**
- **Total white cell count and platelet count are elevated**; absolute basophil count is increased.
- The arterial oxygen saturation is normal in contrast to hypoxic erythrocytosis where it is reduced.
- Bone marrow shows either erythroid hyperplasia or pan hyperplasia.
- Iron stores are depleted.
- Urine and serum levels of erythropoietin are reduced.

Q. Differentiate between primary and secondary polycythaemia.

Ans. Contrasting features of primary and secondary polycythaemia are tabulated in Table 13.3.

Table 13.3 Comparison between primary and secondary polycythemia

Features	Primary polycythemia	Secondary polycythemia
Aetiology	Neoplastic disorder	Caused by hypoxia
Facies	Brick red	Cyanosed
Pruritus	Common	Absent
Oxygen saturation	Normal	Low
Erythropoietin levels	Decreased	Increased
Total white cell count	Increased	Normal
Absolute basophil count	Increased	Normal
Platelet count	Increased	Normal
Leukocyte alkaline phosphatase	Increased	Normal
Vitamin B_{12} levels	Increased	Normal
Bone marrow	Panhyperplasia	Erythroid hyperplasia
Splenomegaly	Present	Absent

Q. Discuss the clinical features and laboratory diagnosis of chronic myeloid leukaemia (CML). (PA18.2)

Ans. CML is a myeloproliferative disease characterized by excessive proliferation of myeloid cells with near normal maturation.

Natural Course

The disease has three phases:

1. **Chronic stable phase**

Clinical features

- Peak incidence in 4th and 5th decades.
- Patients may be asymptomatic in the early stage. Symptoms are mainly due to massive splenomegaly, anaemia and a hypermetabolic state.
- Symptoms due to massive splenomegaly include abdominal distension, dyspepsia, flatulence, reflux oesophagitis, dyspnoea and dragging discomfort in the left hypochondrium.
- Hepatomegaly may be seen.
- Symptoms resulting from the hypermetabolic state include fever, weight loss, night sweats and heat intolerance.
- Anaemia manifests as fatigue, weakness and anorexia.
- Priapism (high counts leading to obstruction of flow in the corpus cavernosum) may be also seen.
- Bleeding tendencies occur late.

Laboratory diagnosis

- ***Peripheral smear*** (Fig. 13.15)
  - Normocytic normochromic anaemia.
  - Leukocyte count is markedly raised, typically between 100×10^9 and 300×10^9/L.
  - Granulocyte precursors ranging from myeloblasts, myelocytes and metamyelocytes to mature neutrophils are seen. Segmented neutrophils and myelocytes predominate.
  - Myeloblasts are less than 10%.
  - Increase in basophils and eosinophils is observed.
  - Platelets are normal or increased.
- ***Bone marrow***
  - Hypercellular with marked proliferation of all granulocytic elements.
  - Twenty to thirty percent of patients show mild bone marrow fibrosis in late stages.

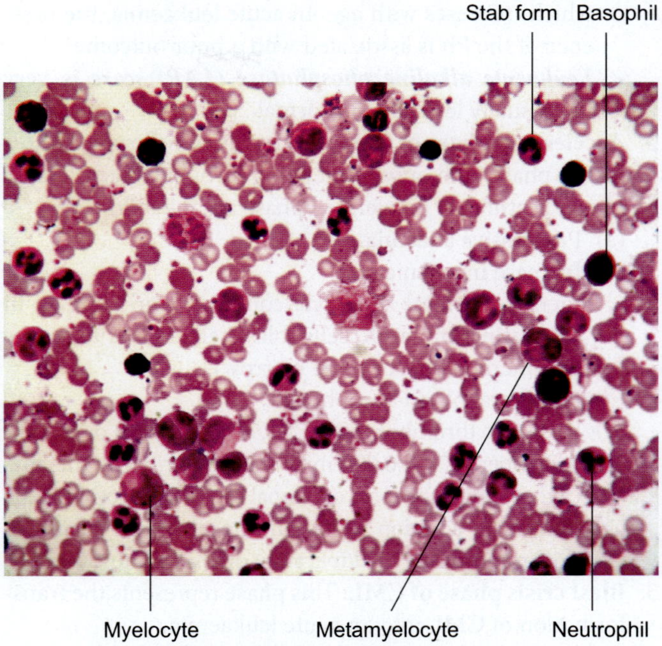

Fig. 13.15 Leishman-stained PBS of CML showing immature cells of myeloid series with a predominance of segmented neutrophils and myelocytes.

- ***Philadelphia chromosome (Ph; Fig. 13.16), a reciprocal translocation between the long arms of chromosome 9 and chromosome 22 (t9; 22),*** is positive in more than 95% of cases, in all three phases. This translocation leads to a juxtaposition of protooncogene *c-abl* (tyrosine kinase encoding gene on chromosome 9) and *bcr* on chromosome 22. The fusion protein p210 bcr–abl is thought to play a role in the malignant transformation of white blood cell precursors in the bone marrow. Ph was the first chromosomal abnormality to be found in leukaemia. It also occurs in acute leukaemia (ALL - 2%–3% of childhood cases; AML - 1% cases). In adults, it is the most common cytogenetic change, the incidence of

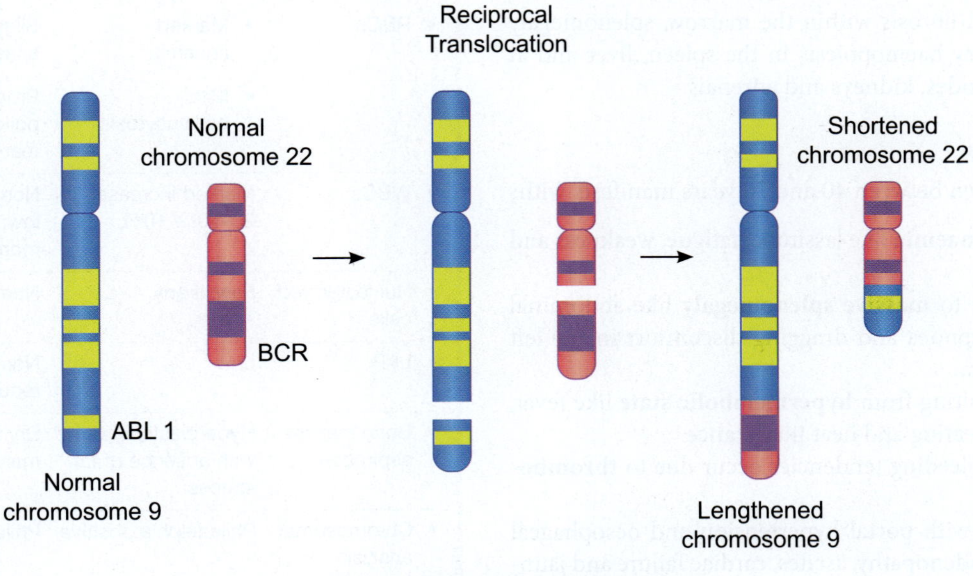

Fig. 13.16 Philadelphia chromosome.

which increases with age. In acute leukaemia, the presence of the Ph is associated with a poor outcome.

- ***Leukocyte alkaline phosphatase (LAP) score*** is very low, usually less than 5 (normal 20–100).

2. **Accelerated phase of CML:** CML may transform itself to a blastic phase with or without going through an accelerated phase. Features of accelerated phase are the following:
   (a) Progressive anaemia.
   (b) Increase in splenic size.
   (c) Increase in total leukocyte count with an increase in circulating immature cells (blast cells 10%–19% in the peripheral blood/or bone marrow).
   (d) Peripheral blood basophilia (>20%).
   (e) Persistent thrombocytosis (>1,000,000/mm^3) or thrombocytopenia (<100,000/mm^3) not responsive to therapy.
   (f) Cytogenetic evidence of clonal evolution (cytogenetic changes in addition to Ph chromosome, e.g. trisomy 8, isochromosome 17q, duplication of Ph chromosome etc.).
3. **Blast crisis phase of CML:** This phase represents the transformation of CML into an acute leukaemia.
   (a) 'Myeloid blast' crises (70%) when the disease transforms into acute myeloblastic leukaemia.
   (b) 'Lymphoid blast' crises (30%) when the disease transforms into acute lymphoblastic leukaemia.

   Blast crisis is characterized by
   - Sudden increase in splenic size.
   - Anaemia and thrombocytopenia.
   - Generalized lymphadenopathy.
   - Peripheral smear and bone marrow showing numerous blast cells (>20%) simulating acute leukaemia.
   - Refractoriness to treatment (treatment of blast crisis is as for acute myeloblastic or lymphoblastic leukaemia).

Q. Outline the clinical features and laboratory diagnosis of primary myelofibrosis (agnogenic myeloid metaplasia).

Ans. Myelofibrosis is a clonal myeloproliferative disorder characterized by JAK2 mutations which result in proliferation of bone marrow (predominantly megakaryocytic and granulocytic), increased fibrosis within the marrow, splenomegaly and extramedullary haemopoiesis in the spleen, liver and at times, in lymph nodes, kidneys and adrenals.

Clinical Features

It is commonly seen between 40 and 70 years manifests with:

- Symptoms of **anaemia** like lassitude, fatigue, weakness and anorexia.
- Symptoms due to **massive splenomegaly** like abdominal distension, dyspnoea and dragging discomfort in the left hypochondrium.
- Symptoms resulting from **hypermetabolic state** like fever, weight loss, sweating and heat intolerance.
- In late stages, bleeding tendencies occur due to **thrombocytopenia**.
- Hepatomegaly with portal hypertension and oesophageal varices, lymphadenopathy, ascites, cardiac failure and jaundice also seen.

Laboratory Diagnosis

- Typical picture is **leukoerythroblastic** (simultaneous presence of erythroid and granulocytic precursors in the peripheral blood). RBCs are usually normocytic normochromic with the presence of a fair number of tear-drop poikilocytes and oval/elliptical cells. Polychromatophils and basophilic stippling may also be seen.
- Platelet count is increased in the early stages, but decreased in the late stages.
- Total leukocyte count may be normal, increased (early stages) or decreased (late stages). Myeloid precursors are abundant but blasts do not exceed 10%.
- ***Bone marrow examination***
  - **Early stage** or **'cellular phase':** The marrow is hypercellular with an increase in all three cell lines, particularly megakaryocytes, which may be large and dysplastic. Fibrosis is minimal.
  - **Late stage** or **'hypocellular phase'**: The marrow is hypocellular with reduction in all cell lines. Marked increase in fibrosis is seen which can be demonstrated by Reticulin stain.
  - **Leukocyte alkaline phosphatase (LAP) score** is elevated.
  - **Philadelphia chromosome** is negative.

Q. Differentiate between CML and myelofibrosis.

Ans. Contrasting features of CML and myelofibrosis are listed in Table 13.4.

Table 13.4 Comparison between CML and myelofibrosis (MF)

Features	CML	MF
Clinical features		
• Splenomegaly	Moderate-to-marked	Marked
• Fever	Common	Uncommon
Laboratory investigations		
• RBCs	• Marked anaemia	Slight-to-moderate anaemia
	• Mild poikilocytosis	Prominent poikilocytosis with tear-drop cells
• WBCs	Marked increase; 20–50 × 10^9/L	Normal, raised, or low; when raised, not more than 50 × 10^9/L
• Nucleated red cells	Few, if any	Numerous
• LAP	Low	Normal, raised, or reduced
• Bone marrow aspiration	Hyperplastic marrow with absence of fat spaces	Dry tap without marrow fragments
• Chromosomal analysis	Philadelphia positive	Philadelphia negative

Q. Write briefly on essential thrombocythemia (ET).

Ans. ET is a clonal myeloproliferative disorder characterized by markedly increased platelet count in the absence of any recognizable stimulatory influence. When the platelet count increases secondary to recognizable stimuli (infections, haemorrhage, iron deficiency, malignancies, collagen vascular disorders and after splenectomy), it is labeled *secondary thrombocytosis*. ET is rare, occurs due to **failure of regulatory mechanisms (activating point mutations in JAK2, MPL or calreticulin,** which render the progenitors thrombopoietin independent leading to excessive proliferation). It is primarily associated with increased platelet count but sometimes may show expansion of cells of other lineages.

Salient Features

- Median age of **50–60 years** at diagnosis, but may occur at any age.
- **Females** are affected more often than males; rarely occurs in children (to rule out hereditary thrombocytosis in these cases).
- More than half of the cases are detected during routine peripheral blood count.
- **Increased proliferation usually confined to megakaryocytes with platelet count >450 × 10⁹/L. PBS shows large platelets and megakaryocytic fragments.**
- **Thrombosis** and **haemorrhage** (due to qualitative and quantitative abnormalities in platelets) alternate with asymptomatic periods.
- May rarely progress to MF.
- Median survival is 10–15 years, hence life expectancy is almost normal.

Diagnostic Criteria (WHO)

1. Sustained platelet count of 450×10^9/L or more in the absence of evidence of reactive thrombocytosis.
2. Megakaryocyte proliferation with large and mature morphology, no or little granulocyte or erythroid proliferation.
3. Does not meet WHO criteria for CML, PV, PMF, MDS, or other myeloid neoplasm.
4. Demonstration of JAK2 V617F or other clonal marker.

Q. Write briefly on myelodysplastic syndrome (MDS).

Ans. The myelodysplastic syndromes are clonal stem cell disorders characterized by progressive cytopenias and ineffective haematopoiesis with production of defective haematopoietic cells of erythroid, myeloid and megakaryocytic series. The bone marrow is replaced by clonal progeny of a neoplastic multipotential stem cell that differentiates but does so in an ineffective manner. These patients are at increased risk of developing acute leukaemias.

Aetiology

In most cases the cause is unknown (idiopathic MDS); however, exposure to radiation, cancer chemotherapy, pesticides and ageing are implicated (secondary MDS). Both primary and secondary MDS are associated with recurrent chromosomal abnormalities like monosomies 5 and 7; deletions of 5q,7q and 20q and trisomy 8.

Table 13.5 Classification of myelodysplastic syndrome (MDS)

Category
MDS with single lineage dysplasia
MDS with ring sideroblasts • MDS with ring sideroblasts and single lineage dysplasia • MDS with ring sideroblasts and multilineage dysplasia
MDS with multilineage dysplasia
MDS with excess blasts
MDS with isolated deletion 5q
MDS unclassifiable

Clinical Features

- Failure of bone marrow to produce normal blood cells leads to anaemia, leucopenia and thrombocytopenia.
- Extramedullary haematopoiesis may occur leading to hepatomegaly and splenomegaly.

Classification (Table 13.5)

Laboratory Diagnosis

- Mild to moderate anaemia with macrocytosis and anisocytosis; dimorphic picture (both hypochromic and normochromic cells) may be seen.
- The WBC count may be normal, increased or decreased. Hypogranular or agranular granulocytes and neutrophils with bilobed Pelger Huet anomaly may be seen.
- Thrombocytopenia (platelets vary in size and some appear hypogranular)
- Marrow is normocellular to hypercellular. Dysplasia of non-lymphoid lineages is seen, namely, erythroid, granulocytic, monocytes and megakaryocytic. Erythroid precursors show dyserythropoiesis accompanied by dysgranulopoiesis and dysmegakaryopoiesis. Immature myeloid cells are present in less well-differentiated subgroups (MDS with excess of blast cells). There is presence of increased iron stores with ring sideroblasts. Cytogenetic analysis is helpful in diagnosis. Several driver mutations overlapping with AML are seen.

Q. Define and classify acute leukaemia? (PA18.2)

Ans. Acute leukaemias are a group of haematological malignancies that usually begin in the bone marrow and manifest with abnormally high leukocyte counts, with the presence of abnormal cells called 'blasts'. Acute leukaemias is classified based on:

1. **Revised FAB (French–American–British) classification:** Blast count for diagnosis of acute leukaemia should be ≥30% in peripheral blood or bone marrow. As per FAB classification, acute leukaemia is categorized into myeloid and lymphoid types, based on its origin (Table 13.6 and 13.7). The revised FAB classification includes the following criteria for classification of acute leukaemia:
   (a) Morphology and cytochemistry of blasts

Table 13.6 Acute myeloid leukaemia (AML)

M0	Minimally differentiated	Undifferentiated by light microscopy; however, myeloid nature is evident on electron microscopy or immunological cell marker studies (presence of one or more myeloid antigens like CD13, CD33 and CD117). B- and T-lymphoid markers are absent and immunophenotyping is essential for differentiating from ALL.
M1	Myeloblastic leukaemia without maturation	Minimal maturation; some blast cells show few granules. Cytochemically ≥3% blasts are peroxidase positive. Immunological cell marker studies reveal expression of at least two myeloid antigens (CD13, CD33, CD117, or MPO).
M2	Myeloblastic leukaemia with maturation	Most frequent subtype. Auer rods (aggregates of azurophilic granules in lysosomes) are commonly seen. There is clear evidence of maturation to promyelocyte stage and beyond. Blasts constitute between 20% and 89% of the nucleated cells in the marrow. Mature cells (promyelocytes to granulocytes) are >10%. Monocytic cells should be less than 20%.
M3	1. Hypergranular promyelocytic leukaemia	Predominance of abnormal promyelocytes, which are hypergranular and show innumerable large azurophilic granules in the cytoplasm. Auer rods are arranged in bundles called *faggots*. Pancytopenia is typical. Myeloperoxidase is strongly positive. There is a formation of a fusion gene *RARa–PML* due to t(15;17) that arrests the maturation of myeloid cells at the promyelocytic stage.
	2. Microgranular variant	Marked leukocytosis with hypogranular promyelocytes having a typical bilobed nucleus.
M4	Myelomonocytic leukaemia	Blasts are >20% of the nucleated cells in the marrow. Monocytic cells and their precursors, and neutrophils and their precursors are each more than 20%. Non-specific esterase is positive in cells of monocytic lineage. Myeloperoxidase is positive in more than 3% blasts. Leukaemic cells express myeloid-associated antigens (CD13 and CD33) and markers of monocytic differentiation (CD14 and lysozyme).
M4Eo	Variant	Shows increase in marrow eosinophils.
M5	Monocytic leukaemia	More than 80% cells in the bone marrow are monocytic (monoblasts, promonocytes and monocytes).
	1. Undifferentiated (monoblastic) M5a	In M5a, 80% or more cells are monoblasts.
	2. Well-differentiated (promonocytic–monocytic) M5b	In M5b, predominant cells are promonocytes and monocytes. Variable expression of myeloid antigens CD33, Cd13, and Cd117 is observed in both M5a and M5b. Monocytic markers CD14, CD36, CD64 and CD11c are positive.
M6	Erythroleukaemia (Di Guglielmo disease)	Predominance of erythroblasts. Two subtypes are: *erythroleukaemia* (>20% of non-erythroid cells are myeloblasts and >50% of all nucleated cells are erythroblasts) and pure *erythroid leukaemia* (>80% of marrow cells are erythroblasts). Erythroblasts may be bizarre looking with bi- and trinucleate forms and megaloblastic nuclear features, and are positive for monoclonal antibody against glycophorin A.
M7	Megakaryoblastic leukaemia	Megakaryoblasts are more than 20% or more in the marrow, resemble lymphoblasts, and show distinct cytoplasmic blebs or pseudopod formation. Cytochemically they are negative for myeloperoxidase and positive for platelet peroxidase. Megakaryoblasts express CD41 (glycoprotein IIb/IIIa) and/or CD61 (glycoprotein IIIa).

Table 13.7 Acute lymphoid leukaemia (ALL)

L1	85%	*Morphology*: L1 blasts are small and homogeneous. The nuclei are round and regular, with little clefting and inconspicuous nucleoli. Cytoplasm is lightly basophilic, scanty and usually without vacuoles *Cytochemistry*: MPO is always negative *Maturation*: pro-B or pre-B lineage
L2	14%	*Morphology*: L2 blasts are large and heterogeneous. The nuclei are irregular and often clefted. One or more, usually large nucleoli are present. The volume of cytoplasm is variable, but often abundant and may contain vacuoles *Cytochemistry*: L2 blasts may have granular PAS positivity. MPO is negative *Maturation*: Pro-B or pre-B and T-cell ALL lineage
L3	Burkitt 1%	*Morphology*: L3 blasts are large in size and homogeneous. The nuclei are regular and round–oval in shape. One or more prominent nucleoli are present. They have moderate-to-abundant deeply basophilic cytoplasm, which contains prominent vacuoles *Cytochemistry*: MPO is always negative. NSE is usually negative but may show focal cytoplasmic positivity. Vacuoles are PAS negative but are classically positive for the neutral lipid stain oil red-O *Maturation*: All L3 leukaemias are surface immunoglobulin (SIg) positive, and are of B-cell lineage

(b) Immunophenotyping
(c) Cytogenetics
(d) Molecular genetics

2. **World Health Organization (WHO) classification:** WHO classification for acute leukaemias differs from the FAB classification as it takes into account not just the morphology and cytochemistry but also the cytogenetic and molecular abnormalities. Blast count for diagnosis of acute leukaemia should be greater than or equal to 20% in peripheral blood or bone marrow (in FAB classification the cut off is 30%; the change has been made subsequent to demonstration that survival pattern of patients with 20%–30% blasts is similar to those with a count of >30%).

(a) **WHO classification of AML**

(i) ***AML with recurrent genetic abnormalities***
A. AML with t(8;21)(q22;q22); AML1/ETO
B. AML with abnormal bone marrow eosinophils inv (16)(p13;q22) or t(16;16)(p13;q22); (CBFb/MYH11)
C. Acute promyelocytic leukaemia AML with t(15;17)(q22;q12)(PML/RARa) and variants
D. AML with t(9;11)(p22;q23); (MLLT3-MLL)
E. AML with t(6;9)(p23;q34); (DEK-NUP 214)
F. AML megakaryoblastic with t(1;22)(p131;q13); RBM15-MKL1
G. AML with mutated NPM1
H. AML with mutated CEBPA

(ii) ***AML with multilineage dysplasia***
A. Following an MDS
B. Without antecedent MDS

(iii) ***AML and MDS, therapy-related***
A. Alkylating agent-related
B. Topoisomerase Type II inhibitor-related
C. Other types

(iv) ***AML not otherwise characterized/specified***
A. AML minimally differentiated (M1)
B. AML without maturation (M2)
C. AML with maturation (M3)
D. Acute myelomonocytic leukaemia (M4)
E. Acute monoblastic and monocytic leukaemia (M5)
F. Acute erythroid leukaemia (M6)
G. Acute megakaryoblastic leukaemia (M7)

(v) ***Myeloid sarcoma***

(vi) ***Myeloid proliferation related to Down syndrome***

(b) **WHO classification of ALL**

(i) ***B lymphoblastic leukaemia/lymphoma***
- B-lymphoblastic leukaemia/lymphoma, not otherwise specified (NOS)
- B-lymphoblastic leukaemia/lymphoma with recurrent genetic abnormalities

A. B-lymphoblastic leukaemia/lymphoma with t(9;22)(q34.1;q11.2); *BCR-ABL1*
B. B-lymphoblastic leukaemia/lymphoma with t(v;11q23.3); *KMT2A* rearranged
C. B-lymphoblastic leukaemia/lymphoma with t(12;21)(p13.2;q22.1); *ETV6-RUNX1*
D. B-lymphoblastic leukaemia/lymphoma with hyperdiploidy
E. B-lymphoblastic leukaemia/lymphoma with hypodiploidy
F. B-lymphoblastic leukaemia/lymphoma with t(5;14)(q31.1;q32.3) *IL3-IGH*
G. B-lymphoblastic leukaemia/lymphoma with t(1;19)(q23;p13.3); *TCF3-PBX1*
H. Provisional: B-lymphoblastic leukaemia/lymphoma, *BCR-ABL1*–like
I. Provisional: B-lymphoblastic leukaemia/lymphoma with *iAMP21*

(ii) ***T lymphoblastic leukaemia/lymphoma***
A. Provisional: Early T-cell precursor lymphoblastic leukaemia
B. Provisional: Natural killer (NK) cell lymphoblastic leukaemia/lymphoma

Q. Write briefly on the aetiopathogenesis of leukaemias. (PA18.2)

Ans. The following factors contributing to the etiopathogenesis of leukaemias:

- **Familial and genetic:** Down syndrome, ataxia telangiectasia, Fanconi anaemia and Bloom syndrome.
- **Drugs and toxins:** Cytotoxic drugs like alkylating agents and exposure to benzene.
- **Retroviruses:** Human T-cell leukaemia-lymphoma virus (human T-cell lymphotropic Type I virus).
- **Ionizing radiation:** Therapeutic irradiation, diagnostic X-rays and nuclear bombs.
- **Immunological:** Immunodeficiency states.

Q. Outline the clinical features and laboratory diagnosis of acute leukaemia. (PA18.2)

Ans. Acute leukaemia is characterized by the replacement of normal marrow elements by immature cells called leukaemic blasts, which ultimately spill over into the peripheral blood. The **clinical presentation** of acute leukaemias is due to one or more of the following:

Anaemia

- Pallor, tiredness, malaise and effort intolerance.
- Cardiorespiratory symptoms in severe anaemia.

Granulocytopenia

Infections at various sites, for example upper respiratory tract, skin, gingiva, lungs and urinary tract. Superficial lymphadenopathy and fever are common.

Thrombocytopenia

- Causes bleeding from gum, nose (epistaxis), skin (purpura, ecchymoses, petechiae and easy bruising), GIT, renal tract and uterus. Bleeding into eye and ear is also seen.
- Intracranial bleeding is a serious and fatal complication.

Myeloid Proliferation

Causes expansion of marrow leading to bone pains and sternal tenderness.

Leukaemic Infiltration Into Organs

- Common in liver, spleen and lymph nodes; results in hepatosplenomegaly and generalized lymphadenopathy.

- Involvement of the central nervous system results in infiltration of brain parenchyma and meninges ('**leukaemic meningitis**').
- Other areas of leukaemic infiltration include mouth, gums (causing gingival hypertrophy), skin, testes, ovaries, eyes and bone.
- Localized proliferation of myeloblasts outside marrow produces solid tumours called **chloromas**.

Laboratory Diagnosis

- **Morphological examination of blood** (Fig. 13.17A,B) **and bone marrow**
  - Severe anaemia of the normocytic normochromic type.
  - A markedly raised TLC (range 1×10^9/L to 500×10^9/L).
  - Numerous blast cells in the peripheral smear.
  - Markedly decreased platelet count.
  - Hypercellular bone marrow with replacement of normal elements by leukaemic blast cells.
- **Cytochemical stains in acute leukaemias**
  - Myeloperoxidase (MPO) is used for identification of primary or azurophilic granules in myeloid precursors. Positive in AML-M1, -M2, -M3 and -M4.

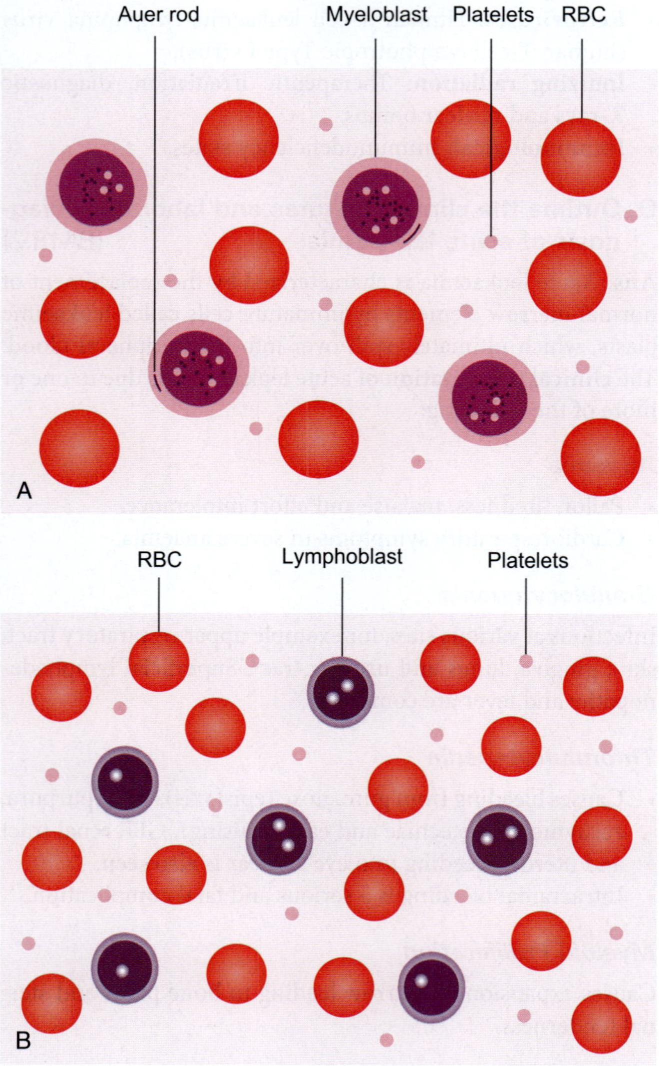

Fig. 13.17 (A and B) Morphological examination of blood and bone marrow in (A) AML and (B) ALL (schematic representation).

Table 13.8 Common cytogenetic abnormalities in acute leukaemias

Chromosomal abnormality	Type of leukaemia	Prognosis
t(8;21)(q22;q12)	AML-M2	Favourable
t(15;17)(q22;q12)	AML-M3	Favourable
Inv(16)(p13;q32)	AML-M4E0	Favourable
Abnormalities of 11q23	AML monocytic	Intermediate
{I7,del(7q), {I5,del(5q), +8, +9, del(11q)	AML with multilineage dysplasia, therapy-related AML	Unfavourable
t(9;22)(q34;q11.2)	Precursor B-ALL	Unfavourable
t(4;11)(q21;q23)	Precursor B-ALL	Unfavourable
t(1;19)(q23;q13.3)	Precursor B-ALL	Unfavourable
t(12;21)(q13;q22)	Precursor B-ALL	Favourable
Hyperdiploidy	Precursor B-ALL	Favourable
Hypodiploidy	Precursor B-ALL	Unfavourable

  - Staining with Sudan black B (SBB) and chloroacetate esterase (CAE) is mostly similar to myeloperoxidase. These stain the phospholipids in the membrane of neutrophilic granules.
  - Non-specific esterase (NSE) is present in large quantities in monocytic cells and is positive in AML-M4 and -M5.
  - Periodic acid-Schiff (PAS) shows granular positivity in the erythroblasts of M6 as well as block positivity in blasts of L1 and L2 subtypes of ALL.
  - Acid phosphatase shows a strong focal positivity in T-cell ALL.
- **Immunophenotyping in acute leukaemias**
  Primary panel (to distinguish AML from ALL and classify B-ALL and T-ALL)
  - Myeloid: CD13, CD33 and CD117
  - B Lymphoid: CD19, CD79a(cyt), CD22(cyt) and CD10
  - T Lymphoid: CD3(cyt), CD2 and C7
  - Non-lineage restricted (primitive stem cell): HLA-R, TDT and CD34

  Secondary panel (to diagnose AML of monocytic, erythroid, megakaryocytic lineage and further subtyping of B and T-cell ALL)
  - Myeloid: CD14, CD64, lysozyme, glycophorin A, CD41 and CD61
  - B Lymphoid: cytIgM, surface Ig (κ/λ)
  - T Lymphoid: CD1a, membrane CD3, CD5, CD4 and CD8
- **Cytogenetics and molecular genetics:** The common cytogenetic abnormalities in acute leukaemias are listed in Table 13.8.

Q. Differentiate between acute lymphoblastic and acute myelogenous leukaemia (or differentiate between lymphoblast and myeloblast). (PA18.2)

Ans. Differences between acute lymphoblastic and acute myelogenous leukaemia are listed in Table 13.9.

Table 13.9 Differences between acute lymphoblastic and acute myelogenous leukaemia

Features	Acute lymphoblastic leukaemia (ALL)	Acute myelogenous leukaemia (AML)
Clinical features		
1. Age group	Children	Adults
2. Lymphadenopathy	Prominent	Less prominent
3. Hepatosplenomegaly	50%–75%	Less common
4. CNS involvement	More common	Less common
5. Gum involvement	Not seen	Gum hypertrophy; common in M5 type
6. Testicular involvement	In 10%–20%	Not seen
7. Eye involvement	More common	Less common
8. Bleeding manifestations	Less common	More common
Investigations		
1. Leukaemic blasts	Lymphoblasts	Myeloblasts
2. Size	Smaller, 10–15 μm	Larger, 12–20 μm
3. N/C ratio	High	Low
4. Chromatin	Clumped	Spongy, skein like
5. Nucleoli	<2; indistinct	2–5; distinct
6. Nuclear membrane	Irregular, convoluted	Regular
7. Auer rods	Not present	Present in 10%–20%
8. TdT (terminal deoxynucleotidyl transferase)	Often positive	Negative
Cytochemical staining		
1. Myeloperoxidase	Negative	Positive
2. Sudan black B	Negative	Positive
3. Chloroacetate esterase	Negative	Positive
4. PAS	Positive (shows block pattern)	Positive in <25% of cells

PAS, Periodic acid–Schiff.

Q. Define subleukaemic or aleukaemic leukaemia. (PA18.2)

Ans. In some patients with acute leukaemia, the total leukocyte count is normal or less than normal but abnormal cells are seen in the peripheral blood; this is termed **subleukaemic leukaemia**. In about 10% of the patients with acute leukaemia, total leukocyte count is normal or less than normal and there are no abnormal cells in the peripheral blood. This is called **aleukaemic leukaemia.** Diagnosis is confirmed by examining the bone marrow, which shows a larger number of leukaemic cells.

Q. Write briefly on normal histology of lymph node.

Ans. While bone marrow and thymus are the primary lymphoid organs, lymph nodes are secondary lymphoid organs responsible for mounting an immune response against foreign antigens and phagocytosis. The lymph node is a bean-shaped organ surrounded by a thin fibrous connective tissue covering called a **capsule**, which is thicker at the **hilus** where it penetrates the lymph node as **fibrous trabeculae**. Several afferent lymphatics enter the node at the convex surface of the capsule and drain into the **subcapsular sinus**.

Cortex is the peripheral part of the lymph node located in the immediate subcapsular region. It contains a large number of follicles (primary and secondary). A **primary follicle** is a rounded aggregate of small, darkly staining inactive (naïve) B lymphocytes, within a network of follicular dendritic cell processes, usually located just under the capsule. It does not contain a **germinal centre.** A **secondary follicle** arises from a primary follicle consequent to antigenic stimulation of B cells and production of antibodies. The pale staining germinal centre is surrounded by **mantle zone** and **marginal zone** lymphocytes. The germinal centre contains predominantly B lymphocytes (including centroblasts and centrocytes), along with scattered follicular T helper cells, T regs, follicular dendritic histiocytes, antigen-presenting **Langerhans cells** (earlier called tingible-body macrophages) and endothelial cells. Sequence of maturation of follicular lymphoid cells is given in Figure 13.18. **The mantle zone** is composed of tightly packed small B lymphocytes. The **marginal zone** contains a mixture of postfollicular memory B cells (derived from stimulation of naïve B cells by T-cell–dependent antigens) and is not well developed in lymph nodes.

Paracortex is the tissue between cortex and medulla. It mainly contains dark-staining mature T cells along with B immunoblasts, interdigitating dendritic cells, plasmacytoid dendritic cells, histiocytes and high endothelial venules (postcapillary venules). Paracortex has a coarse network of reticulin fibres and usually expands during cell-mediated immunological reactions. The *medulla* is located close to the hilum and contains medullary cords, sinuses and blood vessels. *Medullary cords* are found between the sinuses and are composed mostly of small B and T lymphocytes, plasmacytoid lymphocytes, plasmablasts and plasma cells. The *medullary sinuses* carry lymph from afferent to efferent lymphatics. The subcapsular sinus is lined by macrophages and contains mast cells and plasma cells.

The follicles, mantle zone and the interfollicular space are predominantly B-cell zones. The medulla on the other hand is predominantly a T-cell zone.

Q. What is reactive lymphadenitis? (PA19.1)

Ans. Infections and non-infectious inflammatory stimuli can cause lymphadenitis, which may be classified as:

Acute Non-specific Lymphadenitis

- May be confined to a local group of lymph nodes draining a focal infection.
- May be generalized in systemic bacterial or viral infections.

Gross Morphology

- Tender and fluctuant in case of abscess formation.
- Involvement of the overlying skin can produce draining sinuses.

Microscopy

- Large germinal centres.
- A neutrophilic infiltrate is seen about the follicles and within lymphoid sinuses in pyogenic infections.
- In severe infections, centres of the follicles undergo necrosis resulting in formation of an abscess.

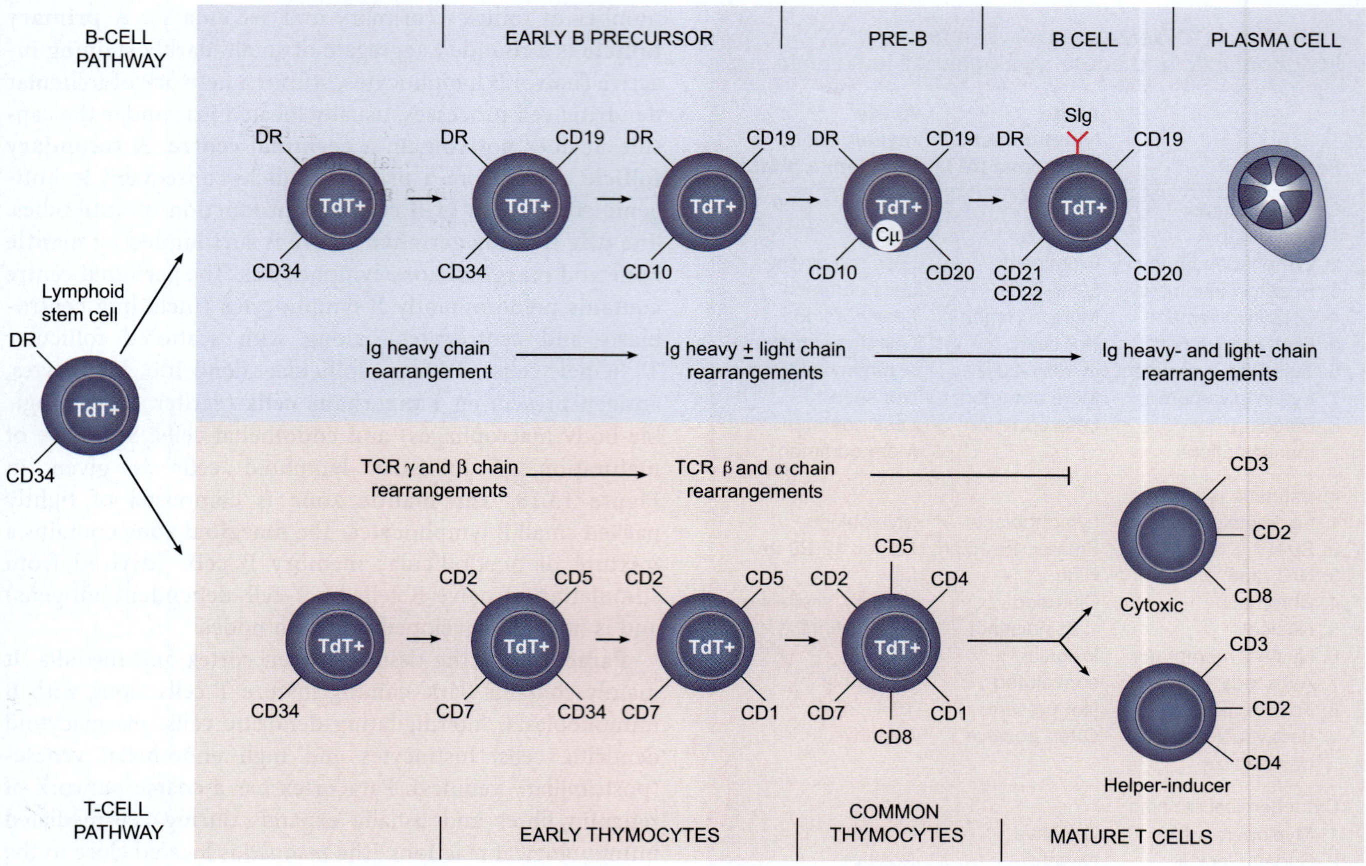

Fig. 13.18 Sequence of maturation of follicular lymphoid cells. (*Source*: Kumar, Abbas, Fausto, et al., *Robbins Basic Pathology: The Hematopoietic and Lymphoid Systems*, 8 ed, Figure 12.13, Elsevier, Saunders, 2007.)

Chronic Non-specific Lymphadenitis

Assumes three patterns depending on the causative agent, namely, follicular hyperplasia, paracortical hyperplasia and sinus histiocytosis

1. **Follicular hyperplasia** (Fig. 13.19)
   (a) Associated with infections and inflammations, which activate B cells.
   (b) Follicles are enlarged with prominent germinal centres.
   (c) Cells in the reactive follicles include activated B cells, scattered macrophages containing nuclear debris **(tingible body macrophages)** and follicular dendritic cells.
   (d) May be confused with follicular lymphomas.

   Features favouring a diagnosis of follicular hyperplasia over a follicular lymphoma
   - Preservation of lymph node architecture with normal areas between germinal centres.
   - Variation in shape and size of lymphoid nodules.
   - Mixed population of lymphocytes at various stages of differentiation.
   - Prominent phagocytic and mitotic activity in germinal centres.
2. **Paracortical hyperplasia**
   (a) Reactive changes in the T-cell regions.
   (b) Encountered in viral infections (EBV), following vaccinations (small pox) and in drug reactions (phenytoin).
3. **Sinus histiocytosis** (Fig. 13.20)

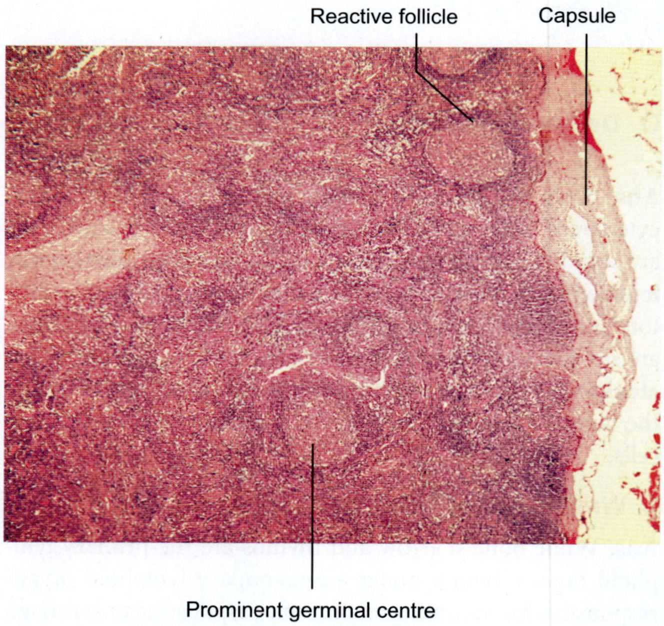

Fig. 13.19 Section from a reactive lymph node showing enlarged follicles with prominent germinal centres (H&E; 100×).

   (a) Distension of the lymphatic sinusoids.
   (b) Hypertrophy of lining endothelial cells and increase in the number of macrophages.
   (c) Often seen in lymph nodes draining cancers (immune response to tumour and its products).

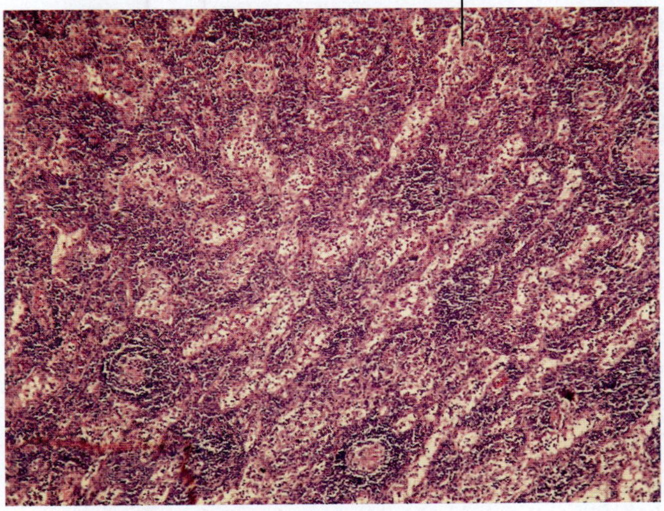

Fig. 13.20 Section from sinus histiocytosis showing distension of the lymphatic sinusoids, hypertrophy of lining endothelial cells, and increase in the number of macrophages (H&E; 100×).

Q. Enumerate the causes of generalized lymphadenopathy.

Ans. ***Causes of generalized lymphadenopathy***

- Disseminated tuberculosis.
- HIV-associated lymphadenopathy.
- Secondary syphilis.
- Infectious mononucleosis.
- Brucellosis.
- Systemic lupus erythaematosus and rheumatoid arthritis.
- Lymphomas.
- Leukaemias (ALL and CLL).

Neoplastic Proliferations of Lymph Nodes

WHO classifies all lymphoid neoplasms into the following broad categories:

1. Hodgkin Lymphoma (HL).
2. B-cell malignancies.
3. T/natural killer (NK)-cell malignancies.
4. Histiocytic and dendritic neoplasms.
5. Posttransplant lymphoproliferative disorders.

Q. Write in detail on Hodgkin lymphoma (HL).

PA19.4, 19.5)

Ans. HL has a bimodal age incidence; affects young adults (15–35 years) and older adults (45–75 years). **Reed–Sternberg (RS) cells** are the diagnostic hallmark of HL.

Classification (Table 13.10)

HL is classified into two broad categories:

1. **Classical HL (95% of HL):** Cell of origin is a germinal centre or post germinal centre B cell, which is PAX5, CD15 and CD30 positive and negative for other markers. Classical HL includes the following entities:
   a. Nodular sclerosis (NS).
   b. Mixed cellularity (MC).

Table 13.10 Classification of Hodgkin Lymphoma (HL)

Subtypes	Morphology	Immunophenotype	Clinical features
NS	Frequent 'lacunar cells' and occasional diagnostic RS cell; in a background of T lymphocytes, eosinophils, macrophages, and plasma cells. Collagenous or fibrous bands divide cellular areas into nodules; cells are arranged in syncytial sheets with interspersed necrosis; rarely the entire lymph node may be replaced by the collagen	RS cells are CD15 and 30 positive; and EBV negative	• Mediastinal involvement is commonly seen • Most patients present in Stage I or II of the disease • Females are more commonly affected than males; usually affects young adults • Constitutes 65%–75% of HL
MC	Frequent 'mononuclear' and 'diagnostic RS cells' with a background infiltrate rich in T lymphocytes, eosinophils, macrophages and plasma cells (Fig. 13.23)	RS cells are positive for CD15, CD30, and EBV; EBV positivity is seen in 70% cases	• More than 50% patients are present in Stage III or IV disease • Usually involve neck nodes • Males are more commonly affected than females and this subtype has a biphasic age distribution (seen in young adults and after 55 years) • Constitutes 20%–25% of HL
LR	Frequent 'mononuclear' and 'diagnostic RS cells', in a background rich in T lymphocytes	RS cells are positive for CD15, CD30, and EBV; EBV positivity is seen in 60% cases	• Uncommon subtype • Males are more commonly affected than females • Affects older adults
LD	• *Reticular variant*: Many 'diagnostic RS cells' and 'variants' with paucity of background reactive cells • *Diffuse fibrosis variant*: Hypocellular fibrillar background with scattered 'diagnostic RS cells' and 'variants', and a few reactive cells	RS cells are positive for CD15, 30, and EBV	• Affects older males • Frequent association with HIV infection • Usually present with advanced disease • Constitute <5% cases of HL

(*Continued*)

Table 13.10 Classification of Hodgkin Lymphoma (HL) (*Cont.*)

Subtypes	Morphology	Immunophenotype	Clinical features
NLP	Nodular growth pattern; frequent 'L and H (popcorn) cells' in the background of follicular dendritic cells and reactive B cells; may transform into a large B-cell lymphoma	RS cells are CD20, CD45, and EMA positive, CD15 negative, CD30 negative, EBV negative and BCL6 positive (BCL6 is a germinal centre–specific transcription factor) indicating an origin from germinal centre B cells	• Affects young males • Causes cervical and axillary lymphadenopathy • Rarely involves mediastinal lymph nodes

c. Lymphocyte rich (LR).
d. Lymphocyte depleted (LD).

2. **Nodular lymphocyte predominant (NLP; 5% of all HL):** Cell of origin is a germinal centre B cell which is positive for CD20 and BCL6 and negative for CD15 and CD30.

Classic RS Cell (Fig. 13.21)

- Large cell (15–45 μm) with abundant cytoplasm.
- Classically has a bilobed mirror image nucleus.
- Multiple nuclei or single nucleus with multiple lobes may be seen.
- Nucleus typically has a large inclusion-like nucleolus of the size of a small lymphocyte (5–7 μm).

Variants of RS Cells (Fig. 13.22)

- **Mononuclear variants (Hodgkin cells):** Single atypical round-to-oblong nucleus with a large inclusion-like nucleolus.
- **Lacunar cells:** Predominantly seen in NS subtype, these cells have a delicate, folded and multilobated nucleus with abundant pale cytoplasm, often disrupted while cutting sections. The nucleus appears to be sitting in a hole (lacuna).
- **L and H variants:** RS cells undergo mummification (shrinkage and pyknosis of nucleus) to give rise to cells with polypoid nuclei resembling popcorn, have inconspicuous nucleoli, and moderate-to-abundant cytoplasm. They are usually seen in the lymphocyte-predominant (LP) subtype.
- **Pleomorphic/anaplastic variant:** Highly pleomorphic cell with a bizzare nucleus.

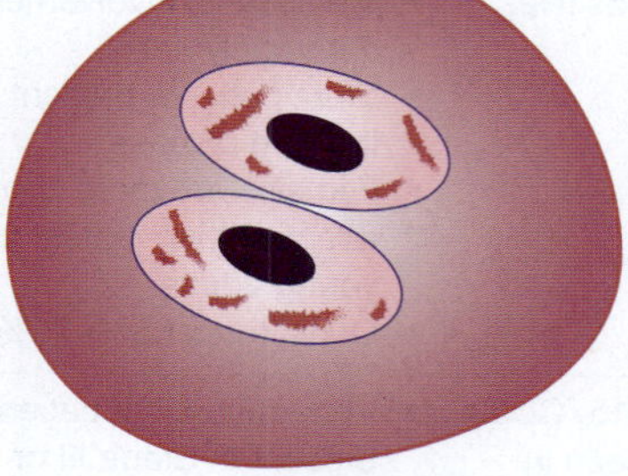

Fig. 13.21 Schematic diagram of a classical RS cell showing abundant cytoplasm, a bilobed mirror image nucleus and a large inclusion-like nucleolus of the size of a small lymphocyte.

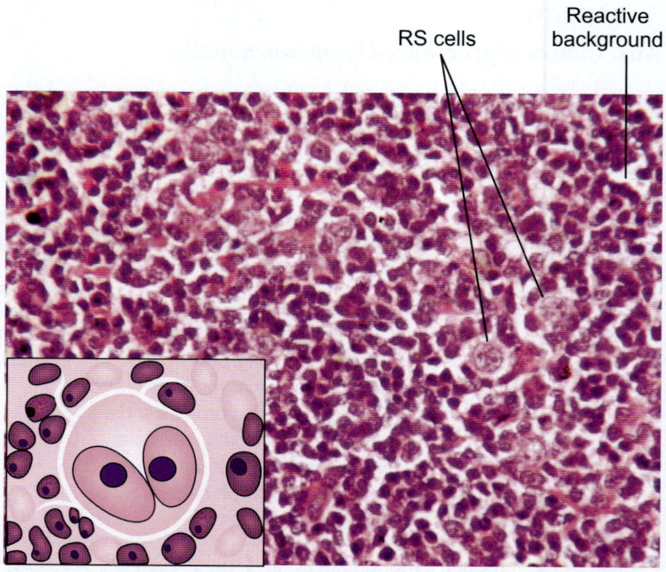

Fig. 13.23 Frequent 'mononuclear' and 'diagnostic Reed–Sternberg (RS) cells' with a background infiltrate rich in lymphocytes, eosinophils, macrophages, and plasma cells in a photomicrograph from HL-mixed cellularity (MC) subtype (H&E; 400×).

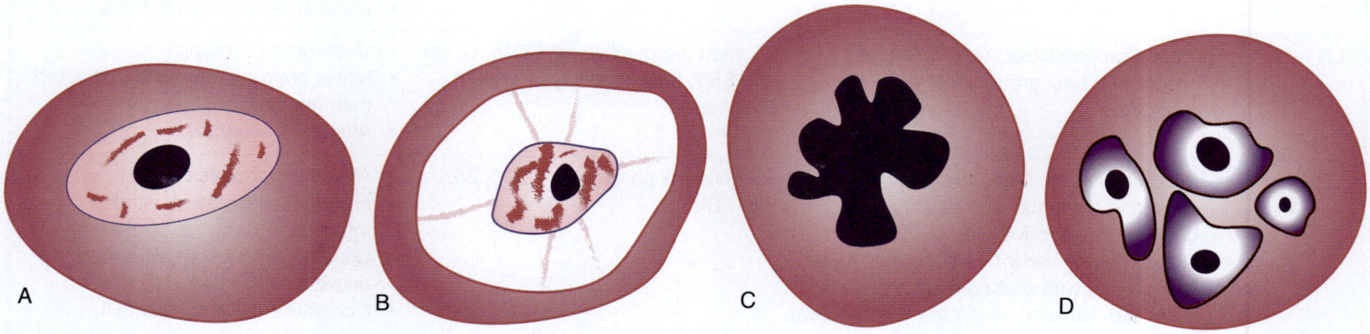

Fig. 13.22 Variants of RS cells. (A) Mononuclear variants (Hodgkin cells), (B) Lacunar cells, (C) L and H variants, (D) Pleomorphic/anaplastic variant.

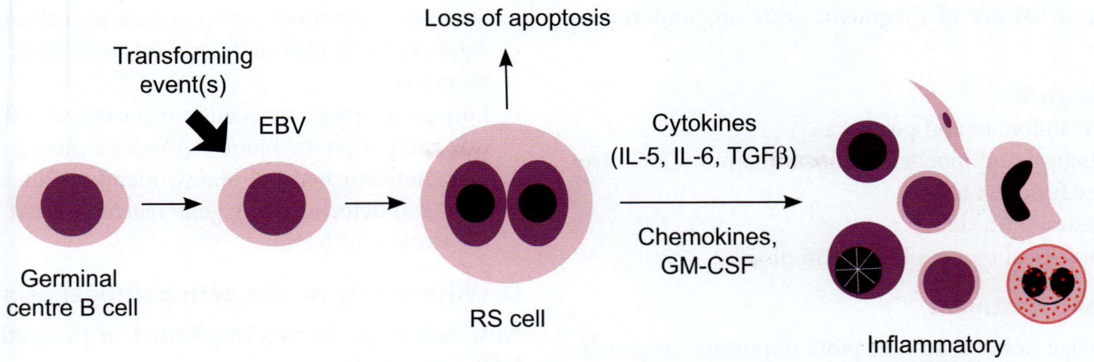

Fig. 13.24 Pathogenesis of HL.

Note: RS-like cells may be seen in solid cancers, NHL, and infectious mononucleosis. For diagnosing 'HL', RS cells must be present in a background of non-neoplastic cells (lymphocytes, plasma cells and eosinophils).

Aetiology and Pathogenesis (Fig. 13.24)

- The cell of origin of RS cells is thought to be a germinal centre or postgerminal centre B lymphocyte. Despite their B cell origin they fail to express most B cell specific genes including Ig genes. This is thought to be because of reprogramming of gene expression, which possibly results from widespread epigenetic changes.
- Rarely (1%–2% cases) RS cells have TCR rearrangements suggesting origin from transformed T cells.
- EBV episomes are frequently present in RS cells. EBV-positive tumour cells express latent membrane protein or LMP-1 (a protein encoded by EBV genome that has transforming activity).
- LMP-1 upregulates NF-kB (transcription factor responsible for lymphocyte activation).
- NF-kB activation appears to be a common event in classical EBV-positive HL (NF-kB activation in EBV-negative cases occurs by acquired mutation in a negative regulator IKB).
- NF-κB activation possibly rescues cells from apoptosis.
- Accumulation of reactive cells is thought to be in response to cytokines released by RS cells, for example IL-5, IL-6, IL-13, TNF and GM CSF. There is a predominance of Th2 cells in the T cell population.
- IL-5 attracts eosinophils, which produce TGF-beta (transforming growth factor beta), which is responsible for the fibrosis.
- Expression of FasL in most RS cells plus loss of FasL expression in the follicular dendritic cells (FDC) of the germinal centre suggests a disturbed FDC microenvironment that may contribute to its pathogenesis. RS cells are aneuploid and demonstrate diverse clonal aberrations including copy number gains in REL proto-oncogene on chromosome 2p and genes encoding PD-L1 and PD-L-2 located on chromosome 9p, both of which are immune check point proteins that inhibit antitumour T cell responses.

Clinical Features

- **Painless enlargement of lymph nodes** (cervical, axillary, supraclavicular, inguinal, paraaortic), which are **discrete, non-tender and rubbery.** Pain and abdominal discomfort due to **splenomegaly** may be seen in half the patients. **Hepatomegaly** is less common.
- Localized disease (stages I and II) in > 60% of patients. Mediastinal involvement in ~60% (mostly nodular sclerosing subtype).
- **'Constitutional or B symptoms'** (fever, night sweats, unexplained weight loss of greater than 10% body weight) are observed in 20%–40% cases, more commonly with disseminated disease (Stages III and IV) and mixed cellularity or lymphocyte depletion subtypes.
- Classical **'Pel–Ebstein' fever** (fever showing cyclical pattern; several days or weeks of fever alternating with afebrile periods) is rare.
- An uncommon paraneoplastic symptom involves occurrence of pain in affected lymph nodes on consumption of alcohol.
- Cutaneous anergy due to depressed cell-mediated immunity may be seen. Cutaneous manifestations include pruritus, pigmentation and purpura.
- Marrow involvement will cause bone pain.

Clinical Staging (Ann Arbor); (Table 13.11).

Ann Arbor staging system is used to quantitate the extent of disease in HL. For staging, besides complete physical

Table 13.11 Clinical (Ann Arbor) staging of HL

Stage	Distribution of disease
I	Involvement of single lymph node region (I) or involvement of a single extralymphatic organ or site (IE).
II	Involvement of two or more lymph node regions on the same side of diaphragm, alone (II) or with involvement of limited contiguous extralymphatic organs or tissue (IIE).
III	Involvement of lymph node regions on both sides of diaphragm, which may include spleen (IIIS) and/or limited contiguous extralymphatic organ/site (IIIE, IIIES).
IV	Multiple or disseminated foci of involvement of one or more extralymphatic organs or tissues with or without lymphatic involvement.

Note: All stages are further divided into (A) and (B) on the basis of the presence or absence of systemic symptoms.
(*Source*: *Robbins & Cotran Pathologic Basis of Disease*, Tenth Edition: Vinay Kumar, Abul K. Abbas, Jon C. Aster, Table 13.9, Page 615, Elsevier Inc., 2021).

examination, a variety of diagnostic tests are undertaken that include:

1. Chest radiograph.
2. CT scan of abdoman and pelvis.
3. Haematological and biochemical examination (CBC, liver and kidney function tests).
4. Bone biopsies, both sides.
5. Histopathological typing of Hodgkin disease.

Prognosis and Treatment

- Tumour stage rather than type more important prognostic factor.
- With current treatment protocols, cure rates of **Stages I** and **II A**—90%.
- **Advanced stage** associated with a 60%–70% disease-free survival for 5 years.
- **Complications of long-term chemotherapy and radiotherapy:**
  - **Neoplastic complications:** Increased rates of myelodysplastic syndrome, acute leukaemia, lung cancer, NHL, breast and gastric carcinoma, sarcomas and malignant melanoma.
  - **Non-neoplastic complications:** Pulmonary fibrosis and accelerated atherosclerosis.

Q. Differentiate between HL and non-Hodgkin lymphoma (NHL). (PA19.4)

Ans. Differences between HL and NHL are given in Table 13.12.

Q. Write briefly on the epidemiology of non-Hodgkin lymphoma (NHL).

Ans. NHL is characterized by clonal proliferation of immune cells; 65% of NHL is of B-lymphocyte origin, 35% T-lymphocyte origin, and 2% of NK-cell origin. This malignant neoplasm of the immune system has the following salient features:

- It constitutes approximately 60% of malignant lymphomas (remaining 40% are HL).
- Most primary NHLs arise in the lymph nodes; few are extranodal in origin.
- Stomach is the most common primary extranodal site.
- Approximately 60% of the patients with NHL are men over 50 years.
- Low-grade lymphomas often metastasize to the bone marrow and peripheral blood (leukaemic phase).
- Immunohistochemical stains, identification of translocation, and detection of *Ig* gene rearrangement are useful in the workup of NHL.

Table 13.12 Clinical differences between HL and non-Hodgkin lymphoma (NHL)

Features	HL	NHL
Nodal involvement	More often localized to a single axial group of nodes	Usually involves multiple peripheral nodes
Pattern of extranodal spread	Orderly spread by contiguity	Non-contiguous spread
Involvement of mesenteric nodes and Waldeyer ring	Rarely involved	Commonly involved
Extranodal involvement	Extranodal involvement uncommon	Extranodal involvement common
Prognosis	Better	Worse

Q. Write briefly on the aetiopathogenesis of NHL.

Ans. Aetiologic factors implicated in the pathogenesis of NHL are as follows:

- **Infections**
  - *Helicobacter pylori* (MALT lymphoma of stomach).
  - EBV (Burkitt lymphoma, post-transplant lymphoma).
  - Human T-cell leukaemia virus Type I (adult T-cell lymphoma/leukaemia).
  - HIV (Diffuse large B-cell lymphoma, Burkitt lymphoma).
  - Hepatitis C (Lymphoplasmacytic lymphoma).
- **Immunodeficiency diseases:** Various inherited (ataxia telangiectasia, Wiskott–Aldrich syndrome) and acquired immunodeficiency diseases, for example AIDS, iatrogenic immunosuppression induced by chemo or radiotherapy are implicated.
- **Autoimmunity:** Sjögren syndrome, non-tropical sprue and rheumatoid arthritis are associated with a higher incidence of NHL.
- **Chemical and drug exposure:** Long-term exposure to phenytoin, agriculture chemicals, radiotherapy and chemotherapy.
- **Cytogenetic abnormalities:** Chromosomal translocations, for example overexpression of BCL-2 protein.

Q. Classify NHL.

Ans. Classification systems used for classification of NHL:

- REAL
- WHO

  Updated REAL (Revised European-American classification)/WHO classification (2008): In 1994 REAL classification was proposed, however in view of the fact that it showed poor reproducibility, it is not used anymore. Since 1995, members of the European and American haematopathology societies have been collaborating on a new World Health Organization (WHO) classification of haematological malignancies. WHO classification uses an updated version of the REAL classification for lymphomas and extends the principles of the REAL classification to the classification of myeloid and histiocytic neoplasms. The latest (2017) WHO classifications recognize three major categories of lymphoid malignancies that can be defined on the basis of a combination of morphology and special studies that identify cell lineage: B-cell neoplasms, T-cell/natural killer (NK)-cell neoplasms and Hodgkin disease/Hodgkin lymphoma (HD). A schematic diagram in Fig. 13.25 depicts the immunophenotype of various B- and T-cell malignancies.

  1. B-cell neoplasms
     (a) Precursor B-cell neoplasm: Precursor B-lymphoblastic leukaemia/lymphoma (B-ALL).

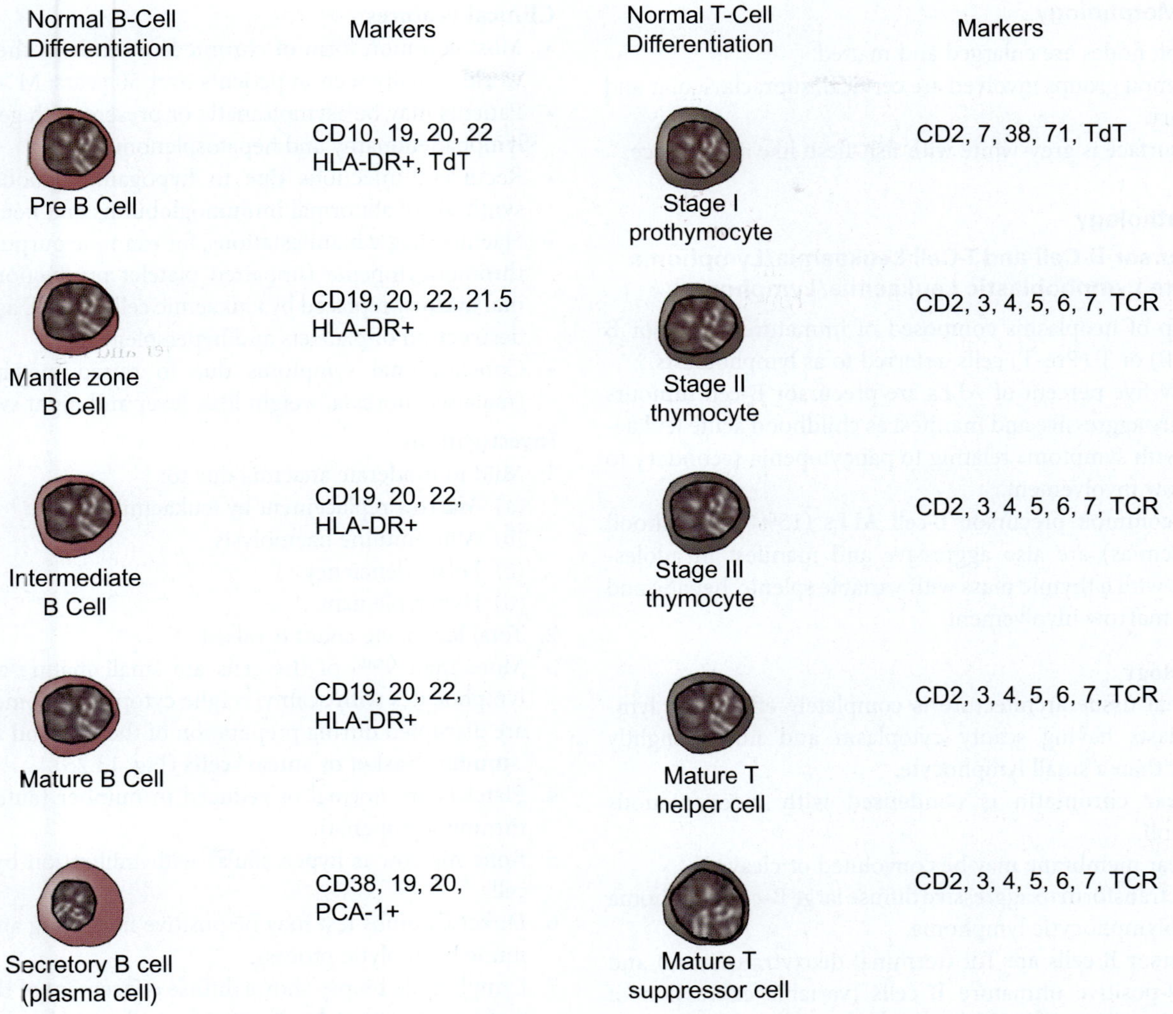

Fig. 13.25 Schematic diagram depicting the immunophenotype of various B- and T-cell malignancies. (*Source*: Modified with permission from Jaffe, 1990, with additional data from Uckun, 1990; *Atlas of Diagnostic Oncology*: Hodgkin Disease and Non-Hodgkin Lymphomas, Figure 16.37, Pages 571–639, Elsevier, Mosby, 2010.)

(b) Mature (peripheral) B-cell neoplasms
- (i) B-cell chronic lymphocytic leukaemia/small lymphocytic lymphoma.
- (ii) Lymphoplasmacytic lymphoma.
- (iii) Splenic marginal zone lymphoma (± villous lymphocytes).
- (iv) Hairy cell leukaemia.
- (v) Plasma cell myeloma/plasmacytoma.
- (vi) Extranodal marginal zone B-cell lymphoma of MALT type.
- (vii) Mantle cell lymphoma.
- (viii) Follicular lymphoma.
- (ix) Nodal marginal zone B-cell lymphoma (± monocytoid B cells).
- (x) Diffuse large B-cell lymphoma (NOS).
- (xi) Diffuse large B cell lymphoma associated with chronic inflammation.
- (xii) Primary effusion lymphoma.
- (xiii) Burkitt's lymphoma.

2. T-cell and NK-cell neoplasms

(a) Precursor T-cell neoplasm: Precursor T-lymphoblastic lymphoma/leukaemia.

(b) Mature (peripheral) T-cell neoplasms
- (i) T-cell prolymphocytic leukaemia.
- (ii) T-cell granular lymphocytic leukaemia.
- (iii) Chronic lymphoproliferative disorder of NK cells.
- (iv) Adult T-cell lymphoma/leukaemia (HTLV1+).
- (v) Extranodal NK/T-cell lymphoma and nasal type.
- (vi) Enteropathy-type T-cell lymphoma.
- (vii) Primary cutaneous T cell lymphoproliferative disorder.
- (viii) Mycosis fungoides/Sézary syndrome.
- (ix) Anaplastic large cell lymphoma.
- (x) Peripheral T-cell lymphoma; unspecified (NOS).
- (xi) Angioimmunoblastic T-cell lymphoma.

Q. Write in detail about the gross and microscopic pathology of NHL.

Ans. Diagnosis made reliably on **lymph node biopsy**; FNAC not adequate for typing of NHL.

Gross Morphology

1. Lymph nodes are enlarged and matted.
2. Common groups involved are cervical, supraclavicular and axillary.
3. Cut surface is grey-white with fish-flesh like appearance.

Histopathology

I. Precursor B-Cell and T-Cell Leukaemia/Lymphoma (Acute Lymphoblastic Leukaemia/Lymphoma):

- Group of neoplasms composed of immature precursor B (Pre-B) or T (Pre-T) cells, referred to as lymphoblasts.
- Eighty-five percent of ALLs are precursor B-cell tumours that are aggressive and manifest as childhood acute leukaemia with symptoms relating to pancytopenia secondary to marrow involvement.
- Less common precursor T-cell ALLs (15% of childhood leukaemias) are also aggressive and manifest in adolescence with a thymic mass with variable splenic, hepatic and bone marrow involvement.

Morphology

- Normal tissue architecture is completely effaced by lymphoblasts having scanty cytoplasm and nuclei slightly larger than a small lymphocyte.
- Nuclear chromatin is condensed with inconspicuous nucleoli.
- Nuclear membrane may be convoluted or cleaved.
- Some transform to aggressive diffuse large B-cell lymphoma or prolymphocytic lymphoma.
- Precursor B cells are Tdt (terminal deoxytransferase) and CD19-positive immature B cells (variable expression of other B-cell markers).
- Precursor T cells are Tdt-positive immature T cells (CD2-, 7-positive and variable expression of other T-cell markers).

Karyotype

- Ninety percent have non-random karyotypic abnormalities.
- Hyperdiploidy (>50 chromosomes) most common; associated with a good prognosis.
- Poor outcome in pre-B-cell tumours is associated with translocation involving the MLL gene on chromosome 11q23 or Philadelphia chromosome positivity.
- Fifty-five to sixty percent of pre-T-cell tumours have activating point mutations in NOTCH1 (transmembrane receptor whose activity is essential for normal T-cell development, that is proliferation and survival of pre-T cells).

II. Mature Peripheral B-Cell Malignancies

1. **Small lymphocytic lymphoma (SLL)/chronic lymphocytic leukaemia (CLL):** CLL is characterized by a persistent lymphocytosis of at least 10×10^9 with infiltration of the bone marrow, spleen and lymph nodes. SLL is essentially a nodal disease (CLL and SLL are morphologically and genotypically similar; differ only in terms of peripheral blood involvement, in the absence of which, a diagnosis of SLL is rendered).

Types

More than 95% of the cases are B-CLL; 5% are T-CLL.

Clinical Features

- Most common form of chronic leukaemia in the Western world, usually seen in patients over 50 years; M > F.
- Patients may be asymptomatic or present with generalized lymphadenopathy and hepatosplenomegaly.
- Recurrent infections due to hypogammaglobulinaemia/ synthesis of abnormal immunoglobulins and neutropenia.
- Haemorrhagic manifestations, for example purpura, due to thrombocytopenia (impaired platelet production as normal marrow replaced by leukaemic cells, as well as immune destruction of platelets and hypersplenism).
- Constitutional symptoms due to raised metabolic rate (malaise, anorexia, weight loss, fever and night sweats).

Investigations

1. Mild to moderate anaemia due to:
   (a) Marrow replacement by leukaemic cells.
   (b) Autoimmune haemolysis.
   (c) Folate deficiency.
   (d) Hypersplenism.
2. Total leukocyte count is raised.
3. More than 95% of the cells are small mature-appearing lymphocytes with scanty, fragile cytoplasm. Some of these are disrupted during preparation of the film and are called **'smudge, basket or smear' cells** (Fig. 13.26).
4. Platelets are normal or reduced in number (autoimmune thrombocytopenia).
5. Bone marrow is hypercellular with infiltration by tumour cells.
6. Direct Coombs test may be positive indicating an autoimmune haemolytic process.
7. Lymph node biopsy shows diffuse effacement of the lymph node architecture by sheets of small round lymphocytes (tumour cell is a resting lymphocyte with a dark staining nucleus and scanty cytoplasm showing minimal cytological atypia and mitoses).
8. Serum folate levels are low.

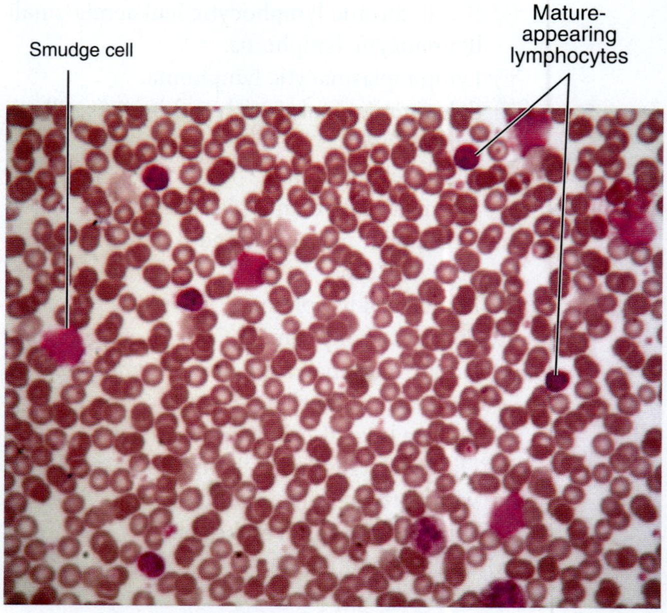

Fig. 13.26 Leishman-stained PBS of CLL showing mature-appearing lymphocytes with scanty, fragile cytoplasm, at places forming 'smudge' cells.

Clinical Staging (Binet Classification)

- Stage A
  - No anaemia or thrombocytopenia.
  - Less than three areas of lymphoid enlargement.
- Stage B
  - No anaemia or thrombocytopenia.
  - Three or more areas of lymphoid enlargement.
- Stage C
  - Anaemia and/or thrombocytopenia present, regardless of the number of areas of lymphoid enlargement.

Note: Lymphoid enlargement includes cervical, axillary, inguinal lymph nodes, liver and spleen.

2. **Follicular lymphoma**
   (a) More common in the western world than in Asian population.
   (b) Affects older age group.
   (c) Presents as painless generalized lymphadenopathy with or without visceral involvement.
   (d) Lymph nodes effaced with a nodular appearance.
   (e) Tumour cells resemble normal follicular centre B cells (centrocyte like with cleaved nuclear contours or nuclear infoldings, coarse chromatin and scanty cytoplasm). A few centroblast-like cells that have vesicular chromatin, several nucleoli and moderate cytoplasm, also seen.
   (f) Pan B markers, CD19, CD20, CD10 and BCL6 (transcription factor required for follicular centre formation) and BCL2-positive.
   (g) Majority of tumours have a characteristic translocation t(14;18).
   (h) Natural course of disease is prolonged (median survival from 7 to 9 years); but not easily curable due to increased levels of BCL2, which blocks apoptosis to increase survival of tumour cells.
   (i) In 40% patients, follicular lymphomas progress to a diffuse large B-cell lymphoma.
3. **Mantle cell lymphoma**
   (a) Four percent of all NHLs.
   (b) Presents in the 5th and 6th decades with lymphadenopathy and involvement of bone marrow, liver, spleen and bowel (multifocal submucosal nodules resembling polyps called lymphomatoid polyposis).
   (c) Lymph nodes show diffuse or vaguely nodular pattern of effacement.
   (d) Composed of B cells that resemble the cells in the mantle zone of normal lymphoid follicles.
   (e) Tumour cells are slightly larger than normal lymphocytes with an irregular nucleus and inconspicuous nucleoli and express IgM, IgD, CD19, CD20 and CD5.
   (f) Translocation (11;14) is commonly seen and results in fusion of Cyclin D1 gene on chromosome 11 to the IgH locus on chromosome 14 inducing dysregulation of expression of Cyclin D1 and increased levels of the same.
   (g) Aggressive with a median survival of 3–5 years.
4. **Diffuse large B-cell lymphoma**
   (a) Accounts for 50% of adult NHLs.
   (b) Median age 60 years; slight male predominance.
   (c) This category includes several forms of NHL, which share the following features:
      (i) B-cell phenotype.
      (ii) Diffuse growth pattern.
      (iii) Aggressive nature (disseminate widely).
   (d) Pan B-cell markers positive along with surface IgM and IgG with variable expression of CD10.
   (e) Tumour cells are largely composed of cells that resemble **centroblasts** (3–4 times the size of resting lymphocytes, round, irregular-cleaved nuclear contours, dispersed chromatin, distinct nucleoli and moderate pale cytoplasm) as well as a few cells that resemble **immunoblasts** (large round to multilobated vesicular nucleus, 1–2 centrally placed prominent nucleoli and pale to intensely staining abundant cytoplasm).
   (f) Some patients have t(14;18); these tumours may represent 'transformed' follicular lymphomas.
   (g) A few cases show rearrangements/mutation in Bcl 6 gene leading to inappropriate increase in Bcl 6 protein.
   (h) Fatal if untreated; complete remission can be achieved in 60%–80% patients by combination chemotherapy.
   (i) Several clinicopathological subtypes:
      (i) Diffuse large B-cell lymphoma that arises in the setting of AIDS and iatrogenic immunosuppression.
      (ii) Diffuse large B-cell lymphoma arising in the post-transplant setting.
      (iii) Kaposi Sarcoma herpes virus (KSHV) or Human herpes virus type 8 (HHV-8) associated 'primary effusion lymphomas' in the pleura, pericardium or peritoneum.
      (iv) Mediastinal large B-cell lymphomas (arise in young females and frequently spread to abdominal viscera and central nervous system).
5. **Burkitt lymphoma**
   (a) This is a high-grade, non-Hodgkin lymphoma having small non-cleaved cells.
   (b) Endemic in some parts of Africa and sporadic in the United States.
   (c) EBV plays an important aetiological role.
   (d) Majority of the cases occurs in children; usually in extranodal sites.
   (e) In African patients, involvement of mandible and maxillary bones manifests with deformity, loosening of teeth and proptosis with loss of vision.
   (f) The North American type preferentially involves the abdomen (bowel, retroperitoneum and ovaries).
   (g) Tumour cells are uniform with round to oval nuclei (approximately, the size of nuclei of macrophages), 2–5 nucleoli and moderate amount of basophilic or amphophilic cytoplasm.
   (h) Neoplasm characterized by a high mitotic rate and cell death leading to the presence of numerous macrophages with debris. These macrophages are often surrounded by a clear space creating a characteristic **'starry sky' appearance.**
   (i) Tumour cells express surface IgM, kappa and lambda light chains and pan B-cell markers (CD19, CD20 and CD10).

(j) Chromosome analysis may show 8; 14 or 2; 8 or 8; 22 translocations. Most translocations fuse MYC with IgH gene on chromosome 14 resulting in dysregulation and overexpression of MYC protein.
(k) Antibodies to EB viral capsid antigen may be present.

6. **Mucosa-associated lymphoid tissue (MALT) lymphoma (extranodal marginal zone lymphoma)**
(a) Low-grade mature B-cell tumour that arises from mucosa-associated lymphoid tissue (MALT).
(b) Seen in salivary glands, stomach, small and large bowel, lungs, orbit and breast.
(c) Gastric type of MALT lymphoma is associated with *Helicobacter pylori* infection. Salivary gland MALT is associated with Sjögren syndrome indicating sustained antigenic stimulation may contribute to development of these lymphomas.
(d) It is mainly seen in elderly patients with median age of 60 years.
(e) MALT lymphomas may remain localized to the organ from which they arise or may spread to the surrounding lymph nodes.
(f) Bone marrow involvement is uncommon and occurs in only 15% cases. Distant metastasis is possible.
(g) Prognosis is good in most cases (5-year survival of 75%).

Common Mature Peripheral T-Cell Malignancies

1. **Mycosis fungoides and Sézary syndrome**
(a) Cutaneous T-cell lymphomas composed of neoplastic CD4+ T cells that home to the skin.
(b) The patient presents with chronic erythrodermic rash manifesting as a localized plaque-like lesion (plaque phase), which later becomes nodular and ulcerated (tumour phase).
(c) Histological findings include infiltration of the epidermis and upper dermis by neoplastic T cells, which have a cerebriform nucleus characterized by marked infolding of the nuclear membrane.
(d) In some cases, a leukaemic phase called **Sézary syndrome** appears, which is characterized by:
(i) Generalized exfoliative erythroderma
(ii) Tumour cells in the peripheral blood
(e) Patients with erythrodermic phase of mycosis fungoides usually survive for many years; survival less (1–3 years) for patients in tumour phase of the disease, visceral disease and Sézary syndrome.

2. **Adult T-cell lymphoma/leukaemia**
(a) Caused by a retrovirus, human T-cell lymphotropic virus-I (HTLV-I).
(b) Patients are infected through transplacental transmission, blood transfusion or sexual contact.
(c) Most patients have an aggressive disease characterized by lymphadenopathy, hepatosplenomegaly, skin infiltration, hypocalcaemia and lytic bone lesions.
(d) Peripheral smear usually reveals characteristic, pleomorphic abnormal CD4-positive cells with indented nuclei.
(e) Leukaemic cells express high levels of CD25 (The IL2 receptor α chain).
(f) Extremely aggressive disease with a median survival of 8 months. A few patients have long, chronic course.
(g) Combination chemotherapy may prolong life but does not produce remissions.

3. **Anaplastic large cell lymphoma (ALCL)**
(a) These typically show anaplastic cytology, constant membrane expression of the CD30 antigen (an activation marker for B or T cells), and rearrangements of ALK gene on chromosome 2p23.
(b) Tumour cells are large, highly anaplastic, with abundant cytoplasm and horseshoe-shaped nuclei.
(c) Clinical features include frequent cutaneous and extranodal involvement, young age at presentation and male predominance.

4. **Peripheral T-cell lymphoma (Unspecified)**
(a) Refers to a group of diseases that do not fit into any of the other subtypes of PTCL (CD4 and CD8+, CD4> CD8; antigen loss frequent—CD7, CD5, CD4/CD8, CD52; CD30 –/+, CD56 –/+, CD10 –, BCL6 –, CLCX13 –, PD1 –).
(b) It constitutes 25% of all PTCLs.
(c) Most commonly presents with peripheral lymphadenopathy; extranodal disease present in 60%. Most common extranodal sites: skin, GIT; lungs and CNS. Majority present with advanced stage disease associated with secondary involvement of marrow, liver, spleen and other extranodal sites.
(d) Histopathology shows paracortical or diffuse infiltrate by medium to large-sized cells with pleomorphic nuclei, vesicular chromatin, prominent nucleoli and frequent mitoses. Reed–Sternberg-like cells can be seen. It has the following types:
(i) TBX21 subtype associated with a polymorphous inflammatory background composed of small lymphocytes, eosinophils, plasma cells, large B cells and epithelioid histiocytes.
(ii) GATA3 subtype associated with monomorphic morphology with minimal inflammatory background.

Lymphoepithelioid variant (Lennert lymphoma) shows an infiltrate of small CD8+ cells with minimal nuclear atypia and epithelioid histiocytes (correlates with TBX21 molecular subtype).

Universal Laboratory Findings in NHL

1. Anaemia of normocytic normochromic type
2. Advanced disease with marrow infiltration →neutropenia, thrombocytopenia and leucoerythroblastic picture
3. Leukaemic conversion of NHL
4. Hyperuricaemia and hypercalcaemia late in the disease

Q. Enumerate various plasma cell disorders.

Ans. Plasma cell disorders are monoclonal neoplasms developing from common progenitors in the B-lymphocyte lineage. Also called paraproteinemias and plasma cell dyscrasias; they include the following diseases:

- Monoclonal gammopathy of undetermined significance (MGUS).

- Heavy chain disease (HCD).
- Multiple myeloma (MM).
- Waldenström macroglobulinemia.
- Immunoglobulin-related amyloidosis.

Monoclonal gammopathy of undetermined significance: MGUS is the most common of a spectrum of diseases called plasma cell dyscrasias. The term MGUS denotes the presence of a monoclonal immunoglobulin (Ig), also called 'M protein', in the serum or urine of persons without definite evidence of MM, Waldenström macroglobulinemia, immunoglobulin-related amyloidosis, or other lymphoproliferative disorders.

Heavy chain diseases: HCDs are rare B-cell proliferative disorders characterized by the synthesis and secretion of incomplete immunoglobulin heavy chains. These disorders were initially recognized as gammopathies due to the presence of monoclonal proteins in the patient's serum or urine. This is associated with a diverse group of disorders including lymphoplasmacytic lymphoma and some marginal zone lymphomas.

Waldenström macroglobulinemia: Waldenström macroglobulinemia, one of the malignant monoclonal gammopathies, is a chronic, indolent, lymphoproliferative disorder characterized by the presence of a high level of a macroglobulin or immunoglobulin M (IgM), elevated serum viscosity, and the presence of a lymphoplasmacytic infiltrate in the bone marrow. A clonal disease of B lymphocytes, Waldenström macroglobulinemia is considered to be a lymphoplasmacytic lymphoma, as defined by the WHO classification.

Immunoglobulin-related amyloidosis: Immunoglobulin-related amyloidosis is a monoclonal plasma cell disorder in which the secreted monoclonal immunoglobulin protein forms insoluble fibrillar deposits in one or more organs. In nearly all cases, the deposits contain immunoglobulin light (L) chains. In a few reported patients, the amyloid deposits have contained immunoglobulin heavy (H) chains; these are termed H chain-type amyloidosis (AH).

Q. Write in detail on the pathology, clinical features and laboratory diagnosis of multiple myeloma (MM). (PA20.1)

Ans. MM results from **clonal proliferation of plasma cells induced by the cytokine IL-6, which is secreted by fibroblasts and macrophages present in the bone marrow stroma.** The plasma cells produce immunoglobulins with only one type of light chain (kappa or lambda). The light chains are produced in excess, and not the whole immunoglobulin molecule. These excess light chains are low molecular weight and appear in the urine as **Bence–Jones proteinuria.** The immunoglobulin produced is called a **'paraprotein' (M-protein).** It appears on electrophoresis as a clear-cut band (**M-band or M-component;** Fig. 13.27). The most common M-component is IgG (60%), followed by IgA (20%–25%); only rarely it is IgM, IgD, or IgE. In the remaining cases, the plasma cells produce κ- or λ-light chains only. Around 1% myelomas are non-secretory.

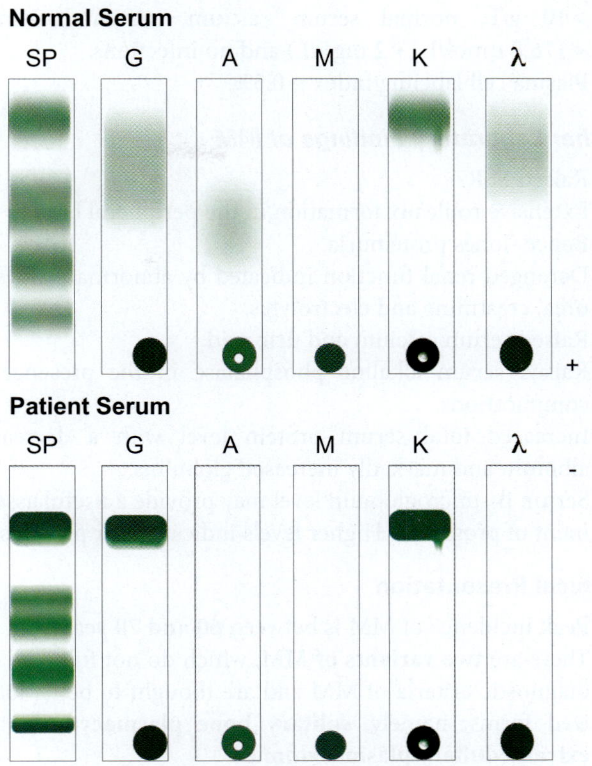

Fig. 13.27 Serum electrophoresis showing monoclonal gammopathy (M protein spike). (*Source*: *Robbins Basic Pathology,* Tenth Edition: Vinay Kumar, Abul K. Abbas, Jon C. Aster, Fig. 13.18, Page 600, Elsevier Inc., 2018.)

Laboratory Diagnosis

Major Criteria

1. Plasmacytoma on tissue biopsy.
2. Bone marrow with greater than 30% plasma cells.
3. Monoclonal globulin spike (M band) on serum protein electrophoresis with an IgG peak of >3.5 g/dL, IgA peak of >2 g/dL, or urinary κ- or λ chain excretion of >1 g/24 hours in absence of amyloidosis.

Minor Criteria

1. Bone marrow with 10%–30% plasma cells.
2. Monoclonal globulin spike is present, but less than major criteria 3.
3. Lytic bone lesions.
4. Hypoglobulinemia of normal proteins: IgM <500 mg/L, IgA <1 g/L or IgG <6 g/L.

Diagnostic: 1 Major criteria and 1 minor criteria.
Diagnostic: 0 Major criteria and 3 minor criteria.

Patients with these criteria associated with one of those listed further are categorized as having indolent myeloma and do not require immediate therapy.

- Absent or limited bone lesions (three or fewer lytic lesions), no compression fractures.
- Stable paraprotein levels: IgG <70 g/L and IgA <50,000 mg/L (<50 g/L).
- No symptoms and associated disease features, including Karnofsky performance status >70%, haemoglobin

>10 g/L, normal serum calcium, serum creatinine <176.8 μmol/L (<2 mg/dL) and no infections.
- Plasma cell labeling index ≥0.5%.

Other Laboratory Findings of MM

- Raised ESR.
- Extensive rouleaux formation in the peripheral blood.
- Bence–Jones proteinuria.
- Deranged renal function indicated by abnormal values of urea, creatinine and electrolytes.
- Raised serum calcium and uric acid.
- Raised serum alkaline phosphatase in the presence of complications.
- Increased total serum protein level with a decreased albumin and markedly increased globulins.
- Serum β_2-microglobulin level may provide a useful assessment of prognosis. Higher levels indicate poor prognosis.

Clinical Presentation

- Peak incidence of MM is between **60 and 70 years.**
- There are **two variants of MM**, which do not fulfill all the diagnostic criteria of MM and are thought to be its localized forms, namely, **solitary bone plasmacytoma** and **extramedullary plasmacytoma.**
- **Solitary bone plasmacytoma** is a single lytic bone lesion without marrow plasmacytosis. It presents as a punched-out lesion involving the flat bones (vertebrae, skull, sternum, ribs, and clavicle) and manifests with bone pain, pathological fractures, and compressive myelopathy (due to vertebral collapse and compression).
- **Extramedullary plasmacytoma** is a lesion of soft tissue (mainly upper respiratory tract) without associated marrow plasmacytosis.
- Those with **skeletal plasmacytomas** develop full-blown MM over a period of 5–10 years, whereas, extra osseous plasmacytomas spread less commonly and are often cured by local resection.
- **MGUS** is the **most common plasma cell dyscrasia** and has the following features:
  - Serum M protein levels <3 g/dL
  - Marrow plasmacytosis <10%
  - No evidence of any other B-cell proliferative disorder
  - No evidence of MM-like tissue damage (bone lysis, renal failure, etc.)
- Osteoclasts are stimulated, resulting in bone resorption and generalized osteoporosis.
- Serum uric acid is elevated due to increased cell turnover.
- Mobilization of calcium from bone results in hypercalcaemia, hypercalciuria and nephrocalcinosis.
- **Renal involvement** is seen in the form of Bence–Jones proteinuria, amyloidosis, hypercalcaemia and hyperuricaemia, eventually resulting in renal damage and renal failure.
- **Immune system involvement** (hypogammaglobulinemia and neutropaenia with granulocyte dysfunction) results in increased susceptibility to infections, particularly of the respiratory system and urinary tract.
- **Hyperviscosity syndrome** results from increased viscosity of blood and may cause blurred vision with retinal venous congestion, papilledema, headache, vertigo, nystagmus, postural hypotension, congestive cardiac failure and clotting problems (purpura, epistaxis and gastrointestinal bleeding). M-components may interact specifically with clotting factors, leading to defective coagulation.
- MM may also present with **neurological manifestations** (amyloid peripheral neuropathy, carpal tunnel syndrome, compressive myelopathy and radiculopathy).
- **POEMS syndrome** is seen in 1% cases of MM. It typically manifests with polyneuropathy, organomegaly, endocrinopathy, MM and skin changes.

Revised International Staging System (RISS) for MM

This revised classification system has been adopted by the International Myeloma Working Group (IMWG). The RISS proposes three disease stages by combining the ISS with high-risk cytogenetic abnormalities or elevated lactate dehydrogenase levels:

- Stage I: Beta-2-microglobulin <3.5 mg/L, albumin ≥3.5 g/dL, no high-risk cytogenetics, and normal serum lactate dehydrogenase levels.
- Stage II: Not stage I or III.
- Stage III: Beta-2-microglobulin ≥5.5 mg/L and high-risk cytogenetics t(4;14), t(14;16) or del(17p), or elevated serum lactate dehydrogenase levels.

Pathology (Fig. 13.28)

- Bone marrow is infiltrated heavily with atypical plasma cells. Gradual replacement of the marrow by plasma cells leads to anaemia, leukopaenia and thrombocytopenia.
- In majority of patients, plasma cells are seen in the peripheral blood in small numbers. In a few patients, however, they may be seen in significant numbers (more than 2000/μL), and this condition is known as **'plasma cell leukaemia'.**

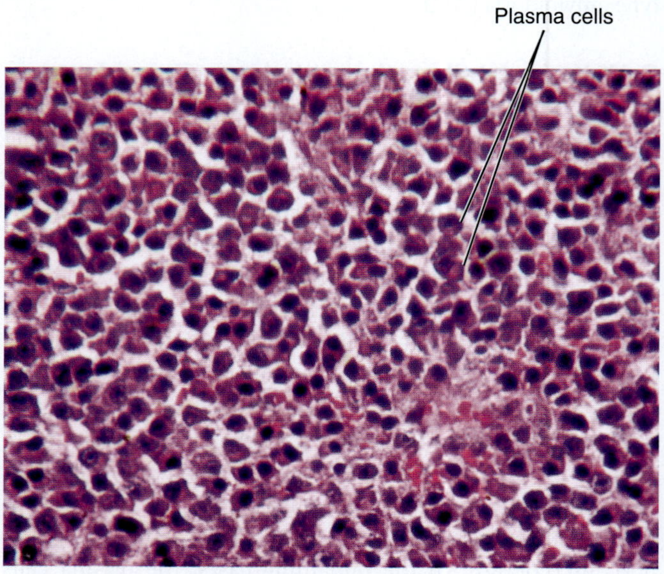

Fig. 13.28 Bone biopsy of multiple myeloma (MM) showing sheets of plasma cells and precursors (H&E; 200×).

Q. Enumerate the common histiocytic disorders.

Ans. The histiocytoses are a group of diverse disorders all characterized by the infiltration of macrophages and dendritic cells in various affected tissues. Normal histiocytes originate from pluripotent stem cells in the bone marrow. Under the influence of GM-CSF, TNF-alpha, IL-3, IL-4, these precursor cells differentiate to become committed stem cells which mature to become antigen-processing cells, with some possessing phagocytic capabilities (macrophages, monocytes, dendritic cells, interdigitating reticulum cells and Langerhans cells).

Classification

Class I: Langerhans cell histiocytosis (LCH)
Class II: Histiocytosis of mononuclear phagocytes other than Langerhans cells
Class III: Malignant histiocytic disorders

LCH can be localized when it manifests as pain or may even be asymptomatic, as in isolated bone lesions. LCH can also involve multiple organs and systems, when it manifests clinically with significant symptoms and consequences. Despite the variation in morphology and clinical features, all the variants of LCH have in common the expression of antigens S100, CD1a, and HLA-DR and presence of *Birbeck granules* demonstrated on electron microscopy. **Birbeck granules** are rod-shaped structures containing dilated tennis racket like terminal ends. They are thought to originate by receptor-mediated endocytosis of **'Langerin'**, a protein present in epidermal cells which is responsible for Birbeck granule synthesis.

Eosinophilic granuloma is the most common type of LCH. It mainly affects children and young adults and presents as a unifocal lytic lesion; common affected sites include femur, skull, vertebrae, ribs and pelvis. Histopathology shows numerous macrophages, lymphocytes, plasma cells, neutrophils, variable number of eosinophils, and Langerhans cells. Langerhans cells are 12–15 µm in diameter and have abundant, pale eosinophilic cytoplasm, irregular and elongated nuclei with prominent nuclear grooves and folds (coffee bean appearance), fine chromatin, and indistinct nucleoli. Occasionally multinucleated cells are seen.

Other forms of LCH include a **chronic disseminated form (Hand–Schüller–Christian disease)** that includes a classic triad of skull lesions, exophthalmos, and diabetes insipidus; *and* **an acute disseminated form (Letterer–Siwe disease)** that affects multiple organs and has a poor prognosis. Histopathology shows a mix of eosinophils, giant cells, neutrophils, foam cells, lymphocytes, plasma cells, fibrosis, and necrosis.

Q. Enumerate the common causes of splenomegaly. (PA19.5)

Ans. *Causes of splenomegaly*

- **Mild splenomegaly** (weight less than 500 g): Acute splenitis, acute splenic congestion, enteric fever, infectious mononucleosis, brucellosis, septicaemia, SLE, infective endocarditis, syphilis and parasitic infestations, for example malaria, kala-azar.
- **Moderate splenomegaly** (weight 500–1000 g): Lymphomas, portal hypertension, acute leukaemias, chronic lymphocytic leukaemia, chronic myeloid leukaemia, haemolytic anaemias (hereditary spherocytosis and thalassaemia major), amyloidosis, Niemann–Pick disease, tuberculosis, sarcoidosis, typhoid, metastatic carcinoma and sarcoma.
- **Massive splenomegaly** (weight more than 1000 g): Chronic myeloid leukaemia, myelofibrosis, hairy cell leukaemia, tropical splenomegaly, kala-azar, portal hypertension, Gaucher disease, lymphomas, cysts and tumours of spleen.

Q. Write briefly on tropical splenomegaly. (PA19.5)

Ans. Seen in residents of malaria endemic areas.

- Presents with low-grade fever and massive hepatosplenomegaly.
- High levels of antimalarial antibodies are found in the blood. IgM levels are markedly raised.

Q. Write briefly on hypersplenism. (PA19.5)

Ans. This is a term used to indicate anaemia, leucopenia and thrombocytopenia associated with prominent splenomegaly and a normal or hypercellular bone marrow (enlarged spleen removes excessive numbers of the formed elements of blood). Leucopenia and thrombocytopenia result from excessive sequestration of these cells in the large spleen. Anaemia is believed to be dilutional, resulting from an increase in total plasma volume.

Criteria for Diagnosis of Hypersplenism

1. Anaemia, leukopaenia, and/or thrombocytopenia.
2. Prominent splenomegaly.
3. Normal or hypercellular bone marrow.
4. Improvement in cytopenias after splenectomy.

Common Causes

- Primary hypersplenism: No detectable cause.
- Secondary hypersplenism: Portal hypertension, malaria, kala-azar; topical splenomegaly syndrome and myeloproliferative disorders.

14 Bleeding and Clotting Disorders

Q. What are the components of normal haemostatic mechanisms? (PA21.1)

Ans. Regulation of normal haemostasis and blood flow involves complex interactions between blood cells (platelets and leukocytes), the endothelial lining of blood vessels and the coagulation cascade (Figure 14.1). The following series of events are observed consequent to injury:

1. **Arteriolar vasoconstriction,** due to reflex neurogenic mechanisms and 'endothelin' (a potent vasoconstrictor secreted by the endothelium).
2. **Activation of the platelets and coagulation pathways** by various mechanisms:
   (a) Endothelial injury exposes the highly thrombogenic subendothelium, which initiates platelet adherence and activation. Platelet adherence to the vessel wall is facilitated by:
      (i) von Willebrand factor (vWF) which is a glycoprotein synthesised and stored in Weibel-Palade bodies of endothelial cells and α-granules of platelets.
      (ii) Binding of vWF to platelet GpIb receptors mediates the adhesion of platelets to the injured endothelium. When platelets come across the injured endothelium they change shape, release granules and become 'sticky'.

Platelet activation results in the discharge of granule contents and formation of thromboxane A_2 from arachidonic acid, by the action of cyclooxygenase and thromboxane synthetase. Thromboxane A_2 is a potent stimulant of platelet aggregation and leads to formation of a haemostatic plug **(primary haemostasis),** which is mediated by **GpIIb/IIIa-receptor** and fibrinogen. Also released are adenosine diphosphate (ADP), which attracts more platelets to the affected area, and serotonin, which is a potent vasoconstrictor. There are several physiologic and

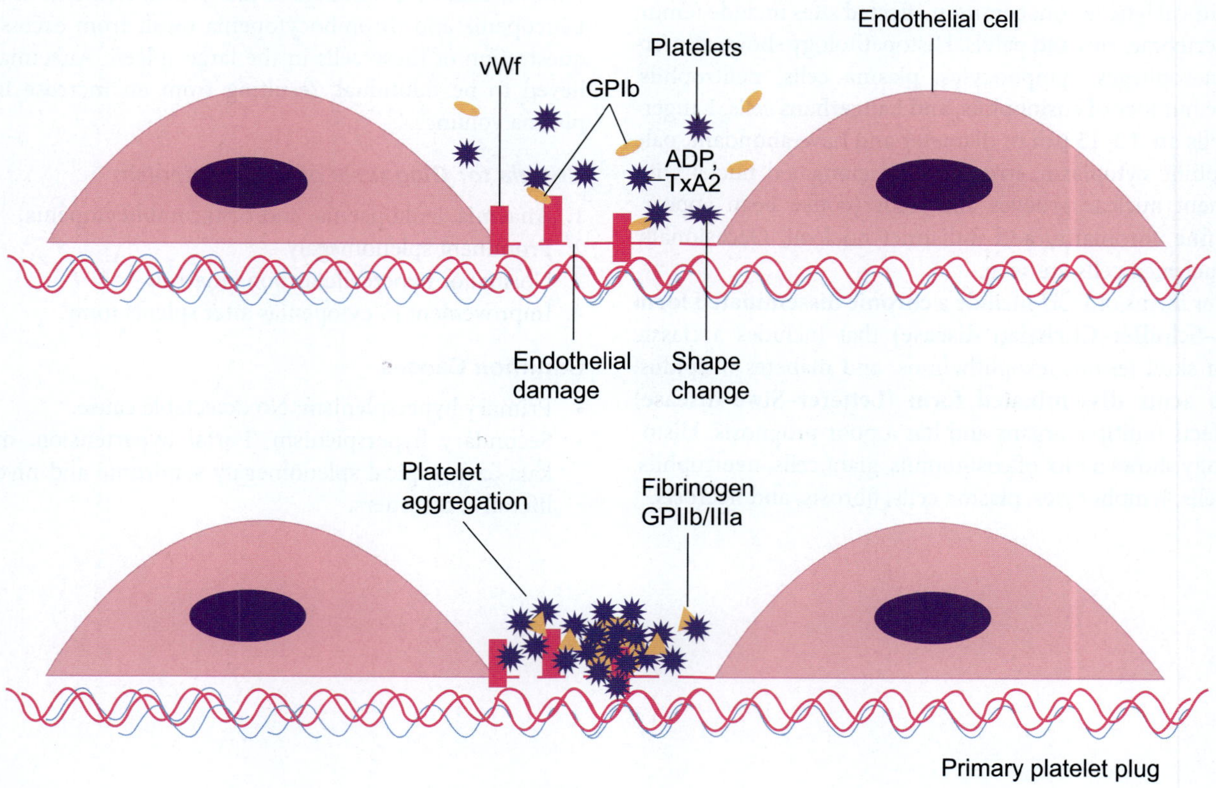

Fig. 14.1 Formation of a primary haemostatic plug.

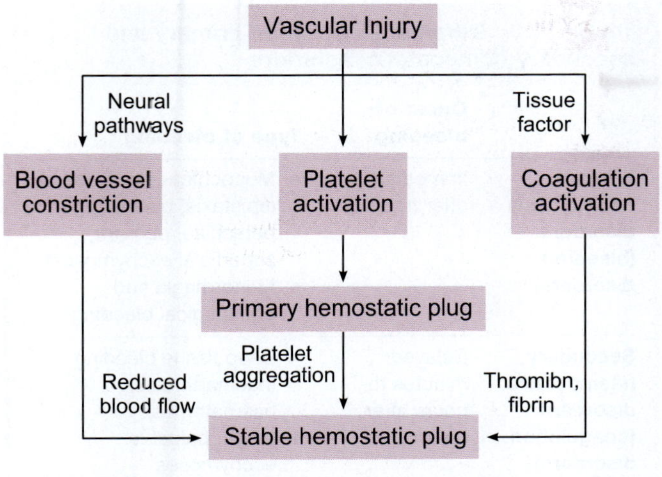

Flowchart 14.1 Formation of a primary haemostatic plug.

pathologic inhibitors of primary haemostasis (Flowchart 14.1).

- **Physiologic**: Endothelial prostacyclin (PGE12) and nitric oxide, both of which inhibit platelet activation. They also form a physical barrier, preventing platelets from being exposed to thrombogenic subendothelial matrix proteins.
- **Pathologic**: High concentrations of fibrin(ogen) degradation products can inhibit platelet aggregation (fragments D and E have a high affinity for platelet membranes and compete with fibrinogen for platelet receptors, thus impairing aggregation) as can paraproteins (high concentrations of monoclonal immunoglobulins with multiple myeloma inhibit platelet aggregation, adhesion and phospholipid exposure).

(b) **Tissue factor (TF),** also released at the site of injury, augments the action of secreted platelet factors to initiate the coagulation cascade. TF activates thrombin, which converts circulating soluble fibrinogen to insoluble fibrin and induces further platelet recruitment and granule release **(secondary haemostasis)**.

(c) Polymerised fibrin and platelet aggregates form a **solid, permanent plug** to prevent any further bleeding.

(d) Simultaneously tissue plasminogen activator (t-PA) and vascular endothelial cells are activated to restrain the haemostatic plug to the site of injury only. This entails release of proteins of the **fibrinolysis cascade**. The physiological function of the fibrinolytic system is to digest deposits of fibrin (thrombi).

(e) In most diseased states, there is a predominance of procoagulant mechanisms and inhibition of anticoagulant and fibrinolytic mechanisms.

The important coagulation factors involved in the intrinsic, extrinsic, and common pathways are enlisted in Table 14.1.

Table 14.1 Coagulation factors

Factors	Traditional name
I	Fibrinogen
II	Prothrombin
V	Proaccelerin
VII	Proconvertin
VIII	Antihaemophilic factor
IX	Christmas factor
X	Stuart–Prower factor
XI	Plasma thromboplastin antecedent
XII	Hageman factor
XIII	Fibrin stabilising factor

Prekallikrein: Fletcher factor.
HMW kininogen: Fitzgerald factor.

Coagulation Factor Inhibitors

Coagulation factor inhibitors are basically antibodies that neutralise the function of a clotting factor. They could be **alloantibodies** (when they occur in patients with inherited factor deficiency) or **autoantibodies** (when they arise in patients without an inherited factor deficiency). The most commonly encountered circulating inhibitor in clinical practice is against factor **VIII. Coagulation factor inhibitors** can be seen in several conditions including connective tissue disorders (RA, SLE, myasthenia gravis), drugs (e.g. penicillins, sulpha, interferons), graft-vs-host disease, malignancy (lymphoproliferative disorders, prostate, renal, lung or colon cancer) and pregnancy. They can also be seen without any identifiable cause, particularly in older adults.

Fibrinolytic System

This system regulates fibrin deposition and its removal. The fibrin-cleaving enzyme **plasmin** is present in the circulation as its inactive precursor form, **plasminogen**, which is activated by proteolytic cleavage. The main plasminogen activators in humans are **t-PA** and **urokinase (u-PA).** The **fibrin-degradation products (FDPs)** released by the action of plasmin on fibrin are useful in diagnosing disseminated intravascular coagulation (DIC). The amino-terminal lysine residues in plasminogen and t-PA are removed for conversion to plasmin by a carboxypeptidase, which in turn is activated by thrombomodulin-bound thrombin referred to as **thrombin-activated fibrinolysis inhibitor (TAFI).**

Plasminogen activator inhibitor-1 (PAI-1) produced by endothelial cells, hepatocytes, platelets and placenta is a potent inhibitor of t-PA. Also, a second **inhibitor PAI-2** has been isolated from human placenta, but its function and mechanism of action is not clear as of now.

α2-Antiplasmin is the main physiological inhibitor of plasmin and it inhibits plasmin function by forming plasmin–antiplasmin complexes.

Deficiencies of the fibrinolytic system, although rare, can be associated with a predisposition to thrombosis or haemorrhage.

Inhibitors of Coagulation (Table 14.2)

Under normal circumstances, in vivo clotting is prevented by several endothelial antithrombotic properties and naturally

Table 14.2 Inhibitors of coagulation

Inhibitor	Target protein
Tissue factor pathway inhibitor (TFPI)	Tissue factor
Antithrombin	Factor II and X
Protein C-protein S	Factor V and VIII
Thrombin activatable fibrinolysis inhibitor (TAFI)	Fibrin
Plasminogen activator inhibitor-1 (PAI-1)	Tissue plasminogen activator (t-PA)

occurring inhibitors of coagulation. The aim is to limit the fibrin clot to the site of injury and not allow it to propagate elsewhere.

1. **Tissue factor pathway inhibitor (TFPI):** It combines first with factor Xa so that coagulation is thereafter dependent on the small amount of thrombin that has been generated. The Xa–TFPI complex can also subsequently inhibit the FVIIa–TF complex.
2. **Antithrombin (AT):** This is a non-vitamin K-dependent protease that inhibits coagulation by neutralising the enzymatic activity of thrombin. Responsible for approximately 70% of thrombin-inactivating capacity in the plasma; it belongs to the serpin group of proteins, and binds to factor IIa forming an inactive thrombin–AT complex, which is subsequently cleared from the circulation by the liver.
3. **Proteins C and S:** Factors Va and VIIIa are the target coagulation factors for protein C and protein S is a cofactor for activated protein C. **Protein C** forms the activated protein C complex together with its cofactor protein S (APC complex) which **inhibits factors Va and VIIIa hereby** inhibiting the coagulation cascade. It is produced in the and its synthesis requires vitamin K.

Endothelial Antithrombotic Properties

1. Intact endothelium prevents platelets and plasma coagulation factors from coming in contact with the highly thrombogenic subendothelial extracellular matrix.
2. Platelets which are activated after focal endothelial injury are prevented from adhering to the uninjured endothelium by endothelial prostacyclin (PGI) and nitric oxide (NO), both were being potent vasodilators and inhibitors of platelet aggregation.
3. Antithrombotic effects are also mediated by endothelial membrane-associated **heparin-like molecules** and **thrombomodulin,** a specific thrombin receptor. The 'heparin-like molecules' are cofactors that interact with *antithrombin III* to inactivate thrombin, factor Xa, and other coagulation factors.

Role of Thrombin in Coagulation

- Cleaves fibrinogen to fibrin, activates factor XIII, and directly induces platelet aggregation and secretion.
- Activates endothelium to generate leukocyte adhesion molecules, t-PA (fibrinolytic), NO, PGI 2 (vasodilators) and PDGF (cytokine).

Table 14.3 Differences between primary and secondary homeostatic disorders

	Onset of bleeding	Type of bleeding
Primary haemostasis disorders (bleeding disorders)	Immediately after trauma	• Mucocutaneous bleeding (epistaxis, bleeding gums, petechiae, purpura, superficial ecchymoses) • Menorrhagia and postsurgical bleeding
Secondary haemostasis disorders (coagulation disorders)	Delayed; minutes to hours after trauma	• Deep tissue bleeding (haemarthrosis, haematomas) • Large, palpable ecchymoses

- Activates inflammatory cells (lymphocytes, plasma cells and macrophages).
- **Thrombomodulin** binds to thrombin, converting it from a procoagulant to an anticoagulant capable of activating *protein C*. Activated protein C, in turn, inhibits clotting by proteolytic cleavage of factors Va and VIIIa; it requires *protein S*, synthesised by endothelial cells, as a cofactor for the same.

Q. Differentiate between primary and secondary homeostatic disorders.

Ans. Differences between primary and secondary homeostatic disorders are enlisted in Table 14.3.

Q. Write briefly on bleeding disorders. (PA21.2)

Ans. Abnormal bleeding can result from abnormalities of platelets or of blood vessels, as well as disorders of the coagulation system (Table 14.4), all of which can be acquired or hereditary. **'Bleeding disorders'** are essentially those which result from abnormalities of platelets and blood vessels). These differ from **disorders of coagulation** in several ways (Table 14.5). The major causes of bleeding disorders are given in Box 14.1.

- **Thrombocytopenia: diminished production** as seen in hereditary thrombocytopenias, viral infections; bone marrow failure—aplastic anaemia, leukaemias, marrow infiltrative disorders, myelofibrosis, megaloblastic anaemia, drug intake, alcoholism; **increased destruction** caused by drugs; heparin; autoantibodies (idiopathic thrombocytopenia purpura, pregnancy, disorders like SLE, AIDS, CLL, etc.); **sequestration** in an enlarged spleen; **dilution loss** in massive transfusion of stored blood; and **increased consumption** in DIC, thrombotic thrombocytopenia purpura, giant haemangiomas, and microangiopathic haemolytic anaemia.
- **Nonthrombocytopenic vascular purpura:** seen in autoimmune diseases, infections, structural malformations like 'Osler–Weber–Rendu disease' or 'inherited disorders of connective tissue matrix like Ehler–Danlos disease and Marfan syndrome'.
- **Rare autosomal recessive disorders: Glanzmann thrombasthenia** and **Bernard–Soulier syndrome** affecting platelet

Table 14.4 Evaluation of haemostasis

Test	Significance
Investigations for vascular and platelet disorders (bleeding disorders)	
Blood smear	For platelet count and platelet morphology.
CBC	For absolute platelet count and haemoglobin/haematocrit values (anaemia may indicate excessive bleeding).
Bleeding time	It is defined as the time taken for a standard skin wound to stop bleeding. Bleeding time measures the ability of platelets to form a primary homeostatic plug to arrest bleeding and therefore measures platelet number and function, as well as the capillary function. Normal range is 3–8 min. A prolonged bleeding time is seen in thrombocytopenia, disorders of platelet function, von Willebrand disease, vascular abnormalities (Ehler–Danlos disease), and severe deficiency of factor V and XI.
Platelet function tests	Evaluate platelets' ability to adhere (retention in a glass bead, etc.) and aggregate (turbidometric techniques using ADP, collagen, and ristocetin) Also include measurement of platelet granule release. If abnormal, indicate presence of either **inherited platelet function** disorders like **von Willebrand disease** (decreased production or dysfunction of von Willebrand factor resulting in reduced platelet adherence; **Glanzmann thrombasthenia** (affects platelets' ability to aggregate); **Bernard–Soulier syndrome** (shows reduced platelet adhesion); **storage pool disease** (affects platelets' ability to release substances that promote aggregation); and **acquired platelet dysfunction,** which may be due to **uraemia, MDS,** and von **Willebrand disease.**
Investigations for coagulation disorders and disorders of the fibrinolytic system	
Clotting time	Clotting time is the time taken by a sample of blood to coagulate in vitro under standard conditions. In order for blood to clot, the enzyme thrombin must be generated from precursor prothrombin. Thrombin converts soluble fibrinogen into insoluble fibrin to form a clot. Generation of thrombin involves the sequential activation of a number of other plasma clotting factors, in the presence of calcium and by factors released by platelets and damaged tissues. If the plasma concentration of these coagulation factors is low or if the factor is absent, or functionally inactive, clotting time will be prolonged. The normal range for clotting time is 4–10 min.
PT	PT determines the time taken by plasma to clot after addition of TF (usually brain extract) and calcium and is a general screening test that detects deficiency of factors II, V, VII, X and fibrinogen **(extrinsic pathway).** Prolonged PT may indicate coagulation factor deficiency or dysfunction, presence of specific factor inhibitor, oral anticoagulant therapy, liver disease, vitamin K deficiency, and DIC, and should be followed by other tests. The test is repeated after adding a small volume of normal plasma to patient plasma; if the clotting time is corrected the abnormality is because of factor deficiency; if not, due to presence of inhibitors.
aPTT	aPPT determines the time taken by plasma previously incubated with kaolin (an activator) to clot after addition of platelet lipid substitute and calcium. Normal range is 30–40 s. A value greater than 10 s longer than control time is considered abnormal. It evaluates factors VIII, IX, XII, XI, PK and high-molecular weight kininogen **(intrinsic pathway of coagulation).** Common causes of prolonged aPTT include heparin injections, DIC, liver disease, and circulating inhibitors.
TT	TT determines the time taken by plasma to clot after addition of solution of thrombin; the concentration of the thrombin solution being adjusted to obtain a clotting time of 15 s. A clotting time of greater than 18 s is considered abnormal. TT is prolonged in the presence of inhibitors (heparin) or FDP (fibrinogen levels <100 mg/dL; normal: 160–415 mg/dL).
Fibrinogen activity	A semiquantitative estimation of fibrinogen can be made by TT. Levels may be low when production is decreased or in DIC and may be high in infection and inflammation, as it is an acute phase reactant.
D-dimer (specific type of cross-linked FDP) assay	FDP are protein fragments of various sizes that result from degradation of fibrinogen and fibrin by plasmin. These are increased in fibrinogenolysis, recent thromboembolism, and DIC. Latex agglutination test (agglutination of latex particles coated with antibody to fibrinogen) or immunoassays (for plasmin degradation products of cross-linked fibrin) are used to assess fibrinolytic activity. Immunoassays are more sensitive and specific. To differentiate between fibrin and fibrinogen degradation products, measurement of fibrinopeptides and specific FDP like D dimer can be done.
Coagulation factor assays	Decreased activity of one or more factors may indicate factor deficiency or presence of a specific factor inhibitor. Mixing studies can be undertaken to determine if there is actual factor deficiency or inhibitor presence.
Factor inhibitor assay	If present, may cause specific factor deficiencies and excessive bleeding.
vWF antigen	If low, may indicate platelet-related acquired condition or von Willebrand disease, increased risk of bleeding.
Ristocetin cofactor	Abnormal in von Willebrand disease.
TEG	Evaluation of functional status of platelets, coagulation cascade, and fibrinolytic activity.

[a]PTT, Activated partial thromboplastin time; CBC, complete blood count; DIC, disseminated intravascular coagulation; FDP, fibrin degradation product; MDS, myelodysplastic syndrome; PK, prekallikrein; PT, prothrombin time; TEG, thromboelastography; TF, tissue factor; TT, thrombin time; vWF, von Willebrand factor.

Table 14.5 Differences between clinical features of bleeding (platelets/vessel wall) and coagulation disorders

Features	Bleeding or purpuric disorders (platelets and vessel wall diseases)	Coagulation disorders
Mucosal bleeding	Common	Rare
Petechiae	Characteristic	Rare
Deep dissecting haematomas	Rare	Characteristic and common
Superficial ecchymoses	Typical; usually small and multiple	Common; large and solitary
Haemarthrosis	Rare	Typical
Bleeding from superficial cuts and scratches	Persistent and profuse	Minimal
Delayed bleeding	Rare	Typical
Family history	Present	Rare
Gender affected	Females more commonly affected	Mostly males

membrane glycoproteins (GPs) and causing abnormal platelet binding and aggregation.

- **Henoch–Schönlein purpura** or **anaphylactoid purpura:** self-limited vasculitis seen in children and young adults; manifests with purpuric rash on the extensor surface of limbs and buttocks with hematuria, colicky abdominal pain, polyarthralgia and acute nephritic syndrome; histopathology shows leukocytoclastic vasculitis; circulating immune complexes composed of IgA, C3, and fibrin are seen; activation of alternate complement pathway is thought to be the underlying mechanism.
- **Haemolytic uremic syndrome** (a clinical syndrome characterised by progressive renal failure that is associated with microangiopathic haemolytic anaemia and thrombocytopenia; HUS is the most common cause of acute kidney injury in children).
- **Liver disease and cirrhosis** (decreased synthesis of clotting factors and thrombocytopenia).
- **Vitamin K deficiency** (decreased synthesis of clotting factors).
- **Septic shock or malignancies** (due to DIC with microvascular thrombosis; bleeding occurs due to massive consumption of coagulation factors or damage to vessel walls).
- **Renal disease** (platelet dysfunction and reduced aggregation).
- **Circulating autoantibodies to coagulation factors** (as seen in lymphoma, systemic lupus erythematosus) or to platelets (as in immune thrombocytopenic purpura).
- **Vitamin C deficiency** (defective collagen synthesis and vessel wall abnormality).
- **Ageing** (increased vessel wall fragility).
- **Prolonged steroid use** (increased vessel wall fragility).

Box 14.1 Classification of Disorders of Primary Haemostasis (Bleeding Disorders)

I. Platelet disorders
  1. Quantitative (Thrombocytopenia)
     (a) ***Decreased platelet survival***
        (i) Immune thrombocytopenia
        (ii) Idiopathic
        (iii) Drug induced
        (iv) Collagen vascular disorders
        (v) Sarcoidosis
        (vi) Non-immunemediated
        (vii) Disseminated intravascular coagulation
        (viii) Thrombotic thrombocytopenia purpura, Haemolytic uraemia syndrome
        (ix) Microangiopathic haemolytic anaemia
        (x) Giant haemangioma
     (b) ***Decreased platelet production***
        (i) Bone marrow failure (aplastic anaemia - congenital and acquired)
        (ii) Bone marrow infiltration (leukaemia, lymphoma, metastasis, granulomatous disease, myelofibrosis)
        (iii) Selective impairment of platelet production (drug induced-alcohol, thiazides, cytotoxic drugs; infections - measles, HIV)
        (iv) Ineffective haematopoiesis (megaloblastic anaemia, MDS)
     (c) ***Splenic sequestration***
        (i) Hypersplenism
     (d) ***Dilutional thrombocytopenia***
        (i) Massive blood transfusions
  2. Qualitative (platelet function) disorders
     (a) ***Congenital/inherited***
        (i) Glanzmann thrombasthenia
        (ii) Wiskott Aldrich syndrome
        (iii) Bernard Soulier syndrome
     (b) ***Acquired***
        (i) Drug-induced
        (ii) Liver disease
        (iii) Alcoholism
        (iv) Uraemia

II. Vessel wall disorders (non-thrombocytopenic purpura)
  1. Congenital disorders
     (a) ***Hereditary haemorrhagic telangiectasia***
     (b) ***Ehlers-Danlos syndrome***
     (c) ***Marfan syndrome***
  2. Acquired disorders
     (a) ***Connective tissue damage*** *(senile purpura, scurvy, Cushing syndrome, steroid therapy)*
     (b) ***Vasculitis*** *(infections, drug reactions, Henoch-Schonlein purpura)*
     (c) ***Amyloidosis***
     (d) ***Simple easy bruising***

- **Polycythemia vera** and **essential thrombocythemia** (demonstrate both thrombotic tendency and bleeding).

Q. Enumerate the clinicopathological features of idiopathic thrombocytopenic purpura. (ITP, PA21.2)

Ans. ITP, also known as primary immune thrombocytopenic purpura and autoimmune thrombocytopenic purpura, is defined as thrombocytopenia in the absence of other causes of thrombocytopenia.

Pathogenesis

- In ITP, an abnormal autoantibody, usually IgG with specificity for one or more platelet membrane glycoproteins (GPs), binds to circulating platelet membranes. In persons with chronic ITP, approximately 75% of autoantibodies are directed against platelet GPIIb/IIIa or GPIb/IX complexes.
- Autoantibody-coated platelets induce Fc receptor-mediated phagocytosis by macrophages in the spleen. Spleen is an important organ because platelet autoantibodies are also formed in the white pulp.

Clinical Features

- It commonly manifests as a bleeding tendency - easy bruising (purpura); extravasation of blood from capillaries into skin and mucous membranes (petechiae and ecchymoses) or epistaxis. Bleeding from gums, haematuria, menorrhagia, metrorrhagia and melena are also seen.
- Cerebral haemorrhage is the most common cause of death in severe thrombocytopenia.
- ITP can be of two types, an acute self-limiting type and a chronic recurrent type.
- Adults may be affected at any age, but most cases are diagnosed in women aged 30–40 years. Peak age in children is 2–6 years.

Laboratory Diagnosis

- **Haemogram** shows thrombocytopenia with a **normocytic normochromic anaemia** (consequent to bleeding).
- **Peripheral blood smear** shows **large/giant platelets**, reflecting the early release of megakaryocytic fragments into the circulation. Platelets lack granules or have an abnormal colour. **Lymphocytosis** and **eosinophilia** are common (Fig 14.2A).
- Assays for **platelet-associated immunoglobulin** or **antiplatelet antibodies** are positive.
- Bone marrow shows an **increase in the number of megakaryocytes** and **their precursors** which may show an **abnormal morphology**. There may be decreased cytoplasmic granularity, variable staining, vacuolisation of the cytoplasm and hypolobulation of the nuclei (Fig 14.2B). Myelopoiesis is normal. Normoblastic erythroid hyperplasia may be seen in response to the anaemia which develops as a consequence of bleeding.
- Bleeding time is prolonged, clotting time, PT and PTTK are within normal range.

Table 14.6 Differences between acute and chronic ITP

Features	Acute ITP	Chronic ITP
Peak age affected	Children, 2–6 years	Adults, 20–40 years
Sex predilection	None	Female to male ratio 3:1
Prior infection	Common (1–3 weeks prior to onset)	Uncommon
Onset of bleeding	Abrupt	Insidious
Haemorrhagic bullae in the mouth	Present	Absent
Platelet count	$<20 \times 10^9/L$	$30–80 \times 10^9/L$
Eosinophilia and lymphocytosis	Common	Rare
Duration	2–6 weeks	Months to years
Spontaneous remission	Occurs in majority	Uncommon

Q. Differentiate between acute and chronic ITP. (PA21.2)

Ans. Differences between acute and chronic ITP are listed in Table 14.6.

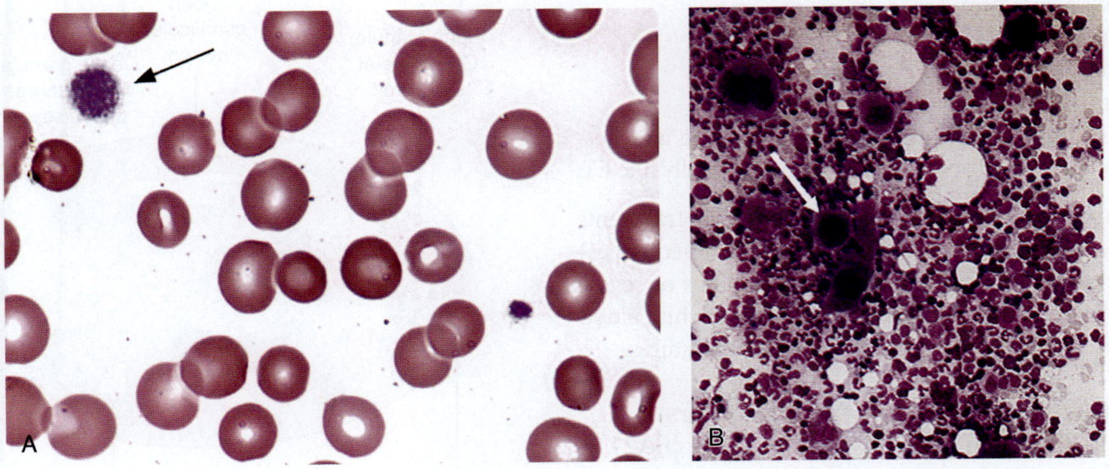

Fig. 14.2 (A and B) Blood and marrow aspirate from child with idiopathic thrombocytopenic purpura. (A) Blood smear shows large platelets. (B) Bone marrow aspirate shows increased numbers of megakaryocytes, many of which appear immature. (Source: *Pediatric Clinics of North America*: Childhood Immune Thrombocytopenic Purpura: Diagnosis and Management, Victor Blanchette and Paula Bolton-Maggs, Volume 55, Issue 2, April 2008, Pages 393–420, Elsevier.)

Q. Define thrombocytosis and enumerate its causes. (PA21.2)

Ans. Thrombocytosis, also called thrombocythemia, is defined as a platelet count **greater than 450,000/μL** (>450 x 109/L). It is categorised into **(1) autonomous (primary) thrombocytosis** and **(2) reactive (secondary) thrombocytosis. Autonomous thrombocytosis** may occur secondary to myeloproliferative disorders, myelodysplastic disorders, or rarely as a result of a hereditary condition. **Reactive thrombocytosis** is most often a transient physiologic response to an underlying condition (e.g. infection). It is important to differentiate between these two categories as autonomous thrombocytosis can be associated with an increased risk for thrombotic or haemorrhagic complications whereas reactive thrombocytosis is not.

Persistent thrombocytosis can result in haemorrhage or thrombotic events. Platelet counts that exceed 1,500,000/μL have an increased risk of bleeding, whereas counts less than 1,000,000/μL are more often associated with thrombosis. Microvascular thrombi may form due to thrombocytosis and may manifest with erythromelalgia (pain and warmth with erythema or mottling of the skin), headache and paresthesias.

A. Reactive (secondary) thrombocytosis

Self-limiting condition that resolves with the resolution of the underlying condition. Common causes include:

1. Tissue damage (due to surgery, infection, malignancy, etc.)
2. Iron deficiency anaemia
3. Asplenia
4. Chronic inflammatory disorders
5. Acute blood loss
6. Exercise

Reactive thrombocytosis may be sometimes be a result of a subclinical disorder or occult cancer. Therefore, asymptomatic patients with thrombocytosis must have a comprehensive physical evaluation for malignancy or other potentially treatable disease.

B. Autonomous (primary) thrombocytosis

1. Myeloproliferative disorders
   (a) Polycythemia vera
   (b) Chronic myeloid leukaemia
   (c) Chronic idiopathic myelofibrosis
   (d) Essential thrombocythemia
2. Hereditary thrombocytosis is an extremely rare and heterogeneous genetic disorder that presents clinically like ET.

Causes of **spurious thrombocytosis** include cell fragments (leukaemia), red cell inclusions (such as Pappenheimer bodies) or schistocytes, as seen in the setting of haemolysis or severe burns. In cryoglobulinaemia, platelet counts and white blood cells rise when samples are prepared at cool temperatures.

Q. Write briefly on platelet function disorders. (PA21.2)

Ans. Clinical evidence of bleeding or a prolonged bleeding time in the setting of a normal platelet count and coagulation studies suggests qualitative platelet disorders. They are most commonly acquired, but can be inherited.

1. **Drug-induced platelet dysfunction:** Drug-induced platelet dysfunction is an important cause of an acquired bleeding diathesis. The most common drugs responsible are aspirin, clopidogrel, ticlopidine, and glycoprotein IIb/IIIa inhibitors. Non-steroidal anti-inflammatory drugs (NSAIDs) inhibit cyclooxygenase reversibly. Ethanol use and aspirin therapy have synergistic effects.
2. **Uremia:** Uremic bleeding syndrome is incompletely understood and may be multifactorial in origin.
3. **Liver disease:** Hepatic disease is associated with platelet dysfunction that is again multifactorial in origin. Increased FDP levels from activation of the fibrinolytic pathway compromise platelet function and impair release of platelet factor III from platelets.
4. **Acquired von Willebrand disease:** Acquired von Willebrand disease (AvWD) is frequently seen in association with drugs, solid tumours, monoclonal gammopathies, lymphoproliferative, myeloproliferative and autoimmune disorders. There are many hypotheses to origin of AvWD - development of autoantibodies directed against von Willebrand factor (vWF) which accelerates clearance of vWF from the circulation and/or inactivation of plasma vWF; absorption or adsorption of plasma vWF on to malignant cells; and drug-induced or cell-mediated proteolysis of plasma vWF.
5. **Paraneoplastic platelet dysfunction:** Platelet dysfunction has also been associated with plasma cell dyscrasias and is believed to be related to coating of the platelet membrane by monoclonal proteins.
6. **Myelodysplastic and myeloproliferative syndromes** may result in platelet dysfunction (e.g. through an acquired glycoprotein IIb/IIIa deficiency).Other conditions associated with qualitative platelet disorders include cardiopulmonary bypass or valvular defects, autoimmune disorders, and severe iron or folate deficiency.
7. **Inherited platelet disorders:**
   These include the common **von Willebrand disease** and the less common **Glanzmann thrombasthenia** and **Bernard-Soulier syndrome** (Fig. 14.3).

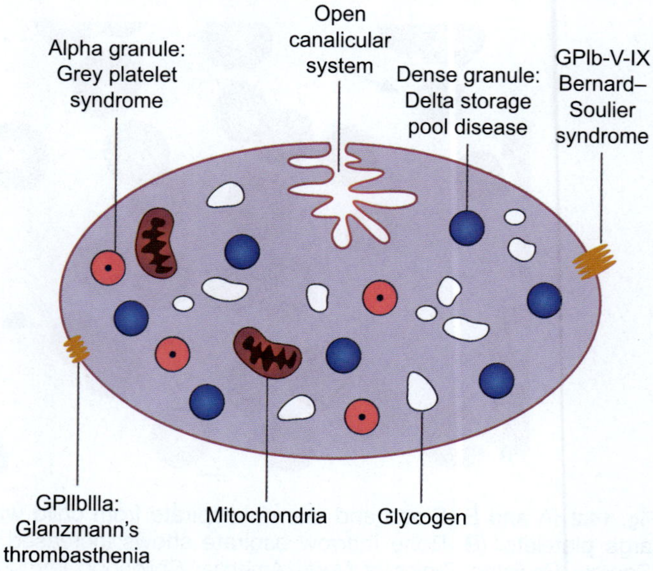

Fig. 14.3 Platelet function defects.

Q. Classify hereditary coagulation disorders. (PA21.3)

Ans. Coagulation disorders have a lesser incidence as compared to bleeding disorders. They can be hereditary or acquired. The major causes of hereditary and acquired coagulation disorders are given in following sections.

Classification of Hereditary Coagulation Disorders

Hereditary deficiencies have been identified for each of the clotting factors. Deficiencies of factor VIII (haemophilia A) and of factor IX (Christmas disease or haemophilia B) are transmitted as sex-linked recessive disorders. Most others follow autosomal pattern of transmission. These hereditary disorders typically involve a single clotting factor.

1. **X linked recessive traits**
   (a) Haemophilia A
   (b) Haemophilia B
2. **Autosomal recessive traits**
   (a) Factor XI deficiency
   (b) Prothrombin deficiency
   (c) Factors V/VII/X/XII/XIII deficiency
   (d) Afibrinogenemia/hypofibrinogenemia
3. **Autosomal dominant traits**
   (a) von Willebrand disease
   (b) Dysfibrinogenemias
   (c) Passovoy factor deficiency
4. **Combined**
   (a) Associated with haemophilia
   (b) Involving vitamin K-dependent factors
5. **Miscellaneous**
   (a) Prekallikrein deficiency
   (b) HMW kininogen deficiency

Haemophilia A and **von Willebrand disease**, two of the most common inherited disorders of bleeding, are caused by qualitative or quantitative defects involving the factor VIII–vWF complex. Plasma factor VIII–vWF is a complex made up of two separate proteins (factor VIII and vWF) that can be characterised according to functional, biochemical and immunologic criteria. Circulating factor VIII is non-covalently associated with very large vWF multimers containing up to 100 subunits. vWF also interacts with several other proteins involved in haemostasis, including collagen, heparin, and platelet membrane GPs (Ib-IX and IIb). GP Ib-IX serves as the major receptor for vWF. The most important function of vWF in vivo is to promote the adhesion of platelets to subendothelial matrix. vWF multimers serve as a carrier for factor VIII and are important for its stability. The half-life of factor VIII in the circulation is 12 h if vWF levels are normal, but only 2.4 h if it is deficient or abnormal (as in patients with von Willebrand disease). The two components of the factor VIII–vWF complex are encoded by separate genes and synthesised in different cells. vWF is produced by endothelial cells and megakaryocytes and can be demonstrated in platelet α-granules. Endothelial cells are the major source of subendothelial and plasma vWF. Factor VIII is made in several tissues; sinusoidal endothelial cells and Kupffer cells in the liver and glomerular and tubular epithelial cells in the kidney appear to be particularly important sites of synthesis.

Q. Write briefly on the pathophysiology, clinical features and laboratory diagnosis of haemophilia.

Ans. Haemophilia is a frequently fatal haemorrhagic diathesis classified into two types depending whether there is deficiency of factor VIII or Factor IX (haemophilia A and haemophilia B).

Haemophilia A (Classic Haemophilia)

Haemophilia A is an X linked, recessive disorder caused by deficiency of functional plasma clotting factor VIII (FVIII), which may be inherited or arise from spontaneous mutation. Rarely, development of autoantibodies to FVIII results in acquired haemophilia A.

Incidence

Incidence of haemophilia is 1 in 20,000 persons.

Pathophysiology

- Factor VIII normally circulates in the plasma bound to a much larger molecule VWF (VIII C along with VWF is called **Factor VIII complex**).
- Functional attribute of Factor VIII is VIII C.
- Examination of haemophilia genes has revealed seven different mutations.

Carrier Detection

- Demonstration of subnormal levels of Factor VIII C by immunoassays.
- Ratio of VIII C to VWF normally 0.74–2.2; in carriers, 0.18–0.9.
- Abnormally low ratios of VIIIC/VWF may be seen in stress
- Falsely high ratios of VIII C/VWF are seen in pregnancy, oral contraceptive intake and contamination of plasma samples with thrombin or proteolytic enzymes.

Haemophilia in Females

Haemophilia in females is seen in the following circumstances:

- Minority of heterozygous carriers in whom X-chromosome inactivation has occurred.
- Mating between affected male and carrier female.
- Due to a new mutant gene in a carrier.

Clinical Manifestations

- Excessive haemorrhage from a trivial injury.
- Haemarthrosis most common and debilitating manifestation; usually preceded by 'Aura' (tingling before haemarthrosis).
- Haemorrhage → organisation and inflammation → chronic proliferative synovitis → chronic haemophilic arthropathy (may lead to fibrous or bony ankylosis).
- Pain, muscle spasm and limitation of mobility.
- Subcutaneous, intramuscular haematomas, psoas and retroperitoneal haematomas.
- Gastrointestinal and genitourinary bleeding.
- Others: Epistaxis, oral mucosal haemorrhage, haemoptysis, haematoma leading to airway obstruction, and excessive bleeding with routine dental procedures.
- Splenomegaly (40% patients).

Laboratory Diagnosis

- Anaemia with neutrophilia.
- Megakaryocytes are normal or increased in number.
- PTT is prolonged; abnormal results of PTT only when Factor VIII C levels fall to <20%–25% of normal. Bleeding and clotting time are abnormal.
- Biological or immunological assays are used to determine the levels of factor VIII. Factor VIII C level deficiency is classified as:
  - Severe deficiency: Factor VIII C level <0–2 U/dL.
  - Moderate deficiency: Factor VIII C level 2–5 U/dL.
  - Mild deficiency: Factor VIII C level >5 U/dL.
- FVIII inhibitor assay.

Haemophilia B (Christmas Disease)

- Inherited, X linked, recessive disorder that results in deficiency of functional plasma coagulation factor IX.
- Manifests with similar clinical features as haemophilia A but constitutes only 20% cases of haemophilia.
- Coagulation studies show normal bleeding time and PT and normal or prolonged aPTT.
- About 50% of these cases have factor IX levels greater than 1% as demonstrated by factor IX assay. The disease is said to be mild when the level is over 5%; moderate when 1%–5%; and severe when below 1%.

Q. Write briefly on von Willebrand disease.

Ans. von Willebrand disease is also called angiohaemophilia and pseudohaemophilia. It is second only to haemophilia A in frequency.

Pathophysiology and Genetics

The gene for vWF is located on chromosome 12. In most cases, this disease is transmitted as an autosomal dominant disorder, but several rare autosomal recessive variants have been identified. More than 20 variants of von Willebrand disease have been described, which can be grouped into two major categories:

- **Type 1 and type 3 von Willebrand disease:** These are associated with **a reduced quantity of circulating vWF**. Type 1, an autosomal dominant disorder, accounts for approximately 70% of all cases and is relatively mild. Type 3 (an autosomal recessive disorder) is associated with extremely low levels of functional vWF, and the clinical manifestations are correspondingly severe. As a severe deficiency of vWF has a marked affect on the stability of factor VIII, some of the bleeding characteristics resemble those seen in hemophilia.
- **Type 2 von Willebrand disease:** This is characterised by qualitative defects in vWF; there are several subtypes, of which type 2A is the most common. It is inherited as an autosomal dominant disorder. Due to missense mutations, the vWF formed is abnormal, leading to defective multimer assembly.

Clinical Manifestations

Mild bleeding, easy bruising, epistaxis, and bleeding following minor procedures.

Laboratory Diagnosis

- **Prolonged BT** and **CT**→ mild bleeding, easy bruising, epistaxis and bleeding following minor procedures.
- **Factor VIII C assay** → levels decreased.
- **von Willebrand factor immunoassay** → levels decreased; As vWF stabilises factor VIII by binding to it, a deficiency of vWF gives rise to a secondary decrease in factor VIII levels. This may be reflected by a prolongation of the PTT in von Willebrand disease types 1 and 3.
- **Ristocetin-induced platelet aggregation delayed** → The plasma level of active vWF, measured as the ristocetin cofactor activity, is reduced (ristocetin induces platelet agglutination followed by secondary aggregation and release reaction; this process depends on binding of vWF to platelet membrane).

Q. Differentiate between haemophilia A, haemophilia B and von Willebrand disease.

Ans. Differences between haemophilia A, haemophilia B and von Willebrand disease are summarised in Table 14.7.

Q. Write briefly on acquired coagulation disorders. (PA21.3)

Ans. Acquired coagulation disorders may result from:

1. **Deficiency of vitamin K-dependent factors**
   (a) Haemorrhagic disease of newborn.
   (b) Liver disease (cirrhosis, fulminant hepatitis, acute fatty liver of pregnancy, biliary obstruction; decompensated liver disease also causes excessive fibrinolysis and bleeding due to decreased hepatic synthesis of α2-antiplasmin).
   (c) Malabsorption of vitamin K.
   (d) Nutritional deficiency.
   (e) Drugs
      (i) Coumarins
      (ii) Broad spectrum antibiotics
      (iii) Cholestyramine.
2 **Accelerated destruction of coagulation factors**
   (a) Disseminated intravascular coagulation (DIC).
   (b) Fibrinogenolysis (liver disease, thrombolytic agents, tumours postsurgery).
3. **Circulating inhibitors of coagulation**
   (a) Specific inhibitors.
   (b) Lupus anticoagulant.
   (c) Antithrombins.
   (d) Paraproteins.
4. **Miscellaneous causes**
   (a) After massive transfusion.
   (b) After antibiotics and antineoplastic agents.
   (c) Congenital heart disease, amyloidosis, nephrotic syndrome, Sheehan syndrome, Gaucher disease and leukaemias.

Q. Write briefly on thrombophilia (Hypercoagulability).

Ans. Thrombophilia is a collective term used to describe a group of conditions in which there is disturbance in the normal homeostatic mechanisms resulting in an increased

Table 14.7 Comparison between haemophilia A, haemophilia B and von Willebrand disease

Features	Haemophilia A	Haemophilia B	von Willebrand Disease
Mode of inheritance	X linked	X linked	Autosomal dominant
Location and pattern of bleeding	Muscle and joints; following trauma or postsurgery	Muscle and joints; following trauma or postsurgery	Mucocutaneous; following trauma and postsurgery
Bleeding time	Normal	Normal	Prolonged
PT	Normal	Normal	Normal
aPTT	Prolonged	Prolonged	Prolonged
von Willebrand factor levels	Normal	Normal	Reduced
Factor VIII levels	Low	Normal	Low (vWF is the carrier molecule for factor VIII and prevents it from premature destruction)
Factor IX levels	Normal	Low	Low
Ristocetin-induced platelet aggregation	Normal	Normal	The plasma level of active vWF, measured as the ristocetin cofactor activity, is reduced (reduced ristocetin induces platelet agglutination followed by secondary aggregation and release reaction; this process depends on binding of vWF to platelet membrane)

tendency for clotting or thrombosis. Patients affected have repeated clotting events. Causes include the following:

1. Genetic mutations, such as Factor V Leiden (activated protein C resistance), proteins C and S deficiency, antithrombin III deficiency, and prothrombin 20210A mutations.
2. Acquired conditions, such as antiphospholipid syndrome (which can occur alone or as a manifestation of an autoimmune disorders, such as systemic lupus erythematosus), disseminated malignancy, immobilisation, inflammatory conditions, pregnancy, oral contraceptives, obesity, diabetes, hormone replacement therapy, and sickle cell anaemia.
3. Inherited disorders of fibrinolytic pathway (dysfibrinogenemia, dysplasminogenemia).
4. Increased prothrombin production.

Q. Write briefly on the aetiopathogenesis, clinical features and laboratory findings in disseminated intravascular coagulation. (DIC, PA21.4, 21.5)

Ans. Also called 'defibrillation syndrome' or 'consumption coagulopathy', DIC is a complex disorder involving intravascular thrombosis, as well as bleeding.

Incidence

1 in 1000 persons.

Causes

- **Obstetric complications**
  - Abruptio placenta.
  - Septic abortion/intrauterine death.
  - Chorioamnionitis.
  - Amniotic fluid embolism.
  - Severe eclampsia.
  - Degenerated Hydatidiform mole and leiomyomas.
  - Fetomaternal blood passage.
- **Infections**
  - Viral: HSV, rubella, smallpox, hepatitis, CMV and epidemic haemorrhagic fever.
  - Bacterial: Meningococcaemia and septicaemia (Gram-positive).
  - Mycotic: Histoplasmosis and aspergillosis.
  - Protozoal: Malaria, kala-azar and trypanosomiasis.
  - Metazoal: Heartworm disease in dogs.
- **Neoplasms**: Carcinoma prostate, ovary, pancreas, breast, lung, carcinoid, rhabdomyosarcoma, neuroblastoma and acute promyelocytic leukaemia.
- **Others:** PNH, incompatible transfusions, fresh water submersion and drug induced.

The above-mentioned conditions induce tissue injury resulting in the release of tissue factor, which in turn activates coagulation. They may also result in endothelial damage causing generalized platelet adhesion and aggregation leading to formation of disseminated microvascular thrombi (thrombotic phase). This is followed by a phase of consumption of coagulation factors and platelets (consumption coagulopathy). A compensatory activation of the fibrinolytic system then ensues and results in increased levels of FDPs. Excessive fibrinolysis may result in bleeding manifestations (bleeding phase).

1. **Acute DIC**

   Clinical findings
   - Multiple bleeding sites.
   - Ecchymoses of skin and mucous membranes.
   - Visceral haemorrhage.

Laboratory abnormalities: Consumption of clotting factors and platelets and intravascular haemolysis (microangiopathic haemolytic anaemia). Abnormalities include:

- Decreased levels of Factors II, V and VIII.
- Fibrinogen level below 1.0 g/L.
- Increased FDP (fibrin degradation products, e.g. FDP, D dimer).
- Platelet count below 100×10^9 /L.
- Prolonged thrombin time (deficiency of fibrinogen and increased FDP levels which inhibit thrombin activity), prolonged prothrombin time (PT) and activated partial thromboplastin time (PTTK).
- Evidence of haemolysis.

2. **Chronic DIC**

Clinical findings

- Signs of deep venous or arterial thrombosis/embolism and
- Superficial venous thrombosis.

Laboratory abnormalities

- Modestly increased prothrombin time in some patients.
- Shortened or lengthened partial thromboplastin time.
- Normal thrombin time in most patients.
- High, normal or low fibrinogen level.
- High, normal or low platelet count.
- Increased levels of FDP (e.g., on testing for FDP, D dimer).

SECTION III

CLINICAL PATHOLOGY AND LABORATORY MEDICINE

Anticoagulants

15

Q. Enumerate the various types of blood specimens used for different diagnostic tests.

Ans. The three main types of blood specimens used for different diagnostic tests are whole blood, plasma and serum. Earlier, serum was the preferred assay specimen for determining extracellular concentrations of constituents in the blood, however, now plasma is preferred for many laboratory tests, as the constituents in plasma more reliably reflect the pathology in a patient than serum.

1. **Whole blood**
   (a) It is a venous, arterial or capillary blood sample, which has the same constitution and properties as blood in *in vivo* state.
   (b) If testing is delayed, *in vitro* anticoagulation can be used to stabilize the constituents in a whole blood sample for a certain period of time.

   Uses

   Complete blood counts (CBC) or haemogram, erythrocyte sedimentation rate (ESR), osmotic fragility test, foetal haemoglobin (HbF) estimation, haemoglobin electrophoresis, blood sugar and urea estimation, and Coomb's test.
2. **Plasma**
   (a) Whole blood anticoagulated with citrate, EDTA or heparin is collected and centrifuged for 15 minutes at 3000 g to give three layers (from top to bottom) cell free supernatant plasma, leucocytes (buffy coat) and erythrocytes.
   (b) Plasma is aspirated and transferred to a centrifuge tube taking care that the cell layers are not disrupted.

   Uses
   - Coagulation studies including coagulation factor assays
   - Confirmation of haemoglobinemia (red coloured plasma as seen in Paroxysmal Nocturnal Haemoglobinuria or PNH).
3. **Serum**
   (a) Whole blood is collected in commercially available plain (i.e. non-anticoagulated), evacuated collection tubes or plain vials and left undisturbed for about 1 hour at room temperature.
   (b) The clot thus formed is loosened gently from the container wall using a thin plastic or glass rod without any agitation in order to prevent any cell lysis.
   (c) A clot activator and a gel (as used in serum separator tubes) can be used to accelerate the clotting.
   (d) The tubes are then centrifuged for 10 minutes at about 1200 g. The supernatant serum then is pipetted into another tube and centrifuged again for 10 minutes at about 1200 g.
   (e) The supernatant (serum) thus obtained is then transferred to fresh tubes for conducting tests or can be stored for delayed testing (4°C for testing within a week, −20°C for up to 3 months, and at −40°C or less for longer time).
   (f) 15%–20% less volume of serum than of plasma is isolated from the same volume of blood. The difference between plasma and serum are tabulated in Table 15.1.

   Uses
   - Estimation of bilirubin, creatinine, uric acid and proteins.
   - Enzyme assays.

Q. Enumerate different anticoagulants. Write briefly on their uses and disadvantages. PA13.2

Ans. The *in vivo* state of constituents of blood must remain unchanged after withdrawal from the body to obtain a valid laboratory investigation result. Anticoagulants are compounds that prevent blood from clotting and maintain the concentrations of the constituents of blood as close to the *in vivo* state as possible. An anticoagulant selected for use in haematological investigations must have the following qualities:

- It must keep the blood in fluid state.
- It must not cause any significant cellular size alterations.
- It must not induce haemolysis.
- It must have a minimal effect on platelet aggregation.
- It must ensure minimal disruption of morphology and staining characteristics of leukocytes.
- It must be readily soluble in water and blood.

Classification of anticoagulants is given in Flowchart 15.1.

The salient features of different commonly used anticoagulants are summarized below:

1. **Ethylene diamine tetra acetic acid** (EDTA)
   (a) Also known as sequestrene or Versenate, EDTA is available as sodium, potassium and lithium salts, all of which can be used for routine haematological investigations.
   (b) It acts by chelating the calcium molecules in blood (calcium ions must be present for the thrombin system to initiate coagulation).

Table 15.1 Differences between plasma and serum

Features	Plasma	Serum
Preparation	Plasma is obtained by centrifugation of anticoagulated blood directly after sample collection	Serum can only be processed after allowing the blood to clot (after 30 minutes to 1 hour)
Composition	• Contains all the clotting factors • Does not show alteration in platelet components as no clotting involved • Does not show alteration in concentration of any constituents, as there is no cellular metabolism or coagulation process • Minimal or no cell lysis is seen as blood is anticoagulated	• Devoid of fibrinogen and clotting factors like XI, VIII, IX, X, V, VII and II which have got used up during clotting • Shows increase in concentrations of platelet components (e.g. potassium, phosphate, lactate dehydrogenase, serotonin, etc.) • Shows decrease in the concentration of certain constituents (glucose, total protein, platelets) as a result of cellular metabolism and the coagulation process • Cell lysis of erythrocytes and leukocytes is activated in non-coagulated blood
Uses	It is mainly used for clotting studies	Serum is used for estimation of bilirubin, creatinine, uric acid and proteins as well as for enzyme assays

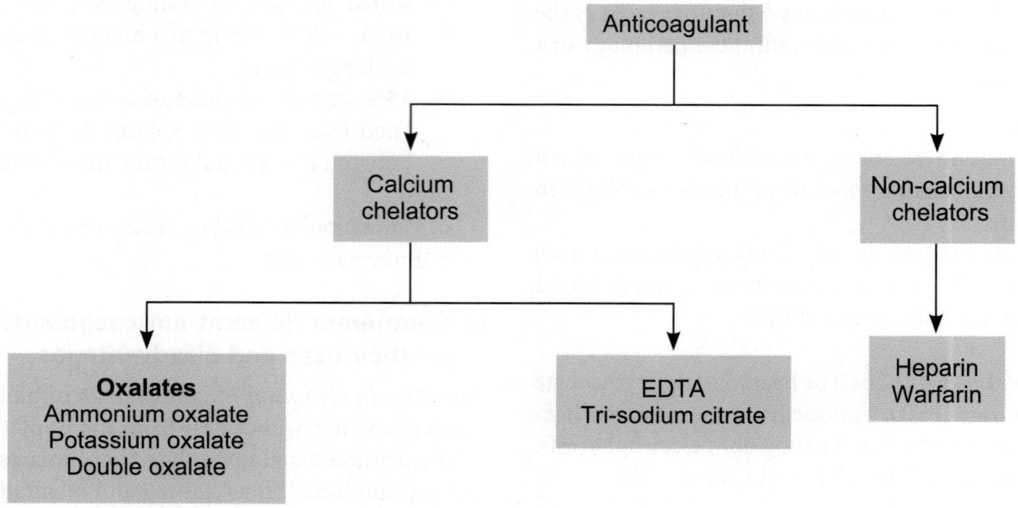

Flowchart 15.1 Classification of anticoagulants.

(c) EDTA should ideally be used in a concentration of 1.2 mg of the anhydrous EDTA salt per ml of blood (1.50 ± 0.25 mg/mL). A concentration more than 2 mg/mL can induce unwanted changes in blood cells (shrinkage and degeneration) leading to incorrect results.

(d) The dipotassium salt of EDTA is preferred over the disodium salt as the former is much more water-soluble and causes minimal changes.

(e) The dilithium salt of EDTA, also less water soluble than the dipotassium salt, has the advantage that the same sample of blood can be used for chemical investigations as well.

(f) EDTA can also be used as a tripotassium salt dispensed in liquid form, however, this is not generally preferred as the blood delivered into the tripotassium salt solution is slightly diluted and the tripotassium salt also produces some shrinkage of red cells.

(g) EDTA is the most commonly and widely used anticoagulant owing to its properties and relatively lower price.

Uses

- Estimation of haemoglobin, packed cell volume (PCV) and erythrocyte sedimentation rate (ESR) by Wintrobe method.
- Can also be used for total cell counts (RBC, WBC and platelet); differential leukocyte count (DLC) as well as peripheral smear (PS) analysis (as it maintains cell morphology).

Disadvantages

- Contraindicated for coagulation studies or analysis of calcium and iron (as it chelates calcium).
- May cause satellite adherence of platelets to neutrophils.
- Induces stranding of fibrin on a blood smear as it interferes with the function of fibrinogen.
- Inhibits alkaline phosphatase, creatinine kinase and leucine amino peptidase activity through chelation of the metallic cofactors.
- Can induce the following changes:
  - Shrinkage of red cells.
  - Distortion of WBCs and platelets.

- Significant decrease in PCV.
- Increase in mean cell haemoglobin concentration (MCHC).
- Platelet swelling and disintegration, leading to an artificially high platelet count because the fragments are counted as normal platelets.
- Leucoagglutination affecting both neutrophils and lymphocytes.

2. **Trisodium citrate**
   (a) Calcium chelating liquid anticoagulant, which removes calcium ions by forming a soluble calcium citrate complex.
   (b) Its most important use is in coagulation studies (9 volumes of blood are added to 1 volume of a 3.8% solution of sodium citrate).
   (c) It is also used for ESR estimation by Westergren method wherein 4 volumes of blood are added to 1 volume of the 3.8% sodium citrate solution.
   (d) It is crucial to get the right ratio of anticoagulant to blood, as osmotic effects, and changes in free calcium ion concentration can affect coagulation test results.

   Uses
   - Used for coagulation studies, ESR estimation, reticulocyte count and Heinz body detection.
   - The formal citrate solution (Dacie's solution) is used as diluent in the counting of RBCs and platelets (3.13 g of trisodium citrate is dissolved in 100 mL of water, 1 mL of formaldehyde is added to every 99 mL of the solution).

   Disadvantages
   Trisodium citrate cannot be used to study haemoglobin, total blood counts, differential leukocyte count (DLC) and PCV because it is always used in solution form, which will alter the concentration of blood, altering the actual values of the above parameters.

3. **Heparin**
   - It is a naturally occurring acid mucopolysaccharide anticoagulant produced by basophils and mast cells that prevents the formation of thrombin from prothrombin, thus inhibiting formation of fibrin from fibrinogen.
   - Lithium or sodium salt of heparin at a concentration of 10–20 IU (0.1–0.2 mg) per mL of blood is used for serum chemistry and gas analysis.
   - It is the ideal anticoagulant for osmotic fragility tests, as it does not alter the size of the cellular components especially red cells.

   Uses
   - Heparin is mainly used for enzyme studies, cell cultures, osmotic fragility testing and immunophenotyping.

   Disadvantages
   - Expensive.
   - Should not be used for blood counts because it often induces platelet and leukocyte clumping.
   - It should not be used for making blood films because it gives faint blue background coloration when the films are stained by Romanowsky dyes, especially in the presence of abnormal proteins.
   - It should not be used in polymerase chain reaction (PCR) with restriction enzymes, because it inhibits enzyme activity.

4. **Sodium fluoride**
   (a) Sodium fluoride acts as a weak anticoagulant by forming calcium fluoride.
   (b) It is used in a concentration of 30 mg of the powder per 5 mL of blood.
   (c) It exerts its preservative action by inhibiting the enolase enzyme involved in glycolysis and is therefore the anticoagulant of choice for measuring blood glucose levels.

   Uses
   - Used for estimation of blood glucose.

   Disadvantages
   - Fluoride acts as an inhibitor of serum enzyme.
   - In large quantities can affect urease, which is used in measuring blood urea nitrogen (BUN).
   - To be used as an anticoagulant, increased concentration/ml would be needed; at such concentrations inhibition of the glycolytic cycle would cause fluid shifts.

5. **Oxalates**
   (a) Sodium, potassium, ammonium and lithium oxalates are the available anticoagulants with potassium oxalate being the most widely used.
   (b) These act by forming an insoluble complex with calcium ions.
   (c) They are used in the concentration of about 1–2 mg/mL.
   (d) Ammonium salt causes swelling of RBCs and potassium salt cause shrinkage; thus double oxalate (a mixture of ammonium and potassium oxalate in the ratio of 3:2; arnmonium-potassium oxalate or Heller and Paul double oxalate) is preferred over the single salts to maintain normal shape and size of the red cells.

   Uses
   - Double oxalate used for estimation of ESR by Wintrobe method.
   - Sodium or potassium oxalate used for estimation of blood urea and specific gravity of blood

   Disadvantages
   - Sodium and lithium oxalates can cause shrinkage of red cells by drawing water into the plasma causing a 10% reduction in the haematocrit and a 5% reduction in the concentration of plasma constituents.
   - Oxalates inhibit the enzymes acid and alkaline phosphatase, amylase and LDH.

Q. Enlist the anticoagulants of choice for different analytical procedures.

Ans. Anticoagulants of choice for different analytical procedures are tabulated in Table 15.2.

Q. Enumerate the various effects of storage on the blood cells.

Ans. Various changes take place in anticoagulated blood when it is stored at room temperature. The changes occur regardless of the anticoagulant, and become evident about 3 hours post collection; by 12 hours post collection the changes become prominent. When blood is kept at 4°C it can be preserved without any significant changes for up to

Table 15.2 Anticoagulants of choice for different analytical procedures

Analytical procedure	Anticoagulant of choice
1. ESR estimation	***Westergren method—*** Trisodium citrate. 3.8% solution (Proportion of blood: citrate = 4:1) ***Wintrobe's method—***EDTA or double oxalate as dried powder
2. Coagulation profile	Trisodium citrate. 3.8% solution (Proportion of blood: citrate = 9:1) Heparin at a concentration of 15 to 20 IU/mL of blood Collection of blood is done in either siliconised vials or tubes (glassware coated with 10 mL silica per litre of water) or commercially prepared vials containing trisodium citrate
3. Osmotic fragility test, cell culture and enzyme studies	Heparin
4. Blood urea and specific gravity of blood	Sodium or potassium oxalate in a concentration of 2 mg/mL
5. Blood sugar	Sodium or potassium fluoride
6. Long-term preservation of red cells for certain tests and for transfusion purposes	Citrate is used in combination with dextrose in the form of ACD, CPD or Alsever's solution

24 hours. The following are the changes induced by storage in blood cells:

- Lobes of neutrophilic nuclei become separated, and their cytoplasmic margins become less well defined and ragged. Cytoplasmic vacuoles are commonly seen.
- Lymphocytes and monocytes show small vacuoles in the cytoplasm; their nuclei stain more homogenously than usual and may later undergo budding resulting in lobulation.
- Red blood cells start deterioration about 6 hours post collection; this manifests as progressive crenation and sphering.
- The RBC, WBC, platelet count and red cell indices are usually stable for up to 8 hours following blood collection. After 8 hours the red cells start to swell leading to an increase in the PCV and MCV, the osmotic fragility increases and the ESR decreases.
- It is best to count leukocytes and especially platelets within 2 hours of sample collection. It should be noted that the decrease in leukocyte count and a progressive decrease in the absolute lymphocyte count may become marked within a few hours, especially if there is an excessive amount of EDTA (>4.5 mg/mL).
- Haemoglobin concentration remains unchanged for days, but infection and high ambient temperatures may cause the blood to lyse, resulting in a decrease in the RBC count and PCV, and an increase in MCH and MCHC.
- It is recommended that coagulation tests must be carried out within 2 hours when the blood or plasma is stored at 22–24°C, 4 hours at 4°C, 2 weeks at −20°C and 6 months at −70°C.
- For a serum or plasma test blood should be centrifuged within 5 hours of collection.

Routine Haematology Techniques 16

Q. Write briefly on estimation of haemoglobin. (PA13.4)

Ans. Haemoglobin is a major constituent of the red cell cytoplasm, accounting for approximately 90% of the dry weight of the mature cell. Haemoglobin molecule is a tetramer consisting of two pairs of similar polypeptide chains called globin chains. A haeme molecule, which is a complex of iron in ferrous form and protoporphyrin, is attached to each of the four chains. Haemoglobin types Portland, Gower I and Grower II, also called embryonic haemoglobins, are present in early foetal life. Foetal haemoglobin (Hb F) dominates the late foetal life; by the 12th week embryonic haemoglobin is replaced by Hb F, which is slowly replaced after birth by two types of adult haemoglobin, Hb A and Hb A2.

In adults these haemoglobin molecules make up the following percentages of total haemoglobin:

- Hb A—95% to 98%
- Hb A2—2% to 3%
- Hb F—0.8% to 2%

In infants and children these haemoglobin molecules make up the following percentages of total haemoglobin:

- Hb F (newborn)—50% to 80%
- Hb F (over 6 months)—1% to 2%

Each of the above types of haemoglobin consist of two different pairs of peptide chains, Hb A ($\alpha 2\ \beta 2$) has two α chains and two β chains, Hb A2 ($\alpha 2\ \delta 2$), has two α chains and two δ chains, and Hb F ($\alpha 2\ \gamma 2$), has two α chains and two γ chains. The haemoglobinopathies consist of structural haemoglobin variants (the most important of which are the sickling disorders) and thalassemias (hereditary defects in the synthesis of either α or β globin chains).

Haemoglobinometry is defined as the estimation of the haemoglobin content in a sample of blood. The following are the different methods for haemoglobin determination:

Visual Methods

Haemoglobin is estimated based on the intensity of colour developed on addition of certain substances to blood. These methods include:

1. Sahli-Hellige method
2. Dares method
3. Halden's method
4. Taliquist method
5. Wintrobe's method

Sahli's Method

It is the most well known visual method of estimation of haemoglobin.

Principle: Haemoglobin present in a sample of blood is converted into acid haematin by addition of N/l0 HCl and its haemoglobin content is determined by matching the solution colour against non-fading glass having a standard colour.

Apparatus: Sahli's haemoglobinometer, N/10 HCl, and distilled water. Sahli's haemoglobinometer (Fig. 16.1) consists of:

1. A comparator box: It has colour standards on either side with a space for keeping the diluting tube in the middle. The standard is a non-fading, yellowish-brown tinted glass, the colour of which is that of acid haematin obtained by treating blood containing 14.5 g of haemoglobin per dL, with 0.1 N HCl and diluting it 100 times.
2. A special diluting haemoglobin tube: It is graduated in gm/dL scale on one side (2–24), and percentage scale on the other side (20–140; 14.5 g/dL corresponds to 100%).
3. A haemoglobin pipette: It is a capillary pipette with a single 20 cu.mm (0.02 mL) marking. It has no bulb.
4. A glass stirrer: It is a thin glass rod used for stirring.
5. N/10 HCl: Prepared by mixing 3.6 g or 3 mL of concentrated HCl in 997 mL of distilled water.

Procedure

1. Take N/10 HCl up to the lowest mark in the diluting tube (2 g%).
2. Place the diluting tube in the space provided in the box.
3. Collect blood from a finger prick or use an EDTA mixed venous sample.
4. Suck the blood in to the haemoglobin pipette up to the 20 cu.mm mark avoiding any air bubbles. Wipe off any blood sticking to the tip of the pipette using cotton.
5. Transfer the blood immediately into the acid taken in the diluting tube.
6. Mix and keep it undisturbed for 10 minutes to allow the haemoglobin to convert to acid haematin.
7. After 10 minutes dilute the contents by adding distilled water drop by drop. After adding each drop mix the contents with a stirrer till the colour matches the colour of the standard.
8. Take the reading both in gram scale and percentage scale by noting the lower meniscus.

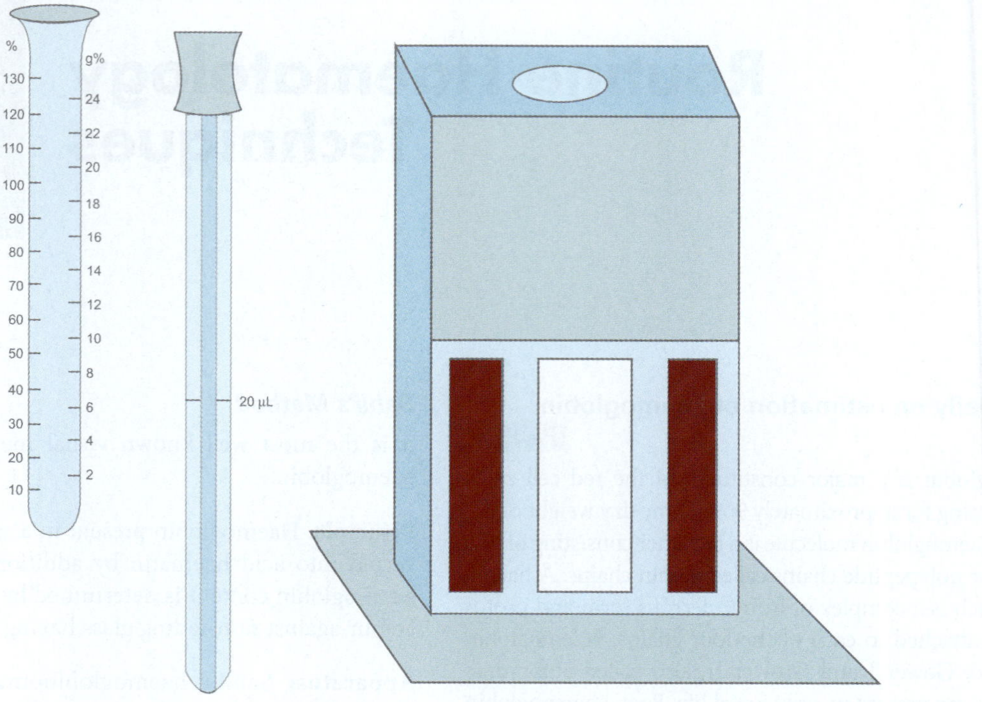

Fig. 16.1 Sahli's hemoglobinometer.

Precautions

1. There should not be any air bubble in the column in the pipette.
2. Blood should be transferred immediately from the pipette to the diluting tube to prevent clotting in the pipette.
3. Wipe off the excess blood sticking to the sides and tip of the pipette.
4. The glass rod should be lifted out of the solution before colour matching and taking the reading, but at no stage should it be taken out of the tube (In doing so, the solution sticking to the stirrer will be lost and will give a false low result. Also, if the stirrer remains in the solution, the colour of the solution will appear lighter).
5. Take the reading without delay, as the solution changes colour over time.
6. Comparison should always be done by keeping the solution at eye level, at arm's length and against natural light.

Advantages

1. Easy to perform and convenient.
2. Cost effective.
3. Less time consuming.

Disadvantages

1. Subjective variations in colour matching are common.
2. Colour of the standard fades with time.
3. There is incomplete conversion of haemoglobin to acid haematin. Sulphhaemoglobin (SHb), methaemoglobin (Hi), and carboxyhaemoglobin (HbCO) do not form acid haematin.
4. Presence of proteins and lipids in the plasma will interfere with colour matching.
5. Acid haematin is not a true solution; it always has some degree of precipitate which interferes with the colour matching and estimation.

Gasometric Method

This is the most accurate method but is not frequently used because it is very complex and time consuming. It uses the Van Slyke apparatus and is based on the fact that one molecule of oxygen binds one iron atom (in other words one molecule of haemoglobin binds four molecules of oxygen). Thus oxygen-combining capacity indirectly measures the amount of haemoglobin. It is estimated that 1 g of haemoglobin binds about 1.34 mL of oxygen. Based on this the haemoglobin concentration can be calculated by using the following formula:

$$\text{Hb in g/dL} = \frac{O_2 \text{ binding capacity / dL of blood}}{1.34}$$

Spectrophotometeric Method

(a) Haemiglobincyanide (HiCN; cyanmethaemoglobin) method

Principle: It is the most widely used automated method. To perform this method, blood is mixed with **Drabkin's solution,** a solution that contains ferricyanide and cyanide. The ferricyanide oxidizes the iron in the haemoglobin, changing haemoglobin to methaemoglobin. Methaemoglobin then unites with the cyanide to form cyanmethaemoglobin. Cyanmethaemoglobin produces a colour, which is measured in a spectrometer at a wavelength of 540 nm or in a photoelectric colorimeter with a yellow–green filter (Fig. 16.2). The colour relates to the concentration of haemoglobin in the blood. Hi, and HbCO, but not SHb, are converted to HiCN.

Diluent: The original Drabkin's reagent, which had a pH of 8.6, was found to cause turbidity from precipitation of plasma proteins and required a long conversion time. Now, a modified

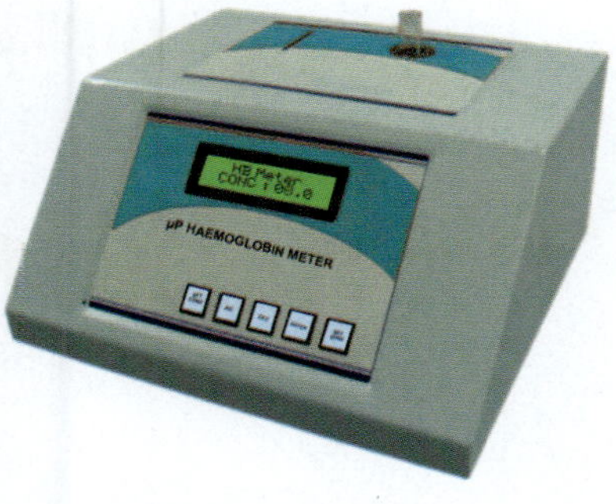

Fig. 16.2 Spectrometer.

solution (Drabkin-type reagent), is being recommended by the International Committee for Standardization in Haematology. It has potassium phosphate instead of potassium bicarbonate, as it minimizes turbidity and also has a shorter conversion time (3–5 min). The following are the constituents of the modified solution,

- Potassium ferricyanide 200 mg
- Potassium cyanide 50 mg
- Potassium dihydrogen phosphate 140 mg
- Non-ionic detergent 1 mL
- Distilled or deionized water to 1 L

The pH of the diluent should be 7.0–7.4, and it should be clear and pale yellow in colour. When spectrometrically measured against water as a blank, at a wavelength of 540 nm, the absorbance should be zero.

Hemiglobincyanide Reference Standard

With the advent of HiCN solution, which is stable for many years, other standards have become less important. A World Health Organization (WHO) International Standard has been established, and a comparable reference material is also available from the European Community Bureau of Reference (BCR). Preparations that conform to these international specifications are available commercially. They contain 550–850 mg of haemoglobin per litre, and the exact concentration is indicated on the label.

Method

1. Add 20 μL of blood to 4 mL of diluent (1 in 201 dilution).
2. Stopper the tube containing the solution and invert it several times.
3. Let the test sample stand at room temperature for at least 5 min (to ensure the complete conversion of haemoglobin). Pour it into a cuvette and read the absorbance in a spectrometer at 540 nm, or in a photoelectric colorimeter with a suitable filter against a reagent blank.

Calculation: Hb concentration in the test sample (g%)

$$= \frac{\text{Absorbance of test}}{\text{Absorbance of standard}} \times \frac{\text{Hb concentration of standard (mg/dL)} \times \text{Dilution factor}}{100\ \text{mg/g}}$$

Advantages

1. A major advantage of the HiCN method is the availability of a stable and reliable reference preparation.
2. Visual error in matching the colour is eliminated.
3. It allows direct comparison with the reference standard, and the readings need not be made immediately after dilution, thus batching of samples is possible.
4. All forms of haemoglobin, except SHb, are readily converted to HiCN. The rate of conversion of blood containing HbCO is markedly slow, but this difficulty can be overcome by prolonging the reaction time to 30 minutes before reading.

Disadvantages

1. The HiCN reagent contains cyanide (in very small quantities), which may be potentially hazardous. Alternative non-hazardous reagents that have been proposed are sodium azide and sodium lauryl sulphate. These convert haemoglobin to haemiglobinazide and haemiglobinsulphate, respectively.
2. Abnormal plasma proteins or a high leukocyte count may result in turbidity when the blood is diluted in the Drabkin-type reagent. The turbidity can be avoided by centrifuging the diluted sample, or by increasing the concentration of potassium dihydrogen phosphate in the reagent.

(b) Oxyhaemoglobin (HbO_2) method

Ammonium hydroxide is used to haemolyse the red cells and converts the haemoglobin to oxyhaemoglobin, which is measured in the spectrophotometer.

Automated Haemoglobinometry

Haemoglobin estimation by an automated procedure that applies the same principle as that described by the manual methods.

Non-automated Haemoglobinometry

Disposable, self-measuring micropipettes are available for haemoglobin estimation, for example The Unopette System in which one such pipette is attached to a plastic holder. The pipette fills by capillary action and empties the blood into an attached reservoir. Here it mixes with the modified Drabkin's reagent, and is then read in a spectrophotometer.

Other Methods

Alkali-Haematin Method

In this method haemoglobin is converted to alkali haematin, which is in a true solution form. The alkaline-haematin method gives a true estimate of total Hb as it measures HbCO, Hi, and SHb; plasma proteins and lipids have little effect on the development of colour. The original method was more cumbersome and less accurate than the HiCN or HbO_2 methods, but a modified method has been developed in which blood is diluted in an alkaline solution with non-ionic detergent and read in a spectrometer at an absorbance of 575 nm against a standard solution of chlorohaemin.

Specific Gravity Method

The copper sulphate specific gravity method is the traditional method used for donor screening at many blood centres.

Though a cheap and easy method, it is not accurate. It involves placing a drop of blood into a test tube with copper sulphate solution; if the drop of blood sinks to the bottom in 10–15 seconds (donor haemoglobin above 12.5 g/dL) the donor qualifies. If the drop of blood floats or takes too long to sink the donor is deferred (donor haemoglobin below 12.5 g/dL). The density of the drop is directly proportional to the donor haemoglobin. If the drop is denser than the specific gravity of the solution, it will sink, otherwise it will float.

Direct Reading Portable Haemoglobinometers (Colour Comparators)

These are simple clinical devices that compare the colour of blood against a range of colours representing haemoglobin concentrations. The HemoCue is an example of a rugged, portable, and accurate haemoglobinometer available for anaemia screening.

Non-invasive Screening Tests

Methods are being developed for using near infrared spectroscopy at body sites, mainly a finger, to identify the spectral pattern of haemoglobin in an underlying blood vessel and derive a measurement of haemoglobin concentration.

Q. Write briefly on manual cell counts using counting chambers. (PA13.4)

Ans. Manual Cell Counts Using Counting Chambers:

White Blood Cell Count

Principle: A sample of whole blood is mixed with a weak acid solution that lyses non-nucleated RBCs and stains the WBCs. Following adequate mixing the sample is introduced into a counting chamber where the leukocytes are counted.

Apparatus: Haemacytometer (kit includes a WBC pipette, counting chamber, and a special cover slip), diluting fluid and microscope.

WBC Pipette (Fig. 16.3): It is a bulb pipette having a long stem and the bulb contains a white bead inside. A small rubber tube with a mouthpiece, is connected to the small narrow portion above the bulb, for sucking blood and fluid into the pipette. The pipette has three markings on it, 0.5, 1 and 11. The total volume of the pipette is 11 parts, of which one part is in the stem and 10 parts in the bulb. A column of diluting fluid is contained in the stem of the pipette and it is not considered when calculating o the dilution (i.e. 11−1 = 10). Thus blood sucked up to the 0.5 mark will have a dilution of 0.5 in 10 or 1 in 20.

Other Uses of the WBC Pipette

1. Cell count in different body fluids like cerebrospinal, peritoneal, pleural and synovial.
2. Sperm count in seminal fluid.
3. Absolute eosinophil count (AEC).
4. RBC count in severe anaemia.
5. Platelet count when it is low.

Counting chambers (Fig. 16.4): The most commonly used counting chamber is the Levy chamber, which has improved

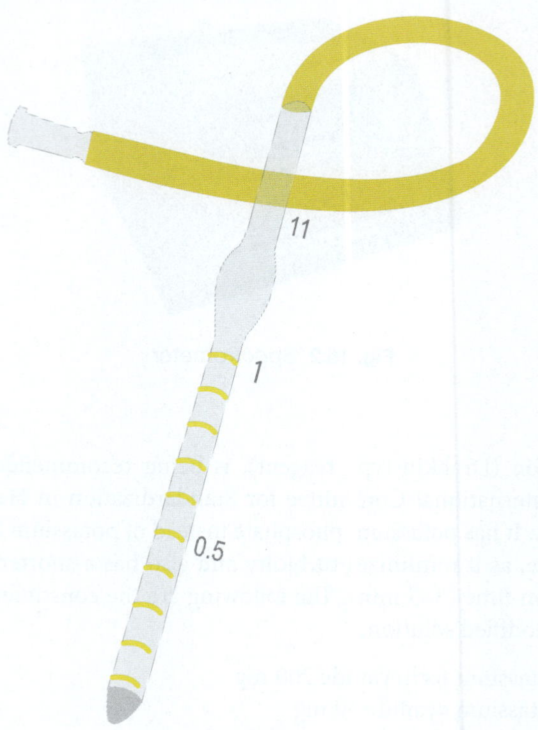

Fig. 16.3 WBC pipette.

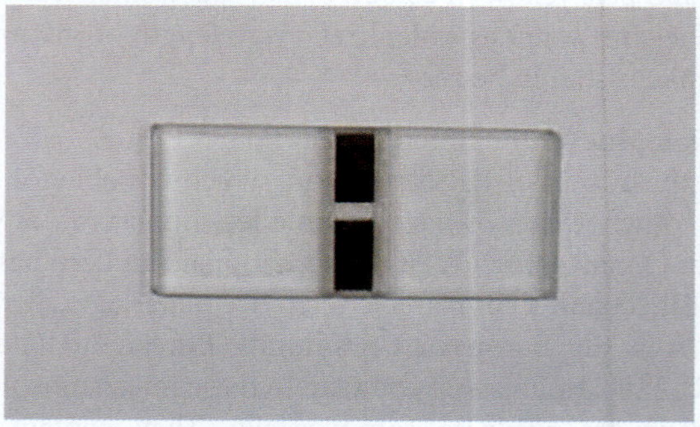

Fig. 16.4 Improved Neubauer Chamber.

Neubauer ruling. The chamber is divided into two central platforms by an H-shaped groove. The central area of the chamber is slightly lower than the sides, such that when a coverslip is put over the chamber the coverslip and the central platform are one-tenth of a millimetre apart (depth of the chamber is 0.1 mm. The counting area is in the form of a central ruled area, which is 3 mm × 3 mm and divided into 9 equal squares. Of these, the four corner squares are used for WBC counting. Each WBC square of 1 mm side is again divided into sixteen smaller squares each of 0.25 mm side. The central 1 mm × 1 mm square is divided into 25 equal small squares of 0.20 mm side, by means of triple lines of which the four corner ones and the central one are used for RBC counting. Each of these squares is subdivided into 16 smaller squares each of 0.20 mm sides. The depth of the grooved area is 0.1 mm.

Diluting fluid: The ideal diluting fluid while diluting the blood should destroy RBCs, and stain the nuclei of WBCs. The most commonly used diluting fluid is Turks fluid; it has the following composition:

1. 1% aqueous solution of gentian violet or methyl violet —0.5 mL.
2. Glacial acetic acid—1.5 mL.
3. Sodium chloride—0.9 g.
4. Distilled water up to 100 mL.

Gentian violet stains the nuclei of WBCs; glacial acetic acid destroys the RBCs and their stroma by haemolysis. The dilution fluid should be regularly filtered to remove any moulds.

Procedure

1. Clean and dry the chamber and cover slip, and place the cover slip over the chamber. Mount the assembly on the mechanical stage of the microscope, and focus any one of the four corner squares under low power.
2. Using a sterile lancet make a sufficiently deep prick such that blood flows freely.
3. Discard the first drop, as it may contain tissue fluid.
4. Place the WBC pipette on the drop and suck in blood up to the 0.5 mark followed by the diluting fluid up to the 11 mark.
5. Allow the blood and diluting fluid to mix well by rolling the pipette horizontally between the palms. Keep the pipette undisturbed for 10 minutes (or lysis of RBCs and staining of WBC nuclei).
6. Charge the counting chamber using a small drop of the diluted blood by touching the tip of the pipette to the edge of the cover slip on the chamber.
7. Keep the counting chamber undisturbed for 2–3 minutes to allow the cells to settle down on the ruled area. Next count the cells under high power.
8. Draw a chart of the four large (1 mm^2) squares, count the number of cells in each square and record the number.
9. The cells touching the left and lower borders should be counted, while those touching the right and upper borders should be omitted. This is to prevent counting the same cells twice.

Precautions

1. Counting chamber, pipette, and lancet should be clean and dry.
2. Blood should not be allowed to clot in the pipette.
3. No air bubble should be present in the pipette or the counting chamber.
4. There should be no undershooting or overshooting with the required amount of blood or diluting fluid.
5. The tip of the pipette should be wiped clean of blood.
6. The diluent should not be cloudy or contain debris.
7. The blood and diluent should mix properly.
8. Always discard the initial two or three drops from the pipette tip before charging the haemocytometer.
9. Avoid overflowing the chamber (causes erroneously high counts).
10. Cells should not be moving while counting. They should be uniformly distributed.

Note: In cases where the WBC count is exceptionally high, as in leukaemia, dilution should be made in the RBC diluting pipette. If nucleated erythrocytes are present, the count is corrected by the following formula:

$$\text{Corrected count} = \frac{\text{Observed count} \times 100}{100 + \text{nucleated RBCs per 100 WBCs}}$$

The percent of nucleated erythrocytes is obtained from the differential count, which is discussed in another course.

Calculation

- Volume of four corner squares = $(1 \times 1 \times 0.1) \times 4$ mm^3 = 0.4 mm^3
- Number of WBCs in four corner squares = N
- Dilution factor = 20
- Number of WBCs in 0.4 mm^3 = $N \times 20$
- Number of WBCs in 1 mm^3 volume = $N \times 20/0.4 = N \times 50$

RBC Count

Apparatus: Haemocytometer (includes an RBC diluting pipette, a counting chamber, a special cover slip), RBC diluting fluid and a microscope.

RBC pipette (Figure 16.5): A bulb pipette having a long stem, which contains a red bead. The pipette has three markings on it, 0.5 mark in the middle of the stem, 1 mark at the junction between the stem and the bulb, and 101 mark above the bulb. The total volume of the pipette is 101 parts of which one part is in the stem and 100 parts in the bulb.

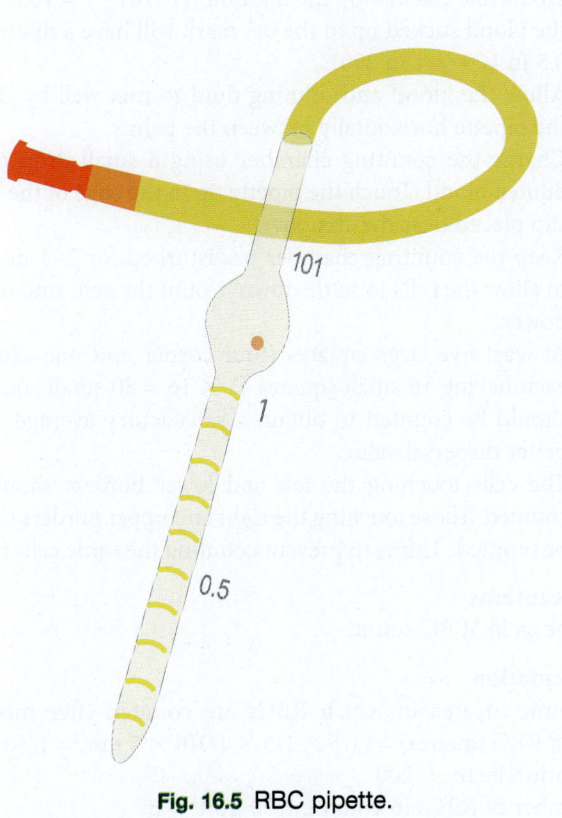

Fig. 16.5 RBC pipette.

Other uses of the RBC pipette

1. WBC count in leukaemias
2. Platelet count

RBC diluting fluids

1. **Hayem's fluid:** It is a commonly used diluting fluid, and is composed of,
   (a) Sodium chloride 0.5 g
   (b) Sodium sulphate 2.5 g
   (c) Mercuric perchloride 0.25 g
   (d) Distilled water 100 mL
   Sodium chloride and sodium sulphate together keep the isotonicity of the fluid. Sodium sulphate also prevents the clumping of red cells. Mercuric perchloride fixes the cells and acts as a preservative.
2. **Dacie's fluid or formol citrate solution:** Stock solution is composed of:
   (a) Trisodium citrate 35.0 g
   (b) Commercial formaldehyde 1.0 mL
   (c) Distilled water to100 ml
   Stock solution is diluted one in ten before use. RBC diluting fluid is isotonic with blood hence haemolysis does not take place. Formalin acts as a preservative and prevents bacterial and fungal growth. Sodium citrate prevents coagulation of blood and maintains the correct osmotic pressure.

Procedure

1. Taking complete aseptic precautions, use a sterile lancet to make a sufficiently deep prick such that blood flows freely.
2. Discard the first drop; it may contain tissue fluid.
3. Suck in blood up to the 0.5 mark of the pipette followed by the diluting fluid up to the 101 mark (The column of diluting fluid contained in the stem of the pipette is not considered while calculating the dilution (i.e. $101-1=100$). Thus the blood sucked up to the 0.5 mark will have a dilution of 0.5 in 100 or 1 in 200).
4. Allow the blood and diluting fluid to mix well by rolling the pipette horizontally between the palms.
5. Charge the counting chamber using a small drop of the diluted blood. Touch the pipette tip to the edge of the cover slip placed over the chamber.
6. Keep the counting chamber undisturbed for 2–3 minutes to allow the cells to settle down. Count the cells under high power.
7. At least five large squares (four corner and one central), each having 16 small squares ($5 \times 16 = 80$ small squares), should be counted to obtain a satisfactory average and a better dispersal value.
8. The cells touching the left and lower borders should be counted. Those touching the right and upper borders should be omitted. This is to prevent counting the same cells twice.

Precautions

Same as in WBC count.

Calculation

Volume of area in which RBCs are counted (five medium sized RBC squares) = $(1/5 \times 1/5 \times 1/10) \times 5\ mm^3 = 1/50\ mm^3$

Dilution factor = 200

Number of RBCs in volume $1/50\ mm^3$ = n

Number of RBCs in $1\ mm^3 = n \times 200 \times 50 = n \times 10{,}000$

RBC count per mm^3 (μL) = $n \times 10{,}000$

Discussion

Normal RBC Count

Adult male: 5–5.5 million/mm^3

Adult female: 4.5–5 million/mm^3

Variation in RBC Count

1. **Polycythemia (erythrocytosis):** It is characterized by neoplastic proliferation of erythroid, granulocytic and megakaryocytic elements. Symptoms are mainly due to absolute increase in the red cell mass. Polycythemia may be relative or absolute.
   (a) **Relative** Polycythemia: Due to haemoconcentration caused by reduced plasma volume, as in dehydration (low fluid intake, vomiting, diarrhoea and excessive sweating). The red cell mass is within normal range.
   (b) **Absolute Polycythemia:** Associated with an increased red cell mass and can be of two types, primary or secondary.
      (i) ***Primary (Polycythemia Vera Rubra):*** Absolute polycythemia of unknown aetiology associated with decreased erythropoietin levels.
      (ii) ***Secondary (erythrocytosis):*** Increased production of erythropoietin as a consequence of hypoxia leading to erythrocytosis as observed in high altitudes, cyanotic congenital heart disease, chronic obstructive pulmonary disease, and erythropoietin producing tumours, for example cerebellar haemangioblastomas, renal tumours, hepatocellular carcinoma and pheochromocytoma.
2. **Anaemia (Erythropenia)**
   (a) Due to decreased production of RBCs.
   (b) Due to increased destruction of RBCs.

Total (Absolute) Eosinophil Count (AEC)

AEC can be estimated based on the values of TLC and DLC. A more precise absolute count can be obtained with a counting chamber using the eosinophil diluting fluid '**Dunger's solution**' having the following constituents:

- **2% aqueous solution of eosin or phloxine (Acid dye):** 10 mL (Stains the granules of eosinophil pink or red).
- **Acetone (Reagent grade):** 10 mL (Helps in preservation of the cellular configuration of eosinophils).
- **Distilled water:** 80 mL (Acts as a lytic agent for red cells and other leukocytes. Lysis of red cells and leukocytes other than eosinophils is completed within 2–3 minutes).

The fluid is filtered and can be refrigerated at 4°C for 3–4 weeks.

Method

Blood is sucked up to the 0.5 mark in a WBC pipette either from a finger prick or an EDTA mixed sample. Eosinophil diluting fluid is then sucked up to the 11 mark and is well mixed by rolling movements between the fingers. After mixing for 1–2 minutes the first few drops are discarded and the Neubauer chamber is then charged. The eosinophils in the four large corner squares are then counted under a high power objective.

Calculation

Number of eosinophils contained in 0.40 mm^3 diluted blood = N
Number of eosinophils contained in 1 mm^3 undiluted blood = N × 0.40 × 20 (dilution) = N × 50
Normal eosinophil count = 50–450 per cmm of blood.

Platelet Count

1. **Direct methods:** Glassware and the diluting fluid must be scrupulously clean and dust free. Two mL of blood is collected from a vein with the help of a dry plastic syringe without frothing. After detaching the needle add contents into a tube containing dipotassium **EDTA** (used for platelet count as it prevents clumping of the platelets). Mix sample gently.
   (a) **Haemacytometer method using ordinary microscope:** Using an RBC pipette the anticoagulant mixed blood is diluted 1:200 with the diluent (formol-citrate and 1% ammonium oxalate solution may be used as diluents). Mixing is done by tilting for 2–3 minutes. The first few drops are discarded and then the Neubauer counting chamber is charged. The counting chamber is placed in a moist enclosure for at least 20 minutes to allow the platelets to settle properly. Platelets appear as highly refractile, small particles under the microscope.
   Number of platelets in five squares = (1/5 × 1/5 × 0.1) × 5
   Number of platelets in 1 × 1/5 × 0.1 mm^3 volume = N
   Number of platelets in 1 mm^3 = N × 50
   Dilution factor = 200
   Platelet count per mm^3 = N × 50 × 200 = N × 10,000
   (b) **Method using phase contrast microscope:** Counting of platelets can also be done using a phase contrast microscope with the same technique as mentioned earlier. This yields better results because of ease in identification.
   (c) **Method using electronic counter:** Use of a coulter counter or other electronic autoanalyzers for platelet counting, either directly from blood or from platelet rich plasma, provides even better results.
2. **Indirect method:** Platelet count based on peripheral smear findings (a proportional count of platelets in relation to red cells) can also be undertaken but the result is poorer.

Discussion

Normal range: 150–400 × 10^9/L.
Causes of thrombocytosis: Post-operative phase, pregnancy, post-partum phase, shock, after burn injury and post-haemorrhagic phase.
Causes of thrombocytopenia: Acute leukaemia and idiopathic thrombocytopenic purpura (ITP).

Reticulocyte Count

Reticulocytes are juvenile red cells that contain remnants of basophilic ribonucleoprotein in their cytoplasm. On staining with certain dyes (**brilliant cresyl blue or new methylene blue**) they show blue precipitate in the form of granules or filaments. The reaction is better observed in vitally stained smears without fixation.

Staining solution: 1 g 'brilliant cresyl blue' or 'new methylene blue' is dissolved in 100 mL of sodium citrate solution (one part 3% sodium citrate to four parts of 0.9% sodium chloride solution).

Method: Two to three drops of staining solution is mixed with three to four drops of EDTA mixed blood, and incubated at 37°C for 20 minutes. Cells are resuspended after gentle mixing, smears are prepared, air-dried and examined under oil immersion objective without fixation and counterstaining. Reticulocyte percentage is expressed in terms of red blood cells.

Example

Assume number of reticulocytes in 150 fields = 50
Total number of red cells in 150 fields = 3000
Reticulocyte percentage = 50/3000 × 100 = 1.6%
For a more precise value, reticulocytes can be counted by fluorescent microscopy stained with **'acridine orange solution'**. RNA shows orange-red fluorescence while DNA appears yellow.

Discussion

Normal reticulocyte count
Adult and children—0.2% to 2.0%
Infants (full term)—2.0% to 6.0%

Causes of reticulocytosis
1. Haemolytic anaemia
2. Anaemia on therapy (regenerating phase of anaemia)

Causes of reticulocytopenia
1. Hypoplastic/aplastic anaemia
2. Myelofibrosis
3. Radiation sickness
4. Cytotoxic drug therapy

Q. Write briefly on methods of estimation of erythrocyte sedimentation rate.

Ans. Normally red blood cells remain suspended uniformly when in circulation. If blood is mixed with an anticoagulant and allowed to stand in vertical tube gravity causes the red cells to settle down over time leaving a supernatant layer of clear plasma. The rate at which the red cells settle down per unit time is called the ESR. Red cells settle down because their specific gravity is greater than that of plasma.

Phases in erythrocyte sedimentation: The sedimentation of red cells over a period of 1 hour takes place in three phases.

1. **Phase of rouleaux formation:** This consists of the initial period of 10 minutes when RBCs stack and form rouleaux without much sedimentation.
2. **Phase of settling:** Settling of the rouleaux occurs at a relatively constant rate over the next 40 minutes.
3. **Phase of packing:** Settling slows down and packing of the RBCs occurs at the bottom of the tube over the last 10 minutes.

ESR is governed by the balance between pro-sedimentation factors and factors resisting sedimentation namely:
1. **Rouleaux formation or stacking of RBCs** (Fig. 16.6): When the degree of rouleaux formation is more (the ratio of surface area to mass of red cells is less) ESR is more. Rouleaux formation is influenced by different factors such as:
   (a) Shape of RBCs; the biconcave disc shape of the RBCs favours rouleaux formation.

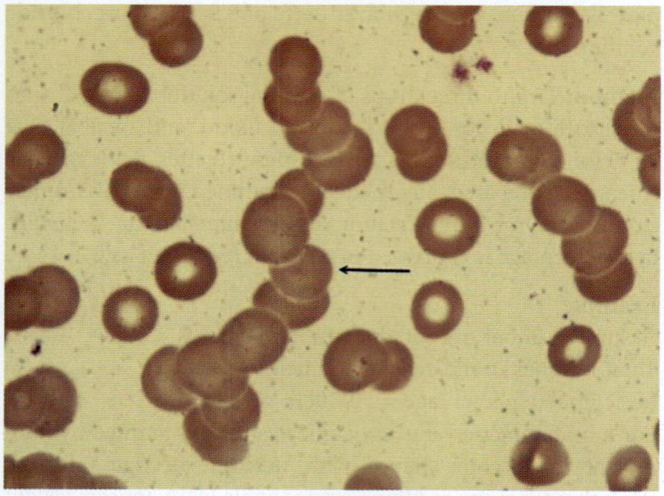

Fig. 16.6 Peripheral smear showing rouleaux formation.

(b) Plasma proteins affect rouleaux formation (albumin reduces rouleaux formation while fibrinogen favours it. During an inflammation, the ESR count is increased, this is due to the increased proportion of fibrinogen in the blood which causes red cells to stick to each other, increasing stacking of RBCs, causing them to settle faster. Also increase in fibrinogen induces colloidal changes in the plasma leading to increased plasma viscosity. Accelerated rouleaux formation can also occur in association with some lymphoproliferative disorders in which there is an increase in the serum immunoglobulin levels.

(c) Products of tissue destruction and inflammation favour rouleaux formation by decreasing the negative charge on the red cells (zeta potential).

2. **Size of RBCs:** Larger size (macrocytosis) means faster sedimentation.
3. **Length and bore of ESR tube:** If the length of the tube is more the RBCs have to travel a longer distance and ESR is more. If the bore of the tube is more the negative charge which keeps the RBCs apart will be less leading to increased ESR.

Different Methods for Estimation of ESR Include

1. **Westergren method**

Apparatus

(a) **Westergren's pipette** (Fig. 16.7): It is a long, cylindrical glass tube with a length of 30 cm and an internal bore diameter of 2.5 mm. It is open at both ends and is graduated from 0 to 200 in the millimetre scale from top to bottom.

(b) **Westergren's stand:** It is a rack with cushioning at the base on which the lower end of the pipette is made to rest. This stand can hold more than one pipette at a time and has adjustable levelling screws, which fix the tubes in a vertical position.

Procedure: The patient is asked to report fasting (a high protein diet may affect plasma protein concentration and alter ESR). Take 1.6 ml of the patient's blood and mix it with 0.4 mL of the anticoagulant (3.8% solution of trisodium citrate). Well mixed anticoagulated venous blood is drawn in a Westergren-Katz tube up to the 200 mm mark. The tube is

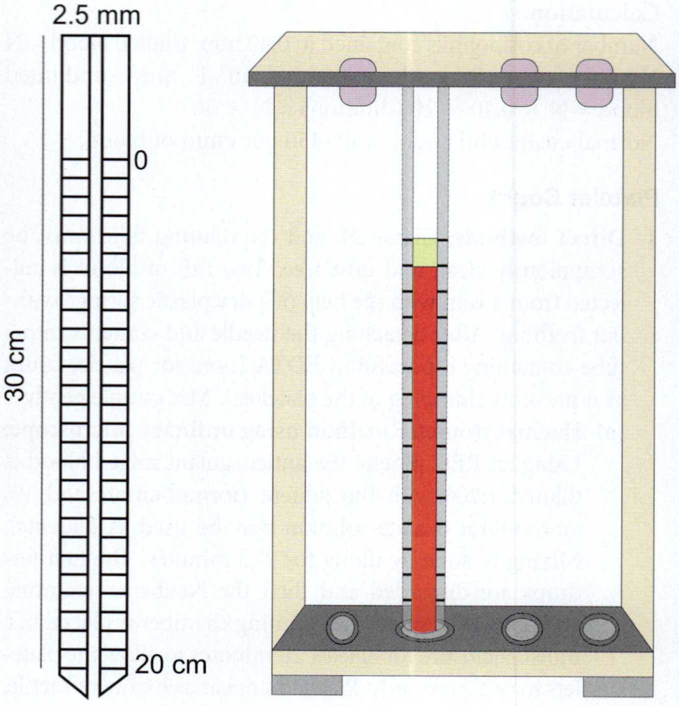

Fig. 16.7 Westergren's pipette.

then placed in a rack in a strictly vertical position for 1 hour at room temperature at which time the distance from the lowest point of the surface meniscus to the upper limit of the red cell sediment is measured. The distance of fall of erythrocytes, expressed as millimetres in the first hour, is the ESR.

Precautions

1. The test should be done within 2 hours of collection of the specimen and at room temperature.
2. There should not be any air bubbles in the blood column.
3. The top level of the blood column should exactly correspond to zero level.
4. The pipette should be mounted vertically.
5. The test must be read at exactly 60 minutes.

Normal values

Males: 3–5 mm in the first hour.

Females: 4–7 mm in the first hour.

2. **Wintrobe method:** Wintrobe's tube (Fig. 16.8) is a short tube closed at one end with graduations on both sides (0–10 on one side and 10–0 on the other). The tube is 110-mm-long and has an internal bore diameter of 2.5 mm. Solid crystals of either EDTA (1–2 mg/mL) or double oxalate (ammonium and sodium or potassium oxalate, 2–3 mg/mL) can be used as an anticoagulant. One mL of blood is mixed with the anticoagulant. The anticoagulated blood is loaded in the tube up to the '0' mark with a Pasteur pipette and the tube is then placed on the Wintrobe's stand. The reading is taken after one hour. The patient is also asked to report fasting. Wintrobe's tube is also used for determining packed cell volume (PCV).

Normal values:

Males: 0–7 mm in the first hour.

Females: 0–15 mm in the first hour.

Comparison of Westergren and Wintrobe methods

Feature	Westergren's method	Wintrobe's method
Quantity of blood required	Greater	Lesser
Dilution of blood with anticoagulant	This method involves usage of liquid anticoagulant causing dilution of blood affecting the ESR value	There is no dilution with anticoagulant as it is solid
Pipetting	Involves mouth pipetting and is therefore not encouraged	Pipetting is done using a Pasteur pipette
Sensitivity	More sensitive particularly with higher values of ESR because sedimentation involves a longer second phase (sinking of RBCs occurs better with a longer tube giving more accurate results of ESR)	The shorter column makes the Wintrobe's method less sensitive. It is more sensitive when ESR is low and less sensitive with higher values of ESR
Estimation of PCV	Not possible	Possible

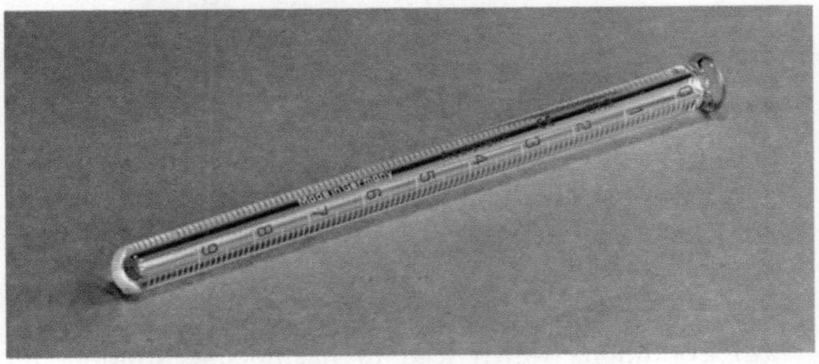

Fig. 16.8 Wintrobe's tube.

3. **Micro ESR method:** This method can be used for both capillary and venous blood. It is primarily for the paediatric population and in patients in whom venepuncture is not possible. A capillary tube 230-mm-long with an internal bore diameter of 1 mm is used. It is graduated 1 mm apart for up to 50 mm. Non-graduated, heparinized capillary tubes can also be used. The tube is filled with 0.2 mL of EDTA mixed blood and the reading is taken as in the Westergren's method.
4. **Zeta sedimentation method (ZSR):** 0.2 mL of EDTA blood is filled in a capillary tube and centrifuged in a Zetafuge 4 times for 45 seconds each. The capillary tube is mechanically rotated to 180 degrees and centrifuged in a reverse direction 4 times for 45 seconds each. RBCs form rouleaux and travel down the tube by alternate compaction and dispersion. ZSR is expressed in percentage and the normal range is 40%–54%. ZSR has an edge over other methods because it requires a smaller amount of blood, and is quicker and more sensitive than the Westergren's method. However, it requires special and expensive apparatus and is difficult to standardize.

Causes of increased ESR

1. Physiological conditions like menstruation and pregnancy.
2. Pathological conditions like infections (tuberculosis and rheumatic fever), collagen vascular diseases (rheumatoid arthritis and SLE), malignancies (multiple myeloma increased secretion of large amounts immunoglobulins) and anaemia.

Causes of decreased ESR

1. Physiological (in newborns).
2. Pathological—Polycythemia, spherocytosis, sickle cell anaemia, and afibrinogenemia.

Clinical significance of ESR: ESR is used as a diagnostic and prognostic tool in the assessment of several pathological conditions some of which are listed earlier. Abnormal ESR alone is not diagnostic of any condition, but with other evidences it may aid in the diagnosis. ESR also helps in assessing disease prognosis (course taken by a disease in response to treatment).

Packed Cell Volume (PCV)

PCV or haematocrit is the volume of packed red cells expressed as a percentage of the volume of whole blood in a sample. Heparin, oxalate, or EDTA is used as the anticoagulant. There are two methods of PCV estimation:

1. **Macrohaematocrit or Wintrobe's method:** Wintrobe's tube is marked in two directions. The ascending marking is for determination of PCV and the descending marking is for ESR. Wintrobe's tube is filled with well-mixed anticoagulated blood using a long Pasteur pipette up to the mark '0' or '10'. The tube is centrifuged at 3000 rpm for 30 minutes. The upper level of the column of packed red cells is read along the markings in ascending order (expressed as a percentage of total volume of blood). Three zones are seen following centrifugation (Fig. 16.9):
   (a) The lowermost zone of packed red cells (PCV) normally 45%–50%.
   (b) A thin intermediate layer of WBCs and platelets called 'buffy coat' normally 2%–3%. Any increase or decrease in the thickness of the buffy coat should be noted. The buffy coat is usually less than 1 mm wide and white in colour.
   (c) Uppermost layer of plasma normally 48%–52%.

   Sources of error
   (a) Improper mixing of blood.
   (b) Inadequate centrifugation.
   (c) Reading of haematocrit without excluding the buffy coat.
2. **Microhaematocrit method:** Capillary tubes 75 mm in length and having an internal diameter of about 1 mm are used for this method. The tubes may be coated with 1 IU of heparin for the direct collection of capillary blood, or uncoated for use with anticoagulated blood samples. Blood is allowed to enter the tube by capillary action and at least

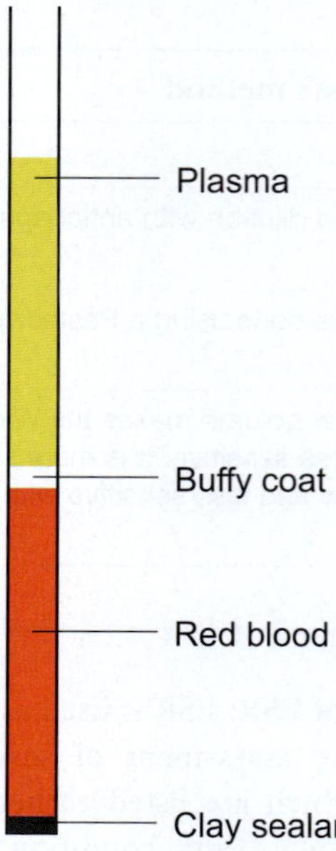

Fig. 16.9 Zones formed following centrifugation in Wintrobe's tube (Buffy coat formation).

15 mm is left unfilled. The tube is then sealed by a plastic seal. The tubes are centrifuged in a microhaematocrit centrifuge at a centrifugal force of 12,000 g for 5 minutes. The proportion of cells to the whole column (i.e. the PCV) is then measured using a reading device. When the PCV is greater than 0.5 it may be necessary to centrifuge further for 5 minutes.

Advantages

(a) The microhaematocrit method is the most accurate means of determining PCV and should be used whenever feasible.
(b) It requires very small quantities of blood so is ideal for the paediatric population and in patients with haemoconcentration, for example burns.
(c) It is not time consuming.
(d) It can be used for a large number of samples at the same time, so can be used for mass surveys.

Precautions

(a) K_2-EDTA is recommended over K_3-EDTA as K_3-EDTA causes shrinkage of the red cells thus reducing the PCV by about 2%.
(b) Anticoagulant concentration should not exceed 2.2 mg/mL as it may cause a false low PCV value due to cell shrinkage.
(c) White cells and platelets (the buffy coat) must be excluded as far as possible from the reading of the packed red cells.

Causes of reduced haematocrit

(a) Pregnancy
(b) Excessive water intake
(c) Anaemia
(d) Conditions which cause expansion of plasma volume, for example hyperaldosteronism.

Causes of increased haematocrit

(a) High altitude (due to hypoxia)
(b) Newborns

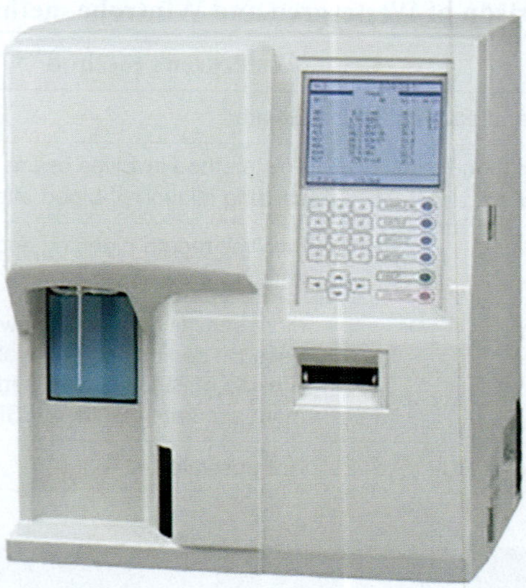

Fig. 16.10 Automated haematology counter.

(c) Excessive sweating
(d) Congenital heart disease
(e) Emphysema
(f) Polycythemia
(g) Conditions which lead to haemoconcentration, for example severe vomiting and diarrhoea

Automated Haematology (PA13.4)

Automation is synonymous with any repetitive task. In haematology, many tasks are repetitives making automation useful. Determination of cell parameters by the haematology analyzer from analysis of electrical impedance and/or light scattering data forms the basis of automated haematology. The automated haematology analyzers (Fig. 16.10) provide results by electrical and light signals generated when blood cells pass through the sensing zone of the machine. Data is recorded in the computer and is also represented graphically. Precision of a measurement system is also called reproducibility. It is the degree to which repeated measurements under unchanged conditions show the same results. This feature is seen to improve with automation. In automation, the processing time is much shorter as compared to manual methods and the numbers of events, which are analyzed are far more. Automation has two phases, a **pre analytical phase** (this phase includes patient registration, sample collection, sample transport, worksheet generation and analyzer programming) and an **analytical phase** (progress in technology has evolved this to a very sophisticated level. The various tasks involved are sample introduction, addition of reagent, mixing of sample and reagent, incubation, detection, calculation and result reporting). Automated counters can be based on the principle of:

1. **Electrical impedance counting** (Wallace coulter 1956): Blood cells are suspended in different isotonic solutions. There are two electrodes, internal and external, and direct current flows through the transducer chambers from the internal to the external electrodes. As the blood cell passes through apertures of known dimensions it causes displacement of some conducting diluents and change in

resistance of the conductive fluid. In this way a pulse is generated, which is recorded by an oscillograph, the height of which is proportional to cell volume. This is the way in which different blood cells are sized and counted.

2. **Light scatter method:** In this technique diluted blood samples pass in sheathed flow through a light source in a single file, and light is scattered as the cell passes through the light beam. Amount of light scattered is detected by a photo multiplier, which converts it into electrical impulses the height of which is proportional to the cell volume.

Principles of different instruments

RBC evaluation: After the counts have been measured by the analyzer the rest of the data is calculated from them. Mean cell volume (MCV) and red cell distribution width (RDW) are derived from the RBC histogram. RDW is the coefficient of variation of the RBC distribution histogram and is a quantitative measure of variation in red blood cell size (anisocytosis). The RDW is elevated in iron deficiency anaemia, myelodysplastic syndromes, macrocytic anaemia secondary to vitamin B12 or folate deficiency, and some malignancies. In contrast, the RDW is usually normal or only mildly elevated in the microcytic anaemia of thalassemia. Haematocrit is calculated from MCV and RBC count.

Hct (L/L, %) = RBC (cells/L) × MCV (L/cell)

MCH and MCHC are calculated from RBC count, MCV and haemoglobin concentration. In unusual circumstances, the automated haematology analyzer produces cell counts which are falsely increased or decreased. Fortunately in almost all these cases the instruments 'flag' the specimen as abnormal so that the operator can verify the results manually or perform necessary corrections.

Causes of spurious results include:

- Hyperlipidemia, fat droplets (from hyperalimentation), hypergammaglobinemia, cryoglobulinemia and leukocytosis (>50 × 10^9/L) can result in spurious elevations of haemoglobin concentration.
- Very small red blood cells (microcytosis) may be counted as large platelets and result in a falsely decreased RBC count.
- Autoagglutination or cryoglobulins lead to RBC clumping, which may falsely increase the RBC count.
- In patients with severe hyperglycaemia (glucose >600 mg/dL) osmotic swelling of the red blood cells may spuriously elevate the MCV.

WBC evaluation: The total WBC count includes all circulating nucleated haematopoietic cells with the exception of nucleated red blood cells (NRBCs). The WBC evaluation is useful in patients with haematologic and infectious diseases. RBCs are removed by lysis and the total WBC count is measured by electrical impedance or light scatter techniques.

Causes of spurious results include:

- Unlysed RBCs
- NRBCs
- Platelet clumps or large platelets
- Cryoglobulins

Differential Leukocyte Count (DLC): Haematology analyzers are more accurate than performing a manual count for DLC. The analyzers can generate a five-part differential, based on the electronic impedance, conductivity and light-scatter measurements. Cell counting with these instruments is rapid, objective and not subject to the slide distributional bias of the manual count. However, the analyzers cannot correctly identify all abnormal white blood cells, and manual examination of the peripheral smear is needed for blasts and immature cells.

Platelet evaluation: A decreased platelet count (thrombocytopenia) can result from a hypocellular marrow or a peripheral platelet destructive process. Elevated platelet counts (thrombocytosis) can result from a reactive or neoplastic process. EDTA-anticoagulated blood is preferred for platelet counts, but the specimen must be thoroughly mixed to prevent platelet clumping and falsely decreased platelet counts (spurious thrombocytopenia). Fragments of red and white blood cells may cause spurious thrombocytosis.

- An instrument problem is differentiated from a specimen-related problem by running a control. If the control results are acceptable the problem is probably specimen-related. Check for clots, haemolysis and lipemia. If the control shows similar problems, it indicates an instrument problem.
- A reagent problem is indicated as a precipitate in the reagent tubing. In the less obvious cases, the most effective way of detecting a problem is by keeping a log of the lot numbers with the opening and expiration dates of the reagents in use, and knowing how each reagent affects the data.

17 Bone Marrow Examination

Q. Enumerate the indications and describe the findings in bone marrow aspiration and biopsy. (PA17.2)

Ans. Bone marrow examination is the pathologic examination of a sample of bone marrow, which is indicated when a disease cannot be diagnosed and classified on the basis of the blood counts and peripheral blood smear examination alone. In some cases, examination of the bone marrow is required for monitoring the course of therapy, for example in leukaemia; performing special studies, such as cytogenetics and microbiological analysis or flow cytometry. Bone marrow can be obtained through:

1. Bone marrow aspiration
2. Bone biopsy

Indications for bone marrow aspiration

- Evaluation of unexplained leukocytopenia, thrombocytopenia, and/or anaemia.
- Diagnosis of aplastic anaemia, myelodysplastic syndrome, chronic myelogenous leukaemia, myelofibrosis and essential thrombocythaemia.
- Evaluation of monoclonal hypergammaglobulinaemia.
- Diagnosis and evaluation of idiopathic thrombocytopenic purpura.
- Diagnosis and management of acute leukaemia and subleukaemic leukaemia.
- Staging of lymphomas.
- Evaluation of pyrexia of unknown origin, unexplained lymphadenopathy and hepatosplenomegaly.
- Diagnosis of infectious diseases, such as leishmaniasis, disseminated fungal disease or HIV.

A bone marrow biopsy and aspiration may also be ordered at intervals when a person is being treated for a cancer, to evaluate whether marrow function is being suppressed and, if it is, when its function begins to recover.

Contraindications for bone marrow aspiration: Absolute contraindications to bone marrow aspiration or biopsy include haemophilia and related coagulation disorders. If there is a skin or soft tissue infection over the hip, a different site should be chosen for bone marrow examination. Bone marrow aspiration and biopsy can be safely performed even in the setting of thrombocytopenia.

Sites for bone marrow aspiration

1. The **sternum** is considered a good site for aspiration because in this site the cortical bone is thin and the marrow contains abundant cells and little fat. However, one has to be careful that the needle is correctly inserted in the sternum, or else, there is a danger of perforating the inner cortical layer and damaging the underlying large blood vessels and right atrium, with serious consequences. Penetration of the underlying mediastinal organs can result in mediastinitis, pulmonary embolism, pneumothorax, cardiac tamponade and cardiac tissue injury, and for these reasons, biopsies are not to be performed from the sternum. Also, this site should not be used in children as the bone is very thin and the marrow cavities are small.
2. The **posterior iliac crest** is optimal for reasons of safety and ease of performance. The **iliac spines** have the advantage that if no material is aspirated, a trephine biopsy can be performed immediately. These sites, however, are difficult to aspirate from in patients with morbid obesity, in which case puncture of the sternum may be necessary. Performance of bilateral iliac biopsies is thought to increase the probability of detecting focal lesions when there is patchy bone involvement, as in carcinoma and lymphoma staging. With the availability of positron emission tomography (PET) for staging of lymphomas and the current inclusion of PET-positive bone disease as indicative of bone involvement in lymphoma, bilateral bone marrow biopsies are rarely done.
3. **Spinous processes of the lumbar vertebrae** may also occasionally be used for aspiration.
4. In infants and children younger than 2 years the medial side of the upper end of **tibia** is considered the site of choice.

Aspiration technique

- Consent for the procedure is obtained.
- The patient is positioned as follows:
  - Lateral decubitus position, knees flexed, and pillow under head, for posterior iliac crest aspiration.
  - Supine position hips and knees flexed, for anterior iliac crest aspiration.
  - Supine position, for a sternal puncture.
- The skin over the chosen site is sterilized with 70% alcohol or 0.5% chlorhexidine.
- The skin, subcutaneous tissue and periosteum overlying the selected site is then infiltrated with a local anaesthetic such as 2–5 mL 2% lignocaine.
- A skin incision is made with a small surgical blade, through which the bone marrow aspiration needle, with a stylet locked in place, is inserted. The most common reusable needles are the **Salah** and **Klima** needles (Fig. 17.1). The

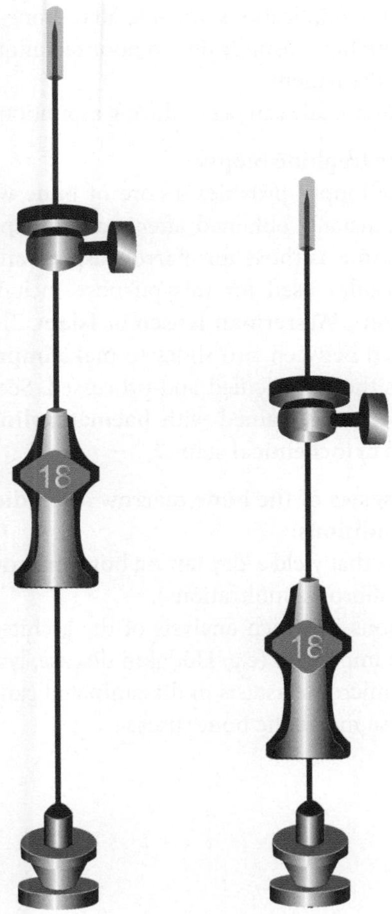

Fig. 17.1 Bone marrow aspiration needles.

needle is passed perpendicularly by slowly rotating clockwise and counter clockwise into the cavity of the ilium at the centre of the oval posterior superior iliac spine or 2 cm posterior and 2 cm inferior to the anterior superior iliac spine or second intercostal space in the midline for sternal aspiration. When the needle is firmly in place and a slight give in pressure is felt, the cavity has been entered.

- After penetrating the bone, the stylet is removed, a 1 or 2 mL syringe is attached, and marrow contents are sucked up for making films.
- If a larger sample is needed (e.g. for cytogenetic or immunophenotypic analysis), a second 5 or 10 mL syringe is attached and a second sample is aspirated.

Preparation and interpretation of smears

- The marrow is poured onto slides placed at an angle of 30 degree so that the blood present in the marrow can be drained off. Films should be made very quickly from the aspirated material, as bone marrow tends to clot faster than blood.
- By using a smooth-edged glass spreader, smears are made of the aspirated marrow, by dragging the marrow fragments behind the spreader. Most of the blood is quickly sucked off from the edge of the drop with the marrow syringe or a fine plastic pipette.
- The remaining material can be stored in EDTA and used later to make more films. Heparin should be used for **immunophenotyping** or **cytogenetic studies**. Formalin for a Cytoblock preparation (clot).
- The smears can be fixed in absolute methanol as soon as they are dry, for subsequent staining by **Romanowsky, Perls** or **cytochemical stains.**
- The preparation is considered satisfactory when marrow particles and free marrow cells can be seen in stained films. The differential counts should be made in the cellular trails, commencing from the marrow fragment and working back towards the head of the film.
- A well-spread film with easily identifiable particles is picked. Several particles are examined with a low-power (×10) objective to estimate the cellularity of the marrow (whether the marrow is hypocellular, normocellular or hypercellular). A cellular area of the film where the nucleated cells are well stained and well spread is chosen and the cells in this area are then examined under higher power (×40).
- At least 500 cells are counted and percentages of different cells are calculated. The **myeloid:erythroid** (M:E) ratio (proportion of myeloid and erythroid cells) is determined; normal M:E ratio varies between 2:1 and 4:1.
- **Maturation of erythroid cells** is classified as normoblastic, megaloblastic or dyserythropoietic.
- **Leukocytic maturation** is looked at and **megakaryocytic number, maturation sequence** and **morphology** are noted.
- Attempt is made to identify **abnormal cells** (as seen in metastatic carcinomas, lymphomas and metabolic disorders).
- **Macrophages** are examined at higher power for evidence of infection (presence of malarial pigment, parasites, bacteria or fungi).
- Areas of **bone marrow necrosis** are looked for. Bone marrow necrosis may occur in sickle cell disease, lymphomas, leukaemia, myeloproliferative diseases, metastatic carcinoma, septicaemia and tuberculosis.
- **Iron content** of macrophages is assessed by Perls stain. At least seven particles should be examined to optimally assess a bone marrow aspirate for iron stores.
- A sample for **bone marrow histology** should ideally be obtained at the same time as bone marrow aspiration, particularly in the case of a 'dry tap'. A dry tap or failure to aspirate marrow suggests bone marrow fibrosis or infiltration.

Cell counts on aspirated bone marrow

- For practical purposes, the degree of marrow cellularity can be assessed as increased, normal, or reduced by inspection of a stained film containing marrow particles. As a rough guide, if less than 25% of the particle is occupied by haemopoietic cells, it is hypocellular, and if more than 75%–80% is occupied, it is hypercellular.
- A 200–500 cell differential can be undertaken and the cells can be classified as erythroid, myeloid, lymphoid and plasma cells.
- Sometimes it may be important to specifically count one cell type (e.g. blasts in acute leukaemia for assessing response to chemotherapy).

Sources of error in cell counts

- **Age of the patient:** The cellularity of the marrow is affected by age. In adults, a smaller proportion of the marrow cavity is occupied by haemopoietic marrow compared with children, and the proportion of fat cells to cellular marrow is increased.
- **Distribution of the marrow cells:** Irregular distribution of the marrow cells in films is an established source of error. For example, megakaryocytes are irregularly distributed in marrow preparations and tend to be carried to the tail of the film. Rarely, aspiration of a lymphoid follicle can result in an abnormally high percentage of lymphocytes in the differential count.
- **Dilution with blood:** This can be overcome by aspirating only a small volume and counting cells in the trails left behind marrow particles as they are spread on the slide.
- **Marrow fibrosis:** In the presence of increased reticulin, some cell types resist aspiration or remain embedded in marrow fragments and may not be adequately represented in the differential count.

Complications of bone marrow aspiration

Albeit extremely rare, complications from bone marrow aspiration and biopsy include:

1. Infection and bleeding.
2. Even rarer complications include iliac bone perforation and haemorrhage, usually due to poor technique and positioning of the patient.
3. Cardiac tamponade can occur during aspiration of sternum.

Bone marrow trephine biopsy

Bone marrow biopsy provides a core of bone with marrow spaces and is usually obtained after marrow aspiration. The sites are the same as those for marrow aspiration (except the sternum). Needles used for this purpose include **Jamshidi** (most common)**, Westerman Jensen** or **Islam**. The tissue obtained is rolled between two slides to make **imprint smears.** The biopsy is then decalcified and processed. Sections of the marrow are cut and stained with **haematoxylin** and **eosin, reticulin** and **cytochemical** stains.

Trephine biopsies of the bone marrow are indicated in the following conditions:

1. Conditions that yield a 'dry tap' on bone marrow aspiration (e.g. myelofibrosis, infiltrations).
2. In conditions in which analysis of the architecture of the marrow is important (e.g. Hodgkin disease, lymphoma).
3. To detect micrometastasis in disseminated cancer.
4. To diagnose metabolic bone disease.

18 Urine Examination

Q. Enumerate and describe the different methods of collection of urine. (IM25.7, PE21.11)

Ans. Different urinary specimens may be required for different estimates in the urine. To obtain a representative specimen, regulation of certain aspects of specimen collection is often necessary. These special conditions include time, duration, and method of collection, along with supervision of the patient' intake. Urine should be collected in a clean dry container. Voided specimens must be fresh (should be examined within two hours of voiding). If analysis is delayed, urine specimens should be refrigerated or preserved. The desired volume of urine to be collected is 50–60 mL (as the quantity of urine required for estimation of specific gravity alone may be 30 mL).

Types of Urinary Specimens

1. **Random specimen:** This is the most commonly received specimen in a laboratory and can be collected at any time.
   Indication: Useful for routine screening tests.
   Disadvantage: It may show erroneous results depending on the dietary, fluid, or medicinal intake; metabolic state of the patient; and physical activity, just before collection.
2. **First morning specimen:** *The first morning specimen*, or 8-hour specimen, is a concentrated specimen, thereby ensuring detection of chemicals and formed elements that may not be present in a dilute random specimen. It is also relatively free of dietary influences and changes due to physical activity. The patient should be instructed to collect the specimen immediately on arising and to deliver it to the laboratory within 2 hours.
   Note: A *fasting specimen* differs from a first morning specimen by being the second voided specimen after a period of fasting.
   Indications
   (a) Ideal screening specimen for proteins, nitrites, microscopic analysis and cytology (preferred because of large volume and concentrated urine).
   (b) Important for preventing false-negative pregnancy tests (because this specimen is most concentrated with human chorionic gonadotropin and other elements).
   (c) Useful for evaluating orthostatic proteinuria.
3. **24-hour (timed) urinary specimen:** When the concentration of the substance to be measured changes with daily activities such as exercise, meals and metabolism, a 24-hour collection is required.
   Indications: Optimum for quantitative protein, sugar and urobilinogen level estimation.
   Method of collection: The patient is instructed to empty bladder at 8:00 a.m. and discard the urine. All subsequent samples are collected, including that morning sample collected at 8:00 a.m. Urine should be pooled and thoroughly mixed prior to analysis. The total volume should be accurately measured and recorded. All specimens should be refrigerated or chemically preserved.
4. **Midstream clean-catch specimen**
   Indication: This specimen is recommended for microbiological culture and antibiotic susceptibility testing because of the reduced incidence of cellular and microbial contamination compared with the voided specimen. It is a safer and less traumatic method than catheterization for obtaining urine for bacterial culture and routine urinalysis.
   Method of collection: By using complete aseptic precautions, separate labia, expose urethral orifice (labia kept separated throughout the collection), clean the area surrounding the meatus with soap balls and then the meatus itself, allow the initial stream of urine to drain, and catch the subsequent mid-stream sample. In males, glans exposed, thoroughly cleaned with a mild antiseptic solution and dried, foreskin retracted, area thoroughly cleaned, mid-stream sample is collected.
5. **Catheterized specimen:** Urine is collected under sterile conditions by passing a catheter (hollow tube) through the urethra into the urinary bladder.
   Indications
   (a) The most commonly requested test on a *catheterized specimen* is bacterial culture. In case a routine urinalysis is also asked for, the culture should be the first to be performed in order to prevent contamination.
   (b) Catheterized specimen is best for cytological examination as it is free of seminal fluid, vaginal cells, inflammatory cells and microorganisms.
   (c) Less commonly, a catheterized specimen may be used to measure functions of individual kidneys. Specimens from the right and left kidneys are collected separately by passing catheters through the ureters of the respective kidneys.
6. **Suprapubic aspiration:** Collection of urine by introduction of a needle through the abdominal wall into the urinary bladder.
   Indications
   (a) Because the bladder is sterile under normal conditions, *suprapubic aspiration* is indicated when a sample is

required for bacterial culture (free of extraneous contamination).
(b) The specimen can also be used for cytological examination.

7. **Prostatitis specimen:** The *three-glass collection* procedure is used to determine prostatic infection. Instead of discarding the first urine passed while collecting a mid-stream specimen, it is collected in a sterile container. Next, the mid-stream portion is collected in another sterile container. The prostate is then massaged so that prostate fluid will be passed with the urine, and this is collected in a third container. Urethral infection or inflammation is tested for by the first container and urinary bladder infection by the second container. The prostatic secretions are cultured and examined for white blood cells (WBCs). More than 10–20 WBCs per high-power field is considered abnormal.
8. **Paediatric specimens:** These can be collected in clear plastic bags provided with hypoallergenic skin adhesive to attach to the genital area of children. The inside of the bag must not be touched while applying it. Sterile specimens may be obtained by catheterization, suprapubic aspiration or by using a clean-catch procedure and a sterile collection bag. Bags that allow a tube to be attached and excess urine transferred to a larger container are available for quantitative testing.
9. **Drug specimen collection:** It is imperative that correct collection procedures and documentation are followed to ensure that the results are those of the specific individual submitting the specimen. One must be careful that no tampering of the specimen occurs such as substitution, adulteration or dilution.

Q. Enumerate the various physical, chemical and microscopic changes, which occur in a urine specimen on standing.

Ans. The various physical, chemical and microscopic changes, which occur in a urine specimen on standing are enumerated below:

- Colour changes (due to breakdown of chromogens).
- Odour changes (due to bacterial growth).
- Increased turbidity (due to bacteriuria, crystalluria, or presence of amorphous material).
- A falsely reduced pH (due to bacterial breakdown of urea into ammonia, as well as loss of carbon dioxide).
- A falsely reduced glucose level (due to utilization by bacteria).
- A falsely negative ketone (to volatilization of acetone and breakdown of acetoacetate by bacteria.
- Bilirubin may be destroyed by light and oxidized to biliverdin.
- Falsely increased nitrites (due to reduction of nitrates by bacteria).
- Disintegration of cells/casts may occur in hypotonic and alkaline urine.

Q. Enumerate the various chemical and cytological preservatives used for preservation of a urinary sample.

Ans. Reliable results can be obtained on a specimen if it has been properly refrigerated, up to 48 hours. Preservatives can be added if the sample needs to be kept for a longer time. These include the following:

1. **Chemical preservatives**
   (a) Mineral acids and vitamin C (lower pH).
   (b) Benzoic acid, boric acid, phenol, thymol, toluene, chloroform, formaldehyde, and mercury compounds (to prevent bacterial growth).
   (c) Sodium fluoride is used for glucose estimation in a concentration of less than 0.5 g/3–4 L urine (decreases glycolysis in cells and bacteria).
2. **Cytological preservative:** Equal volume of 50% alcohol is most often used.

Q. Write briefly on the steps in physical examination of urine. (PA23.1, IM4.12, 25.7, PE21.11)

Ans. Physical examination of urine includes examination of:

1. **Colour:** The specimen must be examined under a good light source, looking down through the container against a white background. The yellow colour of urine is caused by the presence of a pigment called 'urochrome'. Two additional pigments, 'uroerythrin' and 'urobilin', are present in the urine in much smaller quantities and contribute little to the colour of normal, fresh urine. Aberration of urine colour includes the following:
   (a) Pale urine may be seen with high fluid intake.
   (b) Dark yellow/amber urine usually signifies normal concentrated urine, dehydration or increased amounts of bilirubin.
   (c) Causes of cloudy urine include presence of mucus; precipitation of phosphates or urates (wherein, turbidity disappears on addition of acetic acid); bacterial growth; or contamination with semen, faeces, radiographic contrast media, talcum powder, and vaginal creams.
   (d) Red urine indicates the presence of haemoglobin, red blood cells (RBCs), myoglobin, porphyrins, beets, rifampin, or phenolphthalein.
   (e) Black urine may be seen in the presence of homogentisic acid (alkaptonuria), melanin, and medications such as levodopa, methyldopa, phenol derivatives, or metronidazole.
   (f) Blue/green urine colour is limited to bacterial infections, including urinary tract infection by *Pseudomonas* species.
   (g) Milky urine may be seen in pyuria, lipiduria, or chyluria.
2. **Odour:** Normal urine has a faint aromatic odour. Aberrations in odour include the following:
   (a) Ammoniacal fetid odour due to bacterial contamination of urine.
   (b) Mousy odour in phenylketonuria.
   (c) Fruity sweet odour in diabetic ketoacidosis.
   (d) Maple syrupy odour in maple syrup urine disease.
   (e) Rancid odour in tyrosinaemia.
3. **Volume:** Normal volume of urine is 1200–1500 mL per 24 hours.
   (a) **Polyuria** is defined as passage of more than 2000 mLof urine in 24 hours (causes include excessive fluid intake, diuretic therapy, chronic kidney disease, diabetes insipidus, mental disorders, diabetes mellitus, and primary aldosteronism).

(b) **Nocturia** is defined as passage of more than 500 mLof urine with a specific gravity of less than 1.018 at night.

(c) **Oliguria** is defined as passage of less than 500 mLof urine in 24 hours (seen in dehydration, acute glomerulonephritis, shock, toxic nephropathy, and obstruction to urinary flow).

(d) **Anuria** is defined as complete suppression of urine formation.

4. **Specific gravity:** Specific gravity is defined as the density of a solution compared with the density of a similar volume of distilled water at a similar temperature. Because urine is actually water that contains dissolved chemicals, the specific gravity of urine is a measure of the density of the dissolved chemicals in the specimen. Normal range for specific gravity of urine is 1.016 to 1.022.

(a) **Low specific gravity (hyposthenuria)** is defined as a specific gravity of less than 1.007 (seen in excessive fluid intake, diuretic therapy, chronic kidney disease, and diabetes insipidus).

(b) **Low fixed specific gravity (isosthenuria)** is defined as a specific gravity fixed at 1.010 (seen in chronic renal failure as the concentrating power of kidney is lost due to tubular damage).

(c) **Increased specific gravity** is defined as a specific gravity of more than 1.022 (seen in dehydration, glycosuria, renal artery stenosis, heart failure, inappropriate antidiuretic hormone secretion, and proteinuria).

Methods of estimation of specific gravity:

(a) **Urinometer** (Fig. 18.1)

Principle: Specific gravity changes depending on the number, density, and weight of the solute particles in a solution and is used to measure of the concentrating power of the kidney. The specific gravity of urine is its density compared with the density of distilled water that is fixed as 1.000 at 20°C. The urinometer consists of a weighted float attached to a scale that has been calibrated in terms of urine specific gravity. The level to which the urinometer sinks represents the specimen' mass or specific gravity.

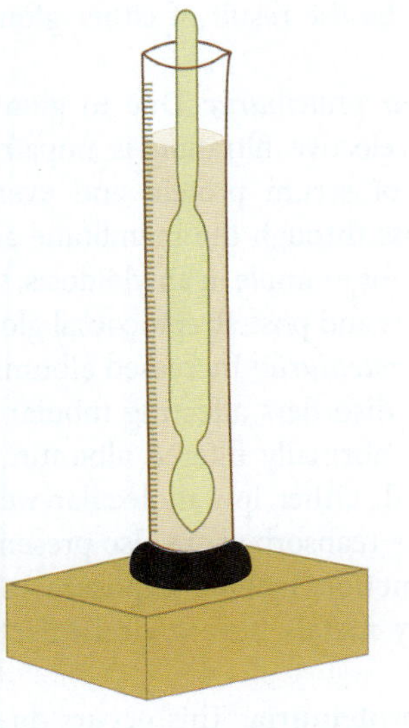

Fig. 18.1 Urinometer.

Method: Fill three-fourth of the cylinder of the urinometer with urine (minimum volume required is 15 mL). Gently lower the urinometer in the cylinder and set the urinometer in spinning motion (should be free floating; not touching sides; there should be no air bubbles). Read the bottom of meniscus. The urinometer should be calibrated with variations in:

(i) Temperature (0.001 for each 3°C above or below 20°C).

(ii) 1 g of protein per decilitre of urine raises the urine specific gravity by 0.003, and 1 g glucose per decilitre adds 0.004 to the reading. Consequently, for each gram of protein present, 0.003 must be subtracted from the specific gravity reading, and 0.004 must be subtracted for each gram of glucose present.

Advantages

(i) Is a relatively simple method.

(ii) Can be calibrated with variations in temperature and solute content.

Disadvantages

(i) Urinometry is less accurate than the other methods currently available and is not recommended by the Clinical and Laboratory Standards Institute.

(ii) Urinometer requires a large volume (10–15 mL) of specimen.

(b) **Refractometer**

Principle: Refractometers are instruments that correlate density of a solution to its specific gravity. They work on the principle that when light passes from a transparent medium of one density to that of another density, it changes its velocity and therefore the direction in which the beam of light is moving. The concentration of solute in the solution determines the velocity and angle at which light passes through a solution. Clinical refractometers make use of this principle and use a prism to direct a specific (monochromatic) wavelength of daylight against a manufacturer-calibrated specific gravity scale.

Advantages

(i) It requires only a few drops of urine.

(ii) Temperature corrections are not necessary because the light beam passes through a temperature compensating liquid prior to being directed at the specific gravity scale.

Disadvantage

(i) Corrections for glucose and protein are still calculated, although refractometer readings are less affected by particle density than are urinometer readings.

(c) **Reagent strips ('urine dipsticks'**– an indirect colorimetric method for estimating specific gravity): This method uses a pad that contains a complex, pre-treated electrolyte that undergoes a pH change based on the ionic concentration of the urine. This change results in a change of colour of the pad. This estimate of specific gravity is rapid and simple and requires no special equipment.

5. **pH:** pH of urine indicates the ability of kidneys to maintain normal hydrogen ion concentration in plasma and extracellular fluid. Metabolic activity produces non-volatile acids such as sulphuric, phosphoric, hydrochloric, pyruvic, lactic and citric, as well as, ketones. These are normally

excreted and bicarbonates reabsorbed. Normal pH ranges from 4.6 to 8 and is usually measured by reagent strips. Urine pH is of clinical significance in the following conditions:

(a) Renal calculi formation.
(b) Precipitation/identification of crystals.
(c) Treatment of urinary tract infections.
(d) Respiratory or metabolic acidosis/ketosis.
(e) Respiratory or metabolic alkalosis.

Q. Write briefly on reagent strips (Fig. 18.2).

Ans. These provide a simple, rapid means for performing analysis of urine, including pH; presence of protein, glucose, ketones, blood, bilirubin, urobilinogen, nitrite, and leukocytes; and specific gravity.

Principle: Reagent strips consist of chemical-impregnated absorbent pads attached to a plastic strip. A colour-producing chemical reaction takes place when the absorbent pad comes in contact with urine. The reactions are interpreted by comparing the colour produced on the pad with a chart supplied by the manufacturer. By careful comparison of the colours on the chart and the strip, a semi-quantitative measurement is also possible.

Technique: Testing includes dipping the reagent strip into a well-mixed specimen (formed elements such as RBCs and WBCs sink to the bottom of the specimen and will be undetected in an unmixed specimen). Excess urine is removed from the strip by running its edge on the container while withdrawing it from the urine. A colour comparison is done against the manufacturer' chart after waiting for the specified duration for reactions to take place.

Recommendations

1. Protect from moisture and heat and store in a cool, dry area.
2. Do not refrigerate; check for discolouration and manufacturer' directions.
3. Test urine as soon as possible (allowing the strip to remain in the urine for an extended duration may cause leaching of reagents from the pads).
4. Remove only enough strips for immediate use and recap tightly.
5. Test a well-mixed, unspun urine sample at room temperature.
6. Do not touch the test area with fingers.

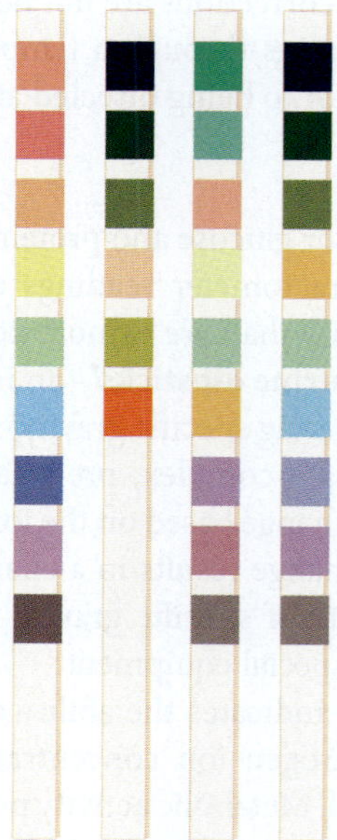

Fig. 18.2 Reagent strips.

Q. Write briefly on the steps in chemical examination of urine. (PA23.1, IM4.12, 25.7, PE21.11)

Ans. Chemical examination of urine includes testing for proteins, glucose, ketones, bile derivatives and blood.

Protein

Proteinuria is frequently seen in early renal disease, making the urinary protein test an important part of any chemical examination. **Normal urine contains very little protein (less than 10 mg/dL or 100 mg/24 hours)** mainly constituted by low-molecular-weight serum proteins, such as albumin, and small amounts of microglobulins, Tamm–Horsfall protein (produced by the tubules), and proteins from prostatic, seminal and vaginal secretions.

Clinical Significance: Proteinuria ≥30 mg/dL has clinical significance. The causes of proteinuria are varied and can be grouped into three major categories: *pre-renal, renal,* and *post-renal,* based on the origin of the protein.

- **Pre-renal proteinuria:** Pre renal proteinuria is caused by conditions affecting the plasma prior to its reaching the kidney. This condition is caused by increased levels of low-molecular-weight plasma proteins such as **haemoglobin, myoglobin, and the acute phase reactants** associated with infection and inflammation. The increased filtration of these proteins exceeds the normal reabsorptive capacity of the renal tubules, resulting in an overflow of the proteins into the urine. Because reagent strips detect primarily albumin, pre-renal proteinuria is usually not discovered in a routine urinalysis.
- **Renal proteinuria:** Proteinuria associated with true renal disease may be the result of either glomerular or tubular damage.
  - *Glomerular proteinuria:* Due to glomerular membrane damage, selective filtration is impaired, and increased amounts of serum protein and eventually RBCs and WBCs pass through the membrane and are excreted in the urine, for example in amyloidosis, systemic lupus erythematosus and post-streptococcal glomerulonephritis.
  - *Tubular proteinuria:* Increased albumin level is also observed in disorders affecting tubular reabsorption, because the normally filtered albumin can no longer be reabsorbed. Other low-molecular-weight proteins that are usually reabsorbed are also present. Causes of tubular dysfunction include exposure to toxic substances and heavy metals, severe viral infections and *Fanconi syndrome.*
- **Post-renal proteinuria:** This occurs due to abnormalities of the lower urinary tract (ureters, bladder, urethra, prostate

and vagina). Bacterial and fungal infections as well as presence of blood as the result of injury or menstrual contamination contributes protein, as does the presence of prostatic fluid and large amounts of spermatozoa.

Benign proteinuria: It is usually transient and can be produced by conditions such as strenuous exercise, high fever, dehydration and exposure to cold.

Orthostatic (postural) proteinuria: It occurs following periods spent in a vertical posture and disappears when a horizontal position is assumed. Increased pressure on the renal vein when in the vertical position is believed to account for this condition.

Microalbuminuria: The onset of diabetic nephropathy is first predicted by detection of *microalbuminuria.* It is defined as excretion of 30–300 mg of albumin/day and requires collection of a 24-hour urine specimen. Other ways to test for microalbuminuria include immunochemical assays for albumin or albumin-specific reagent strips that also measure creatinine to determine an albumin:creatinine ratio.

Bence–Jones proteinuria

- Bence–Jones proteins are monoclonal immunoglobulin light chains **produced by plasma cells. They are sufficiently small to be excreted by the kidney. They are found in the urine of most patients with multiple myeloma, macroglobulinaemias, and amyloidosis and can be used for diagnosis of the disease as well as monitoring the response to treatment.**
- Bence–Jones proteinuria may eventually result in renal failure by two mechanisms:
  - Direct toxicity to epithelial cells.
  - Combination with the Tamm–Horsfall protein under acidic conditions may form large tubular casts, which can obstruct the lumen and also induce peritubular inflammatory reaction (cast nephropathy).
- Bence–Jones proteinuria can be detected by:
  - Heat coagulation test (Bence–Jones proteins coagulate at temperatures between 40°C and 60°C and dissolve when the temperature reaches 100°C. Therefore, a specimen that appears turbid between 40°C and 60°C and clear at 100°C can be suspected of containing Bence–Jones proteins).
  - Immunoelectrophoresis (more sensitive method; it detects even minute quantity of the protein).

Qualitative Tests for Protein

1. **Heat coagulation test**
   Principle: Proteins in urine are coagulated by heat, and the degree of coagulation is directly proportional to the amount of proteins present.
   Procedure: Pour 2–3 mL of urine into a 13 mm × 100 mm glass tube and hold it by using a tube holder. Heat the upper half of the column of urine in a flame until it boils, keeping the lower half as control (if the lower half is heated, convection currents are set up, which make the whole tube hazy and traces of protein may be missed).

Table 18.1 Semi quantitative assessment of urinary protein content with heat coagulation test

Cloudiness	Quantity of protein
No cloudiness	Negative
Faint cloudiness (may be observed only if the tube is held against a black background)	Trace
Definite cloud without granular flocculation	1+
Heavy and granular cloud without flocculation	2+
Dense cloud without marked flocculation	3+
Thick curdy flocculation	4+

Table 18.2 Semi quantitative assessment of urinary protein content with sulphosalicylic method

Concentration of proteins	Turbidity reported as
<0.01 g%	Trace
0.01–0.05 g%	1+
0.05–0.2 g%	2+
0.2–0.5 g%	3+
>0.5 g%	4+

   Appearance of cloudiness in the upper portion indicates the presence of proteins. Add 2–3 drops of 3% acetic acid to the precipitate and observe. If the precipitate disappears, it indicates the presence of phosphates and carbonates. Persistence of the precipitate indicates presence of albumin. This test may be used as a **semi-quantitative test**, as follows (Table 18.1).
2. **Sulphosalicylic acid (SSA) method**
   Principle: Urine proteins are precipitated by SSA, which gives a white precipitate, and the degree of the precipitate is proportional to the protein level.
   Procedure: To 2 mLof acidic urine in a glass tube, add equal volume of 3% SSA. Mix gently. Invert to mix, and leave for 10 minutes at room temperature. This test may be used as a **semi-quantitative test**, as follows (Table 18.2).
3. **Heller' nitric acid test:** Take 5 mL of concentrated nitric acid in a test tube, and add a few drops of urine along the walls of the test tube. A whitish ring of precipitate appears at the junction of the two fluids due to formation of acid metaprotein when albumin is present.

Quantitative Estimation of Protein

Esbach' method

Principle: Picric acid is used to precipitate proteins, and the amount of protein precipitate is measured by volume.

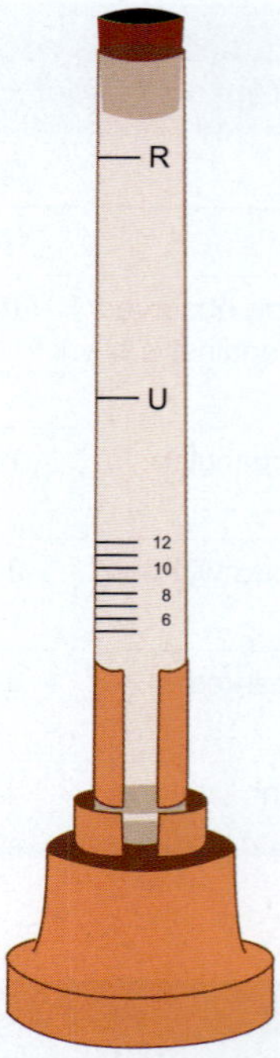

Fig. 18.3 Esbach' albuminometer.

Reagents and equipment

1. **Esbach' albuminometer** (Fig. 18.3)**:** It is a thick-walled glass tube graduated in grams of dried albumin per 1000 mL of urine. It has two marks: 'R' above and 'U' in the middle.
2. **Esbach' reagent**
   - **Picric acid**—10 g (precipitates albumin)
   - **Citric acid**—20 g (dissolves phosphates)
   - **Distilled water**—1000 mL

Procedure

- The albuminometer is filled with urine up to the mark 'U' and Esbach' reagent is added up to the mark 'R'.
- After proper mixing, the tube is corked and kept vertically in a stand for 24 hours.
- The urine may be diluted to get more accurate values and the dilutions are made on the basis of the specific gravity.
- The level of precipitate formed is measured against the graduation on the tube, and the reading is given in grams per litre of urine. This value is multiplied by the dilution factor to get the result in grams percent.

Normal range: 100–150 mg/24 h

Glucose

Causes of glycosuria: Diabetes mellitus, pregnancy, renal glycosuria, alimentary glycosuria, intravenous infusion of glucose and increased intracranial tension.

Clinical significance: Normally, almost all the glucose filtered by the glomerulus is reabsorbed in the proximal convoluted tubule; therefore, urine contains only minute amounts of glucose. Tubular reabsorption of glucose occurs by active transport in response to the body' need to maintain an adequate concentration of glucose. In case of high blood glucose level (**hyperglycaemia**), as occurs in diabetes mellitus, the tubular transport of glucose ceases, and glucose appears in the urine. The blood level at which tubular reabsorption stops (**renal threshold**) for glucose is approximately 160–180 mg/dL. **Glycosuria can also be non-diabetic.** Non-diabetic glycosuria can be renal glycosuria or alimentary (lag storage) glycosuria. **Renal glycosuria** is defined as glycosuria that occurs due to a lowered renal threshold for glucose in the absence of hyperglycaemia. There is transient abnormal increase in blood glucose level following a meal, when the concentration of blood glucose exceeds the normal renal threshold. During this time, glucose spills into the urine. This is labelled **alimentary glycosuria** and usually occurs in patients undergoing gastric surgery resulting in rapid gastric emptying, hyperthyroidism or hepatic disease.

Qualitative Tests for Glucose

1. **Copper reduction tests:** These tests rely on the ability of glucose and other substances to reduce copper sulphate to cuprous oxide in the presence of alkali and heat. A colour change progressing from a negative blue ($CuSO_4$) through green, yellow and orange/red (Cu_2O) occurs when the reaction takes place. The classic **Benedict' and Fehling' tests** are based on this principle.

   (a) **Fehling' test:** Fehling' solution should always be prepared fresh. It is prepared initially as two separate solutions, known as Fehling' A and Fehling' B. Fehling' A is a blue aqueous solution of copper sulphate, while Fehling' B is a clear solution of aqueous potassium tartarate (or Rochelle salt) and a strong alkali (sodium hydroxide).

   Procedure: Take equal volumes of Fehling' solution 'A' and 'B' in a test tube and add eight drops of urine to it. Boil for 3–5 minutes. Formation of yellow or brownish-red precipitate indicates presence of reducing sugar (the blue alkaline cupric hydroxide present in Fehling' solution, when heated in the presence of reducing sugars, gets reduced to yellow or red cuprous oxide).

   (b) **Benedict' test:** Benedict' qualitative solution contains cupric sulphate (17.3 g), sodium carbonate (100 g), and sodium citrate (173 g) in 1000 mL of distilled water. Benedict' quantitative solution contains cupric sulphate (18 g), sodium carbonate (100 g), sodium citrate (200 g), potassium ferrocyanide solution (5%; 5 mL) and potassium sulphocyanate (125 g) in 1000 mL of distilled water.

   Procedure: Five millilitres of Benedict' reagent is taken in an 18 mm × 150 mm glass tube and boiled for 1 minute. Add eight drops (0.5 mL) of urine, mix well, and boil for 2–3 minutes. Cool the tube and observe for any colour change. This test may be used as a **semi-quantitative test**, as follows (Table 18.3).

Note: Quantitative estimation of glucose in the urine can be done by titrimetric method using Benedict quantitative agent.

Another method that employs Benedict' principle is testing by the **Clinitest** tablet, which contains copper sulphate, sodium carbonate, sodium citrate and sodium hydroxide. Upon addition of the tablet to water and urine, heat is pro-

Table 18.3 Semiquantitative assessment of urinary sugar content with Benedict' method

Colour change	Quantity
No change in the original colour	Negative
Pale green and slightly cloudy	Trace (<0.5 g/dL)
Green precipitate	1+ (1 g/dL)
Yellow to orange precipitate	2+ (1–1.5 g/dL)
Orange to red precipitate	3+ (1.5–2 g/dL)
Brick red precipitate and clear supernatant	4+ (>2 g/dL)

duced by the hydrolysis of sodium hydroxide and its reaction with sodium citrate, and carbon dioxide is released from the sodium carbonate to prevent room air from interfering with the reduction reaction. **Clinitest, like Benedict' test, is subject to interference from other reducing substances.** Therefore, both do not provide a confirmatory test for glucose. **False-positive reaction** can be seen with galactose, lactose, fructose, maltose, pentoses, ascorbic acid, certain drug metabolites, antibiotics such as cephalosporins, homogentisic acid, creatinine and uric acid. The dipstick technique (based on glucose oxidase test) is specific for glucose and eliminates the false-positive reaction due to the substances mentioned earlier.

2. **Reagent strip glucose oxidase test:** Reagent strips that are impregnated with the enzyme **glucose oxidase detect only glucose.** These strips use the following double sequential enzyme reaction:

   Reaction A:

   $$\text{Glucose} + O_2 \xrightarrow{\text{Glucose oxidase}} \text{Gluconic acid} + H_2O_2$$

   Reaction B:

   $$H_2O_2 + \text{Chromogen peroxidase} \rightarrow \text{Oxidized chromogen}$$

   The chromogen that is used varies among the different reagent strips.

Ketones

Fat metabolism involves production of three intermediate products—**acetone, acetoacetic acid and β-hydroxybutyric acid**. Normally, all the metabolized fat is completely broken down into carbon dioxide and water and identifiable amounts of ketones do not appear in the urine, however, when there is depletion of available carbohydrate as the major source of energy, body stores of fat are metabolized to supply energy. This leads to production of excessive quantities of fatty acids that cannot be metabolized completely by tissues, resulting in ketonuria.

Causes of ketonuria

- Diabetes mellitus and glycogen storage diseases (there is inability to metabolize carbohydrates, leading to increased fat metabolism).
- Starvation/fasting, high-protein and low-carbohydrate diets, or prolonged vomiting (there is inadequate intake of carbohydrates or loss of carbohydrates).
- Hypermetabolic states, such as fever, pregnancy, or lactation; during acute illness; or severe stress.

Urinary ketone monitoring is required for:

- Diagnosing and treating diabetic ketoacidosis.
- Monitoring of insulin dosage.
- Evaluation of malabsorption disorders, pancreatic disorders and inborn errors of carbohydrate and amino acid metabolism.

Tests for Urine Ketones

1. **Ketostix, acetotest and other commercial strips** are available for detection of acetoacetic acid and acetone. One end of these strips, which is impregnated with a buffered mixture of sodium nitroprusside and glycine, is dipped in fresh urine. The colour produced is compared with the colour chart provided.
2. **Rothera' test:** It is based on the principle that acetone and acetoacetic acid react with sodium nitroprusside in the presence of an alkali to produce a purple colour.
   Procedure: Take 5 mL of urine in a glass tube, and saturate it with ammonium sulphate or ammonium chloride. Add a crystal or 0.5 mL of 20% aqueous solution of sodium nitroprusside to it. Mix well, and then add 2–3 mL of concentrated ammonia carefully down the side of the tube so that it layers on top of the urine. If acetone and acetoacetic acid are present, a purple colour ring will form at the junction of the two layers within 30–60 seconds. The result can be graded from trace to 3+ on the basis of the intensity of the colour formed, as detailed below:
   No change in colour: Negative
   Pinkish ring: +
   Red ring: ++
   Deep purple ring: +++
   Note: β-hydroxybutyric acid is not normally detected by Rothera' test and has to be oxidized to acetoacetic acid by adding hydrogen peroxide to urine in order to detect it.
3. **Gerhardt' test:** Ten percent ferric chloride solution is added drop by drop to 5 mL of urine until all phosphates are precipitated. An excess of ferric chloride is then added; if a reddish colour develops, the urine is considered positive for ketones.

Urinary Pigments

1. **Bilirubin:** The appearance of bilirubin in urine can provide an early indication of liver disease. It is often detected in extra-hepatic obstructive jaundice and hepatic jaundice.
   Tests for Bilirubin
   (a) **Foam test for bilirubin:** This is the simplest test for demonstration of bilirubin. When normal urine is shaken, there is formation of white coloured foam, while in the presence of bilirubin, the foam appears yellow or greenish-yellow. The results of this test should always be confirmed by chemical tests.

(b) **Reagent strip test:** The most routine testing for bilirubin utilizes reagent strips (Multistix and Chemistrip) based on a diazochemical reaction. The strip is typically impregnated with stabilized diazotized salt, such as 2,4-dichloroaniline diazonium salt, and gives a brown colour with presence of bilirubin in urine.

(c) **Fouchet' test:** When ferric chloride in acid solution is added to a precipitate of urine containing bilirubin, a green colour is produced as the bilirubin in the urine is oxidized to biliverdin.

Procedure: To 10 mL of urine in a test tube, add 3 mL of 10% barium chloride, followed by three drops of saturated ammonium sulphate. Mix well, allow to stand for a few minutes, and filter. Add 1–2 drops of **Fouchet' reagent** (trichloroacetic acid, ferric chloride, and distilled water) to the precipitate and examine for any colour change. Appearance of a green or blue colour indicates a positive reaction.

(d) **Gmelin' test:** Filter 5 mL of urine, and dry the filter paper. Add a few drops of fuming nitric acid to the filter paper. Formation of a green ring indicates the presence of bile pigment.

2. **Urobilinogen:** A 24-hour urine collection from a normal adult contains approximately 1–4 mg of urobilinogen. Increased urine urobilinogen (>1 mg/dL) is observed in liver disease and haemolytic disorders. Measurement of urine urobilinogen level is valuable in the detection of early liver disease. Impairment of liver function decreases the ability of the liver to process the urobilinogen recirculated from the intestine. The excess urobilinogen remaining in the blood is filtered by the kidneys and appears in the urine. Decreased amounts of urinary urobilinogen can result from severe diarrhoea and kidney insufficiency. The absence of urobilinogen is observed in patients with complete obstruction of the bile duct.

Ehrlich' test for urobilinogen

Ehrlich' reagent: Dissolve 2 g of para-dimethyl aminobenzaldehyde in 100 mL of 20% hydrochloric acid. When stored at 25°C–35°C in an amber-coloured bottle, it is stable for 6 months.

Procedure: To 10 mL of urine taken in a test tube, add 1mL of Ehrlich' reagent. Mix well, allow it to stand for 3–5 minutes, and observe for any colour change.

Result: A faint pink colour indicates normal urine, whereas a cherry red colour indicates the presence of increased amounts of urobilinogen. The tube test is modified to differentiate among urobilinogen, porphobilinogen and Ehrlich-reactive compounds (Watson–Schwartz differentiation test).

3. **Haemoglobin and myoglobin:** Haemoglobinuria may result from lysis of RBCs in the urinary tract, particularly in dilute, alkaline urine or intravascular haemolysis and the subsequent filtering of haemoglobin through the glomerulus. Myoglobin, a haem-containing protein found in muscle tissue, reacts positively with the reagent strip test for blood and produces clear red-brown urine. The presence of myoglobin should be suspected in patients with muscle destruction or rhabdomyolysis, as in, trauma, crush syndromes, prolonged coma, convulsions, muscle-wasting diseases, alcoholism, heroin abuse, excessive exertion, and in patients taking the cholesterol-lowering medications (statins).

Differences between haemoglobinuria and myoglobinuria:

(a) Observe a fresh morning urine specimen or one voided after exercise. Urine with myoglobinuria is characteristically red when fresh and turns black upon standing.

(b) Dissolve 2.8 g of ammonium sulphate in 5 mL of urine. A normal-coloured supernatant indicates that the precipitated pigment is haemoglobin. If the supernatant is coloured, it is evidence of myoglobin. This is based on the fact that larger haemoglobin molecules will precipitate and the smaller myoglobin molecules will remain in the solution.

(c) Other methods that can be used to differentiate the two pigments are immunodiffusion, haemagglutination inhibition and immunoelectrophoresis.

Q. Write briefly on the steps in microscopic analysis of urine. (PA23.1, IM4.12, 25.7, PE21.11)

Ans. Microscopic examination of urine aids majorly in the detection of renal and urinary tract diseases. Microscopy detects those cellular and non-cellular elements of urine that do not give distinct chemical reactions. Centrifuged urine sediment contains all the insoluble materials (*formed elements*) that come into the urine following glomerular filtration and during passage of fluid through the renal tubules and lower urinary tract. In general, randomly collected urine specimens are satisfactory for microscopic evaluation; however, it is recommended that examination take place when the sample is fresh, particularly if no preservative has been added. Cells and casts begin to lyse within 2 hours of collection. Refrigeration (2°C–8°C) helps prevent the lysis of pathologic entities; however, this may increase the precipitation of various amorphous and crystalline materials. Mid-stream collection is recommended for females to reduce contamination from vaginal elements.

- Centrifuge 12 mL of urine for 5 minutes at a relative centrifugal force (RCF) of 400 (this produces an optimum amount of sediment with the least chance of damaging the elements).
- Remove supernatant leaving behind a few drops.
- Mix sediment with a drop or two of the supernatant and resuspend.
- Smear and examine.

Examination of the Sediment

The microscopic examination should include observation of a minimum of 10 fields under both low and high power. The slide is first examined under low power to detect the general composition of the sediment. When elements such as cells, casts, or crystals, which require identification, are encountered, the setting is changed to high power. If the conventional glass slide method is being used, casts have a tendency to locate near the edges of the coverslip, making low-power scanning essential.

1. **RBCs**
   (a) Under high power, unstained erythrocytes (RBCs) appear as pale biconcave disks that may vary somewhat in size but are usually about 7 µm in diameter (Fig. 18.4).
   (b) Normal urinary RBC count ranges between 0 and 2/high-power fields (HPFs) or 3–12/µL.
   (c) In hypotonic urine, RBCs appear as faint, colourless circles due to dissolution of haemoglobin (also called shadow cells or ghost cells). Hypertonic urine may induce crenation of RBCs.
   (d) RBCs may be confused with yeast cells (yeast cells show budding; also, on adding a few drops of acetic acid RBCs lyse but not yeast cells).
   (e) Distorted RBCs are called dysmorphic erythrocytes (presence of these indicates haematuria of renal origin).
   (f) The observation of microscopic haematuria can be critical to the early diagnosis of glomerular disorders, malignancy of the urinary tract, and presence of renal calculi.

   Causes of haematuria: Haematuria of non-pathological significance is observed following strenuous exercise and during menstruation. Pathological haematuria is most closely related to disorders of renal or genitourinary origin and can occur as a result of lesions at various levels:

   Kidney: Polycystic kidney, hereditary nephritis, tuberculosis, acute nephritic syndrome, tumours (renal cell carcinoma and Wilm' tumour), infarction, pyelonephritis, immunoglobulin A nephropathy, and trauma.

   Ureters: Ureteric calculi and neoplasms.

   Urinary bladder: Rupture, cystitis, tuberculosis, transitional cell carcinoma, calculi, *Schistosoma haematobium* infection.

   Prostate: Prostatitis, nodular hyperplasia prostate, carcinoma prostate.

   Urethra: Rupture, urethritis, stricture, calculi, and transitional cell carcinoma.

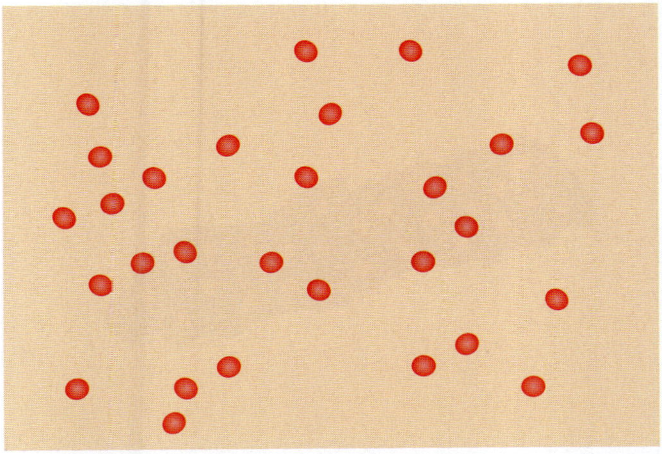

Fig. 18.4 Schematic diagram of high power view of red cells in urinary sediment.

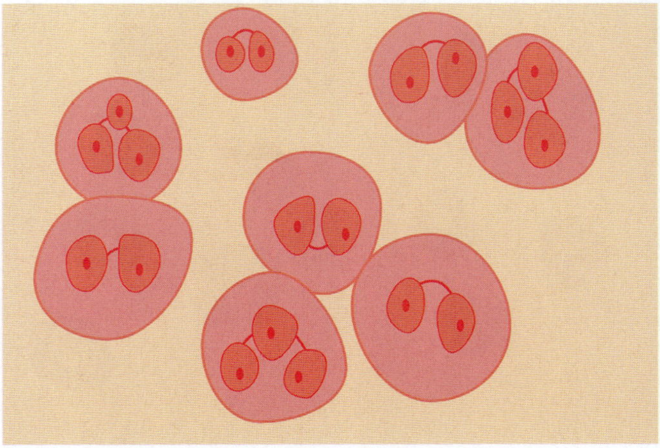

Fig. 18.5 Schematic diagram of high power view of urinary sediment showing polymorphs.

   Haematuria can also result from **systemic conditions**, such as bleeding disorders and collagen diseases and **drugs** (salicylates, cyclophosphamides and anticoagulants).

2. **WBCs** (Fig. 18.5)
   (a) An increase in urinary WBC numbers is called **pyuria** and indicates the presence of an infection or inflammation in the genitourinary system, such as pyelonephritis, cystitis, prostatitis, and urethritis. However, pyuria can also be present in non-bacterial disorders, such as glomerulonephritis, lupus erythematosus, interstitial nephritis, and tumours.
   (b) **More than 20 WBCs/HPFs** are considered **abnormal** and **more than 30/HPFs** are indicative of **acute infection.**
   (c) WBCs measure an average of approximately 12 µm in diameter (larger than RBCs). Neutrophils are the most common leukocyte found in urinary sediment. They are easy to identify because they contain granules and multilobed nuclei. Adding 2% acetic acid yields better nuclear morphology.
   (d) Neutrophils absorb water in hypotonic urine. Brownian movement of the granules in these swollen cells produces a sparkling appearance, thereby justifying the name **'glitter cells'**.
   (e) Presence of **leukocyte casts** is suggestive of renal infection or involvement.
   (f) Mononuclear leukocytes can be confused with renal tubular epithelial (RTE) cells, which are larger than WBCs and more polyhedral in shape, with an eccentric nucleus. A 0.5% solution of toluidine blue, a metachromatic stain, provides enhancement of nuclear detail and can be used to differentiate WBCs and RTE cells.

3. **Epithelial cells:** Three types of epithelial cells are seen in urine: **squamous, transitional (urothelial) and renal tubular cells. Squamous cells** (Fig. 18.6) are the largest cells found in the urine sediment. The distal one-third of the urethra is lined by squamous epithelial cells, and in the urine, these cells appear as large and flat, with abundant cytoplasm and small, round central nuclei. Their margins are often folded. When stained with crystal violet–safranin, nuclei appear purple and cytoplasm appears pink to violet. Many of the squamous cells

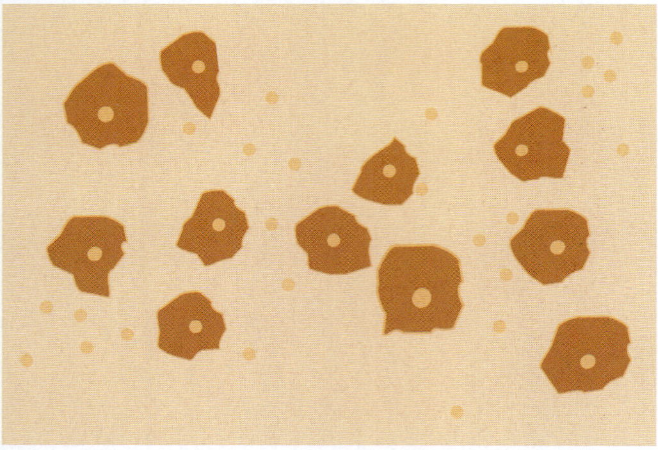

Fig. 18.6 Schematic diagram of high power view of squamous epithelial cells in urine.

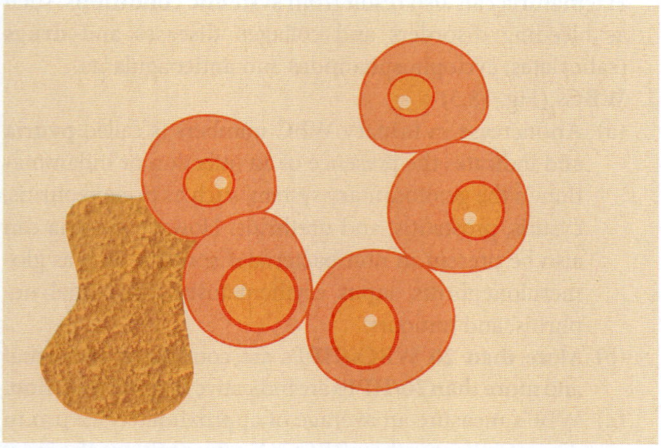

Fig. 18.7 Schematic diagram of high power view of transitional epithelial cells in urine.

present in female urine may be derived from the vagina or vulva.

Transitional epithelial cells (Fig. 18.7) are smaller than squamous cells and have distinct, centrally located nuclei. They line the urinary tract from the renal pelvis to the lower third of the urethra. RTE cells vary in size and shape depending on the area of the renal tubules from which they originate. The cells from the proximal convoluted tubule are larger than other RTE cells and have a coarsely granular cytoplasm. Cells from the distal convoluted tubule are smaller than those from the proximal convoluted tubule and are round or oval. The presence of more than two RTE cells per HPFs indicates tubular injury, and such specimens should be referred for cytologic urine testing.

4. **Lipids:** When triglycerides, neutral fats, and cholesterol pass across the glomerular membrane, there is appearance of free fat droplets, lipid-containing cells and casts in the urinary sediment. The lipid stains—Oil Red O and Sudan III—and polarizing microscopy can be used to confirm the presence of these elements.
5. **Casts:** The major constituent of casts is **Tamm–Horsfall protein**, a glycoprotein excreted by the RTE cells of the distal convoluted tubule (DCT) and upper collecting ducts

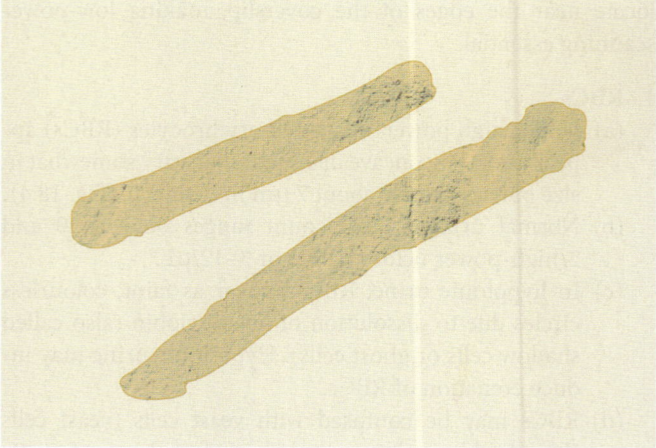

Fig. 18.8 Hyaline casts.

(CD). Under normal conditions, Tamm–Horsfall protein is excreted at a relatively constant rate. The rate of excretion appears to increase under conditions of stress and exercise. Other protein components of cast matrix are albumin and immunoglobulins. Casts which are unique to the kidney are formed within the lumens of the DCT and CD and can be of many types:

(a) **Hyaline casts** (Fig. 18.8) are the most frequently occurring casts in urine. They are composed almost entirely of Tamm–Horsfall protein and are colourless, homogeneous, and transparent. The presence of 0–2/low power field is considered normal (seen following strenuous exercise, dehydration, heat exposure, and emotional stress). Pathological hyaline casts are observed in acute glomerulonephritis, pyelonephritis, chronic renal disease, and congestive heart failure.

(b) **RBC casts** (Fig. 18.9) indicate renal haematuria. RBC casts may appear brown to almost colourless and are usually diagnostic of glomerular disease.

(c) **WBC casts** (Fig. 18.10) are present in renal infection (pyelonephritis) and in non-infectious inflammation. They mainly comprise neutrophils. **Bacterial casts**

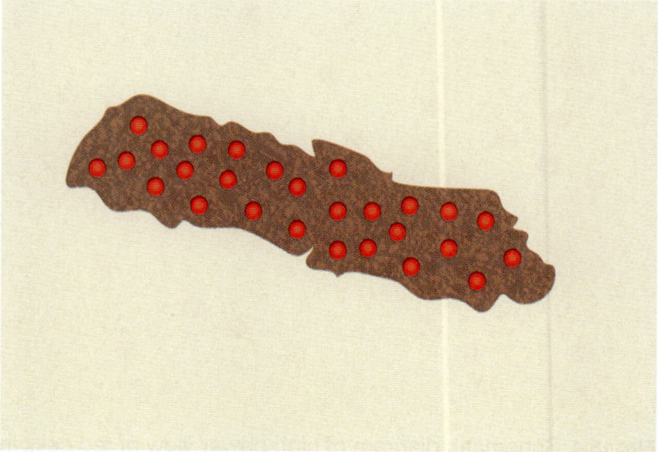

Fig. 18.9 RBC cast.

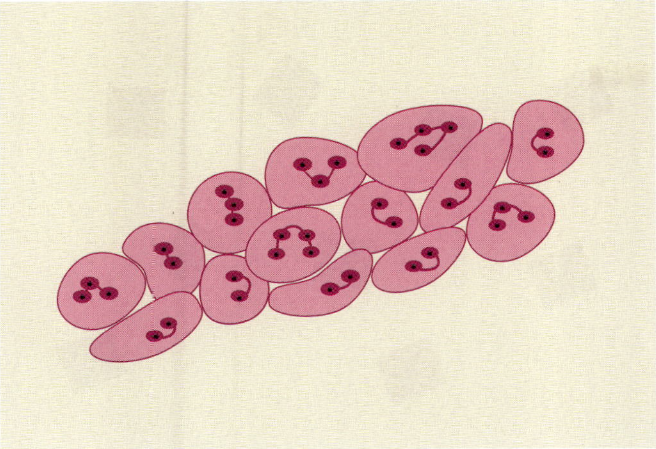

Fig. 18.10 WBC cast.

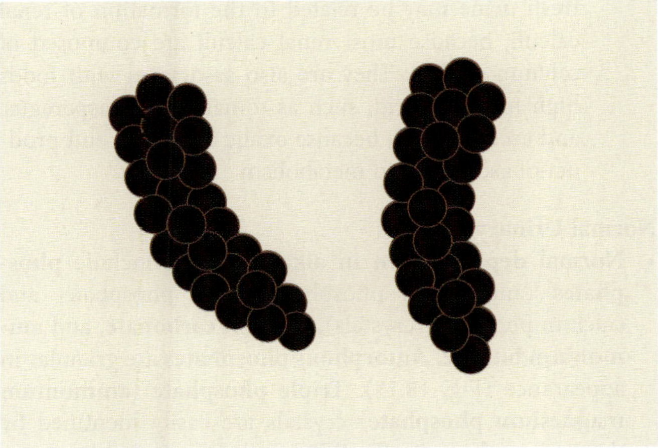

Fig. 18.11 Granular cast.

containing bacilli both within and bound to the protein matrix are seen in pyelonephritis.

(d) **Granular casts** (Fig. 18.11) almost always indicate significant renal disease. However, granular casts may be present in the urine for a short time following strenuous exercise. Granular casts that contain fine granules may appear grey or pale yellow, whereas those containing larger coarse granules are darker. These casts often appear black because of the density of the granules.

(e) **Epithelial casts** (Fig. 18.12) contain RTE cells and represent advanced tubular destruction (heavy metal or drug-induced toxicity, viral infections, allograft rejection, and severe pyelonephritis). They are rarely seen in urine because renal disease that primarily affects the tubules is infrequent.

(f) **Waxy casts** (Fig. 18.13) result from extreme urinary stasis and are found in patients with severe chronic renal failure, malignant hypertension, and diabetic nephropathy. Waxy casts appear yellow, grey, or colourless. They frequently occur as short, broad casts, with blunt or broken ends and often have cracked or serrated edges.

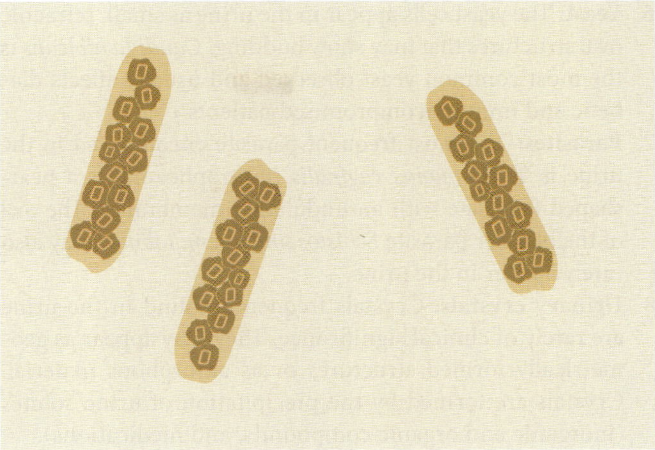

Fig. 18.12 Epithelial cast.

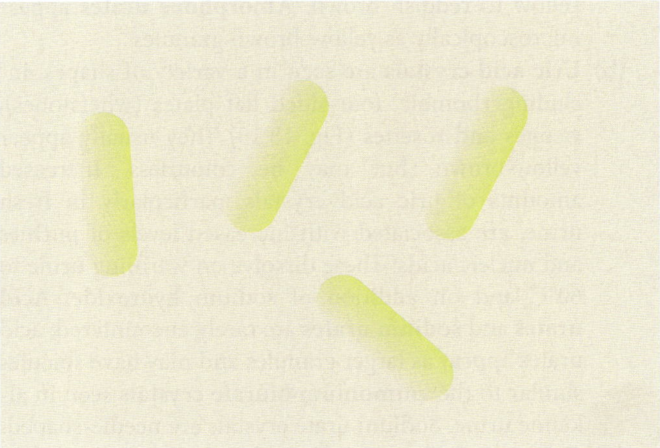

Fig. 18.13 Waxy cast.

(g) **Fatty casts** (Fig. 18.14) are seen when there is fatty degeneration of the tubular epithelium, as in degenerative tubular disease. Fatty casts also result from nephrotic syndrome, lupus, and toxic renal poisoning.

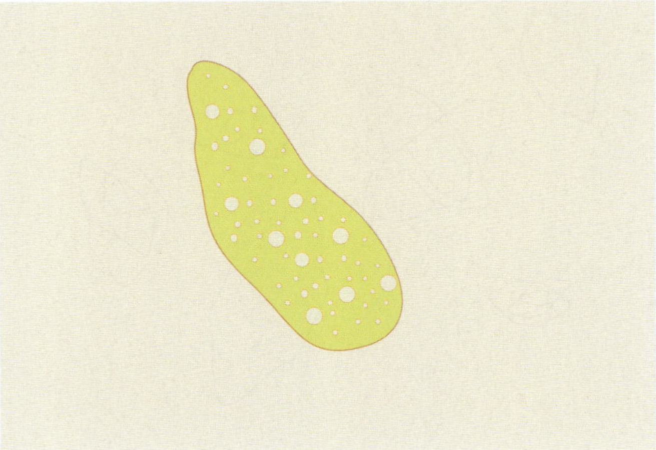

Fig. 18.14 Fatty cast.

6. **Yeast:** The yeast cells appear in the urine as small, refractile oval structures that may show budding. *Candida albicans* is the most common yeast observed and usually affects diabetic and immunocompromised patients.
7. **Parasites:** The most frequent parasite encountered in the urine is *Trichomonas vaginalis* (its trophozoite is a pear-shaped flagellate with an undulating membrane). The ova of the bladder parasite *Schistosoma haematobium* may also rarely appear in the urine.
8. **Urinary crystals:** Crystals frequently found in the urine are rarely of clinical significance. They may appear as geometrically formed structures or as amorphous material. Crystals are formed by the precipitation of urine solutes (inorganic and organic compounds, and medications).
   (a) **Normal deposits seen in acidic urine** include **urates (amorphous urates, uric acid, and sodium urate crystals)**. Microscopically, most urate crystals appear yellow to reddish brown. **Amorphous urates** appear microscopically as yellow-brown granules.
   (b) **Uric acid crystals** are seen in a variety of shapes, including rhombic, four-sided flat plates (whetstones), wedges and rosettes (Fig. 18.15) They usually appear yellow-brown, but may be colourless. Increased amounts of uric acid crystals, particularly in fresh urine, are associated with increased levels of purines and nucleic acids. These dissolve on warming urine to 60°C and on addition of sodium hydroxide. **Acid urates** and **sodium urates** are rarely encountered; acid urates appear as larger granules and may have spicules similar to the **ammonium biurate crystals** seen in alkaline urine. Sodium urate crystals are needle-shaped.
   (c) **Calcium oxalate** crystals are frequently seen in acidic urine, but they can be found in neutral urine and even rarely in alkaline urine. The most common form of calcium oxalate crystals is the dihydrate that is easily recognized as a colourless, octahedral envelope or as two pyramids joined at their bases (Fig. 18.16). Monohydrate calcium oxalate crystals are oval or dumbbell shaped. The finding of clumps of calcium oxalate crystals in fresh urine may be related to the formation of renal calculi, because most renal calculi are composed of calcium oxalate. They are also associated with foods high in oxalic acid, such as tomatoes and asparagus, and ascorbic acid, because oxalic acid is an end product of ascorbic acid metabolism.

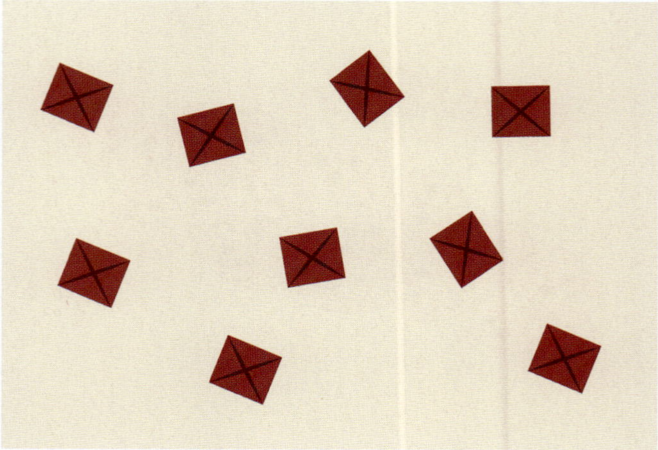

Fig. 18.16 Calcium oxalate crystals.

Normal Urinary Crystals

- **Normal deposits seen in alkaline urine** include **phosphates** (amorphous phosphate, triple phosphate, and calcium phosphate crystals), **calcium carbonate**, and **ammonium biurate. Amorphous phosphates** are granular in appearance (Fig. 18.17). **Triple phosphate (ammonium magnesium phosphate)** crystals are easily identified by their prism shape ('coffin lid') or feathery fern appearance (Fig. 18.18). They are often seen in urine associated with the presence of urea-splitting bacteria. **Calcium phosphate crystals** appear as colourless, flat rectangular plates or thin prisms (Fig. 18.19). **Calcium carbonate crystals** are small and colourless, with dumbbell or spherical shapes. **Ammonium biurate crystals** appear as yellow–brown 'thorny apples' (spicule-covered spheres; Fig. 18.20) and are usually

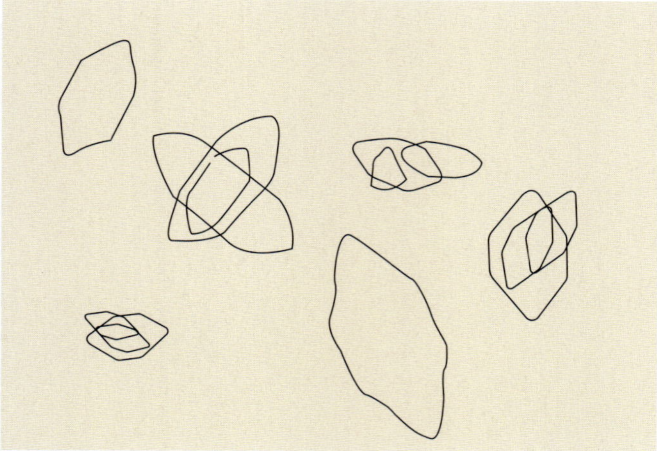

Fig. 18.15 Uric acid crystals.

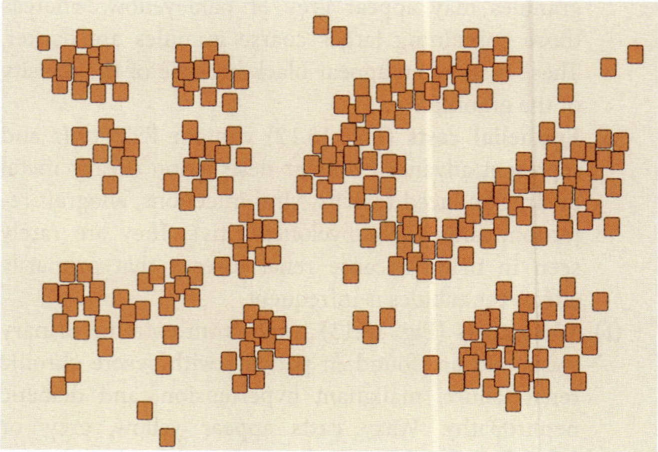

Fig. 18.17 Amorphous phosphates.

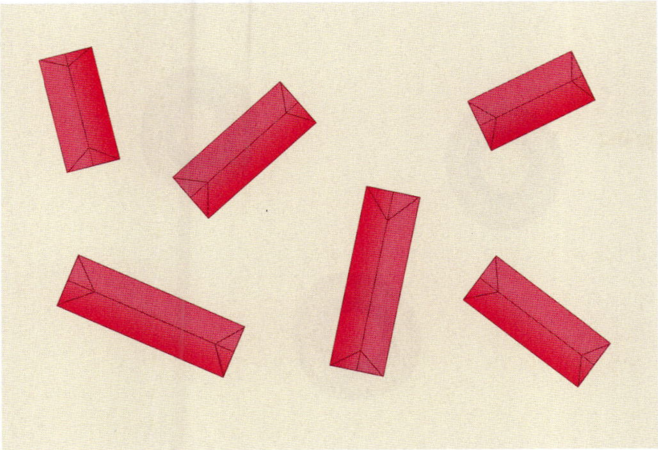

Fig. 18.18 Triple phosphate (ammonium magnesium phosphate).

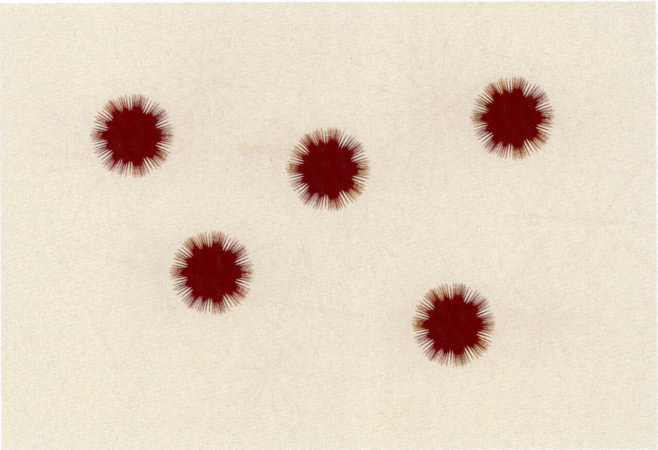

Fig. 18.20 Ammonium biurate crystals.

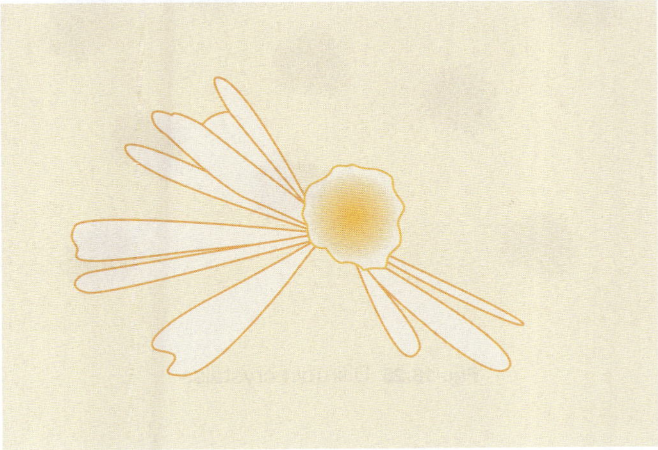

Fig. 18.19 Calcium phosphate crystals.

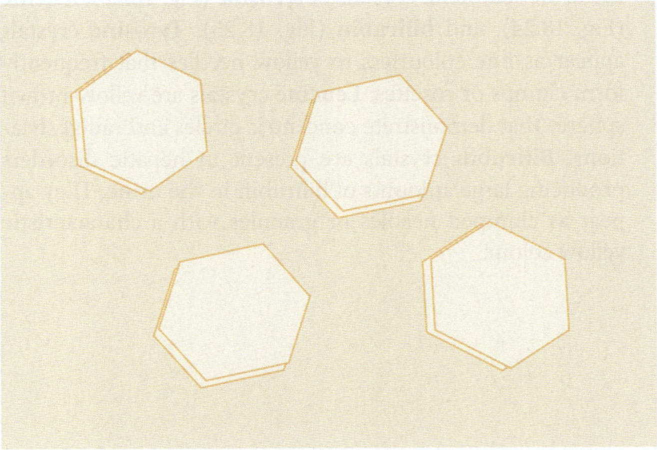

Fig. 18.21 Cystine crystals.

encountered in urine infected with ammonia produced by urea-splitting bacteria.

Abnormal Urine Crystals

Abnormal urine crystals are found in acidic urine or rarely in neutral urine and include the following:

- **Cystine crystals:** These are found in the urine of persons who inherit a metabolic disorder that prevents reabsorption of cystine by the renal tubules (cystinuria). Cystine crystals appear as colourless, hexagonal plates (Fig. 18.21).
- **Cholesterol crystals:** These are rarely seen unless specimens have been refrigerated, because the lipids remain in droplet form. They appear as rectangular plates with a notch in one or more corners and are associated with disorders producing lipiduria (Fig. 18.22).

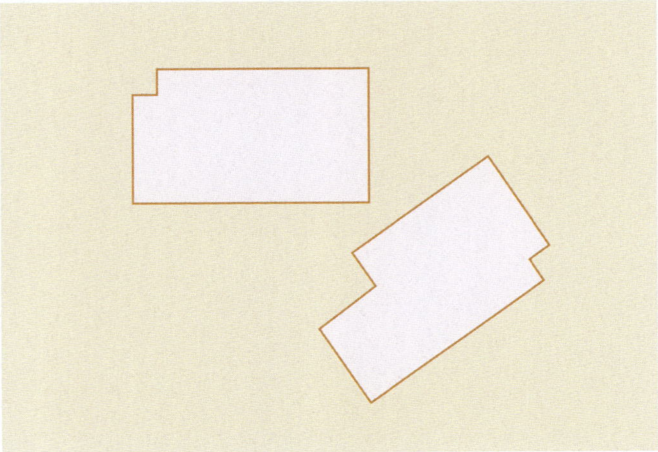

Fig. 18.22 Cholesterol crystals.

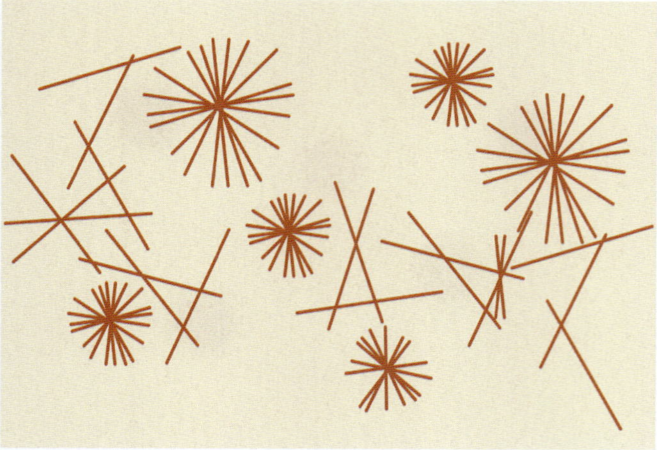

Fig. 18.23 Tyrosine crystals.

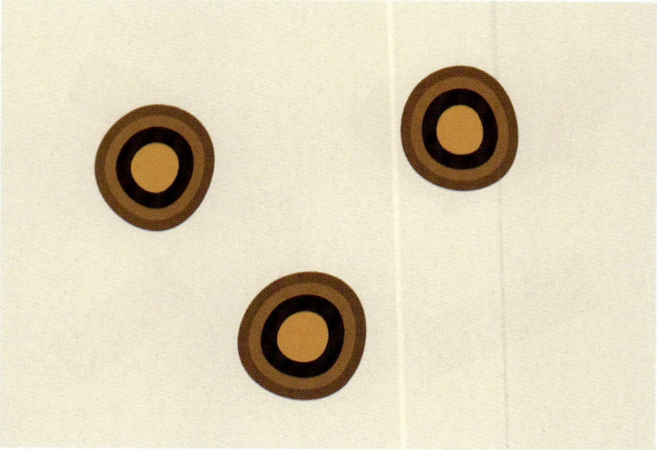

Fig. 18.24 Leucine crystals.

- **Crystals associated with liver disorders:** In the presence of severe liver disorders, three types of crystals may be found in the urine sediment: crystals of **tyrosine** (Fig. 18.23), **leucine** (Fig. 18.24), and **bilirubin** (Fig. 18.25). **Tyrosine** crystals appear as fine colourless to yellow needles that frequently form clumps or rosettes. **Leucine** crystals are yellow-brown spheres that demonstrate concentric circles and radial striations. **Bilirubin** crystals are present in hepatic disorders producing large amounts of bilirubin in the urine. They appear as clumped needles or granules with a characteristic yellow colour.

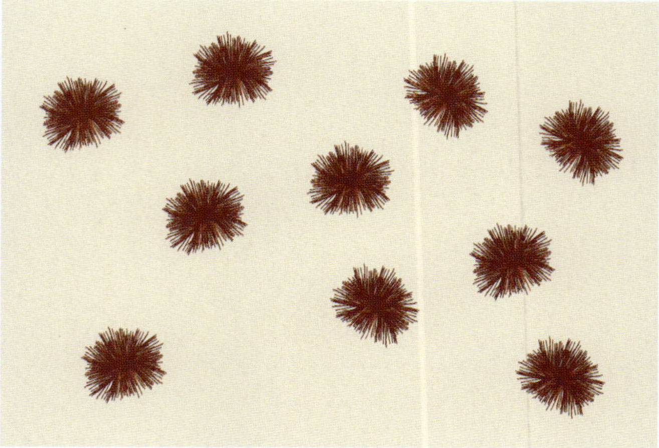

Fig. 18.25 Bilirubin crystals.

Examination of Body Fluids

19

Q. Write briefly on the steps in examination of synovial fluid.

Ans. Synovium refers to the tissue lining joint spaces, tendon sheaths, and bursae. It is composed of a 1–4 cell layer thick lining of synoviocytes (intima) overlying vascularised connective tissue (sub-intima). The intimal cells are of two types, fibroblast like synovial cells or type B cells and macrophage-like synovial cells or type A cells. The fibroblastic synovial cells (derived from mesenchyme) manufacture hyaluronan together with a molecule called lubricin, which lubricates the joint surfaces. The macrophage-like synovial cells (derived from monocytes in blood) are responsible for the removal of undesirable substances from the synovial fluid. The synoviocytes also contribute to the local production of cytokines and proteolytic enzymes that degrade the extracellular matrix (components of the inflammatory rheumatoid arthritis pathways).

Synovial fluid is an ultrafiltrate of blood plasma combined with hyaluronic acid produced by the synovial cells. Small ions and molecules like Na^+, K^+, glucose, urea can readily pass through into the joint space and are, therefore, similar in concentration to plasma, while large molecules are absent or present in trace amounts. Synovial fluid acts as a lubricant and adhesive and provides nutrients for the avascular articular cartilage.

Arthrocentesis is the removal of synovial fluid from a joint. A local anaesthetic is applied and then a needle is inserted into the space between the bones, and synovial fluid is collected. The specimen should ideally be separated into three parts: 3–10 mL into a sterile heparinized tube or syringe for microbiological studies; 2–5 mL in an anticoagulant tube (sodium heparin or liquid EDTA [ethylenediaminetetraacetic acid]) for microscopic examination; and approximately 5 mL into a plain (no anticoagulant) tube for chemical analysis (normal synovial fluid does not clot since fibrinogen is absent).

Indications

1. To diagnose the cause of joint inflammation, such as in infective, degenerative (osteoarthritis), inflammatory or autoimmune arthritis (rheumatoid arthritis and systemic lupus erythematosus [SLE]) (Table 19.1).
2. To diagnose crystallopathies such as gout and pseudogout.
3. Sometimes performed to monitor a patient with a known joint condition.
4. May be performed to drain excess synovial fluid to relieve pressure in the joint and for introduction of corticosteroids into the joint to help reduce inflammation and relieve pain.

Physical Characteristics

1. **Volume:** The average volume of synovial fluid in a joint is 0.1–2.0 mL.
2. **Colour:** Normal synovial fluid is straw-coloured. Purulent synovial fluid (in septic arthritis) appears yellowish-green. Reddish synovial fluid indicates the presence of red blood cells (RBCs).

Table 19.1 Categorization of disease based on findings of synovial fluid examination

		Category			
Finding	**Normal**	**Group I Non-inflammatory**	**Group II Inflammatory**	**Group III Infectious**	**Group IV Haemorrhagic**
Clarity	Transparent	Transparent	Transparent or opaque	Opaque	Opaque
Colour	Clear to pale yellow	Xanthochromic	Xanthochromic	White	Red-brown or xanthochromic
WBCs/mL	0–150	<3000	3000–75,000 Sodium fluoride can be used for glucose estimation.	50,000–200,000	50–10,000
Polymorphonuclear leukocytes (%)	<25	<30	>50	>90	<50
Glucose (blood/synovial fluid difference mg/dL)	0–10 (0–0.56 mmol/L)	0–10 (0–0.56 mmol/L)	0–40 (0–2.2 mmol/L)	20–100 (1.11–5.5 mmol/L)	0–20 (0–1.11 mmol/L)

WBC, White blood cell.

3. **Viscosity:** Viscosity is assessed by dropping the synovial fluid from a glass pipette. Normal synovial fluid produces a string effect, with a long tail owing to high viscosity. A raindrop pattern with a short tail is due to low viscosity. Inflammatory arthritis is associated with decreased viscosity (due to depolymerization of the hyaluronate chain), whereas a non-inflammatory effusion is characterized by increased viscosity.
4. **Clarity:** Normal synovial fluid is transparent and clear. A cloudy synovial fluid indicates the presence of microorganisms, white blood cells (WBCs), or crystals.
5. **Mucin clot test:** If synovial fluid is mixed with a few drops of 2% acetic acid, a mucin clot appears. A well-formed mucin clot is seen in normal and non-inflammatory effusions, and a friable mucin clot is characteristic of inflammatory, purulent and haemorrhagic arthritis (friability is due to fragmentation of hyaluronate–protein complexes).

Chemical Examination

1. **Glucose levels** in synovial fluid are typically equal or lower than blood and may be significantly lower in inflammation and infection. Glucose levels in synovial fluid are estimated by using the method used for estimation of blood sugar level.
2. **Protein levels** in synovial fluid are increased in inflammatory joint disease and bacterial infection and are estimated by biuret method. Normal levels range from 1.07 to 2.13 g/dL.
3. **Lactate dehydrogenase (LDH) levels** are increased in rheumatoid arthritis, infectious arthritis and gout.
4. **Uric acid levels** are increased in gout.

Microscopic Examination

Normal synovial fluid contains <150 cells/μL, mainly comprising synovial cells, chondrocytes, mononuclear cells and polymorphs. Total cell count is conducted by using haematological counting chambers. WBC counting method is used, but the acetic acid in WBC fluid is replaced by isotonic saline solution as the former precipitates the hyaluronate–protein complexes. For a differential count, the specimen is centrifuged at 2000 rpm for 10 minutes and a smear is prepared from the sediment and stained with Giemsa.

- **Non-inflammatory effusions** have a WBC count of <3000 cells/μL as seen in degenerative/osteoarthritis, traumatic arthritis, neuropathic arthropathy, pigmented villonodular synovitis, early rheumatoid arthritis, early bacterial infections, viral arthritis and early rheumatic fever. In viral arthritis, the WBC count in the synovial fluid is increased with predominantly mononuclear cells.
- **Inflammatory arthropathies** have a WBC count >3000 cells/μL as seen in rheumatoid arthritis, SLE, Reiter's syndrome, rheumatic fever, acute crystal-induced arthritis and psoriatic arthritis.
- **Bacterial (septic) arthritis**, gout, and rheumatoid arthritis are characterized by WBC counts exceeding 60,000 cells/μL. Bacterial, fungal and tuberculous joint infections constitute this group.
- **Synovial fluid in rheumatoid arthritis** commonly shows presence of cells called **'ragocytes'** (polymorphonuclear leukocytes, with cytoplasmic inclusions of aggregated immunoglobulin G, fibrin and complement). *Rheumatoid factor* is found in synovia of approximately 60% of rheumatoid arthritis patients, usually at a titre equal to or slightly lower than the serum titre. *Antinuclear antibodies* are found in the synovial fluid of approximately 70% of patients with systemic lupus erythematosus and 20% of patients with rheumatoid arthritis. Neither is specific enough for practical use.
- **Presence of RBCs** may indicate recent traumatic aspiration, traumatic arthritis, pigmented villonodular synovitis, synovial haemangioma and haematologic disorders (haemophilia, thrombocytopenia, anticoagulant therapy).
- Synovial fluid should be evaluated under polarized light to identify and to distinguish the types of **crystallopathy** that is present. Needle-like monosodium urate (MSU) crystals are associated with gout, and rhomboidal calcium pyrophosphate crystals are associated with pseudogout. MSU crystals show negative/yellow birefringence in compensated polarized light.

  Calcium pyrophosphate crystals show positive/blue birefringence in compensated polarized light.
- **Gram stain** and **culture testing** is ordered to determine the type of microorganism; susceptibility testing against certain antibiotics can be performed to guide antimicrobial therapy. An acid–fast bacilli smear and culture is done for diagnosing tuberculosis.

Q. Write briefly on the steps in examination of cerebrospinal fluid. (PA35.1)

Ans. Cerebrospinal fluid (CSF) is formed by the choroid plexus, presumably through the process of ultra-filtration and secretion. It protects the brain and spinal cord, circulates nutrients and collects waste. **Blood–brain barrier** is the barrier between the brain and the blood. It consists of two morphologically unique components: a layer of capillary endothelium held together by intercellular tight junctions, and the choroid plexus, where specialized choroidal ependymal cells are bound by tight junctions overlies fenestrated capillaries.

Specimen Collection

CSF is collected for diagnostic or therapeutic purposes by a technique called **'lumbar puncture,'** which involves the insertion of a spinal needle into the subarachnoid space of the region between the third and fourth lumbar vertebrae (lumbar region is most often used as it allows the needle to be inserted below the end of the spinal cord). After measuring the opening pressure, collect a few millilitres of fluid in three separate collection tubes under strictly sterile conditions. Label tubes in order of sampling (Tube #1: chemical tests, Tube #2: microbiological examination, and Tube #3: cell counts).

Note: Do not remove more than a total of 15–20 mL.

Precautions

The patient should not be on any anticoagulant therapy, and the platelet count should be >50,000/mm³.

Indications

CSF examination is used for the diagnosis of:

1. Bacterial, fungal, tubercular and viral meningitis (Table 19.2).

Table 19.2 Pathological findings in different types of meningitis

Feature	Normal cerebrospinal fluid (CSF)	Acute pyogenic (bacterial) meningitis	Acute lymphocytic (viral) meningitis	Chronic (tuberculous) meningitis
Naked eye appearance	Clear and colourless	Cloudy or frankly purulent	Clear or slightly turbid	Slightly turbid; forms fibrin coagulum on standing
CSF pressure	60–150 mm H_2O	Elevated (>180 mm H_2O)	Elevated	Elevated
Protein level	15–45 mg/dL	Markedly raised due to increased permeability of blood–CSF barrier	Raised	Raised
Glucose level	50–80 mg/dL	Markedly reduced due to impaired glucose transport and increased glucose utilization by white blood cells and microorganisms	Normal	Reduced
CSF cytology	0–4 lymphocytes/μL	10–10,000 neutrophils/μL	10–100 lymphocytes/μL	100–1000 lymphocytes/μL

2. Carcinomatous meningitis (metastatic carcinoma, leukaemia/lymphoma).
3. Encephalopathy.
4. Subarachnoid haemorrhage.
5. Spinal canal blockage.
6. CNS syphilis.

Physical Characteristics of CSF

- **Daily production** of CSF is approximately 500 mL, and its total volume is 100–150 mL.
- **Normal opening pressure** in lateral decubitus position in adults is 75–200 mm H_2O and in children 10–100 mm H_2O.
- **Causes of elevated opening pressure** include poliomyelitis, encephalitis, congestive heart failure, meningitis, superior vena cava syndrome, cerebral oedema and a mass lesion. **Decreased opening pressure** is observed in spinal–subarachnoid block, dehydration, circulatory collapse and CSF leakage.
- Normally CSF is clear and colourless. Turbidity appears when the cell count is >500/μL.
- Normal CSF does not show clot formation. Increased protein level may lead to spontaneous clotting of the specimen.
- Coloured CSF is abnormal and usually occurs after a traumatic tap, in which case there is less blood staining in the second and third tubes. Uniform red colouring of all three tubes suggests recent bleeding into the subarachnoid space. **Xanthochromia** (increased CSF bilirubin level) may be seen within 12 hours of a subarachnoid haemorrhage and may persist for up to 3 weeks. It may also be seen in any condition in which CSF protein level is very high and in patients with jaundice.

Microscopic Examination of CSF

- Transfer well-mixed fluid into the counting chamber of the haemocytometer. CSF total leukocyte count is done like the total blood WBC count.
- Cell count must be done within one hour after removal of CSF since the cells start disintegrating after that. Normal CSF has 0–8 lymphocytes/μL, without any erythrocytes or granulocytes. Greater than 10 cells /μL is considered abnormal.
- Neutrophilic leukocytosis is usually associated with bacterial (pyogenic) meningitis, cerebral abscess, and central nervous system haemorrhage. Mixed leukocytosis may be seen in tuberculosis. Lymphocytic leukocytosis is characteristic of viral infections, meningismus, brain tumour and multiple sclerosis.

Microbiological Examination

- Gram stain, bacterial culture and antigen detection studies.
- India ink preparation and antigen detection test for *Cryptococcus.*
- Serological testing for specific diseases, for example syphilis.
- Nucleic acid probes after polymerase chain reaction amplification for detection of *Mycobacterium tuberculosis*, herpes simplex virus, enteroviruses, cytomegalovirus and *Toxoplasma gondii.*
- Viral culture.

Chemical Examination

Protein

- CSF total protein level can be measured by turbidometric or colorimetric methods.
- Normal protein content of CSF is 15–45 mg/dL. Infants have higher values, presumably because of the immaturity of blood–brain barrier.
- Elevated protein level is seen in acute meningitis, subarachnoid haemorrhage, and **'Froin's syndrome'** (generally due to loculation or presence of a tumour; is a combination of very high protein level, xanthochromia and lymphocytic pleocytosis).
- Increased CSF gamma globulin level may be seen when the total protein level is within normal limits (e.g. multiple sclerosis, neurosyphilis, leukoencephalitis, and some degenerative diseases). This fraction can be determined by protein electrophoresis.

Glucose

- The normal CSF glucose levels vary between 50–80 mg/dL (60%–80% of serum glucose levels).
- Elevated CSF glucose level is observed in diabetes mellitus. Decreased levels are generally associated with bacterial

meningitis and meningeal dissemination of tumours (rapid glycolysis by bacteria, leukocytes and tumour cells).

Other tests

- **Chloride:** Normal: 120–128 mEq/L; may be low in tuberculosis. This is probably a non-specific change and has no diagnostic significance.
- **Enzymes:** Levels of 'creatinine kinase' may be elevated in cerebral infarction.
- **Lactic acid:** Levels of lactic acid are inversely proportional to glucose levels.
- **Cytology:** May be undertaken for detection of malignant cells.

Q. Write briefly on the steps in examination of pleural fluid. (IM4.12)

Ans. The pleural cavity is a potential space lined by mesothelium of the visceral and parietal pleura. The pleural cavity normally contains a small amount of fluid that facilitates movement of the two membranes against each other. An accumulation of fluid is called an **effusion**, which results from an imbalance of fluid production and reabsorption. A sample of pleural fluid can be obtained by a procedure called **thoracocentesis (pleural tap)**. **Indications** for thoracocentesis include:

1. Evaluation of the cause of effusion (Table 19.3).
2. Differentiate a transudate from exudate.
3. Symptomatic treatment of a large pleural effusion.

Procedure

Pleural tap is an invasive procedure, which removes fluid from the pleural space for diagnostic or therapeutic purposes. A cannula, or hollow needle, is carefully introduced into the thorax, along the mid-axillary line, in the ninth intercostals space, generally after administration of local anaesthesia. It is critical that patients hold their breath to avoid piercing of the lung. The aspiration should not exceed 1 L, as there is a risk of development of pulmonary oedema.

Contraindications

1. An uncooperative patient.
2. Uncorrected coagulation disorder.
3. Emphysema; using mechanical ventilation, and only one functioning lung (relative contraindications).
4. Chest wall cellulitis at the site of puncture.

Table 19.3 Cellular differential of pleural effusions

Neutrophilia (>50%)

- Acute bacterial pneumonia
- Pulmonary infarction
- Acute pancreatitis
- Subphrenic abscess
- Early stage of tuberculosis

Lymphocytosis (>50%)

- Tuberculosis
- Viral infection
- Malignancy
- Chylothorax
- Autoimmune diseases (Rheumatoid pleuritis and systemic lupus erythematosus)
- Uraemia

Pleural fluid (5 mL) is collected in a green-top (heparin) tube for evaluation of levels of amylase, cholesterol, glucose, lactate dehydrogenase (LDH), pH, protein, and triglycerides; lavender-top (EDTA) tube for cell count; sterile containers for microbiology specimens; and 200–500 mL of fluid in a clear container with anticoagulant for cytology (ensure that there is an equal amount of fixative and fluid in the container for cytology).

Complications

Major complications of this procedure include:

1. Pneumothorax.
2. Haemorrhage.
3. Hypotension (due to a vasovagal response).
4. Pulmonary oedema.

Minor complications include a dry tap, subcutaneous *haematoma*, dyspnoea, and cough (after removing large volume of fluid). The use of ultrasound for needle guidance can minimize the complication rate.

Normal pleural fluid is a clear ultra-filtrate of plasma with the following characteristics:

- Normal amount is 50 mL.
- Red blood cells (RBCs) are absent.
- White blood cell (WBC) count is less than 1000 WBCs/mm^3.
- Protein level is less than 1–2 g/dL.
- Glucose level ranges between 70 and 100 mg/dL.
- Amylase level ranges from 138 to 404 units/L.
- pH is about 7.6.
- LDH level is less than 50% of plasma.
- Sodium, potassium and calcium concentrations are similar to that of the interstitial fluid.

Exudates and transudates are distinguished based on total protein concentrations being above (exudates) or below (transudates) 3.0 g/dL. However, using total protein alone misclassifies both exudates and transudates in a substantial number of cases (30%). It is now well accepted that test combinations increase sensitivity and improve accuracy, and these are the basis for the well-established **Light's criteria (1972)**, as given below.

Transudative effusions are caused by a combination of increased hydrostatic pressure and decreased oncotic pressure in the pulmonary or systemic circulation, for example **heart failure, cirrhosis and hypoalbuminaemia, usually from the nephrotic syndrome**. A transudative effusion is characterized by the following:

- Pleural fluid/serum protein ratio <0.5 or absolute value <3 g/dL.
- Pleural fluid/serum LDH ratio <0.6 or absolute value <0.45 upper normal serum limit.
- Pleural fluid specific gravity <1.018.

Exudative effusions are caused by local pathology leading to increased capillary permeability, for example, **tuberculosis,**

pyogenic infections (pneumonia, lung abscess, bronchiectasis), viral and fungal infections, neoplasms, trauma to chest wall, osteomyelitis, post-myocardial infarction syndrome, amoebic liver abscess, acute pancreatitis, systemic disorders (systemic lupus erythematosus, rheumatoid arthritis and septicaemia). An **exudative effusion** is characterized by the following:

- Pleural fluid/serum protein ratio >0.5 or absolute value >3 g/dL.
- Pleural fluid/serum LDH ratio >0.6 or absolute value >0.45 upper normal serum limit.
- Pleural fluid specific gravity >1.018.

Gross Examination

- Transudates are typically clear or straw-coloured.
- Malignancy, tuberculosis, trauma, pulmonary infarction and pancreatitis may result in a haemorrhagic effusion.
- Bacterial infections or empyema induce a cloudy, turbid pleural effusion.
- Milky white effusion is the result of lymphatic obstruction.
- Greenish effusion results from infection with pseudomonas, streptococcus and pneumococcus.

Microscopic Examination

- RBC count >100,000 cells/ mm^3 may be due to malignancy, trauma, pulmonary embolism and bleeding diathesis.
- If WBC count is elevated with neutrophils >50%, acute pleuritis or other pyogenic infections should be suspected.
- If WBC count is elevated with lymphocytes >90%, a tuberculous pathology, lymphoma or epithelial malignancies should be suspected.
- If WBC count is elevated with eosinophils >10%, asbestos effusion, parasitic infections or pneumothorax are the differentials.

Bacteriological Examination

- Gram stain and culture establishes aetiology of infection.
- Sensitivity testing guides therapy.
- Acid–fast smears and cultures can identify tuberculosis.

Cytological Examination

- Sample is collected in a 50 mL heparinized bottle. Taking three samples maximizes correct results.
- Cytology is positive in approximately 60% of malignant pleural effusions. Negative test results are related to factors such as the type of tumour (commonly negative with mesothelioma, sarcoma and lymphoma), the tumour burden in the pleural space, and the expertise of the cytologist.

Chemical Analysis

Protein

The measurement of pleural fluid total protein or albumin level has little clinical value except when combined with other parameters to differentiate exudates from transudates.

Glucose

The glucose level of normal pleural fluid, transudates and most exudates is similar to serum levels. Decreased pleural fluid glucose level, accepted as a level below 60 mg/dL or a pleural fluid/serum glucose ratio less than 0.5, is most consistent and dramatic in rheumatoid pleuritis and grossly purulent pneumonic exudates. Low pleural fluid glucose level may also be present in malignancy, tuberculosis, lupus pleuritis and oesophageal rupture.

Others

- **Antinuclear antibodies or ANA** (a ratio of pleural fluid ANA to serum ANA >1.0 suggests systemic lupus erythematosus).
- **Rheumatoid factor** >640 U/mL suggests rheumatoid-related effusion.
- **Adenosine deaminase** >70 IU/L suggests tuberculosis.
- A high **amylase** level (twice the serum level or absolute value greater than 160 Somogy units) in the pleural fluid is indicative of either acute or chronic pancreatitis, or pancreatic pseudocyst that has dissected or ruptured into the pleural space, cancer or oesophageal rupture.

Q. Write briefly on the steps in examination of ascitic fluid. (IM4.12)

Ans. Ascites is the presence of excess fluid in the peritoneal cavity. Up to 50 mL of fluid is normally present in the peritoneal cavity. Aspiration of ascitic fluid for diagnostic and therapeutic purpose is called **ascitic tap.**

Procedure: Obtain 50–100 mL of ascitic fluid by diagnostic paracentesis from the linea alba region, 2 cm below the umbilicus, by using a 22-gauge needle. Routine evaluation includes gross inspection; analysis for total protein, albumin and glucose levels; total and differential cell counts; culture; and cytology. In some instances, ascitic amylase, lactate dehydrogenase (LDH), and triglyceride levels also need to be analyzed.

Indications

- **Diagnostic paracentesis** (patients with ascites of unknown aetiology, patients with suspected infections).
- **Therapeutic paracentesis** is indicated when ascites fluid has accumulated enough to cause respiratory compromise, abdominal pain, or worsening of existing inguinal or umbilical hernias.

Contraindications

1. Severe coagulopathy not correctable by vitamin K, fresh frozen plasma, etc.
2. Inability of physician to demonstrate ascites fluid on physical examination.
3. Lack of patient cooperation.

Precautions

1. Prothrombin and partial thromboplastin time must be performed prior to paracentesis.
2. Very large amounts of fluid should not be removed in one instance to avoid hypotension.
3. If ascites fluid leaks persistently from the puncture site, the patient should be made to remain supine with the site angled directly upwards, until the leak stops spontaneously.

Complications

1. Abdominal wall haematoma (rare, only approximately 2% of cases in some studies).
2. Infection (also extremely rare).

Classification of Ascites

1. **Based on aetiology:**

   Increased hydrostatic pressure
   - Cirrhosis
   - Hepatic vein occlusion (Budd–Chiari's syndrome)
   - Inferior vena cava obstruction
   - Constrictive pericarditis
   - Congestive heart failure

   Decreased colloid osmotic pressure
   - End-stage liver disease with diminished protein synthesis
   - Nephrotic syndrome with protein loss
   - Malnutrition
   - Protein-losing enteropathy

   Increased permeability of peritoneal capillaries
   - Tuberculous and bacterial infections
   - Malignancies

   Miscellaneous causes
   - Pancreatic ascites (leakage of fluid from a pancreatic pseudo cyst)
   - Myxoedema
   - Ovarian disease (Meig's syndrome)
   - Chronic haemodialysis

2. **Based on composition of fluid:** Ascites fluid is traditionally categorized as either 'exudative' or 'transudative' on the basis of laboratory analysis. Transudative ascites (LDH <200 units/L, ascites/serum protein ratio <0.5, ascites/serum LDH ratio <0.6) is caused mainly by cirrhosis, that is, increased portal venous pressure or decreased portal venous colloid osmotic pressure. Exudative ascites (values outside the above range) is generally non-cirrhotic in its pathophysiology and may be due to peritoneal membrane permeability defects.

   Transudative ascites
   - Cirrhosis
   - Congestive heart failure
   - Hepatic vein obstruction (Budd–Chiari's syndrome)
   - Nephrotic syndrome
   - Meig's ovarian tumour syndrome
   - Constrictive pericarditis
   - Inferior vena cava obstruction
   - Viral hepatitis with submassive or massive hepatic necrosis

   Exudative ascites
   - Neoplastic diseases involving the peritoneum
   - Tuberculous peritonitis
   - Pancreatitis
   - Post-surgical peritonitis

Gross Appearance

- **Normal ascitic fluid is clear to pale yellow.** **Milky/chylous ascites may be a manifestation of** lymphoma, tuberculosis, parasitic infection and lymphatic obstruction.
- **Cloudy/turbid fluid is a feature of** spontaneous bacterial peritonitis, perforated bowel, appendicitis and pancreatitis.
- **Haemorrhagic ascites may develop in association with neoplasms, ha**emorrhagic pancreatitis and perforated peptic ulcer.

Biochemistry

- **Normal protein level ranges between 0.3 and 4.0 g/dL. Protein level is elevated in tuberculous pathology.**
- **Glucose:** In uncomplicated ascites, glucose level is similar to that in the serum. The levels can drop drastically in spontaneous bacterial peritonitis, particularly in late stages, secondary to bacterial consumption.
- **Serum–ascites albumin gap (SAAG):** SAAG is calculated by subtracting the ascitic fluid albumin value from the serum albumin value, and it correlates directly with portal pressure. It is the best single test for classifying ascites into portal hypertensive (SAAG >1.1 g/dL) and non-portal hypertensive (SAAG <1.1 g/dL) causes. Non-portal hypertensive causes include peritoneal carcinomatosis, inflammation of the pancreas or biliary system, nephrotic syndrome, and peritonitis.
- **Triglyceride concentration** may be elevated is chylous ascites.

Cell Count

Normal ascitic fluid contains fewer than 500 leukocytes/μL and fewer than 250 polymorphonuclear leukocytes or neutrophils/μL. A count greater than 250 cells/μL is highly suggestive of bacterial peritonitis. In tuberculous peritonitis and peritoneal carcinomatosis, lymphocytes usually predominate. When the red blood cell count is >50,000/μL, it denotes haemorrhagic ascites, which is usually due to malignancy, tuberculosis, or trauma.

Cytology

Cytology smears are reported to be 58%–75% sensitive for detection of malignant ascites.

Gram Stain and Culture

Culture has 92% sensitivity for the detection of bacteria in ascitic fluid, and Gram stain is only 10% sensitive for visualizing bacteria in bacterial peritonitis.

Semen Analysis

20

Q. Write briefly on the steps in examination of semen. (PA23.3)

Ans. Conventional semen analysis includes measurement of sperm concentration, motility and morphology, identification and quantification of cells other than spermatozoa (Table 20.1).

Normal semen comprises spermatozoa suspended in secretions from the testis and epididymis, which are also mixed at the time of ejaculation with secretions from the prostate, seminal vesicles and bulbourethral glands. Semen analysis is used for the evaluation of reproductive dysfunction, that is, infertility, for selection of donors for therapeutic insemination and also to monitor the success of varicocelectomy and vasectomy.

Specimen collection: Examination of seminal fluid is done for investigating male infertility. The following instructions for sample collection and delivery are given to the subject:

- The sample should be collected after a minimum of 48 hours and no longer than 7 days of sexual abstinence. Multiple semen specimens should be analyzed for a reliable evaluation of male infertility.
- Ideally, the sample should be collected near the laboratory. If not, it should be delivered to the laboratory within 1 hour of collection. The sample should be examined immediately after liquefaction and within 1 hour of ejaculation and should be protected from extremes of temperature.
- The sample should be collected in a clean, wide-mouthed glass or plastic container. Incomplete samples should be not analyzed, particularly if the first portion of the ejaculate is lost.

Macroscopic Evaluation

- A normal sample is **grey–opalescent** in colour, homogenous and **liquefies within 30 minutes at room temperature** under the influence of enzymes of prostatic origin. The liquefaction time should be recorded, as it may suggest functional disturbance of the prostate. Semen acquires a yellowish tint with ageing. Presence of blood in semen (haematospermia) leads to a brownish or red coloured ejaculate. Brown semen may also be due to infection/inflammation of the prostate, urethra, epididymis or seminal vesicles. The sample may appear clear if the sperm concentration is too low.
- The semen sample should be well mixed. Incomplete mixing can lead to errors in calculating the sperm counts.
- The **viscosity** of the liquefied sample can be estimated by aspiration into a 5-mL pipette and then allowing the semen to drop by gravity and observing the length of the thread formed. A normal sample leaves the needle as small discrete drops, while in cases of abnormal consistency, the drop will form a thread of >2 cm. Increased consistency may be related to prostate dysfunction due to chronic inflammation.
- The **volume** of the ejaculate is approximately 2–6 mL. A low ejaculate volume can reflect abnormalities in accessory sex gland fluid synthesis/secretion or physical obstruction somewhere in the reproductive tract. Large volumes can be found in association with varicocele or after relatively long periods of sexual abstinence.
- The **pH** is determined by acidic secretions of the prostate and alkaline secretions of the seminal vesicles. It should normally be in the range of 7.2–8.0.

Microscopic Examination

Sperm morphology: Ideally, a sperm should have a regular oval head, with a connecting mid-piece and a long straight tail (Fig. 20.1). Abnormalities of sperm morphology include round heads, pinheads, very large heads, double heads and absent tails. A normal sample should have at least 15% normal forms (which means even up to 85% abnormal forms is considered to be acceptable).

The sperm concentration can be estimated roughly during the initial examination. A fixed volume of semen (not more

Table 20.1 Normal values of semen variables

Standard tests	
Volume	>2.0 mL
pH	7.2–8.0
Sperm concentration	20×10^6 spermatozoa/mL or more
Total sperm count	$>15 \times 10^6$ spermatozoa per ejaculate or more
Motility	*50% or more with forward progression or 25% or more with rapid progression within 60 minutes of ejaculation
Morphology	30% or more with normal forms
Vitality	75% or more live
White blood cells	Fewer than 1×10^6/mL
Immunobead test	Fewer than 20% spermatozoa with adherent particles
Mixed antiglobulin reaction test	Fewer than 10% spermatozoa with adherent particles

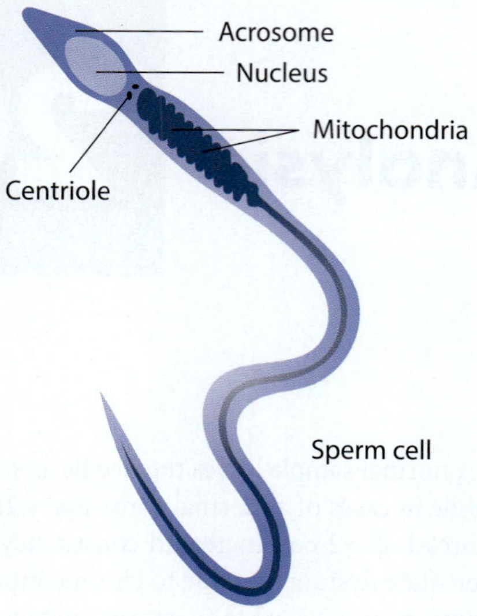

Fig. 20.1 Sperm cell.

than 10 mL) is delivered onto a clean glass slide and covered with a 22 mm × 22 mm coverslip. The microscopic field is scanned for the count and motility of spermatozoa.

Sperm count: This can be done by using the haemocytometer method. In this procedure, a 1:20 dilution from each well-mixed sample is prepared by diluting 50 mL of liquefied semen with 950 mL diluent. The latter is prepared by adding 50 g of sodium carbonate ($NaHCO_3$), 10 mL of 35% formalin, and, optionally, 0.25 g of trypan blue or 5 mL of saturated aqueous gentian violet to distilled water and making up the solution to a final volume of 1000 mL. A count less than 10×10^6 spermatozoa/mL is labelled **oligospermia**. Absence of sperms is called **azoospermia**. Cells other than spermatozoa include polygonal cells from the urethral tract, germ cells, spermatogonia and white blood cells (WBCs). While a few WBCs (pus cells) in the semen are considered normal, many suggest the presence of seminal infection. Pus cells can be confused with sperm precursor cells (which are normally found in the semen).

Sperm motility: Motility is described as the percentage of sperms demonstrating flagellar motion viewed on a bright-field or phase-contrast microscope. Normal motility is defined as more than 60% of sperm having normal movement, and the WHO 2010 lower reference limit (5th percentile) is 40%. Motility is graded as follows:

- Grade 0: No movement
- Grade 1: Sluggish movement
- Grade 2: Slow movement in a poorly defined direction
- Grade 3: Slow or curved forward movement
- Grade 4: Fast movement straight forward

Another way to measure motility is based on *motility grade*, where the motility of sperm is divided into four different grades:

- Grade a: Sperm with progressive motility. These swim fast in a straight line. Sometimes it is also denoted motility IV.
- Grade b: (non-linear motility): These also move forward but tend to travel in a curved or crooked motion. Sometimes also denoted motility III.
- Grade c: These have non-progressive motility. The tails move but there is no forward movement. Sometimes also denoted motility II.
- Grade d: These are immotile and fail to move at all. Sometimes also denoted motility I.

Sperm agglutination: Under the microscope, this is seen as the sperms clumping together. Agglutination impairs sperm motility.

If the sperm test is abnormal, it will need to be repeated 3–4 times over a period of 3–6 months to confirm whether the abnormality is persistent or not.

Sperm viability: Vital staining of the spermatozoa is done for measuring the fraction of viable sperms independently of their motility. Live and dead sperm are distinguished by adding one drop of eosin Y stain to one drop of semen and smearing the mixture on a microscopic slide. If the stain has passed through the membrane, the cell is considered dead, if it remains unstained, the cell is considered alive. This staining technique makes it possible to differentiate spermatozoa that are immotile but alive from those that are dead.

Immunological tests: The most specific antibodies to assess immunologic infertility are the ones binding to head or tail antigens. These antibodies are usually of the IgA (most significant) or IgG classes, and rarely of the IgM class and can be demonstrated by **direct or indirect mixed agglutination reaction (mixed antiglobulin reaction or MAR) tests** for IgG and IgA or by **immunobead assay**, which detects all classes but with varying sensitivity. Both tests require motile sperm. The direct MAR test can be performed on fresh semen, and the result can be read within a few minutes with a light microscope. Semen is mixed with latex particles coated with non-specific human IgG. Monospecific antisera to human IgG is added. The anti-IgG bridges the sperm-bound IgG, if present, and particle-bound IgG, to form mixed agglutinates. In the absence of sperm-bound IgG, the anti-IgG agglutinates only the latex particles. Under light microscopy, the localized binding of the particles identifies the antibody as being specific to head, tail or any other region of the sperm structure. An indirect test can also be done with this reagent to detect the presence of sperm antibody in semen, cervical mucus, or serum.

Computer-Aided Semen Analysis (CASA)

CASA is a semi-automated technique that uses a video camera and computer to analyze sperm concentration and movement. It measures the following parameters:

- Curvilinear velocity: The average distance per unit time between successive sperm positions.
- Straight-line velocity: The speed of forward movement.
- Linearity: The straight-line velocity divided by the curvilinear velocity.
- It also measures the average path velocity, the amplitude of lateral head displacement, and the flagellar beat frequency, and it is used to evaluate for evidence of hyperactivation.

Though CASA produces excellent results it is mainly used for research purposes due to cost constraints.

Immunohaematology

21

Q. What are blood groups? Enumerate the important blood group systems (PA22.1).

Ans. Blood groups are genetically determined antigens that can be detected on the RBC surface by specific antibodies (Table 21.1).

Q. What is the clinical significance of the ABO blood group system? (PA22.1)

Ans. The ABO system (Table 21.2) is the product of one gene locus situated on chromosome 9, which determines the expression of ABO blood groups on RBCs, endothelial cells and some epithelial cells.

- The basic precursor substance in ABO antigens has a short chain of sugars.
- There are two types of chains: Type I and Type II chains, which differ from each other in the way the terminal galactose joins the *N*-acetyl glucosamine residue.
- The basic precursor substance is converted to **H substance** by **L-fucosyltransferase** (**H gene** codes for this transferase that attaches fucose to the terminal end of the precursor substance to produce **H antigen**).
- The **A gene** codes for a transferase that attaches ***N*-acetyl-galactosamine** to the precursor substance, thereby producing A antigen (blood group A).
- The **B gene** codes for a transferase that attaches **galactose** to the precursor substance to produce **B antigen** (blood group B).
- The **O gene** is inactive; hence, neither A, nor B antigens are present on the surface of blood group O RBCs.

Table 21.1 Important blood group systems

Name of blood group system	Name of antigens
ABO	H, A_1, A_2 and B
Rh	D, C, E, c and e
P	P and p
MNS	M, N, S and s
Lutheran (Lu)	Lu^a and Lu^b
Lewis (Le)	Le^a and Le^b
Duffy (Fy)	Fy^a and Fy^b
Kidd (JK)	JK and JK

- **Group AB** individuals have H antigen that carries both A or B active sugars.
- An individual receives one blood group antigen from the mother and one from the father.
- Antibodies belonging to ABO system are naturally occurring, IgM type, complete antibodies (capable of agglutinating RBCs in saline suspension).
- The A group contains about twenty subgroups, of which A1 and A2 are the most common. A1 makes up 80% of all A type blood while A2 makes up for the rest.

Q. What is the clinical significance of the Bombay Phenotype (hh)? (PA22.1)

Ans. Some individuals do not inherit the H gene and are not able to express substance H on their RBCs and thus, do not produce A or B antigens. Instead, they produce antibodies to substance H and both A and B antigens. They can receive blood only from other hh donors but can donate like group O individuals.

Q. Write briefly on 'routine ABO blood grouping'. (PA22.2)

Ans. Routine ABO grouping

- Includes both cell and serum testing.
- ABO testing should be done at room temperature or lower.
- Controls should always be run during ABO grouping.

There are two types of grouping:

- **Forward type** identifies the blood group antigen on the surface of RBCs by using anti-A and anti-B test serum.
- In **reverse grouping**, group A and B red cells are allowed to react with patient serum to identify the isohaemagglutinins that correspond with the blood group.

Table 21.2 ABO blood group

Blood group	Antigen on cell surface	Antibody in serum
A	A	Anti-A
B	B	Anti-B
AB	A and B	Neither
O	Neither anti-A or anti-B	Anti-A, B

- Before transfusion, the ABO system must be appropriately matched between recipient and donor.
- For example, a blood group A person, who has anti-B IgM antibodies, can receive only A or O blood.
- Individuals with blood group O can receive only O blood owing to the presence of anti-A IgM, anti-B IgM and anti-A,B IgG in their serum, which would destroy cells with A or B antigen on their surface.
- Individuals with blood group AB (universal recipient) may receive blood from any group, since they have no isohaemagglutinins to destroy the transfused cells.

Q. Write briefly on different blood group systems besides ABO system. (PA22.1)

Ans. Blood group systems besides ABO system include:

1. **Rh antigen system**
   (a) The Rh antigen system has three closely linked gene loci, coding for D antigen (there is no d antigen), C and/or c antigen and E and/or e antigen.
   (b) Thus, the antigens produced are C, D, E, c and e.
   (c) An individual may have similar or different sets of these three Rh antigens on each chromosome; for example, CDE/cde, cde/cde, or CdE/cdE (each person inherits one trio gene from each parent).
   (d) Individuals who are positive for D antigen are considered Rh-positive (85% of the population) and those who lack it are Rh-negative.
   (e) Individuals with a weak variant of D antigen, called the **Du variant,** are also considered Rh-positive.
   (f) **Alloimmunization** (formation of an antibody against an antigen) occurs if a person is exposed to an Rh antigen that is not on the patient's RBCs (e.g. an Rh-negative person exposed to Rh-positive RBCs may develop anti-D antibodies).
   (g) The majority of clinically important antibodies that produce a transfusion reaction are warm-reacting (IgG) antibodies (e.g. anti-D, anti-Kell) rather than cold-reacting (IgM) antibodies.
2. **Duffy antigen system:** African-Americans commonly lack **Duffy (Fy) antigens** on their RBCs, which protect their cells from *Plasmodium vivax* infestation, since *P. vivax* requires Duffy antigen as a receptor to bind to the RBCs.
3. **I antigen system:** May be associated with cold-reacting IgM antibodies against i antigen or I antigens leading to a cold autoimmune haemolytic anaemia (e.g. anti-i is associated with infectious mononucleosis and anti-I with *Mycoplasma pneumoniae* infection).
4. **Lewis antigens** are closely related to ABH antigens and are produced in body secretions. Naturally occurring IgM antibodies develop against these antigens, but they are generally weak antibodies of no clinical importance.

Q. Write briefly on the principles of blood transfusion. (PA22.2)

Ans. Blood transfusion involves the collection, storage and infusion of a donor's blood to a recipient. Routinely, ABO and Rh typing is done on donor blood, atypical antibodies, (e.g. anti-D, anti-Kell) are tested for using the indirect Coombs test, serology is done for syphilis, hepatitis B, hepatitis C, HIV-1 and -2 and HTLV-1.

Indications for Blood Transfusion

- Traumatic haemorrhage
- Gynaecological blood loss
- Surgical blood loss
- Severe anaemia
- Coagulation disturbances
- Leukaemias
- Haemolytic anaemias
- Thalassaemia
- Peripheral circulatory failure/shock
- Burns

Blood Storage

- Plasma potassium, ammonia and phosphate increase during storage while RBC 2,3-bisphosphoglycerate (BPG) and plasma pH decrease during storage.
- The basic purpose of efficient blood storage is to increase the shelf life of preserved blood and to maintain high intra-erythrocyte BPG levels for the optimal oxygen exchange with tissue.
- **CPDA** (citrate–phosphate–dextrose–adenine) preserves cells for 35 days owing to the action of citrate as an anticoagulant, phosphate and adenine as substrates for ATP synthesis and dextrose as the source of anaerobic glycolysis in RBCs.

Crossmatch

The **standard pretransfusion tests** on the recipient consist of ABO group and Rh typing, an antibody screen for atypical antibodies (indirect Coombs test), a direct Coombs test (to identify IgG antibodies on RBCs) and a major crossmatch. The **major crossmatch** is accomplished in a test tube by mixing a sample of the recipient's serum with a sample of RBCs from the donor unit. The purpose of this crossmatch is to detect atypical (not naturally occurring) antibodies present in the recipient's serum that may be directed against foreign antigens on the RBCs in the donor unit.

Q. Write briefly on blood component therapy. (PA22.4)

Ans. Different types of blood components:

- **Packed RBCs** are useful in the treatment of anaemia, since they have less volume and a higher haematocrit than whole blood. Each unit of packed RBCs should raise the Hb by 1 g/dL and the haematocrit by 3%.
- **Platelet transfusions** are generally indicated when patients have a platelet count <50,000 cells/μL and have clinical evidence of bleeding or are candidates for a surgical or invasive procedure. Each unit of platelets infused should raise the platelet count by 5000–10,000 cells/μL.
- **Granulocyte transfusions** are reserved for patients who have severe sepsis associated with an absolute neutropenia <500 cells/μL that has not responded appropriately to antibiotics within 48 h.

- **Fresh-frozen plasma** (FFP) contains all the coagulation factors and is the component of choice in bleeding associated with multiple factor deficiencies as seen in severe liver disease, Warfarin overdose and disseminated intravascular coagulation.
- **Cryoprecipitate** contains Factor VIII, fibrinogen, Factor XIII and fibronectin and is the component of choice in the treatment of mild von Willebrand disease and fibrinogen deficiency.
- **Factor VIII concentrates** are primarily used in the treatment of haemophilia A.
- **Albumin, plasma protein fraction** (PPF), **crystalloid solutions**, (e.g. normal saline, Ringer lactate containing sodium, chloride, potassium, calcium and lactate) and **colloid substitutes**, for example dextran and hydroxyethyl starch are utilized as volume expanders.
- **Immune serum globulin** is useful in the treatment of hypogammaglobulinaemia.

Q. What are transfusion reactions? (PA22.5, 22.6)

Ans. Transfusion reactions include:

Immediate Reactions

- **Febrile reactions:** The most common early reactions and are due to the cytokines (IL1, IL6, IL8 and TNF) produced by leukocytes during storage. Characterized by fever, chills and headache, febrile reactions can be reduced in frequency by depletion of leukocytes.
- **Allergic reactions:** Flushing, urticaria, fever, tachycardia, wheezing, dyspnoea and cyanosis are secondary to antibodies directed against plasma proteins in the donor unit including IgA (Type I hypersensitivity reaction).
- **Acute haemolytic transfusion reactions:** Usually due to mismatched transfusion, these reactions are characterized by hypotension, heat and burning at the site of transfusion, fever, pain in the lower back or chest, bleeding due to DIC, oliguria due to renal failure. They may be intravascular or extravascular.
  - **Intravascular haemolytic transfusion reactions** are due to an **ABO mismatch** (type II hypersensitivity reaction).
  - **Extravascular haemolytic transfusion reactions** are due to presence of an atypical antibody in the recipient (e.g. antiKell) that was undetectable (too low a titre) in the initial antibody screen.
- **Circulatory overload:** Rapid transfusion of blood may lead to congestive heart failure. Particularly prone are patients with severe anaemia and previous history of heart disease.
- **Endotoxic shock and fever due to bacterial contamination of blood.**

Delayed Transfusion Reactions

- **Delayed haemolytic transfusion:** Occur 3–10 days after the infusion of blood and are most often due to extravascular haemolysis from an atypical antibody reaction against donor RBCs.
- **Transfusion haemosiderosis** due to chronic or multiple transfusions.
- **Graft versus host reaction** due to granulocyte or WBC transfusion in immune-deficient patients.

Q. Write briefly on autologous blood tranfusion. (PA22.7)

Ans. Autologous blood transfusion is defined as tranfusion of blood collected from a single patient and retransfusion back to the same patient as and when required. This is in contrast to allogenic blood transfusion where blood from unrelated donors is transfused to the recipient.

There are three methods of autologous transfusion:

i. Cell salvage: blood is collected from suction, surgical drains, or both and retransfused back to the patient after filtration or washing.
ii. Preoperative autologous donation (PAD): blood is collected in advance of an elective procedure, stored in the blood bank and transfused back to the patient when required.
iii. Acute normovolaemic haemodilution (ANH): blood is collected immediately before surgery and blood volume is restored by crystalloid or colloid. The blood is then retransfused at the end of surgery once haemostasis is achieved.

Advantages of autologous transfusions

1. Reduced risk of transmission of infection and transfusion reactions.
2. Safer transfusion in patients with rare blood groups and multiple auto-antibodies.

Disadvantages of autologous transfusions

1. Wastage of unused blood.
2. Increased risk of bacterial contamination.

22 Liver Function Tests

Q. Write briefly on liver function tests.
(PA25.6, IM5.14, 15.9, PE26.9)

Ans. Liver has to perform different kinds of biochemical, synthetic and excretory functions, so no single biochemical test can detect the global functions of liver. All laboratories usually employ a battery of tests for initial detection and management of liver diseases and these tests are frequently termed as 'liver function tests (LFTs)', they help in the following:

- Screening and identification of the pattern of liver disease.
- In assessing the severity of liver disease.
- In the follow up of patients affected by liver disease.

Liver disease is classified broadly into two categories of injury: cell necrosis and cholestasis. A classification of liver disease that best facilitates effective laboratory test strategy and interpretation of results is as follows:

Cell Necrosis

Acute: Viral hepatitis, toxic hepatitis, alcoholic hepatitis, ischaemic necrosis.

Chronic: Chronic active hepatitis, autoimmune hepatitis, cirrhosis.

Cholestasis: The cholestasis occurs when bile flow into the duodenum is reduced. It is usually due to obstruction, but adverse effects of medications, genetic defects or autoimmune processes may also interfere with the bile flow. **Extrahepatic biliary obstruction** occurs either within the biliary system from stones or stricture or from extrinsic compression such as from malignant lymphadenopathy. **Intrahepatic cholestasis** occurs either from direct canalicular injury or from compression due to hepatocyte swelling, as in severe hepatitis. Most likely causes of cholestasis include:

- Gall stones
- Tumours
- Medications (erythromycin, phenytoin, amoxicillin-clavulanic acid, combined oral contraceptive pill, some antipsychotics)
- Pregnancy
- Primary biliary cirrhosis
- Systemic sepsis

Intrahepatic causes

Diffuse: Drugs, primary biliary cirrhosis.

Focal: Metastatic tumour, granuloma, intrahepatic cholelithiasis.

Extrahepatic Causes: Stone, tumour.

LFT can be classified into:

A. **Tests of the liver's capacity to transport organic anions and to metabolize drugs**—Serum bilirubin, urine bilirubin and urobilinogen.

B. **Tests that detect injury to hepatocytes (serum enzyme tests)**—Aminotransferases, alkaline phosphatase, glutamyl transpeptidase, 5 nucleotidase and leucine aminopeptidase.

C. **Tests of the Liver's biosynthetic capacity**—Serum proteins, albumin, ceruloplasmin, α-1 antitrypsin, α-feto protein and prothrombin time.

1. **Serum Bilirubin**
   (a) Serum bilirubin is an indicator of excretory function of the liver.
   (b) It is an endogenous anion derived from degradation of hemoglobin released from red cells.
   (c) Levels must exceed 2.5 mg/dL to produce clinical jaundice.
   (d) Increased serum bilirubin is seen in hepatocellular and obstructive liver disease and haemolysis.
   (e) Types of bilirubin include:
      (i) **Total bilirubin:** This is measured as the amount, which reacts in 30 minutes after addition of alcohol. Normal serum bilirubin level is 0.3–1.0 mg/dL.
      (ii) **Direct bilirubin:** This is the water-soluble fraction and is measured by the reaction with diazotized sulfanilic acid in 1 minute and this gives estimation of conjugated bilirubin. Normal level <0.3 mg/dL. **Indirect bilirubin** is calculated by the difference of the total and direct bilirubin and is a measure of unconjugated fraction of bilirubin.
   (f) **Increased unconjugated bilirubin** results from overproduction, impaired uptake and conjugation
   (g) **Increased conjugated bilirubin** results from impaired intrahepatic excretion or regurgitation of unconjugated or conjugated bilirubin from hepatocytes of bile ducts.
   (h) **Mild elevations in bilirubin levels** are seen in liver diseases, physiological jaundice and inherited hyperbilirubinemias, haemolysis, ineffective erythropoiesis, haematoma formation, etc.

(i) **Moderate elevations in bilirubin levels** are seen in extra and intra hepatic biliary atresia, drugs, viral hepatitis and inherited hyperbilirubinemias.

2. **Bilirubin in the urine**
   (a) Normally, bilirubin cannot be detected in urine. Unconjugated bilirubin is tightly bound to albumin and not filtered by the glomerulus and thus not present in the urine.
   (b) Since conjugated bilirubin is water soluble, bilirubinuria in a jaundiced patient points to **conjugated hyperbilirubinemia (hepatobiliary disease).**
3. **Urine urobilinogen**
   (a) Urinary urobilinogen is detected by **Ehrlich's test.**
   (b) Urobilinogen is absent in urine in obstructive/cholestatic jaundice.
   (c) Markedly increased urobilinogen is observed in urine in haemolytic disease (bilirubinuria).
   (d) An increase in the urobilinogen in urine is a sensitive indicator of hepatocellular dysfunction, for example alcoholic liver damage, cirrhosis or hepatocellular malignancy. In viral hepatitis it appears early in urine.
4. **Liver enzymes**
   (a) **Aminotransferases**
      (i) The aminotransferases (formerly transaminases) are the most frequently utilized and specific indicators of hepatocellular necrosis and include aspartate aminotransferase (AST, SGPT) and alanine aminotransferase (ALT, SGOT).
      (ii) ALT is more specific for hepatocellular damage because the activity of ALT outside the liver is low and it is found primarily in the liver. AST is also found in heart and muscle.
      (iii) Whereas the AST is present in both the mitochondria and cytosol of hepatocytes, ALT is mainly localized to the cytosol.
      (iv) Normal value of AST ranges between 5 and 40 IU/L and of ALT between 10 and 55 IU/L.
      (v) Aminotransferase levels are useful to differentiate between hepatocellular jaundice and obstructive jaundice. Marked elevations seen in severe viral hepatitis, drug-induced injury and circulatory shock. Mild elevations seen in neonatal hepatitis, extra hepatic biliary atresia, fatty liver, cirrhosis, NASH (non-alcoholic steatohepatitis) and drug toxicity.
      (vi) Ratio of AST and ALT can be useful in differential diagnosis.
      (vii) **AST: ALT =1** is associated with ischaemia (congestive cardiac failure, ischaemic necrosis and hepatitis).
      (viii) **AST: ALT >2.5** is associated with severe skeletal muscle trauma, alcoholic hepatitis and alcohol-induced deficiency of pyridoxal phosphate.
      (ix) **AST: ALT <1** is seen in hepatocellular necrosis due to viral hepatitis, ischaemic necrosis and toxic hepatitis.
   (b) **Alkaline phosphatase or ALP (indicator of cholestasis)**
      (i) Serum contains ALP activity, derived from liver and bone. ALP from the liver, bone and kidney are thought to be from the same gene but that from intestine and placenta are derived from different genes.
      (ii) Normal serum level is 3–13 KA units. In liver, alkaline phosphatase is found in the microvilli of bile canaliculi and on the sinusoidal surface of hepatocytes.
      (iii) The mechanism by which alkaline phosphatase reaches the circulation is uncertain; leakage from the bile canaliculi into hepatic sinusoids may result from leaky tight junctions. The other hypothesis is that the damaged liver fails to excrete alkaline phosphatase made in bone, intestine and liver.
      (iv) In **hepatocellular jaundice,** very little ALP is liberated from the cells and the rise in ALP is less than threefold, in **obstructive jaundice,** due to obstruction of biliary tract, new ALP that is synthesized escapes into blood. Hence, ALP levels are markedly raised in obstructive jaundice.
      (v) **Causes of raised ALP:**
         - Hepatic causes: It usually indicates cholestasis or obstruction and is a sensitive indicator of mild biliary obstruction. Hepatic causes of increased ALP include tumours and viral hepatitis.
         - Bone-related causes: These include osteomalacia, bone metastasis, Paget's disease, rickets, rapid bone growth in adolescents and children.
         - Pregnancy-related increase (non-pathological): Released into serum from placenta in late pregnancy.
         - Blood type O and B (non-pathological): Released form small intestine after a fatty meal.
   (c) **Gamma-glutamyl transpeptidase or GGT**
      (i) GGT is an indicator of cholestasis. If the source of ALP is not clear, the levels of two enzymes, **gamma glutamyl transferase** and **5'nucleotidase** can be determined. The latter are more specific for liver disease. Raised levels occur in biliary obstruction and parenchymal damage. GGT is also raised in acute and chronic alcoholism.
      (ii) The other enzyme that may be estimated to detect cholestasis but is not routinely used is **leucine aminopeptidase.**
      (iii) Increased levels of serum GGT correlates with ALP levels and may result from the following:
         - **Hepatic causes:** Moderate elevation is seen in hepatocellular injury and alcohol ingestion. Rapid and marked increase is seen in obstructive jaundice and metastatic infiltration (which may be associated with obstruction).
         - **Other causes** include pancreatitis, brain tumours, renal, prostatic and cardiac disease.

5. **Plasma proteins**
   (a) Plasma protein levels are an indicator of the synthetic ability of liver.
   (b) **Albumin** is synthesized in liver. Normal serum albumin level is 3.5–4.5 g/dL. In chronic liver diseases like cirrhosis and chronic active hepatitis, serum albumin levels are reduced (<3 g/dL).
   (c) **Globulins** are synthesized by the reticuloendothelial system. Normal serum globulin level is 1.5–3 g/100 mL. Their levels rise in chronic liver disease. Chronic active hepatitis and cryptogenic cirrhosis show an elevation of mainly IgG. Alcoholic liver disease and biliary cirrhosis are associated with a primary increase in IgA and IgM respectively.
6. **Coagulation factors**
   (a) Coagulation factor levels are also an indicator of the synthetic ability of the liver.
   (b) Liver synthesizes 11 coagulation factors and activates some in the presence of vitamin K.
   (c) Prothrombin time (PT) is prolonged in liver disease (PT depends on factors I, II, V, VII and X, and gets prolonged when the plasma concentration of any one of these falls below 30% of normal).
7. **Bromsulphthalein (BSP) clearance** BSP clearance is delayed in Dubin–Johnson syndrome

Summary of LFT

1. **Indicators of cell necrosis:** AST, ALT, AST:ALT ratio, LDH.
2. **Indicators of cholestasis:** ALP, GGT.
3. **Indicators of organic anion metabolism:** Total and direct bilirubin.
4. **Indicators of synthetic function of liver:** Protein synthesis (albumin, prothrombin time, coagulation factor levels).
5. **Immunologic markers of liver disease:** Total globulin, immunoglobulins, auto-antibody screen, for example antinuclear antibody (ANA), anti-mitochondrial antibody (AMA), anti-smooth muscle antibody (SMA), anti-LKM-1, AMA, viral markers (total HAV, IgM HAV, HBsAg, total anti-HBc, IgM anti-HBc, anti-hepatitis C antibody, CMV and EBV).
6. **Specific markers**
   (a) **Hereditary haemochromatosis:** Transferrin saturation, serum ferritin, C282Y/H63D mutations and hepatic iron index.
   (b) **Wilson's disease:** Serum ceruloplasmin, urinary copper.
   (c) **α1-antitrypsin deficiency:** Serum electrophoresis and phenotypic analysis.
   (d) **Hepatocellular carcinoma:** α fetoprotein levels, imaging (ultrasound and CT are non-invasive and help in detecting structural abnormalities, Doppler test can be used to assess the condition of the blood vessels) and liver biopsy.
   (e) **Autoimmune hepatitis:** Immunoglobulin quantitation, anti-nuclear antibody, smooth muscle antibody, type 1 liver-kidney microsomal antibody.
   (f) **Primary biliary cirrhosis:** Immunoglobulin quantitation, antimitochondrial antibody.

Renal Function Tests

23

Q. Write briefly on kidney function tests. (IM10.16, 10.17)

Ans. The kidneys excrete metabolic waste products and regulate the serum concentration of a variety of substances. At some stage during the course of renal disease, the routinely measured substances often become abnormal and the extent of the abnormality generally depends on the severity of the disease. Patients with kidney disease have few signs and symptoms early in disease course and laboratory evaluation may be only way of detecting disease. Renal function tests include:

1. **Urine examination (See Chapter 18)**
   (a) Physical and chemical examination
   (b) Microscopic examination
   (c) Bacteriologic examination
2. **Blood examination**
   (a) Blood urea (BUN)
   (b) Serum creatinine
   (c) Serum electrolytes
   (d) Serum protein
   (e) Serum cholesterol
   (f) Serum uric acid
3. **Renal clearance tests (CT)**
   Tests for glomerular function:
   (a) Inulin CT
   (b) Creatinine CT
   Tests for tubular function:
   (a) Urea CT
   (b) Para-amino hippuric (PAH) CT
4. **Concentration and dilution tests**
   (a) Concentration test (fluid deprivation test)
   (b) Dilution test (excess fluid intake test)
5. **Others**
   (a) Intravenous pyelography
   (b) Ultrasonography
   (c) Arteriography
   (d) FNAC/renal biopsy

1. **Urinalysis**
   (a) Urine specimens are examined in a routine manner by semiquantitatively estimating the concentrations of components like glucose, ketones, bilirubin, urobilinogen, protein, haemoglobin, and pH; measurement of specimen volume, determination of specific gravity or osmolality and microscopic examination of the urine sediment for cells, casts and crystals.
   (b) The entire group of tests is clinically useful for evaluating a wide variety of pathologic conditions, and the following are particularly useful for evaluating renal diseases.
      (i) Specific gravity
      - It is measured for the purpose of determining concentrating ability of kidneys. Normal specific gravity of a concentrated urine specimen is greater than 1.025 (range 1.005 to 1.030). The specific gravity of a urine specimen from a fluid deprived patient with severe renal disease (with loss of concentrating ability) is 1.010.
      - In the last stage of renal disease, specific gravity becomes fixed at 1.010 regardless of fluid intake.
      - Specific gravity is much easier to measure than is osmolality and generally the two results correlate well.

      (ii) Osmolalty
      - Osmolality is a measure of the number of particles dissolved in a solution. **Osmolality in blood** is created by protein, glucose, chloride, sodium, bicarbonate and urea dissolved in the plasma.
      - It is used to assess the patient's fluid status and identify any ADH abnormalities **(normal value is 285–298 mOsm/kg)**. Increased values are seen in alcoholism, aldosteronism, diabetes insipidus, high protein diet, dehydration, hypercalcaemia, hyperglycaemia, hypernatraemia and hyperkalaemia.
      - Decreased values are seen in fluid overload, hypernatraemia, liver failure with ascites and Addison's disease.
      - **Urine osmolality (normal: 500–800 mOsm/kg H_2O)** varies based on the patient's fluid status and metabolic waste products being excreted. It is affected by the concentration ability of kidneys, ADH levels and serum levels of protein, urea, glucose, sodium, bicarbonate and chloride.
      - Increased values are seen in dehydration, Addison's disease, diabetes mellitus, diarrhoea, hyperglycaemia, hypernatraemia and cirrhosis; decreased values are seen in overhydration,

hyponatraemia, hypocalcaemia, aldosteronism and diabetes insipidus.
  - Normal kidneys can concentrate urine so that the concentration of osmotically active substances is 3–4 times greater than that of plasma. When concentrating ability is completely lost, the osmolality of urine can be no greater than that of serum.

2. **Serum creatinine and urea**
   - Concentrations of **serum creatinine and urea** change inversely with changes in glomerular filtration rate (GFR). Disadvantage of BUN/Creatinine is that they are insensitive measurement of renal function. Changes are usually not evident till there is a 50%–75% decrease in GFR.
   - Changes in serum creatinine concentration more reliably reflect changes in GFR than do changes in serum urea concentrations. Creatinine is disposed almost entirely by glomerular filtration. **Normal range of serum creatinine is 0.5–1.5 mg/dL.**
   - Urea formation is influenced by a number of factors such as liver function, protein intake and rate of protein catabolism. Urea excretion also depends upon hydration status and the extent of water reabsorption as well as upon GFR. It is a major nitrogenous end product of protein and amino acid catabolism; produced by the liver and distributed throughout intracellular and extracellular fluid. Urea is excreted from the body primarily by the kidneys and in small proportions by sweat or intestinal bacteria. It is freely filtered but reabsorbed in proximal and distal nephron. **Normal BUN values are 8–20 mg/dL.**
3. **Serum uric acid**
   - Uric acid is end product of protein metabolism and excreted by kidneys and bowels. Increase in serum uric acid may result from ingestion of food high in purine (meat, fish, etc.), strenuous exercise or heavy alcohol ingestion. **Normal value in males is 3.6–8.5 mg/dL, and in females 2.3–6.6 mg/dL.**
   - Increased levels are also seen in gout, shock, renal failure, diabetic ketoacidosis, leukaemia, lead poisoning, polycythemia vera, acute alcohol ingestion, psoriasis, pernicious anaemia and toxaemia of pregnancy. Decreased values are seen in Hodgkin's disease and multiple myeloma.
4. **Protein**
   - Levels *in serum* can generally be maintained at concentrations above the lower limit of normal by increased hepatic protein synthesis so long as protein loss is less than about 3 g/day.
   - Spot urine specimens can be used to detect and monitor proteinuria.
   - First morning specimens are preferred method; screening for proteinuria can be accomplished with either standard urine dipsticks (total proteinuria) or albumin-specific dipsticks.
   - Patients with positive dipstick tests should have confirmation with quantitative measurement (albumin-creatinine ratio, protein-creatinine ratio, or 24-hour collection).
5. **Measurement of GFR**
   - GFR cannot be measured directly; it is remarkably constant in a single individual under constant conditions, however, there are large variations between individuals.
   - Determination of **clearance**, from measurement of a substance concentration in both a 24-hour urine collection and a serum specimen, provides a clinically useful estimate of GFR.
   - **Clearance (C)** is defined as the rate at which an indicator substance is removed from plasma per unit concentration (volume from which all of a substance is removed per unit time). For a substance *Z* cleared by renal elimination:

     $Cz\_Uz\ xV\ /\ Pz$, where Uz is urinary concentration of z, Pz is plasma concentration of Z, and V is urine flow rate.

     If substance z is freely filtered and only excreted by GFR, then: $GFR\ \_\ Uz\ xV/Pz$.
   - Thus, plasma concentration of indicator is inversely related to GFR and GFR can be assessed from plasma concentration.

Characteristics of an ideal marker for GFR measurement

- Constant rate of production (or for exogenous marker can be delivered intravenously at a constant rate).
- Freely filterable at the glomerulus (minimal protein binding).
- No tubular reabsorption or secretion.
- No extrarenal elimination or metabolism.
- Availability of an accurate and reliable assay.
- For exogenous marker: safe, convenient, readily available, inexpensive, and does not influence GFR.

Use of exogenous markers to measure GFR

- Most commonly used exogenous marker is **inulin** (it is a fructose polymer, freely filtered, neither reabsorbed nor secreted by tubules, and physiologically inert).
- Other markers, which can be used include **radionuclide-labelled markers** (125_{I}-iothalamate and 51Cr-ethylenediaminetetra-acetic acid or EDTA) and **radiocontrast markers** (Iothalamate sodium, iohexol).

Use of endogenous markers to determine GFR

- **Creatinine** is the most commonly used endogenous marker.
- It is generated in muscle by non-enzymatic conversion of creatine and phosphocreatinine and the generation is proportional to muscle mass and is relatively constant.
- Levels vary according to diurnal and menstrual variations, race and diet; it is not an ideal marker as it also is excreted by tubular secretion.
- Because of reciprocal relationship between GFR and serum creatinine (SCr), a large change in GFR is initially required to raise SCr levels from normal; however, once SCr is elevated, small changes in GFR will raise it exponentially.
- Glomerular filtration rate is estimated, in clinical practice, from the creatinine clearance which is calculated from measurements of serum creatinine concentration

(Crs), urine creatine concentration (Cru), and the urine volume (V) collected over a time period (t, usually expressed in minutes):
Creatinine Clearance = (Cru × V/t)/Crs.
(Normal range is for males is 85–125 mL/min and females is 75–115 mL/min).

- Glomerular filtration rate is proportional to body surface area and the above range is for the average adult with a surface area of 1.73 square meters. The 'corrected' creatinine clearance is obtained by multiplying the measured creatinine clearance X 1.73 and dividing by actual body surface area.

6. **Hyperphosphatemia, hyperuricaemia and metabolic acidosis**
   - These do not develop until there is 70%–80% loss of renal functional capacity, so that measurements of serum phosphate, uric acid or bicarbonate, do not provide a very sensitive indication of the possibility of renal disease.
   - However, measurement of serum phosphate and uric acid is useful for monitoring the effect of therapy during chronic renal disease and/or the effects of attempts to minimize increased serum concentrations by restricting dietary intake of phosphate and nucleotides. Acidosis is generally mild and without pathophysiologic consequences until the uremic stage.
7. **Calcium:** Deficiency of calcium in chronic renal disease (because of deficient renal activation of vitamin D), does not usually result in frank hypocalcaemia because secondary hyperparathyroidism develops as a compensatory response to maintain serum calcium concentrations within the normal range.
8. **Sodium and potassium**
   - Sodium and potassium levels are maintained till renal dysfunction is sufficiently severe to cause oliguria.
   - Electrolyte determinations are, therefore, not useful for detecting or assessing the progression of renal disease.
   - Evaluation of renal sodium reabsorption is, however, valuable for assessing tubule function and is useful for distinguishing whether rapidly developing azotemia is due to acute renal failure or to prerenal azotemia from a compensatory decrease in renal blood flow due to hypovolaemia.

Laboratory findings in specific renal syndromes

1. **Nephrotic syndrome**
   - Proteinuria >3 g/day.
   - Hypoproteinaemia with plasma albumin levels <3g/dl.
   - Generalized oedema.
   - Hyperlipidemia and lipiduria.
2. **Nephritic syndrome**
   - Haematuria and red cell casts.
   - Proteinuria (<2 g/day) with or without oedema.
   - Azotemia.
   - Hypertension.
3. **Tubulointerstitial disease**
   - White cell casts.
   - Proteinuria (<1 g/day).
   - Azotemia.
4. **Acute renal failure**
   - Sudden oliguria.
   - Rapidly developing azotemia (serum creatinine increases at a maximum rate of about 2 mg/dL per day).
   - Broad waxy casts (renal failure casts).
   - Urine sodium concentration >40 mEq/L.
   - Normal serum calcium, increased phosphate and potassium and decreased sodium.
   - Normal serum parathormone levels.
5. **Chronic renal failure**
   - Progressive and irreversible deterioration of renal function due to slow destruction of renal parenchyma.
   - Manifests with azotemia and acidosis.
   - Low serum calcium, markedly increased phosphate and potassium and decreased sodium.
   - Increased serum parathormone levels.
   - Normocytic normochromic anaemia; in case of blood loss microcytic hypochromic anaemia.

SECTION IV

SYSTEMIC PATHOLOGY

Diseases of Blood Vessels

24

The blood supply of heart comprises three major vessel types: **arteries** (carry blood from the heart to the systemic circulation), **capillaries** (responsible for exchange of water and chemicals between the blood and tissues) and **veins** (carry blood from capillaries back towards the heart).

Arteries

The **arteries** and **veins** have a similar structure with **three layers, from inside to outside**:

1. ***Tunica intima (thinnest layer):*** It is composed of a single layer of flattened cells (lining endothelium) held together by a polysaccharide matrix composed of collagen, proteoglycans and elastin. Outside this is present a thin layer of connective tissue (subendothelial connective tissue) and circularly arranged elastic bands called internal elastic lamina, which separates the intima from the media.
2. ***Tunica media (thickest layer):*** This is limited on the inside by the internal elastic lamina and on the outside by another thick elastic band called external elastic lamina (the latter separates the media from the adventitia). Tunica media is constituted by connective tissue and polysaccharide substances and is rich in vascular smooth muscle (especially arteries), which controls the calibre of the vessel.
3. ***Tunica adventitia:*** It is made of loose connective tissue and elastic fibres and contains nerves that supply the vessel as well as nutrient capillaries (vasa vasorum). The inner part of the tunica media receives nourishment by direct diffusion of nutrients and oxygen from the lumen, whereas the outer part of the media is nourished by the vasa vasorum.

Veins

Veins are different from arteries in the following ways (Figs 24.1, 24.2):

1. They have a thinner wall.
2. The three tunicae are less well defined.
3. The elastic tissue is scanty and not well organized into internal and external elastic laminae.
4. The media is richer in collagen and contains less smooth muscle.

Capillaries

These are 7–8 microns in diameter and are lined by endothelial cells which form their tunica intima (inner layer) with pericytes forming their tunica adventitia (outer layer).

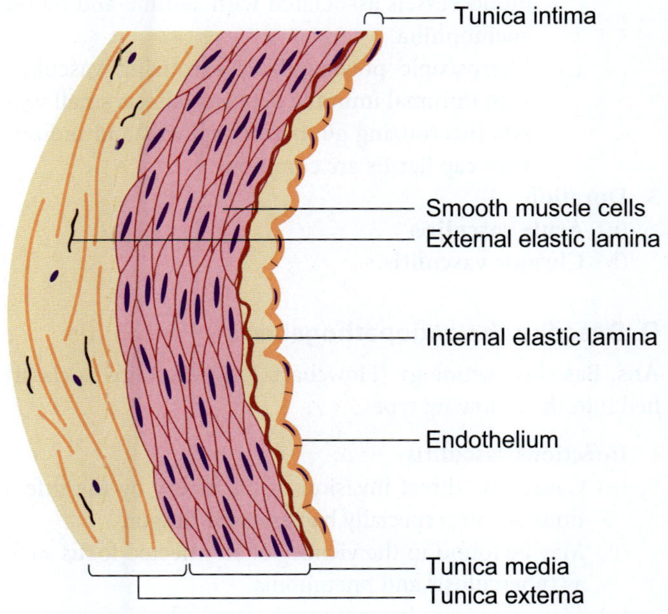

Fig. 24.1 Structure of an artery.

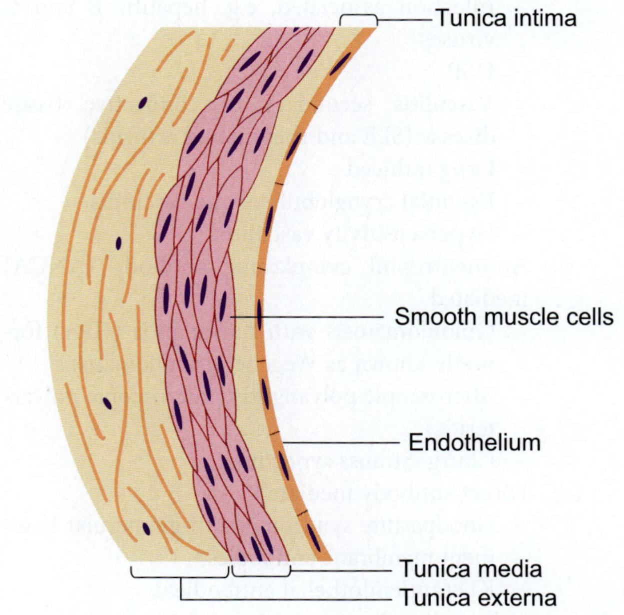

Fig. 24.2 Structure of a vein.

Arterioles

They are the smallest branches of the arterial tree which have a diameter less than 100 microns. The intima of an arteriole is composed of endothelial cells which rest on a basement membrane. Larger arterioles may have a fine internal elastic lamina. The arteriolar media is composed of one or two layers of smooth muscle cells and the adventitia is insignificant.

DISEASES OF BLOOD VESSELS

Q. Define vasculitis.

Ans. Vasculitis (angiitis) is an inflammatory process involving vessels. Depending on the vessel involved, vasculitis is labelled as arteritis, capillaritis or venulitis. Vessel lumen may get compromised leading to possible ischemia and necrosis. Vasculitis be confined to one single organ (i.e. skin), or may simultaneously involve several organ systems. The most common forms of systemic vasculitis in children are Henoch–Schönlein purpura (HSP) and Kawasaki disease (KD). Vasculitis can also occur secondary to another disease. Diseases associated with secondary vasculitis include infection, malignancy, collagen vascular disease (e.g. systemic lupus erythematosus [SLE], dermatomyositis) and drug hypersensitivity.

Q. Classify vasculitis.

Ans. Vasculitis is classified based on the following:

1. **Etiopathogenesis**
   (a) **Direct infection**
      (i) Bacterial, e.g. caused by *Neisseria*, streptococci, staphylococci, *M. tuberculosis* and *M. leprae*
      (ii) Rickettsial, e.g. Rocky Mountain spotted fever
      (iii) Spirochaetal, e.g. syphilis
      (iv) Fungal, e.g. aspergillosis and mucormycosis
      (v) Viral, e.g. herpes zoster and varicella.
   (b) **Immunological**
      (i) Immune complex mediated
         - Infection associated, e.g. hepatitis B and C viruses
         - HSP
         - Vasculitis secondary to connective tissue disease (SLE and rheumatoid arthritis)
         - Drug induced
         - Essential cryoglobulinaemic vasculitis
         - Hypersensitivity vasculitis.
      (ii) Antineutrophil cytoplasmic antibody (ANCA) mediated
         - Granulomatosis with polyangiitis (GPA) formerly known as Wegener granulomatosis
         - Microscopic polyangiitis (microscopic polyarteritis)
         - Churg–Strauss syndrome.
      (iii) Direct antibody mediated
         - Goodpasture syndrome (anti-glomerular basement membrane antibodies)
         - KD (antiendothelial antibodies).
      (iv) Cell mediated
         - Organ allograft rejection.
      (v) Unknown
         - Giant cell arteritis
         - Polyarteritis nodosa (PAN)
         - Takayasu arteritis.
2. **Size of the vessel involved** (International Chapel Hill Consensus Conference on the Nomenclature of Vasculitis; Fig. 24.3)
   (a) **Large vessel vasculitis**
      (i) Giant cell (temporal) arteritis: Granulomatous arteritis of the aorta and its major branches, with predilection for extracranial branches of the carotid artery.
      (ii) Takayasu arteritis: Granulomatous inflammation of the aorta and its major branches.
   (b) **Medium-sized vessel vasculitis**
      (i) PAN (classic): Necrotizing inflammation of medium-sized or small arteries without glomerulonephritis or vasculitis in arterioles, capillaries or venules.
      (ii) KD: Arteritis involving large, medium-sized or small arteries, associated with mucocutaneous syndrome, usually seen in children.
      (iii) Primary central nervous system vasculitis.
   (c) **Small-vessel vasculitis**
      (i) ANCA-associated vasculitis: Patients with circulating antibodies to neutrophilic cytoplasmic antigens.
      (ii) Granulomatosis with polyangiitis (Wegener, abbreviated GPA): Granulomatous inflammation involving the respiratory tract with necrotizing vasculitis affecting small to medium-sized vessels; necrotizing glomerulonephritis is common.
      (iii) Churg–Strauss syndrome (eosinophilic granulomatosis with polyangiitis [EGPA]): Eosinophil-rich granulomatous inflammation involving the respiratory tract and necrotizing vasculitis affecting medium- and small-sized blood vessels associated with asthma and blood eosinophilia.
      (iv) Microscopic polyangiitis: Necrotizing vasculitis with minimal immune deposits; affects small vessels (necrotizing glomerulonephritis and pulmonary capillaritis are common).
3. **Duration**
   (a) **Acute vasculitis**
   (b) **Chronic vasculitis.**

Q. Describe the aetiopathogenesis of vasculitis.

Ans. Based on aetiology (Flowchart 24.1) vasculitis is classified into the following types:

1. **Infectious vasculitis**
   (a) Caused by direct invasion of the artery by the infectious agents, especially bacteria and fungus.
   (b) May be found in the vicinity of an infected focus such as tuberculosis and pneumonia.
   (c) May arise from haematogenous spread of infection, as in infective endocarditis or septicaemia.

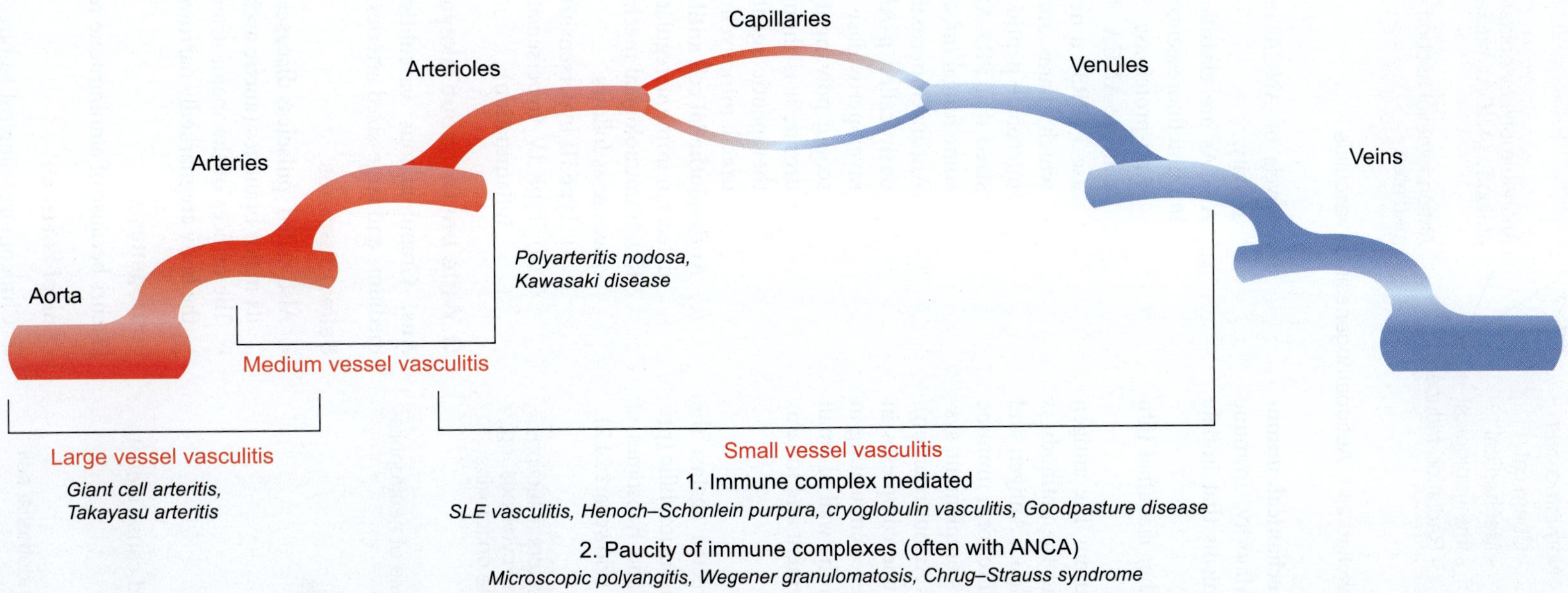

Fig. 24.3 **Nomenclature of vasculitis.** (*Source: Robbins & Cotran Pathologic Basis of Disease,* Tenth Edition: Vinay Kumar, Abul K. Abbas, Jon C. Aster, Figure 11.24: Marc K. Halushka, Richard N. Mitchell, Elsevier Inc., 2021.)

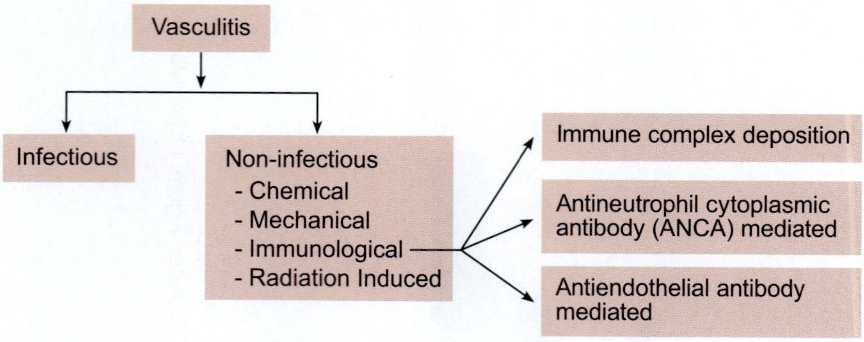

Flowchart 24.1 Aetiopathogenesis of vasculitis.

2. **Non-infectious vasculitis (chemical, mechanical, immunological and radiation induced):** Majority, immune mediated. Main immunological mechanisms that initiate non-infectious vasculitis are as follows:
   (a) **Immune complex deposition:** Further classified into two types:
      (i) Local immune complex formation: The antigen diffuses into the vessel wall and the antibody is brought from the circulating blood. Antigen and antibody react in the vessel wall to form immune complexes, which activate the complement system (seen in PAN and simulates Arthus reaction).
      (ii) Deposition of circulating immune complexes in the vessel wall: Immune complexes circulating in the blood may get deposited in the wall of small blood vessels to activate complement and inflammatory cells (seen in SLE).
   (b) **ANCA**
      (i) ANCAs are autoantibodies directed against the enzymes mainly found within the azurophilic (primary) granules in neutrophils and lysosomes of monocytes and endothelial cells (Flowchart 24.2).

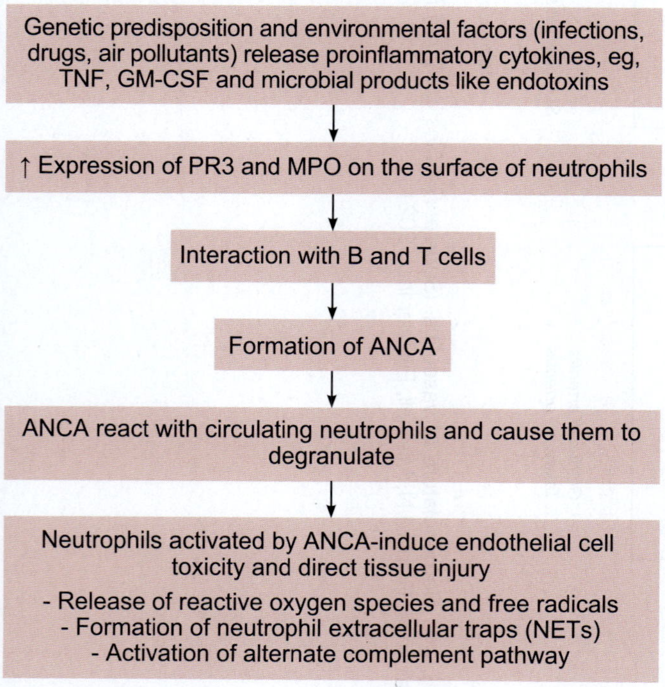

Flowchart 24.2 Mechanism of ANCA-induced vasculitis.

      (ii) Levels of ANCA reflect the degree of disease activity.
      (iii) ANCAs are classified into two types based on immunofluorescence patterns:
         – Anti-proteinase 3 (PR3-ANCA): Previously called **c-ANCA**. The target antigen is proteinase 3 **(PR3)**, a neutrophil granule constituent which shares antigenic structure with some microbial peptides. It is therefore hypothesized that PR3-ANCA is generated following some fungal infections.
         – Antimyeloperoxidase (MPO-ANCA): Previously called **p-ANCA**. The target antigen is myeloperoxidase (**MPO**); seen in microscopic polyangiitis and Churg–Strauss syndrome, it is thought to be induced by some therapeutic agents (hydralazine, propylthiouracil, minocycline).
   (c) **Antiendothelial cell antibodies:** These are induced by defects in immune regulation, and are seen in SLE and KD. Immunological mechanisms responsible for most cases are as follows:
      (i) Type III hypersensitivity
      (ii) Type IV hypersensitivity (as in granulomatous inflammation).

Q. Write briefly about Takayasu arteritis.

Ans. Granulomatous vasculitis which typically involves medium- and large-sized arteries.

Salient Features

- Also called '**pulseless disease**', chiefly affects the aorta and its major branches (**aortic arch syndrome**).
- The orifices of the major arteries to the upper portion of the body are markedly narrowed or obliterated.

Pathogenesis

Occurs because of autoimmune reaction to aortic tissue.

Clinical Features

- Clinicomorphological features overlap with those of giant cell arteritis; however, unlike the latter, which is usually seen in women older than 50 years, Takayasu arteritis affects younger women.
- Early disease manifests with non-specific symptoms (fever, weight loss and fatigue); marked lowering of blood pressure

and weaker pulses in upper extremities along with ocular disturbances and neurological deficit are late manifestations. More distal involvement leads to claudication of the legs.

Gross Pathology

Irregularly thickened aortic wall with wrinkling of intima.

Microscopy

Severe transmural granulomatous inflammation with giant cells and patchy necrosis in the tunica media.

Q. Write briefly about temporal (giant cell) arteritis.

Ans. Inflammatory disease involving arteries of the head.

Salient Features

- Typically causes granulomatous inflammation of medium- and large-sized arteries.
- Cranial (temporal, ophthalmic and common carotid), axillary, brachial and femoral arteries are commonly involved.
- Affects adults older than 70 years, with a slight female preponderance.

Pathogenesis

Attributed to T-cell–mediated immunological reaction against arterial wall components.

Clinical Features

Symptoms vary from being non-specific (fever, fatigue and weight loss) to severe headache and blindness (caused due to ophthalmic artery involvement).

Gross Pathology

The affected arteries are thickened and cord like, with narrowing of the lumina.

Microscopy

- Sections show chronic granulomatous reaction, usually around the internal elastic lamina, typically involving the entire circumference of the vessel wall.
- Internal elastic lamina is fragmented with the presence of giant cells of foreign body or Langhans type.
- Eccentric or concentric intimal cellular proliferation may cause luminal narrowing.

Q. Write briefly about polyarteritis nodosa (PAN).

Ans. PAN is a systemic necrotizing vasculitis involving small- and medium-sized muscular arteries.

Salient Features

- Affects adults (males more commonly affected than females).
- Kidneys, heart, liver, GIT, muscle, pancreas, testes, nervous system and skin usually involved with sparing involvement of pulmonary or glomerular vessels.
- Most people present with hypertension.

Pathogenesis

Deposition of immune complexes and hepatitis B antigenaemia is implicated.

Clinical Features

Ischaemia and infarction of the affected tissues and organs results in:

- Fever, malaise, weakness and weight loss.
- Renal manifestations (albuminuria and haematuria).
- Abdominal pain and melena.
- Peripheral neuritis.

Gross Pathology

- Transmural (involvement of whole thickness of the vessel wall) and segmental (involvement of only a portion of the vessel circumference) vasculitis of small- and medium-sized muscular arteries.
- Predilection for bifurcations and branching points.
- Segmental erosion with weakening of arterial wall may cause aneurysmal dilation or localized rupture.

Microscopy

- ***Acute stage:*** Transmural inflammation (chiefly neutrophils and eosinophils) with fibrinoid necrosis.
- ***Healing stage:*** Fibroblastic proliferation with chronic inflammation (lymphocytes, plasma cells and macrophages).
- ***Healed stage:*** Thickened arterial wall due to dense fibrosis (haemosiderin-laden macrophages and organized thrombi may be seen).

All stages of inflammation can be present at the same time.

Q. Write briefly about Kawasaki disease (KD).

Ans. Originally reported in Japan, KD the foremost cause of heart disease affecting children.

Salient Features

- Self-limiting acute febrile illness of childhood (majority of patients are younger than 4 years).
- Affects large- to medium-sized to small arteries.

Pathogenesis

The pathogenesis of KD is unknown; infectious agents are thought to trigger the disease in genetically predisposed individuals.

Clinical Features

- Conjunctival and oral erythema, and erythema of palms and soles.
- Oedema of hands and feet.
- Desquamative rash and cervical lymph node enlargement **(mucocutaneous syndrome)**.
- Commonly involves the coronary arteries to form aneurysms which may rupture, resulting in acute myocardial infarction.

Pathology

- Transmural inflammation similar to that in PAN; however, less fibrinoid necrosis.
- Most changes in the cardiovascular system; segmental erosion with weakening of arterial wall may cause aneurysmal dilation, thrombosis or localized rupture.

Q. Write briefly about microscopic polyangiitis.

Ans. Necrotizing vasculitis, also known as hypersensitivity or leucocytoclastic vasculitis.

Salient Features

- Characterized by inflammatory involvement of venules, capillaries and arterioles of skin, mucous membrane, lungs, brain, heart, GIT, kidneys and muscles.
- Necrotizing glomerulonephritis and pulmonary capillaritis are much more common than in PAN. Also, microscopic polyangiitis affects smaller vessels and all its lesions are in the same histopathological stage, unlike PAN, wherein all stages of inflammation can be present at the same time.

Pathogenesis

It is thought to be because of an immunological response to an antigen that may be bacteria (streptococci), viruses, malarial parasite, drugs (penicillin) and chemicals. Antibodies are formed leading to immune complex formation or development of secondary ANCA-associated immune responses.

Clinical Features

Depending on the vessel involved, the patient may present with the following:

- Haemoptysis, albuminuria and haematuria.
- Abdominal pain and melena.
- Muscle pain and weakness.
- Palpable purpura.

Pathology

Segmental and focally transmural lesions which involve the smallest vessels, sparing medium-sized and large arteries. Two histological forms are seen:

- ***Leucocytoclastic vasculitis:*** Vasculitis is caused due to immune complex deposition. There is fibrinoid necrosis with neutrophilic infiltrate in the vessel wall. Many neutrophils appear fragmented.
- ***Lymphocytic vasculitis:*** Vascular injury occurs because of lymphocyte–macrophage–mediated delayed hypersensitivity.

Q. Write briefly about Churg–Strauss syndrome (also called 'allergic granulomatosis and angiitis' and 'eosinophilic granulomatosis with polyangiitis' [EGPA]).

Ans. Churg–Strauss syndrome, now called EGPA, is a rare small-vessel vasculitis.

Salient Features

- Multisystem disease characterized by vasculitis with granulomas and eosinophilic necrosis.
- Has a strong association with allergic rhinitis, bronchial asthma, lung infiltrates and eosinophilia.
- Commonly affects vessels in the lungs, heart, spleen, peripheral nerves and skin. Renal disease is less frequent.
- Coronary arteritis and myocarditis are the main causes of death.

Pathogenesis

It is thought to result from hyper-responsiveness to an allergic stimulus. ANCAs are positive in 50% of cases.

Clinical Features

- Palpable purpura (due to involvement of skin).
- Gastrointestinal bleeding.
- Focal and segmental glomerulosclerosis.
- Cardiomyopathy (in >50% of patients).

Pathology

- Infiltration of vessels and perivascular tissue by eosinophils without overt vasculitis in the early phase.
- Intravascular and extravascular granulomas with vasculitis in the later stage.

Q. Write briefly about Wegener granulomatosis (granulomatosis with polyangiitis [GPA]).

Ans. GPA is a necrotizing vasculitis characterized by a clinicopathological triad of:

1. Necrotizing granulomas of the upper respiratory tract (ear, nose, sinuses and throat) and/or lower respiratory tract (lungs).
2. Focal necrotizing granulomatous vasculitis of the small- to medium-sized vessels.
3. Focal necrotizing crescentic glomerulonephritis.

Pathogenesis

- May represent a T-cell-mediated hypersensitive response to some inhaled infectious or environmental agent.
- Characterized by the presence of immune complexes (in vessel wall and glomeruli) and PR3-ANCA, which is a good marker of the disease.

Clinical Features

- It usually affects adult males, in the fifth decade; multiple organ involvement may be seen.
- Clinical manifestations include:
  - Persistent pneumonitis with bilateral infiltrates in the lungs.
  - Chronic sinusitis and nasopharyngeal ulceration.
  - Chronic renal disease, skin rashes, muscle pain and articular involvement.
- GPA without renal involvement is labelled 'limited form' of the disease.
- If left untreated, 80% of the patients die within a year.

Pathology

- Necrotizing vasculitis (segmental or circumferential) of small and sometimes large vessels.
- Granulomatous inflammation with geographic pattern of necrosis with extensive infiltration by neutrophils, mononuclear cells, epithelioid cells, multinucleate giant cells and fibroblasts.
- Dispersed granulomas may coalesce to form nodules that undergo cavitation.
- Renal lesions may be focal or diffuse, namely focal necrotizing (acute focal proliferation and necrosis in the glomeruli with thrombosis) and diffuse crescentic glomerulonephritis.

Q. Write briefly about Raynaud phenomenon.

Ans. Raynaud phenomenon is not a true vasculitis, but a functional vasospastic disorder chiefly affecting small arteries and arterioles of the extremities of young healthy females.

- Clinically, it presents with pallor, redness and cyanosis of the digits and tips of nose or ears.
- Cause is not known; it is thought to be due to vasoconstriction mediated by autonomic stimulation of the affected vessels.
- Ischaemic effect is provoked by cold (emotions, trauma, hormones and drugs also play a role).
- No pathological change is observed in the vessel wall except mild intimal thickening later in the course of the disease.
- Raynaud phenomenon can be primary or secondary. The latter occurs because of an underlying cause, e.g. atherosclerosis, connective tissue disease, multiple myeloma and Buerger disease. Primary Raynaud phenomenon differs from secondary Raynaud phenomenon in having symmetrical involvement of the extremities.

Q. Write briefly about Buerger disease.

Ans. Also called thromboangiitis obliterans, it is characterized by acute and chronic, segmental, thrombosing, inflammatory involvement of the small- and medium-sized arteries and veins of extremities.

- It usually affects men younger than 35 years, particularly the heavy smokers.
- Intermittent claudication due to ischaemia manifests as intense pain in the limbs.
- Fibrous tissue cuffs may form around arteries, veins and nerves leading to gangrene.

Aetiopathogenesis

- Heavy cigarette smoking directly damages the endothelium leading to hypercoagulability and thrombosis.
- An immune response to some constituents of tobacco smoke has also been implicated.
- Familial occurrence, ethnic distribution and HLA association point to a possible genetic basis.

Pathology

- **Early stage:** Polymorphs in all the layers of vessels accompanied by thrombosis in the lumen.
- **Advanced stage:** Mononuclear infiltrate with fibrosis.

Q. Describe the salient features of phlebothrombosis (thrombophlebitis).

Ans. Phlebothrombosis occurs when a thrombus forms in a vein in the absence of inflammation of the vein (*phlebitis*). *Thrombophlebitis* indicates thrombosis with venous inflammation. Phlebothrombosis has the following salient features:

- Deep leg veins are involved in more than 90% of cases followed by periprostatic venous plexus in males and pelvic venous plexus in females.
- Cardiac failure, genetic hypercoagulability syndromes, neoplasia, pregnancy, obesity, postoperative state, prolonged bed rest and immobilization are the most important clinical predispositions.
- Migratory thrombophlebitis (**Trousseau sign**) is seen in adenocarcinomas of pancreas, colon and lung. Hypercoagulability may occur as part of a paraneoplastic syndrome. The resultant venous thrombosis has a tendency to appear in one site only to disappear, followed by thromboses in other veins (migration).
- Thrombi in the legs present with the following:
  - Local manifestations
    - Oedema distal to an occluded vein
    - Cyanosis
    - Dilatation of superficial veins
    - Heat, tenderness, redness, swelling and pain

      Note: The above-mentioned features may be absent in bedridden patients. In these patients, pain is elicited by applying pressure over affected veins, squeezing the calf muscles or forced dorsiflexion of foot (**Homans sign**).
  - Pulmonary embolism
    - This is a common and serious manifestation (not infrequently may be the first manifestation). It is caused due to the contraction of the surrounding vessels, which tends to displace the thrombi from their attachment.

Q. Write briefly about superior vena cava syndrome.

Ans. This is usually caused by a neoplasm that compresses and invades the superior vena cava, most commonly bronchogenic carcinoma and mediastinal lymphoma. It manifests as dusky cyanosis and dilatation of veins of the head, neck and arms. Pulmonary vessels may also get compressed causing respiratory distress.

Q. Write briefly about inferior vena cava syndrome.

Ans. Many neoplasms, e.g. hepatocellular and renal cell carcinoma, show a striking tendency to grow within veins with ultimate extension into the inferior vena cava (occasionally into the right atrium). It manifests with marked oedema of legs, distension of superficial collateral veins of the lower abdomen and massive proteinuria (due to renal vein involvement).

Q. Write briefly about lymphangitis and lymphoedema.

Ans. Primary lymphangitis is an extremely uncommon primary disorder of the lymphatic vessels. Secondary lymphangitis and lymphoedema develop in association with inflammation and cancer. **Lymphangitis** may be acute or chronic depending on its duration.

Acute lymphangitis is caused by bacterial infections, most commonly β-haemolytic streptococci (Flowchart 24.3).

Chronic lymphangitis results from the persistence of acute lymphangitis or chronic infections, e.g. tuberculosis, syphilis and actinomycosis.

- **Primary (idiopathic) lymphoedema** may occur as an **isolated congenital defect** (simple congenital lymphoedema), as **Milroy disease** (heredofamilial congenital lymphoedema) or as **lymphoedema praecox** (affects young females; presents with oedema of unknown cause, which usually begins in the feet and slowly accumulates to cause swelling β-haemolytic streptococcal infection

↓

Lymphatics become dilated with exudate (neutrophils and histiocytes), which extends through the wall into perilymphatic tissue

↓

Cellulitis or focal abscess formation (clinically, manifests as painful subcutaneous red streaks that extend along the course of lymphatics with painful enlargement of lymph nodes)

Flowchart 24.3 Pathogenesis of acute lymphangitis.

of the involved extremity to many times normal size with superimposed infections and chronic ulceration).

- **Obstructive (secondary) lymphoedema:** It occurs secondary to occlusion of lymphatic drainage because of spread of malignant tumours, radical surgical procedures, e.g. radical mastectomy with axillary dissection, postirradiation fibrosis, filariasis and postinflammatory thrombosis, and scarring.
- **Chylous ascites, chylothorax and chylopericardium** is caused by rupture of dilated lymphatics into the respective cavities.
- Persistence of lymphoedema leads to subcutaneous interstitial fibrosis with enlargement of the affected part and induration, called **'peau d'orange'** appearance.

Q. Define aortic dissection. Describe in brief its pathology and clinical consequences.

Ans. Aortic dissection (dissecting haematoma) is a catastrophic illness characterized by the forceful separation of the planes of the media with the formation of an intramural haematoma within the vessel wall, which may rupture outside causing massive haemorrhage.

Salient Features

- Unlike an aneurysm, aortic dissection may or may not be associated with dilatation of the vessel (therefore, the older term **'dissecting aneurysm'** is discouraged).
- Most common site is ascending **aorta**.
- It affects two age groups:
  - Hypertensive men aged between 50 and 70 years.
  - Younger patients with a connective tissue abnormality, which affects the aorta, e.g. Marfan syndrome (genetic defect in fibrillin, a connective tissue protein responsible for elastic tissue formation).
- Aortic dissection can be iatrogenic in origin (trauma during cardiac catheterization or bypass surgery).
- Rarely, dissection of aorta occurs during or following pregnancy (due to haemodynamic stress of pregnancy-induced vascular remodelling).

Types

- Aortic dissections are generally classified into two types:
  - Type A: More common and more serious proximal lesions involving ascending aorta only or ascending and descending aorta (types I and II of DeBakey classification; Fig. 24.4).
  - Type B: Distal lesions not involving the ascending part and beginning distal to the subclavian artery (type III of DeBakey classification; Fig. 24.4).

Clinical Effects

- Aortic dissection presents with sudden severe pain, beginning in the anterior chest and radiating to the back.
- It may rupture leading to haemorrhage into body cavities (pleural, pericardial or peritoneal).
- Retrograde dissection into the aortic root can cause disruption of the aortic valve.
- Cardiac tamponade, aortic insufficiency and myocardial infarction may be seen.
- Compression of spinal arteries may cause transverse myelitis.

Pathological Changes

- The most common histopathological lesion is **cystic medial degeneration.**
- Dissection is seen between the outer and middle third of aortic media, so that blood separates the intima and inner two-thirds of the media on one side from the outer one-third of the media and the adventitia on the other.
- In 10% of dissecting aneurysms, a second intimal tear is seen in the distal part of the dissection, so that the blood enters the false lumen through the proximal tear and re-enters the true lumen through the distal tear **(double barrel aorta).**
- If the patient survives, the false lumen may develop endothelial lining **(chronic dissection).**

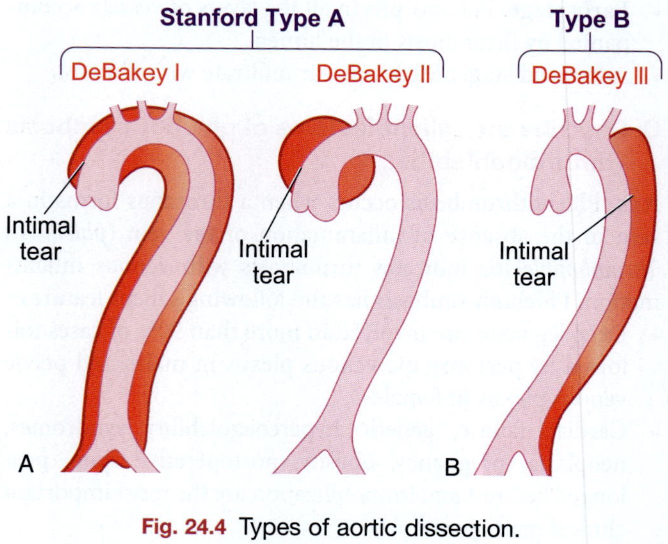

Fig. 24.4 Types of aortic dissection.

Q. Define and classify aneurysms. Summarize their morphology and clinical consequences. (PA27.2)

Ans. An aneurysm is a permanent abnormal dilatation of a blood vessel occurring because of congenital or acquired weakening or destruction of the vessel wall. It is commonly seen in large elastic arteries, especially aorta and its major branches.

Classification

1. **Depending on the composition of the wall** (Fig. 24.5)
   (a) True aneurysm: Composed of all the layers of the vessel wall or thinned-out wall of the heart.
   (b) False or pseudoaneurysm: A breach in the vascular wall leads to the formation of an intravascular haematoma, which has a fibrous wall, and occurs secondary to trauma.
2. **Depending on the shape** (Fig. 24.5)
   (a) Saccular: Large spherical outpouching.
   (b) Fusiform: Spindle-shaped dilatation.
   (c) Cylindrical: Continuous parallel dilatation.
   (d) Serpentine or varicose: Tortuous dilatation.
   (e) Racemose: Mass of intercommunicating small arteries and veins.
3. **Based on pathogenetic mechanisms**
   (a) Atherosclerotic (arteriosclerotic) aneurysm (most common type).
   (b) Syphilitic (luetic) aneurysm (found in the tertiary stage of syphilis).
   (c) Dissecting aneurysm (dissecting haematoma) in which blood enters the wall of the vessel.
   (d) Mycotic aneurysm (weakening of the arterial wall by microbial infection).
   (e) Berry aneurysm (malformation located in the circle of Willis in the base of the brain).

Aneurysms most commonly encountered in clinical practice are as follows:

1. **Abdominal aortic aneurysm (AAA)**
   - Most common form of aortic aneurysms, usually seen in males older than 50 years.
   - Most frequent location is the abdominal aorta (other common locations are thoracic aorta [ascending and arch of aorta], iliac artery and large systemic arteries).
   - Most common cause is atherosclerosis.

   Pathogenesis
   - **Severe atherosclerosis** (thinning and destruction of the medial elastic tissue causes atrophy and weakening of the vessel wall, eventually leading to aneurysm formation).
   - **Genetic predisposition** (genetic defects lead to inadequate or abnormal synthesis of connective tissue component as in Marfan and Ehlers–Danlos syndromes).
   - **Abnormality in matrix metalloproteinases** (decreased level of tissue inhibitors of metalloproteinases, i.e. TIMP), which disturbs the balance between collagen synthesis and degradation.
   - **Infections** (bacterial, mycotic leading to suppuration or syphilitic leading to endarteritis obliterans and ischaemia).

   Pathology
   - Variable sized, usually larger than 5–6 cm.
   - Most frequently fusiform or saccular.
   - Lumen may contain a mural thrombus.
   - Two variants of AAA:
     - Inflammatory: Less frequent; characterized by dense periaortic fibrosis containing lymphocytes, plasma cells and macrophages; thought to be caused due to a localized immune response to the wall of abdominal aorta.
     - Mycotic: Infected by circulating organisms which cause suppuration.

   Clinical features
   - Presents as a palpable pulsatile abdominal mass.
   - May rupture into the peritoneal cavity causing fatal haemorrhage.
   - Vascular obstruction of a branch of aorta, e.g. renal, mesenteric and vertebral may lead to ischaemic injury in the kidney, GIT and spine, respectively.
   - Embolization may occur from an atheroma or mural thrombus.
   - Compression of the ureter or erosion of a vertebra presents as pain, which is deep, boring, visceral and felt most prominently in the lumbosacral region.

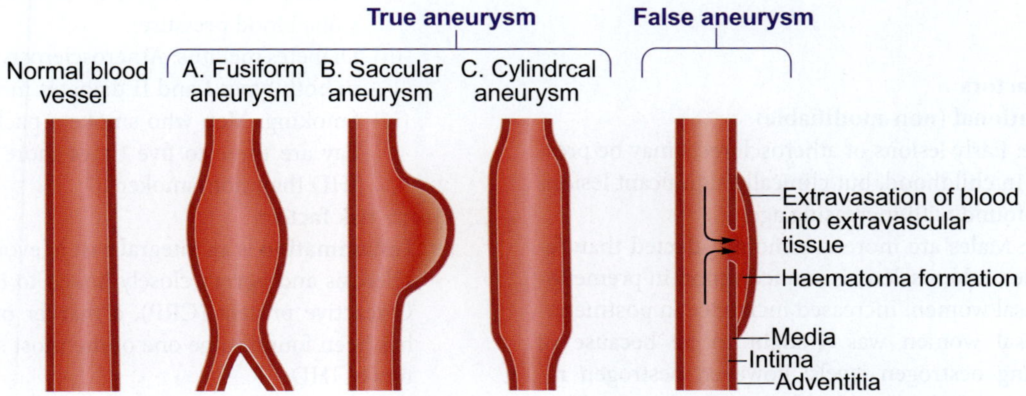

Fig. 24.5 Types of aneurysm.

2. **Thoracic aortic aneurysms**

Pathogenesis
- Most commonly associated with hypertension.
- May also be associated with connective tissue disorders, e.g. Marfan syndrome.

Pathology
- Weakening of the vessel wall leading to progressive dilatation.

Clinical features
- Breathing difficulty (due to compression of the lung and airways).
- Difficulty in swallowing (due to compression of the oesophagus).
- Chronic cough (due to compression of the recurrent laryngeal nerve).
- Costovertebral pain (due to erosion of a rib or vertebra)
- Heart failure (due to aortic valvular dilation and insufficiency).
- Catastrophic blood loss (due to rupture).

Q. Define arteriosclerosis. (PA27.1)

Ans. The term **'arteriosclerosis'** is synonymous with 'hardening of the arteries', which indicates reduced elasticity and thickening of arterial walls. Arteriosclerosis has three main histopathological patterns:

1. **Atherosclerosis:** is the most common and clinically significant pattern of arteriosclerosis in which there is formation of intimal fibrofatty plaques.
2. **Monckeberg medial calcific sclerosis:** is an entity in which there are calcific deposits in muscular arteries of the elderly. These deposits are often visible on imaging but do not narrow the vessel lumen and therefore have little clinical significance.
3. **Hyaline** and **hyperplastic arteriolosclerosis:** affect small arteries and arterioles and are mostly seen associated with hypertension and diabetes mellitus.

Q. Define atherosclerosis. Enumerate the risk factors involved in the pathogenesis of atherosclerosis.

Ans. Atherosclerosis is characterized by the formation of the **fibrofatty plaques** affecting primarily the intima of large- and medium-sized muscular arteries (aorta, coronary and cerebral).

Risk Factors

1. **Major risk factors**
   (a) **Constitutional (non-modifiable)**
      (i) Age: Early lesions of atherosclerosis may be present in childhood, but clinically significant lesions are found with increasing age.
      (ii) Sex: Males are more commonly affected than females; atherosclerosis is uncommon in premenopausal women. Increased incidence in postmenopausal women was thought to be because of falling oestrogen levels; however, oestrogen replacement therapy in older women has not been found to decrease the cardiovascular risk.
      (iii) Genetic factors: Hereditary genetic derangements of lipoprotein metabolism, which predispose the individual to high blood lipid level such as familial hypercholesterolaemia, have been implicated.
      (iv) Familial and racial factors: The established predisposition to ischaemic heart disease (IHD) is multifactorial in origin and is related to the presence of other risk factors such as diabetes and hypertension which show familial clustering. Blacks have less severe atherosclerosis than whites.

   (b) **Acquired (potentially modifiable)**
      (i) Hyperlipidaemia
      - Major classes of lipoproteins are chylomicrons, very low-density lipoproteins (VLDL), low-density lipoproteins (LDL) and high-density lipoproteins (HDL).
      - LDL delivers cholesterol to peripheral tissues (bad cholesterol) and HDL removes cholesterol from the tissues to deliver it to the liver to finally be excreted in the bile (good cholesterol).
      - Diets containing large quantities of saturated fats raise the plasma cholesterol levels. Also, transfats which form because of artificial hydrogenation of polyunsaturated oils (as in baking) are immensely harmful.
      - Diets rich in polyunsaturated fats and omega-3 fatty acids lower the plasma cholesterol levels.
      - Most evidence implicates hypercholesterolaemia:
        - Atherosclerotic plaques contain cholesterol and cholesterol esters.
        - Individuals with hypercholesterolaemia, e.g. patients of diabetes mellitus, myxoedema and nephrotic syndrome, have increased risk of developing atherosclerosis.
        - Dietary regulation and cholesterol-reducing drugs have beneficial effects.

      Note: Main lipids in blood are cholesterol (normal 140–200 mg/dL; borderline, 240 mg/dL) and triglycerides (normal <160 mg/dL). Elevation of serum cholesterol >260 mg/dL in men and women causes three times higher risk of heart disease.

      (ii) Hypertension: Major risk factor at all ages; increased risk is related to both systolic and diastolic blood pressure.
      (iii) Diabetes mellitus: Atherosclerosis manifests faster in both types I and II diabetes mellitus.
      (iv) Smoking: Men who smoke a pack of cigarettes a day are three to five times more likely to die of IHD than non-smokers.

2. **Minor risk factors**
   (a) **Inflammation** is an integral part of evolution of atherosclerosis and is very closely linked to its development. C-reactive protein (CRP), a marker of inflammation, has been found to be one of the most sensitive predictors of IHD.
   (b) **Obesity:** Abdominal/central obesity has been found to be an important risk factor.

(c) **Metabolic syndrome:** It is characterized by insulin resistance, glucose intolerance, hypertension, central obesity, dyslipidaemias, endothelial dysfunction, increased oxidative stress and a systemic inflammatory state, which predisposes to thrombosis.

(d) **Lipoprotein(a) levels:** Lipoprotein(a) is an aberrant form of LDL that has the apolipoprotein B-100 portion of LDL linked to apolipoprotein A. Increased levels predispose to cardiovascular events.

(e) **Factors affecting haemostasis:** Several factors associated with coagulation and fibrinolysis are important predictors of cardiovascular events, e.g. increased levels of thrombin, plasminogen activator inhibitor and fibrinogen are associated with increased risk of myocardial infarction and stroke.

(f) **Physical inactivity and lack of exercise:** A sedentary lifestyle predisposes to atherosclerosis.

(g) **Lifestyle:** Type A behaviour characterized by aggressiveness, competitiveness and drive has increased risk.

(h) **Hyperhomocystinaemia and homocystinuria:** High levels of circulating homocysteine may lead to endothelial injury and vascular disease.

Q. Write in brief about the pathogenesis of atherosclerosis.

Ans. The exact pathogenesis of atherosclerosis is not known; it is thought to be a multifactorial disease. Many theories have been put forward:

- **Encrustation hypothesis proposed by Rokitansky in year 1852:** Atheroma represents lipid encrustation on the arterial wall and formation of thrombus by components of blood (platelets, fibrin and leucocytes).
- **Insudation hypothesis proposed by Virchow in year 1856:** There is cellular proliferation of intimal cells because of increased imbibing of lipids from blood ('lipid theory').
- **Currently, the most accepted theory in circulation is reaction/response-to-injury hypothesis** (Flowchart 24.4). This theory identifies atherosclerosis as a chronic inflammatory and healing response to endothelial injury.

Q. Describe the pathological features and clinical consequences of atherosclerosis.

Ans. Early lesions show diffuse intimal thickening. Fatty streaks are the forerunners in the evolution of atherosclerotic plaques.

1. **Fatty streaks and dots**

   Salient features
   - Start by themselves and are harmless, but are considered earliest precursors of atheromas.
   - Usually begin in the first year of life, and are present in all children older than 10 years.
   - Especially prominent in the aorta and other major arteries and are associated with the known risk factors of atherosclerosis.

   Gross morphology: Multiple, flat or slightly elevated, yellow intimal spots less than 1 mm in diameter, which coalesce into elongated streaks, 1 cm or longer.

   Microscopy: Composed of lipid-laden macrophages (foam cells) and a few T lymphocytes.

2. **Atheromatous plaques** (Fig. 24.6): Fully developed lesions, also called fibrous plaque, fibrofatty plaque or atheroma.

   Gross morphology: White to yellowish-white, 1- to 2-cm lesion raised above the luminal surface; has a grey-white fibrous cap and a central core of yellowish white, soft, grumous lipid.

   Microscopy: Depends on the age of the lesion.
   - **Superficial (luminal) part of fibrous cap** is composed of smooth muscle cells and collagen.
   - **Cellular area under and to the side of the fibrous cap (shoulder of the lesion)** is more cellular and composed of foamy macrophages, T lymphocytes and few smooth muscle cells.
   - **Deeper (central) soft core** is located deep to the cap and is composed of extracellular lipid material, cholesterol clefts (needle-shaped, cleft-like spaces), fibrin, necrotic debris and lipid-laden foam cells.
   - **Older advanced lesions** show dense hyalinized collagen, fibrous tissue and smooth muscle cells.

Clinical Features of Atherosclerosis

- Most often and most severely affected are elastic arteries, such as abdominal aorta, carotids and iliac; and large- and medium-sized muscular arteries, such as coronary and popliteal.
- Symptomatic plaques most often involve arteries supplying the heart, brain, kidneys and lower extremities.
- Major clinical consequences of atherosclerosis are as follows:
  - Myocardial infarction (heart attack).
  - Cerebral infarction (stroke).
  - Intermittent claudication and peripheral vascular disease (gangrene) of lower extremities.
  - Ischaemic bowel disease, infarction and ischaemic strictures of the intestine.
  - Renovascular hypertension.

Complications of Atherosclerosis

1. **Calcification:** Occurs in advanced plaques, especially in aorta and coronaries. The diseased intima crackles like egg shell when incised.
2. **Ulceration:** Layers covering the soft pultaceous material of an atheroma may ulcerate due to trauma or haemodynamic force.
3. **Thromboembolization:** Thrombosis occurs because of ulceration of the plaque and endothelial damage. Emboli composed of lipid material and debris may arise from the thrombi.
4. **Haemorrhage:** It originates either from the luminal blood or rupture of thin capillaries in adventitia.
5. **Aneurysm formation:** Severe atherosclerosis causes atrophy and thinning of the media with fragmentation of the internal elastic lamina resulting in weakening of the vessel wall and aneurysm formation.
6. **Progressive plaque growth:** It causes critical stenosis and obstruction of the vessel.

Endothelial cell injury

↓

Endothelial dysfunction or denudation due to hyperlipidaemia, hypertension, toxins in cigarette smoke, viruses and other infective agents, haemodynamic disturbances, immune complex deposition, irradiation, homocysteine, etc.

↓

Platelet aggregation and platelet release reaction

↓ ↑VCAM-1, IL-1 and TNF

Circulating monocytes and lymphocytes (both CD4+ and CD8+ T cells) adhere to the area of injury and emigrate into the vessel wall (monocytes become macrophages)

↓

The above cells release various cytokines (growth factors) some of which induce smooth muscle proliferation and direct chemotaxis of the smooth muscle cells to the intimal area of the vessel

↓

Macrophages, lymphocytes and smooth muscle cells imbibe LDL-containing cholesterol and become foam cells with subsequent development of fatty streaks (reversible lesions)

↓

Injured endothelial cells and macrophages also produce free radicals, which induce formation of oxidized LDL, a potent enhancer of the atherosclerotic process (oxidized LDL acts to attract, proliferate, immobilize and activate monocytes and is cytotoxic for endothelium and smooth muscle cells; it is ingested by macrophages through scavenger receptors different from LDL receptors)

↓

Fatty streaks continue to enlarge and eventually disrupt the endothelial surface

↓

Platelets adhere to the damaged endothelium overlying the fatty streaks and increase PDGF, which further contributes to smooth muscle proliferation

↓

Over time, the proliferating smooth muscle cells located at the base of the fatty streak begin to synthesize collagen, elastin and proteoglycans, which subsequently produce fibrous plaques

↓

Fibrous plaques undergo dystrophic calcification, haemorrhage, thrombosis, fissuring and ulceration to form a complicated atheromatous plaque

Flowchart 24.4 Reaction/response-to-injury hypothesis.

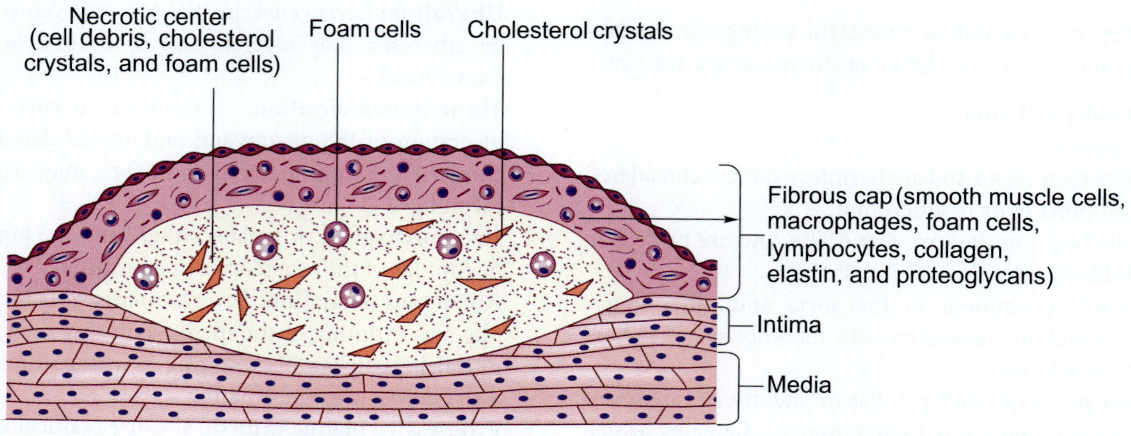

Fig. 24.6 Diagrammatic representation of an atheroma.

Table 24.1 Differences between fatty streak and atheroma

Features	Fatty streak	Atheroma
Age affected	Starts in children as young as 1 year	Affects older individuals
Composition	Lipid accumulation is mainly intracellular (lipid-filled foam cells); T lymphocytes and extracellular lipid are present in small amounts	Large core of extracellular lipid
Gross appearance	• Multiple yellow, flat lesions less than 1 mm in diameter • Do not encroach upon the lumen	• Whitish yellow, raised, usually eccentric lesions, measuring 0.5–1.5 cm in diameter • Encroach upon the lumen
Vasculature involved	May be distributed in areas other than those generally affected by atherosclerosis	Primarily affects elastic as well as large- and medium-sized muscular arteries
Geographic distribution	May be seen in geographic areas which have a low incidence of atherosclerosis	Common in the Western world and developed countries
Clinical consequences	Does not generally cause any obstruction to blood flow	May cause myocardial and cerebral infarction, aortic aneurysms and peripheral vascular disease

Q. Differentiate between fatty streak and atheroma.

Ans. Differences between fatty streak and atheroma are summarized in Table 24.1.

Q. Classify hypertension. Write briefly about the factors regulating blood pressure and describe its morphological effects.

Ans. High blood pressure or hypertension is a common worldwide disease, which causes tremendous morbidity and mortality. Although it could be systemic, pulmonary, or portal in origin, the term "hypertension" invariably indicates systemic hypertension. Sustained systemic hypertension causes end organ damage and is a major risk factor for atherosclerosis. It therefore predisposes the individual to multi-infarct dementia, stroke, myocardial infarction, hypertensive heart disease resulting in congestive heart failure, aortic dissection, peripheral vascular disease, and chronic kidney disease. The clinical classification of hypertension is given in Table 24.2.

- Blood pressure varies with many factors such as age, exercise and emotional disturbances, e.g. fear and anxiety, so should be measured twice during two separate examinations under least stressful conditions.
- Industrialized countries have a higher prevalence of hypertension.
- Hypertension is more common among males and Afro-Americans.
- The control of hypertension reduces mortality due to stroke and coronary artery disease.
- Systolic blood pressure correlates with stroke volume and the compliance of the aorta.
- Factors determining **systolic pressure** include **preload** (volume of blood in the left ventricle), **afterload** (resistance against ejection of blood from the left ventricle) and **contractility of the heart**. The ability of the aorta to expand during systole is labelled **compliance**. Compliance is directly related to elasticity of the vessels which tends to decrease with age. This is the mechanism underlying systolic hypertension which develops with ageing.
- **Diastolic blood pressure** is directly dependent on the amount of blood in the aorta during diastole which in turn is determined by the **peripheral vascular resistance** and the **heart rate**. Increased diastolic pressure is caused by peripheral vasoconstriction, increase in blood viscosity as in leukaemias and polycythaemia and increase in heart rate. Factors that cause peripheral vasoconstriction by contracting the arteriolar smooth muscle include α-adrenergic stimuli (increased circulating catecholamines and angiotensin II, and increased total body sodium). **Excess sodium increases** plasma volume which increases systolic pressure and induces vasoconstriction of arterioles (increases **calcium-mediated contraction of the smooth muscle**).

Table 24.2 Clinical classification of hypertension

Category	Systolic (mm Hg)	Diastolic (mm Hg)
Normal	90–119	60–79
Prehypertension	120–139	80–89
Hypertension		
1. Stage I	140–159	90–99
2. Stage II	>160	>100
Malignant hypertension	>200	>140
Isolated systolic hypertension	>140	<90

Aetiological Classification of Hypertension

- Hypertension is classified into two types:
  - ***Primary or essential or idiopathic*** *(90%–95%):* Wherein cause of increased blood pressure is unknown.
  - ***Secondary hypertension*** *(5%–10%)*: Hypertension secondary to diseases of kidneys, endocrines or other organs.

- Both primary and secondary hypertension can be benign or malignant:
  - ***Benign hypertension*** is characterized by a moderate elevation of blood pressure slowly rising over many years. Patients have a long and asymptomatic life, unless myocardial infarction or a cerebrovascular accident occurs.
  - ***Malignant hypertension*** is typically associated with a marked and rapid increase in blood pressure to 200/120 mm Hg or more. Patients present with papilloedema, retinal haemorrhages, hypertensive encephalopathy and renal failure. Life expectancy after diagnosis is generally less than 2 years, if not treated effectively.

Essential (Primary) Hypertension

- ***Both genetic and environmental factors are thought to play a role in its development.***
  - ***Genetic factors:*** Familial clustering and prevalence in twins has been observed, indicating a role of genetic factors. Mutations in single genes can cause Mendelian or monogenic forms of hypertension. More than ten genes have been implicated. These mutations are thought to alter blood pressure by altering renal regulation of sodium levels. Multiple genome-wide association studies (GWAS) have revealed gene loci in already established pathways of hypertension as well as some immune-related novel genes. It has been suggested that the hypertension can be the result of cumulative genetic polymorphisms. Epigenetic alterations, such as DNA methylation and histone modification, have also been implicated in increasing susceptibility to hypertension.
  - ***Racial and environmental factors:*** Essential hypertension has been found to be more prevalent among blacks than among whites. Environmental factors such as high salt intake, obesity, occupation (skilled population is more affected than unskilled), higher living standards and high levels of stress are also implicated.
- ***There are some risk factors which modify the course of essential hypertension. These include:***
  - ***Age:*** *Ageing* increases predisposition to hypertension probably due to reduction in vascular compliance resulting from stiffening of the arteries. Younger the age at which hypertension is seen, lower the life expectancy, particularly if it is left untreated.
  - ***Sex:*** Females with hypertension appear to do better than males.
  - ***Atherosclerosis:*** Hypertension increases the incidence of atherosclerosis-related complications.
  - ***Other risk factors:*** These include excess of alcohol intake and diabetes mellitus.

Secondary Hypertension

Secondary hypertension can result from conditions affecting different organs:

- **Renal causes:** Renal *parenchymal abnormalities* like acute glomerulonephritis, chronic renal failure, polycystic disease, pyelonephritis, interstitial nephritis, amyloidosis, diabetic nephropathy, renin-producing tumours, Liddle syndrome [gain of function mutation in the epithelial Na^+ channel protein which increases absorption of sodium in the distal convoluted tubule (DCT)] and *renovascular* causes like renal artery stenosis, vasculitis, and collagen vascular diseases. Renovascular causes result in decreased glomerular blood flow in the afferent arterioles and release of renin.
- **Endocrine causes:** Cushing syndrome, hyperaldosteronism, oral contraceptives, oestrogens, pregnancy-induced, pheochromocytoma, acromegaly, primary hypothyroidism, thyrotoxicosis and hyperparathyroidism.
- **Cardiovascular causes:** Coarctation of aorta (causes systolic hypertension in the upper part of the body) and PAN.
- **Neurological causes:** Acute stress, increased intracranial pressure and psychogenic.
- **Miscellaneous causes:** Alcohol, obesity, NSAIDs, cocaine, nicotine, erythropoietin, cyclosporine, tacrolimus, adrenergic medications, decongestants, and pregnancy (preeclampsia).

Renal Regulation of Blood Pressure

The kidneys and heart interact to regulate the vascular tone and blood volume by altering sodium balance. The various regulatory mechanisms involved are as follows:

1. ***Activation of renin–angiotensin system:*** Renin is an enzyme that is produced by renal juxtaglomerular cells that are present in the proximity of afferent glomerular arterioles. It is released in response to decreased blood pressure in the afferent arterioles, increased levels of circulating catecholamines or low sodium levels. Renin cleaves angiotensinogen to angiotensin I, which undergoes peripheral catabolism to produce angiotensin II. Angiotensin II regulates blood pressure by:
   - Increasing vascular smooth muscle tone.
   - Stimulating secretion of aldosterone.
   - Regulating renal sodium and water resorption (reduction in glomerular filtration rate due to reduced blood flow results in increase in proximal tubular reabsorption of sodium).
2. ***Release of vasodepressor material:*** A number of vasodepressor materials and antihypertensives, e.g. prostaglandins and nitrous oxide, counterbalance the vasopressor effect of angiotensin II.
3. ***Natriuretic factors:*** Atrial and ventricular myocardium secretes natriuretic peptides which inhibit the renin–angiotensin system, thereby causing sodium excretion, diuresis and vasodilatation. Increased stretching of atria and ventricles of the heart due to increased BP induces the release of natriuretic factors.

Role of Cardiac Output and Peripheral Resistance in Regulation of Blood Pressure

Arterial blood pressure is a product of cardiac output and peripheral vascular resistance, both of which are regulated by various genetic and environmental factors. Cardiac output is dependant on stroke volume and heart rate. Stroke volume is in turn determined by the filling pressure, which is essentially controlled by sodium hemostasis. Heart rate is controlled by the prevailing

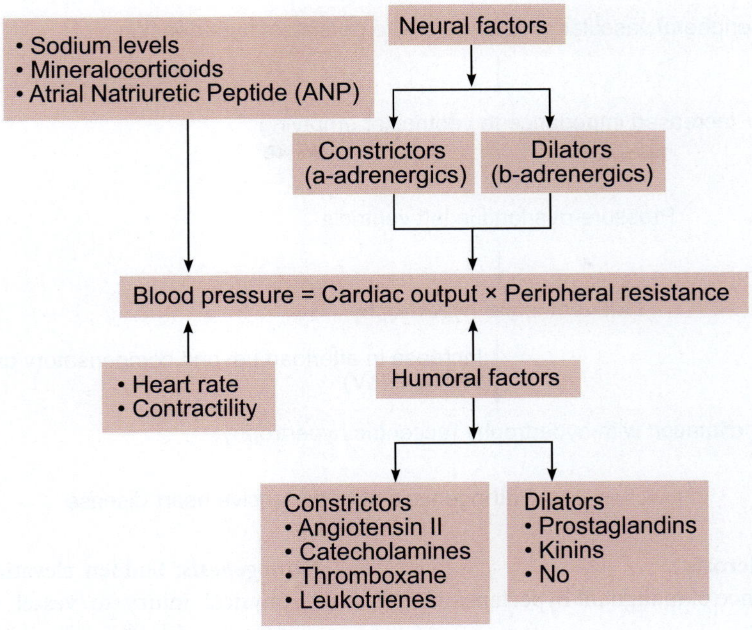

Flowchart 24.5 Role of cardiac output and peripheral resistance in regulation of blood pressure.

adrenergic activity. The factors affecting cardiac output therefore include sodium intake, renal function, and mineralocorticoid levels. Peripheral vascular resistance is dependent upon the sympathetic activity, humoral factors (vasoconstrictors like angiotensin and catecholamines and vasodilators like prostaglandins and kinins), and local autoregulation (vasoconstriction consequent to increased blood flow in an organ to prevent its hyperperfusion).

The vascular endothelium is a very important determinant of blood pressure as it synthesizes various vasodilating and constricting mediators. These mediators include angiotensin II, bradykinin, endothelin, nitric oxide, and growth factors like platelet-derived growth factor, fibroblast growth factor, and insulin growth factor. Endothelin and angiotensin II are potent vasoconstrictors and growth factors that may be major players in the pathogenesis of hypertension. Nitric oxide is a potent vasodilator that is involved in local autoregulation.

Role of cardiac output and peripheral resistance in regulation of blood pressure is depicted in Flowchart 24.5.

Effects of Hypertension

The major effects of systemic hypertension are noted in the following organs:

- Heart
- Blood vessels
- Kidneys
- CNS
- Retina

Effects on Heart (Hypertensive Heart Disease)

- It is usually seen in association with systemic hypertension of prolonged duration, and is the second most common form of heart disease after IHD.
- Death in hypertensive patients is due to congestive heart failure, IHD, cerebrovascular accident (stroke) and renal failure.

Pathogenesis: Pressure overload in systemic hypertension induces left ventricular hypertrophy. Extreme hypertrophy eventually leads to cardiac dilatation and failure (decompensation). Pulmonary hypertension due to primary lung disorders can lead to right-sided heart failure or cor pulmonale. (see Flowchart 24.6).

Gross pathology: Marked hypertrophy of the left ventricle, which in the initial stages is without dilatation (concentric) and later accompanied by dilatation (eccentric hypertrophy). The thickness of the left ventricular wall may reach 2 cm or beyond. This decreases the ventricular filling resulting in left atrial dilatation. The weight of the heart may increase.

Microscopic findings: Enlargement and degeneration of myocardial fibres with areas of myocardial fibrosis, which impairs the diastolic filling.

Effects on Blood Vessels (Hypertensive Arteriolosclerosis)

Hypertension affecting blood vessels has three main pathological patterns, namely:

1. **Hyaline arteriosclerosis**
   This pattern may be:
   - Physiological in origin when it occurs as a result of ageing.
   - Pathological in origin when it occurs because of hypertension or diabetes mellitus.

   Pathogenesis: Chronic haemodynamic stress of hypertension induces leakage of components of plasma and deposition of immunoglobulins, complement, fibrin and lipid in the vessel wall. In diabetes, non-enzymatic glycosylation of the basement membrane of small vessels makes them permeable to proteins, which leak through into the vessel wall to produce hyaline change.

   Pathology (Fig. 24.7): Vessel walls are thickened and lumina narrowed and eosinophilic hyaline material is deposited in the intima and media.

Increased peripheral vascular resistance due to persistent hypertension

↓

Increased impedance to ventricular emptying

↓

Pressure overload in left ventricle

↓

Left ventricular hypertrophy

↓ Increase in afterload beyond compensatory capacity of left ventricle (LV)

LV dilatation with hypertrophy (eccentric hypertrophy)

Flowchart 24.6 Pathogenesis of hypertensive heart disease.

2. **Hyperplastic arteriolosclerosis**

This is usually a consequence of malignant hypertension or toxaemia of pregnancy.

Pathogenesis: Increase in blood pressure causes endothelial injury, which in turn leads to increased vascular permeability and leakage of plasma components. This is thought to stimulate smooth muscle proliferation and basement membrane duplication.

Pathology: Vessels typically show intimal thickening, which may manifest as follows:

- *Onion skinning*: Concentric layers of hyperplastic intimal smooth muscle cells (Fig. 24.8).
- *Mucinous intimal thickening*: Deposition of anhydrous ground salts.
- *Fibrous intimal thickening*: Laying down of collagen, elastic fibres and hyaline deposits in intima.

3. **Necrotizing arteriolitis**

This pattern of arteriosclerosis is typically associated with severe or malignant hypertension.

Pathogenesis: Sudden elevation of pressure causes direct physical injury to vessel wall leading to endothelial damage with fibrin deposition and wall necrosis.

Pathology: Hyaline sclerosis and fibrinoid necrosis of vessel wall, along with an infiltrate of neutrophils in adventitia.

Effects on Kidneys (Hypertensive Renal Disease)

Hypertensive renal disease may present as any of the following morphological patterns:

1. **Benign nephrosclerosis:** It is the spectrum of renal changes associated with the benign phase of hypertension. Benign nephrosclerosis is the most common form of renal disease in persons older than 60 years (common autopsy finding), and its severity increases in the presence of diabetes mellitus.

Clinical features

- Variable elevation of blood pressure.
- Headache and dizziness.
- Palpitations and nervousness.

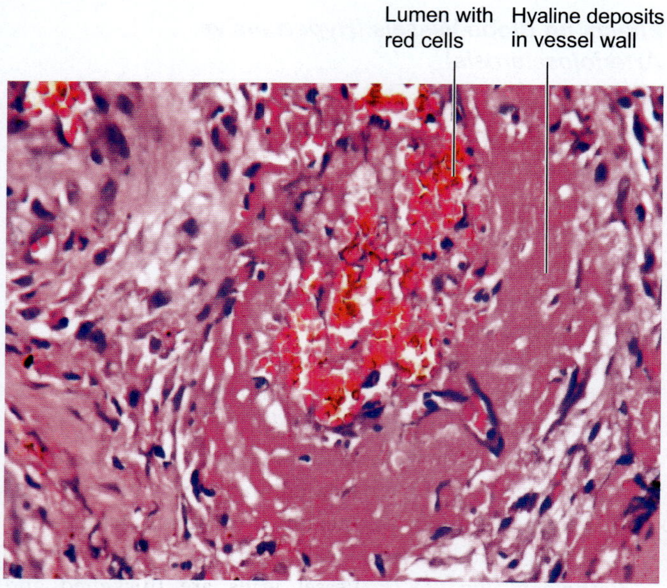

Fig. 24.7 Hyaline arteriosclerosis showing thickening of the vessel wall and deposition of hyaline material (H&E; 100×).

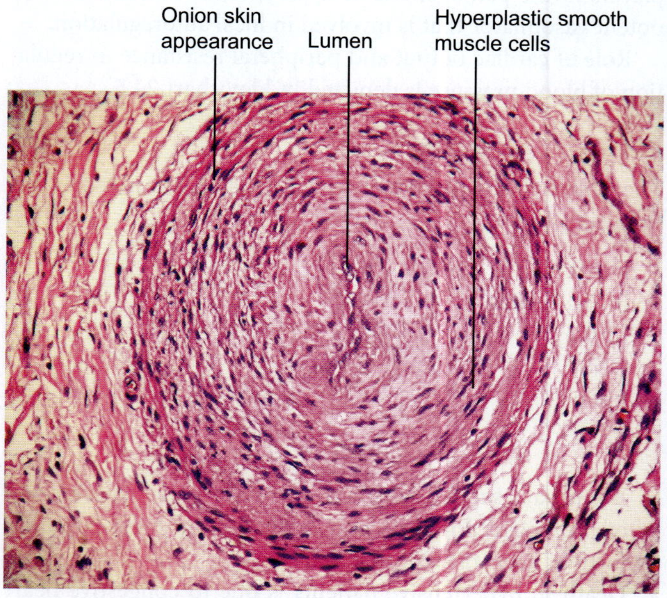

Fig. 24.8 Hyperplastic arteriolosclerosis showing onion skinning (H&E; 100×).

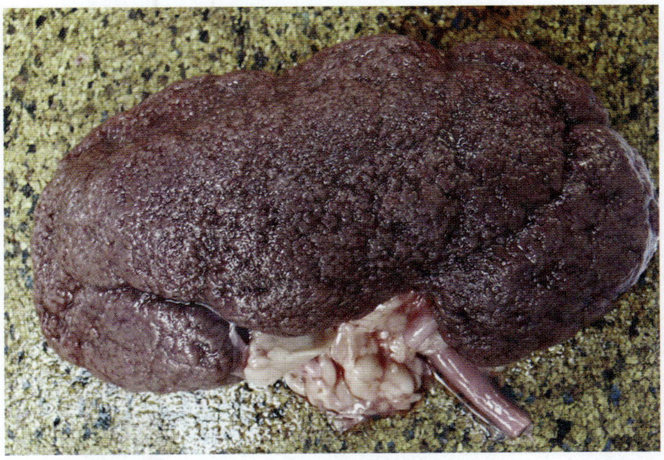

Fig. 24.9 Gross image of a contracted kidney from a patient of benign nephrosclerosis showing fine cortical scarring. The capsule is adherent to the cortical surface, and the latter shows fine granularity (grain leather appearance). (*Source: Uropathology: High-yield Pathology,* Figure 4, Pages 254–255, Elsevier, Saunders, 2012.)

- Renal function tests and urine examination may be normal in the early stage; however, the patient may manifest with mild proteinuria and presence of hyaline and granular casts in the late stage.

Gross pathology (Fig. 24.9)

- Both kidneys are reduced in size and weight because of cortical scarring (small contracted kidneys).
- The capsule is adherent to the cortical surface, which appears finely granular and resembles leather grain.

Microscopic findings (Fig. 24.10)

- *Vascular changes*
  - *Hyaline arteriolosclerosis:* Homogeneous eosinophilic thickening (hyalinization) of the walls of small arteries and arterioles.
  - *Intimal thickening:* Proliferation of smooth muscle cells in the intima of the arcuate and interlobular arteries along with medial hypertrophy and reduplication of the internal elastic lamina.

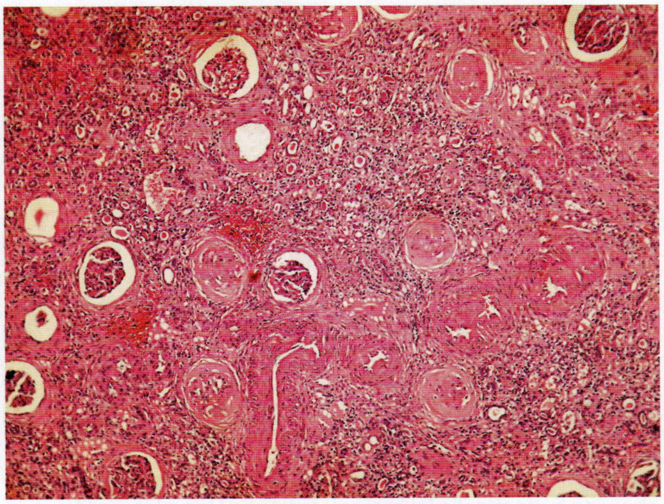

Fig. 24.10 Photomicrograph of end-stage kidney disease showing homogeneous eosinophilic thickening (hyalinization) of the vessel walls (H&E; 100×).

- *Parenchymal changes*
  - Glomerular shrinkage.
  - Deposition of collagen in Bowman's space.
  - Periglomerular fibrosis and complete sclerosis of the glomerulus.
  - Tubular atrophy and fine interstitial fibrosis.

2. **Malignant nephrosclerosis:** A manifestation of malignant or accelerated hypertension, this pattern is uncommon and usually occurs as a superimposed complication in 5% of cases of pre-existing benign hypertension; it can occur in pure form also.

Clinical features

- It presents with headache, dizziness, impaired vision, papilloedema and deranged renal function.
- Urine findings include haematuria and proteinuria.

Gross pathology (Fig. 24.11)

- If superimposed on pre-existing benign hypertension, kidneys are small, shrunken and reduced in size.
- In pure form, kidneys enlarge and show pinpoint petechial haemorrhages on the cortical surface (**flea-bitten**

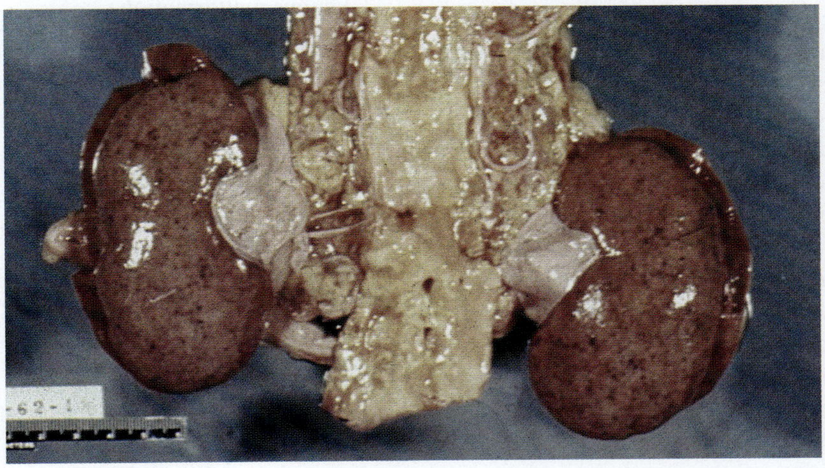

Fig. 24.11 Gross image of kidneys in malignant nephrosclerosis showing pinpoint petechial hemorrhages on the cortical surface (flea-bitten kidney). (*Source: Diagnostic Atlas of Renal Pathology: A Companion to Brenner & Rector's The Kidney,* 9ed, Figure 2.92, Pages 303–375, Elsevier, Saunders, 2012.)

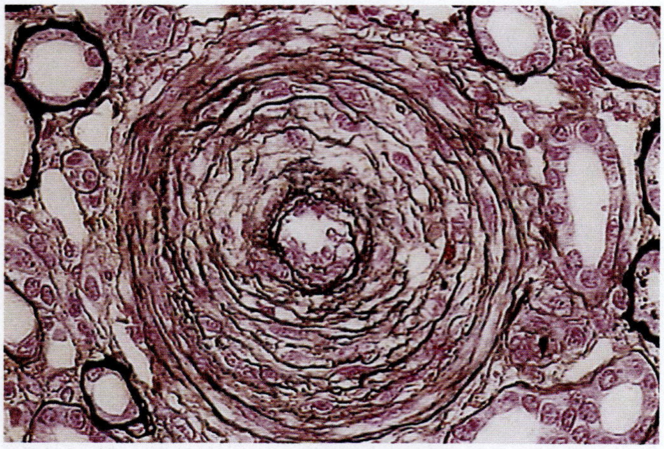

Fig. 24.12 Microscopic image of malignant nephrosclerosis showing hyperplastic intimal sclerosis or onion-skin proliferation (reticulin; 200×). (*Source: Comprehensive Clinical Nephrology: Thrombotic Macroangiopathies, Including Hemolytic Uremic Syndrome,* Figure 28.7, Pages 344–355, Elsevier, Saunders, 2010.)

kidney) because of rupture of arterioles and glomerular capillaries.

Microscopic findings (Fig. 24.12)

- *Necrotizing arteriolitis:* Fibrinoid necrosis, a few acute inflammatory cells and small haemorrhages.
- *Hyperplastic intimal sclerosis or onion-skin proliferation:* Concentric laminar proliferation of smooth muscle cells, collagen and basement membrane material.
- *Ischaemic changes:* Tubular loss, fine interstitial fibrosis and foci of infarction.

Effects on CNS

- Stroke (cerebral haemorrhage and lacunar infarction).
- Carotid atheromas and transient ischaemic attacks.
- Subarachnoid haemorrhage.
- Hypertensive encephalopathy (neurological symptoms such as disturbances in speech, vision, paraesthesias, fits and loss of consciousness).

Effects on Retina (Hypertensive Retinopathy)

- Focal spasm of the arterioles followed by progressive sclerosis (arteriolar walls become opaque with narrow light reflex).
- Chronic hypertension leads to intimal thickening, media wall hyperplasia and hyaline degeneration of arterioles.
- Severe hypertension causes necrosis of vascular smooth muscle and endothelial cells resulting in exudate formation ('soft exudates' are ill-defined and result from microinfarctions, whereas 'hard exudates' are due to leakage of protein from increased vessel permeability).
- Persistent increased pressure in the arterioles may result in the formation of microaneurysms, which may rupture leading to 'flame haemorrhages'.
- Impeded arteriolar circulation results in a compression of venules and ultimately dilatation because arteriole and venous basement membranes are adherent with shared collagen fibres at the crossing points.
- There is development of a depression in the wall of the venule (arteriovenous nicking).
- Papilloedema (swelling of the optic disk) occurs.

Keith–Wagener–Barker classification of hypertensive retinopathy

Grade I: Focal narrowing of the arterioles, mild arteriovenous nicking.

Grade II: Arteriole narrowing, copper wiring present, arteriovenous nicking more accentuated.

Grade III: Arteriole narrowing, silver wiring present, haemorrhages, soft and hard exudates, disappearance of the vein under the arteriole, disk normal.

Grade IV: Arterioles fine fibrous cords; same as grade III except papilloedema is present.

Laboratory Workup of Essential Hypertension and Its Consequences

- Heart disease, e.g. ECG, chest X-ray for cardiomegaly and ECHO for left ventricular hypertrophy.
- Renal disease, e.g. urine analysis, serum blood urea nitrogen (BUN), creatinine, renal ultrasound and angiography.
- Mineralocorticoid excess states, e.g. serum electrolytes.
- Pheochromocytoma, e.g. urinary catecholamines.
- Diabetes mellitus, e.g. serum glucose.
- Lipid abnormalities, e.g. lipid profile.

Q. Classify vascular anomalies.

Ans. Classification of vascular anomalies:

1. **Vascular tumours**

   Benign

   Hemangioma (infantile, congenital, rapidly involuting congenital, non-involuting congenita, tufted angioma ± Kasabach-Merritt phenomenon)

   Intermediate malignancy

   Epithelioid haemangioma

   Malignant

   Kaposiform Hemangioendothelioma (± KMP)
   Spindle cell hemangioendothelioma
   Epithelioid hemangioendothelioma
   Angiosarcoma

2. **Vascular Malformations**

   Slow-flow:

   Capillary malformation
   Venous malformation
   Lymphatic malformation

   Fast-flow:

   Arterial malformation
   Arteriovenous malformation
   Combined vascular malformation (a mix of any of the above)

Q. Describe the clinicopathological features of haemangiomas.

Ans. Haemangiomas are common benign tumours of infancy and childhood. These are difficult to differentiate from malformations or hamartomas.

1. **Capillary haemangioma** (Fig. 24.13)
   (a) Vascular tumour believed to be a proliferation of vascular endothelial cells. It is composed of capillary channels with RBCs.
   (b) It is most commonly found in the skin, subcutaneous tissue and mucous membranes of the oral cavities and

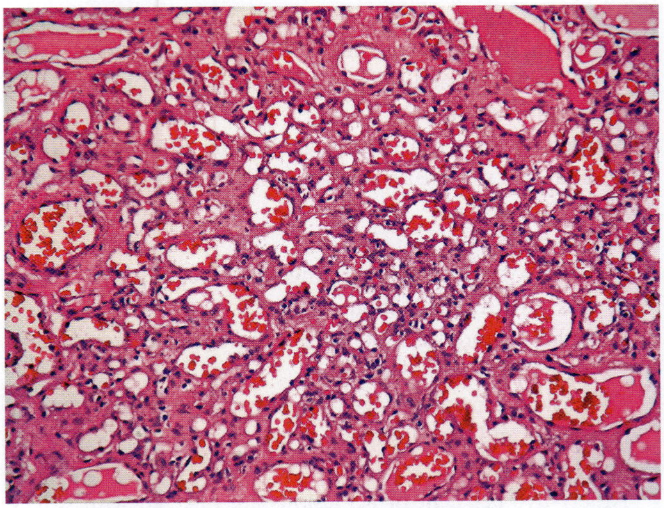

Fig. 24.13 Microscopic image of capillary hemangioma showing numerous small capillary channels containing RBCs (H&E; 200×).

lips; it presents as a red to reddish-purple raised lesion. It may also be seen in the liver, spleen and kidneys.

(c) **'Strawberry type'** of capillary haemangioma is very common and tends to regress by 7 years of age in 75%–90% of cases.

(d) Capillary haemangioma may cause cosmetic disturbance or manifest with bleeding due to traumatic ulceration.

2. **Pyogenic granuloma (lobular capillary haemangioma or polypoid capillary haemangioma)**
   (a) It typically presents as a red/pink to purple nodule, smooth or lobulated, which may follow trauma.
   (b) It shows a striking resemblance to exuberant granulation tissue with oedema and acute and chronic inflammation (Fig. 24.14).
   (c) **'Granuloma gravidarum'** is a pyogenic granuloma occurring in 10% of the pregnant women (regresses after delivery).
3. **Cavernous haemangioma**
   (a) Usually involves deeper structures.

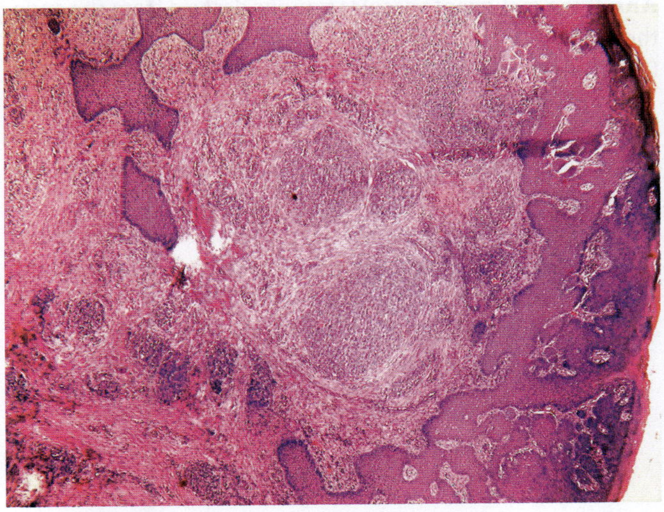

Fig. 24.14 Microscopic image of granuloma pyogenicum showing a polypoidal lesion composed of lobules of proliferating capillary channels with hyperplastic overlying epithelium.

   (b) Locally destructive large lesions, which show no tendency to regress.
   (c) Red-blue, soft, spongy, 1–2 cm in diameter.
   (d) Rare giant forms that affect large subcutaneous areas of face or extremities.
   (e) Sections show a poorly defined unencapsulated lesion, composed of large cavernous vascular spaces separated by scant connective tissue stroma.

Q. Describe the clinicopathological features of lymphangiomas.

Ans. Lymphangioma is a benign lymphatic counterpart of haemangioma. It is of two types:

1. **Capillary lymphangioma** (also called **lymphangioma circumscriptum**)
   (a) It is millimetres to centimetres in diameter.
   (b) It tends to occur subcutaneously in head and neck region and axilla.
   (c) It is distinguished from capillary channels by the absence of blood cells.
   (d) Lobulated but unencapsulated aggregates of thin-walled lymphatics, separated by scant connective tissue stroma, comprise the lesion.
2. **Cavernous lymphangioma** (also called **cystic hygroma**)
   (a) Occurs in children in neck and axilla and rarely retroperitoneal region.
   (b) Histopathology shows massively dilated cystic lymphatic spaces lined by endothelial cells and separated by connective tissue stroma that often contains lymphoid aggregates.
   (c) Margins not well-defined and therefore difficult to remove.

Q. Describe the clinicopathological features of glomus tumour.

Ans. Glomus tumour (glomangioma) is an exquisitely painful tumour arising from modified smooth muscle cells of the glomus body (a specialized arteriovenous anastomosis involved in thermoregulation).

- It manifests as a small (<1 cm in diameter), red-blue, firm nodule usually located in the distal portion of digits.
- Histopathology shows aggregates and nests of specialized glomus cells (small, round to oval with scanty cytoplasm) lying in connective tissue stroma containing branching vascular structures (Fig. 24.15).

Q. Write briefly on Kaposi sarcoma (KS).

Ans. KS was first described by Kaposi in 1872 and is frequently associated with AIDS. There are four known forms of the disease:

(a) **Chronic/classic/European KS**
   (i) Mostly affects older men of Eastern European or Mediterranean descent.
   (ii) Not associated with HIV.
   (iii) Presents with multiple red to purple skin plaques or nodules on extremities.
   (iv) Viscera and mucosa involved in 10% of cases.

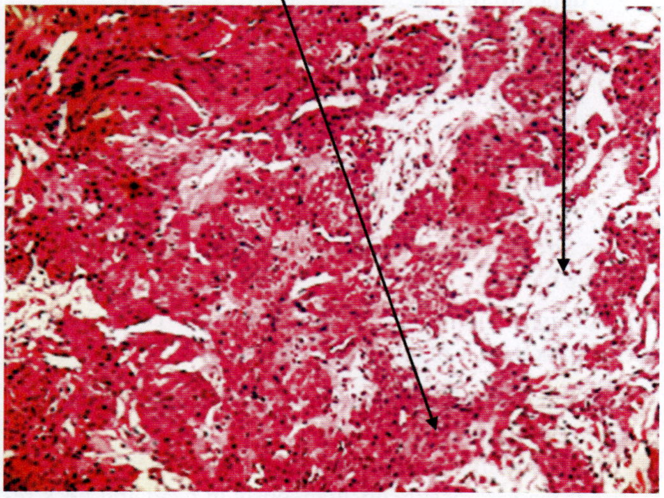

Fig. 24.15 Microscopic image of glomus tumour (glomangioma).

(b) **Lymphadenopathic/African/endemic KS**
   (i) Particularly prevalent among young Bantu children of South Africa.
   (ii) Presents with localized or generalized lymphadenopathy.
   (iii) Aggressive disease course and strong association with AIDS.

(c) **Transplant (immunosuppression)-associated KS**
   (i) It occurs several months to a few years post-transplant in patients receiving high doses of chemotherapy.
   (ii) It is aggressive, and involves lymph nodes, mucosa and visceral organs (usually fatal).
   (iii) Skin lesions may be absent.

(d) **AIDS-associated KS**
   (i) KS is the most common AIDS-associated cancer in the United States.
   (ii) Involvement of lymph nodes and the gut and wide and early dissemination is the hallmark of the disease.
   (iii) Most patients, however, succumb to AIDS-associated opportunistic infections rather than consequences of KS.

Morphology of KS: Three stages are identified:

- **Patch stage:** Pink to red, solitary to multiple macules in the distal lower extremities are seen at this stage.
  Microscopy: Dilated, irregular and angulated blood vessels lined by endothelial cells with an interspersed infiltrate of lymphocytes, plasma cells and macrophages.
- **Plaque stage:** Patch lesion over time converts into larger, violaceous and raised plaques.
  Microscopy: Dilated, jagged and dermal vascular channels lined by plump cells accompanied by perivascular aggregates of spindle cells; scattered between vascular channels are haemosiderin-laden macrophages, lymphocytes, plasma cells and pink hyaline globules of uncertain origin.
- **Nodular stage:** At a later stage, lesions become distinctly nodular and may be accompanied by involvement of lymph nodes and viscera.
  Microscopy
  - Sheets of plump proliferating spindle cells in the dermis and subcutaneous tissue.
  - Small scattered slit-like vessels in a background containing RBCs and pink droplets.
  - Marked haemorrhage, haemosiderin-laden macrophages and lymphocytes.

Pathogenesis of KS

- Ninety-five per cent of KS lesions are infected with KSHV (KS-associated herpes virus, also called human herpesvirus-8 [HHV-8]).
- Immunosuppression is an important cofactor in the pathogenesis and clinical expression of the disease.
- KSHV proteins disrupt the control of cellular proliferation and prevent apoptosis of endothelial cells, through the production of P53 inhibitors and a viral homologue of cyclin D.

Q. Write briefly about vascular neoplasms of intermediate malignancy.

Ans. Haemangioendotheliomas are a group of vascular neoplasms showing histological features intermediate between benign haemangioma and frankly malignant angiosarcomas. They usually affect adults, 60% of which are women. Most common site is extremities followed by head and neck, mediastinum, and trunk.

A representative of this group is epithelioid haemangioendothelioma. It occurs in medium-sized and large veins in soft tissue; well-defined vascular channels are conspicuous and tumour cells are plump epithelial like with intracytoplasmic vacuoles representing small vascular lumina.

Q. Write briefly about angiosarcoma.

Ans. It is a malignant vascular tumour derived from the endothelium.

(a) Angiosarcomas vary from highly differentiated tumours to those resembling epithelial neoplasms such as carcinomas and melanomas. They stain positive for CD31, CD34 or VW factor and are seen in older adults, most commonly in skin, soft tissue, breast and liver.
(b) They may arise in the setting of lymphoedema, radiation exposure or foreign material introduced into the body iatrogenically or accidentally.
(c) Local invasion and distal metastatic spread is common. Outcome is poor with very few surviving 5 years.

25 Diseases of the Heart

NORMAL HEART

- The weight of a **normal heart** averages approximately 250–300 g in females and 300–350 g in males.
- It is enclosed in a double-walled sac called **pericardium**. The pericardium consists of an outer fibrous layer called the parietal pericardium and an inner layer called the visceral pericardium or the epicardium.
- The wall of the human heart is composed of three layers. The outer layer is the **epicardium**; the middle layer is called **myocardium** and the innermost layer is called **endocardium**.
- The **endocardium** merges with the endothelium, which lines the blood vessels and covers heart valves (valvular endocardium). The usual thickness of the free wall of the right ventricle is 0.3–0.5 cm and that of the left ventricle is 1.3–1.5 cm.
- Structure of the normal heart is depicted in Fig. 25.1. An increase in cardiac weight or size is termed *cardiomegaly*. Thickening of the ventricular wall is called *hypertrophy*, and an enlarged chamber size indicates *dilation*.
- The *myocardium* is composed of specialized muscle cells called *cardiac myocytes*. The basic contractile unit of the cardiac muscle is called the *sarcomere*, which is composed of thick and thin filaments containing *myosin* and *actin*, respectively, along with regulatory proteins troponin and tropomyosin. The striated appearance of cardiac myocytes is because of a specific arrangement of sarcomeres. The sliding of the actin filaments between the myosin filaments towards the centre of each sarcomere is the mechanism responsible for the contractility of the cardiac muscle.
- Besides myocytes, other cells that are present in the heart include endothelial cells and fibroblasts. Cardiac myocytes contain structures called *intercalated discs* that join individual cells to allow mechanical and electrical coupling.

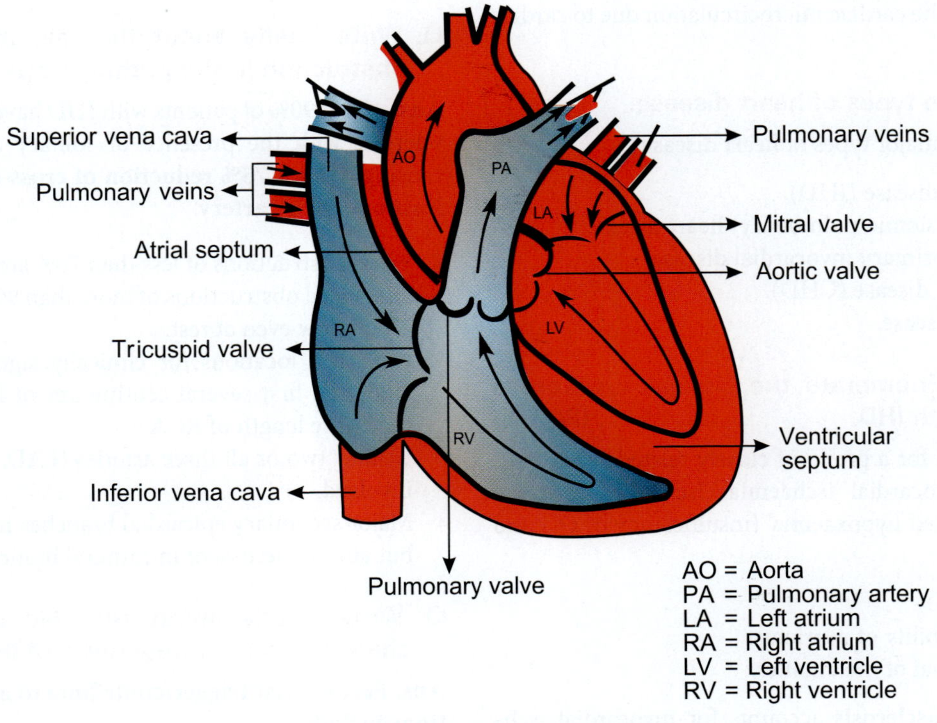

Fig. 25.1 Pictorial representation of normal structure of the heart.

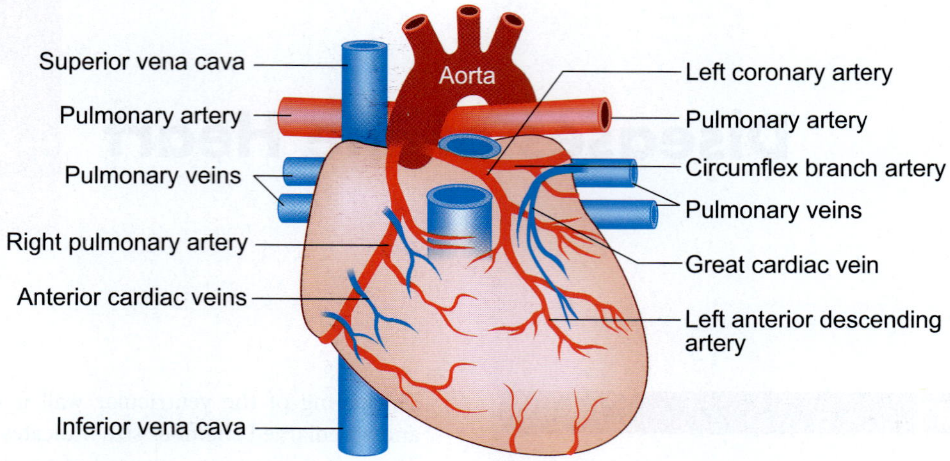

Fig. 25.2 Vascular supply of the heart.

VASCULAR SUPPLY OF THE HEART (FIG. 25.2)

The three major epicardial coronary arteries that perfuse the heart are as follows:

1. Anterior descending branch of the left coronary artery (left anterior descending artery [LAD]), which supplies most of apex of the heart, the anterior wall of the left ventricle and the anterior two-thirds of the ventricular septum.
2. Circumflex branch of the left coronary artery (left circumflex artery [LCX]), which gives rise to patent ductus arteriosus (PDA) and thereby perfuses the posterior third of the septum.
3. Right coronary artery (RCA), which supplies the right atrium, right ventricle, interventricular septum and sino-atrial node (SA) and atrioventricular (AV) nodes.

Majority of the perfusion of the myocardium by the coronary arteries occurs during ventricular diastole, when there is no compression of the cardiac microcirculation due to cardiac contraction.

Q. Enumerate the types of heart disease.

Ans. There are five major types of heart disease:

- Ischaemic heart disease (IHD).
- Hypertensive (systemic/pulmonary) heart disease.
- Non-ischaemic primary myocardial disease.
- Congenital heart disease (CHD).
- Valvular heart disease.

Q. Define IHD. Enumerate the clinical syndromes associated with IHD. (PA27.5)

Ans. IHD is a term for a group of closely related syndromes resulting from myocardial ischaemia. Ischaemia is more harmful than 'isolated hypoxaemia' (insufficiency of O_2) and is characterized by:

- Insufficiency of O_2.
- Decreased availability of nutrients.
- Decreased removal of metabolites.

Coronary atherosclerosis accounts for myocardial ischaemia in more than 90% of cases of IHD; therefore, IHD is also called **coronary artery disease**. The various **clinical syndromes associated with IHD** are as follows:

1. Myocardial infarction (MI).
2. Angina pectoris.
   (a) Stable.
   (b) Prinzmetal or variant.
   (c) Unstable or crescendo.
3. Chronic IHD with heart failure.
4. Sudden cardiac death.

The above-mentioned clinical syndromes are a result of a complex dynamic interaction between:

- Fixed atherosclerotic narrowing.
- Intraluminal thrombosis overlying a disrupted atherosclerotic plaque.
- Platelet aggregation and vasospasm.

Q. Write briefly about the role of fixed coronary obstruction in the pathogenesis of IHD.

Ans. About 90% of patients with IHD have underlying atherosclerosis with the presence of solitary or multiple lesions, causing **at least 75% reduction of cross-sectional area of at least one major artery**.

- Fixed obstructions of less than 70% are usually asymptomatic. Fixed obstructions of more than 90% cause inadequate blood flow even at rest.
- Common locations for clinically significant stenosis include the first several centimetres of LAD and LCX, and the entire length of RCA.
- Usually two or all three arteries (LAD, LCX and RCA) are involved.
- Major secondary epicardial branches may also be involved but atherosclerosis of intramural branches is rare.

Q. Write briefly about the role of acute plaque change in the pathogenesis of IHD.

Ans. Factors that trigger/contribute to acute plaque alterations include:

- Adrenergic stimulation.

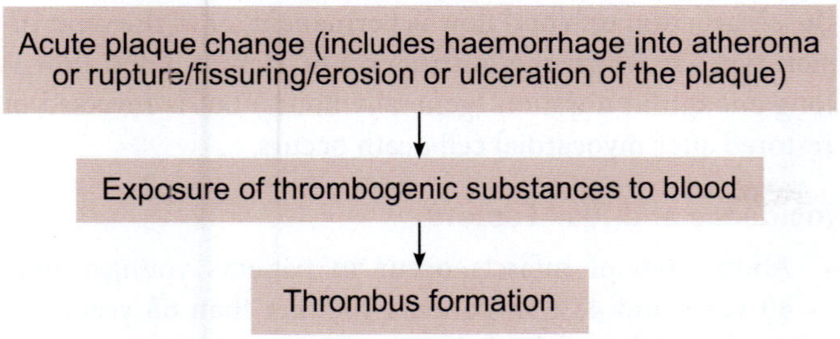

Flowchart 25.1 Role of acute plaque change in the pathogenesis of IHD.

- Structure and composition of plaque (eccentric location, large soft core and thin fibrous cap predispose to plaque alterations, whereas plaques with dense collagen, thick fibrous caps, minimal inflammation and scant necrosis are called 'stable plaques' because they are less likely to rupture).
- **Moderately stenotic (50%–60% stenosis) lipid-rich atheromas are the most dangerous lesions** (plaques causing >60% obstruction reduce blood flow, thus decreasing mechanical stress in the vessel wall and reducing chances of its disruption; **slowly developing occlusions, even if they are high grade, are less dangerous because they stimulate collateral vessel formation**).

Role of acute plaque change in the pathogenesis of IHD is summarized in Flowchart 25.1.

Q. Write briefly about the role of coronary thrombosis in the pathogenesis of IHD.

Ans. Acute transmural MI is usually caused by superimposition of a thrombus on a disrupted, previously partially stenotic plaque, causing total occlusion.

Thrombus formation is aided by:

- Thromboxane A_2 and other platelet constituents.
- Fibrinogen.
- Lipoprotein(a), which inhibits fibrinolysis.

Q. Write briefly about the role of vasoconstriction in the pathogenesis of IHD.

Ans. Vasoconstriction/spasm may contribute to the pathogenesis of Prinzmetal angina as well as acute MI. It is induced by:

- Circulating adrenergics.
- Release of platelet contents.
- Impaired secretion of endothelial cell relaxing factors, e.g. nitrous oxide.
- Release of mediators from perivascular cells such as mast cells.

Q. Write briefly about the role of inflammation in the pathogenesis of IHD.

Ans. Role of inflammation in IHD is depicted in Flowchart 25.2.

Note: Inflammation is thought to have an established role in the pathogenesis of atherosclerosis and proteins involved in inflammation are considered potential markers of CAD, e.g. C-reactive protein (CRP).

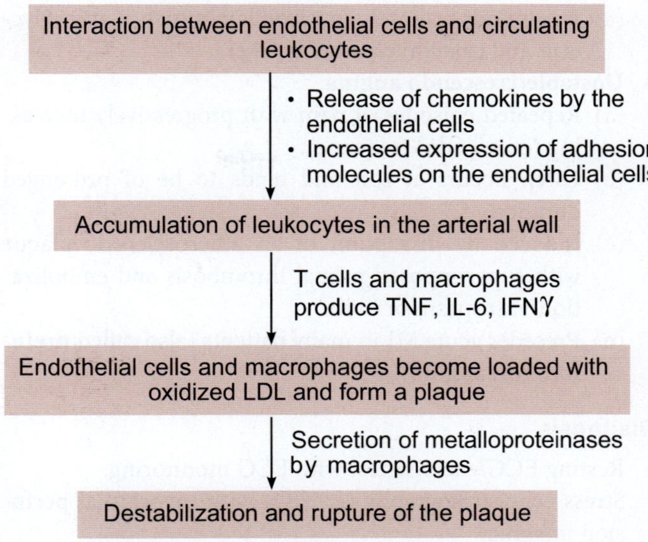

Flowchart 25.2 Role of inflammation in IHD.

Q. Define and classify angina pectoris. Write briefly about the different types of angina.

Ans. Angina pectoris is defined as a symptom complex of IHD characterized by paroxysmal recurrent attacks of substernal or precordial chest discomfort (constricting, squeezing and choking, knife-like) caused by transient (from 15 seconds to 15 minutes) myocardial ischaemia that falls short of inducing cellular necrosis that defines infarction.

Three Overlapping Patterns

1. **Stable/exertional/classical angina**
   (a) Reduction of coronary perfusion due to chronic stenosing fixed coronary atherosclerosis, aortic stenosis or hypertension with concentric left ventricular hypertrophy (oxygen supply inadequate for the thickened ventricular wall).
   (b) Decreased coronary flow causes subendocardial ischaemia.
   (c) The heart is vulnerable to ischaemia whenever there is an increased demand, i.e. physical activity and emotional excitement.
   (d) There is exercise-induced chest pain, which may be accompanied by shortness of breath, diaphoresis, numbness and pain in the inner arm, shoulder and arm.
   (e) It is relieved by rest/decreased demand and nitroglycerin (decreases cardiac work by dilating peripheral vasculature).
   (f) Stress test shows ST segment depression of >1 mm.
2. **Prinzmetal variant angina**
   (a) It is an uncommon pattern of episodic angina that occurs at rest and is due to coronary artery spasm with or without underlying coronary atherosclerosis.
   (b) The vasoconstriction is usually caused by an increase in thromboxane A_2.
   (c) Attacks are unrelated to physical activity, heart rate or blood pressure.
   (d) Elevation of ST segment (indicative of transmural ischaemia) is typically seen on stress test.

(e) It responds promptly to vasodilators such as nitroglycerin and calcium channel blockers.

3. **Unstable/crescendo angina**
   (a) Repeated episodes of pain with progressively increasing (crescendo) frequency.
   (b) Often occurs at rest and tends to be of prolonged duration.
   (c) Induced by disruption of an atherosclerotic plaque with superimposed partial thrombosis and embolization/vasospasm or both.
   (d) Precedes acute MI in many patients (also called **preinfarction angina**).

Diagnosis

- Resting ECG/exercise test with ECG monitoring.
- Stress echocardiography (ECHO) with myocardial perfusion imaging.
- Computed tomography (CT) calcium scoring (scores >75% are associated with increased risk of MI).
- Coronary angiography.
- MRI for demonstrating motion wall abnormalities of the myocardium and to differentiate a stunned myocardium from a non-viable myocardium.

Q. Differentiate between stable angina, Prinzmetal variant angina and unstable/crescendo angina.

Ans. Differences between stable angina, Prinzmetal variant angina and unstable/crescendo angina are summarized in Table 25.1.

Q. What is myocardial infarction (MI)? Write briefly about the aetiopathogenesis, clinical features and morphological evolution of an acute MI.

Ans. MI is defined as myocardial ischaemia that induces cellular necrosis. It is a leading cause of death in industrialized nations. The injury is irreversible and results in significant segmental necrosis of the myocardium (generally >1 cm). The term 'acute' indicates infarction less than 3–5 days old, when the inflammatory infiltrate is primarily neutrophilic. Acute MI may be either of the non-reperfusion type, in which case the obstruction to blood flow is permanent, or of the reperfusion type, in which the obstruction or lack of blood flow is long enough in duration (generally hours) but is reversed or restored after myocardial cell death occurs.

Incidence and Risk Factors

- About 10% of infarcts occur in patients younger than 40 years and 45% in patients younger than 65 years (increasing risk with increasing age).
- Males are more commonly affected than females (the latter show increasing risk with decreasing oestrogen levels).
- Hypertension, diabetes mellitus, hyperlipoproteinaemias, increased apolipoprotein B, increased lipoprotein(a), increased CRP and hyperhomocystinuria are established risk factors for acute MI.

Evolution of Coronary Arterial Occlusion (See Flowchart 25.3)

Coronary artery occlusion causes heart tissue damage due to ischaemia and can lead to myocardial infarction. The immediate and common cause of artery obstruction is the formation of a thrombus or a ruptured plaque. In 10% of cases, MI is not associated with atherosclerosis and is caused by other mechanisms:

1. **Vasospasm:** Intense, relatively prolonged, vasospasm with or without coronary atherosclerosis and platelet aggregation can induce acute MI.

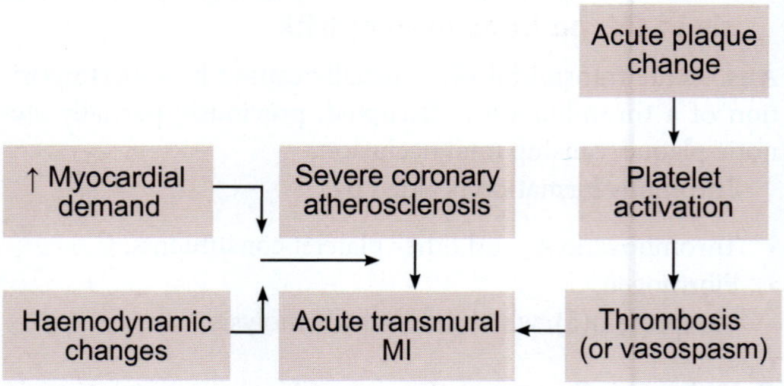

Flowchart 25.3 Evolution of coronary arterial occlusion.

Table 25.1 Differences between stable angina, Prinzmetal variant angina and unstable/crescendo angina

Features	Stable angina	Prinzmetal variant angina	Unstable/crescendo angina
Cause	Fixed coronary atherosclerotic narrowing	Due to coronary artery spasm	Induced by disruption of an atherosclerotic plaque with superimposed partial thrombosis and embolization/vasospasm or both (dynamic stenosis)
Precipitating factors	Heart vulnerable to ischaemia whenever increased demand, i.e. physical activity and emotional excitement	Occurs at rest, not related to physical activity or emotional excitement	Often occurs at rest and tends to be of prolonged duration
Relieving factors	Relieved by rest/decreased demand and nitroglycerin (decreases cardiac work by dilating peripheral vasculature)	Responds promptly to vasodilators such as nitroglycerin and calcium channel blockers	May respond to vasodilators such as nitroglycerin and calcium channel blockers
Outcome	Responds to medication	Transmural ischaemia, which generally responds to medication	Harbinger of subsequent acute MI in many patients (also called preinfarction angina)

2. **Emboli:** These may arise from left atrium because of atrial fibrillation, left-sided mural thrombosis, vegetative endocarditis, paradoxical embolus from the right side of the heart or peripheral veins.
3. **Unexplained:** In one-third of patients, small intramural coronary vessel disease (such as vasculitis), antithrombin III deficiency, amyloidosis, cocaine abuse, dissection or haematological abnormalities, e.g. haemoglobinopathies and polycythaemia vera, may lead to acute coronary episodes.

Clinical Features of Acute MI

- Squeezing, constricting or burning type of retrosternal chest pain which most often occurs in the early morning hours (attributed to the increase in catecholamine-induced platelet aggregation and increased serum concentrations of plasminogen activator inhibitor-1 post awakening). The pain may radiate up to the neck, shoulder and jaw and down to the ulnar aspect of the left arm).
- Dyspnoea due to pulmonary congestion/pulmonary oedema or impaired contractility of the heart.
- Indigestion, feeling of fullness and gas.
- Apprehension or anxiety.
- Excessive sweating.
- Nausea with or without vomiting.
- Lightheadedness with or without syncope.
- Cough or wheezing.
- Hiccupping (which is thought to be due to irritation of the phrenic nerve or diaphragm).
- Rapid thready pulse.
- May be asymptomatic, discovered on ECG (silent MIs are common in patients with underlying diabetes mellitus and in elderly patients).

Decreased aerobic glycolysis and onset of anaerobic glycolysis

↓

Inadequate production of high-energy phosphates (creatinine phosphate and ATP)

↓

Lactic acidosis

Flowchart 25.4 Biochemical consequences of acute MI.

Myocardial Response

Decreased coronary blood supply induces profound functional, biochemical and morphological changes. The **biochemical consequences** of acute MI are shown in Flowchart 25.4. There are **three main morphological events** which occur after acute myocardial infarction:

1. ATP depletion leading to loss of contractility within a few minutes.
2. Setting in of a state of irreversible injury within 20–40 minutes.
3. Beginning of microvascular injury within 1 hour.

The sequential morphological changes in acute MI are summarized in Table 25.2.

Q. Write briefly about reperfusion injury.

Ans. Infarct modification by reperfusion (restoration of blood flow by thrombolysis, percutaneous intervention and bypass surgery):

- Reperfusion within 15–20 minutes revives everything and prevents all necrosis.

Table 25.2 Morphological changes in acute MI

Time	Gross changes	Microscopic changes
0–4 h	None	Waviness of fibres at border
4–12 h	None (the infarcted area can be highlighted by immersion of the dead tissue in triphenyl tetrazolium chloride, which gives a brick red colour to intact areas which have lactate dehydrogenase activity and does not stain the infracted area because the enzymes have leaked out in the latter due to membrane injury)	Beginning of coagulation necrosis, oedema
12–24 h	Dark mottling	Coagulative necrosis with pyknosis of nuclei (Fig. 25.3); neutrophilic infiltration, myocyte hypereosinophilia; marginal contraction band necrosis
1–3 days	Hyperaemia around a yellow-tan infarct centre	Disintegration of dead myofibrils followed by phagocytosis of dead cells by macrophages at infarct border
3–7 days	Maximally yellow-tan and soft; well-delineated hyperaemic border	Early formation of fibrovascular granulation tissue at margins
7–10 days	Red-grey depressed infarct borders	Well-established granulation tissue with new blood vessels and collagen deposition
10–14 days	Progressive formation of a grey-white scar	Increased collagen deposition with decreased cellularity
2–8 weeks	Scarring complete	Dense collagenous scar forms

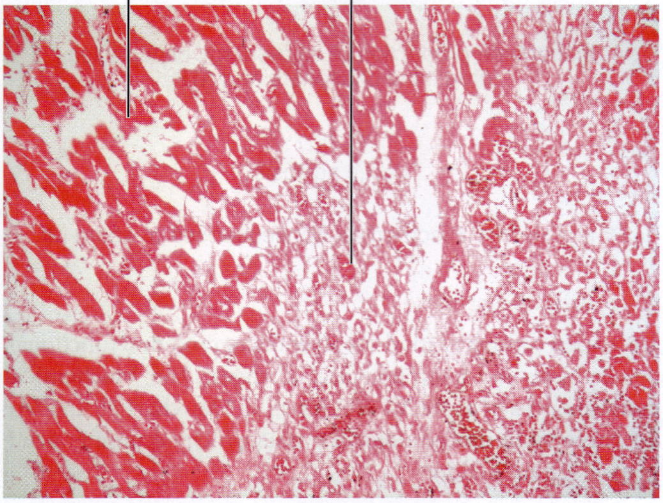

Fig. 25.3 Photomicrograph of a myocardial infarct showing an area of coagulative necrosis surrounded by viable myocardium (H&E; 100×).

- Thrombolysis by tissue plasminogen activator/streptokinase re-establishes blood flow/rescues ischaemic (and not dead) myocardium when given within the first 3–4 hours.
- Anticoagulant therapy with heparin, thrombin inhibitors and factor Xa inhibitors is used to prevent clot propagation.
- Percutaneous transluminal coronary angioplasty (PTCA) relieves some of the obstruction caused by the plaque as well.
- Salvaged tissue is biochemically and functionally altered (stunned myocardium) and may predispose the tissue to **dysrhythmias**.
- Reperfusion can sometimes trigger deleterious effects labelled **'reperfusion injury'**, which could manifest as follows:
  - **Arrhythmias:** These occur because of unstable myocardium.
  - **Haemorrhagic infarct:** A partially completed and reperfused infarct is haemorrhagic (vasculature injured due to ischaemia becomes leaky when the flow is restored).
  - **Contraction bands:** These are intensely eosinophilic transverse bands composed of closely packed hypercontracted sarcomeres (produced by exaggerated contraction of myofibrils due to exposure to high concentration of calcium ions at the instant perfusion is re-established).
  - **Stunned myocardium:** Refers to the persistence of biochemical abnormalities for days to several weeks after rescue from ischaemia by reperfusion.

Q. Enumerate the types of myocardial infarcts. Differentiate between transmural and subendocardial infarcts.

Ans. Depending on the thickness of the myocardium involved, myocardial infarcts are classified as follows:

1. **Transmural infarcts:** These involve the whole thickness of the ventricular wall in the distribution of a single coronary artery. These are also called ST-elevation myocardial infarcts or STEMI. This type of infarct is associated with the appearance of Q waves and increase in cardiac enzymes and has a high mortality rate.
2. **Subendocardial infarcts:** These involve only the inner one-third to one-half of the ventricular thickness. These are also called non-STEMI infants. Q waves are absent. Cardiac enzymes are increased. Non-STEMI infarcts have a lower mortality rate.
3. **Multifocal microinfarcts:** Multifocal microinfarction is seen when small intramural vessels are involved by vasculitis, microembolization or vasospasm.

The differentiating features between transmural and subendocardial infarcts are enlisted in Table 25.3.

Table 25.3 Differences between transmural and subendocardial infarcts

Features	Transmural infarct	Subendocardial infarct
Extent	Involves the whole thickness of the ventricular wall in the distribution of a single coronary artery	Involves only the inner one-third to one-half of the ventricular thickness; may be multifocal and has a circumferential distribution
Frequency	More common (95%)	Less common (5%)
Causes	Associated with coronary atherosclerosis, acute plaque change, superimposed completely obstructive thrombosis	No plaque disruption seen
Epicarditis	Common	Not common
Cardiac aneurysm formation	May be seen	Not seen
ECG changes	Elevation of ST segment	No ST elevation

Q. Enumerate the consequences and complications of acute MI.

Ans. Most deaths occur within 1 hour of onset of an acute MI. Three-fourth of patients have one or more complications. Complications of acute MI include:

1. **Left ventricular contractile dysfunction:** Abnormality in the left ventricular function is proportionate to the size of the infarct and may result in:
   (a) Left ventricular failure with hypotension and pulmonary vascular congestion.
   (b) Pump failure (cardiogenic shock; seen in 10%–15% of cases; caused by a large infarct involving more than 40% of the left ventricle area and is associated with a 70% mortality rate).
2. **Arrhythmias**
   (a) Conduction disturbances due to myocardial irritability (sinus tachycardia, bradycardia, ventricular premature contractions, ventricular tachycardia, ventricular fibrillation and asystole).

(b) Infarcts of inferoseptal region (area lodging the bundle of His), may lead to heart block.

3. **Myocardial rupture**
   (a) Myocardial rupture (due to transmural necrosis) may cause haemopericardium and cardiac tamponade.
   (b) Complete rupture of ventricular wall/septum can lead to formation of a left-to-right shunt.
   (c) Incomplete rupture may result in the formation of a pseudoaneurysm.
   (d) Papillary muscle rupture (most commonly 3–7 days after the onset of the infarct) causes valvular dysfunction (mitral regurgitation).
4. **Pericarditis:** It could be **early pericarditis (fibrinous or fibrinohaemorrhagic)** or **delayed immunologically mediated pericarditis** (**Dressler syndrome**, seen 2–10 weeks after infarction).
5. **Right ventricular infarction:** Isolated right ventricular infarction is rare. It usually accompanies ischaemic injury of the left ventricle and septum.
6. **Infarct extension/expansion:** New necrosis/weakening and disproportionate stretching, thinning or dilatation of infarct lead to its extension/expansion.
7. **Embolism from mural thrombosis** (Flowchart 25.5): Abnormal myocardial contractility leads to endocardial damage, which in turn leads to mural thrombosis and embolism.
8. **Ventricular aneurysm formation**
   (a) Late complication.
   (b) Associated with a large transmural anteroseptal infarct that converts into thin scar tissue.
9. **Papillary muscle dysfunction:** It is the postinfarct mitral regurgitation due to ischaemic injury to the papillary muscle and underlying myocardium; it may later lead to papillary muscle fibrosis.
10. **Progressive late heart failure:** Chronic IHD (also called **ischaemic cardiomyopathy** [CMP]) is caused by postinfarction cardiac decompensation due to exhaustion of compensatory hypertrophy of the non-infarcted myocardium.

Complications occurring within the first 72 hours include cardiogenic shock, arrhythmias, acute pulmonary oedema and cardiac tamponade. Late complications include cardiac aneurysm formation, chronic IHD or ischaemic CMP, congestive heart failure, pulmonary hypertension and delayed pericarditis.

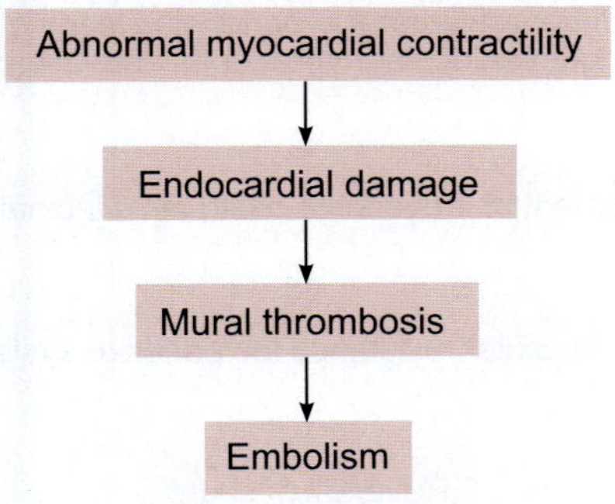

Flowchart 25.5 Pathogenesis of embolization from mural thrombosis.

Q. Write briefly about the laboratory diagnosis of acute myocardial infarction (MI).

Ans. A patient is diagnosed with MI if two (probable) or three (definite) of the following WHO criteria are met with:

- Clinical history of ischaemic type of chest pain lasting for more than 20 minutes.
- Changes in serial ECG tracings such as ST elevation/inverted T wave/appearance of Q wave.
- Rise in levels of serum cardiac biomarkers or enzymes (particularly on serial testing), which leak out of the damaged myocardium into the blood, such as:

1. **Creatinine kinase (CK)**
   (a) **Different isoenzymes of CK include MM** (from skeletal muscle and heart), **MB** (principally from myocardium, particularly MB2) and **BB** (from brain and lung).
   (b) **CK activity:** It begins rising in 2–4 hours, peaks in 24 hours and falls in 72 hours.
   (c) **CKMB:** It is more specific/begins rising in 4–8 hours, peaks in 18 hours and falls in 48–72 hours.
   (d) **CKMB2/CKMB1 ratio >1.5 is a highly sensitive indicator of myocardial injury.**
   (e) CKMB may also be increased in myocarditis, muscular dystrophy, rhabdomyolysis and polymyositis.
2. **Troponins (Tn)**
   (a) Troponins are proteins that regulate calcium-mediated contraction of cardiac and skeletal muscle.
   (b) They are of two types, namely TnI and TnT.
   (c) Troponins are not normally detectable in the serum; their levels are elevated in acute MI (appear within 3–12 hours and peak at 24 hours).
   (d) Troponins of different origins can be distinguished by specific antibodies, which can also be used for quantitative assays.
   (e) These are the **most sensitive and specific cardiac markers, as sensitive and more specific than CKMB** (sensitivity is 84% and specificity is 80%–95%).
   (f) Troponin levels remain elevated for 7–10 days permitting a late diagnosis/evaluation of the progression of the infarct.
   (g) Levels may also be increased in unstable angina, myocarditis, cardiac failure, renal failure and pericarditis.
3. **Lactate dehydrogenase (LDH)**
   (a) LDH1 is myocardium specific.
   (b) It rises 24 hours after an acute MI, reaches a peak in 3–6 days and returns to normal in 14 days.
4. **Myoglobin**
   (a) **First cardiac marker to become elevated.**
   (b) Lacks cardiac specificity.
   (c) Excreted rapidly in the urine.
   (d) Returns to normal within 24 hours of the initiation of MI.

Other investigations for acute MI

- Echocardiogram (to see abnormalities of regional wall motion).
- Radioisotopic studies (radionuclide scan).

- Perfusion scintigraphy (for regional perfusion).
- MRI (for structural characterization).

Q. Write briefly about Dressler syndrome.

Ans. Dressler syndrome (also called post-MI syndrome) is thought to develop consequent to an autoimmune reaction to the necrotic muscle resulting from an episode of acute myocardial infarction. It occurs weeks or months post MI and presents with fever, pericarditis and pleurisy. It is usually treated with aspirin and NSAIDs or corticosteroids.

Q. Define sudden cardiac death.

Ans. Sudden cardiac death is defined as an unexpected death from cardiac cause within 1 hour of onset of symptoms. It may be a consequence of the following:

- IHD.
- Congenital structural abnormality of the heart and blood vessels (aortic valve stenosis/mitral valve prolapse).
- Myocarditis.
- Pulmonary hypertension.
- Abnormality of cardiac conduction system.
- Isolated hypertrophy/increased cardiac mass.

Risk factors include obesity, glucose intolerance, hyperlipidaemias, hypertension, left ventricular hypertrophy, CMPs and a previous non-STEMI. Sudden cardiac death generally occurs secondary to acute disruption of an atherosclerotic plaque or a lethal arrhythmia.

Q. Define congenital heart disease (CHD). Write briefly about its aetiopathogenesis.

Ans. CHD is defined as an abnormality of the heart and blood vessels which is present since birth and is due to faulty embryogenesis during third to eighth gestational weeks (when major cardiovascular structures develop). Faulty embryogenesis can result in:

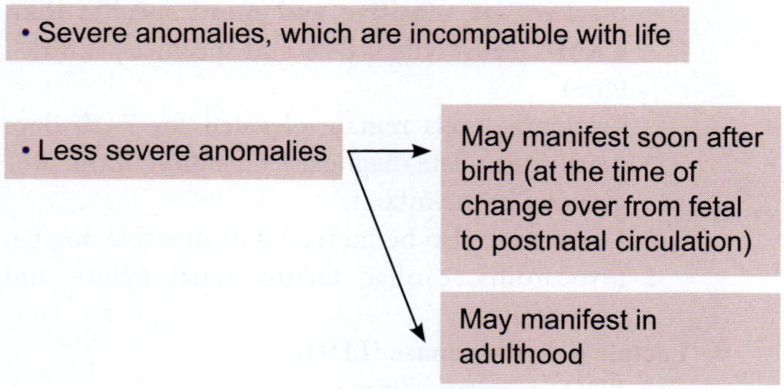

Incidence

- 6–8/1000 live-born full-term infants (most common heart disease in children).
- It is higher in premature infants and stillborns.

Aetiopathogenesis

Both genetic factors and maternal risks are implicated.

Genetic Factors

- ***Single gene mutations*** (genes encoding transcription factors required for normal cardiac development, e.g. GATA4, Tbx5 and genes encoding components of the Notch pathway).
- ***Small chromosomal deletions***, e.g. deletion of chromosome 22q11.2 in DiGeorge syndrome, which leads to abnormal development of the fourth bronchial arch and derivatives of third and fourth pharyngeal pouches responsible for the development of the heart.
- ***Additions and deletions of whole chromosomes***, e.g. trisomy of chromosomes 13, 15, 18 and 21, and Turner syndrome.

Maternal Risks

Rubella, alcohol and drugs (teratogens).

Q. Classify congenital heart disease. Write briefly about the clinicopathological features of the various types of CHD.

Ans. *Classification and clinicopathological features of various types of CHD:*

1. **Malpositions of the heart (dextrocardia):**
   (a) Apex of the heart points to the right of the chest.
   (b) It may be accompanied by situs inversus; so, the heart remains in normal position with respect to the other organs.
   (c) Isolated dextrocardia may be associated with major anomalies, e.g. transposition of aorta and transposition of great vessels.
2. **Shunts:** Abnormal communication between chambers or blood vessels:
   (a) **Left-to-right shunt** (Flowchart 25.6): Under normal circumstances the flow through the systemic and pulmonary circulations is balanced. The same volume of blood circulates through the systemic circulation, then

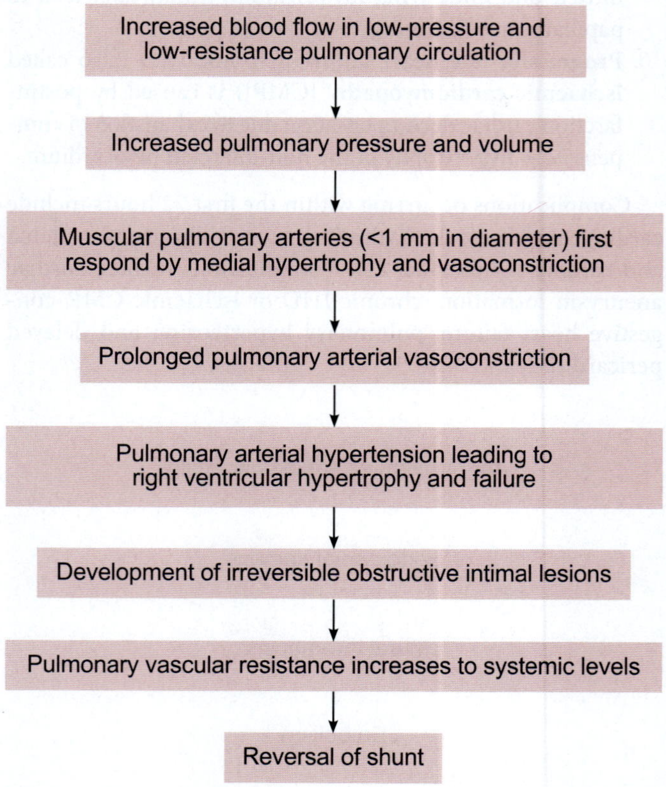

Flowchart 25.6 Consequences of a left-to-right shunt.

the pulmonary circulation, then back to the systemic circulation, and so on. Left to right shunts are characterized by a leak of blood from the systemic to the pulmonary circulation. This causes a larger pulmonary than the systemic flow. As a result, the pulmonary circulation carries not only the blood that entered the right atrium and right ventricle through the superior and inferior vena cava, but also the additional blood entering through a shunt. This causes the blood volume and/or pressure in the pulmonary circulation to become abnormally high. If the shunt is significant, there is progressive damage to the pulmonary vasculature and gradual development of irreversible pulmonary hypertension. Pulmonary vascular resistance increases to systemic levels to cause reversal of shunt which is also called late cyanotic CHD or Eisenmenger syndrome. If significant irreversible pulmonary hypertrophy develops, structural defects of CHD are considered irreparable.

Examples

- Shunts with increased pulmonary blood flow **(atrial septal defect [ASD]).**
- Shunts with increased pulmonary blood flow and pressure **(ventricular septal defect [VSD] and patent ductus arteriosus [PDA]).**

(i) **ASD**

- Abnormal opening in the atrial septum that allows communication of blood between left and right atria.
- Well tolerated and asymptomatic till adulthood.
- Murmur develops because of excessive blood flow through the pulmonary valve.
- Three major types according to the location in the septum (Fig. 25.4):
  - Secundum abnormality (90% of all ASDs): Results from a deficient or fenestrated fossa ovalis.
  - Primum abnormality (5% of ASDs): Occurs adjacent to AV valves; usually associated with a cleft anterior mitral (partial AV septal defect).
  - Sinus venosus defect (5% of ASDs): Located near the entrance of superior vena cava.

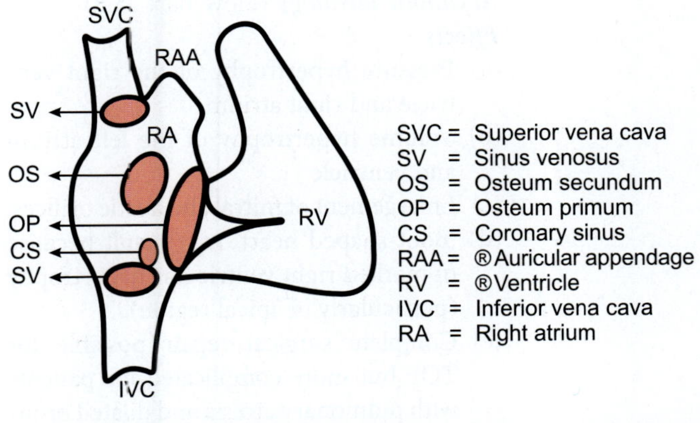

Fig. 25.4 Schematic diagram to show various types of ASD.

Effects of ASD

- Left-to-right shunt at the atrial level with increased pulmonary flow (because the pulmonary vascular resistance is less than the systemic vascular resistance and because the distensibility of the right ventricle is more than that of the left).
- Volume hypertrophy of the right atrium and right ventricle ultimately leading to failure.
- Enlargement and hemodynamic changes of the tricuspid and pulmonary valves.
- Volume atrophy of the left atrium and left ventricle (reduction in muscle mass) with small-sized mitral and aortic orifices.
- Complications: Paradoxical embolization and irreversible pulmonary disease.
- Complete reversal of the abnormal haemodynamics by ASD closure (surgical or catheter based).

(ii) **VSD**

- It is the most common CHD (25% of CHD in children and 10% in adults; 30% occur as isolated anomaly; rest associated with other defects).
- It is recognized early in life.
- Small defects close spontaneously, whereas larger defects remain patent and produce significant effects.

Depending on location, VSD may be of the following types (Fig. 25.5):

- Ninety per cent of cases have a defect in the membranous septum close to the bundle of His (membranous VSD).
- Remaining 10% have VSD in the muscular or trabecular part of the septum. The defect may be located immediately below the pulmonary valve (subpulmonic) or present as multiple defects in the septum (infundibular VSD).

Effects of VSD

- Left-to-right shunt at the ventricular level.
- Increased blood in the right ventricle and pulmonary artery leading to volume

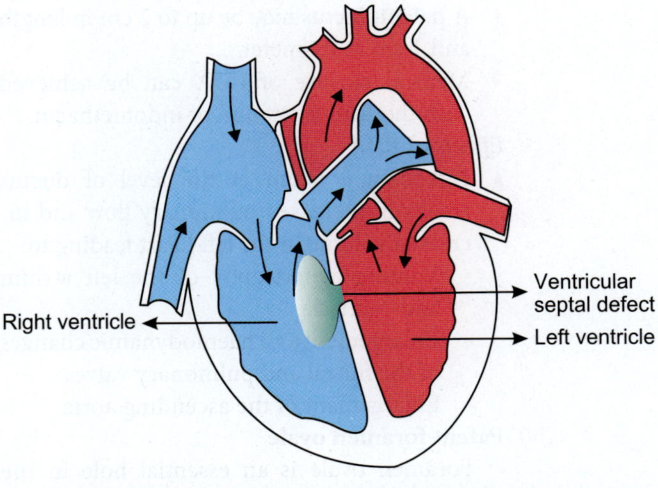

Fig. 25.5 Schematic diagram to depict different types of VSD.

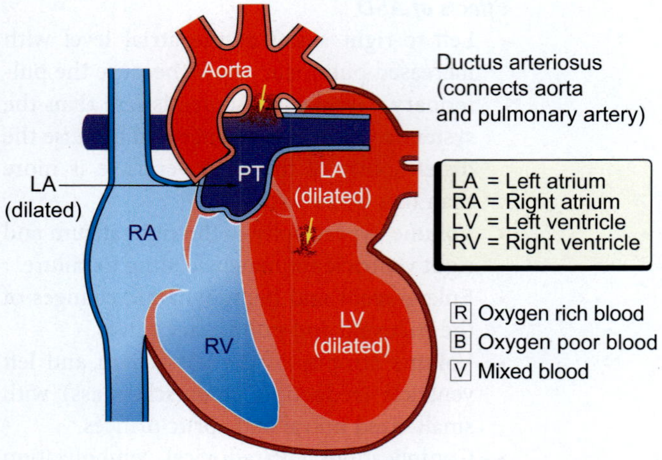

Fig. 25.6 Schematic diagram to show PDA.

hypertrophy of the right ventricle and enlargement and haemodynamic changes in the tricuspid and pulmonary valves.

- Eventually leads to pressure hypertrophy of the right atrium, volume hypertrophy of the left atrium and ventricle and enlargement and haemodynamic changes in the mitral and aortic valves.

(iii) **PDA**

- Ductus arteriosus is the vascular connection between the aorta (descending) and the bifurcation of the pulmonary artery, which normally closes within the first to second day of life.
- Persistence (due to continued synthesis of PGE2) for more than 3 months of age is abnormal and is called PDA (Fig. 25.6).
- It constitutes 10% of congenital malformations of the heart and great vessels.
- Ninety per cent of cases present as an isolated defect; remaining are associated with VSD, coarctation and pulmonary stenosis (PS) and aortic stenosis.
- Characteristic **harsh machinery-like murmur** is heard on auscultation.
- A patent ductus may be up to 2 cm in length and 1 cm in diameter.
- Medical closure of PDA can be achieved with the administration of indomethacin.

Effects of PDA

- Left-to-right shunt at the level of ductus results in increased pulmonary flow and increased volume in the left heart leading to:
  - Volume hypertrophy of the left atrium and ventricle.
  - Enlargement and haemodynamic changes of the mitral and pulmonary valves.
  - Enlargement of the ascending aorta.

(iv) **Patent foramen ovale**

- Foramen ovale is an essential hole in the atrial septum through which oxygenated blood from the placenta travels directly from the right atrium to the left atrium without passing through the immature lungs.
- Under normal circumstances, it closes at birth because of increased pressure in the left side of the heart.
- If the foramen remains patent, a transient increase in the right-sided pressure, as is seen during coughing, sneezing or bowel movements, can produce transient right-to-left shunting and paradoxical embolus.

(b) **Right-to-left shunts**

- Blood from the right side of the heart enters the left side.
- Dusky blueness of the skin and mucous membranes (cyanosis) occurs because of poorly oxygenated blood entering systemic circulation. It is also called **'cyanotic CHD'**.
- 'Bland or septic emboli' arising in peripheral veins bypass pulmonary circulation (where they are normally filtered) and enter systemic circulation. These are called **paradoxical emboli** and may cause brain infarction and abscess.
- **'Clubbing'** of tips of fingers and toes **(hypertrophic osteoarthropathy)** and **'polycythaemia'** result from chronic long-standing cyanosis.

Examples

(i) **Tetralogy of Fallot (TOF)**

- Most common cyanotic CHD
- Four components (Fig. 25.7):
  - VSD usually large (shunt abnormality)
  - Displacement of aorta to the right such that it overrides the VSD
  - PS (obstruction)
  - Right ventricular hypertrophy
- Severity of clinical features proportionate to the extent of PS and size of VSD.
- Two types of TOF exist:
  - ***Cyanotic tetralogy*** (Flowchart 25.7)

    Effects

    (a) Pressure hypertrophy of the right atrium and right ventricle.
    (b) Smaller and abnormal tricuspid valve.
    (c) Smaller left atrium and left ventricle.
    (d) Enlarged aortic orifice.
  - ***Acyanotic tetralogy*** (Flowchart 25.8)

    Effects

    (a) Pressure hypertrophy of the right ventricle and right atrium.
    (b) Volume hypertrophy of the left atrium and ventricle.
    (c) Enlargement of mitral and aortic orifices.
    (d) 'Boot-shaped heart' may result because of marked right ventricular hypertrophy (particularly of apical region).
    (e) Complete surgical repair possible for TOF but more complicated for patients with pulmonary atresia and dilated bronchial arteries.

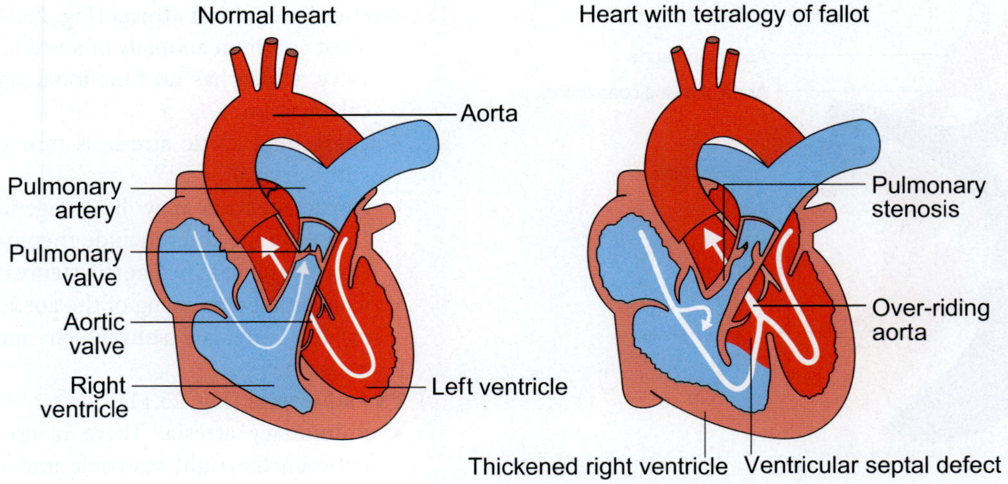

Fig. 25.7 Schematic diagram to demonstrate TOF.

Prominent pulmonary stenosis and mild VSD
↓
More resistance to outflow of blood from right ventricle
↓
Right to left shunt at ventricular level
↓
Cyanosis

Flowchart 25.7 Pathogenesis of cyanotic tetralogy.

VSD larger, pulmonary stenosis mild
↓
Mainly left to right shunt
↓
Increased pulmonary flow
↓
Increased volume in left heart

Flowchart 25.8 Pathogenesis of acyanotic tetralogy.

(ii) **Transposition of great arteries** (Fig. 25.8)
- Complex malformations as regards position of the aorta, pulmonary trunk, AV orifices and position of the atria in relation to ventricles.
- Several forms of transpositions are encountered:
  - **Regular transposition**
    - It is the most common type.
    - Aorta (normally situated to the right and posterior with respect to the pulmonary trunk) is displaced anteriorly and to the right.
    - Aorta emerges from the right ventricle and pulmonary trunk from the left ventricle so there is cyanosis from birth.

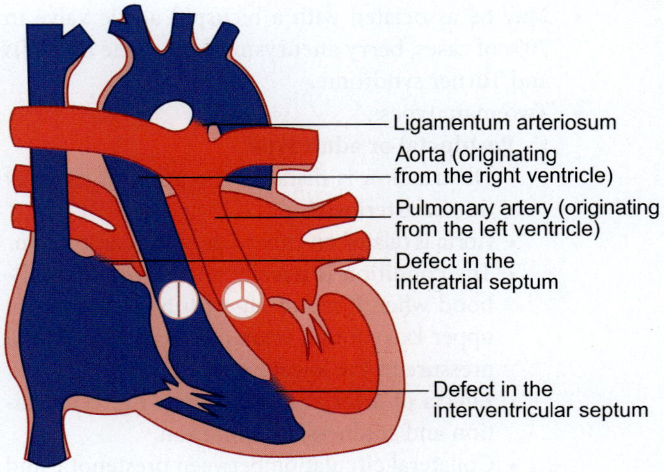

Fig. 25.8 Schematic diagram to demonstrate transposition of great arteries.

  - **Corrected transposition**
    - Transposition of great arteries and veins (pulmonary veins enter the right atrium and systemic veins drain into the left atrium) resulting in 'physiological correction'.

(iii) **Persistent truncus arteriosus**
- Arch separating the aorta from the pulmonary artery fails to develop.
- Single large common vessel receives blood from right and left ventricles.
- Associated VSD is common.
- Left-to-right shunt and early systemic cyanosis are typical.

(iv) **Tricuspid atresia and stenosis**
- Rare; often associated with PS or atresia.
- May be accompanied by an interatrial defect through which right-to-left shunting of blood takes place leading to early cyanosis.

3. **Obstructive CHD**

(a) **Coarctation of aorta** (Fig. 25.9)
- Localized narrowing in any part of aorta commonly located below the origin of the subclavian artery.

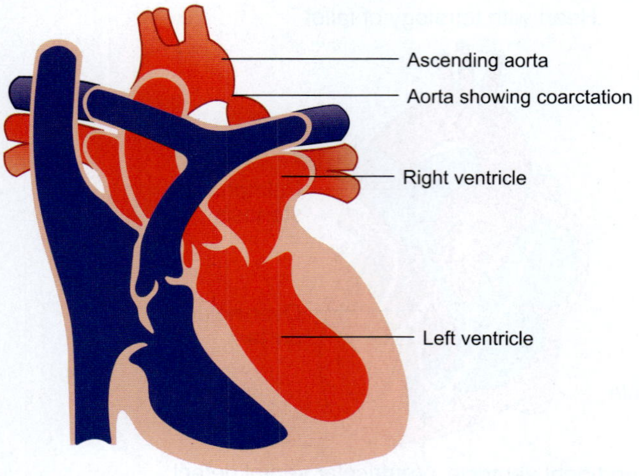

Fig. 25.9 Schematic diagram to demonstrate coarctation of aorta.

- May be associated with a bicuspid aortic valve in 70% of cases, berry aneurysm in the circle of Willis and Turner syndrome.
- Two main types:
  - **Postductal or adult type**
    - Obstruction is distal to the point of entry of ductus arteriosus.
    - Aorta is dilated on either side of the constriction.
    - The condition is usually recognized in adulthood when it manifests with hypertension in upper extremities, weak pulses and low blood pressure in the lower extremities.
    - Effects of arterial insufficiency, e.g. claudication and coldness, are common.
    - Collateral circulation between prestenotic and poststenotic arterial branches leads to enlarged and palpable intercostal arteries.
    - Erosions on the inner surface of ribs may be seen.
  - **Preductal or infantile type**
    - Narrowing proximal to the ductus arteriosus (aortic arch, ascending aorta).
    - Manifests with cyanosis in the lower half of the body; upper half remains unaffected because it is supported by vessels originating proximal to the coarctation.
    - Has a poor prognosis.

(b) **Aortic stenosis and atresia** (Fig. 25.10)
- Most common anomaly of aorta is a bicuspid aortic valve, which has no functional significance except calcification.
- Congenital aortic atresia is rare and incompatible with survival.
- Aortic stenosis may be congenital or acquired. Causes of the latter include rheumatic heart disease (RHD) and calcified aortic stenosis.
- Congenital narrowing of the aortic valve can occur in the valvular, subvalvular and supravalvular locations.

(c) **PS and atresia** (Fig. 25.11)
- Pulmonary atresia: There is no communication between the right ventricle and the lungs. Blood bypasses the right ventricle through interatrial defect.
- PS: It is the commonest form of obstructive CHD, comprising about 7% of all CHDs; it may be an isolated defect or a part of TOF.

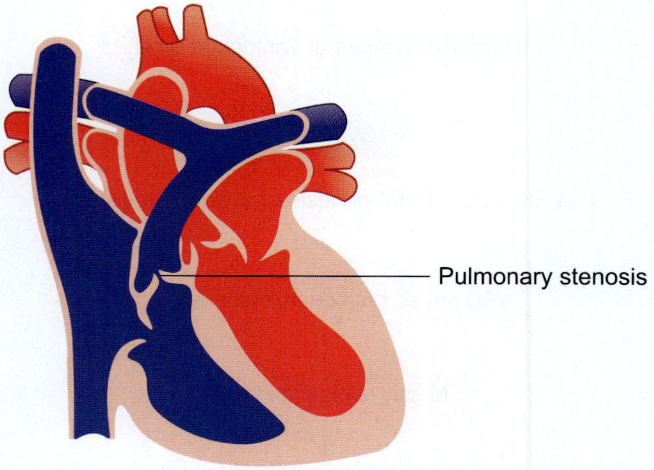

Fig. 25.11 Schematic diagram to demonstrate pulmonary stenosis.

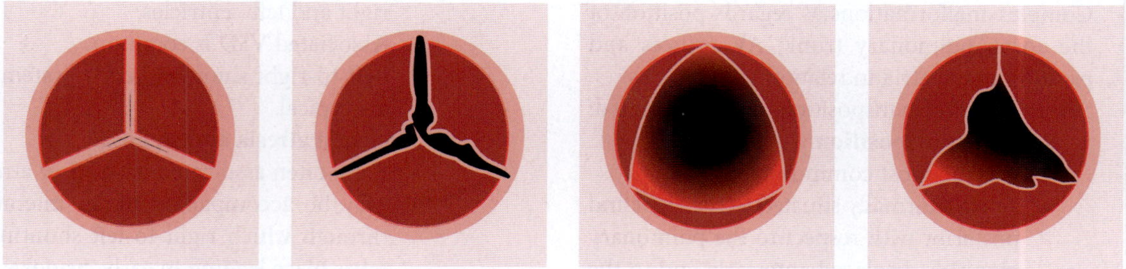

Fig. 25.10 Schematic diagram to demonstrate aortic stenosis.

Q. Write in detail about the aetiopathogenesis, clinical features and laboratory diagnosis of acute rheumatic fever and rheumatic heart disease (RHD). (PA27.4)

Ans. Acute rheumatic fever is an **acute immune-mediated multisystem disease, which primarily involves the heart, joints, central nervous system, skin and subcutaneous tissues**.

- Its peak incidence is between **5 and 15 years** and it is rare in infants and children younger than 5 years.
- It is more common in poor economic conditions and overcrowding.
- **It progresses over course of time to chronic rheumatic heart disease.**

Aetiology

- It is a delayed inflammatory response to pharyngeal infection with group A streptococci.
- The latent period between the pharyngeal infection and the onset of rheumatic fever ranges from 1 to 5 weeks.
- Type 5 strain commonly causes rheumatic fever. The other rheumatogenic serotypes include 1, 3, 6, 14, 18, 19 and 24.
- Antibodies develop against streptococcal antigens but cross-react with cardiac myosin and sarcolemmal membrane protein as well as joints and skin.

Pathology

Acute rheumatic fever is characterized by exudative inflammatory lesions of the connective tissue mainly involving the heart, joints and subcutaneous tissues. These exudative lesions are replaced by scar tissue in the later or healed phase of the disease (chronic rheumatic heart disease). All three layers (endocardium, myocardium and pericardium) of the heart are involved, resulting in **pancarditis**. The following pathological changes are seen in the different layers:

- **Myocardium:** Myocardium shows the pathognomonic myocardial **Aschoff body** (focus of swollen eosinophilic collagen surrounded by lymphocytes, plasma cells, fibroblasts, Aschoff giant cells and large basophilic cells called **Anitschkow cells**, which have abundant cytoplasm, round to oval nuclei with central, slender, wavy, ribbon-like chromatin; therefore, Anitschkow cells are also called caterpillar cells; Fig. 25.12). Aschoff bodies are classically located in the interstitial connective tissue of myocardium, especially in perivascular location, and may persist for many years in chronic rheumatic inflammation, especially in those who develop severe mitral stenosis.
- **Endocardium:** Rheumatic endocarditis produces verrucous lesions, which heal with fibrous thickening and adhesions of valve commissures, leaflets and chordae tendinae, resulting in varying degrees of stenosis and regurgitation. Regurgitant streams produce irregular thickening of the left atrium called **MacCallum plaques**. Mitral valve is the most commonly involved, followed by aortic valve and, rarely, tricuspid valve. Pulmonary valve is almost never involved.
- **Pericardium:** Serofibrinous pericarditis produces a classical '**bread and butter**' appearance.

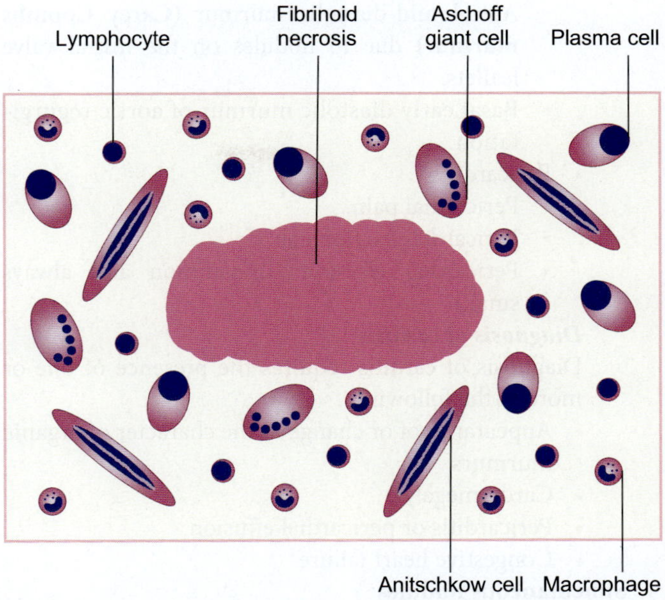

Fig. 25.12 Schematic diagram to demonstrate Aschoff body (focus of swollen eosinophilic collagen surrounded by lymphocytes, plasma cells, fibroblasts, Aschoff giant cells and large basophilic cells called **Anitschkow cells**, which have abundant cytoplasm, round to oval nuclei with central, slender, wavy, ribbon-like chromatin).

Clinical Manifestations

1. **Sore throat:** History of antecedent upper respiratory tract infection in the past 1–5 weeks.
2. **Polyarthritis**
   (a) Arthritis is the most common major manifestation of rheumatic fever (present in nearly 75% of cases).
   (b) Classical presentation is acute migratory or fleeting polyarthritis (most commonly of large joints of the extremities such as knees, ankles and wrists). As pain and swelling subside in one joint, others tend to get involved.
   (c) Involvement of hips, small joints of hands and feet, spine, sternoclavicular and temporomandibular joints is rare.
   (d) Affected joints show signs of inflammation with or without effusion.
   (e) Over a period of time, involved joints heal without any residual deformity.
3. **Carditis**
   (a) Features of carditis develop early (within 3 weeks of onset) and occur in 40%–50% of cases.
   (b) It may be asymptomatic and picked up on ECHO only.
   Manifestations of carditis
   - Myocarditis
     - Tachycardia, disproportionate to fever and persisting during sleep.
     - Arrhythmias of which prolongation of the PR interval is the most common.
     - Features of congestive heart failure and cardiomegaly.
   - Endocarditis
     - Apical systolic murmur of mitral regurgitation.

- Apical mid-diastolic murmur **(Carey Coombs murmur)** due to nodules on the mitral valve leaflets.
- Basal early diastolic murmur of aortic regurgitation.

- Pericarditis
  - Pericardial pain.
  - Pericardial friction rub.
  - Pericardial effusion (uncommon and always small).

Diagnosis of carditis

Diagnosis of carditis requires the presence of one or more of the following:

- Appearance of or change in the character of organic murmurs.
- Cardiomegaly.
- Pericarditis or pericardial effusion.
- Congestive heart failure.

4. **Subcutaneous nodules**
   (a) Associated with severe carditis and tend to occur several weeks after its onset (delayed manifestation).
   (b) Manifest as small, painless nodules over extensor surfaces and bony prominences.
5. **Erythema marginatum**
   (a) Occurs in nearly 10% of cases of acute rheumatic fever.
   (b) Characterized by erythematous macules with a clear centre and serpiginous margins, most commonly seen on the trunk and proximal parts of extremities.
6. **Chorea (Sydenham chorea; chorea minor; Saint Vitus dance)**
   (a) Chorea usually appears following a long latent period (up to 6 months) after the initial streptococcal infection.
   (b) Purposeless, involuntary movements associated with muscle weakness, emotional instability, tics and psychotic features characterize chorea.

Chronic Rheumatic Fever

The average duration of an untreated attack of acute rheumatic fever is approximately 3 months. Chronic rheumatic fever is defined as disease persisting for longer than 6 months and may be a cause of persisting congestive heart failure.

Laboratory Investigations for Acute Rheumatic Fever

1. **Isolation of group A streptococci:** Throat swab cultures positive for group A streptococci.
2. **Streptococcal antibody tests (serological tests)**
   (a) These tests confirm a recent streptococcal infection.
   (b) Common serological tests used for diagnosing acute rheumatic fever are as follows:
      (i) Antistreptolysin O (ASO) levels (single titre of ASO more than 200 Todd units in adults and 300 Todd units in children older than 5 years is taken as positive; however, a rising titre is even more significant).
      (ii) Anti-DNase B levels (elevated titers are found in approximately 80% of acute rheumatic fever cases. An elevated anti-DNase B titer is helpful in diagnosing acute rheumatic fever in the 20% of patients who do not have elevated ASO titers).
      (iii) Antihyaluronidase (AH) levels (antihyaluronidase antibodies usually rise at about the second week of infection and decline for three to five weeks afterward).
      (iv) Antistreptozyme test (ASTZ) levels (very sensitive indicator of recent streptococcal infection; titres more than 200 U/mL are considered positive).
3. **Acute-phase reactants:** The following tests confirm the presence of an inflammatory process, but are non-specific:
   (a) Raised erythrocyte sedimentation rate (ESR).
   (b) Increased CRP.
4. **Haematological abnormalities and levels of serum proteins**
   (a) Neutrophilic leucocytosis.
   (b) Increase in serum complement level.
   (c) Increase in serum mucoproteins and alpha-2 and gamma-globulin levels.
   (d) Anaemia due to suppression of erythropoiesis.
5. **Electrocardiogram:** The most consistent abnormality is prolongation of the PR interval.
6. **X-ray chest:** Evidence of cardiac failure may be seen, such as:
   (a) Cardiomegaly
   (b) Pulmonary congestion
7. **ECHO:** ECHO may show:
   (a) Myocardial dysfunction
   (b) Valvular dysfunction
   (c) Pericardial effusion

Jones criteria for diagnosis of acute rheumatic fever are summarized in Table 25.4.

Table 25.4 Diagnosis of acute rheumatic fever (Jones criteria)

Major manifestations	Minor manifestations
• Carditis	• Fever
• Polyarthritis	• Arthralgia
• Chorea	• Previous rheumatic fever or rheumatic heart disease
• Erythema marginatum	• Raised ESR
• Subcutaneous nodules	• Positive CRP
	• Prolonged PR interval (first-degree AV block)

Supporting evidence of preceding streptococcal infection includes:
- Recent scarlet fever
- Positive throat culture for group A *Streptococcus*
- Increased streptococcal antibodies

Two major manifestations or one major and two minor manifestations, along with at least one supporting evidence, indicate a high probability of rheumatic fever.

Q. Classify endocarditis. Write briefly about the clinicopathological features of the various types of endocarditis. (PA27.6)

Ans. Endocarditis is the inflammatory involvement of the endocardial layer of the heart including valves, chordae and papillae.

Classification

1. **Non-infective**
   (a) Rheumatic endocarditis (see answer to the previous question).
   (b) Atypical verrucous (Libman–Sacks) endocarditis.
   (c) Non-bacterial thrombotic endocarditis (NBTE) or marantic endocarditis.
2. **Infective**
   (a) Bacterial endocarditis.
   (b) Other infective types (tuberculous, syphilitic and fungal).

Atypical Verrucous (Libman–Sacks) Endocarditis

Pathogenesis

This type of endocarditis is characterized by the formation of sterile vegetations in patients with collagen vascular diseases (systemic lupus erythematosus [SLE], systemic sclerosis and thrombotic thrombocytopenic purpura). These lesions are essentially composed of fibrinoid material thought to result from activation of the complement system and recruitment of Fc receptor–bearing cells.

Gross Pathology

- Small (1–4 mm in diameter), single or multiple, granular pink vegetations which are typically seen in the mitral and tricuspid valves.
- Both surfaces of affected valves, adjoining ventricular and atrial endocardium are involved.
- Healed lesions do not produce any significant valvular deformity.

Microscopy

- Verrucae composed of fibrinoid material (fibrin + platelet thrombi) are pathognomonic.
- Valves show areas of necrosis, proliferating capillaries, histiocytes, plasma cells, lymphocytes and neutrophils.

Non-bacterial Thrombotic/Cachectic/Marantic Endocarditis

Pathogenesis

NBTE typically shows the presence of sterile thrombotic vegetations in association with the following conditions:

(a) Chronic debilitating diseases, e.g. cancers, particularly mucin-secreting adenocarcinomas (which show increased blood coagulability or disseminated intravascular coagulation [DIC] due to the procoagulant effect of mucin) and non-mucin-secreting malignancies such as promyelocytic leukaemia (promyelocyte granules contain procoagulant substances).
(b) Hyperoestrogenic states, severe burns or sepsis, which promote hypercoagulability.
(c) Endocardial trauma because of an indwelling catheter.

Gross Pathology

- Small (1–5 mm in diameter) single or multiple vegetations are seen along the line of closure of the leaflets.
- These are more friable than vegetations of RHD.
- Healed vegetations form fibrous nodules.

Microscopy

Bland thrombi (platelets and inflammation) without accompanying inflammatory reaction or bacteria.

Complications

Embolization may result in infarcts in the brain, lung, spleen and kidney.

Bacterial Endocarditis

It is caused by invasion of heart valves or mural endocardium by a microbe and may be classified into acute or subacute types depending on the virulence of the organism and cardiac status of the patient.

(a) Acute bacterial endocarditis
   (i) Destructive, necrotizing and ulcerative invasion by highly virulent bacteria.
   (ii) Usually affects normal valves.
   (iii) Death within days to weeks in 50% of patients, despite antibiotics and surgery.
(b) Subacute bacterial endocarditis
   (i) Caused by less destructive and less virulent microorganisms.
   (ii) Usually affects previously diseased heart.

Predisposing Factors

- Conditions which initiate transient bacteraemia and septicaemia.
  - Periodontal infections.
  - Genitourinary tract infections.
  - Infections of gastrointestinal and urinary tracts.
  - Tonsillectomy, adenoidectomy, bronchoscopy and surgery on respiratory mucosa.
- Underlying heart disease
  - RHD.
  - CHD (VSD, subaortic stenosis, myxomatous mitral value and artificial valves).
- Impaired host defences.
  - Immunodeficiency.
  - Diabetes mellitus.
  - Neutropenia or deficient function of neutrophils.

Causative Agents

- *Staphylococcus aureus* (10%–20% of cases), affects healthy or diseased heart and is the major offender in intravenous drug users.
- *Streptococcus viridans* (50%–60% of cases), causes endocarditis in previously damaged/abnormal valves.
- *Staphylococcus epidermidis* (10% of cases), is the most common cause of prosthetic valve endocarditis.
- Other organisms implicated are the **HACEK group** (*Hemophilus*, *Actinobacillus*, *Cardiobacterium*, *Eikenella* and *Kingella kingae*).

Gross Pathology

- Valves of the left heart, i.e. mitral and aortic, are most frequently affected.
- Vegetations involve atrial surface of AV valves and ventricular surface of semilunar valves.

- Size varies between a few millimetres and centimetres; the vegetations are grey, single or multiple and friable.
- Acute bacterial endocarditis vegetations are bulkier than those of subacute endocarditis.

Microscopy

The vegetations have three recognizable zones:

- Outer layer or cap composed of eosinophilic material (fibrin and platelets).
- Basophilic zone composed of bacterial colonies.
- Deeper zone composed of non-specific inflammatory cells.

Clinical Features

Fever with chills, weakness, malaise and weight loss.

Complications and Sequelae

- Cardiac complications
  - Valvular stenosis or insufficiency.
  - Perforation, rupture and aneurysm formation.
  - Abscess in valve ring extending to myocardium.
  - Suppurative pericarditis.
  - Cardiac failure.
- Extracardiac complications
  - Emboli can arise from the left or right side of the heart (Flowcharts 25.9A and B).
  - Microembolization may result in:
    - **Petechiae** (on the skin and conjunctiva because of involvement of local vessels).
    - **Osler's nodes** (painful tender nodules seen in pulps of fingers, thought to form because of deposition of immune complexes).
    - **Roth's spots** (involvement of retinal vessels may result in circular retinal haemorrhages with pale centres).
    - **Janeway spots** on palms and soles (due to septic emboli in the skin).
    - **Subungual splinter haemorrhages** (due to embolic damage to cutaneous capillaries).
    - **Painful splenomegaly** (due to splenic vessel involvement).

Causes of Death

- Cardiac failure.
- Embolism to various organs.
- Renal failure
- Rupture of mycotic aneurysms in vital organs.

Rarely, infectious endocarditis can also result from tuberculous, syphilitic, fungal, viral and rickettsial infections.

Laboratory Studies

- Normocytic normochromic anaemia of chronic disease with leucocytosis.
- Increased ESR.
- Increased levels of CRP.
- Two sets of positive blood cultures including aerobic, anaerobic and fungal (90% sensitivity) of three specimens taken at intervals of 2–3 hours.
- Deranged coagulation panel.
- Increased BUN and serum creatinine.
- Decreased C3 and C4 levels.
- Proteinuria and microscopic haematuria in 50% of patients.
- Echocardiographic detection of vegetations, valve lesion and chamber dilatation.

Diagnostic Criteria for Infective Endocarditis (Modified Duke's Criteria)

1. Major criteria
   (a) Positive blood culture for infective endocarditis (IE)
      (i) Typical microorganism of IE from two separate blood cultures (*S. viridans*, *Streptococcus bovis* or HACEK group, community-acquired *S. aureus* or enterococci, in the absence of a primary focus), or
      (ii) Microorganisms consistent with IE from persistently positive blood cultures defined as follows:
        - Two positive cultures of blood samples drawn >12 hours apart, or
        - All of three or a majority of four separate cultures of blood (with the first and last samples drawn 1 hour apart).
   (b) Evidence of endocardial involvement
      (i) Positive echocardiogram for IE, or

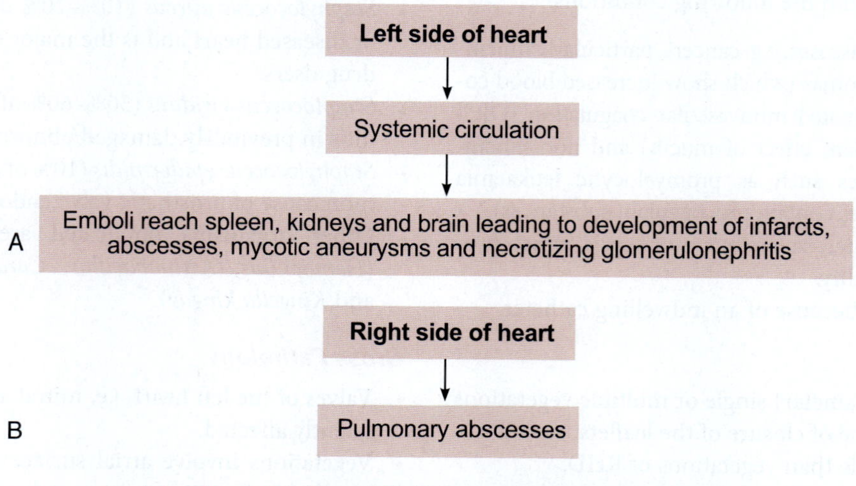

Flowchart 25.9 (A and B) Extracardiac complications.

(iii) Abscess or new partial dehiscence of prosthetic valve, or
(iv) New valvular regurgitation (worsening or changing of pre-existing murmur not sufficient).

2. Minor criteria
   (a) Predisposing valvular lesion.
   (b) Fever.
   (c) Embolic phenomenon.
   (d) Vasculitic phenomenon.
   (e) Microbiological evidence (organism grown but does not meet major criteria).
   (f) Suggestive echocardiographic findings
   Definite endocarditis: Two major or one major and three minor or five minor criteria.
   Possible endocarditis: One major and one minor or three minor criteria.

Q. Enumerate the differences between acute and subacute endocarditis.

Ans. The differentiating features of acute and subacute endocarditis are enlisted in Table 25.5.

Table 25.5 Differentiating features of acute and subacute endocarditis

Features	Acute bacterial endocarditis	Subacute bacterial endocarditis
Duration	<6 weeks	>6 weeks
Causative organisms	*Staphylococcus aureus*, β-streptococci	*Streptococcus viridans*
Virulence of organisms	High	Low
Pre-existing pathology	None	Previously damaged valves
Lesion characteristics	Large, invasive and destructive	Less invasive and destructive
Clinical presentation	Rapid deterioration, usually fatal	Gradual downhill course or recovery

Note: Classification of infective endocarditis into acute and subacute forms is largely discarded because of the availability of antibiotics, which alter the course of the same.

Q. Compare the morphological features of different types of endocarditis.

Ans. The distinguishing features of vegetations in major forms of endocarditis are summarized in Table 25.6.

Q. Write briefly about the aetiology and clinicopathological features of myocarditis.

Ans. Myocarditis is inflammatory involvement of the myocardium, which has diverse causes. It is classified based on aetiology into:

1. **Infective myocarditis**
   (a) Viral (coxsackievirus, echovirus, influenza virus, HIV).
   (b) Chlamydial (*Chlamydophila psittaci*).
   (c) Rickettsial (*Rickettsia typhi*).
   (d) Bacterial (*C. diphtheriae*, *Neisseria meningococcus*, *Borrelia*).
   (e) Fungal (*Candida*).
   (f) Helminthic (*Trichinosis*).
   (g) Protozoal (*Trypanosoma*, *Toxoplasma*).
2. **Immunological myocarditis**
   (a) Connective tissue diseases (rheumatoid arthritis, lupus erythematosus, polyarteritis nodosa and scleroderma).
   (b) Drug hypersensitivity (methyldopa and sulphonamides).
   (c) Postviral.
   (d) Poststreptococcal.
   (e) Transplant rejection.

Table 25.6 Distinguishing features of vegetations in major forms of endocarditis (Fig. 25.13A–D)

Features	Rheumatic	Libman sacks	Bacterial	NBTE
Valves commonly affected	Mitral alone or mitral and aortic combined	Mitral and tricuspid	Mitral, aortic or combined mitral and aortic	Mainly mitral; less commonly aortic and tricuspid
Distribution of vegetations	Occur along lines of closure; atrial surface of A–V valves and ventricular surface of semilunar valves	Occur on cusps/leaflets on either one or both surfaces	On valve cusps, may extend into the chordate	Occur along lines of closure (on one side)
Gross appearance	Small (1–5 mm), multiple, warty, firmly attached, produce thickening, and shortening of leaflets as well as fusion of valve commissures leading to permanent valvular deformity	Small to medium sized, multiple vegetations; generally do not produce much deformity	Large irregular, destructive, friable masses, damage the underlying myocardium	Small but larger than RHD; loosely attached; usually do not damage the valve
Constituents	Fibrin and platelets, no bacteria; adjacent endocardium may show presence of **Aschoff bodies**	Granular, fibrinoid, eosinophilic material; sterile vegetations; may contain **haematoxylin bodies** equivalent to lupus erythematosus (LE) cells	Fibrin and platelets with bacterial colonies and acute inflammatory cells	Fibrin–platelet thrombi, no bacteria
Embolization	Less common	Less common	Friable vegetations; very common	Very common

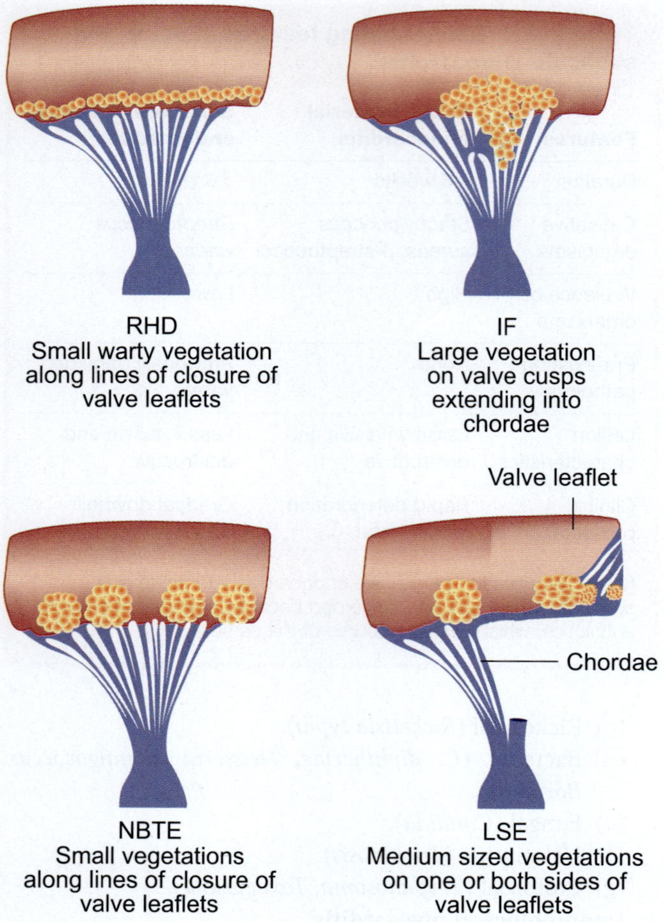

Fig. 25.13 (A–D) Types of endocardial vegetations.

3. **Myocarditis of unknown origin**
   (a) Sarcoidosis.
   (b) Giant cell myocarditis.

Infective Myocarditis

This is the most common type of myocarditis. It results from direct invasion of causative organisms or their toxins into the myocardium or a destructive immune response to their antigens. Common causes include:

- **Viral**
  - Myocarditis is seen in 5% of viral infections because of direct viral cytotoxicity or a destructive cell-mediated immune reaction.
  - Myocardium is pale and flabby; shows focal or patchy necrosis and mural thrombi on gross examination. Microscopy shows oedema and infiltration by neutrophils, which in the later stages are replaced by lymphocytes and macrophages.
- **Bacterial**
  - Myocardium shows abscesses.
  - Exudate is chiefly composed of neutrophils, lymphocytes, plasma cells and macrophages.
  - Coagulative necrosis may be seen.
- **Helminthic:** *Echinococcus granulosus* and *Trichinella spiralis* are generally implicated.
- **Fungal:** Seen in immune deficiency, cancer and chronic debilitating diseases.
- **Protozoal (Chagas disease):** Mixed inflammation around parasitized myofibres is seen.

Q. Enumerate and describe the various types of cardiomyopathies. (PA27.9)

Ans. CMP is a heterogeneous group of diseases associated with mechanical and electrical dysfunction of the myocardium. CMPs may be localized to the heart or may form a part of a systemic disease.

1. **Primary CMP:** Diseases confined to the heart muscle; may be genetic or acquired in origin.
   Three pathophysiological categories are encountered (Table 25.7):
   (a) Dilated (congestive) CMP.
   (b) Hypertrophic (obstructive) CMP.
   (c) Restrictive/obliterative or infiltrative CMP.
   Furthermore, restrictive CMP includes the following entities:
   (i) Cardiac amyloidosis.
   (ii) Endocardial fibroelastosis.
   (iii) Endomyocardial fibrosis.
   (iv) Loeffler endocarditis.
2. **Secondary CMP:** The myocardial involvement is seen as a component of a systemic or a multiorgan disorder, as in the following:
   (a) Nutritional deficiencies (alcoholic CMP and beriberi).
   (b) Toxic chemicals (cobalt, arsenic, lithium and hydrocarbons).
   (c) Drugs (emetine, cyclophosphamide, adriamycin and catecholamines).
   (d) Metabolic diseases (cardiac amyloidosis, hemochromatosis and glycogen storage diseases).
   (e) Neuromuscular diseases (Friedreich ataxia and muscular dystrophies).
   (f) Infiltration by leukaemias and carcinomas.
   (g) Connective tissue diseases (rheumatoid arthritis, systemic sclerosis and drug induced).

Q. Write briefly about diseases of the pericardium. (PA27.7)

Ans. The **visceral pericardium** is a simple layer of mesothelial cells and the **parietal pericardium** is made of fibrous and elastic tissue. Pericardium is about 2 mm thick and well innervated. Diseases of the pericardium are usually secondary to or associated with other cardiac and systemic diseases. Normally, no more than 30–50 mL of thin, clear, straw-coloured fluid is seen in pericardial sac. Pericardial cavity may undergo distension by fluid (effusion), blood (haemopericardium) or pus (purulent pericarditis). When significant fluid accumulates in the pericardial cavity, it can cause cardiac tamponade, which is characterized by rapidly declining cardiac output progressing to cardiogenic shock. Pericarditis (inflammation of the pericardium) may be classified based on the onset (acute or chronic) and aetiology (serous, fibrinous, purulent, haemorrhagic and chylous).

Table 25.7 Types of CMP (Fig. 25.14A–C)

Features	Dilated (congestive) CMP	Hypertrophic (obstructive) CMP	Restrictive/obliterative or infiltrative CMP
Definition	• Systolic dysfunction with dilatation of all four chambers	• Diastolic dysfunction (reduced chamber size and impaired diastolic filling) • 25% of patients have left ventricular outflow obstruction	Diastolic dysfunction (restriction in ventricular filling due to reduction in the volume of ventricles)
Incidence	90% of all CMPs	Less common	Less common
Age affected	20–50 years	25–40 years	Variable

Causes	• **Familial or genetic**
	  • Inheritance is mainly autosomal dominant
	  • X-linked, autosomal recessive or mitochondrial inheritance less common
	  • Inherited mutations seen in proteins such as dystrophin, cardiac α-actin, desmin and nuclear proteins such as lamin A and C
	• **Acquired**
	  • Viral myocarditis (enterovirus and coxsackievirus implicated)
	  • Toxic damage from alcohol (direct toxicity or beriberi heart disease due to thiamine deficiency), cobalt, chemotherapy with doxorubicin and other anthracyclines
	  • Peripartum CMP
	  • Iron overload as in hereditary haemochromatosis
	  • Excessive catecholamines as in pheochromocytoma
	  • Supraphysiological or extreme psychological stress
		Genetic; inherited mutations in sarcomere proteins (β-myosin heavy chain or troponin I and T, myosin-binding protein C and α-tropomyosin)	Idiopathic; or associated with amyloidosis, radiation-induced fibrosis, sarcoidosis, metastatic tumour or inborn errors of metabolism

Clinical features	Slowly progressing heart failure, shortness of breath, easy fatigability, poor exercise tolerance	Usually asymptomatic; symptomatic on heavy physical activity. May manifest with dyspnoea, angina and congestive cardiac failure or sudden death	Presentation dependent on specific type. May manifest with dyspnoea, angina and congestive cardiac failure or sudden death
Gross appearance	• Heart is enlarged; weight may increase up to 1000 g **('flabby hypocontracting heart')** • Dilatation of all four chambers giving rise to a typical globular appearance • Endocardial thickening • Presence of mural thrombi	• Heavy hypercontracting heart • Asymmetric myocardial hypertrophy (interventricular septum more hypertrophied than free walls of the ventricles) • Transverse section: Banana-like appearance	• Ventricles normal or slightly enlarged • Cavities not dilated • Myocardium is firm
Microscopy	• Hypertrophy of some myocardial fibres, and atrophy of others; interstitial fibrosis with focal mononuclear infiltrate • Small subendocardial scars may be seen	• Myocardial cell disorganization in the ventricular septum • Myocardial fibres are irregularly and haphazardly arranged (normally parallel) • Interstitial fibrosis • Individual muscle hypertrophy and presence of large prominent nucleoli (transverse diameter more than 40 cm)	Patchy or diffuse interstitial fibrosis, which varies from minimal to extensive
Outcome	Mitral regurgitation/arrhythmias may be observed; average survival from onset to death is 5 years	Medical treatment to relax ventricles and surgical reduction of septum can be undertaken	Gradually progressive cardiac failure

Classification of Pericarditis

1. **Classification of pericarditis based on onset**
   (a) Acute.
   (b) Chronic.
2. **Classification of pericarditis based on aetiology**
   (a) Acute non-specific (idiopathic).
   (b) Infective (bacterial, viral, tubercular, fungal or other infections).

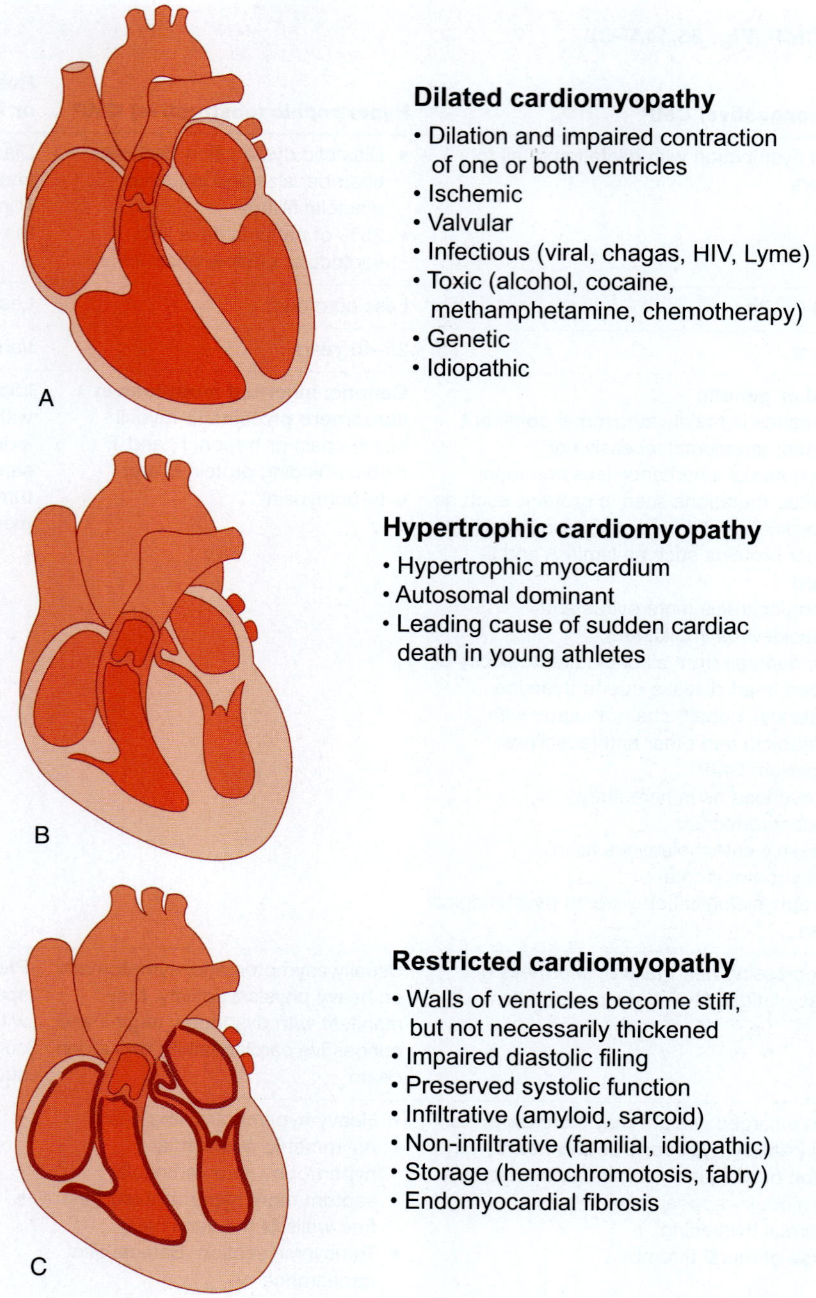

Fig. 25.14 (A–C) Types of cardiomyopathies (CMP).

(c) Immunological (rheumatic fever or other connective tissue disorders).
(d) Neoplastic.
(e) Metabolic (uraemia, myxoedema or gout).
(f) Traumatic (including post–cardiac surgery).

Acute Pericarditis

1. **Serous pericarditis:** Accumulation of serous fluid, which differs from transudate of hydropericardium in having increased protein content and higher specific gravity.

   Causes

   (a) Viral infection, e.g. mumps, coxsackie A or B.
   (b) Rheumatic fever.
   (c) Rheumatoid arthritis, SLE and scleroderma.
   (d) Uraemia.
   (e) Involvement by a malignant tumour.
   (f) Tuberculous pericarditis in early stage.

   Pathology

   - Usually the volume of the fluid does not exceed 50–200 mL.
   - There is infiltration of epicardial and pericardial surfaces by scant neutrophils, lymphocytes and histiocytes.
   - Clear, watery fluid; specific gravity <1.015.

2. **Fibrinous and serofibrinous pericarditis:** Fibrinous **(bread and butter)** pericarditis is the most common type of pericarditis. It may resolve or lead to adhesive

pericarditis. A pericardial frictional rub can be elicited when it is active.

Causes

(a) Acute viral illness.
(b) Uraemia.
(c) MI (postinfarction Dressler syndrome).
(d) Rheumatic fever.
(e) Trauma.
(f) Acute bacterial infections.

Pathology

- Pericardial surface is dry and granular.
- Pericardial fluid appears thick, yellow or cloudy because of abundant leucocytes and erythrocytes.
- During course of evolution, fibrin may get digested or become organized.

3. **Purulent pericarditis:** It is a consequence of the invasion of the pericardial space by infective organisms, which reach by the following routes:
   (a) Direct extension from neighbouring inflammation, e.g. empyema, lobar pneumonia and mediastinal infections.
   (b) Seeding from blood.
   (c) Lymphatic extension.
   (d) Direct introduction during cardiotomy.

   Most common causative organisms are staphylococci, streptococci and pneumococci. The patient presents with high-grade fever, rigors and a pericardial friction rub.

   Pathology

   - Serosa is reddened, granular and coated with exudate (thin creamy pus).
   - Organization of exudate may lead to **constrictive pericarditis.**
4. **Haemorrhagic pericarditis**
   It is characterized by an exudate composed of blood mixed with fibrinous or suppurative material. Its causes include:
   (a) Malignant neoplastic involvement of the pericardium.
   (b) Bacterial infections.
   (c) Bleeding diathesis.
   (d) Tuberculosis.
   (e) Following cardiac surgery.
5. **Chylous pericarditis**
   This type of pericarditis occurs because of lymphatic obstruction.

Chronic Pericarditis

1. **Tubercular/caseous pericarditis:** Pericardial involvement occurs by direct spread from a tuberculous focus in tracheobronchial lymph nodes and usually results in disabling constrictive pericarditis.
2. **Chronic adhesive pericarditis:** Fibrinous, suppurative or haemorrhagic pericarditis heals by organization and leads to the formation of fibrous adhesions between parietal and visceral pericardium. This is usually seen because of infection by pyogenic bacteria and tuberculosis.
3. **Chronic constrictive pericarditis:** Rarely the pericardial space may get filled with fibrous or fibrocalcific tissue, which interferes with normal functioning of the heart. It is usually a consequence of tuberculous, purulent or haemorrhagic pericarditis.

Q. Write briefly about cardiovascular syphilis. (PA27.10)

Ans. Cardiovascular syphilis is now quite rare; however, sporadic cases still occur. It has been reported that 75% of untreated patients develop tertiary syphilis after 15 years, with cardiovascular syphilis being the most common manifestation. *Treponema* lodges in the vasa vasorum and incites an inflammatory reaction leading to aortitis. Patients may subsequently develop aortic insufficiency, coronary ostial stenosis and, less commonly, aortic aneurysms. The aortic aneurysms occur most commonly in the ascending and aortic arch and have a high mortality. Antibiotic therapy should be initiated immediately, followed by surgical therapy.

Q. Define heart failure. Discuss the types, common causes, pathophysiology and clinical features of heart failure. (PA27.3)

Ans. Heart failure is defined as a state in which the ventricles cannot maintain an adequate cardiac output to meet the metabolic needs of the body.

Pathophysiology

- **Cardiac output** is a function of:
  - **Preload**, which refers to the volume and pressure of blood in the ventricles at the end of diastole.
  - **Afterload**, which refers to the pressure against which the left ventricle contracts. The main determinants of afterload are total peripheral resistance and left ventricle size.
  - **Myocardial contractility**, which mainly depends on the levels of circulating catecholamines.
- Heart failure is characterized by a decrease in cardiac output (except in high-output failure), increased preload, as well as afterload, and decreased myocardial contractility.
- **Compensated heart failure:** Compensated heart failure implies that the compensatory changes have prevented the development of overt heart failure; a minor added insult such as an infection may precipitate severe heart failure.
- **Compensatory mechanisms** are mediated through renin–angiotensin system and autonomic nervous system and include:
  - Increased myocardial contractility
  - Myocardial hypertrophy
  - Neurohormonal mechanisms
    (i) Sympathetic stimulation.
    (ii) Activation of renin–angiotensin system.
    (iii) Release of atrial natriuretic peptide.

Types of Heart Failure

- **Systolic and diastolic heart failure**
  - Systolic heart failure is characterized by an abnormality of myocardial contraction.

- Diastolic heart failure is characterized by an abnormality of ventricular relaxation, which causes poor ventricular filling and high filling pressure.

- **Acute and chronic heart failure**
  - Acute heart failure develops suddenly. The sudden reduction in cardiac output results in systemic hypotension without peripheral oedema, e.g. acute MI and rupture of a cardiac valve.
  - Chronic heart failure develops gradually. Here, systemic arterial pressure is well maintained, but oedema develops, e.g. dilated CMP and multivalvular disease.
- **Left-sided, right-sided and biventricular heart failure**
  - Left-sided (left ventricular) heart failure.
    - 'Left side' is a term for the functional unit of left atrium, left ventricle, mitral valve and aortic valve.
    - There is reduction in left ventricular output, increase in left atrial pressure and increase in pulmonary venous pressure.
    - Acute increase in left atrial pressure causes pulmonary congestion and pulmonary oedema, e.g. in MI.
    - Gradual increase in left atrial pressure causes reflex pulmonary hypertension, but no pulmonary oedema, e.g. aortic stenosis.
  - Right-sided (right ventricular) heart failure.
    - 'Right side' is a term for the functional unit of right atrium, right ventricle, tricuspid valve and pulmonary valve.
    - There is reduction in right ventricular output, which results in systemic venous congestion leading to accumulation of fluid in the body, resulting in swelling and oedema.
    - It is seen in cor pulmonale, pulmonary valvular stenosis and multiple pulmonary emboli.
  - Biventricular heart failure: There is failure of both left and right ventricles, e.g. disease processes affecting both ventricles such as dilated CMP and IHD or disease of the left heart leading to chronic elevation of left atrial pressure, pulmonary hypertension and subsequent right ventricular failure.
- **Forward and backward heart failure**
  - *Forward heart failure:* Decreased cardiac output
  - *Backward heart failure:* Normal cardiac output, but marked salt and water retention and pulmonary and systemic venous congestion
- **High-output and low-output heart failure**
  - High-output heart failure is associated with an increased cardiac output, e.g. cardiac failure associated with hyperthyroidism, anaemia, pregnancy, arteriovenous fistulae, beriberi and Paget disease.
  - Low-output heart failure is associated with a low cardiac output, e.g. heart failure associated with IHD, hypertension, CMP, valvular diseases and pericardial disease.

Common Causes of Heart Failure

- ***Failure of myocardial pump***
  - MI.
  - Hypertensive heart disease.
  - Myocarditis.
  - CMPs.
  - Pulmonary embolism.
  - Anaemia, pregnancy and thyrotoxicosis (increased demand).
  - Drugs such as beta-blockers, corticosteroids and NSAIDs.
- ***Obstruction to outflow***
  - Systemic hypertension.
  - Aortic stenosis and PS.
  - Pulmonary hypertension.
- ***Obstruction to inflow:*** Mitral and tricuspid stenosis.
- ***Disorders of cardiac conduction:*** Cardiac arrhythmias.

Clinical Manifestations of Heart Failure

- ***Dyspnoea:*** Dyspnoea is initially exertional, but progressively worsens to a stage of breathlessness even at rest. The mechanisms underlying dyspnoea include:
  - Interstitial pulmonary oedema.
  - Respiratory muscle dysfunction/fatigue due to poor perfusion.
  - Bronchial mucosal oedema and increased bronchial mucus production.
- ***Orthopnoea:*** Dyspnoea occurring in recumbent position (on lying flat) and relieved by sitting up is known as orthopnoea. The mechanisms underlying orthopnoea include:
  - Increased venous return to the lungs in recumbent position.
  - Elevation of the diaphragm.
  - Reabsorption of the peripheral oedema that had accumulated while the patient was ambulant.
- ***Paroxysmal nocturnal dyspnoea (PND)***
  - Severe shortness of breath occurring at night, which awakens the patient from sleep and is relieved by sitting upright.
  - Occurs due to depression of the respiratory centre during sleep and reduced adrenergic stimulation of the myocardium at night resulting in further impairment of myocardial function.
- ***Cyanosis*** of mucosa and nail beds.
- ***Pulse:*** Sinus tachycardia (due to increased adrenergic activity) and pulsus alternans (alternate large and small volume beats with a normal rhythm).
- ***Blood pressure:*** Diminished pulse pressure because of reduced stroke volume.
- ***Jugular venous pressure:*** Raised as a consequence of elevated systemic venous pressure.
- ***Liver (congestive hepatomegaly)***
  - Right upper quadrant pain from stretching of the capsule of the liver.
  - Liver enlarged and tender because of elevated right-sided heart pressures transmitted backward into the portal vein circulation.
- ***Pleural effusion, ascites and pericardial effusion***
  - Right-sided pleural effusion is more common and results from increased pleural capillary pressure and transudation of fluid into the pleural space.

- Ascites results from transudation secondary to elevated pressure in hepatic veins, portal veins and veins draining the peritoneum.

- ***Acute pulmonary oedema***
  - Caused by marked elevation of pulmonary capillary pressure.
  - Clinically, characterized by severe breathlessness, cough with copious, pinkish, frothy expectoration and bilateral crepitations.
  - Seen over dependent parts (gravity dependent) with sparing of face and arms.
  - In ambulatory patients, oedema is seen over the legs, particularly in the pretibial region. It is less in the morning and more towards the evening. Oedema is sacral in bedridden patients.
  - In advanced stage cases, generalized oedema or anasarca may be seen.
- ***Non-specific symptoms***
  - Anorexia, nausea, abdominal pain and fullness (congestion of the liver and portal venous system).
  - Fatigue and weakness (reduced perfusion of skeletal muscles).
  - Low-grade fever (reduced cutaneous flow).

Diagnosis

- Chest radiograph: may show cardiomegaly, prominence of upper lobe veins, **Kerley A and B lines** (cuffing of the areas around the bronchi) and other features of pulmonary oedema.
- ECG: to identify arrhythmias, IHD and right and left ventricular hypertrophy.
- ECHO: for evaluation of ejection fraction, valvular status and chamber size.

26 Diseases of the Lungs

AIRWAYS

Structural hierarchy (Flowchart 26.1): The conducting portion is made up of the trachea, which give rise to two primary bronchii. These then branch successively to give rise to secondary and tertiary bronchii, which further branch to give rise to several orders of progressively smaller airways called bronchioles, the smallest of which are called terminal bronchioles (last component of conducting system). The respiratory component is called the lung acinus (Fig. 26.1) and this has the following components:

1. Respiratory bronchiole.
2. Alveolar duct.
3. Alveolar sac (blind end of respiratory passages and site for gas exchange).

A cluster of three to five terminal bronchioles with its acinus is called a lobule.

Histology

The respiratory tree is lined by pseudostratified tall columnar ciliated epithelium admixed with mucus-secreting goblet cells in the cartilaginous airways. At the transition from bronchi to bronchioles the epithelium changes to a ciliated columnar epithelium, glands and cartilage are absent. The smooth muscle is relatively thicker than in the bronchi. Bronchial mucosa also has neuroendocrine cells that exhibit neurosecretory-type granules, which contain serotonin, calcitonin and gastrin-releasing peptide. The alveolar macrophage is filled with carbon and lying loose in the alveolar spaces.

Alveolar wall

- The alveolar wall (alveolar septum; Fig. 26.2) is composed of the following layers:
  1. Capillary endothelium.
  2. Basement membrane with surrounding interstitial tissue which separates the capillary endothelium from the alveolar lining.
  3. Alveolar epithelium, which is of two principal cell types:
     (a) Flattened type I pneumocytes (cover 95% of the alveolar surface).
     (b) Rounded type II pneumocytes (are a source of pulmonary surfactant and participate in repair wherein they replace the damaged type I pneumocytes).

Bronchi
(have cartilaginous walls lined by pseudostratified ciliated columnar epithelium with mucous-producing goblet cells and submucosal glands)

↓ Dichotomous branching

Bronchioles
(lined by ciliated columnar epithelium; lack cartilage and submucosal glands in their walls)

↓ Further branching

Terminal bronchioles
(bronchioles less than 1 mm in diameter)

↓

Acini
(spherical structures with a diameter of about 3.5 mm)

Flowchart 26.1 Structural hierarchy of airways.

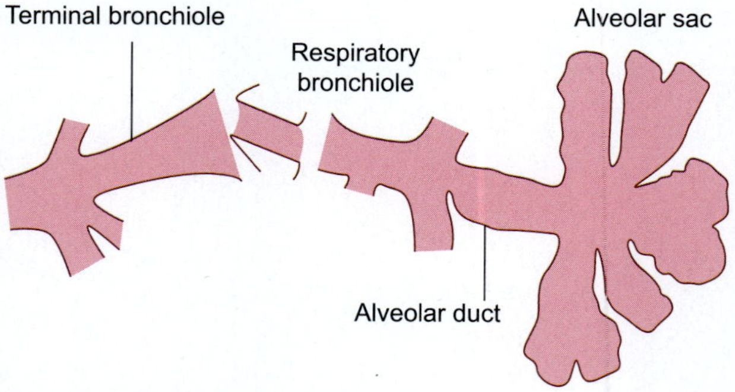

Fig. 26.1 Parts of a normal acinus.

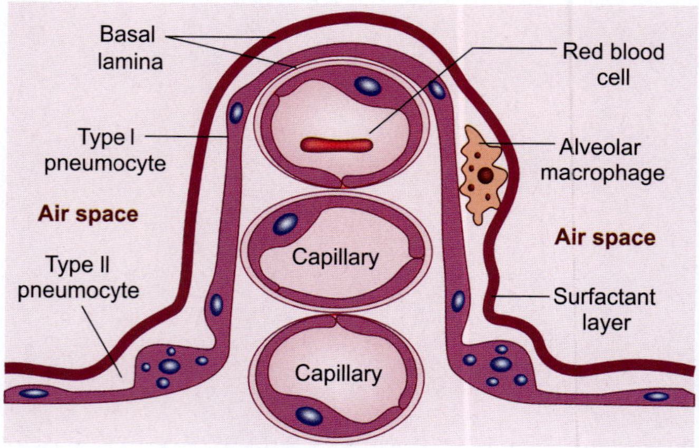

Fig. 26.2 Schematic diagram of the structure of the alveolar septum.

Q. Write briefly about acute respiratory distress syndrome (ARDS).

Ans. ARDS is a manifestation of severe acute lung injury (ALI).

Salient Features

- Also known as **diffuse alveolar damage** or **shock lung.** Diffuse alveolar capillary damage induces leakage of fluid from pulmonary capillaries into the interstitium. Loss of type I pneumocytes allows fluid to accumulate in the alveolar spaces and damage to type II pneumocytes leads to surfactant abnormalities, both of which compromise alveolar gas exchange.
- ARDS presents with rapid onset of severe life-threatening respiratory insufficiency, cyanosis and severe arterial hypoxaemia in the absence of cardiac failure (the respiratory insufficiency may be refractory to O_2 therapy).
- May progress to extrapulmonary multisystem organ failure.

Causes

- **Infections**
  - Sepsis
  - Diffuse pulmonary infections (viral, *Mycoplasma* and *Pneumocystis* pneumonia and miliary tuberculosis)
- **Physical injuries**
  - Head injury
  - Pulmonary contusions
  - Drowning
  - Fractures and fat embolism
  - Burns
  - Ionizing radiation
- **Pulmonary embolization**
- **Inhalation of irritants**
  - Oxygen toxicity
  - Smoke
  - Gases and chemicals such as ammonia, chlorine and nitrogen dioxide
- **Chemical injury**
  - Heroin or methadone or barbiturate overdose
  - Acetylsalicylic acid
  - Thiazides
- **Haematological conditions**
  - Multiple transfusions
  - Disseminated intravascular coagulation (DIC)
- **Others**
  - Pancreatitis
  - Uraemia
  - Cardiopulmonary pass
  - Hypersensitivity reactions

Gross Pathology

Heavy, red, boggy lungs, which ooze fluid on cutting.

Microscopy

- Alveolar lining and pulmonary capillary endothelium are damaged.
- Alveolar walls are lined by a **waxy hyaline membrane** consisting of fibrin-rich oedema fluid mixed with cytoplasmic and lipid remnants of necrotic epithelial cells.
- Type II pneumocytes proliferate to regenerate alveolar lining.
- Fibrin exudates organize and intra-alveolar fibrosis may ensue.

X-Ray

Shows diffuse bilateral infiltrates.

Q. Define atelectasis. Enumerate and describe its various types.

Ans. Atelectasis is defined as complete or partial collapse of a lung or a section (lobe) of a lung. It may be due to incomplete expansion of the lungs at birth (neonatal atelectasis) or collapse of previously inflated lungs produces areas of relatively airless parenchyma (acquired atelectasis).

Types

1. **Resorption atelectasis:** Is a result of complete obstruction of an airway (Flowchart 26.2).
2. **Compression atelectasis:** Develops due to external compression of lungs (Flowchart 26.3).
3. **Contraction atelectasis:** Occurs due to localized or generalized fibrosis of lungs or pleura preventing their full expansion.

Q. Write briefly about chronic obstructive pulmonary disease (COPD). (PA26.3)

Ans. COPD occurs as a result of partial or complete chronic obstruction of airflow. Disorders associated with airflow obstruction include:

1. Emphysema
2. Chronic bronchitis
3. Asthma
4. Bronchiectasis
5. Small airway disease (bronchiolitis)

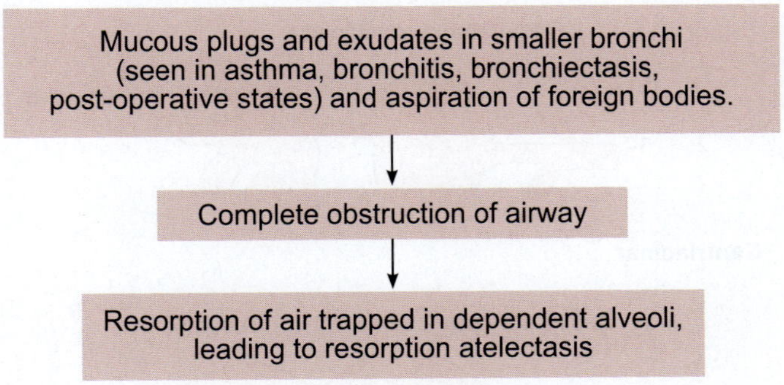

Flowchart 26.2 Mechanism of development of resorption atelectasis.

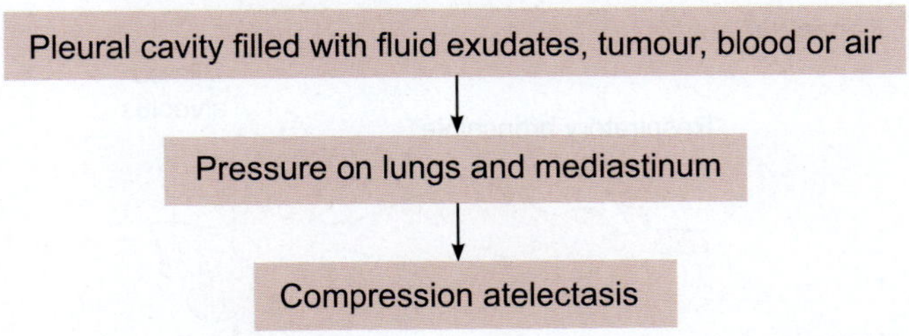

Flowchart 26.3 Mechanism of development of compression atelectasis.

Emphysema

Definition

Abnormal permanent enlargement of the airspaces distal to terminal bronchiole (including respiratory bronchiole, alveolar duct and alveolus), accompanied by destruction of their walls without fibrosis. Dilatation of airspaces without destruction is called **overinflation**.

Types

Emphysema is classified according to the anatomic distribution into four major types (Fig. 26.3):

1. **Centriacinar (centrilobular) emphysema**
   (a) Affects the central or proximal part of acini and spares the distal part (in severe centriacinar emphysema, distal acinus may be involved, making it panacinar).
   (b) More common in upper lobes.
   (c) Predominantly seen in heavy smokers in association with chronic bronchitis.
   (d) May coexist with coal workers' pneumoconiosis (CWP; walls of emphysematous spaces demonstrate large amounts of pigment).
   (e) Peribronchial and bronchiolar spaces commonly show inflammation.

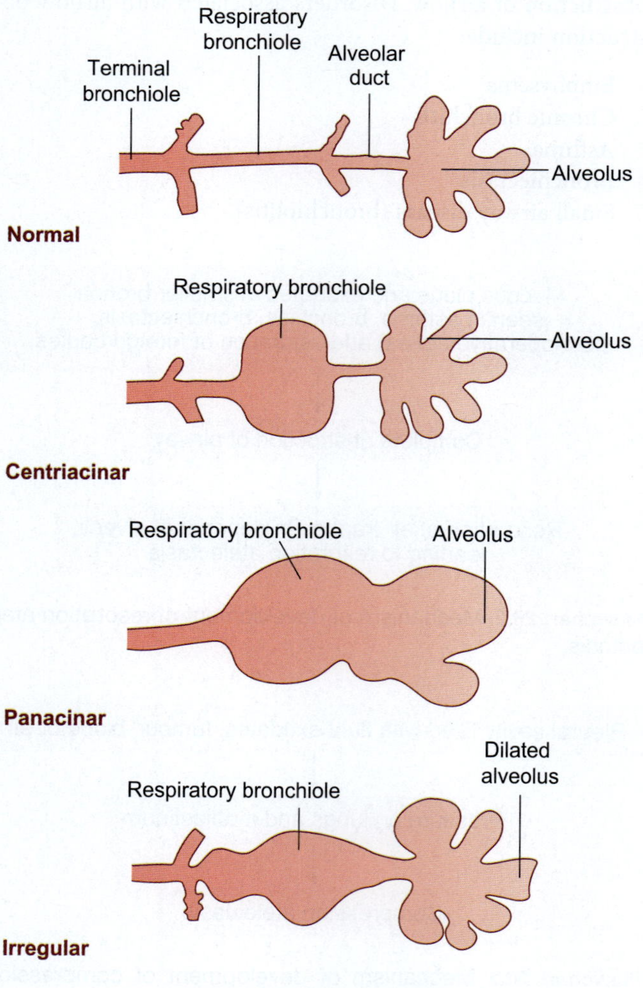

Fig. 26.3 Types of emphysema.

2. **Panacinar (panlobular) emphysema**
   (a) Uniformly enlarged acini from the level of respiratory bronchiole to the terminal blind alveolar sac.
   (b) More common in lower zones and anterior margin of lungs; most severe at the bases.
   (c) Associated with α_1-antitrypsin (α_1-AT) deficiency.
3. **Paraseptal (distal acinar)**
   (a) Involvement of distal acinus with preservation of the proximal part.
   (b) Localization along pleura and perilobular septae.
   (c) Common in the upper part of lungs, adjacent to areas of fibrosis and atelectasis.
   (d) Characteristic finding is the presence of multiple, continuous and enlarged airspaces 0.5–2 cm, forming cyst-like structures (bullae), which may rupture to produce spontaneous pneumothorax.
4. **Irregular (paracicatricial) emphysema**
   (a) Irregular involvement of acinus.
   (b) Usually asymptomatic and clinically insignificant.

Others Types of Emphysema

Sometimes the term 'emphysema' may be applied to certain conditions not conforming strictly to the definition of emphysema, e.g.:

1. **Compensatory emphysema:** Dilatation of alveoli without destruction of septal walls in response to loss/removal of lung substance elsewhere.
2. **Obstructive overinflation:** Expansion of lung because of air trapped within it. Trapping of air could be due to:
   (a) Subtotal obstruction: Air enters in inspiration but cannot exit in expiration (ball valve mechanism).
   (b) Total obstruction: Ventilation occurs through collaterals (pores of Kohn and canals of Lambert), which bring in air behind the obstruction.
3. **Bullous emphysema**
   (a) A form of emphysema that produces large subpleural bullae (blebs >1 cm in size), rupture of which may lead to pneumothorax.
   (b) Usually a consequence of old tuberculous scarring.
4. **Interstitial emphysema**
   (a) Characterized by air entry into connective tissue stroma of lung, mediastinum or subcutaneous tissue.
   (b) Causes include an alveolar tear caused by bronchiolar obstruction accompanied by explosive coughing (whooping cough, bronchitis, etc.) or puncture of the lung due to a chest wound or a fractured rib.

Pathogenesis

- **Role of 'protease–antiprotease' imbalance** and **genetic deficiency of α_1-AT**
  - The main protease involved in emphysema is elastase, released by macrophages, and responsible for breakdown of the lung's fragile elastic lamina (of which elastin is a structural protein component).
  - This is believed to be central in the development of emphysema. Peptides from elastin can be detected in increased quantities in patients with emphysema.

- Normally, the injury caused by proteases is prevented by antiproteases, e.g. α_1-AT.
- Homozygous patients with a genetic deficiency of protease inhibitor α_1-AT have an increased tendency to develop emphysema. Smoking exaggerates this tendency.
- α_1-AT is encoded by a gene in the Pi (protease inhibitor) locus on chromosome 14. It is synthesized in the liver and is present in serum, tissue fluid and macrophages. Normal α_1-AT phenotype is PiMM. α_1-AT-deficient phenotype is PiZZ. Eighty per cent of patients with PiZZ end up with emphysema. Pi null phenotype has no detectable levels of α_1-AT.

- **Role of neutrophils:** Foreign antigens (noxious cigarette smoke) induce inflammatory immune cells (including polymorphonuclear cells, eosinophils, macrophages, CD4- and CD8-positive lymphocytes), which transport the antigens to the bronchus-associated lymphatic tissue layer where the release of neutrophilic chemotactic factors occurs. Neutrophils are a source of the following:
  - Elastase activity.
  - Cellular proteases (proteinase 3 and cathepsin).
  - Matrix metalloproteinases (MMPs).
  - Oxygen-derived free radicals (inactivate native antiproteases by oxidative injury).
- **Role of macrophages**
  - Proteolytic enzymes such as MMPs are mainly released by macrophages. They lead to destruction of the lung's epithelial barrier.
  - Macrophages are found to be 5- to 10-fold higher in the bronchoalveolar lavage fluid of emphysematous patients.
- **Role of T lymphocytes**
  - The T lymphocytes in the sputum of emphysematous smokers are mainly CD8-positive cells. These release chemotactic factors to recruit more cells and growth factors that promote structural change.
  - The inflammation is further amplified by oxidative stress and protease production.
- **Role of smoking:** Smoking enhances elastase activity of macrophages. Macrophage elastase is not inhibited by α_1-AT and it can, in fact, digest the latter. The mucus hyperplasia, bronchiolar oedema and fibrosis in smokers' airways result in the small airway narrowing of less than 2 mm.

Clinical Features

Patients do not become symptomatic until at least one-third of functional parenchyma is damaged. Presenting signs and symptoms of emphysema include:

- Dyspnoea.
- Cough (late onset and with scanty sputum).
- Severe weight loss.
- Barrel-shaped chest.
- Prolonged expiration (key to diagnosis).
- Hunched position and breathing through pursed lips.
- Death may be due to either of the following:
  - Respiratory acidosis and coma.
  - Right-sided heart failure.
  - Massive collapse of lungs secondary to pneumothorax.

Chronic Bronchitis

Definition

Persistent cough with sputum production for at least 3 months in 2 consecutive years. It is **common in habitual smokers and inhabitants of smoke-laden cities and may progress to the following:**

- COPD
- Cor pulmonale and heart failure
- Atypical metaplasia and dysplasia of respiratory epithelium.

Types

1. **Simple chronic bronchitis:** Productive cough but no physiological evidence of airflow obstruction.
2. **Chronic asthmatic bronchitis:** Hyperactive airways with intermittent bronchospasm and wheezing.
3. **Obstructive chronic bronchitis:** Development of chronic airflow obstruction usually with associated emphysema in some patients, e.g. heavy smokers.

Pathogenesis

- Chronic bronchitis may result from repeated attacks of acute bronchitis, or evolve gradually because of heavy smoking or inhalation of air pollutants in the environment.
- Exposure to irritants, such as pollution, chemicals, tobacco smoke, and infections causes bronchial irritation. This initiates the influx of inflammatory cells (neutrophils, macrophages and CD8+ T cells which release chemotactic and proinflammatory cytokines (Flowchart 26.4). Airway epithelial cells also release inflammatory mediators in response to infectious and inflammatory stimuli. Repeated irritation over a period of time leads to goblet cell metaplasia, hyperplasia of submucous glands, mucus hypersecretion and plugging of the bronchiolar lumen, and later fibrosis.
- **Role of cigarette smoking in the pathogenesis of chronic bronchitis:** Cigarette smoking predisposes to chronic bronchitis by:
  - Interfering with ciliary action of respiratory epithelium and function of alveolar macrophages.

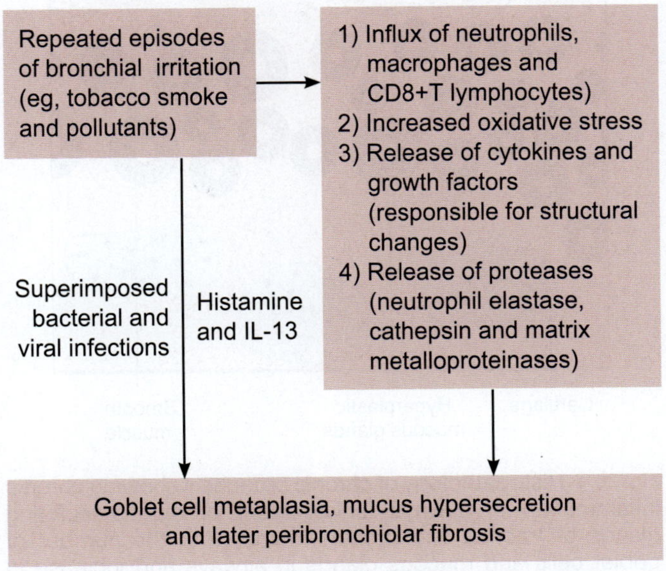

Flowchart 26.4 Pathogenesis of chronic bronchitis.

- Causing direct damage to airway epithelium.
- Leading to hypertrophy and hyperplasia of mucous glands.
- Inhibiting ability of bronchial and alveolar leucocytes to clear bacteria.

- **Role of viral and bacterial infections in bronchitis:** Acute bronchitis can be brought about by infections, such as those caused by *Mycoplasma* species, *Chlamydia pneumoniae, Streptococcus pneumoniae, Moraxella catarrhalis* and *Haemophilus influenzae*, and by viruses, such as influenza, parainfluenza, adenovirus, rhinovirus and respiratory syncytial virus.

Gross Morphology

- Hyperaemia, swelling and oedema of airways.
- Excessive mucinous to mucopurulent secretions in the bronchi and bronchioles.

Microscopy (Fig. 26.4)

- Chronic (predominantly lymphocytic) inflammation of airways.
- Enlargement of mucus-secreting glands of trachea and bronchi.
- Increase in the number of goblet cells and mucous glands in airways.
- Increase in **Reid index** (ratio of thickness of the mucous gland layer to the thickness of the wall between the epithelium and the cartilage [normal 0.4]).
- Squamous metaplasia and dysplasia.

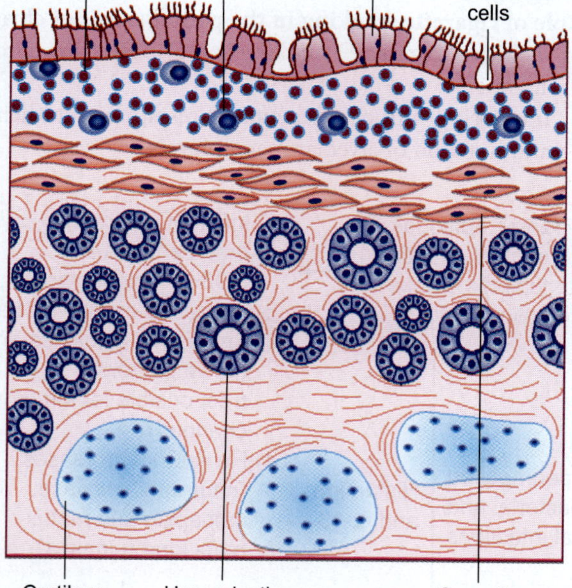

Fig. 26.4 Histopathology of chronic bronchitis showing chronic inflammation of airways, enlargement of mucus-secreting glands of trachea and bronchi, increase in the number of goblet cells and mucous glands in airways and increase in Reid index.

- Thickening of the bronchiolar wall due to oedema, mucous gland hyperplasia, inflammation and fibrosis.
- Obliteration of lumina of bronchioles due to fibrosis (bronchiolitis obliterans).

Histopathological changes in small airways in young smokers include:

- Goblet cell metaplasia with mucus plugging.
- Clustering of pigmented alveolar macrophages and infiltration by inflammatory cells.
- Fibrosis of bronchiolar wall.

Clinical Features

- Persistent cough with production of sputum.
- Later stages, hypercapnia, hypoxaemia and mild cyanosis **(blue bloaters).**
- Death occurs due to severe infection or cor pulmonale and cardiac failure.

Bronchial Asthma

Definition

Asthma is a chronic inflammatory disorder of the airways that causes recurrent episodes of wheezing, breathlessness, chest discomfort and cough particularly at night and/or early morning. It is associated with variable degree of bronchoconstriction, inflammation of the bronchial walls and increased mucus secretion.

Pathogenesis

- The pathophysiology of asthma is complex and involves the following components:
  - Airway inflammation.
  - Intermittent airflow obstruction.
  - Bronchial hyper-responsiveness.
- **Genetic predisposition to type I hypersensitivity (atopy)** and **hyper-responsiveness on exposure to certain environmental triggers (inhaled allergens** such as house dust, mites and pets, **viruses** such as rhinovirus and respiratory syncytial virus, **smoking, drugs** such as beta-adrenergic blockers, **NSAIDS and aspirin hypersensitivity, environmental pollutants** sulphur dioxide, ozone, diesel particulates, **gastroduodenal reflux, exercise** and **emotional stress)** induce bronchial hyper-responsiveness leading to acute and chronic airway inflammation. Susceptibility locus is thought to be on chromosome 5 (5q). Two types of $\mathbf{T_H}$ lymphocytes have been characterized: T_H1 and T_H2. T_H1 cells produce IL-2 and interferon (IFN)-α, which are critical in cellular defence mechanisms in response to infection. T_H2 cells, in contrast, mediate allergic inflammation by secreting cytokines such as IL-4 (which stimulates B cells to produce IgE), IL-5 (which activates eosinophils) and IL-13 (which stimulates mucus secretion from bronchial submucous glands).
- T_H1 cells normally secrete cytokines that inhibit T_H2 cells and vice versa. Imbalance in this reciprocal arrangement can lead to the development of asthma. T_H1 cells produce IFN-γ, which suppresses inflammation in airways. A transcription factor, called **T-bet**, required for $\mathbf{T_H1}$ cell differentiation, is found to be absent from lung lymphocytes in asthmatic

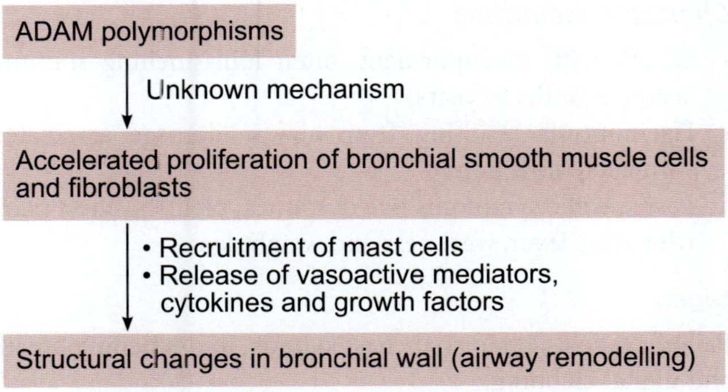

Flowchart 26.5 Airway remodelling due to ADAM polymorphisms.

patients. In the absence of the restraining influence of IFN-γ, T_H2 cells provoke airway inflammation.

- Microenvironment in the bronchial wall may be altered because of **ADAM 33 polymorphisms** (ADAM 33 is expressed by lung fibroblasts and bronchial smooth muscle cells and belongs to a subfamily of MMPs; Flowchart 26.5). Structural changes like deposition of subepithelial collagen, hypertrophy/hyperplasia of the submucous glands and hypertrophy of bronchial smooth muscle are referred to as "airway remodelling").

Types

1. Based on frequency and severity of symptoms
   (a) Mild intermittent
   (b) Mild
   (c) Moderate
   (d) Severe persistent
2. Based on response to steroids
   (a) Steroid dependent
   (b) Steroid resistant
3. Based on initiating factors
   (a) Extrinsic: Induced by an extrinsic antigen and initiated by a type 1 hypersensitivity reaction.
   (b) Intrinsic: Initiated by diverse non-immune mechanisms, e.g. aspirin ingestion, cold, stress and exercise; precipitated by several factors unique to the patient.
4. Based on aetiology
   (a) Atopic asthma (type 1 IgE-mediated response triggered by environmental allergens such as food, dust, pollen and animal dander; most common type of asthma; begins in childhood; positive family history and skin reaction).
   (b) Non-atopic asthma (no identifiable causative external agents; no family history or positive skin test).

Gross Morphology

- Overinflated lungs with small areas of atelectasis.
- Occlusion of bronchi and bronchioles by thick, tenacious mucous plugs.

Microscopy

- Thickening of basement membrane of bronchial epithelium.
- Oedema and inflammation in the bronchial walls (cells involved are eosinophils and mast cells).
- Presence of **Charcot–Leyden crystals** (crystalloids made of eosinophil membrane protein called galectin-10; appear as long or pyramidal, pink structures on H&E sections).
- Mucous plugs in bronchi and bronchioles containing whorls of shed epithelium, which appear like corkscrew-shaped twisted structures composed of condensed thick mucus surrounded by clear material (**Curschmann spirals**).
- Increase in size of submucosal glands and hypertrophy of bronchial wall muscle.

Clinical Features and Diagnosis

- During an asthmatic episode, the patient presents with **chest tightness, dyspnoea, wheezing and cough without production of sputum.**
- The patient may be asymptomatic between asthmatic episodes.
- The most severe form of asthma is labelled **'status asthmaticus'**. This may last for days to weeks, be unresponsive to treatment and lead to severe cyanosis and sometimes death.
- Sputum is viscous, and rich in eosinophils, **Charcot–Leyden crystals** and **Curschmann spirals.**
- **Peripheral blood eosinophilia** can be seen.

Bronchiectasis

Definition

Abnormal and permanent dilatation of proximal and medium-sized bronchi (>2 mm in diameter), caused by destruction of the muscular and elastic components of the bronchial walls.

Causes

- **Congenital bronchiectasis** results from developmental arrest of the bronchial tree, e.g. bronchopulmonary sequestration, which is classified as either intralobar or extralobar and results in chronic lower respiratory tract infections that later lead to bronchiectasis.
- The **more common acquired forms** occur in adults and older children and require an infectious insult, impairment of drainage, airway obstruction and/or a defect in host defence to develop.
  - **Primary infections:** Bronchiectasis may result as a consequence of necrotizing infections that are either poorly treated or not treated at all. Typical offending organisms include *Klebsiella* species, *Staphylococcus aureus*, *Mycobacterium tuberculosis*, *Mycoplasma pneumoniae*, *Mycobacterium avium* complex, fungi (*Aspergillus species*) and certain viruses.
  - **Bronchial obstruction:** Endobronchial tumours, foreign body impaction and right middle lobe syndrome (which results from an abnormal angulation of the lobar bronchus at its origin, predisposing it to obstruction).
  - **Cystic fibrosis (CF):** Bronchiectasis associated with CF is secondary to mucous plugging of proximal airways and chronic pulmonary infection, especially with *P. aeruginosa*.
  - **Young syndrome:** This genetic variant of CF presents with bronchiectasis, sinusitis and azoospermia.

- **Primary ciliary dyskinesia:** It presents with immotile or dyskinetic cilia and/or sperms. This may lead to poor mucociliary clearance, recurrent pulmonary infections and, ultimately, bronchiectasis. A variant of this condition, initially described by **Kartagener**, comprises the clinical triad of situs inversus, nasal polyps, sinusitis and bronchiectasis due to immotile cilia of the respiratory tract.

Gross Morphology

- Bronchiectasis may present as (1) a focal process involving a lobe or a segment of the lung or (2) a diffuse process involving both lungs. The former is the most common presentation of bronchiectasis, whereas the latter is most often associated with systemic illnesses.
- The bronchi and bronchioles are dilated and can be traced up to the pleural surface.
- The wall of the bronchi is thickened because of fibrosis and the lumen may be filled with mucopurulent secretions.
- Reid characterized bronchiectasis as cylindrical, cystic or varicose based on morphology:
  - *Cylindrical bronchiectasis*: Bronchi are dilated minimally and have straight, regular outlines (primarily due to mucosal oedema).
  - *Cystic or saccular bronchiectasis*: Bronchi have a ballooned appearance and demonstrate air–fluid levels (due to ulceration with bronchial neovascularization).
  - *Varicose bronchiectasis*: Bulbous bronchi with dilatations and intervening sites of relative constriction due to scarring.

Microscopy

In an active case, there may be acute and chronic inflammation of the bronchi and bronchioles, desquamation of the epithelium and necrotizing ulceration. In more chronic cases, fibrosis of the bronchial and bronchiolar walls is seen (Fig. 26.5).

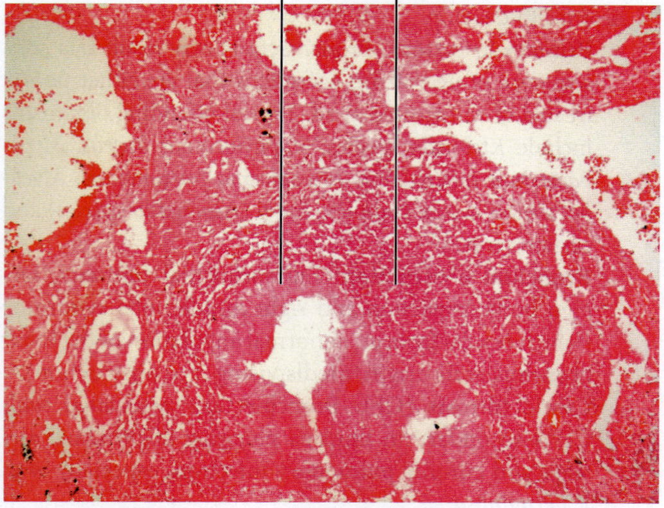

Fig. 26.5 Section showing chronic inflammation of the bronchi and bronchioles (H&E; 200×).

Clinical Presentation

- Cough with mucopurulent, often foul-smelling sputum, lasting months to years.
- Haemoptysis resulting from airway damage associated with acute infection.
- Less specific symptoms like dyspnoea, pleuritic chest pain, wheezing, fever, weakness and weight loss.

Signs

Pallor, cyanosis, abnormal chest sounds, foul-smelling breath and digital clubbing.

Complications

1. Recurrent pneumonias
2. Lung abscess
3. Respiratory failure
4. Cor pulmonale
5. Empyema
6. Amyloidosis

Q. Differentiate between centriacinar and panacinar emphysema. (PA26.3)

Ans. Differences between centriacinar and panacinar emphysema are given in Table 26.1.

Q. Differentiate between chronic bronchitis and emphysema. (PA26.3)

Ans. Differences between chronic bronchitis and emphysema are given in Table 26.2.

Table 26.1 Differences between centriacinar and panacinar emphysema

Features	Centriacinar emphysema	Panacinar emphysema
Distribution	Central or proximal part of acini affected and distal acini spared	Acini uniformly enlarged from the level of respiratory bronchiole to terminal blind alveolar sac
Part of lung involved	More common in upper lobes	More common in lower zones and anterior margin of lungs; most severe at the bases
Aetiology	Predominantly seen in heavy smokers, often in association with chronic bronchitis	Associated with α_1-AT deficiency
Pigment deposition	Walls of emphysematous spaces contain large amounts of pigment (associated with coal workers' pneumoconiosis)	No such findings or association
Inflammation	Inflammation around bronchi and bronchioles is commonly encountered	Not seen
Frequency of occurrence	More common	Less common

Table 26.2 Differences between chronic bronchitis and emphysema

Features	Chronic bronchitis	Emphysema
Age	40–45 years	50–75 years
Dyspnoea	Mild and late	Severe and early
Cough	Early onset with copious sputum	Late onset with scanty sputum
Infections	Common	Occasional
Respiratory insufficiency	Repeated	Terminal
Cor pulmonale	Common	Rare and terminal
Airway resistance	Increased	Normal or slightly increased
X-ray chest	Large heart	Small heart
Physical appearance	Blue bloater	Pink puffer

Q. Differentiate between extrinsic and intrinsic asthma. (PA26.3)

Ans. Differences between extrinsic and intrinsic asthma are given in Table 26.3.

Q. Enumerate the various pulmonary infections.

Ans. Common pulmonary infections include:

1. Acute pneumonia.
2. Healthcare-associated pneumonia.
3. Hospital-acquired pneumonia.
4. Aspiration (inhalation) pneumonia.
5. Chronic pneumonia.
6. Pneumonia in an immunocompromised host.
7. Necrotizing pneumonia and lung abscess.

Table 26.3 Differences between extrinsic and intrinsic asthma

Features	Extrinsic asthma	Intrinsic asthma
Evolution	Induced by a type I hypersensitivity reaction due to an extrinsic antigen; positive skin hypersensitivity tests	Immune mechanism not involved; precipitated by some variable idiosyncratic reactions; negative skin hypersensitivity tests
Family history	Present	Absent
Age group affected	Childhood	Adults
Other allergies, e.g. rhinitis, urticaria, eczema	Present	Absent
Serum IgE	Increased	Normal
Associated emphysema	Rare	Common
Associated bronchitis	Absent	Present

Q. Classify pneumonia and write briefly on its aetiopathogenesis and morphological manifestations.

Ans. See Chapter 9.

Q. Outline the aetiopathogenesis, morphology and complications of lung abscess. (PA26.2)

Ans. A localized suppurative process within the lungs which induces necrosis of lung tissue.

Aetiopathogenesis

Causative Organisms

- *Aerobic* and *anaerobic streptococci.*
- *Staphylococcus aureus.*
- *Bacteroides.*
- *Fusobacterium.*

Predisposing Factors

- Oropharyngeal: Surgical procedures, dental sepsis and sinusitis.
- Bronchial obstruction: Secretions, bronchiectasis and bronchogenic carcinoma.
- Direct and haematogenous spread: Direct trauma and infection from other organs.
- Aspiration of infective material: Gastric contents may be aspirated in comatose patients, alcoholics, patients under anaesthesia, or with sinusitis and depressed cough reflex.
- Antecedent primary bacterial infection particularly in immunosuppressed patients: *S. aureus, Klebsiella pneumoniae, Streptococcus pyogenes* and *Pseudomonas*.
- Septic embolism: From thrombophlebitis (affecting systemic veins) or infective bacterial endocarditis vegetations in the right side of the heart.
- Idiopathic/primary cryptogenic lung abscess: No definite cause found.

Morphology

- Characterized by suppurative destruction of the lung parenchyma with a central area of cavitation.
- May be solitary or multiple.
- Pulmonary abscesses due to aspiration are more common on the right side because of the more vertical right main bronchus; abscesses that develop secondary to pneumonias and bronchiectasis are usually multiple, basal and diffusely scattered.
- Abscesses due to septic emboli and pyaemia are also multiple but may affect any region of the lungs.
- Superimposed saprophytic infections lead to a large, ill-defined, foul-smelling and multilocular cavity (**gangrene of the lung**).

Complications

- Involvement of pleural cavity by extension of the infection (empyema).

- Haemorrhage.
- Metastatic brain abscess or meningitis from septic emboli
- Secondary amyloidosis.
- Clubbing of the fingers and toes.

Q. Write in details about the aetiopathogenesis, morphological (or autopsy) findings, sequelae and complications of pulmonary tuberculosis.

Ans. See Chapter 9.

Q. Classify chronic interstitial lung diseases (ILD). Write briefly about their clinicopathological features.

Ans. Chronic ILD are a heterogeneous group of disorders characterized by the diffuse and chronic involvement of pulmonary connective tissue, principally the alveolar interstitium.

Classification

1. Fibrosing alveolitis
   (a) Usual interstitial pneumonia (UIP) or idiopathic pulmonary fibrosis (IPF).
   (b) Non-specific interstitial pneumonia (NSIP).
   (c) Cryptogenic organizing pneumonia (COP).
   (d) ILD associated with:
      (i) Collagen vascular diseases.
      (ii) Pneumoconiosis.
      (iii) Drug reactions.
      (iv) Radiation injury.
2. Granulomatous ILD
   (a) Sarcoidosis.
   (b) Hypersensitivity pneumonitis.
3. Eosinophilic ILD.
4. Smoking-related ILD
   (a) Desquamative interstitial pneumonia (DIP).
   (b) Respiratory bronchiolitis-associated ILD.
5. Pulmonary alveolar proteinosis (PAP).

Salient Features

- The aetiopathogenesis of many of the above-mentioned conditions is unknown or not clearly understood.
- Patients with ILD usually present with dyspnoea, tachypnoea, end-inspiratory crackles and cyanosis without wheezing (clinical and pulmonary functional changes are those of restrictive rather than of obstructive nature).
- Classical physiological features are decreased carbon monoxide diffusing capacity and reduced lung volume and compliance.
- X-ray chest shows diffuse infiltration by small nodules, irregular lines or ground glass shadows.
- Eventually, the patient goes into secondary pulmonary hypertension and cor pulmonale.
- Scarring or gross destruction of lung leads to end-stage or honeycomb lung.

Pathogenesis

See Flowchart 26.6.

Q. Write briefly about idiopathic pulmonary fibrosis (IPF) or usual interstitial pneumonia (UIP).

Ans. IPF is characterized by progressive interstitial fibrosis leading to lung failure.

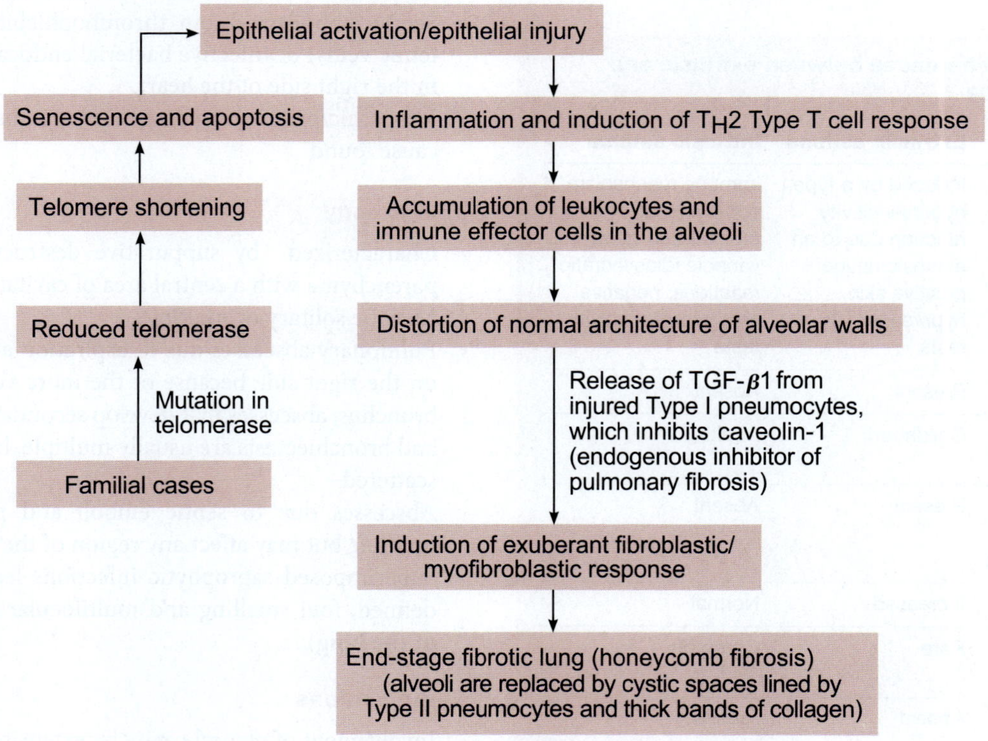

Flowchart 26.6 Pathogenesis of ILD.

Salient Features

- Usually affects individuals older than 50 years.
- Histological picture labelled as UIP but can have overlapping features with other entities (connective tissue disorders, hypersensitivity pneumonia and asbestosis).
- Diagnosis should be based on the complete clinical-radiological picture and morphology.

Pathogenesis

Injury to alveolar epithelium (or pneumocytes) is the key event. Both genetic and environmental factors are implicated.

1. **Environmental factors:** Smoking, gastro-oesophageal reflux, exposure to toxins such as metal fumes and occupational exposure (farming, stone polishing and hair dressing) damage alveolar epithelium and activate immune responses to generate profibrogenic factors, resulting in collagen production and fibrosis. Increased TGF-β1 activity likely has role in abnormal fibrosis.
2. **Genetic factors:** Mutations in gene encoding surfactant proteins SFTPC (surfactant protein C), SFTPA2 (surfactant protein A2), TERT (encoding protein component of telomerase), TERC (encoding RNA component of telomerase) and genetic abnormality leading to increased secretion of MUC5B, an abnormal mucin that predisposes to alveolar epithelial injury, are all implicated. Aberrant Wnt/β-catenin signalling pathway may be related to abnormal remodelling.

Histopathology

- Prominent fibrosis along the interlobular septae and subpleural region with patchy interstitial fibrosis.
- Early lesions are cellular and contain plump fibroblasts, and late lesions are densely collagenized.
- Fibrosis induces distortion of cellular architecture and formation of cystic spaces resulting in a 'honeycomb appearance'.
- Chronic inflammation may be seen in the areas of fibrosis.

Clinical Features

- Insidious onset with progressively increasing dyspnoea and dry cough.
- Hypoxaemia, clubbing and cyanosis are seen in later stages.
- The disease course is variable; mostly the patient worsens despite immunosuppressants.

Q. Write briefly about cryptogenic organizing pneumonia (COP).

Ans. COP is a relatively rare disease of unknown aetiology in which the patient presents with cough and dyspnoea.

Salient Features

- It is thought to be a repair process in response to preceding alveolar injury. Injury to capillary endothelial cells and alveolar epithelial cells results in the leakage of plasma proteins, especially coagulation factors. Intra-alveolar coagulation generates fibrin on alveolar surfaces. Fibroblasts/myofibroblasts migrate into the affected area, proliferate and generate loose fibrosis in the form of a small polyp. IL-6, IL-8 and TGF-β1 may play an important role in the pathogenesis.
- X-ray shows patchy peribronchial and subpleural consolidation.
- Microscopy shows polypoid bits of loose connective tissue in the bronchioles, alveoli and alveolar ducts (**Masson bodies**). No interstitial fibrosis is seen and most patients recover after being given steroids for six months or longer.

Q. Write briefly about pulmonary involvement in autoimmune diseases.

Ans. Lungs can be involved in the following autoimmune diseases:

1. **Rheumatoid arthritis**
   - Involved in 30%–40% of patients.
   - May present as chronic pleuritis, pleural effusion, interstitial pneumonitis or fibrosis and follicular bronchiolitis.
2. **Scleroderma or systemic sclerosis:** Diffuse interstitial fibrosis and pleural involvement.
3. **SLE:** Transient infiltrates, pneumonitis and pleural involvement.

Q. Write in details about the clinicopathological features of sarcoidosis.

Ans. Sarcoidosis is a multisystem disease of unknown origin characterized by the formation of non-caseating granulomas.

Aetiopathogenesis

It is unknown, but consensus is that disordered immune regulation, genetic predisposition and presence of certain environmental agents may all contribute.

Immunological Abnormalities

- An unknown/ unspecified antigen is presented by APCs to CD4+ T cells which results in antigen induced helper T cell proliferation, intra-alveolar and interstitial accumulation of CD4+ T cells, and an increased CD4+:CD8+ T cell ratio.
- Increased levels of T-cell-derived TH1 cytokines, such as IL-2 and IFN-γ, result in T-cell expansion and macrophage activation. Oher cytokines such as IL-8, TNF and macrophage inflammatory protein 1α (MIP- 1α) recruit additional T cells and monocytes, ultimately contributing to the formation of a granuloma.
- Anergy to *Candida* and common skin antigens such as purified protein derivative (PPD) and polyclonal hypergammaglobulinaemia may be seen.

Genetic Association

Familial clustering of cases and association with certain HLA haplotypes (HLA-A1 and HLA-B8).

Environmental Contribution

Several microbes have been implicated in the pathogenesis of sarcoidosis, e.g. *Mycobacteria*, *Propionibacterium acnes*, *Borrelia burgdorferi*, viruses, fungi and *Rickettsia* species.

Morphology

- Involved tissue shows non-caseating granulomas composed of closely packed epithelioid cells with Langhans or foreign body giant cells (lymphocytes are few in number, so granulomas also called **'naked granulomas'**).

- Fibrinoid necrosis may be seen.
- Long-standing granulomas are enclosed within fibrous rims or hyaline scars and may show the following inclusions:
  - Laminated concretions composed of calcium and proteins known as **Schaumann bodies.**
  - Stellate inclusions in giant cells called **asteroid bodies.**
- **Necrotizing sarcoid granulomatosis** is very rare and controversial (usually affects women and has excellent response to steroids and immunosuppressive drugs); It has to be **differentiated from tuberculosis, fungal infections or granulomatosis with polyangiitis (Wegener's granulomatosis).**

The following organs are commonly involved in sarcoidosis:

1. **Lungs**
   (a) Lung is the most commonly involved organ.
   (b) Either no gross lesion or 1- to 2-cm nodules; often in bronchial submucosa, so biopsies are helpful.
   (c) Sections show epithelioid cell granulomas which coalesce to produce small nodules around lymphatics, bronchi, blood vessels and sometimes within alveoli; heal with fibrosis.
   (d) Pleural surfaces are involved in 10% cases.
2. **Lymph nodes**
   (a) Involved in almost all cases; sarcoidosis mainly affects hilar and mediastinal nodes, and may occasionally manifest as generalized lymphadenopathy.
   (b) Nodes are enlarged, discrete, non-tender and sometimes calcified.
   (c) Tonsils may also be involved in some cases.
3. **Spleen**
   (a) Microscopic involvement of spleen is seen in three-fourth of cases but gross enlargement is seen in very few cases.
   (b) It contains scattered granulomas.
4. **Liver**
   (a) Involved less often than spleen.
   (b) Shows scattered granulomas located more often in the portal triads than in the lobular parenchyma.
5. **Bone marrow**
   (a) Typically involves the phalangeal bones creating small-circumscribed areas of lysis.
   (b) Widening of bony shafts and new bone formation on the outer surfaces may be seen.
6. **Skin and mucosa**
   (a) Skin lesions are encountered in about 50% of cases.
   (b) These include discrete subcutaneous nodules, erythematous plaques or red, scaly, flat lesions.
   (c) Lesions may also appear in the mucous membranes of the oral cavity, larynx and upper respiratory tract.
7. **Eye**
   (a) It may cause iritis or iridocyclitis, corneal opacities, glaucoma and total loss of vision.
   (b) Inflammation of lacrimal glands and suppression of lacrimation are commonly encountered.
8. **Salivary glands**
   (a) Bilateral involvement of the salivary glands is usual.
   (b) Combined uveoparotid involvement is labelled **Mikulicz syndrome**.
9. **Muscle:** Involvement of muscle manifests as muscle weakness, tenderness and fatigue.

   Sarcoid granulomas may also be seen in the CNS, endocrine organs, kidneys and heart.

Clinical Features

- It is usually discovered accidentally on routine X-ray or CT scan.
- The onset of respiratory symptoms is insidious (shortness of breath, cough, chest pain and haemoptysis).
- Constitutional signs and symptoms include fever, fatigue, weight loss, anorexia and night sweats.
- It usually presents with peripheral and perihilar lymphadenopathy, diffuse pulmonary disease, cutaneous lesions, eye involvement or hepatosplenomegaly.
- Lungs may show interstitial fibrosis, localized bronchial stenosis, distal bronchiectasis or atelectasis.
- Chronic progressive course or alternating periods of remission (spontaneous or steroid induced) and activity are typical.
- Most resolve spontaneously or after steroid therapy with minimal or no residual manifestations.
- Some succumb to progressive pulmonary fibrosis and cor pulmonale.
- Commonly, there is anergy to skin test antigens with polyclonal hypergammaglobulinaemia.
- Eighty per cent have elevated serum angiotensin-converting enzyme (not a specific finding).
- Sarcoidosis is a diagnosis of exclusion, because there are no specific criteria for disease.
- Infective pathology needs to be excluded by culture and use of special stain.
- **Best prognosis** is hilar lymphadenopathy alone.
- **Worst prognosis** is pulmonary disease without adenopathy.

Q. Write briefly about hypersensitive pneumonitis.

Ans. Hypersensitivity (allergic) pneumonitis is an immunologically mediated response to an extrinsic antigen involving initially immune complex (type III) and later granulomatous (type IV hypersensitivity). It includes the following conditions:

- **Farmer lung** caused by mouldy hay containing actinomycetes (external antigen).
- **Pigeon breeder's disease** or **bird fancier's disease** caused by proteins from serum, excreta or feathers of birds.
- **Humidifier** or **air-conditioner lung** caused by thermophilic bacteria in heated water reservoirs.

Clinical Features

- Acute form: Recurring episodes of fever, dyspnoea, cough and leucocytosis.
- Chronic form: Signs of progressive respiratory failure, dyspnoea, cyanosis and reduced lung compliance.

X-Ray

Diffuse or nodular infiltrates.

Pulmonary Function Tests

These are indicative of a restrictive disorder.

Morphology

Histological changes are mainly seen in bronchioles; these include:

- Interstitial pneumonitis consisting of lymphocytes, plasma cells and macrophages.
- Non-caseating granulomas.
- Interstitial fibrosis and obliterative bronchiolitis (in late stage).

Q. Write briefly about pulmonary eosinophilia.

Ans. Pulmonary eosinophilia includes several entities, e.g. acute eosinophilic pneumonia with respiratory failure, secondary eosinophilia and idiopathic chronic eosinophilic pneumonia.

1. ***Acute eosinophilic pneumonia with respiratory failure:*** It is a steroid-responsive disease which presents with hypoxaemia, fever, dyspnoea and pulmonary infiltrates. The bronchoalveolar lavage fluid contains more than 25% eosinophils and histopathology shows extensive alveolar damage with eosinophilic infiltration.
2. ***Secondary eosinophilia:*** It occurs secondary to bacterial, fungal and parasitic infections, hypersensitivity pneumonitis, drug allergies, asthma, allergic bronchopulmonary aspergillosis and Churg–Strauss syndrome.
3. ***Idiopathic chronic eosinophilic pneumonia:*** Is a diagnosis of exclusion, responds to steroid therapy and manifests with cough, fever, dyspnoea, night sweats and weight loss. There is consolidation of peripheral lung substance which is infiltrated by lymphocytes and eosinophils (inflammatory cells are present within the alveoli and in the alveolar septae).

Q. Write briefly about smoking-associated interstitial disease.

Ans. ILD associated with smoking includes:

1. **DIP:** Airspaces contain aggregates of macrophages which were earlier thought to be desquamated pneumocytes, which is why the entity was named DIP. It presents insidiously between 40 and 50 years in smokers with dyspnoea and cough and is steroid responsive.
2. **Respiratory bronchiolitis-associated ILD:** It is a bronchocentric condition which is typified by peribronchiolar chronic inflammation and fibrosis. Pigment-containing macrophages are present in the respiratory bronchioles and the patient presents with dyspnoea and cough.

Q. Write briefly about pulmonary alveolar proteinosis (PAP).

Ans. PAP results from a defect in pulmonary macrophage function which results in impaired removal of surfactant from the alveolar and bronchiolar spaces.

Salient Features

- It is a rare disease characterized by a defect in GM-CSF or macrophage function.
- There is intra-alveolar or intrabronchiolar accumulation of surfactant.
- The patient presents with cough and expectoration of gelatinous material.
- Histopathology shows consolidation of lung substance because of the presence of surfactant containing PAS-positive precipitate in the alveolar spaces. There is minimal inflammation with the presence of cholesterol clefts.
- PAP may be:
  1. **Autoimmune:** Presence of neutralizing antibodies to GM-CSF (reduced or absent GM-CSF signalling interferes with the terminal differentiation of the alveolar macrophages, which in turn impairs their ability to catabolize the surfactant).
  2. **Secondary:** Occurs secondary to a variety of conditions (haematopoietic disorders, immunodeficiency syndromes, inborn errors of metabolism and acute silicosis).
  3. **Hereditary:** Rare neonatal condition caused by GM-CSF receptor gene mutations.

Q. Describe the clinicopathological features of occupational lung diseases. (PA26.5)

Ans. Occupational lung diseases are a reaction of the lung to inhalation of mineral dusts encountered in the workplace.

- **Factors which determine the extent of damage caused by the inhaled dust:**
  - Size and shape of the particle.
  - Their solubility and physiochemical composition.
  - The amount of dust retained in the lung.
  - The additional effect of other irritants, such as tobacco smoke.
  - Host factors, such as efficiency of clearance mechanism and immune status of the host.
- **Types of tissue response to inhaled dust:**
  - Formation of fibrous nodules.
  - Interstitial fibrosis
  - Hypersensitivity reaction

Diseases Caused by Mineral Dusts and Environmental Pollutants (Table 26.4)

1. **Coal worker's pneumoconiosis (CWP):** Pneumoconiosis is the general term for a class of interstitial lung diseases caused by inhalation of mineral dusts. CWP, the commonest form of pneumoconioses, is caused by inhalation of carbon particles. It may manifest as follows:
   i. **Asymptomatic anthracosis**
      (a) Common, benign and asymptomatic accumulation of carbon dust.
      (b) Incidence has been found to increase with cigarette smoking and atmospheric pollution.
      (c) Alveolar macrophages engulf carbon and accumulate along lymphatics.
   ii. **Simple CWP with little or no pulmonary dysfunction**
      (a) Lungs show coal macules (1–2 mm in diameter) or larger coal nodules. These are basically aggregates of dust-laden macrophages with increase in reticulin and collagen.
      (b) Upper lobes and upper zones of lower lobes are more heavily involved.
      (c) The macules and nodules are commonly seen adjacent to respiratory bronchioles where dilatation of alveoli leads to **centrilobular emphysema**.

Table 26.4 Diseases caused by mineral dusts and environmental pollutants

Agents	Diseases	Exposure
Mineral dusts		
Coal dust	Anthracosis	Coal mining
	Macules	
	Progressive massive fibrosis (PMF)/Caplan syndrome	
Silica	Silicosis, Caplan syndrome	Sand blasting, stone cutting, foundry workers
Asbestosis	Mesothelioma, carcinoma lung, larynx, colon, pleural plaques	Mining, milling, fabrication
Beryllium	• Acute berylliosis • Beryllium granulomas • May cause bronchogenic carcinoma	Mining, fabrication
Iron oxide	Siderosis	Welding
Barium sulphate	Baritosis	Mining
Tin oxide	Stannosis	Mining, metallurgy, porcelain industry
Organic dusts that cause hypersensitivity pneumonitis		
Mouldy hay	Farmer lung	Farming
Bagasse	Bagassosis	Wall board and paper manufacturing
Bird dropping	Bird breeder's lung	Bird handling
Organic dusts that induce asthma		
Cotton, flax, hemp	Byssinosis	Textile manufactures
Chemical fumes and vapours		
NO, SO_2, benzene, NH_3	Bronchitis/ARDS/asthma/pulmonary oedema/poisoning	Occupational and accidental exposure

iii. **Complicated CWP (progressive massive fibrosis [PMF])**
   (a) It requires many years to develop and is characterized by intensely blackened scars 2–10 cm, usually multiple, bilateral and located more often in the upper parts of the lungs.
   (b) These masses may break down centrally because of ischaemic necrosis or secondary tuberculous infection.
   (c) Pleura and regional lymph nodes are blackened and fibrotic. Fibrous lesions are composed of dense collagen and carbon pigment.
   (d) Wall of respiratory bronchioles and pulmonary vessels are thickened, and show scanty inflammatory infiltrate of lymphoid and plasma cells. Alveoli are dilated.

2. **Rheumatoid pneumoconiosis or Caplan syndrome** (rheumatoid arthritis with CWP, silicosis or asbestosis): Lungs have rounded, firm nodules with central necrosis, cavitation or calcification. Sections from the nodules show fibrinoid necrosis enclosed by palisading mononuclear cells and fibroblasts.

Clinical course of pneumoconiosis

- Simple CWP usually has a benign course; PMF may lead to cor pulmonale in a few patients.
- Coal dust exposure increases the incidence of chronic bronchitis and emphysema.

Factors implicated in the development of PMF

- Older age of the miners.
- Amount and duration of exposure to coal dust.
- Coexisting tuberculosis.
- Coexisting silicosis which may further damage the lungs by the following mechanisms:
  - Free radical generation (reactive oxygen species that damage the lung parenchyma).
  - Release of chemotactic factors, which induce infiltration of inflammatory cells into the pulmonary tissue.
  - Release of fibrogenic cytokines – IL-1, TNF and PDGF (platelet-derived growth factor) – which cause healing by fibrosis.

3. **Silicosis (knife grinder's lung disease)**
   i. It is the most prevalent chronic occupational lung disease.
   ii. Silica has two forms: crystalline and amorphous; the crystalline forms (quartz, cristobalite and tridymite) are more fibrogenic and toxic than the non-crystalline forms.
   iii. Prolonged exposure leads to nodular fibrosing pneumoconiosis.

Silica particles reach the alveoli

↓

Engulfed by macrophages

↓

Silica dust is cytotoxic and kills the macrophages, which engulf it, resulting in tissue necrosis

↓

Dying macrophages release silica dust, which induces growth factors such as IL-1, TNF and fibronectin that cause fibroblast proliferation and collagen synthesis

↓

New macrophages engulf the debris (a repetitive cycle of phagocytosis and tissue necrosis ensues)

↓

Silica-laden macrophages reach respiratory bronchioles, alveoli, interstitial tissue, pleural and interlobar lymphatics, and regional lymph nodes to cause pathological changes

Flowchart 26.7 Pathogenesis of silicosis.

Pathogenesis: See Flowchart 26.7.

Pathological changes

Early stages: There are tiny, discrete pale to black nodules in the upper zones of the lungs.

Late stages

- There are hard, collagen-rich scars, some of which may show central cavitation because of superimposed tuberculosis or ischaemia.
- Fibrotic lesions are also seen in the **pleura**.
- Thin sheets of calcification (**'egg shell' calcification**) may be noted in **lymph nodes.**
- Progression with development of PMF ensues.
- Microscopy shows concentric layers of hyalinized collagen surrounded by a dense capsule of more condensed collagen. Polarization shows birefringent silica particles.

Clinical features: The patient manifests mainly with dyspnoea.

Complications

- Pulmonary tuberculosis (silicosis may depress the cell-mediated immunity [CMI]) and increase susceptibility to pulmonary tuberculosis).
- Rheumatoid arthritis/Caplan syndrome.
- Cor pulmonale.
- Lung cancer.

4. **Asbestos-related disease**
   i. Prolonged exposure to asbestos dust produces three types of diseases:
      (a) Asbestosis of lungs (parenchymal interstitial fibrosis).
      (b) Pleural disease (localized fibrous plaques or diffuse fibrosis).
      (c) Tumours (bronchogenic carcinoma, pleural and peritoneal mesotheliomas, laryngeal carcinoma).

Inhaled asbestos fibres are phagocytosed by alveolar macrophages

↓

Reach the interstitium via lymphatics, some reach pleura and regional lymph nodes

↓

Activation of alveolar and interstitial macrophages to produce chemotactic factors and fibrogenic mediators

↓

Generalized interstitial pulmonary inflammation and fibrosis

Flowchart 26.8 Pathogenesis of asbestosis.

   ii. Asbestos is a family of crystalline hydrated silicates that form fibres, which may exist as two distinct geometric forms:
      (a) Serpentine (chrysotile): Curly and flexible fibres (90% of commercial form of asbestos).
      (b) Amphibole: Straight, stiff and brittle fibres.
   iii. Amphiboles are less prevalent but more pathogenic than chrysotile because they are more rigid and less soluble.
   iv. High-risk individuals include miners, millers and fabrication workers.

Pathogenesis (Flowchart 26.8): Asbestos reaches the alveoli easily, and has the ability to penetrate epithelial cells, leading to diffuse interstitial disease rather than nodular deposits as in silicosis. **Asbestos bodies** are carcinogenic, and can act as both initiators and promoters.

Gross pathology

- Affected lungs are small and firm with marked thickening of the pleura.
- Variable degree of subpleural fibrosis is seen; advanced cases may show cystic changes.
- In contrast to CWP and silicosis, asbestosis begins in the lower lobes and subpleurally.

Microscopy

- Non-specific interstitial fibrosis with scattered **asbestos bodies** (asbestos fibres coated with glycoprotein and haemosiderin, which appear as golden brown beaded rods; the coating is most prominent at the ends of the fibers giving these a dumb-bell appearance).
- Emphysematous foci, seen between areas of fibrosis.
- Pleural involvement, which may result in the following:
  - Pleural effusion.
  - Visceral pleural fibrosis.
  - Pleural plaques (most common lesions with asbestos exposure; circumscribed, flat, 1-cm, firm-to-hard bilateral nodules).

Clinical features

- It is a slow insidious illness, which may be asymptomatic for years, the most common clinical manifestations being dyspnoea and dry cough.

- Pulmonary hypertension and cor pulmonale are observed in advanced cases.

5. **Berylliosis:** Occurs due to heavy exposure to dust/fumes of metallic beryllium or its salts used in nuclear, electronic and aerospace industries.
   (a) **Acute berylliosis**
   - Seen after 2–4 weeks of exposure.
   - Manifests with dyspnoea, hypercapnia and chest pain due to filling up of alveoli with protein-rich fluid and formation of hyaline membrane.
   - Complete recovery may be seen.

   (b) **Chronic berylliosis**
   - It is seen after 20 years or more of exposure.
   - Cell-mediated hypersensitivity reaction produces noncaseating granulomas.

Q. Define cor pulmonale. Enumerate the types of cor pulmonale.

Ans. Cor pulmonale is dilatation (with or without hypertrophy) of the right ventricle because of a primary respiratory disorder.

- Hypertrophy is a feature of chronic cor pulmonale, whereas dilatation dominates in acute cor pulmonale.
- Pulmonary hypertension is the common link between heart and lung dysfunction.

Q. What is acute cor pulmonale? Discuss the clinical manifestations of acute cor pulmonale.

Ans. Acute cor pulmonale usually follows acute massive pulmonary embolism, which is sufficient enough to obstruct more than 60% of pulmonary circulation. It leads to acute pulmonary hypertension, acute right ventricular dilatation and failure.

Q. Discuss the aetiopathogenesis and clinicopathological features of chronic cor pulmonale.

Ans. Chronic cor pulmonale is defined as a combination of hypertrophy and dilatation of the right ventricle secondary to pulmonary hypertension, which results from diseases of lung, pulmonary circulation or thorax.

Aetiology

- COPD (including chronic bronchitis and emphysema) is responsible for more than 50% of cases of chronic cor pulmonale.
- Early onset of cor pulmonale is seen in patients with chronic bronchitis (blue bloaters).
- The onset of cor pulmonale is late in patients with emphysema (pink puffers).
- Increased pulmonary vascular resistance and pulmonary hypertension are the central mechanisms in all cases of chronic cor pulmonale.

Clinical Features

- Dyspnoea, because of pulmonary hypertension, not relieved by sitting up.
- Dry cough.
- Chest pain because of dilatation of the root of pulmonary artery.
- Exercise-induced peripheral cyanosis.
- **Signs of overt right heart failure** including peripheral oedema, raised jugular venous pressure, tender hepatomegaly, cardiac enlargement, right ventricular third heart sound and a gallop rhythm.

Q. Classify lung tumours. Briefly describe their aetiopathogenesis and morphology. (PA26.6)

Ans. The new WHO classification makes extensive use of immunohistochemistry and molecular testing to classify lung tumours in an attempt at personalizing treatment strategies for different lung cancer types. Broadly lung tumours are categorized into:

Classification of Tumours of the Lung

- Benign and malignant epithelial tumours (which constitute 90%–95% of lung tumours).
- Bronchial carcinoids (which constitute 5% of all lung tumours).
- Mesenchymal (pulmonary hamartoma, chondroma, PEComas), lymphohistiocytic, ectopic and miscellaneous tumours (which constitute 2%–5% of all lung tumours).

Classification of Malignant Epithelial Tumours

1. **Histological classification (WHO 2015 abridged)**
   (a) Squamous cell carcinoma (preinvasive lesion - squamous cell carcinoma in situ; invasive lesions - keratinizing, non-keratinizing, and basaloid squamous cell carcinoma).
   (b) Adenocarcinoma (most common).
      (i) Preinvasive lesions (atypical adenomatous hyperplasia, adenocarcinoma in situ [AIS] – non-mucinous or mucinous).
      (ii) Minimally invasive adenocarcinoma (MIA; non-mucinous or mucinous).
      (iii) Invasive adenocarcinoma (lepidic, acinar, papillary, solid according to predominant pattern of arrangement of tumour cells).
   (c) Neuroendocrine tumours.
      (i) Small cell carcinoma: Combined small cell carcinoma.
      (ii) Large cell neuroendocrine carcinoma: Combined large cell–neuroendocrine carcinoma.
      (iii) Carcinoid tumour: Typical and atypical.
   (d) Large cell carcinoma.
   (e) Adenosquamous carcinoma.
   (f) Carcinomas with pleomorphic, sarcomatoid or sarcomatous elements.
   (g) Carcinoma of salivary gland origin.
2. **Therapy-based/clinical classification**
   (a) Small cell carcinoma (aggressive; shows a high initial response to chemotherapy).
   (b) Non–small cell carcinoma (has a better prognosis than small cell carcinoma).

Epidemiology

- Lung carcinoma is the most frequently fatal malignancy with a peak incidence between 40 and 70 years.
- Adenocarcinoma is the most common lung carcinoma in females; the overall incidence of adenocarcinoma has increased over the past few years (increase in incidence is thought to be due to increase in the number of female smokers).
- Strongest relationship with smoking is seen in squamous cell and small cell carcinoma.

Aetiology and Pathogenesis

1. **Role of tobacco smoking**
   (a) Invariable statistical association with the following:
   - Amount of daily smoking and tendency to inhale.
   - Duration of habit (heavy smokers smoking more than 40 cigarettes/day for many years have a 20-fold increased risk).
   - Ninety per cent of lung carcinoma occur in smokers. Cigar and pipe smoking is associated with less risk.
   - Cigarette smoking is known to be associated with other cancers, e.g., cancer of lip, tongue, floor of mouth, pharynx, larynx, oesophagus, urinary bladder, pancreas and kidney.

   (b) Documentation of precursor histological changes (basal cell hyperplasia, dysplasia and carcinoma in situ) in the lining epithelium of the respiratory tract in smokers.

   (c) Experimental work has revealed the presence of more than 1200 harmful substances found in tobacco smoke, e.g.:
   (i) Initiators such as polycyclic aromatic hydrocarbons (benzopyrene).
   (ii) Promoters such as phenol derivatives.
   (iii) Radioactive elements – polonium-210, carbon-14 and potassium-40.
   (iv) Arsenic, nickel and moulds.

   Not all people exposed to tobacco smoke, however, develop lung cancer. It is therefore hypothesized that the mutagenic effect of tobacco smoke is dependent on genetic variants (the procarcinogens present in tobacco smoke are converted to carcinogens by P-450 monooxygenase enzyme; specific P-450 polymorphisms have an enhanced ability to activate them, making smokers with these genetic variants more susceptible to lung cancer).
2. **Industrial hazards associated with lung carcinoma**
   (a) Radiation
   (b) Uranium (miners)
   (c) Asbestosis (particularly, when coupled with smoking)
   (d) Nickel, chromates, coal, mustard and arsenic
3. **Indoor and outdoor air pollutants:** Radon, a radioactive gas, is associated with increased risk of lung cancer when exposed in high concentrations. Polycyclic hydrocarbons from fossil fuels and vehicular diesel emission are important outdoor pollutants involved in the pathogenesis of lung cancer.
4. **Role of molecular genetics**
   (a) Loss of tumour suppressor genes such as P53 and RB1, and inactivation of CDK inhibitor P_{16} are seen equally in adenocarcinoma and squamous cell carcinoma. Allelic losses on short arm of chromosomes 3, 9 (leading to loss of CDKN2A gene and thereby inactivation of CDK inhibitor P_{16}) and 17 (loss of P53 gene) may precede invasion in squamous cell carcinoma. Squamous cell carcinomas also show amplification of FGFR1 (fibroblast growth factor receptor tyrosine kinase) and MET.
   (b) P53 and RB1 mutations along with chromosome 3p deletions are common in small cell carcinoma. Small cell carcinomas also commonly demonstrate amplification of genes of MYC family.
   (c) Gain-of-function mutations involving the growth factor receptor signalling pathways (genes encoding receptor tyrosine kinases, e.g. EGFR, BRAF, ERB2/HER2, ALK, ROS, MET and RET), amplifications in epidermal growth factor receptor (EGFR) gene and mutations in KRAS are typically seen in patients with adenocarcinoma.

Precursor Lesions of Lung Cancer

1. Squamous dysplasia and carcinoma in situ.
2. Atypical adenomatous hyperplasia (small, <5-mm lesions, solitary or multiple, composed of dysplastic pneumocytes lining fibrosed alveolar walls).
3. AIS (formerly called bronchioloalveolar carcinoma; it is a lesion smaller than 3 cm; it is constituted by dysplastic cells which grow along alveolar septa).
4. Diffuse idiopathic pulmonary neuroendocrine cell hyperplasia.

Gross Morphology

- Most common location is the hilar region.
- Most lesions arise from the first-, second- and third-order bronchi; few arise from peripheral alveolar septal cells and terminal bronchioles.
- Peripheral tumours are usually adenocarcinomas.

Clinicopathological Features of the Major Types of Lung Carcinoma

1. **Squamous cell carcinoma**
   (a) More common in males and has a strong association with smoking.
   (b) Usually central in location (main to segmental bronchi); there has been a recent increase in the incidence of peripheral lesions.
   (c) May be **peribronchial** in location when the tumour presents as an ulcerated growth which invades the wall of the bronchus to involve the peribronchial tissue. **Intraparenchymal** masses grow as cauliflower-like masses which push the surrounding lung substance. **Endobronchial tumours** present as exophytic masses which project into the lumen of the bronchus and eventually obstruct it (Flowchart 26.9).
   (d) **Well-differentiated lesions** show minimal atypia, intercellular bridges as well as abundant keratin

Starts as a small area of mucosal thickening

↓

Irregular warty growth

↓

Fungates into the bronchial lumen to grow as an intraluminal mass
or
Penetrates the wall of bronchus to grow in peribronchial tissue
or
Grows as an intraparenchymal mass

↓

- May involve pleural or pericardial surface
- Spread to tracheal, bronchial and mediastinal lymph nodes
- Lymphatic and haematogenous spread to adrenals, liver, brain and bone (often metastases is the first presentation of an occult bronchogenic carcinoma)

Flowchart 26.9 Evolution of lung carcinoma.

(keratinization is seen as numerous keratin pearls as well as individual cell keratinization; squamous cells with intracellular keratin demonstrate abundant dense eosinophilic cytoplasm).

(e) **Moderately differentiated lesions** show moderate atypia, individual cell keratinization, occasional keratin pearl, if any, and fewer intercellular bridges (Fig. 26.6).

(f) **Poorly differentiated lesions** are focally keratinized (do not demonstrate keratin easily) and show severe atypia. These lesions are difficult to recognize as squamous in origin.

(g) Squamous metaplasia, dysplasia and squamous cell carcinoma in situ may be seen in the adjacent tissue.

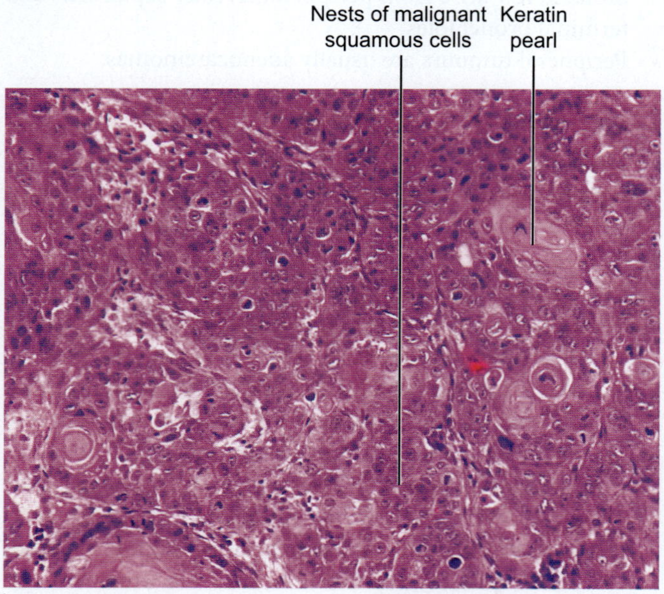

Fig. 26.6 Moderately differentiated squamous cell carcinoma showing moderate atypia, individual cell keratinization and occasional keratin pearl formation (H&E; 200×).

2. **Adenocarcinoma**

(a) **AIS:** These are tumours less than 3 cm with a lepidic growth pattern and no stromal invasion. Formerly known as bronchioloalveolar carcinoma, they arise from the terminal bronchioloalveolar region of the lung and are usually observed as **solitary 'coin' lesions.**

(b) **MIA:** These are tumours less than 3 cm with an invasive component less than 5 mm. They are associated with a peripheral lepidic pattern and scarring without any necrosis, pleural involvement or lymphovascular invasion. Pleural scars representing desmoplastic response to the tumour may be present.

(c) **Invasive adenocarcinoma**
- Most common carcinoma in females and non-smokers.
- Usually peripheral/smaller/slow growing/solitary.
- Tan-white cut surface, may have central area of scar or necrosis, usually well defined but non-encapsulated.
- Shows invasion >5 mm, is named by predominant pattern, has mucinous and non-mucinous subtypes and the following five histological patterns:
  - **Lepidic:** Type II pneumocytes and club cells proliferate to line alveolar walls which tend to maintain their architecture. The tumour lacks architectural complexity; no lymphovascular or perineural invasion is seen.
  - **Acinar:** Gland forming tumour with round/oval glands invading the stroma.
  - **Papillary:** Alveolar lining is replaced by malignant cuboidal/columnar cells lining fibrovascular cores.
  - **Micropapillary:** Tufting that lacks true fibrovascular cores.
  - **Solid:** Sheets of neoplastic cells.

(d) **Well-differentiated adenocarcinomas** show well-formed glands with occasional papillary differentiation and easily demonstrable mucin.

(e) **Poorly differentiated lesions** show minimal gland formation with solid sheets of poorly differentiated cells, which require special stains/immunohistochemistry to demonstrate foci of mucin-producing cells.

(f) **Mucinous adenocarcinoma** spreads easily, forming satellite nodules, comprises glands lined by tall columnar cells with apical mucin vacuoles.

(g) Majority of tumours are positive for **thyroid transcription factor 1 (TTF1)**.

3. **Small cell carcinoma**

(a) It is a highly malignant tumour; it metastasizes widely and has a strong association with cigarette smoking.

(b) It may be hilar/central or peripheral.

(c) Cut surface is soft, friable and grey-white and may show extensive haemorrhage and necrosis.

(d) Epithelial cells are small, round to oval with scanty cytoplasm, appear lymphocyte-like (but twice to thrice the size of a small resting lymphocyte; Fig. 26.7) and are called oat cells (previously called oat cell carcinoma). Occasionally, they may be

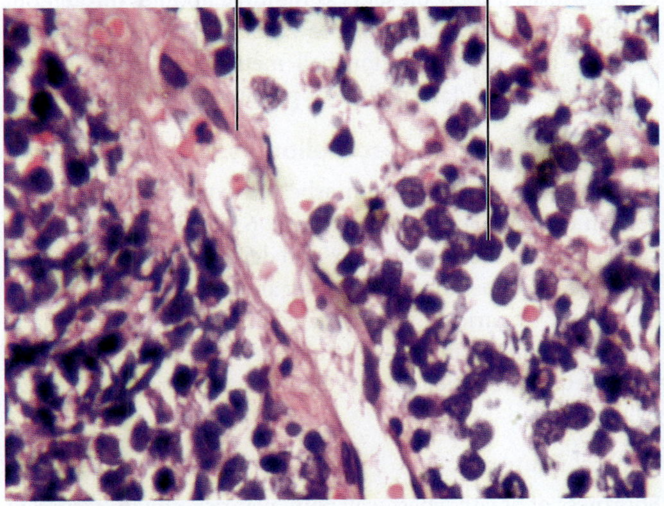

Fig. 26.7 Section from small cell carcinoma of lung showing round-to-oval tumour cells with scanty cytoplasm and hyperchromatic crowded nuclei (H&E; 400×).

spindle shaped or polygonal. Nuclei are hyperchromatic with fine granular salt and pepper chromatin and inconspicuous nucleoli.

(e) Necrosis and mitotic activity are common. Basophilic staining of vessel walls is commonly seen because of smudging by DNA from necrotic cells **(Azzopardi effect)**.

(f) Nuclear moulding is prominent and results from close apposition of tumour cells that have scanty cytoplasm.

(g) Tumour cells demonstrate dense core neurosecretory granules (evidence of origin from neuroendocrine or Kulchitsky cells), and are positive for chromogranin, synaptophysin, CD57, neuron specific enolase (NSE), Phosphotungstic acid haematoxylin (PTAH) and polypeptide hormones.

4. **Large cell carcinoma**

(a) Large anaplastic polygonal cells with vesicular nuclei (thought to be undifferentiated squamous and adenocarcinomas which can no longer be recognized on light microscopy).

(b) ***Variants:*** Giant cell, clear cell, spindle cell and large cell neuroendocrine carcinoma.

About 10% of lung carcinomas have a combined morphology with two or more histological types.

Consequences of Bronchogenic Carcinoma

- **Emphysema** (due to partial obstruction of airways by the tumour).
- **Atelectasis** (due to total obstruction of airways by the tumour).
- **Suppurative/ulcerative bronchitis or bronchiectasis** or **pulmonary abscess** (due to impaired drainage of airways).
- Venous congestion or **dusky head** (due to compression or invasion of superior vena cava).
- **Haemoptysis** (due to haemorrhage from tumour in the airway).
- **Pleural effusion, pericarditis or tamponade** (due to extension of tumour to pleural/pericardial sac).
- Apical tumours invade into brachial or cervical sympathetic plexus causing pain in the region of ulnar nerve or **Horner syndrome (ipsilateral enophthalmos, ptosis, miosis and anhidrosis)**; may be accompanied by destruction of first and second ribs and sometimes thoracic vertebrae **(Pancoast syndrome).**
- **Hoarseness** (due to recurrent laryngeal nerve invasion), **dysphagia** (due to oesophageal invasion) and **diaphragmatic paralysis** (due to phrenic nerve invasion).

Diagnosis of Lung Carcinoma

Common Symptoms

Cough, weight loss, chest pain and dyspnoea.

Investigations

X-ray/CT chest, sputum cytology, bronchoalveolar lavage, bronchial washings and brushings, ultrasound or CT-guided fine needle aspiration cytology (FNAC) or biopsy, and bronchoscopic biopsy.

Paraneoplastic Syndromes Associated With Bronchogenic Carcinoma

Various hormones or hormone-like substances are secreted by bronchogenic carcinoma, e.g.:

- Antidiuretic hormone (ADH) leading to hyponatremia.
- Adrenocorticotropic hormone (ACTH) leading to Cushing syndrome.
- Parathyroid hormone (PTH) or parathyroid hormone related peptide causing hyperkalaemia.
- Calcitonin leading to hypocalcaemia.
- Gonadotropins causing gynaecomastia.
- Serotonin-inducing carcinoid syndrome.

Other Systemic Manifestations of Lung Carcinoma

- **Lambert–Eaton myasthenic syndrome** (a rare autoimmune disorder associated with small cell carcinoma that is characterized by muscle weakness of the limbs resulting from an autoimmune reaction, in which antibodies are formed against voltage-gated calcium channels in the neuromuscular junction).
- **Sensory type of peripheral neuropathy.**
- **Acanthosis nigricans** (brown to black, velvety hyperpigmentation of the skin usually found in body folds).
- **Leukaemoid reactions.**
- **Hypertrophic pulmonary osteoarthropathy** (clinical triad of digital clubbing, arthralgias and ossifying periostitis).

Q. Write briefly on neuroendocrine tumours of the lung.

Ans. Neuroendocrine tumours of the lung are classified into:

1. Benign tumours.
2. Carcinoids.
3. Small cell carcinoma.

Bronchial Carcinoids

1. These constitute 1%–5% of all lung tumours.
2. Patients affected are generally young.
3. There is no relationship with smoking/environmental factors.
4. They present as finger-like or spherical polypoid masses, projecting into the lumen and covered by mucosa. They are rarely more than 3–4 cm.
5. Most carcinoids remain confined to the main stem bronchus; some intraluminal masses show infiltration into the peribronchial tissue (collar button lesion).
6. Microscopy shows a neuroendocrine growth pattern (organoid, trabecular, nested, pseudoglandular, rosette formation). Tumour cells are uniform with a polygonal shape, round to oval nuclei with salt and pepper chromatin and inconspicuous nucleoli, along with moderate to abundant eosinophilic cytoplasm. Typical carcinoids have less than 2 mitoses per 10 high-power fields and absence of necrosis, whereas atypical carcinoids have between 2 and 10 mitoses per high-power field and foci of necrosis.

Q. Write briefly on metastatic tumours of the lung.

Ans. Metastatic tumours of lung have the following salient features:

- The lung is the most common site for metastases for both carcinomas and sarcomas. Local spread may occur from the oesophagus and mediastinum.
- Common sources of epithelial metastases include GIT, breast, thyroid, kidney, pancreas and liver.
- Other tumours which frequently metastasize to lungs include osteogenic sarcoma, melanoma, leukaemia-lymphomas, neuroblastoma and Wilms tumour.
- Metastasis usually presents as multiple nodules throughout the lung substance, more towards the periphery; when large, it is labelled canon ball metastasis. Rarely, it may present as a solitary nodule or pneumonic consolidation.

Q. Write briefly on mesotheliomas. (PA26.7)

Ans. Strong association with asbestos exposure. Usually occurs in elderly patients; median age, 63–70 years. Latent period between asbestos exposure and development of disease of 20–40 years, depending on severity and duration of exposure. Can occur in parietal, visceral, mediastinal or diaphragmatic pleura. Common inactivated tumour suppressors in malignant pleural mesothelioma are BAP1, neurofibromin 2 (NF2), CDKN2A.

Clinical Features

Shortness of breath, chest wall pain, pleurisy, cough, recurrent unilateral pleural effusion (serous to haemorrhagic).

Morphology

- Pleura thickened due to infiltration by neoplastic cells and desmoplastic stromal reaction.
- Malignant mesothelial cells are either epithelioid subtype or spindled (sarcomatoid/desmoplastic) subtype or a combination thereof (biphasic).
- Panel of at least two carcinoma markers – pCEA, TTF1, and two mesothelial markers – WT1, calretinin, CK5, CK5/6, D2-40) recommended for diagnosis.

Diseases of Oral Cavity and Gastrointestinal System

27

ORAL CAVITY

- The process of digestion starts in the oral cavity, which is the beginning of the gastrointestinal tract (GIT). It has many supporting structures, like the lips, teeth and tongue.
- Oral cavity has two main parts: the **outer portion** or, **the vestibule**, and an **inner mouth cavity**. The vestibule (space between the cheeks and the lips) is smaller than the oral cavity proper. The stratified squamous non-keratinised epithelium lining the oral mucosa changes to stratified squamous keratinised epithelium in the lips.
- The boundaries of the oral cavity include the alveolar arches and teeth (lateral and front), the pharynx (behind) and the palate (superiorly).
- The palate consists of two regions: the anterior two-third or bony part, called the **hard palate** and the posterior one-third or fibromuscular part, known as the **soft palate**. The palate is also lined by stratified squamous non-keratinised epithelium.
- The bones that are part of the oral cavity are the maxilla, mandible and the hard palate. The hard palate is formed by the palatine process of the maxilla and the maxillary process of the palatine bones.

Q. Write briefly on benign tumours and tumour-like lesions of oral cavity.

Ans. The oral cavity is a site for numerous benign tumours as well as tumour-like conditions.

- Common **'tumour-like lesions'** of the oral cavity include pyogenic granulomas, fibroepithelial polyps, fibrous epulis, denture hyperplasia and mucoceles.
- **Benign tumours** in the oral cavity may arise from the following:
  - Squamous epithelium
  - Mesenchymal tissue
  - Minor salivary glands
- The most common **benign epithelial neoplasm** is **squamous papilloma**. It is a small, cauliflower-like, sessile or pedunculated lesion having a central fibrovascular core covered by hyperplastic (acanthotic), stratified squamous epithelium. Most of these are viral in origin and show 'koilocytosis'. Koilocytes are defined as cells showing a hyperchromatic nucleus with irregular nuclear membrane surrounded by a clear zone. Other common epithelium-derived neoplasms in this location are **tumours of the minor salivary glands.**
- **Benign mesenchymal tumours** include **haemangioma, lymphangioma, fibroma, lipoma, neural tumours**, etc.
- **Granular cell tumour** (earlier called granular cell myoblastoma) is a mesenchymal tumour of the skin and mucosal surfaces. In the oral cavity, it is most commonly located in the dorsum of the tongue. The tumour comprises large polygonal cells, which have abundant granular cytoplasm containing cytoplasmic inclusions. The epithelium overlying the tumour may show pseudoepitheliomatous hyperplasia.

Q. Write briefly on precancerous lesions of oral cavity.

Ans. The most relevant precancerous lesions of oral cavity are **leukoplakia** and **erythroplakia**. Both are seen in adults (peak age 40–70 years) and both have a multifactorial origin. Tobacco consumption is the most important risk factor.

Leukoplakia

The term leukoplakia is defined by the World Health Organization (WHO) as, 'a well defined white patch/plaque that cannot be scraped off and cannot be characterized clinically or pathologically'. Approximately, 5%–25% of these lesions are premalignant. Thus, until proved otherwise by histological evaluation, all leukoplakic patches must be considered precancerous.

Differential Diagnosis of White Lesions in Oral Cavity

- Reactive epithelial hyperplasias (hyperorthokeratosis, parakeratosis and acanthosis).
- Leukoplakia of infective origin (candida, syphilis and hairy leukoplakia associated with Epstein–Barr virus).
- Lichen planus.
- Oral submucous fibrosis.
- Lupus erythematosus.
- Congenital lesions (e.g. white-sponge nevus, dyskeratosis congenita and pachyonychia congenita).
- Invasive carcinoma.

Morphology

- Leukoplakic patches are mostly seen on the cheek (buccal) mucosa, angles and floor of the mouth, tongue, palate and gingiva.
- They may be solitary or multiple, and are of variable size and shape.

- Microscopic examination shows varied histopathology ranging from hyperkeratosis and/or acanthosis without atypia to lesions with marked dysplasia, sometimes merging into carcinoma in situ or invasive carcinoma.

Erythroplakia

- Erythroplakia indicates a red patch that is difficult to categorise clinically as any established disease entity. It usually presents as, a well-defined, velvety, granular or nodular lesion in the soft palate, floor of mouth, ventral surface of the tongue and retromolar area.
- Erythroplakia almost always presents with superficial erosions; epidermal thickening is unusual.
- Histologically, these lesions are more aggressive compared with leukoplakic lesions and show changes varying from dysplasia, carcinoma in situ, to frankly invasive carcinoma. The red colour of the lesion is due to marked subepithelial inflammation and dilatation of submucosal vessels.

Q. Write briefly on e squamous cell carcinoma of the oral cavity. (PA24.1)

Ans. Squamous cell carcinomas (SCCs) comprise almost 95% of cancers of the head and neck (HNSCCs) and are most commonly located in the oral cavity.

Pathogenesis

- The pathogenesis of SCC is multifactorial; **tobacco products** (betel quid/pan containing areca nut, slaked lime and tobacco), **smoking** (cigarette, beedi, pipe, cheroot smoking), and **alcohol in excess** (can act as a co-carcinogen with tobacco or a promoter) are all implicated.
- Other risk factors include **inherited genomic instability, persistent irritation** (due to ill fitting dentures or jagged teeth), and **human papilloma virus** (HPV types 16, 18 and 33) **infection, radiation exposure, metal refining, diesel exhaust** and **asbestos exposure.**
- SCC evolves through a multistep process in which activation of oncogenes and inactivation of tumour suppressor genes are simultaneously ongoing. **Inactivation** of **p16** and **p53** genes leads to squamous hyperplasia and hyperkeratosis and is seen in almost 80% cases. **Amplification** and **over expression** of **Cyclin D1 gene** constitutively activates the cell cycle.

Morphology

- Oral SCC may present as an **ulcertive, verrucous** or **nodular plaque-like lesion**, often seen developing in a pre-existing leukoplakic or erythroplakic lesion.
- It usually begins as a dysplastic lesion, which progresses to carcinoma in situ and then invasive carcinoma.
- SCCs range from well-differentiated keratinizing neoplasms to poorly differentiated (Fig. 27.1), anaplastic, sometimes sarcomatoid tumours (spindle-cell variant of SCC).
- Local metastasis preferentially occurs in the cervical lymph nodes, while distant metastasis is most commonly noted in mediastinal lymph nodes, lungs, liver and bones.

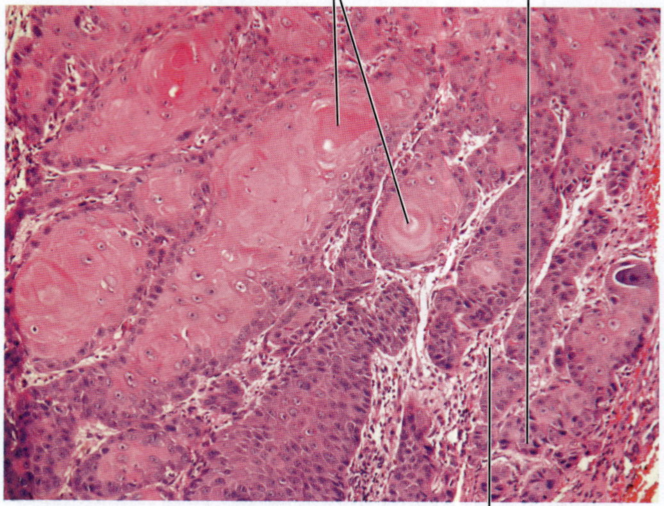

Fig. 27.1 Photomicrograph of a well differentiated squamous cell carcinoma showing keratin pearls and nests of dysplastic squamous cells infiltrating the underlying stroma (H&E; 100×).

Q. Write briefly on verrucous carcinoma of the oral cavity.

Ans. Also called **Ackerman tumour,** verrucous carcinoma is locally invasive, non-metastatic variant of SCC. It constitutes 5% of intraoral carcinomas and is associated with tobacco chewing, snuff dipping and HPV infection. Most common sites include buccal mucosa, gingiva, tongue, palate and tonsillar pillar.

Gross Morphology

- **Exophytic, warty or plaque-like lesion.**
- Granular, red-white, hyperkeratotic; usually 1–10 cm in maximum dimension.
- May invade adjacent soft tissue and bone.

Microscopy (Fig. 27.2)

- Well-differentiated hyperplastic squamous epithelium with orderly maturation showing upwards and downwards proliferation with keratin also in invaginations.
- Broad, blunt, downwards pushing rete pegs are seen.
- There is minimal atypia; mitotic activity is present; lymphoplasmacytic infiltrate may be seen in the underlying lamina propria.

SALIVARY GLANDS

- There are three major salivary glands—**parotid, submandibular** and **sublingual**—as well as innumerable minor salivary glands distributed throughout the mucosa of the oral cavity. All these glands are subject to inflammation or to development of neoplasms.
- Salivary glands are **compound exocrine glands** with **ductal** and **acinar** portions. The **acinar portion may be serous,**

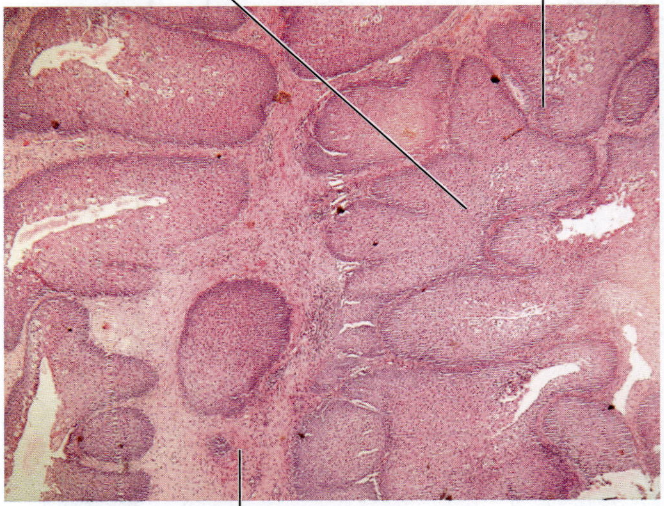

Fig. 27.2 Photomicrograph from verrucous carcinoma of the oral cavity showing well-differentiated hyperplastic squamous epithelium with orderly maturation showing upwards and downwards proliferation with keratin in invaginations (H&E; 100×).

mucinous or **mixed**; and, all **acini** are lined by **luminal cells**, which are enclosed by **myoepithelial cells**.

- Serous acini have dense, basophilic, Periodic acid–Schiff (PAS)-positive intracytoplasmic secretory granules containing amylase and a small central lumen.
- Mucous acini are larger than serous acini; have cells with abundant cytoplasm containing mucin, well-rounded basal nuclei and are arranged around empty lumina; produce acidic **mucins (positive for alcian blue and mucicarmine)** and **neutral mucins (positive for PAS)**.
- **Myoepithelial cells** surround acini and intercalated ducts and mediate contraction.
- **Ducts** are intercalated, striated or interlobular, all with outer basal cells and inner luminal cells. Intercalated ducts have reserve cells that regenerate acinar tissue and terminal duct system.

Q. Write briefly on salivary gland tumours.

Ans. Salivary gland tumours (SGTs) are relatively uncommon; they constitute only about 2% of all head and neck neoplasms. Nearly 80% of these tumours occur in the parotid glands, 15% in the submandibular glands and the remaining 5% in the sublingual and minor salivary glands. Benign neoplasms make up about 80% of parotid tumours, 50% of submandibular tumours and less than 40% of sublingual and minor salivary gland tumours.

Classification

Benign epithelial tumours

- Pleomorphic adenoma (mixed tumours)
- Myoepithelioma
- Adenoma (basal cell, canalicular, sebaceous, lymphadenoma and cystadenoma)
- Warthin tumour
- Oncocytoma
- Ductal papilloma

Malignant epithelial tumours

- Acinic cell carcinoma
- Mucoepidermoid carcinoma
- Adenoid cystic carcinoma
- Polymorphous adenocarcinoma
- Epithelial–myoepithelial carcinoma
- Basal-cell adenocarcinoma
- Salivary duct carcinoma
- Adenocarcinoma; not otherwise specified
- Myoepithelial carcinoma
- Carcinoma expleomorphic adenoma
- Carcinosarcoma
- Others

Pleomorphic Adenoma (Mixed-Parotid Tumour)

- Accounts for more than 90% of the benign tumours of salivary glands.
- Thought to originate from **epithelial/myoepithelial/ductal reserve cells.**.
- Called a **'mixed tumour'** as it shows an admixture of epithelial and stomal elements.
- The term **'pleomorphic'** indicates the variable cell types seen in this tumour.

Clinical Features

- Presents as painless swelling at angle of the jaw.
- Most common location is **superficial lobe of parotid** followed by the **submandibular gland**. It is rare in minor salivary glands.
- Most often diagnosed in the fourth to sixth decades of life, it is uncommon in children. Women are more frequently affected.

Gross Morphology

- Small, well-demarcated, round to bosselated/multilobulated lesion.
- Appears well encapsulated, but on close inspection shows finger-like extensions across the tumour capsule at multiple sites.
- They are typically solid, but cut surface has a variegated appearance; may be grey-white, myxoid, with blue, translucent pseudochondroid areas.

Microscopic Features (Fig. 27.3 A and B)

- Pleomorphic adenomas show both epithelial and mesenchymal differentiation.
- They can undergo secondary malignant change (**carcinoma ex-pleomorphic adenoma**). The secondary malignancy is usually an adenocarcinoma or an undifferentiated malignancy seen arising in the background of a benign pleomorphic adenoma.
- Epithelial component (ductal and myoepithelial cells) forms ducts, acini, tubules, strands or sheets. Ductal cells are cuboidal; myoepithelial cells are plasmacytoid, flattened or spindled.

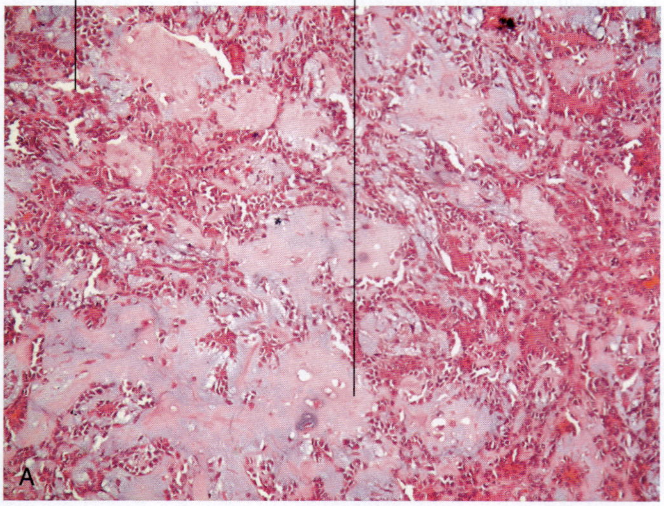

Fig. 27.3 (A) Pleomorphic adenoma showing epithelial and myoepithelial cells lying against a myxoid or pseudochondroid stroma (H&E; 100×).

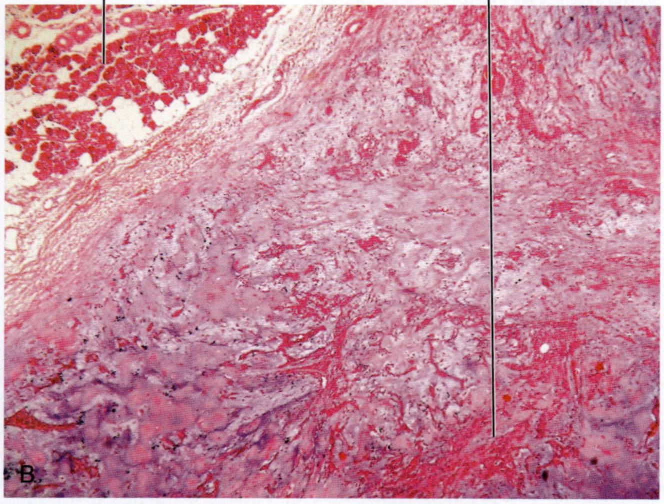

Fig. 27.3 (B) Photomicrograph from a pleomorphic adenoma showing both epithelial and mesenchymal elements. Epithelial components (ductal and myoepithelial cells) are seen forming ducts, acini, tubules, strands or sheets. Ductal cells are cuboidal; myoepithelial cells are flattened or spindled (H&E; 100×).

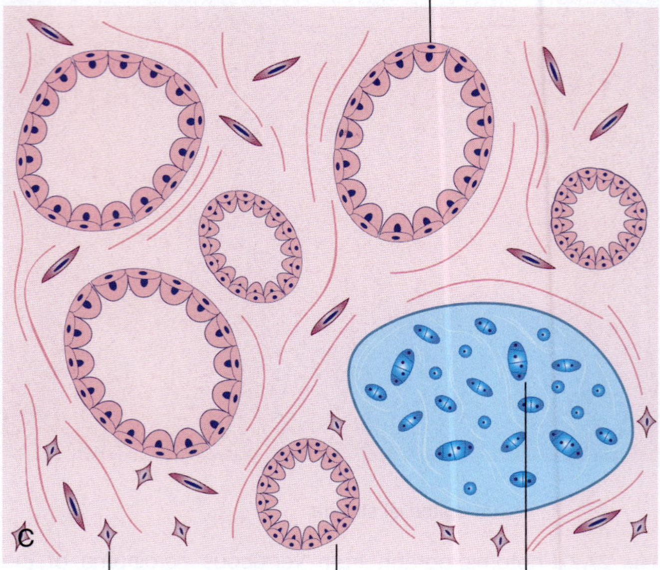

Fig. 27.3 (C) Schematic representation of pleomorphic adenoma.

- Background stroma may be mucoid, myxoid, pseudochondroid or hyaline (Fig. 27.3C).

Warthin Tumour

- Also called papillary cystadenoma lymphomatosum, it is a benign tumour seen exclusively in the parotid gland.
- Warthin is the second most frequent tumour seen in the salivary glands.
- Histogenesis is disputed, but it is thought to arise from heterotopic salivary tissue trapped in a regional lymph node during embryogenesis.

Clinical Features

- Usually affects males in the fifth to seventh decades of life.
- May be multicentric or bilateral.

Gross Morphology

- Arises in superficial parotid gland; is small, round-to-oval, lobulated and encapsulated.
- Mucin-containing narrow cysts or cleft (slit)-like spaces showing papillary projections may be seen on the cut surface.

Microscopic Features (Fig. 27.4A and B)

- Warthin tumour is a biphasic tumour showing epithelial and myoepithelial components, along with a lymphoid stroma.
- Epithelial components include:
  - Glandular or cystic structures lined by double-layer epithelium.
  - The inner cell layer is of columnar cells with abundant, finely granular cytoplasm (oncocytic cells).
  - The outer cell layer is cuboidal to polygonal.
  - Secretory cells are dispersed in inner layer of columnar cells.
  - Spindle-shaped or flattened cells constitute myoepithelial component.
- Lymphoid stroma is present under the epithelium in the form of lymphoid follicles, often with germinal centres.

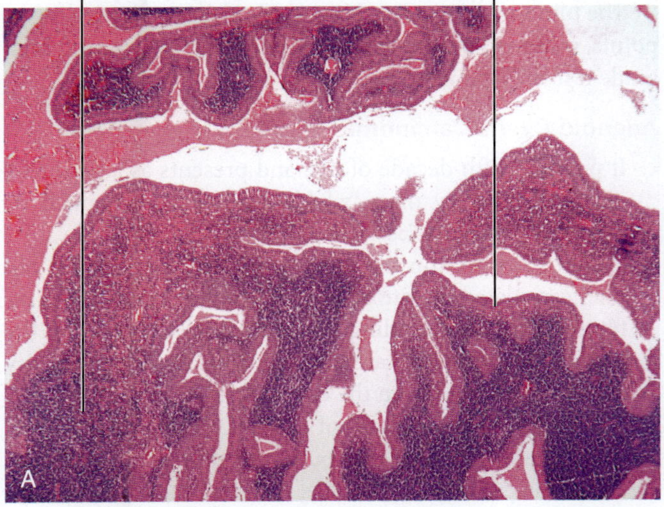

Fig. 27.4 (A) Section from Warthin tumour showing papillary structures lined by oncocytic cells (inner layer) and cuboidal cells (outer layer), lying in a lymphoid stroma (H&E; 40×).

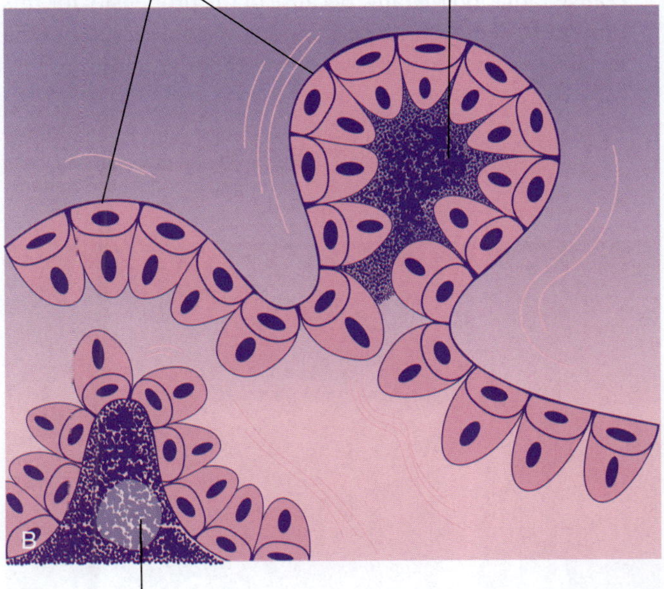

Fig. 27.4 (B) Schematic representation of Warthin tumour.

Monomorphic Adenoma

- This tumour is similar to pleomorphic adenoma, except it **does not contain a mesenchymal stromal component.**
- It is **more common in minor salivary glands** (e.g. upper lip), is bilateral in about 10% cases, and has a very rare malignant potential.
- **Types include:**
  - Basal-cell adenoma (most common)
  - Canicular adenoma
  - Clear-cell adenoma
  - Membranous adenoma
  - Glycogen-rich adenoma

Basal cell adenomas are well-encapsulated, smooth tumours on gross inspection, and are divided into four subtypes based on their microscopic appearance—solid, trabecular, tubular and membranous. The constituent tumour cells are monomorphic basaloid epithelial cells that show peripheral nuclear palisading, and have hyperchromatic, round nuclei and indistinct cytoplasm.

Mucoepidermoid Carcinoma (MEC)

MEC is the most common malignant tumour of the parotid gland and the second most common malignancy (adenoid cystic carcinoma is more common) of the submandibular and minor salivary glands.

Clinical Features

- Majority occur in parotid gland; some also in palate.
- Age range 15–86 years, no gender predominance.
- Low grade: 15% recur, 5 year survival 90%–98% (usually stage I).
- High grade: 25% recur, 5 year survival 50%–56%.

Gross Morphology

- On gross inspection, some MECs appear well circumscribed and may be partially encapsulated. Others are poorly defined and infiltrative.
- The cut surface of the tumour may contain solid areas, cystic areas or both. The cystic spaces contain viscous or mucoid material.

Microscopy (Fig. 27.5A and B)

- These tumours are characterised by presence of three populations of cells—**the mucous cells, intermediate cells** (are squamoid, smaller than regular squamous cells and

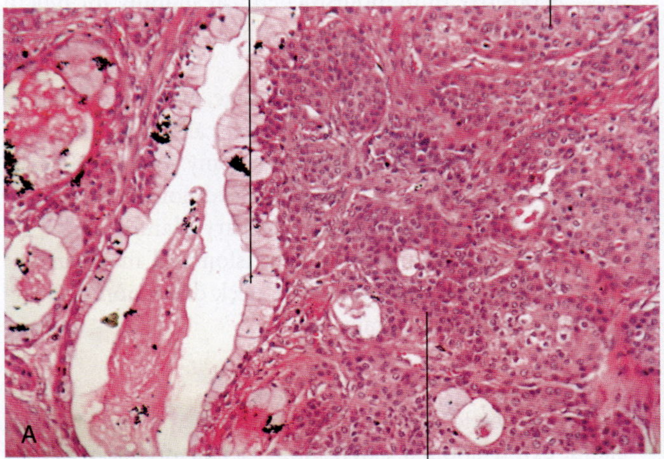

Fig. 27.5 (A) Intermediate grade mucoepidermoid carcinoma displaying both an epidermoid component and cystic spaces lined by mucous cells (H&E; 200×).

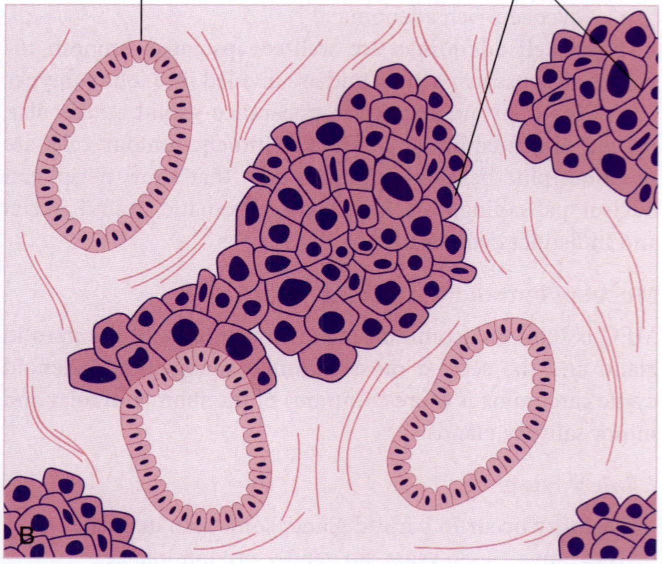

Fig. 27.5 (B) Schematic representation of mucoepidermoid carcinoma (high grade).

may show cytoplasmic mucin vacuoles) and **the epidermoid/squamous cells**, the proportion of mucous cells and epidermoid cells helps to define grade of the tumour. MEC may be low grade (well differentiated) or high grade (poorly differentiated).

- **Low-grade MEC** has prominent cystic structures and proportionally more mucous cells, which may form gland-like spaces and fewer epidermoid cells.
- **Intermediate-grade tumours** display fewer cysts and a substantial solid component. Although mucous cells are still present, there is an increasing proportion of epidermoid cells and occasional keratin pearl formation.
- The **high-grade carcinomas** are solid tumours comprised mainly of epidermoid cells that show prominent cellular atypia and mitoses. These tumours can be mistaken for an SCC. A positive immunohistochemical staining for mucin indicates a high-grade mucoepidermoid carcinoma, rather than an SCC.
- Therapy for MEC depends on the stage, grade and location of the tumour. Stages I and II disease can often be treated by surgical excision alone (parotidectomy with facial nerve preservation, submandibular gland excision or wide local excision of an involved minor salivary gland). Stages III and IV disease require radical excision and may warrant additional intervention such as a neck dissection or postoperative radiation therapy.

Prognostic Factors

- Poor prognostic factors: older age, male, submandibular gland, extraglandular extension, vascular invasion, necrosis, high-mitotic rate, high-histologic grade

  AFIP point system
- 2 points if <20% intracystic component
- 2 points if neural invasion
- 3 points if necrosis
- 3 points if 4+ mitotic figures/10 HPF
- 4 points if anaplasia

The tumour is considered low grade if the total score is 0–4 points, intermediate grade if the score is 5–6 points, and high grade if it is 7+ points.

Adenoid Cystic Carcinoma

- It peaks in fifth decade of life, and presents as a gradually enlarging salivary mass, which may be accompanied by pain and paraesthesias.
- On gross inspection the tumour appears well defined but unencapsulated. In late stages, the tumour can be seen infiltrating the surrounding normal tissue. Contrary to the name, these tumours are solid in consistency and rarely display cystic spaces on the cut surface.
- The tumour is composed of epithelial and myoepithelial cells variably arranged in tubular, cribriform and solid patterns. The cribriform pattern is the most common and easily recognisable. It is often referred to as 'Swiss-cheese' pattern. Tumour cells are arranged in nests around cylindrical spaces that may contain a mucinous or hyalinised material. Cells that are arranged in layers and form ductal structures characterise tubular pattern. The solid pattern contains sheets of tumour cells with no intervening spaces (Fig. 27.6).
- Current treatment recommendations for adenoid cystic carcinoma include complete surgical resection and postoperative radiation therapy. Because of the propensity for this tumour to demonstrate perineural invasion, sacrifice of the facial nerve may be necessary for tumour eradication.

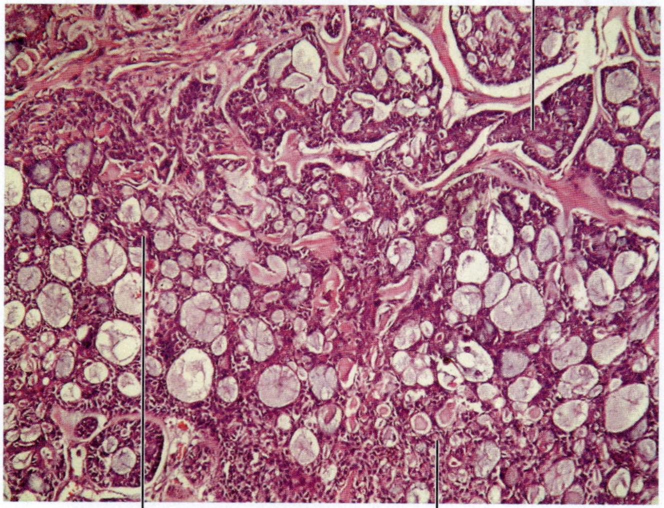

Fig. 27.6 Adenoid cystic carcinoma showing tumour cells arranged in a cribriform pattern around cylindrical spaces that contain mucinous material (H&E; 200×).

Acinic Cell Carcinoma

- Acinic cell carcinoma is a rare tumour that accounts for about 1% of all salivary neoplasms.
- It typically presents in the fifth decade of life, and is more common in women. Bilateral parotid disease occurs in approximately 3% of cases.
- Most common presentation is that of an asymptomatic enlarging mass.
- Gross appearance demonstrates a mass that is well circumscribed but lacks a true capsule.
- Acinic cell carcinoma is a malignant neoplasm demonstrating serous acinar cell differentiation. Acinar cells are large, polygonal with lightly basophilic, granular cytoplasm and round, eccentric nucleus. The cytoplasmic zymogen secretory granules are PAS-positive, resistant to diastase digestion and non-reactive or only weakly reactive to mucicarmine stain.
- This tumour is generally regarded as a low-grade malignancy. Treatment is surgical excision.

Adenocarcinoma

- Adenocarcinomas of the salivary glands are rare but aggressive tumours.
- They are most common in the parotid followed by the minor salivary glands.
- Microscopically there is formation of glandular structures, and based on the degree of differentiation they are described as grades I, II or III tumours. Grade I lesions have well-formed ductal structures, while Grade III lesions have a more solid growth pattern with few glandular characteristics.
- Treatment for adenocarcinoma is aggressive. Complete local excision with facial nerve sacrifice, partial resection of the maxilla or mandible, postoperative radiation therapy and neck dissection is warranted in most cases.

Malignant Mixed Tumours (MMT)

- Carcinoma expleomorphic adenoma is the most common MMT. It occurs when a carcinoma develops from the epithelial component of a pre-existing pleomorphic adenoma. The other two tumours in this category, carcinosarcoma and metastasizing mixed tumour, are much less common.
- In a carcinosarcoma, the metastatic lesions contain both the stromal and epithelial elements. This is different from the carcinoma expleomorphic adenoma in which only the epithelial elements are present in metastasis. The metastasizing mixed tumour refers to an otherwise benign pleomorphic adenoma that develops metastatic deposits of tumour.
- Microscopically, carcinoma expleomorphic adenoma most often is an undifferentiated carcinoma (30%) or adenocarcinoma (25%). This tumour tends to be more aggressive than other salivary malignancies.

OESOPHAGUS

Adult oesophagus is 24–30 cm in length from cricoid to oesophagogastric junction and 38–40 cm from dental incisors. For the purpose of classification, staging and reporting of oesophageal carcinoma, oesophagus is divided into four segments, namely:

(a) **Cervical:** Cricoid to thoracic inlet.
(b) **Upper thoracic segment:** Thoracic inlet to tracheal bifurcation.
(c) **Mid-thoracic segment:** Tracheal bifurcation to 8th cervical vertebra.
(d) **Lower thoracic segment:** 8th cervical vertebra to the stomach.

Histology

- Oesophageal mucosa is lined by non-keratinized stratified squamous epithelium.
- Lamina propria is composed of connective tissue.
- Muscularis mucosae is thicker than in the other parts of GIT.
- Mucous glands are present in the uppermost and lowermost regions; glands in the lowermost region resemble cardiac glands of the stomach.
- Submucosa is composed of branched tubular mucous glands throughout.
- Muscularis externa is composed variably of:
  - Striated muscle (forms pharyngoesophageal sphincter) in the upper one-third.
  - Has both smooth and striated muscles in the middle one-third.
  - Smooth muscle in the lower one-third [forms lower oesophageal sphincter (LES) lower one-third].
  - Muscularis externa has two layers—outer longitudinal and inner circular.
- Adventitia has connective tissue blending with the surrounding tissue.

Q. Write briefly on achalasia cardia.

Ans. Achalasia cardia is caused by a **failure of relaxation of LES** and has the following features:

- **Complete absence of peristalsis** and **elevation of resting LES pressure** or **low amplitude non-peristaltic contractions**
- Increased intraoesophageal pressure.
- Functional obstruction of oesophagus with a dilated fluid and food-filled proximal portion.

Age

20–40 years.

Symptoms

Progressive dysphagia for solids and liquids, regurgitation, chest pain and weight loss.

Aetiology

- **Primary achalasia:** Aetiology unknown (may be neuronal rather than a myopathic disorder). Number of ganglion cells have been found to be decreased in Auerbach's plexus (ganglion cell degeneration).
- **Secondary forms:** Typically seen in Chagas disease (Trypanosoma cruzi infection), polio, diabetic autonomic

neuropathy, infiltrative disorders, for example malignancy, amyloidosis and sarcoidosis. Coexistence with other autoimmune diseases like Sjogren syndrome or thyroiditis indicates that there may be immune-mediated destruction of inhibitory oesophageal neurons.

Pathology

Oesophageal wall is thickened in the distal portion (there is smooth muscle hypertrophy, particularly of inner circular layer); proximal dilated segment is actually thinned out.

Q. Write briefly on gastroesophageal reflux disease (GERD).

Ans. GERD is a chronic diffuse erosive/ulcerative oesophagitis. Normally, the oesophageal lining is protected from acids by:

1. The abundant submucosal glands in proximal and distal oesophagus (which secrete mucin and bicarbonate).
2. The tone of LES which prevents reflux of acidic gastric contents.

Pathogenesis

Both genetic and environmental factors contribute to cause decreased LES pressure which allows reflux.

Predisposing Factors

Pregnancy, ascites, obesity, delayed gastric emptying and peristaltic disorders, for example scleroderma.

Clinical Features

Heartburn, regurgitation, dysphagia/odynophagia, water brash (hypersalivation) and a typical intermittent chest pain.

Complications

Ulceration, haematemesis, melena, stricture formation and Barrett oesophagus.

Diagnosis

X-ray and endoscopy.

Pathology

- One-third patients have a normal appearing mucosa. Erythema and red streaks are earliest markers of disease followed by erosions and ulcers.
- There may be contact bleeding with endoscope indicating increased friability.
- Dilated vessels and inflammatory cells are present.
- Predominance of eosinophils points to a diagnosis of **'eosinophilic esophagitis'** which is seen in patients with atopy with coexisting atopic dermatitis, rhinitis, asthma and eosinophilia. These patients present with dysphagia and symptoms of food impaction.

Q. Write briefly on Barrett's oesophagus.

Ans. Barrett's oesophagus is a complication of long-standing GE reflux. It is seen between 40 and 60 years of age; males are more commonly affected than females. Hallmark is replacement of distal squamous mucosa by metaplastic columnar epithelium as a response to prolonged injury.

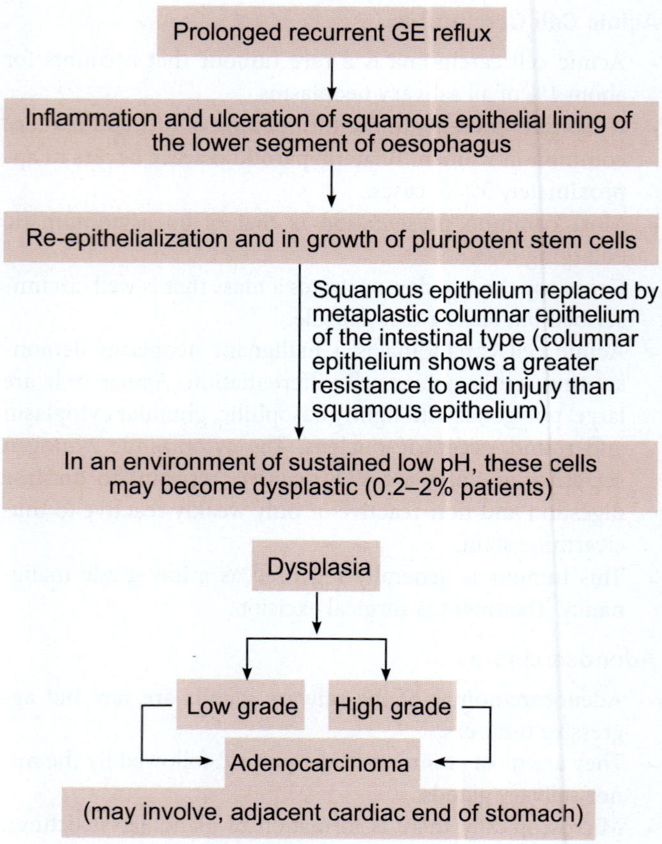

Flowchart 27.1 Pathogenesis and consequences of Barrett's oesophagus.

Pathogenesis (See Flowchart 27.1)

Gross Morphology

Red and velvety mucosa with raised patches, which later form large nodular masses with infiltrative or ulcerative features.

Microscopy

- Normal distal squamous mucosa is replaced by metaplastic columnar epithelium. Goblet cells are seen and are a must for diagnosis).
- Low- or high-grade dysplasia can be seen in the metaplastic epithelium.
- Most important complication is the development of adenocarcinoma (30–40 folds increased risk).
- Most tumours are mucin-producing glandular tumours.
- Occasional development of SCC, adenosquamous or adenocarcinoid tumours supports the concept that Barrett's epithelium arises from pluripotent cells.

Q. Write briefly on carcinoma oesophagus.

Ans. Age group affected in carcinoma oesophagus is more than 50 years; males are more commonly affected than females.

Predisposing Conditions/Factors

1. **Adenocarcinoma:** Incidence is on the rise in Western countries due to **rampant obesity** which in turn is responsible for increasing the incidence of GERD and Barrett mucosa. Other predisposing factors include **tobacco**

use and **prior radiation**. Adenocarcinoma in Barrett's oesophagus arises consequent to certain genetic and epigenetic changes. Genetic changes include mutation or **over expression of p53, amplification of ERBB 2** and **Cyclin genes**. The main epigenetic change is **hypermethylation of p16/INK4a**.

2. **Squamous cell carcinoma:** Most common type worldwide. Predisposing factors include:
   (a) Achalasia
   (b) Plummer–Vinson syndrome
   (c) Strictures, diverticulae and webs
   (d) Alcohol, hot and spicy foods, betel chewing, smoking, aflatoxins and silica
   (e) Diet deficient in vitamins A, C and trace elements
   (f) Diet high in nitrosamines

Clinical Features

Dysphagia/odynophagia, weight loss, iron deficiency, haemorrhage and sepsis from the tumour, chest pain and vomiting.

Gross Morphology

60% polypoidal (fungating) lesions, 25% ulcerative and 15% diffuse infiltrating lesions.

Microscopy

- Majority are SCCs which involve the upper thoracic segment (half occurring in middle third of oesophagus).
- May be superficial (carcinoma limited to mucosa and submucosa) or advanced (infiltrating into muscularis propria). Superficial lesions have a much better prognosis.
- Adenocarcinomas and undifferentiated carcinomas are less common.
- Adenocarcinomas usually arise in oesophageal mucous glands or Barrett's oesophagus and are of the intestinal type.
- Visceral metastasis to liver, lung and kidney is early and frequent.
- Overall prognosis is very poor.

STOMACH

Stomach is a saccular organ with a volume of about 1.5 L. It is divided into five anatomic regions, each of which has different histology and functions. These are:

1. Cardia: Where the contents of the oesophagus empty into the stomach.
2. Fundus: Formed by the upper curvature of the organ.
3. Body: Main central dome-shaped part.
4. Pylorus: Lower part, which empties the contents of stomach into the small intestine.
5. Pyloric sphincter: Stomach demarcated from the duodenum by this muscular sphincter.

Layers of Stomach

- Mucosa: Consists of epithelium, lamina propria and a thin layer of smooth muscle labelled muscularis mucosae.
- Submucosa: Consists of fibrous connective tissue with the Meissner's plexus.

Table 27.1 Cells found in different layers of the deeper glandular component of gastric mucosa

Name	Secretory product	Location in stomach
Mucous cells	Mucous and pepsinogen II	Cardiac and pyloric regions
Brightly eosinophilic parietal (oxyntic) cells	Acid and intrinsic factor	Fundic, cardiac and pyloric regions
Basophilic chief (zymogenic cells)	Pepsinogen I and II	Fundic region
Endocrine (APUD) cells	Gastrin, histamine, endorphins, serotonin, cholecystokinin and somatostatin	Fundic, cardiac and pyloric regions

- Muscularis externa: Three layers of smooth muscle, namely:
  - Inner oblique layer
  - Middle circular layer
  - Outer longitudinal layerAuerbach's plexus is found between the outer longitudinal layer and middle circular layer.

Normal gastric mucosa has two compartments:

1. Superficial foveolar, which is uniform throughout the stomach.
2. Deeper glandular compartment which has different types of cells found in the different layers of these glands (Table 27.1; Fig. 27.7).

Q. Classify gastritis.

Ans. Gastritis is classified based on:

1. **The inflammatory cell type and duration:**
   (a) Acute gastritis (infiltration by neutrophils).

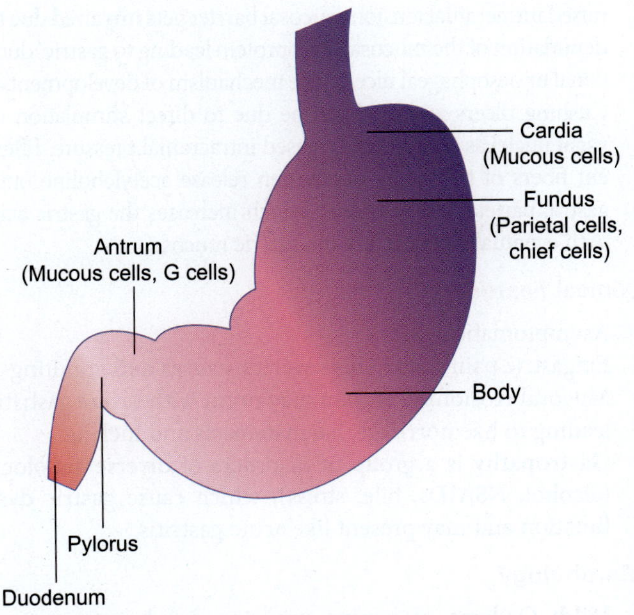

Fig. 27.7 Parts of stomach and their lining cells.

(b) Chronic gastritis (infiltration by lymphocytes and plasma cells).
   (i) *Helicobacter pylori–induced gastritis*
   (ii) Autoimmune gastritis
   (iii) Others

2. **The region involved**
   (a) Antral gastritis
   (b) Corpus gastritis
   (c) Pan gastritis
3. **The presence of premalignant changes**
   (a) Non-atrophic gastritis
   (b) Atrophic gastritis (may progress to carcinoma)

Q. Describe the aetiology, morphology and clinical presentation of acute gastritis.

Ans. Acute transient inflammation of gastric mucosa is labelled acute gastritis.

Aetiology

Acute gastritis occurs when there is a dominance of damaging factors or breakdown of gastroduodenal defence mechanisms. Causes include:

1. Drugs (aspirin, NSAIDs, oral iron therapy) - Reduce prostaglandin and bicarbonate secretion, both of which have a protective effect.
2. Alcohol, smoking, chemotherapy, irradiation, mechanical trauma (nasogastric tube), chemicals, bile reflux - Direct cellular injury to gastric epithelium and inadequate cellular regeneration.
3. Uraemia and infection with urease secreting *H. pylori* - Inhibit gastric bicarbonate transporters.
4. Burns and severe stress (**Curling ulcers**) - Reduced plasma volume in burns leads to ischaemia and cell necrosis (sloughing) of the gastric mucosa. Increased secretion of gastric acid in response to higher secretion of gastrin hormone in patients is thought to be responsible for stress ulceration.
5. Intracranial disease (**Cushing ulcers**) - In severe trauma and raised intracranial tension mucosal barrier gets impaired due to denudation of the mucosal glycoprotein leading to gastric, duodenal or oesophageal ulcers. The mechanism of development of Cushing ulcers is thought to be due to direct stimulation of vagal nuclei as a result of increased intracranial pressure. Efferent fibers of the vagus nerve then release acetylcholine onto gastric parietal cell receptors, which increases the gastric acid with eventual ulceration of the gastric mucosa.

Clinical Features

- Asymptomatic
- Epigastric pain of variable severity, nausea and vomiting
- Mucosal erosion/ulceration may occur with severe gastritis leading to haemorrhage, haematemesis and melena
- **Gastropathy** is a group of disorders of diverse aetiology (alcohol, NSAIDs, bile, stress), which cause gastric dysfunction and may present like acute gastritis.

Morphology

- **Mild:** Oedema of lamina propria, vascular congestion, scattered neutrophils, with intact mucosa.
- **Moderate/severe:** Mucosal erosion/ulceration may occur with severe gastritis leading to haemorrhage **(acute erosive gastritis)**. The lumen shows acute inflammatory infiltrate and a fibrino-purulent exudate. Neighbouring epithelium may show regenerative changes. Foveolar cell hyperplasia with characteristic corkscrew appearance is often seen along with epithelial hyperplasia. Presence of neutrophils in direct contact with epithelial cells above the basement membrane anywhere in GIT is indicative of active inflammation.

Q. Describe the aetiology, morphology and complications of chronic gastritis.

Ans. Chronic inflammation of gastric mucosa and submucosa results in mucosal atrophy, epithelial metaplasia, dysplasia and predisposition to development of carcinoma without accompanying mucosal erosion.

Aetiology

- ***H. pylori* infection**
  - *H. pylori* is a gastric pathogen that has a strong causal association with gastritis and peptic ulcer disease.
  - It is a **Gram-negative, non-invasive, non-sporing rod-shaped bacteria usually found in the mucin of the surface and neck region of foveolar cells.**
  - *H. pylori* attaches to the niche provided by gastric mucus by **flagella**, has **urease** to buffer gastric acid, and **adhesin** to bind to gastric epithelial cells (better binding with cells that express type O antigen).
  - Urease releases ammonia from endogenous urea, which raises the gastric pH. Raised gastric pH increases the bacterial survival as well as acts on gastrin releasing G cells to release gastrin causing hypergastrinaemia.
  - **Mode of spread** is **oro-oral** and **faeco-oral**.
  - **Predisposing factors** include **poverty** and **overcrowding**.
  - *H. pylori* can be demonstrated in 90% patients with chronic gastritis of the pyloric antrum.
  - Chronic infection is seen in approximately 2/3 of the population worldwide, prevalence is decreasing due to improved sanitation and antibiotic use.
  - Acute infection is usually asymptomatic. Symptoms are generally associated with chronic gastritis.
  - Acid secretion may be normal or increased.
  - *H. pylori* mediated gastritis is the result of **combined influence of bacterial enzymes and toxins with release of toxic chemicals from recruited neutrophils.** It has two types of cytotoxic genes, namely, **Cytotoxin associated gene A (cagA)** and **vacuolating agent (vac A)**. There is an association between an infection with a cag positive H. pylori strain and the development of gastric carcinoma. VacA cytotoxin, responsible for epithelial cell damage, is also associated with gastric carcinogenesis.
  - *H. pylori* does not invade tissue under normal circumstances and instead induces release of **pro-inflammatory cytokines like IL-1 beta and tumour necrosis factor** by intestinal mucosal cells. This activates neutrophils and macrophages and impairs the mucosal defence leading to epithelial damage.

- On **gross examination** the mucosa appears red, coarser than normal, and may have thickened rugal folds or thin/flat mucosa in the late stages.
- On **microscopic examination** intraepithelial neutrophils with subepithelial plasma cells are seen. Pit abscesses (accumulation of neutrophils at the bottom of the pits) may be seen.
- **Patterns of inflammation** include non-atrophic antral predominant gastritis, non-atrophic corpus predominant gastritis (associated with proton pump inhibitor use), non-atrophic pangastritis and multifocal atrophic gastritis (with advancing time).
- **Multifocal atrophic gastritis** is characterised by patchy mucosal atrophy, reduced chief and parietal cell mass and acid secretion, and intestinal metaplasia. This type has a greater risk of developing adenocarcinoma.
- Lymphoid aggregates may form with or without germinal centres (induction of mucosa associated lymphoid tissue or MALT). Presence of follicles is strongly associated with *H. pylori*, the density of follicles is highest in the angulus, the most common site of gastric lymphoma.
- **Chronic infection with this pathogen is known to be associated with gastric adenocarcinoma (intestinal type) and low-grade gastric lymphoma.**
- **Diagnosis of *H. pylori* includes non-invasive and invasive tests:**
  - **Non-invasive tests**
    - Laboratory serologic assays for antibodies to *H. pylori* have a sensitivity and specificity of >85% and previously were considered the non-invasive tests of choice for initial documentation of *H. pylori* infection.
    - However, these tests are associated with a high rate of false-positive results. As a result, urea breath testing and stool antigen testing are preferred for initial diagnosis.
    - **Urea breath tests** use an oral dose of ^{13}C- or ^{14}C-labelled urea. In an infected patient, the organism metabolises the urea and liberates labelled CO_2, which is exhaled and can be quantified in breath samples taken 20–30 min after ingestion of the urea. Sensitivity and specificity are >95%. Urea breath tests are well suited for confirming eradication of the organism after therapy. False-negative results are possible with recent antibiotic use or concomitant proton pump inhibitor therapy.
    - **Stool antigen assays** seem to have a sensitivity and specificity near that of urea breath tests, particularly for initial diagnosis.
  - **Invasive tests**
    - Modified Giemsa, Silver stains (Warthin-Starry) and Immunohistochemistry (IHC) can be used to demonstrate *H. pylori* in a gastric biopsy (gold standard).
    - Bacterial culture or DNA detection by PCR can also be done.

- **Autoimmunity:** Presence of autoantibodies, to gastric parietal cells, mainly to the acid-producing enzyme H^+/K^+-ATPase leading to loss of both acid-producing and intrinsic factor-producing cells. The gastric corpus (body) undergoes progressive atrophy. Its sequelae include development of pernicious anaemia, adenocarcinoma and gastric carcinoid.
- **Toxic substances:** Alcohol intake and tobacco smoking.
- **Iatrogenic causes:** Postsurgical (antrectomy and gastroenterostomy).
- **Radiation exposure**: Radiation-induced gastritis is an infrequent cause of gastrointestinal bleeding.
- **Infectious granulomatous gastritis:** Granulomatous gastritis is a rare entity caused by organisms like *M. tuberculosis* and fungi usually in patients who are immunosuppressed.
- **Chronic reactive chemical gastropathy:** Gastritis may result from long-term intake of aspirin or NSAIDs. It also develops when bile-containing intestinal contents reflux into the stomach.
- **Others:** Amyloidosis and graft versus host reactions.

Gross Morphology

Mucosa reddened, coarse with thick rugal folds in early, and thinned with flattened rugal folds in long-standing disease.

Microscopic Features

- Lamina propria is infiltrated by chronic inflammatory infiltrate composed of lymphocytes and plasma cells. (Fig. 27.8).
- Intestinal metaplasia is frequently seen.
- In long-standing disease due to *H. pylori* as well as autoimmune gastritis, there is loss or atrophy of parietal cells, leading to hypochlorhydria or achlorhydria.
- This, in turn, may induce G-cell hyperplasia and hypergastrinaemia.
- *H. pylori,* if present, lies in the superficial mucosal layer among the microvilli of epithelial cells.
- Occasionally, dysplasia may develop.

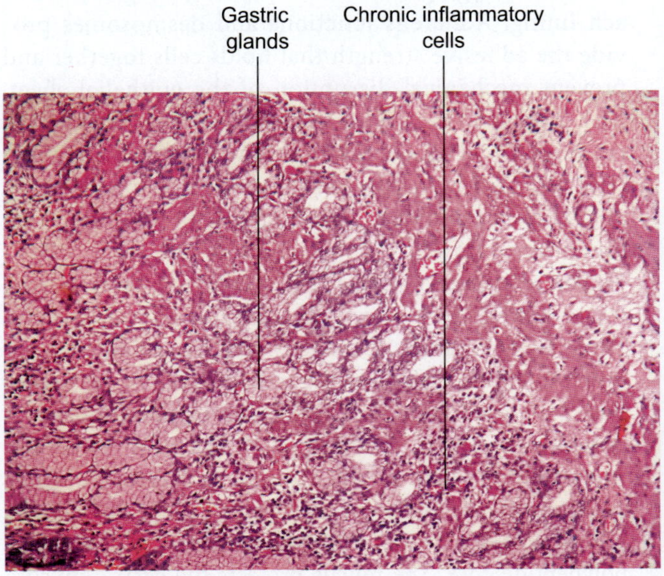

Fig. 27.8 Gastric mucosa showing chronic non-specific inflammation (H&E; 200×).

Clinical Features

- Nausea, vomiting and upper abdominal discomfort.
- ***Mild form***: Hypochlorhydria (not achlorhydria), pernicious anaemia absent and serum gastrin level normal or slightly increased.
- ***Severe form***: Achlorhydria, pernicious anaemia and hypergastrinaemia.

Complications

Peptic ulcer, mucosal atrophy, intestinal metaplasia, dysplasia and gastric carcinoma.

Q. Write briefly on the aetiology, pathology and complications of peptic ulcer. (PA24.2)

Ans. Peptic ulcer is a chronic (remitting and relapsing), often solitary lesion, present in any part of GIT that is exposed to acid and peptic juices; usually, diagnosed in middle to old age.

Sites (in Decreasing Order)

- First portion of duodenum (anterior or posterior wall within a few cos of the pyloric valve).
- Antral region of stomach (98% of the peptic ulcers present in duodenum or stomach; ratio of duodenal and gastric ulcers is about 4:1).
- Gastroesophageal junction.
- Margins of gastrojejunostomy.
- Duodenum, stomach and jejunum in Zollinger–Ellison syndrome.
- Meckel's diverticulum.

Pathogenesis

The gastric mucosal barrier consists of three protective components:

- **A compact epithelial cell lining:** Cells in the epithelium of the stomach are bound by tight junctions that prevent damaging substances from injuring the stomach lining. Adherens junctions and desmosomes provide the adhesive strength that holds cells together and prevent mechanical disruption of the epithelial sheet. Any damage to the gastric epithelial cells is restituted in the presence of adequate blood flow and an alkaline pH. Growth factors and prostaglandins contribute to epithelial regeneration. Prostaglandins also maintain the mucosal flow.
- **Mucus covering:** A special mucus covering, derived from mucus secreted by surface epithelial cells and foveolar cells. This insoluble mucus forms a protective gel-like coating over the entire surface of the gastric mucosa. It is composed of more than 95% water, the organization being provided by long interacting glycoprotein molecules (mucus glycoprotein or mucin). These molecules are largely made up of carbohydrate which is present in large numbers of relatively small oligosaccharide units packed around the polypeptide core. The mucus protects the gastric mucosa from auto-digestion by pepsin and from erosion by acids and other caustic materials that are ingested.
- **Bicarbonate ions** - Secreted by the surface epithelial cells, the bicarbonate ions act to neutralise harsh acids.
- **Rich mucosal blood flow** - This maintains the epithelial barrier providing nutrients, and oxygen, and by removing the toxic metabolites. It also provides bicarbonate ions which neutralises the acid secreted by parietal cells.

Peptic ulcer results whenever defence mechanisms of stomach are impaired and/or damaging factors become predominant.

Gastroduodenal Defence Mechanisms

- Mucous layer on surface
- Bicarbonate secretion into mucosa
- Adequate mucosal blood flow
- Apical surface membrane transport
- Epithelial regenerative capacity
- Prostaglandin secretion

Damaging Factors

Gastric acid and peptic enzyme secretion is aggravated by:

- NSAIDs like aspirin (direct mucosal irritation and reduction in prostaglandin and bicarbonate secretion).
- Cigarette smoking and alcohol (evidence that tobacco use is a risk factor for duodenal ulcers is not conclusive, however, cigarette smoking is known to impair blood flow and healing capacity of the mucosa and accelerate gastric emptying. Also, *H pylori* infiltration is denser in the gastric antrum of smokers).
- Ischaemia and shock (decreased oxygen delivery).
- Iron preparations (direct mucosal damage).
- Viral infections (direct mucosal damage).
- Ageing (reduced mucin and bicarbonate secretion).
- Urease secreting *H. pylori* and gastric injury associated with uraemia (inhibition of gastric bicarbonate transporters by ammonium ions).
- Chemotherapy and chemicals (direct mucosal injury).
- Duodenal-gastric reflux, psychological stress and hyperkalaemia.

Role of H. pylori in Peptic Ulceration

- It secretes **urease, protease** and **phospholipase**.
  - Urease generates free ammonia that binds with H^+ and decreases acidity; thus, colonisation and survival of the organism is favoured.
  - Proteases damage the glycoprotein of gastric mucous.
  - Phospholipases damage surface epithelial cells and also release leukotrienes and eicosanoids.
- *H. pylori* increases production of proinflammatory cytokines, for example IL-1, IL-6, TNF and IL-8 (chemotactic to neutrophils).
- May cause thrombotic occlusion causing ischaemia.
- Epithelial injury is induced by VacA (a vacuolating toxin) regulated by CagA (cytotoxin- associated gene).

H. pylori **is associated with duodenal ulcer in 80%–90% patients and gastric ulcer in 60% patients.** Virulence of the infecting strain determines development of peptic ulcer in an individual infected with *H. pylori*.

Clinical Features

Approximately, 70% of peptic ulcers are asymptomatic. Patients with silent peptic ulcers may later present with ulcer related complications. Between 43% and 87% of patients with bleeding peptic ulcers present without antecedent dyspepsia or other heralding gastrointestinal symptoms.

- **Dyspepsia** or upper abdominal pain or discomfort is the most prominent symptom in patients with peptic ulcers. Approximately 80% of patients with endoscopically diagnosed ulcers have epigastric pain. Occasionally, the discomfort localises to the right or left upper quadrants of the hypochondrium. Radiation of pain to the back may occur. Burning, a feeling of fullness, bloating or belching and chest discomfort may accompany the pain.
- **Haematemesis or melena** resulting from gastrointestinal bleeding.
- Rarely, a briskly bleeding ulcer can present as **haematochezia**.
- Symptoms consistent with **anaemia** (e.g. fatigue, dyspnea) may be present.
- Sudden onset of symptoms may indicate **perforation**.
- NSAID-induced gastritis or ulcers may be silent, especially in elderly patients.

Alarming features that warrant prompt gastroenterology referral include the following:

- Bleeding or anaemia.
- Early satiety.
- Unexplained weight loss.
- Progressive dysphagia or odynophagia.
- Recurrent vomiting.
- Family history of gastrointestinal cancer.

Nearly three-quarters of people with peptic ulcers don't have symptoms. Less often, ulcers may cause more severe signs or symptoms such as difficulty in breathing and unexplained weight loss.

Gross Morphology

- Small, round-to-oval, sharply punched-out ulcers, varying in size between 2 and 4 cm.
- Usually, solitary with a straight wall, and overhanging mucosa (mucosa may overhang the base).
- Gastric mucosal folds can be traced up to the margin of the ulcer in a benign ulcer. The radiating folds of mucosa from the ulcer appear like spokes of a wheel.
- Base—clean and smooth (due to peptic digestion).

Microscopic Features (PA24.3)

In an active ulcer, four distinct zones are appreciated (**Askanazy zones**; Fig. 27.9A and B):

1. Zone of fibrinoid necrosis.
2. Zone of non-specific inflammatory infiltrate (predominantly neutrophils).
3. Zone of granulation tissue (proliferating blood vessels, fibroblasts and mononuclear cells).
4. Zone of fibrosis (collagenous or fibrous scar formation).

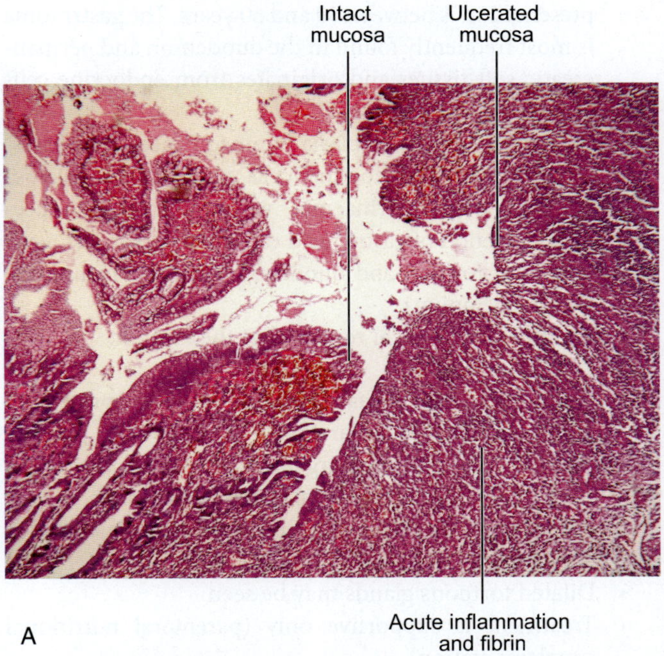

Fig. 27.9 (A) Section shows both intact (*left*) and ulcerated mucosa (*right*). The superficial layer of the ulcer is represented by acute inflammation and fibrin and the base shows inflammatory granulation tissue (H&E; 100×).

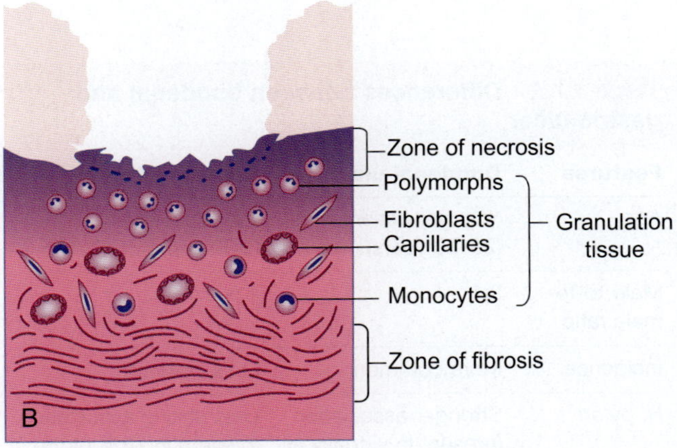

Fig. 27.9 (B) Schematic diagram showing an active gastric ulcer with four Askanazy zones.

Complications

- ***Bleeding***: Most frequent complication (seen in 15%–20% of the patients); may be life threatening, and sometimes, is the first indication of presence of peptic ulcer.
- ***Perforation***: Life-threatening late presentation (responsible for two-third of the deaths due to ulcers); may result in acute peritonitis and subphrenic abscess; may involve adjacent organs.
- ***Gastric outlet obstruction:*** Occurs due to oedema or scarring.

Q. Write briefly on hypertrophic gastropathies.

Ans. Hypertrophic gastropathies include:

1. **Zollinger–Ellison (ZE) syndrome:**
   - This syndrome presents with hypergastrinaemia due to a gastrinoma (gastrin-producing tumour); usual age of

presentation is between 50 and 60 years. The gastrinoma is most frequently found in the duodenum and peripancreatic soft tissues and originates from endocrine cells of both gut and pancreas.

- Gastrin induces hyperplasia of mucous neck cells (causing diarrhoea), endocrine cells and oxyntic mucosa (causing hypergastrinaemia which in turn induces hypersecretion of gastric acid causing ulcers in the usual sites like stomach and duodenum and also in unusual sites like jejunum).
- Treatment is surgical resection of the tumour.

2. **Menetrier disease**
   - Patient aged 30–60 years presents with hypoproteinaemia, weight loss and diarrhoea.
   - There is cerebriform enlargement or hypertrophy of the rugal folds due to epithelial hyperplasia which mainly affects mucous cells in the body and fundus. This is attributed to increased TGF-alfa.
   - Dilated tortuous glands may be seen.
   - Treatment is supportive only (parenteral nutritional supplementation).

Q. Differentiate between duodenal and gastric ulcer.

Ans. Differences between duodenal and gastric ulcer are listed in Table 27.2.

Table 27.2 Differences between duodenal and gastric ulcer

Features	Duodenal ulcer	Gastric ulcer
Age	Younger patients (20–50 years)	Older patients (>60 years)
Male-to-female ratio	3:1	1.5–2:1
Incidence	More common	Less common
H. pylori	Stronger association (present in virtually all patients of duodenal ulcer); hypersecretion of acid pepsin is important in pathogenesis	Less strong association (present in 70% of the cases of gastric ulcer); disruption of mucosal barrier is most important pathogenetic factor
Favoured location	First part of duodenum (anterior wall)	Along lesser curvature and pyloric antrum
Acid level	Usually high	Usually normal; increased only if gastrin level is increased
Pain	Relieved after intake of food	Aggravated after intake of food
Night pain	Common	No night pain
Melena	More common	Less common
Vomiting and haematemesis	Less common	More common
Weight loss	No weight loss	Marked weight loss

Table 27.3 Differences between benign and malignant peptic ulcer

Features	Benign ulcer	Malignant ulcer
Age	Comparatively younger age	Older age
Sex	Clear-cut male predominance	Slight male predominance
Site	Usually along lesser curvature of pylorus and antrum	Along greater curvature of stomach
Size	Benign ulcers are generally less than 4 cm (however, size is not an absolute criterion for differentiation between benign and malignant ulcers)	Generally more than 4 cm
Ulcer base	Clear; rarely haemorrhagic	Necrotic debris may be present
Mucosal folds	Radiating from the ulcer crater	Interrupted; flattening of the rugae around the ulcer due to infiltration by malignant cells
Margins	No or minimal heaping	Heaping prominent
Barium meal	Sharply punched-out lesion	Irregular lesion

Q. Differentiate between benign and malignant peptic ulcer.

Ans. Differences between benign and malignant peptic ulcer are listed in Table 27.3.

Q. Classify tumours of stomach.

Ans. Classification of tumours of stomach

1. **Non-epithelial/mesenchymal tumours**
   (a) Gastrointestinal stromal tumours (GISTs)
   (b) Leiomyoma and leiomyosarcoma
   (c) Lipoma
   (d) Schwannoma
   (e) Granular cell tumour
   (f) Lymphoma
2. **Epithelial tumours**
   (a) Intraepithelial gastric neoplasia (adenoma)
   (b) Adenocarcinoma (most common malignancy; may be further sub-typed into: papillary, tubular, mucinous, signet ring, adenosquamous and undifferentiated types)
   (c) Small cell carcinoma
   (d) Neuroendocrine tumours

Q. Write briefly on the epidemiology, aetiopathogenesis, clinical features, gross and microscopic features of gastric adenocarcinoma. (PA24.4)

Ans. Worldwide, **gastric adenocarcinoma** constitutes 8% of all cancers, and is responsible for more deaths than lung cancer. The incidence of gastric cancer has declined in the past decade. 90% of malignant tumours in stomach are carcinomas.

Epidemiology

- High incidence in Japan, Chile, Northern Italy, China, Portugal, Russia.
- Males more commonly affected.
- More prevalent in lower socioeconomic groups.
- Occurrence in young patients is usually associated with radiation therapy or chemotherapy for other malignancies.
- 90% of malignant tumours in stomach are carcinomas.
- Most gastric carcinomas are adenocarcinoma; other carcinoma types are rare.

Predisposing Factors

Gastric carcinogenesis is a multistep and multifactorial process. While the intestinal type of gastric cancer is often related to environmental factors such as *H pylori* infection, diet and life style, the diffuse type is more often associated with genetic abnormalities.

Dietary Factors

- Foods containing nitrites or their precursor nitrates.
- Smoked, salted foods, and pickled items (contain benzopyrene).
- Less intake of fresh fruits and vegetables.
- High complex carbohydrate consumption and low dietary fat or protein.

Host Factors

- *H. pylori* infection and chronic gastritis manifest with multifocal mucosal atrophy and intestinal metaplasia (the former causes hypochlorhydria which favours *H. pylori* colonisation and the latter predisposes to intestinal type of gastric carcinoma).
- Partial gastrectomy (results in reflux of irritant biliary contents and chronic gastritis).
- Gastric dysplasia and adenomas.
- Cigarette smoking.
- Menetrier's disease.
- Barrett's oesophagus.
- Low socioeconomic status.
- Rubber and coal workers.

Genetic Factors

- Blood group A.
- Familial gastric cancers are due to mutations in CDH1, which encodes E-cadherin, responsible for the epithelial intercellular adhesion (loss of E-cadherin is usually associated with diffuse gastric cancer).
- Mutations in β-catenin, microsatellite instability and hypermethylation of several genes like TGFβRII, BAX, IGFIIR and p16INK4α are noted in sporadic intestinal type gastric cancer.

Racial Factors

More common in Blacks, Americans and Indians.

Geographical Influence

More prevalent in Japan, Finland and Iceland.

Pathogenesis

Three oncogenic pathways that are deregulated in the majority (>70%) of gastric cancers are the proliferation/stem cell, NF-κβ, and Wnt/beta-catenin pathways (Fig. 27.10).

- Ten to 15% of gastric cancers show familial clustering but only 1%–3% are related to identified inherited predisposition

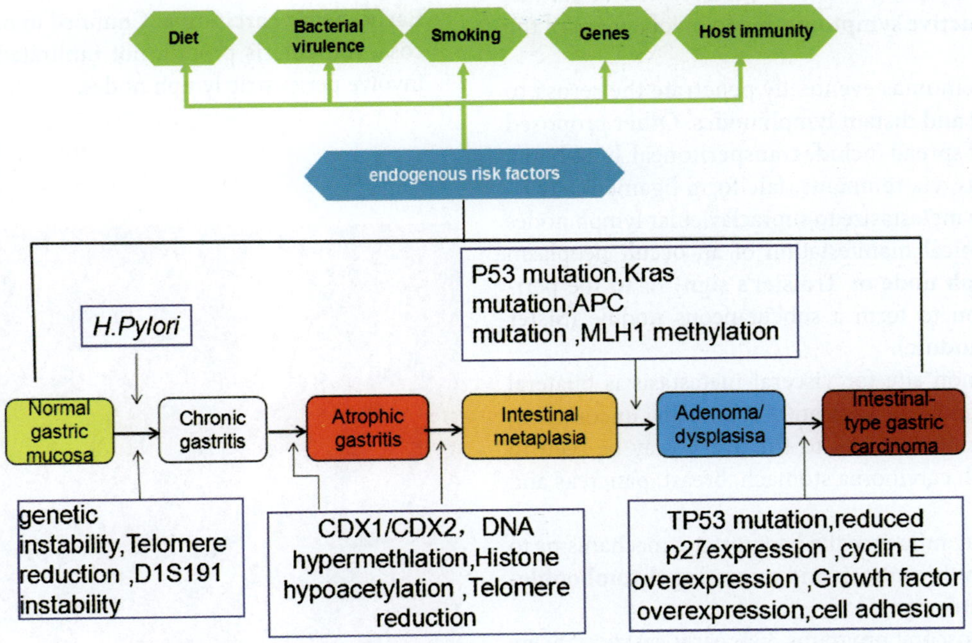

Fig. 27.10 The pathogenesis of intestinal-type and diffuse-type gastric cancer. Intestinal-type gastric cancer (top half of diagram) develops through a series of well-characterised events, whereby Helicobacter pylori infection promotes the differentiation of the normal gastric mucosa to chronic gastritis, which then progresses to atrophic gastritis. As a consequence of chronic inflammation and glandular regeneration, metaplasia often occurs in intestinal-type GC. The metaplasia-neoplasia-carcinoma sequence is driven by additional mutations in genes, including Tp53, p27, cyclin E. (*Source:* The application of transgenic and gene knockout mice in the study of gastric precancerous lesions: Qi Wang, Hua-feng Pan, Wei Liu, Zi-ming Zhao, *Journal PRP,* Vol. 214: 12, Fig. 2, Elsevier GmbH, 2018.)

syndromes such as **hereditary diffuse gastric cancer, hereditary non-polyposis colon cancer (Lynch syndrome), familial adenomatous polyposis, Peutz-Jeghers syndrome, Li-Fraumeni syndrome,** or **familial breast** and **ovarian cancer.**

- One of the **defining criteria of hereditary diffuse gastric cancer** is the presence of a ***CDH1*(E-cadherin) germline mutation.*CDH1*mutations have only been found in hereditary and sporadic diffuse type gastric cancer, but not in intestinal type.**
- In contrast, gastric cancer in patients with **microsatellite instability (MSI)**, that is, **deficiency or inactivation of one of the DNA mismatch repair genes (MMR) coding for MLH1, MSH2, MSH6 or PMS2 proteins (hereditary non-polyposis colon cancer patients) show intestinal type morphology** in 79% of patients.
- **Sporadic intestinal type cancers** are associated with **mutations increasing the signalling of the Wnt pathway mostly due to loss of functional mutations in the APC (Adenomatous Polyposis Coli) tumour suppressor gene and gain of function mutations in the gene encoding β-catenin.**
- **Mutations in Tp53** are seen in most of **sporadic gastric cancers (both intestinal and diffuse type).**
- **Loss of function mutations in other tumour suppressor genes like BAX** (involved in apoptosis) and **CDKN2A** (involved in cell cycle control).

Clinical Features

- May remain asymptomatic until late; symptoms include **weight loss, abdominal pain, nausea, vomiting and altered bowel habits.**
- There may be **dysphagia** due to involvement of cardiac end and **obstructive symptoms** due to involvement of the pylorus.
- All gastric carcinomas eventually penetrate the serosa to spread to local and distant lymph nodes. Other proposed mechanisms of spread include transperitoneal, lymphatic, haematogenous, via remnants, falciform ligament, etc.
- May frequently metastasize to supraclavicular lymph nodes as the first clinical manifestation of an occult neoplasm **(Virchow lymph node or Troisier's sign)** or to the periumbilical region to form a subcutaneous nodule **(Sister Mary Joseph nodule).**
- Another common site for visceral metastasis is bilateral ovaries **(Krukenberg tumour).** Although uncommon, metastatic adenocarcinoma to the ovary may be seen in association with carcinoma stomach, breast, pancreas and gallbladder.
- The tumour may influence the haemostatic mechanisms to cause **deep vein thrombosis** and **migrating thrombophlebitis (Trousseau's sign).**
- With mass endoscopy programs 35% early gastric cancers could be detected in Japan.
- There has been a steady decrease in the overall prevalence of gastric adenocarcinoma due to decreased prevalence of *H. pylori* and decreased intake of dietary carcinogens. However, an increase in the incidence of cardiac lesions has been observed which can be attributed to Barrett oesophagus, chronic GERD and obesity.
- Chromo-endoscopy may increase the detectability of small-sized cancers.

Location

- Pylorus and antrum (50%–60%)
- Cardia (25%)
- Body and fundus (15%–25%)

Lesser curvature is involved more often as compared to greater curvature and most common location is lesser curvature of antropyloric region.

Classification

Based on Histology (Lauren classification)

1. **Intestinal type (Fig. 27.11A)**
   (a) Polypoid bulky masses with or without ulceration.
   (b) Tumour cells form glands resembling colonic adenocarcinoma (this type of tumour arises from intestinal metaplasia).
   (c) Cells have apical mucin vacuoles.
   (d) Growth is expansile (grows as a cohesive mass along broad fronts).
2. **Diffuse/gastric type** (Fig. 27.11B)
   (a) Infiltrating tumours.
   (b) Cells show signet-ring appearance (nucleus pushed to periphery due to presence of large intracytoplasmic mucin vacuoles).
   (c) No gland formation is seen.
   (d) Scattered individual cells or small cell nests permeate the gastric wall (infiltrative pattern).

Based on Depth of Invasion (Fig. 27.11C)

1. **Early gastric carcinoma:** Confined to mucosa and submucosa, muscularis propria not infiltrated; may or may not involve perigastric lymph nodes.

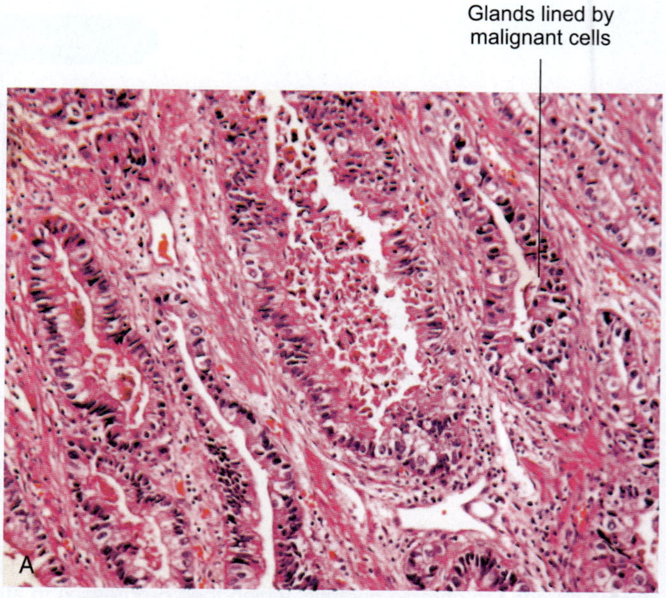

Fig. 27.11 (A) Intestinal type adenocarcinoma stomach showing tumour cells with apical mucin vacuoles forming glands resembling colonic adenocarcinoma (H&E; 100×).

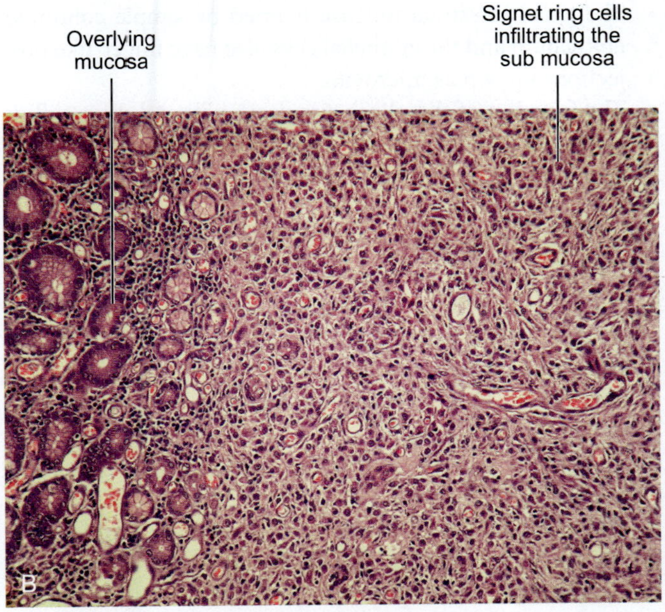

Fig. 27.11 (B) Scattered individual cells or small cell nests permeate the gastric wall (infiltrative pattern; H&E; 100×).

2. **Advanced gastric carcinoma:** Infiltrates muscularis propria.

Based on Gross Appearance

1. **Exophytic/polypoid/fungating**: A cauliflower-like tumour mass (Fig. 27.11D) protruding into lumen.
2. **Flat/depressed/infiltrative:** No obvious tumour mass in the mucosa. In the later stages, the infiltration of a part or entire stomach by individual infiltrating tumour cells giving it a 'leather bottle' appearance **(linitis plastica).**
3. **Excavated:** Shallow crater in early stages to large malignant ulcer in advanced lesions. Resemble chronic peptic ulcers with heaped up, beaded, shaggy, irregular margins and necrotic base.

Q. Write briefly on gastrointestinal stromal tumours (GISTs).

Ans. Gastrointestinal stromal tumour (GIST):

- Most common mesenchymal tumour of GIT; most common location is **stomach.**

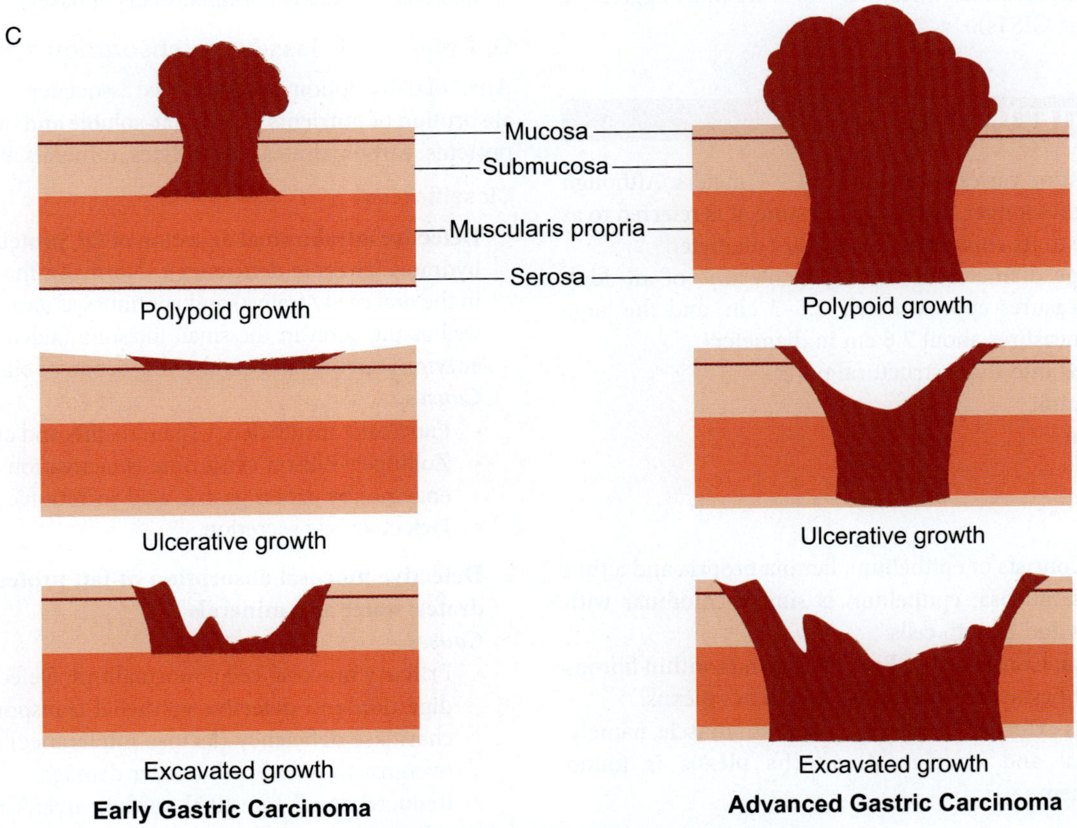

Fig. 27.11 (C) Early and advanced carcinoma of stomach.

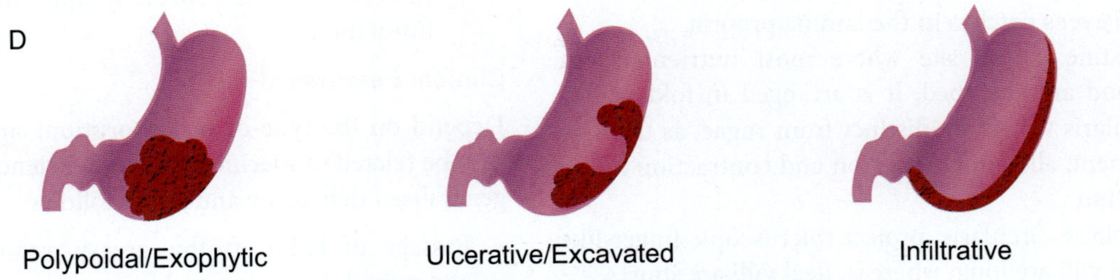

Fig. 27.11 (D) Gross types of gastric carcinoma.

- It is **male predominant**; is seen in the **fifth and sixth decades** and can present as a triad called **Carney's triad** (gastric GIST, paraganglioma and pulmonary chondroma).
- Origin from **interstitial cells of Cajal** (which are the pacemaker cells for gut peristalsis and are located in muscular propria).
- Associated with a **gain of function mutation of the gene encoding for tyrosine kinase c-kit** (receptor for stem cell factor). This leads to constitutional **activation of c-KIT** which in turn activates the **RAS pathway** to promote cell proliferation.
- Patient usually presents with an abdominal mass. CT is the best diagnostic modality.
- GISTs may be as large as 30 cm, solitary, well-circumscribed, fleshy, submucosal or subserosal masses. When large they may cause ulceration of the overlying mucosa.
- Sections show mainly spindle cells or epithelioid cells or an admixture of the two cell types. Tumour cells express **c-KIT (CD117)** and **CD 34.**
- Prognosis of the tumour is dependant on **tumour size** (recurrence and metastasis associated with a size >5 cm); **mitoses** and **location** (intestinal GISTs are more aggressive than gastric GISTs).

SMALL INTESTINE

- Small intestine varies in length from 4–7 meters. Although it is 4–5 times longer than large intestine, it is referred to as 'small' due to its comparatively smaller diameter.
- The average diameter of the small intestine of an adult human measures approximately 2.5–3 cm, and the large intestine measures about 7.6 cm in diameter.
- It is divided into three structural parts:
  - Duodenum
  - Jejunum
  - Ileum

Duodenum

- **Mucosa:** Consists of epithelium, lamina propria and a thin muscularis mucosa; epithelium is simple columnar with goblet cells and Paneth cells.
- **Submucosa:** Composed of Brunner's glands within fibrous connective tissue, which also has Meissner's plexus.
- **Muscularis externa:** Two layers of smooth muscle, namely, longitudinal and circular. Auerbach's plexus is found between them.

Jejunum and Ileum

- Lack Brunner's glands.
- Ileum has Peyer's patches in the lamina propria.
- Small intestine is the site where most nutrients from ingested food are absorbed. It is arranged in folds called plicae circularis which are distinct from rugae, as they are not permanent, allowing distention and contraction of the small intestine.
- From the plicae circularis, project microscopic finger-like villi. Jejunal villi are long; whereas, ileal villi are short.
- The small intestinal mucosa is lined by simple columnar epithelium and the epithelial cells also have finger-like projections known as microvilli.
- The function of the plicae circularis, villi and microvilli is to increase the amount of surface area available for secretion of enzymes and absorption of nutrients.

COLON

- It consists of the ascending, transverse, descending and sigmoid colon. Colon from caecum to the splenic flexure (the junction between the transverse and descending colon) is also known as the right colon. The remainder is known as the left colon.
- There is increase in the thickness of mucosa from caecum to rectum.
- Surface epithelium is composed of absorptive tall columnar epithelium with goblet cells and endocrine cells.
- Columnar cells and goblet cells are present in the ratio of approximately 4:1.
- Paneth cells are most prominent in the caecum and proximal colon (usually confined to crypt bases).

Q. Define and classify malabsorption syndrome.

Ans. Malabsorption syndrome is associated with impaired absorption of nutrients like fat, fat-soluble and other vitamins, proteins, carbohydrates, electrolytes, minerals and water.

Classification

1. **Defective intraluminal digestion of fat, proteins and carbohydrates (enzyme deficiency):** Normally, the process starts in the oral cavity (saliva) and continues as gastric digestion as well as digestion in the small intestine (aided by pancreatic enzyme secretion and emulsifying action of bile).
   Causes
   - Pancreatic insufficiency (pancreatitis and cystic fibrosis).
   - Zollinger–Ellison syndrome (inactivation of pancreatic enzymes by excess gastric acid secretion).
   - Defective bile secretion.
2. **Defective mucosal absorption of fat, proteins, carbohydrates, water and minerals**
   Causes
   - Primary mucosal cell abnormalities: Defective terminal digestion and defective epithelial transport, e.g. disaccharidase deficiency (lactose intolerance) and bacterial overgrowth with brush border damage.
   - Reduced small intestinal surface area: Crohn disease, celiac sprue and surgery.
   - Lymphatic obstruction: Lymphoma and tuberculosis.
   - Infections: tropical sprue, Whipple disease and parasitic infestation.

Clinical Features

Depend on the type of malabsorption; signs and symptoms may be related to specific nutrient deficiency or may be due to generalised deficiency and are as follows:

- Passage of bulky, frothy, greasy, yellow or grey stools, abdominal distension and flatus.

- Weight loss and muscle wasting.
- Anaemia from iron, pyridoxine, folate or vitamin B_{12} deficiency.
- Bleeding (petechiae and purpura) due to vitamin K deficiency.
- Oedema due to protein deficiency.
- Dermatitis, mucositis and hyperkeratosis due to vitamin A, zinc, essential fatty acids and niacin deficiency.
- Osteopenia and tetany due to defective calcium absorption.
- Amenorrhea, impotence and infertility from generalised malnutrition.
- Hyperparathyroidism due to protracted calcium and vitamin deficiency.

Q. Differentiate between celiac (non-tropical) sprue and environmental or tropical enteropathy.

Ans. Differences between celiac and tropical sprue are listed in Table 27.4.

Q. Enumerate the morphologic features of celiac sprue.

Ans. Morphological features of celiac sprue:

- Diffuse enteritis with atrophy or total loss of villi.
- Vacuolar degeneration of surface epithelium, loss of microvilli and increased number of intraepithelial CD8+ T lymphocytes.
- In an attempt to maintain mucosal thickness, crypts become hyperplastic, elongated and tortuous and also show increased mitotic figures.
- Plasma cells, lymphocytes, macrophages, and mast cell infiltration in lamina propria.

Note: The above pathological findings are characteristic of celiac sprue but non-specific and can be seen in tropical sprue as well. Mucosal histology reverts to normal after excluding gluten from the diet.

Q. Enumerate the ulcero-inflammatory diseases of small and large intestine.

Ans. Ulcero-inflammatory diseases of small intestine include:

- Crohn disease
- Typhoid ulcer
- Tuberculous ulcer
- Ulcers due to *Campylobacter spp.*
- Drug-induced ulcers

Ulcero-inflammatory diseases of large intestine include:

- Ulcerative colitis
- Shigella-induced ulcers
- Ulcers due to *Campylobacter spp.*
- Amoebic ulcers

Q. Write briefly on the pathology and complications of intestinal tuberculosis. (PA24.5)

Ans. Intestinal tuberculosis may be **primary** (caused by *Mycobacterium bovis* ingested via unpasteurised milk) or **secondary** (in a patient of active pulmonary tuberculosis, swallowing of coughed up material can result in secondary tuberculosis of intestine).

Table 27.4 Differences between celiac and tropical sprue

Features	Celiac sprue	Environmental or tropical enteropathy (tropical sprue)
Other names	Gluten-sensitive enteropathy, non-tropical sprue	Post-infectious sprue; may occur in epidemic or endemic forms
Pathogenesis	Immune-mediated disease due to sensitivity to gluten and related proteins (water insoluble gliadin) present in wheat, oat, barley and rye. No organism implicated. Gladden peptides induce secretion of IL 15, which activates CD8+ intraepithelial lymphocytes. These lymphocytes express NKG2D, a natural killer cell marker and receptor for MHC class I polypeptide-related sequence (MIC-A). Epithelial cells which express surface MIC are recognized and attacked by NKG2D expressing lymphocytes.	Infectious disease. Occurs exclusively in patients living in or visiting the tropics. No specific causal agent implicated. Enterotoxigenic bacterial (cyclospora and *E. coli*) overgrowth is found
Genetic predisposition	HLA (DQ2 and DQ8) association accounts for almost half of the genetic component of celiac disease. The remaining genetic factors include polymorphisms of immune regulatory genes like IL-2 and IL-21	None
Distribution	Affects mainly the proximal part of small intestine (higher gluten exposure than distal part)	Affects the distal small bowel
Associated clinical conditions	Dermatitis herpetiformis and neurological disorders	Frequent folate or vitamin B_{12} deficiency (due to involvement of distal small bowel) leading to atypical enlargement of nuclei of epithelial cells (megaloblastic change)
Secondary malignancy	Intestinal lymphoma, small intestinal adenocarcinoma and oesophageal squamous cell carcinoma	No such predisposition
Treatment	Gluten-restricted diet	Broad-spectrum antibiotics

Salient Features

- Intestinal tuberculosis mainly occurs in **terminal ileum**; colon is rarely involved.
- **Primary tuberculosis** of intestine mainly involves **mesenteric lymph nodes**, which are en**larged, caseous and matted, and usually heal by fibrosis and calcification.**
- **Intestinal lesions are more prominent than nodal lesions in secondary tuberculosis**. Lesion starts as a **small ulcerative lesion, which progressively enlarges to form a large transverse ulcer, perpendicular to the long axis of the bowel** (as intestinal tuberculosis spreads through lacteals or lymphatics, which are transversely oriented). Serosa may also exhibit tubercles.
- **Hyperplastic caecal tuberculosis** is a variant of secondary intestinal tuberculosis involving **caecum** (sometimes ascending colon), which is commonly **palpable as a lump** (called hyperplastic because the tuberculous granulation tissue formed in this lesion masquerades as a lump).

Complications

- **Tuberculous peritonitis** may occur as a part of disseminated tuberculosis or result from a tuberculous lesion in close proximity to the peritoneum. It may manifest as effusion or as fibrosis **(doughy abdomen)**.
- The **transverse or circumferential ulceration** is eventually replaced by a **fibrous stricture,** which in turn may result in **intestinal obstruction.**

Q. Differentiate between tuberculous and typhoid ulcer of intestine.

Ans. Differences between tuberculous and typhoid ulcer are listed in Table 27.5.

Q. Define inflammatory bowel disease (IBD). Write briefly on its aetiopathogenesis. (PA24.6)

Ans. IBD is a chronic relapsing inflammatory disorder of unknown origin, which results from an abnormal immune response to normal flora of gut/self-antigens, in genetically susceptible individuals. Pathogenesis of IBD involves genetic susceptibility, immune dysregulation and triggering by microbial flora (Fig. 27.12).

Genetic Predisposition

- Sporadic in 85%–90% cases.
- Higher incidence in relatives of patients who are known cases of IBD. Genetic factors contribute less to the pathogenesis of ulcerative colitis than Crohn disease.
- IBD is linked to specific HLA types; **(ulcerative colitis with HLADRB1 and HLADR7 and Crohn disease with HLADQ4).**
- Association with non-HLA genes, namely, **NOD2/CARD15** (nucleotide-binding oligomerisation domain-2) and a mutant form of **IL23**, is well known.
- NOD2 is an intracellular receptor for **muramyl dipeptidase**, a component of the cell wall in many bacteria, which plays an important role in host responses to these bacteria. It is expressed in **Paneth cells.**
- NOD2/CARD15 protein prevents entry of microbes into intestinal wall and regulates innate immune response.
- The mutant form is defective in its response to the bacteria, thus allowing chronic infection to be established in the intestine and promoting inflammatory reactions.
- Alternately, the disease-associated mutant form may promote excessive host response to the intestinal bacteria.
- Other susceptibility genes include **ATG16L1** (autophagy related 16-like) and **IRGM** (immunity related GTPase M). These also play an important role in host responses to intestinal pathogens.
- IL-23 promotes production of IL17 by T cells and IL17 has been implicated in inflammatory reactions seen in IBD and other chronic diseases.

Defective Immune Response

Immune reactions may be directed against self-antigens of the intestine or bacterial antigens. Primary damaging cells appear to be CD4+ T cells.

1. **Innate immunity**
   (a) The innate immune response represents our first line of defence against pathogens. It is non-specific and

Table 27.5 Differences between tuberculous and typhoid ulcer

Features	Tuberculous ulcer	Typhoid ulcer
Causative organism	*Mycobacterium tuberculosis*	*Salmonella typhi*
Site	Anywhere in small intestine; most common in terminal ileum and caecum, rarely colon	Most common in terminal ileum (Peyer's patches); may occur in jejunum
Orientation of the ulcer	Perpendicular to long axis of bowel (transverse ulcer) due to spread by lacteals (lymphatics)	Parallel to long axis of bowel (longitudinal ulcer) due to involvement of Peyer's patches
Microscopic features	Epithelioid cell granulomas with or without caseous necrosis	Lymphoplasmacytic infiltrate with histiocytes some of which show erythrophagocytosis
Fibrosis and stricture formation	Common; intestinal tuberculosis may present with subacute or acute intestinal obstruction	Rare
Perforation	May be present	Common
Bleeding	Absent	Present

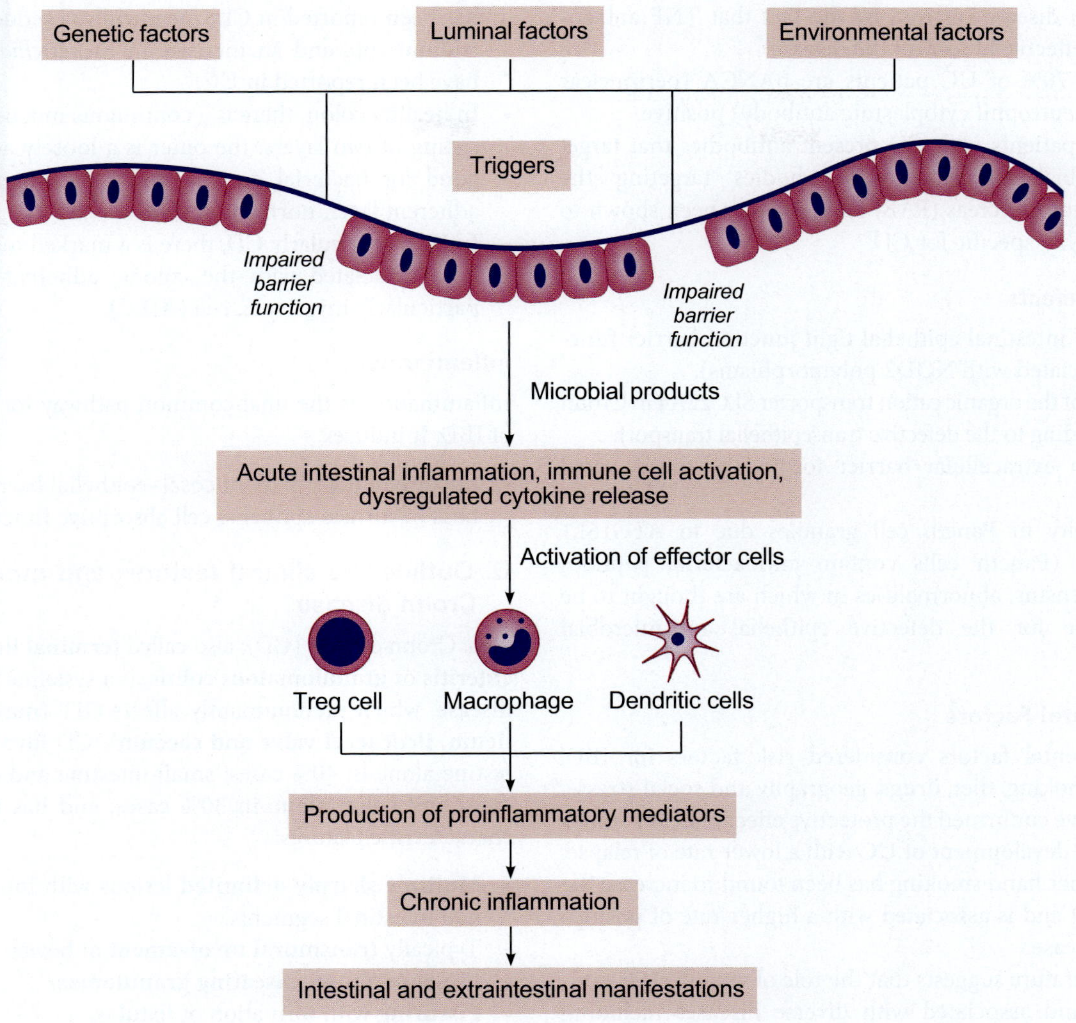

Fig. 27.12 The intestinal microbiota, environmental factors and food antigens either cause a leaky barrier or penetrate through a barrier leak into deeper, submucosal tissue layers. In the genetically susceptible host, epigenetic modifications, and a dysregulation of the innate and adaptive immune response occurs and manifests with chronic intestinal inflammation.

quick (onset within minutes or hours) and is mediated by epithelial cells, neutrophils, dendritic cells, monocytes, macrophages and natural killer cells.

(b) Innate immunity is largely based on the sensing of lipopolysaccharide (LPS) on bacterial cell wall of both commensals and pathogens. Upon the sensing process, the cytoplasmic Nuclear Factor-κB (NF-κB) signalling complex is unleashed from its inhibitor and allowed to bind the promoter regions of pro-inflammatory cytokine genes, including interleukin (IL)-2.

(c) Microbial antigen recognition is mediated by pattern recognition receptors including toll-like receptors or TLRs on the cell surface and NOD-like receptors in the cytoplasm). The expression and function of both TLRs and NOD proteins have been found to be altered in IBD.

(d) In CD patients, mucosal neutrophil recruitment and production of IL-1β and IL-8 are selectively reduced in CD patients but not in UC patients. NOD2 mutations (most commonly associated with CD) induce a defective ability of the gut to respond to LPS inducing disease susceptibility.

(e) NOD2 mutations may lead to reduced activation of NF-κB (resulting in reduced antibacterial activity), and lack of inhibition of TLR2 stimulation (leading to activation of inflammatory pathways and excessive Th-1 responses).

2. **Adaptive immunity**
   (a) Adaptive immunity is specific, late in onset (takes several days to respond) and depends on the type and number of T cells.
   (b) Th1 cells, induced by IL-12, produce a high amount of IFN-γ, whereas Th2 cells release IL-4, IL-5 and IL-13.
   (c) An abnormal Th1 immune response is thought to cause intestinal inflammation in CD while UC has been considered as a Th2-mediated disease.
   (d) Tissue inflammation may be the result of secretion of IL17 by a recently discovered subset of CD4+ T cells called **T_H17 subset.**

(e) **TNF** may play an important role in the pathogenesis of Crohn disease (proven by the fact that TNF antagonists effectively control the disease).

(f) Some 70% of UC patients are pANCA (perinuclear anti-neutrophil cytoplasmic antibody) positive.

(g) Most patients with CD present antibodies that target microbial antigens. Autoantibodies targeting the exocrine pancreas (PAB) have recently been shown to be highly specific for CD.

Epithelial Defects

- Defects in intestinal epithelial tight junction barrier function (associated with NOD2 polymorphisms).
- Mutation of the organic cation transporter SLC22A4 in Crohn disease leading to the defective transepithelial transport.
- Defects in extracellular barrier formed by the secreted mucin.
- Abnormality in Paneth cell granules due to ATG16L1 mutations (Paneth cells contain antibacterial peptides called defensins, abnormalities in which are thought to be responsible for the defective epithelial anti-microbial function).

Environmental Factors

- Environmental factors considered risk factors for IBD, include smoking, diet, drugs, geography and social stress.
- Studies have confirmed the protective effect of heavy smoking on the development of UC with a lower rate of relapse. On the other hand smoking has been found to increase the risk of CD and is associated with a higher rate of postoperative disease.
- Recent literature suggests that the role of vitamin D is multifarious and associated with diverse diseases including IBD.
- Aspirin and NSAIDs may have an effect in triggering onset or relapse of IBD. High dose, prolonged using duration and frequent use of NSAIDs had been associated with an increased risk of CD and UC.
- Use of antibiotics is an important environmental factor, influencing the risk of IBD through their effect on the microbiome.
- Stress, including depression and anxiety, may worsen IBD.
- Recent evidence suggests that air pollution may contribute to the risk of CD and UC. It has been found that high levels of NO_2 and SO_2 correlate with the increased risk of CD and UC.

Microbial Factors

- Microbes provide an antigenic trigger to a basically dysregulated immune system.
- The human gut microbiome is a 10 to the power14 microorganism population mainly dwelling within the colon.
- Gut microbiome gets established within the first 2 weeks of life and remains stable thereafter.
- There is a significantly reduced biodiversity and stability in faecal microbiome in IBD patients compared to healthy controls.
- Firmicutes and Bacteroidetes phyla predominate in healthy intestines, whereas, the microbiota in IBD is characterised by a relative lack of the same. An increase in enterobacteria has been reported in CD; meanwhile, a reduction in Clostridium spp. and an increase in *Escherichia coli* (*E. coli*) have been reported in UC.
- In healthy colon, there is a continuous mucus coating consisting of two layers: the outer is a loosely adherent layer, good for bacterial growth; while the inner is a tightly adherent layer, normally sterile.
- In IBD, particularly CD, there is a marked increase in bacteria associated with the colonic adherent mucus layer particularly invasive *E. coli* (AIEC).

Inflammation

Inflammation is the final common pathway for pathogenesis of IBD. It induces

- Impaired integrity of mucosal–epithelial barrier.
- Loss of surface epithelial cell absorptive function.

Q. Outline the clinical features and morphology of Crohn disease. (PA24.6)

Ans. Crohn disease (CD), also called **terminal ileitis, regional enteritis** or **granulomatous colitis,** is a systemic inflammatory disease, which predominantly affects GIT (**mainly terminal ileum, ileocaecal valve and caecum).** CD involves small intestine alone in 40% cases; small intestine and colon in 30% cases and colon alone in 30% cases, and has the following characteristic features:

- **Multiple sharply delimited** lesions with intervening normal intestinal segments.
- Typically **transmural involvement** of bowel.
- Presence of **non-caseating granulomas.**
- **Fissuring** with formation of **fistulas.**

Clinical Features

- May affect any age, but major **peaks in the second and third decades** of life.
- Presents with recurrent episodes of **diarrhoea, crampy abdominal pain, fever and melena.**
- **Remissions and relapses are common.**
- Patients may develop **malabsorption, fistulae** and **intestinal stricture** or **obstruction. Fistula may form to other loops of bowel, urinary bladder, vagina and perianal skin.**
- **Extraintestinal manifestations** include uveitis, sacroiliitis, migratory polyarthritis, erythema nodosum, bile duct inflammatory disorder, obstructive uropathy and nephrolithiasis.

Gross Morphology (Fig. 27.13)

- Serosa is dull, opaque and granular with creeping fat appearance (the subserosal fat appears firm and contracted over the involved areas and may encircle along the antimesenteric border).
- Mesentery is thickened, oedematous or fibrotic **(hosepipe appearance).**
- Intestinal wall is rubbery and thick due to oedema and inflammation in the early stages and fibrosis and hypertrophy of muscularis propria in the later stages.

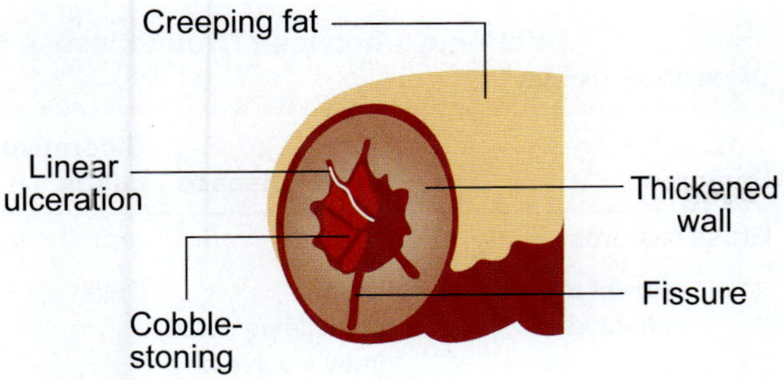

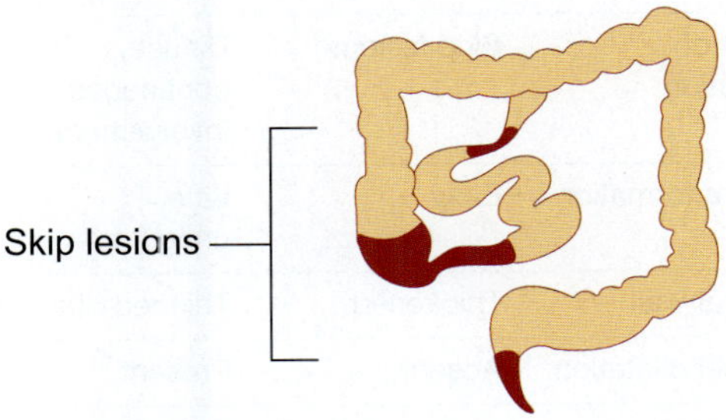

Fig. 27.13 Dull, opaque and granular serosa with creeping fat appearance (figure on top; the subserosal fat appears firm and contracted over the involved areas and may encircle along the antimesenteric border). Schematic diagram showing skip lesions (bottom).

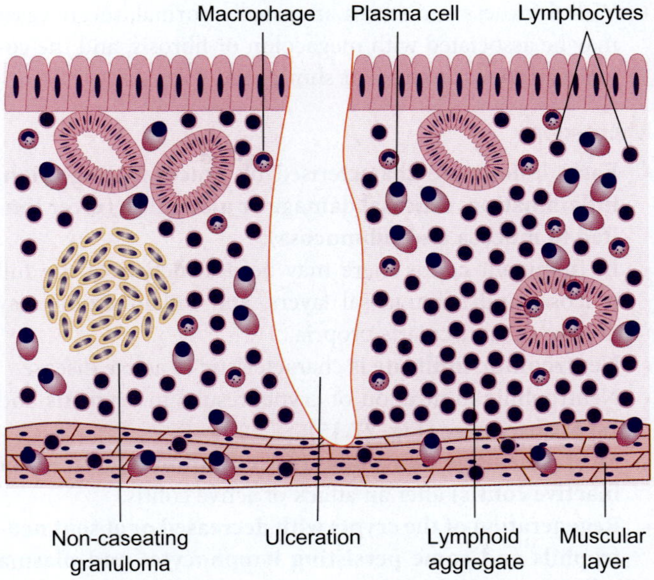

Fig. 27.14 Transmural inflammation affecting all layers with formation of lymphoid aggregates, more prominent in submucosa and serosa, with relative sparing of muscularis propria. Neutrophils are focally present. Non-caseating granulomas are seen.

- Lumen is narrowed **(string sign on X-ray).**
- **Skip lesions are characteristic** (sharp demarcation of the involved segment from the uninvolved).
- **Aphthous linear ulcers)** is the earliest manifestation. Multiple aphthae coalesce longitudinally to form **linear snake-like ulcers** oriented along the long axis of the bowel. The ulcers may become deeper to result in the formation of or **sinus tracts** and **fistulae.**

Microscopy (Fig. 27.14)

- There is **mucosal oedema** and **loss of normal folds.**
- Active Crohn disease shows **abundant neutrophils** in the **lamina propria** and **crypts** which damage the crypt epithelium and form **crypt abscesses.** Ulceration is frequent.
- Areas of aphthous ulceration with intervening normal mucosa gives rise to the typical **cobblestone appearance.**
- Repeated cycles of crypt damage and regeneration lead to **architectural distortion** of the mucosa. **Branching crypts with abnormal shapes** replace the normally straight and parallel crypts.
- Gland dropout is frequent. Forked glands and shortened glands that fail to reach the muscularis mucosae are often seen.
- Lamina propria fibrosis may be present with thickening of muscularis mucosae indicating the initiation of chronicity in the lesion.
- **Transmural inflammation** affecting all layers can be demonstrated.
- Lymphoid aggregates are present at all levels. Infiltrate in some cases is more prominent in submucosa and serosa, with relative sparing of muscularis propria.
- Intramural inflammatory infiltrate is largely lymphohistiocytic. Neutrophils may be focally present.
- **Non-caseating granulomas** and **fibrosis** are common.
- Granulomas can also be seen in the **mesenteric lymph nodes. Cutaneous nodules** form which also show non-caseating granulomas (earlier labelled metastatic Crohn disease).
- Epithelial metaplasia (pyloric and Paneth cell) develops as a consequence of chronic injury. Paneth cells are rare in the normal left colon.
- Neural hyperplasia may be present in submucosa and muscularis propria. May contain ganglion cells.

Q. Describe the clinical features, morphology and complications of ulcerative colitis. (PA24.6)

Ans. Ulcerative colitis is an ulceroinflammatory disease limited to colon. It usually affects only the mucosa and submucosa except in very severe forms. It peaks between 20 and 25 years and is more common in females.

Gross Morphology

Early Active Colitis

- The lesion extends in a retrograde and continuous fashion from rectum to proximal parts of colon; **no skip lesions are seen.** Involvement of a few centimetres of ileum when the entire colon is involved can be seen and is termed **'backwash ileitis'.**
- The mucosa is red, granular and friable and bleeds easily.
- Broad-based mucosal ulcers; aligned along the long axis of the colon and pseudopolyps (due to bulging of regenerating mucosa) are a common sight.
- No mural thickening is seen and the serosa is normal.

Chronic Colitis

- Extensive ulceration along bowel axis but usually not serpentine as in Crohn's disease; have pseudopolyps (isolated islands of regenerating mucosa) and flat mucosa.

- Wall thickness and serosa are usually normal; severe cases may be associated with megacolon or fibrosis, and the colon may appear narrow or shortened.

Microscopy

- **Early lesions** are characterised by **mucosal congestion, inflammation, mucosal damage or ulceration (ulcer limited to mucosa and submucosa)**.
- In fulminant colitis there may be destruction of the full mucosal and submucosal layers, and inflammation may involve the muscularis propria.
- **Neutrophilic infiltrate** is characteristic of active disease.
- Neutrophilic infiltration of crypts results in **cryptitis** and **crypt abscessese (Fig. 27.15).**
- Most patients go into a **phase of resolution (Quiescent of inactive colitis)** after an attack of active colitis.
- **Regeneration of the crypts with decreased or absent neutrophils and some persisting lymphocytes and plasma cells is generally seen.**
- **Chronic ulcerative colitis** is associated with **epithelial regeneration with loss of goblet cells** and **mucin depletion**.
- A diffuse, predominantly mononuclear infiltrate is seen in the lamina propria comprising lymphocytes, plasma cells, histiocytes and eosinophils. Basal lymphoplasmacytic aggregates may be present. **Granulomas are not seen.**
- Even after healing, **mucosal architectural disarray, colonic gland atrophy and submucosal fibrosis** may be seen.
- **Paneth cell metaplasia** and **epithelial dysplasia** are common.
- **UC lacks the fibrosis typical of Crohn disease**. May be associated with **toxic megacolon**.

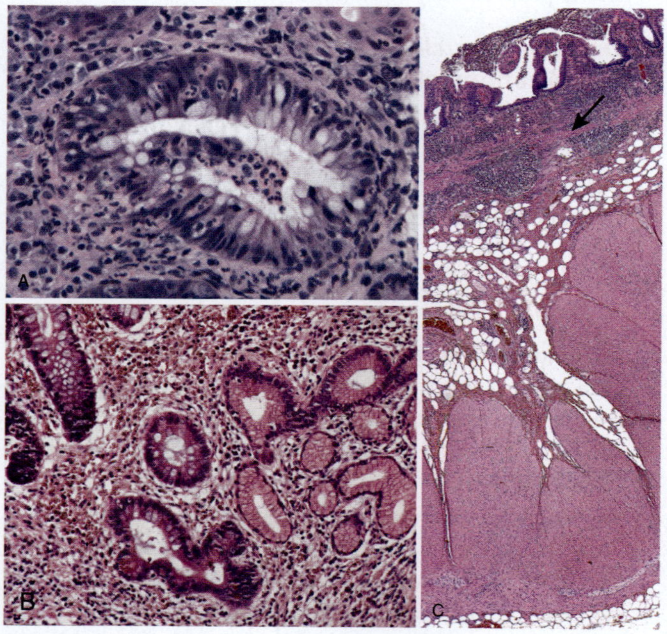

Fig. 27.15 Microscopic pathology of ulcerative colitis. (A) Crypt abscess. (B) Pseudopyloric metaplasia (bottom). (C) Disease is limited to the mucosa. (*Source: Robbins and Cotran Pathologic Basis of Disease - Systemic Pathology,* Volume 2, First Bangladesh Edition: Vinay Kumar, Abul K. Abbas, Jon C. Aster, Fig. 17-37, Page 802, Elsevier Inc., 2017.)

Table 27.6 Differences between Crohn disease and ulcerative colitis

Features	Crohn disease	Ulcerative colitis
Gross features		
Bowel region affected	Ileum, sometimes colon (may involve any part of GIT)	Colon
Pattern of distribution	Skip lesions	Diffuse, continuous involvement
Stricture formation	Early	Late, uncommon
Intestinal wall	Thickened	Thinned out
Intestinal dilatation	Absent	Present
Progression	Antegrade	Retrograde
Microscopic features		
Ulcers	Deep linear	Superficial
Pseudo polyps	Absent	Present
Lymphoid reaction	Marked	Mild
Fibrosis	Marked	Mild
Serositis	Marked	Absent or mild
Granulomas	Present in 50% of the cases	Absent
Fistula/sinus	Present	Absent
Clinical features		
Fat/vitamin malabsorption	Present	Absent
Malignant potential	Less	More
Response to surgery	Poor	Good

Complications

- Toxic megacolon (caused by neuromuscular shutdown due to damage to muscularis propria and neural plexus).
- Perianal fistula.
- Development of colonic carcinoma.
- Bleeding.
- Perforation (damage to muscularis propria leads to perforation and pericolonic abscess formation).

Q. Differentiate between Crohn disease and ulcerative colitis.

Ans. Differences between Crohn disease and ulcerative colitis are summarized in the Table 27.6.

Q. Write briefly on amoebic colitis. Differentiate between amoebic and ulcerative colitis.

Ans. Amoebic colitis is caused by the protozoan *Entamoeba histolytica.*

- The life cycle of ***E. histolytica*** has the following stages:
  - Trophozoite stage: Spherical to oval trophozoites can be demonstrated in the stool of patients who exhibit acute symptoms.
  - Precyst stage: The trophozoite converts into a precyst form in the colon of the patient.
  - Cyst stage: Amoebic cysts have a thick chitinous wall and four nuclei. Infection occurs by the faecal route due to ingestion of food contaminated with the faeces containing the cysts.
- The cysts are resistant to gastric acid and are passed as it is to the colon where they colonise the epithelial surface to release trophozoites. Most frequent location of colonisation is caecum and ascending colon.
- Trophozoites produce a lytic substance, which aids in invasion of the crypts. They then burrow laterally into the lamina propria to form a superficial **flask-shaped ulcer** with a narrow neck and wide base.
- Trophozoites may reach the liver by invading blood vessels to produce an **amoebic liver abscess** in about 40% cases.
- Clinically, patient in the **acute stage** presents with abdominal pain and bloody diarrhoea. **Amoebic liver abscess** typically manifests with right upper quadrant pain, low-grade fever and weight loss.
- Trophozoites can microscopically be demonstrated in the surface of the ulcer, which shows both acute and chronic inflammation.
- Thickening of the intestinal wall with napkin ring-like constriction (**ameboma**) may occasionally occur and can be confused with malignancy.
- Diagnosis is based on stool examination, serology and radiology.

Differences between amoebic and ulcerative colitis are listed in Table 27.7.

Q. Classify polyps of the intestine and describe their clinicopathological features.

Ans. Polyps of the intestine are classified into:

1. **Non-neoplastic polyps: Include inflammatory, hamartomatous and hyperplastic polyps.**
   (a) **Inflammatory polyps**
      (i) Present with a clinical triad of rectal bleeding, mucous discharge and a lesion in the anterior rectal wall.
      (ii) The lesion is due to an abnormal anorectal sphincter that leads to recurrent abrasion and ulceration of the overlying rectal mucosa.
      (iii) Recurrent injury and healing causes some degree of mucosal prolapse and formation of the inflammatory polyp.
      (iv) Microscopically, the polyp shows epithelial and fibromuscular hyperplasia and a mixed inflammatory infiltrate in the lamina propria.
   (b) **Hamartomatous polyps:** Occur sporadically and as part of genetic or acquired syndromes, examples are:
      (i) Juvenile polyps
      - Focal malformations of mucosal epithelium and lamina propria, which usually occur in children less than 5 years of age.
      - Majority occurs in rectum and present with rectal bleeding or prolapse.
      - May be sporadic or syndromic.
      - Sporadic juvenile polyps are usually solitary lesions and are called retention polyps.
      - Individuals with autosomal dominant inheritance have 3–100 or more polyps. Most common mutation is of SMAD4 (which encodes an intermediate in TGF-β pathway). The juvenile polyposis syndrome is associated with a higher risk of colonic adenocarcinoma.

Table 27.7 Differences between amoebic and ulcerative colitis

Features	Amoebic colitis	Ulcerative colitis
Cause	Infective; caused by *Entamoeba histolytica*	Unknown; may result from dysregulated immune responses, in genetically susceptible individuals
Pathogenesis	Transmission by faecal-oral route (infection is spread through ingestion of cyst form of the parasite, a resistant structure that is found in stools)	Genetic predisposition with immunologic dysregulation
Distribution	Localized to caecum and ascending colon, sigmoid, rectum and appendix in decreasing order. In severe cases, entire large intestine may be involved	Involves rectum and extends proximally to involve whole colon in severe cases
Ulcer	Pin-head to large-sized ulcers seen. Muscularis propria acts as a barrier to trophozoites. The ulcer fans out laterally just above the muscularis propria, to form discrete flask-shaped ulcers (narrow neck and broad base). Intervening mucosa is normal	• Broad-based ulcers with continuous involvement; no intervening normal mucosa. • Usually, superficial: limited to mucosa and submucosa
Morphology	Liquefactive necrosis; few inflammatory cells; mainly neutrophils	Diffuse mononuclear infiltrate, crypt abscesses
Pseudopolyps	Absent	Present
Risk of cancer	Nil	Present

- Microscopically, cystically dilated glands filled with mucin and inflammatory cells are seen in a background of lamina propria with mixed inflammation.

(ii) Peutz–Jeghers polyps
- Peutz–Jeghers polyps are hamartomatous polyps seen in the small intestine, colon and stomach that occur as part of the rare autosomal dominant syndrome called Peutz–Jeghers syndrome.
- Also seen in this syndrome is melanotic mucosal and cutaneous pigmentation and increased risk of several malignancies including cancer of colon, pancreas, breast, lung, ovaries, uterus and testicles. It is caused by a germ-line mutation in LKB1/STK11 gene that encodes a serine/threonine protein kinases.
- Present as large and pedunculated polyps with a lobulated appearance.
- Histologically characterised by extensive connective tissue and smooth muscle arborisation (intermixing) throughout the polyp; the glands being lined by normal looking intestinal epithelium.

(iii) Cowden syndrome
- Hamartomatous polyps in GIT associated with an increased risk of neoplasms of thyroid, breast, uterus and skin.
- Caused by a germline mutation in PTEN (phosphatase and tensin homologue) tumour suppressor gene.
- PTEN encodes a phosphatase that acts as an inhibitor of signals from several tyrosine kinase receptors and favours apoptosis through the BAD/BCL2 pathways.

(iv) Cronkhite–Canada syndrome
- Non-hereditary polyposis seen in individuals over 50 years who present with diarrhoea, weight loss, abdominal pain and weakness.
- Hamartomatous polyps are seen in stomach, small intestine and colorectum.
- Polyps are histologically similar to juvenile polyps.
- Intervening non-polypoidal mucosa also shows crypt dilatation, oedema and inflammation in the lamina propria.
- Other manifestations include nail atrophy or splitting, hair loss and hypo- and hyperpigmentation of the skin.

(c) **Hyperplastic polyps**

(i) Epithelial proliferations that are thought to result from delayed shedding of surface epithelial cells lead to piling of goblet and absorptive cells.

(ii) Hyperplastic polyps do not have a malignant potential.

(iii) The crowding gives rise to a serrated surface (histological hallmark).

(iv) A sessile serrated adenoma, which is histologically similar but has malignant potential, needs to be differentiated from a hyperplastic polyp.

(v) Classically, less than 5 mm and seen in left colon.

(vi) May be single or multiple.

2. **Neoplastic polyps (adenomas of the small and large intestine)**

(a) Are **variable in size** and may be **pedunculated or sessile**; show a progressive increase in incidence with increasing age (peak incidence after 60 years).

(b) **Familial predisposition present**; males and females are equally affected.

(c) **All adenomas are a result of proliferative epithelial dysplasia and may give rise to invasive carcinomas.**

(d) Adenomas are classified into four types based on epithelial architecture:
(i) **Tubular adenomas**
(ii) **Villous adenomas**
(iii) **Tubulovillous adenomas**
(iv) **Sessile serrated adenomas**

(e) Malignant transformation depends on polyp size, histological architecture and severity of epithelial dysplasia. Villous adenomas greater than 4 cm in diameter are likely to undergo malignant transformation.

Tubular Adenomas

- May **arise anywhere in the colon; about half found in the rectosigmoid.**
- May be **solitary** or **multiple.**
- Large adenomas usually have a slender stalk 1–2 cm long with a raspberry-like head.

Histology

- **Stalk covered by normal colonic mucosa whereas the head is composed of branching glands lined by dysplastic epithelium, which may or may not be mucin secreting (Fig. 27.16).**
- All degrees of atypia may be encountered. **Cancer may be limited to mucosa (intramucosal carcinoma)** or be **frankly invasive, extending into the submucosa of the stalk.**

Villous Adenomas

- **Finger-like polyps**, which are larger than most epithelial polyps.
- Usually seen in the **rectosigmoid**; generally, **sessile, broad-based** and **velvety or cauliflower-like.**

Histology

- **Filiform extensions of mucosa covered by dysplastic epithelium (Fig. 27.17).**
- All degrees of dysplasia may be encountered.
- **Invasive carcinoma is seen in about 40% of these lesions.**

Tubulovillous Adenomas

- Show an admixture of tubular and villous areas.
- They are intermediate between tubular and villous adenomas in terms of their histology and behaviour.

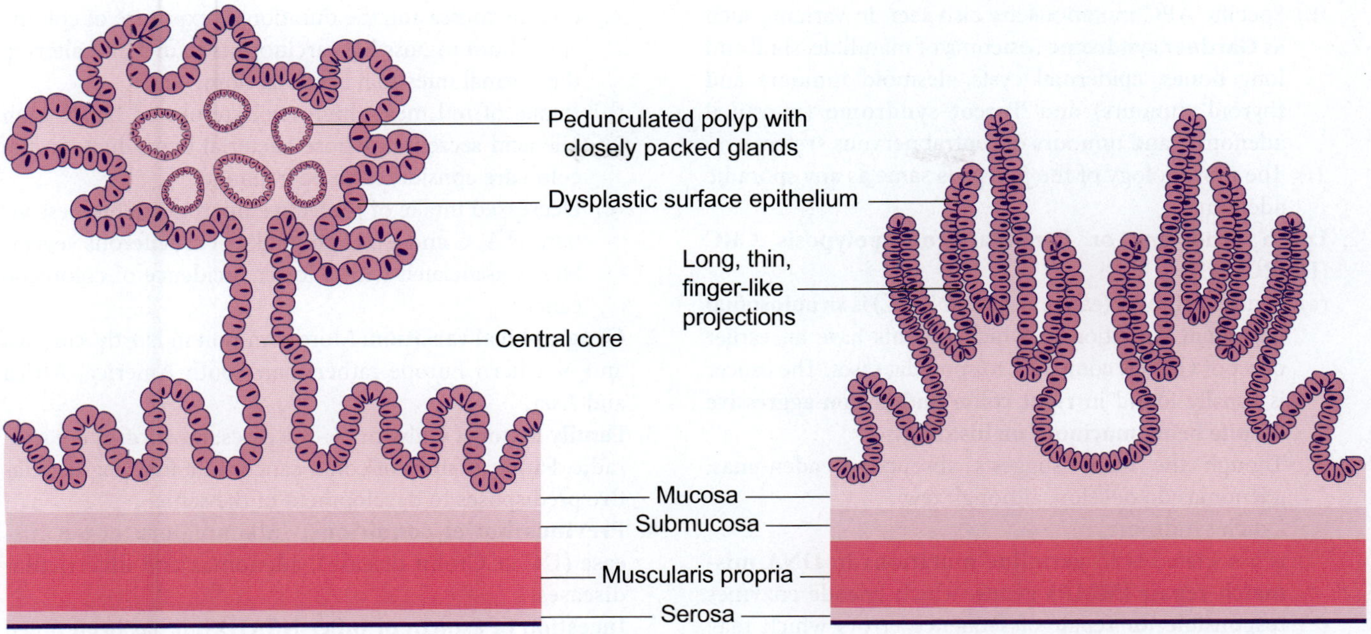

Fig. 27.16 (Left) Tubular adenoma comprising a stalk covered by normal colonic mucosa and a head composed of branching glands lined by dysplastic epithelium.
Fig. 27.17 (Right) Villous adenoma comprising filiform extensions of mucosa covered by dysplastic epithelium.

Sessile Serrated Adenomas

- **Premalignant sessile lesions of colon.**
- More common in the **right colon.**
- Overlap histologically with hyperplastic polyps but unlike hyperplastic polyps have a serrated architecture through the entire length of the gland (in hyperplastic polyps the serrated architecture is limited to the surface of the gland).

Q. Differentiate between tubular and villous adenomas.

Ans. Differences between tubular and villous adenomas are listed in Table 27.8.

Q. Write briefly on hereditary cancer syndromes of colon. (PA24.7)

Ans. Gastrointestinal polyps can develop as sporadic lesions or as part of hereditary polyposis syndromes. The most common colonic cancer-associated syndromes include:

1. **Familial adenomatous polyposis (FAP)**
   (a) This is an **autosomal dominant disorder with a genetic defect** (inactivating mutations) **localised to the APC gene on chromosome 5q21.**
   (b) APC is a tumour suppressor gene involved in cell cycle control and downregulation of beta-catenin through the Wnt signalling pathway. The APC protein is normally involved in apoptosis of colonic epithelial cells and its mutations may cause uncontrolled proliferation of the crypt base cell population, including crypt stem cells. Mutant crypt stem cells may clonally expand to form adenomas and carcinomas.
   (c) Patients with FAP typically develop a **large number of polyps**, which carpet the entire colon.
   (d) **A minimum number of 100 are required for the diagnosis.**
   (e) Adenomas may also be present in other parts of the intestine, for example duodenum.
   (f) Polyps manifest as early as adolescence or early adulthood.
   (g) Conversion to colonic cancer is 100% by middle age.

Table 27.8 Differences between tubular and villous adenomas

Features	Tubular adenoma	Villous adenoma
Architecture	>75% tubular architecture	>50% villous architecture
Incidence	90%–95% (most common)	1% of all adenomas
Distribution	90% cases in colon	More in rectum and rectosigmoid
Age	Early	Late
Gross	Small; pedunculated	Large, sessile or cauliflower-like
Histology	Stalk has fibromuscular tissue and prominent blood vessels; covered by non-neoplastic mucosa. Head region shows tubule-like structures lined by dysplastic cells (instead of the normal mucin-secreting colonic mucosa)	Villiform mucosa covered by dysplastic, disorderly columnar epithelium
Risk of malignancy	Low	High

(h) Specific APC mutations are also seen in variants such as **Gardner syndrome** (osteoma of mandible, skull and long bones, epidermal cysts, desmoid tumours and thyroid tumours) and **Turcot syndrome** (intestinal adenomas and tumours of central nervous system).

(i) The morphology of the polyps is same as any sporadic adenoma.

2. **Lynch syndrome or hereditary non-polyposis CRC (HNPCC)**

(a) Lynch syndrome (earlier called HNPCC) is an **autosomal dominant** condition in which patients have an earlier onset of CRC as compared to sporadic cases. The cancer is usually found in **right colon and is non-aggressive despite being mucinous on histology**.

(b) Though the name suggests absence of adenomas; adenomas do develop, although few.

(c) Lynch syndrome.

(d) is associated with **germline mutations in DNA mismatch repair (MMR) genes,** which encode enzymes responsible for repair of sequence errors which may occur during DNA replication. An important diagnostic feature of MMR-deficient tumours is the high rate of mutations that accumulate in repetitive nucleotide regions and these mutations are known as **microsatellite instability (MSI)**.

(e) Based on the micro satellite length MSI is divided into three groups, namely, MSI-high (MSI-H), MSI-low and MSI-stable (MSI-S).

(f) Six MMR genes have been identified and are designated as hMSH2, hMSH6, hMLH1, hMLH3, hPMSH1 and hPMSH2.

(g) **Germline mutations in MSH2 or MLH1 are most common**; germline mutations in MSH6 or PMS2 are less frequent.

(h) Mutations in EPCAM (epithelial cellular adhesion molecule)/TACSTD1 (tumour-associated calcium signal transducer 1) gene may result in Lynch syndrome: EPCAM gene is adjacent to MSH2 and mutations in EPCAM may result in MSH2 promoter hypermethylation and subsequent inactivation of MSH2.

(i) Most common hereditary colorectal carcinoma syndrome (accounts for 2%–5% of all colorectal carcinomas); 80% patients with Lynch syndrome develop colorectal carcinoma.

(j) **Extracolonic cancers associated with Lynch syndrome include: cancers of stomach, small intestine, endometrium, ovary and urinary bladder.**

Q. Write briefly on the aetiopathogenesis, morphology and staging of colorectal carcinoma.

(PA24.7)

Ans. Adenocarcinoma of colon is the most common malignant tumour of colorectal region.

Aetiopathogenesis

1. **Dietary factors**

(a) High content of refined carbohydrate and low content of dietary fibre reduces bulk, increases transit time, thereby increasing the duration of exposure of colonic epithelium to possible carcinogens in diet and altering the normal intestinal bacterial flora.

(b) Intake of red meat (high cholesterol and hence high bile acid secretion, whose bacterial byproducts in the colon are considered to be irritants).

(c) Decreased intake of protective micronutrients (less vitamins A, C and E). High intake of cruciferous vegetables is associated with a lower incidence of colorectal cancer.

2. **Geographical variation:** More common in North America and Northern Europe rather than South America, Africa and Asia.
3. **Family history:** Only in 1%–3% cases; most cases are sporadic. Family history of colon cancer in a first degree relative predisposes to development of the same.
4. **Previous bowel conditions:** Inflammatory bowel disease (UC > Crohn disease), adenomas and diverticular diseases.
5. **Ingestion of aspirin or other NSAIDS:** It has been noted that aspirin and other NSAIDs may have a protective role in colorectal carcinogenesis as they inhibit cyclooxygenase-2 (COX-2) which is expressed in 90% colorectal cancers. COX-2 is instrumental in production of PGE-2 which is thought to be responsible for epithelial proliferation.
6. **Others:** Physical inactivity, obesity specially abdominal, smoking, excessive alcohol and sugar consumption.

CRC results from the progressive accumulation of multiple genetic and epigenetic aberrations within cells. The progression from colorectal adenoma to carcinoma is caused by three major pathways: Microsatellite instability, chromosomal instability and CpG island methylator phenotype. Two distinct molecular pathways have been implicated in CRC and they are:

1. **Adenoma-carcinoma sequence (APC β-catenin pathway; Flowchart 27.2):**

(a) This pathway is responsible for 80% sporadic colonic cancers and involves a series of genetic alterations accompanying the progressive conversion of normal mucosa to malignancy.

(b) **APC** is the chief negative regulator of β-catenin, which in turn forms a part of the **Wnt signalling pathway.**

(c) APC protein binds to and degrades **β-catenin.**

(d) The latter accumulates if there is loss of APC and moves to the nucleus where it complexes with the DNA-binding factor TCF to induce transcription of genes like MYC and Cyclin D1, which promote cellular proliferation. Both copies of APC must be inactivated by mutation or epigenetic events for accumulation of β-catenin.

(e) The **KRAS gene** belongs to the *RAS* gene family involved in signalling pathways that regulate cellular proliferation, differentiation or survival. Several studies have reported an association between *KRAS* mutations, and poor prognosis of CRC. In contrast, several other studies reported that *KRAS* mutations were strong independent predictors of survival in patients with CRC. These contradictory

Normal mucosal epithelium

↓

Germline (inherited) or somatic (acquired) mutation of cancer suppressor 'gatekeeper' APC (adenomatous polyposis coli) gene located at 5q21 (first hit)

↓

Hyperproliferative epithelium

↓

Methylation abnormalities or inactivation of normal alleles of APC, β-catenin, and MutS Homolog 2 or MSH2 (second hit)

↓

Early adenoma

↓

Mutation in proto-oncogene (K-RAS at 12p12)

↓

Intermediate adenoma

↓

Homozygous loss of additional cancer suppressor genes-LOH at 18q21 (Mothers against decapentaplegic homolog 2 or SMAD2 and SMAD4 genes, which affect TGF-β-signalling)

↓

Late adenoma

↓

- Homozygous loss of additional cancer suppressor gene p53 at 17p13.
- Additional mutations and gross chromosomal alteration of many genes

↓

Carcinoma

Flowchart 27.2 Adenoma–carcinoma sequence (APC β-catenin pathway).

findings may be explained by the differences in the distribution of specific *KRAS* mutations, stage at diagnosis or other characteristics. *KRAS* mutations have emerged as an important predictive marker of resistance to anti-epidermal growth factor receptors (*EGFR*) agents, including panitumumab and cetuximab. Activating *KRAS* mutations have been identified in 35%–45% of CRC cases.

(f) **Allelic loss at chromosome 18q** is detected in 70% of CRC in the late carcinogenic process, and is considered as a poor prognosis marker in patients with CRC. The high frequency of allelic deletions involving chromosome 18q suggests the presence of candidate tumour-suppressor genes whose inactivation may serve a significant role in CRC, including *SMAD2* and *SMAD4* (Mothers against decapentaplegic homolog 2 and 4). These *SMAD* genes encode downstream signal transducers for transforming growth factor-β (*TGF-β*), and their alterations may confer resistance to TGF-β and contribute to tumourigenesis.

(g) **TP53 loss of function** has been reported in 50–75% of CRC cases, much higher compared with that in adenoma, indicating its role in the transition from an adenoma to carcinoma. Majority of the TP53 mutations reported in CRC are missense mutations followed by point mutations that are transitions at CpG sites. CpG sites are regions in some genes that include the promoter and transcriptional start site. Cytosines in CpG nucleotides are normally unmethylated. Methylation of cytosine causes gene silencing.

(h) Most adenomas do not demonstrate **telomerase activity** whereas CRCs demonstrate increasing telomerase activity as the lesion progresses.

2. **Microsatellite instability pathway (defective DNA repair):**
   (a) Microsatellites are repeated sequences of 1–6 nucleotides in the genome. They may undergo insertion or deletion of bases during normal cellular replication and these are corrected by DNA mismatch repair (MMR) genes.
   (b) Deficiency in cellular MMR leads to widespread mutagenesis and neoplastic development.
   (c) An important diagnostic feature of MMR-deficient tumours is the high rate of mutations that accumulate in repetitive nucleotide regions and these mutations are known as microsatellite instability (MSI).
   (d) A standard panel of markers to test for MSI in tumours has been recommended and efficiently separates tumours into those with high, low or no microsatellite instability (MSI-H, MSI-L or MSS).
   (e) There is a minority of CRCs with MSI in which the MMR genes do not demonstrate any mutations. These tumours instead have hypermethylation of MLH1 promoter region and may show mutations in BRAF oncogene. Theses are labelled 'CpG island hypermethylation phenotype (CIMP)'.

Gross Morphology (Fig. 27.18A)

Can be found anywhere in the colon and are typically seen as **exophytic polypoid and annular constricting growths in the right-sided and left-sided colon respectively.** The latter are also referred to as **'apple core'or'napkin-ring' lesions.** Right-side colonic tumours grow along the wall of the caecum and colon and rarely cause obstruction, whereas, left-sided tumours are associated with intestinal obstruction and desmoplasia. Diffusely infiltrating tumours mimicking linitis plastica of stomach may also be seen.

Microscopic Features

- Ninety-eight percent of all colonic cancers are **adenocarcinomas**, which vary in differentiation from well differentiated (Fig. 27.18B) to poorly differentiated anaplastic tumours.
- Mucin-producing tumours have a poorer prognosis (mucin facilitates spread of tumours as it dissects through the gut wall).
- Signet-ring appearance of tumour cells and endocrine differentiation may be seen.
- Anal carcinomas are usually squamous in origin.

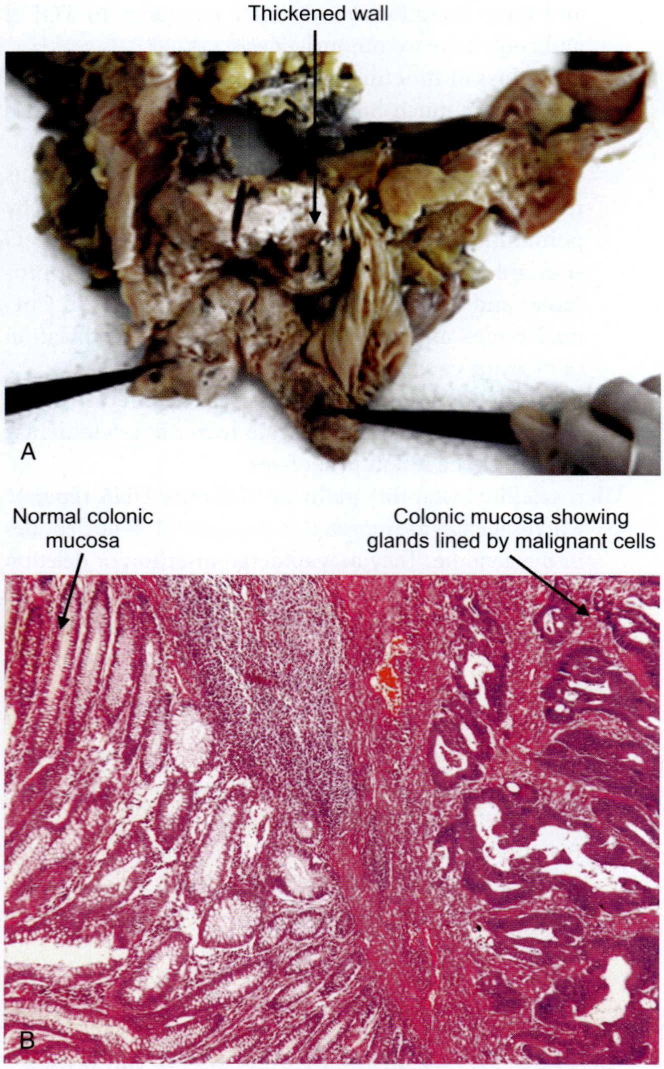

Fig. 27.18 (A) Gross picture of adenocarcinoma colon showing an infiltrating growth pattern. (B) Section from adenocarcinoma colon showing junction of normal (left) and neoplastic (right) mucosa (H&E; 200×).

Spread of Tumour

- Direct spread.
- Lymphatic spread to local lymph nodes, regional and distant lymph node groups.
- Haematogenous spread to liver, lungs, brain, bones and ovaries.

Prognosis

Most important prognostic criteria for colorectal carcinoma are:

- Depth of invasion (invasion into muscular propria is associated with an adverse prognosis).
- Presence or absence of lymph node metastasis (lymph node metastasis reduces the survival rate).
- Poor differentiation/mucinous tumours (are associated with a bad prognosis).

The earlier used Dukes and Kirklin and Astler–Coller staging systems have been replaced by TNM and American Joint Committee on Cancer (AJCC) staging systems.

Q. Enumerate the various modalities for diagnosing colorectal carcinoma.

Ans. Modalities for diagnosing colorectal carcinoma:

1. Digital rectal examination.
2. Testing for occult blood loss in stool by Guaiac test.
3. Double contrast barium enema (apple-core appearance), sigmoidoscopy or colonoscopy and endoscopy-directed biopsy.
4. Computed tomography and other radiographic techniques to look for the primary as well as the spread.
5. Serum markers like CEA (has little diagnostic value as levels become significantly elevated only after the tumour has achieved a considerable size; CEA levels also elevated in carcinoma of lung, breast, ovary, urinary bladder and prostate and non-neoplastic disorders like alcoholic cirrhosis, pancreatitis and ulcerative colitis).
6. Molecular detection of APC mutations in epithelial cells from stool is being considered as a diagnostic tool.

Q. Differentiate between right-sided and left-sided colonic carcinoma.

Ans. Differences between right-sided and left-sided colonic carcinoma are listed in Table 27.9.

Q. Describe the clinicopathological features of carcinoid tumour of GIT.

Ans. Salient features of carcinoid tumour of GIT:

- Derived from cells of neuroendocrine origin, which are normally present throughout the GI mucosa.
- Constitute about 2% of colorectal malignancies and almost half of the small intestinal malignant tumours.

Table 27.9 Differences between right-sided and left-sided colonic carcinoma

Features	Right-sided colonic carcinoma	Left-sided colonic carcinoma
Site	Caecum and ascending colon	Descending colon and sigmoid
Gross appearance	Fungating polypoid carcinoma. Large cauliflower-like soft friable mass projecting into lumen	Ulcerative or ulceroinfiltrative lesions producing a napkin-ring constriction (annular ring). May show central ulceration with slightly elevated margins
Clinical features	Bleed readily; fatigue, weakness, iron deficiency anaemia. Obstructive symptoms less common due to a larger area available for the tumour to expand	Occult bleeding, change in bowel habits, crampy lower left quadrant discomfort, constipation and obstructive symptoms more prominent
Diagnosis	Late	Early (due to early onset of obstructive symptoms)

- Release peptide and non-peptide hormones, which are responsible for their clinical manifestations.
- Usually arise in the pancreas, peripancreatic tissue, lungs, biliary tree and liver. In the GIT, appendix is the most common site followed by ileum, rectum, stomach and colon.
- No age is exempt, peak incidence during sixth decade.
- Cut surface is solid and yellow-tan.
- The tumour cells have argentaffin granules which stain positive with silver stains.
- Carcinoids are slow-growing tumours with different characteristics and growth patterns and can be subdivided based on the following features:
  - Growth pattern (trabecular, glandular, undifferentiated and mixed).
  - Hormone produced (bradykinin, serotonin, histamine and prostaglandins).
  - Site of origin: foregut (pancreas, stomach and duodenum), midgut (jejunum, ileum, appendix and ascending colon) or hind gut (transverse colon, descending colon and rectum).

Gross Morphology

- Small button-like submucosal elevation with intact or ulcerated overlying mucosa.
- Ileal and gastric carcinoids are multiple, whereas appendiceal carcinoids are solitary and usually involve the tip of the organ.

Microscopic Features

- Tumour cells are uniform and *monotonous* in appearance, forming discrete islands, glands, cords or trabeculae (Fig. 27.19).
- They have scanty cytoplasm and round-to-oval nucleus with fine stippled (salt and pepper) chromatin.
- Mitoses is infrequent and cellular atypia is uncommon.
- Other features: Presence of membrane-bound secretory granules (or dense core granules), containing chromogranin A, synaptophysin, neuron-specific enolase, etc. These can be demonstrated with immunohistochemical stains.

Characteristic Features of Carcinoids in Specific Locations

Terminal Ileum

- Peak involvement in seventh decade.
- Female predominance.
- Multicentric.
- Metastasize widely.

Appendix

- Most common gut carcinoid.
- Affects patients in the third and fourth decades of life.
- Usually solitary.
- Behave like locally malignant tumours/metastasis is rare (rectal and appendiceal carcinoids, almost never metastasize).

Hind Gut Carcinoids

- Constitute 10%–20% of all cases.
- Involve mainly rectum and colon.

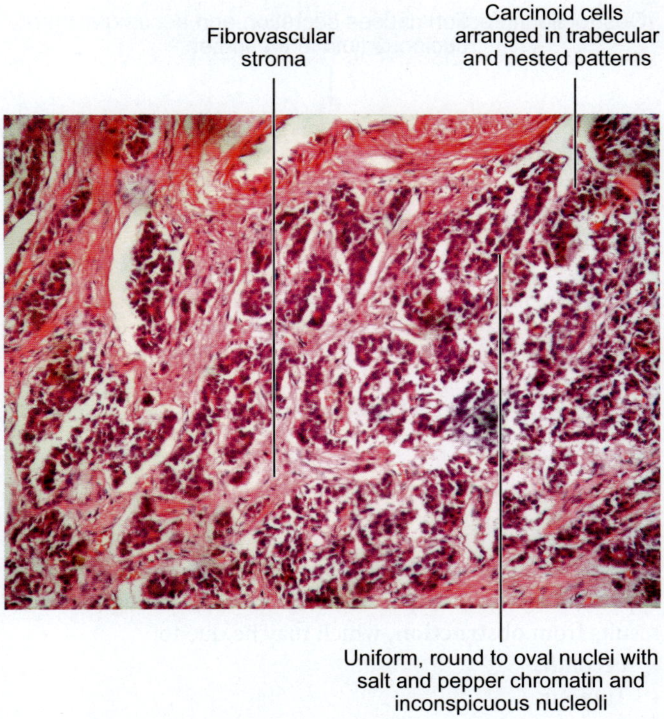

Fig. 27.19 Carcinoid tumour comprising uniform and monotonous appearing tumour cells forming discrete islands, glands, cords or trabeculae and having scanty cytoplasm and round-to-oval nucleus with fine stippled chromatin (H&E; 100×).

Foregut Carcinoids

- Argentaffin-negative.
- Seen in stomach, duodenum and oesophagus.

Carcinoid Syndrome

Salient Features

- It is present in 1% of all carcinoid tumour patients.
- More common in patients in whom the tumour has widely metastasized, particularly to the liver. Loss of liver function is essential for the syndrome to manifest, as liver normally converts active 5-HT (5-hydroxytryptamine or serotonin) into its inactive form 5-HIAA (5-hydroxy indole acetic acid).
- **Secretory product** mainly responsible for the syndrome is **5-HT;** histamine, bradykinin, prostaglandins, etc., may also contribute.

Clinical Presentation

- Cutaneous flushes and cyanosis *(vasomotor disturbances).*
- Diarrhoea, cramps, nausea and vomiting *(due to intestinal hyper motility).*
- Cough, dyspnoea and wheezing *(asthmatic bronchoconstrictive attack due to released mediators).*
- Hepatic metastasis causing nodular liver *(hepatomegaly)* in some patients.
- *Systemic fibrosis* involving heart (right-sided valvular stenosis and endocardial fibrosis), retroperitoneal and pelvic fibrosis in other patients.

Obstruction/infection causes secretion and accumulation of mucinous fluid in the lumen

↓

Increased intraluminal pressure

↓

Impairs venous drainage by compressing veins

↓

Ischaemic injury and bacterial proliferation result in further inflammation, oedema, exudation and ischaemic injury to appendix

Flowchart 27.3 Pathogenesis of acute appendicitis.

Q. Describe the clinicopathological features of acute appendicitis.

Ans. Acute appendicitis is defined as acute inflammation of appendix. It is generally seen in children and young adult and results from **obstruction,** which may be due to:

- Fecolith.
- Tumour.
- Foreign body.
- Oxyuris vermicularis.
- Diffuse lymphoid hyperplasia.

Other Causes

- Inappropriate intake of roughage.
- Haematogenous spread of infection to appendix.
- Vascular occlusion.
- Idiopathic.

Pathogenesis (See Flowchart 27.3)

Morphology

The histological hallmark for the diagnosis of acute appendicitis is neutrophilic infiltration of the muscularis propria.

Normal Appendix

- Serosa is glistening and thin.
- No neutrophilic infiltrate observed in the muscle layer.

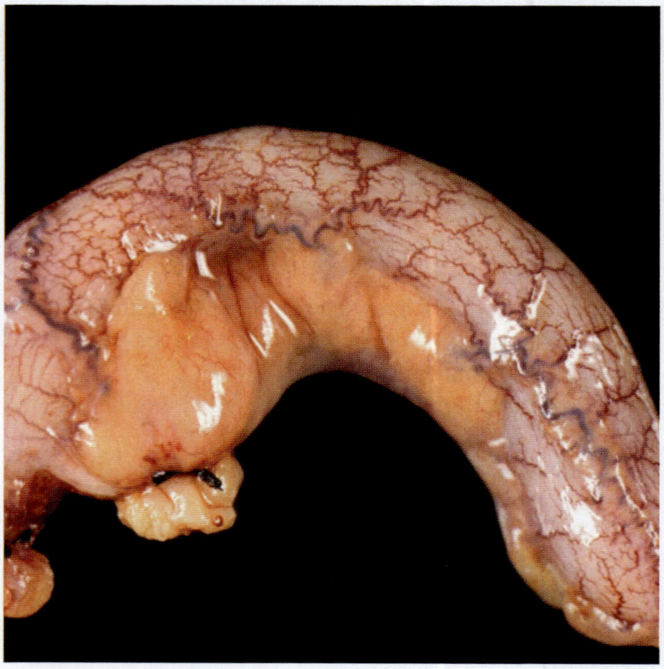

Fig. 27.20 Gross specimen of swollen appendix with a hyperaemic, dull and granular mucosa and congested subserosal vessels. (*Source: Diagnostic Pathology: Gastrointestinal,* 2ed.: Gregory Y. Lauwers, Amitabh Srivastava, Joel K. Greenson, et. al., Acute Appendicitis, Elsevier Inc., 2016.)

Acute Appendicitis (Fig. 27.20)

- Organ swollen with a hyperaemic, dull and granular mucosa.
- Neutrophilic infiltration in mucosa, submucosa and muscularis propria.
- Subserosal vessels congested.

Acute Suppurative Appendicitis

- Serosa is coated with a fibrinopurulent exudate.
- Prominent ulceration and necrosis in the mucosa.

Diseases of Hepatobiliary System and Pancreas

28

LIVER

- Largest solid organ in the body (1200–1500 g).
- Divided into right and left lobes by the falciform ligament, the fissure of ligamentum teres and the fissure of ligamentum venosum.
- Surgical division into **right and left hemilivers** by the middle hepatic vein, which lies between the inferior vena cava and the gallbladder, and passes through the porta hepatis.
- The right and left hemilivers are further subdivided into a total of eight segments in accordance with subdivisions of hepatic vasculature.
- Each segment is made up of histological units called **'lobules'**; each lobule is composed of a central vein, radiating sinusoids, separated from each other by plates of hepatocytes containing bile canaliculi and peripherally located portal tracts (Fig. 28.1). Hepatocytes are large polyhedral cells arranged as flat, anastomosing plates, one cell thick. Venous sinusoids have **kupffer cells** that are liver macrophages. Between the sinusoids and the hepatocytes are seen storage cells called **Ito cells**.
- The portal tracts contain branches of hepatic artery, portal vein, bile ducts and hepatic lymphatics, and comprise the main connective tissue stroma of the liver.
- Different regions of the lobule are referred to as **'periportal', 'mid-zonal' and 'centrilobular'.**
- Using the hepatic vasculature as reference, the liver architecture is divided into **'acini'.**
- On the basis of distance from the portal vessels, acinus is divided into **'zone 1' (closest to the portal vessels), 'zone 2' and 'zone 3' (farthest from the portal vessel).**
- Bile flows in the opposite direction along the **biliary canaliculi into terminal bile ductules (cholangioles)** and then **interlobular bile ducts** located in the portal tracts.

Q. Enumerate the important functions of liver.

Ans. Functions of liver

1. **Metabolic**
   - Metabolism of carbohydrates, proteins and lipids
2. **Synthetic**
   - Albumin
   - Coagulation factors
   - Complement
   - Haptoglobin
   - Ceruloplasmin
   - Transferrin
   - Protease inhibitors
3. **Storage**
   - Iron
   - Copper
   - Vitamins A, D and B_{12}
4. **Excretion**
   - Bile salts
   - Bilirubin

Q. Write briefly on bilirubin metabolism. (PA25.1)

Ans. Metabolism of bilirubin (Figure 28.2; Flowchart 28.1):

- **80%–85%** of bilirubin is derived from the catabolism of the haemoglobin of senescent red blood cells.
- **15%–20%** is derived from the bone marrow, destruction of maturing cells, liver and the turnover of haem and haem-containing precursors (cytochromes, myoglobin, etc.).

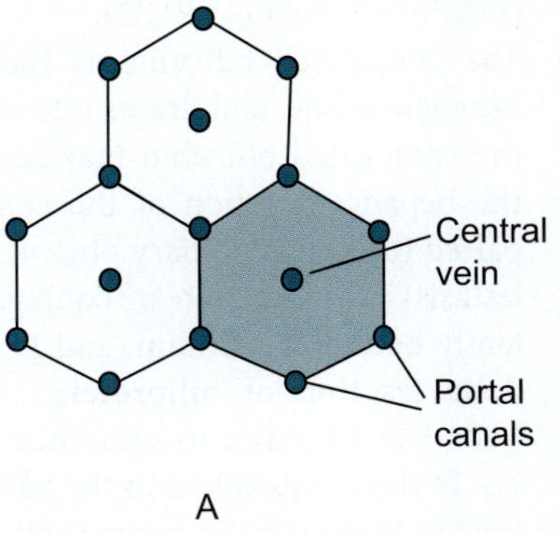

Fig. 28.1 Schematic diagram of a (A) Lobule and (B) Acinus.

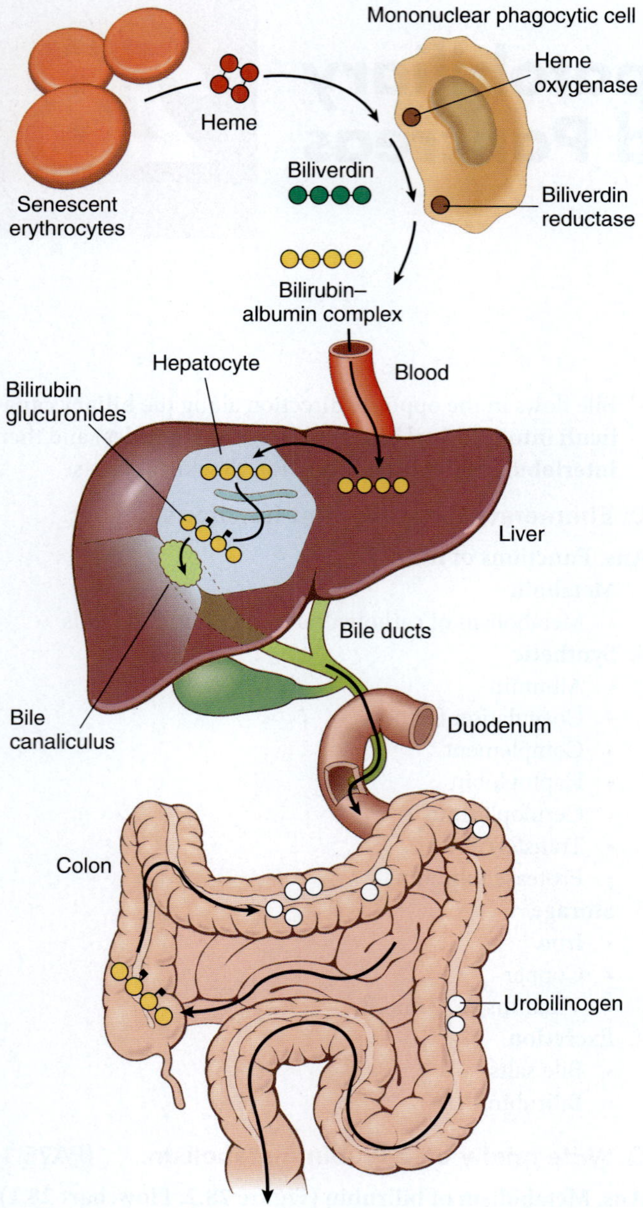

Fig. 28.2 Bilirubin metabolism. (*Source: Robbins & Cotran Pathologic Basis of Disease,* 10ed: Vinay Kumar, Abul K. Abbas, Jon C. Aster, Fig. 18.26: Sanjay Kakar, Ryan M. Gill, Elsevier Inc., 2021.)

- Heme is a ring of four pyrroles joined by carbon bridges and a central iron atom.
- Bilirubin is generated by a by a two-stage degradation reaction that mainly takes place in the cells of the reticuloendothelial system (spleen and the Kupffer cells of the liver).
- The enzyme **heme oxygenase** acts on heme to liberate the chelated iron and leads to the formation of the green pigment, **biliverdin**. This is the rate-limiting step in bilirubin production.
- This green pigment is acted upon further by the nicotinamide adenine dinucleotide phosphate (NADPH) dependent enzyme, **biliverdin reductase** leading to formation of an orange-yellow pigment known as **bilirubin**.
- Bilirubin, being insoluble in aqueous solution, is carried in circulation bound to **albumin,** which is a reversible and covalent type of bonding.
- The binding affinity of albumin for bilirubin is extremely high, and under ideal conditions, no free (non-albumin bound) unconjugated bilirubin is seen in the plasma. To a lesser degree, especially in states of hypoalbuminaemia, binding also occurs with high-density lipoprotein.
- When the albumin-bilirubin complex reaches the liver, it gets dissociated.
- Bilirubin is then taken up into the hepatocytes from the liver sinusoids by two different mechanisms: **passive diffusion** and **receptor-mediated endocytosis**. The process of passive diffusion is not energy-consuming and as a result, follows a concentration gradient. Active transporter uptake is mediated by carrier proteins 1A and 1B (members of the organic anion transporting polypeptide family or OATP). These polypeptides are encoded by the genes: *SLCO1B1* and *SLCO1B3*. Within the hepatocyte bilirubin binds to cytosolic proteins known as **glutathione-S-transferases (Ligandins)**. Conjugated bilirubin that escapes reuptake into the hepatocyte is excreted in the urine.
- Conjugation renders bilirubin soluble in aqueous solutions and facilitates its secretion across the canalicular membrane for excretion into bile. Bilirubin is conjugated within the hepatocyte to glucuronic acid by a family of enzymes, termed **uridine-diphosphoglucuronic glucuronosyltransferase (UDPGT)**. Many different isoforms of UDPGT exist, but the physiologically important isoform in bilirubin glucuronidation is **UDPGT1A1**.
- Under normal conditions, bilirubin diglucuronide is the predominant molecule synthesised. However, if the conjugation system is overwhelmed under conditions of excessive bilirubin synthesis, the majority of bilirubin may be conjugated as bilirubin monoglucuronide. The ratio of mono-conjugated to the diconjugated pigment in bile is 1:4.
- Conjugated bilirubin is actively transported across the bile canalicular membrane of the hepatocyte. There are at least four known canalicular transporters that participate in excretion of conjugated bilirubin. However, the **multidrug resistance-associated protein 2 (MRP2)** appears to play the dominant role in the canalicular secretion of conjugated bilirubin. A portion of conjugated bilirubin is transported into the sinusoids and portal circulation by MRP3, which can undergo hepatocyte reuptake via the sinusoidal proteins, organic anion transport protein 1B1 and 1B3 (OATP1B1 and OATP1B3).
- The conjugated bilirubin is then actively secreted into canalicular bile, and drains into the small intestine. Part of the conjugated bilirubin may accumulate in serum when the hepatic excretion of the conjugated bilirubin is impaired (prolonged biliary obstruction or intrahepatic cholestasis). This fraction of conjugated bilirubin gets covalently bound to albumin, and is called **delta bilirubin** or **delta fraction** or **biliprotein**. As the delta bilirubin is bound to albumin, its clearance from serum takes about 12–14 days (equivalent to the half-life of albumin) in contrast to the usual 2–4 hours (half-life of bilirubin). Unconjugated bilirubin is partially reabsorbed across the lipid membrane of the small intestinal epithelium and undergoes

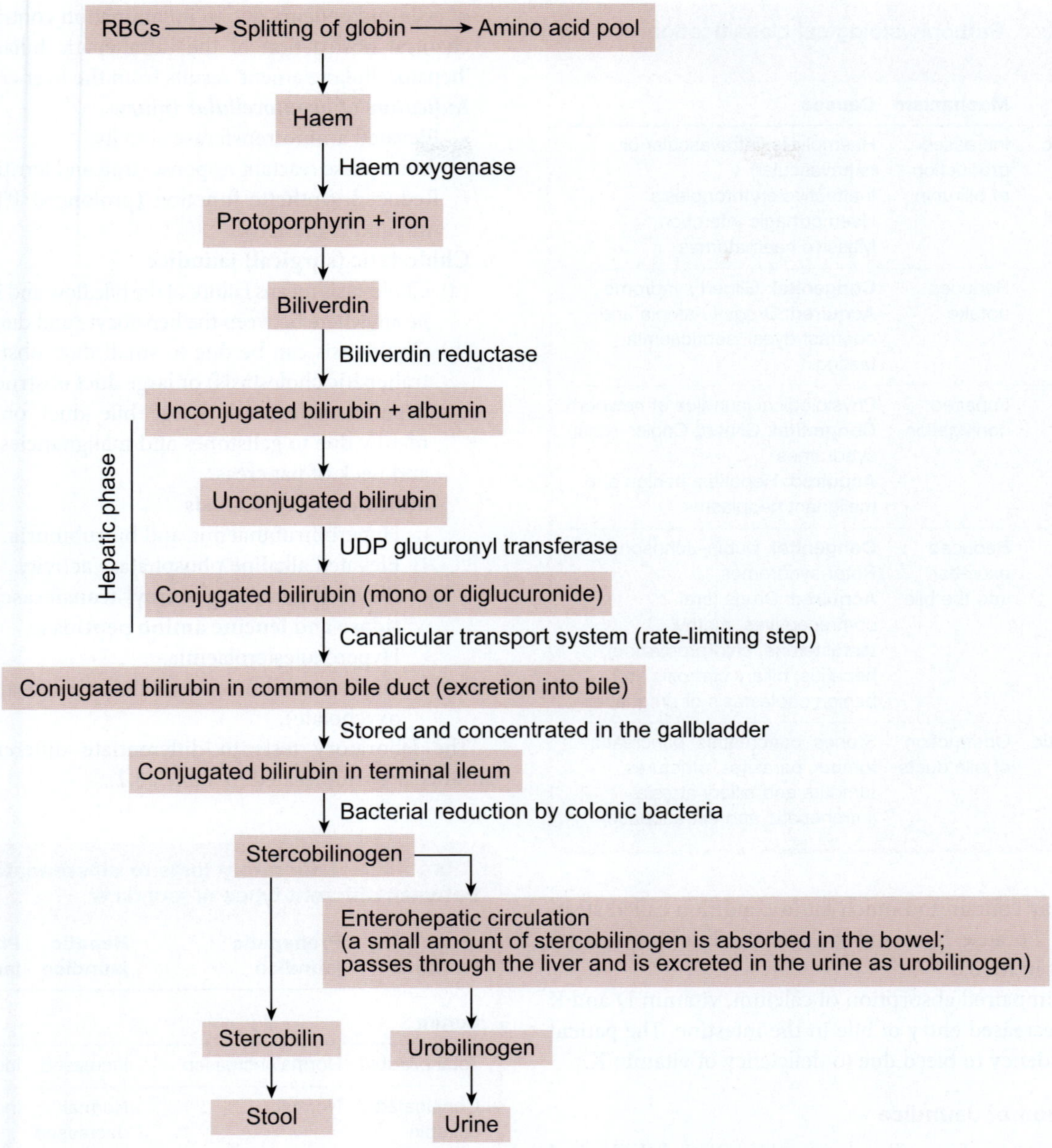

Flowchart 28.1 Bilirubin metabolism.

enterohepatic circulation. The conjugated bilirubin reaches the distal ileum and colon where it is rapidly reduced and deconjugated by colonic flora to a series of molecules termed **urobilinogen**.

- The major urobilinoids seen in stool are known as urobilinogen and stercobilinogen. These substances are colourless but turn orange-yellow after oxidation to **urobilin**, giving stool its distinctive colour.
- Unconjugated bilirubin tightly bound to albumin cannot be filtered by the glomeruli and is not excreted in the urine. Conjugated bilirubin is filtered by the glomeruli and is excreted in the urine.

Q. Define and classify jaundice. (PA25.1, 25.6)

Ans. Bilirubin and cholesterol have low-water solubility and cannot be excreted into urine. Bile is the primary pathway for elimination of both. Hepatocellular damage leads to a disruption in bile metabolism and manifests clinically as *jaundice* (yellowish pigmentation of skin and mucous membranes) and *icterus* (yellow discolouration of sclera). The latter occurs because bilirubin has a special affinity for elastin which is present abundantly in the sclera. Yellow discolouration is also prominent in the palpebral conjunctiva, sublingual mucosa and lower abdominal skin.

Clinical Features of Jaundice

- Jaundice (excess bilirubin deposited in the skin and mucosae).
- Dark urine (results from excess bilirubin excreted by the kidneys).
- Light-coloured stools (passage of bilirubin into the intestine is blocked).
- Generalised itchiness (retention of bile products in the skin may cause itching, with subsequent scratching and skin damage).

Table 28.1 Pathophysiological classification of jaundice

Type	Mechanism	Causes
Prehepatic	Increased production of bilirubin	Haemolysis (intravascular or extravascular) Ineffective erythropoiesis Haemorrhagic infarction Massive haematomas
Hepatic	Reduced uptake	**Congenital**: Gilbert syndrome **Acquired**: Drugs (rifampin and contrast dyes), septicaemia, fasting
	Impaired conjugation	Physiological jaundice of newborn **Congenital**: Gilbert, Crigler–Najar syndromes **Acquired**: Hepatitis, benign and malignant neoplasms
	Reduced excretion into the bile	**Congenital**: Dubin–Johnson and Rotor syndromes **Acquired**: Drugs (oral contraceptives, methyl testosterone, chlorpromazine), hepatitis, biliary cirrhosis and benign cholestasis of pregnancy
Posthepatic	Obstruction of bile ducts	Stones, pancreatitis, pancreatic tumour, parasites, strictures, tumours and biliary atresia (intrahepatic and extrahepatic)

- Stools may contain too much fat (a condition called steatorrhoea) because bile cannot enter the intestine to help digest fat in foods.
- There is impaired absorption of calcium, vitamin D and K due to decreased entry of bile in the intestine. The patient has a tendency to bleed due to deficiency of vitamin K.

Classification of Jaundice

The classification of jaundice is based on the **pathological mechanisms** underlying it (Table 28.1):

1. **Haemolytic jaundice**
   (a) Increased destruction of red blood cells or their precursors, resulting in a predominant increase in unconjugated bilirubin.
   (b) Absence of bilirubin in urine.
   (c) Urinary urobilinogen is increased (more than 4 mg/24 h).
   (d) Other liver function tests are normal.
   (e) Evidence of haemolytic anaemia (increased reticulocyte count, or presence of fragmented red cells or Schistocytes in the peripheral blood film, decreased haptoglobin, increased LDH and positive direct Coombs test).
2. **Hepatocellular jaundice:** In hepatocellular jaundice, concentration of both unconjugated and conjugated bilirubin is increased. It has two elements, an 'obstructive element', causing impaired uptake of unconjugated bilirubin into the cell and of conjugated bilirubin into biliary canaliculi. Swelling of cells and oedema due to inflammation contribute to mechanical obstruction of the intrahepatic biliary tree. The 'hepatocellular element' results from the liver cell damage.
   Indicators of hepatocellular injury:
   - Elevated aminotransferase activity.
   - Acute phase reactant response (iron and ferritin elevation).
   - Reduced synthetic function (prolonged PT, low albumin and cholesterol).
3. **Cholestatic (surgical) jaundice**
   (a) Cholestasis means failure of the bile flow and its cause may lie anywhere between the hepatocyte and duodenum.
   (b) Cholestasis can be due to small duct obstruction (intrahepatic cholestasis) or large duct obstruction (extrahepatic cholestasis). Large bile duct obstruction is mainly due to gallstones and malignancies of the head and neck of pancreas.
   Indicators of cholestasis
   - Hyperbilirubinaemia and bilirubinuria.
   - Elevated alkaline phosphatase activity.
   - Elevated **gamma glutamyl transferase, 5′ nucleotidase** and **leucine amino peptidase.**
   - Hypercholesterolaemia.
   - High-serum bile salts (mainly cholate and chenodeoxycholate).

The laboratory tests to differentiate different types of jaundice are enumerated in Table 28.2.

Table 28.2 Laboratory tests to differentiate between different types of jaundice

Features	Prehepatic jaundice	Hepatic jaundice	Posthepatic jaundice
Serum			
Total bilirubin	Normal/increased	Increased	Increased
Conjugated bilirubin	Normal	Normal/ decreased	Increased
Unconjugated bilirubin	Increased	Normal/ increased	Normal
Urobilinogen	Increased	Normal/ Increased	Decreased/ negative
Urine			
Bilirubin in urine	Absent	Absent	Present
Urinary urobilinogen	Increased (more than 4 mg/24 h)		
Peripheral smear	Evidence of haemolysis (increased reticulocyte count, schistocytes or fragmented red cells in the peripheral blood film, decreased haptoglobin, increased LDH and positive direct Coombs test)	Not seen	Not seen

Q. Write briefly on congenital non-haemolytic hyperbilirubinaemias.

Ans. Congenital non-haemolytic hyperbilirubinaemias include:

Gilbert Syndrome

- Autosomal recessive inheritance.
- Mild deficiency of UGT1A1 (Uridine diphosphate-glucuronyltransferase); Levels are reduced to 10%–35% of normal and result in unconjugated hyperbilirubinaemia.

Crigler–Najjar Syndrome—Type I

- Autosomal recessive inheritance.
- Complete absence of UGT1A1 activity.
- Severe unconjugated hyperbilirubinaemia and kernicterus leading to neonatal death.

Crigler–Najjar Syndrome—Type II

- Autosomal dominant inheritance.
- Partial deficiency of UGT1A1.
- Jaundice is milder than type I, kernicterus is occasionally seen.

Dubin–Johnson Syndrome

- Autosomal recessive inheritance.
- Decreased canalicular excretion of bilirubin into biliary canaliculi.
- Conjugated hyperbilirubinaemia and bilirubinuria.
- The degree of hyperbilirubinaemia may be increased by intercurrent illness, oral contraceptives and pregnancy.
- The syndrome is due to defective **MRP2** (multidrug resistance-associated protein 2), which is required for secretion of conjugated bilirubin from the hepatocytes into canaliculi.
- **BSP (bromsulphthalein) retention test shows impaired clearance with a reflux back into blood in 90 min.**
- Hepatomegaly with a **dark pigment** in centrilobular hepatocytes (derived from polymerised epinephrine metabolites).

Rotor Syndrome

- Autosomal recessive inheritance.
- Due to poor uptake and storage of bilirubin by liver cells.
- Mild jaundice, conjugated hyperbilirubinaemia and bilirubinuria.
- BSP retention test shows impaired clearance but there is no reflux back into blood.
- Liver biopsy is normal and does not show dark pigment.

Q. Outline the aetiology, epidemiology, clinical features and laboratory diagnosis of viral hepatitis. (PA25.3)

Ans. Viral hepatitis is defined as viral infection of the hepatocytes leading to inflammation of the liver.

Types of Viral Hepatitis

1. Hepatitis A caused by hepatitis A virus (HAV).
2. Hepatitis B caused by hepatitis B virus (HBV).
3. Delta hepatitis caused by hepatitis D virus (HDV).
4. Hepatitis C caused by hepatitis C virus (HCV).
5. Hepatitis E caused by hepatitis E virus (HEV).
6. Hepatitis G virus.
7. Hepatitis caused by other viruses (cytomegalovirus, Epstein–Barr virus, Herpes simplex virus and yellow fever virus).

1. **Hepatitis A**

   Aetiology

   Caused by hepatitis A virus (HAV), an RNA virus belonging to the Picornavirus group. The hepatocytic receptor for HAV is HAVcr-1 or TIM-1, a glycoprotein. The mechanism of hepatocellular injury involves cytotoxic T lymphocytes and NK cells that kill hepatocytes infected with the virus. HAV is not a cytopathic virus.

   Epidemiology

   - Incubation period is 2–6 weeks.
   - HAV is transmitted almost exclusively by the faeco-oral route (infected persons excrete the viruses in their faeces for two weeks before the onset and one week after the onset of the illness). Source of the infection is contaminated water, milk and raw or steamed-shell fish.
   - Can rarely spread by blood transfusions and homosexual activity.
   - Does not cause chronic liver disease or carrier state; rarely causes fulminant hepatitis (0.1% case fatality). Extrahepatic manifestations include immune complex-mediated complications like arthralgia, vasculitis, glomerulonephritis, and skin rash. Infection with HBVA can be prevented by its vaccine.
   - It is more common in children and rare in adults.

2. **Hepatitis B**

   Aetiology

   - Caused by an enveloped DNA virus called hepatitis B virus (HBV), belonging to the group of **hepadnaviruses.**
   - HBV is a 42 nm **'Dane particle'** composed of:
     - A **surface envelope** (antigen expressed on it is called hepatitis B surface antigen, **HBsAg**).
     - A **nucleocapsid core** containing DNA (antigen expressed on its surface is called hepatitis B core antigen or **HBcAg**).
     - Another soluble antigen in the nucleocapsid is called hepatitis B e-antigen or **HBeAg**.
     - A **DNA polymerase enzyme (pol)** that exhibits reverse transcriptase activity.
     - A protein from the X region, **HBX** necessary for viral replication; HBX controls gene transcription and thus acts as a gatekeeper for hepatocyte check points in cell cycle.
   - The corresponding antibodies are:
     - Anti-HBs
     - Anti-HBc
     - Anti-HBe

   ***Serological diagnosis* (Fig. 28.3):**

   - HBV enters hepatocytes by binding of HBsAg to the bile salt transporter, NTCP (sodium taurocholate cotransporting polypeptide). The viral genome is seen in the nucleus as a covalently closed circular DNA (cccDNA). HBV replication occurs by reverse transcription.

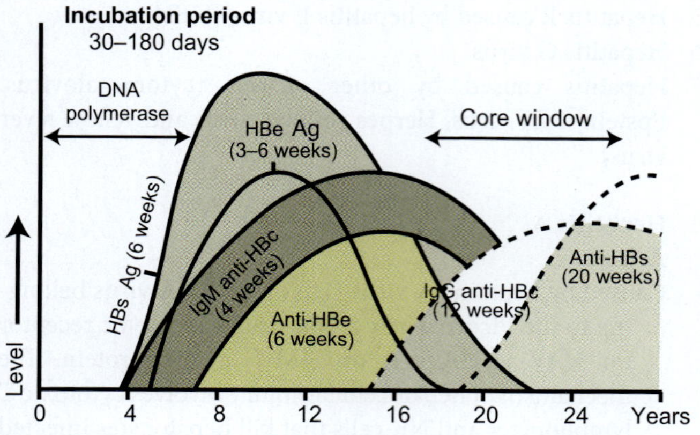

Fig. 28.3 Serological diagnosis of hepatitis B.

- Serum HBsAg is the first serum virological marker to appear. It appears in the later part of the incubation period or in the early prodrome of hepatitis B. Peak levels are reached during acute disease and the levels decline to undetectable levels in 3–6 months. Antibody to HBsAg is detected in the serum after HBsAg disappears.
- HBeAg, HBV–DNA and DNA polymerase are detected in the serum immediately after the appearance of HBsAg. Their presence indicates active viral replication.
- IgM anti-HBc appears in serum just before the patient manifests with acute disease (it is the earliest antibody to appear and is replaced by IgG anti-HBc over a period of few months.
- Persistence of detectable HBsAg beyond 6 months suggests chronic hepatitis B infection. In such cases, anti-HBs becomes negative but anti-HBc remains detectable.
- **Indicators of chronic replication:**
  - Persistence of circulating HBsAg, HBeAg and HBV DNA.
  - Presence of anti-HBc and occasionally anti-HBs.

Epidemiology

- Incubation period is about 1–4 months.
- Asymptomatic carriers or persons with acute hepatitis or chronic liver disease are the source of infection. It is present in all body fluids except stool.
- The main route of transmission of Hepatitis B is parenteral (commonly occurs after transfusion of infected blood or blood products, injections with contaminated needles, dialysis, tattooing and acupuncture). It spreads through body fluids like saliva, urine, semen and vaginal secretions.
- Mother-to-child spread (vertical or perinatal transmission) is also common.
- High-risk groups include spouses of persons having acute infection, homosexuals, healthcare workers, dentists and haemophiliacs.
- The incidence of a chronic carrier state in HBV infection varies between 1% and 20%.
- Acute HBV infection is mild in majority of patients with some patients having constitutional symptoms (anorexia, fever, jaundice, abdominal pain. May be associated with immune complex mediated vasculitis (PAN) and glomerulonephritis. Acute liver failure occurs in 0.1–0.5% acutely infected patients. Vaccination is highly effective.

3. **Delta hepatitis (hepatitis D)**

Aetiology

- It is caused by hepatitis D virus (HDV), which is a defective RNA virus. The RNA genome is encapsulated or covered by an outer coat of hepatitis B surface antigen.
- It requires hepatitis B virus for replication and expression.
- Incubation period is 1–4 months.
- HDV RNA is detectable in the blood and liver just before and during acute symptomatic disease.
- HDV can infect a person simultaneously with HBV **(coinfection)** or it may super infect a person who is already a chronic carrier of HBV **(super infection).**
- Acute coinfection by HBV and HDV is best suggested by presence of IgM against both HDAg and HBcAg.

Epidemiology

Two epidemiological patterns exist:

- Predominant transmission by non-parenteral route, especially close personal contact **(endemic areas).**
- Predominant transmission by parenteral route, that is persons exposed frequently to blood and blood products, mainly intravenous drug addicts and haemophiliacs **(non-endemic).**

4. **Hepatitis C**

Aetiology

- Formerly called blood-borne, non-A and non-B hepatitis, it is a single-stranded RNA virus belonging to the family *Flaviviridae.* It shows a lot of genomic instability and antigenic variability, thereby making it difficult to develop a vaccine against it.
- HCV has a single open reading frame that codes for a polyprotein which later gives rise to several functional proteins (two envelope proteins, E1 and E2, and five core proteins, p7, NS2, NS3/4a (a protease), NS5A (a replication complex) and NS5B (RNA polymerase). These viral proteins are targeted for developing drug antagonists for HCV.
- HCV RNA can be detected in the course of infection, well before the appearance of antibodies to HCV (Fig. 28.4).

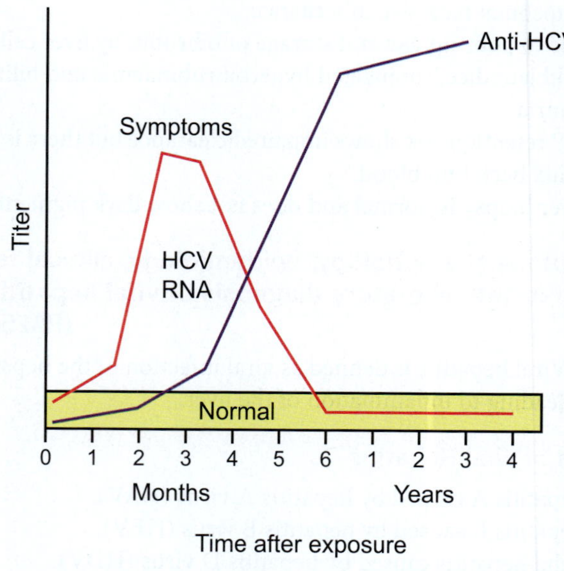

Fig. 28.4 Serological diagnosis and viral markers of hepatitis C.

Epidemiology

- Incubation period is 6–8 weeks.
- HCV is the cause of greater than 90% cases of post-transfusion hepatitis. Perinatal and sexual transmission can occasionally be seen.
- Carrier state is quite common with hepatitis C infection.
- HCV is rarely symptomatic but is the most common cause of chronic viral hepatitis. Anti-HCV antibody is found to be positive in more than 50% cases of unexplained cirrhosis or hepatocellular carcinoma.

5. **Hepatitis E**

Aetiology

- It is a non-enveloped single-stranded RNA virus belonging to the Hepevirus genus.
- It is responsible for 40%–60% cases of acute hepatitis in India. HEV antigen can be identified in the cytoplasm of hepatocytes during active infection. The virus itself can be isolated from the stools of the patient and anti-HEV IgG and IgM antibodies can be detected in serum.

Epidemiology

- Incubation period is 4–5 weeks.
- Primary mode of transmission is enteric (epidemic, water-borne hepatitis). Source of infection is animal reservoirs (monkeys, dogs, pigs and cats).
- A characteristic feature of HEV infection is the high-mortality rate among pregnant women.

6. **Hepatitis G**

- HGV is similar to viruses in the *Flaviviridae* family.
- Can be transmitted by blood transfusion.
- HGV coinfection is observed in 6% of chronic HBV infections and in 10% of chronic HCV infections; however, *whether HGV is actually pathogenic in humans remains unclear*.

Clinically, viral hepatitis evolves through the following phases: (*1*) asymptomatic, (*2*) acute and (*3*) chronic.

Asymptomatic Phase

Patients are identified incidentally based on elevated aminotransferases or presence of serological markers.

Acute Viral Hepatitis

Acute viral hepatitis is further subdivided into the following clinical stages:

1. *Incubation period:* The incubation period varies depending on the type of viral hepatitis.
2. *Symptomatic preicteric phase*: Also called prodromal phase, it lasts for a few days up to 2 weeks before the onset of jaundice, and manifests with fever, headache, malaise, anorexia, nausea, vomiting, diarrhoea, distaste for cigarettes and upper abdominal pain (due to stretching of liver capsule). Patients with HBV infection occasionally have a 'serum sickness-like syndrome' with skin rashes and polyarthralgia.
3. *Symptomatic icteric phase*: This is characterise by conjugated hyperbilirubinaemia with passage of dark urine and yellowish discolouration of the sclera. The constitutional symptoms diminish with the onset of clinical jaundice when the patient develops tender hepatomegaly. With progressively increasing obstruction to biliary canaliculi, jaundice worsens, stools become paler, urine becomes darker and liver becomes more palpable (cholestatic phase). Icteric phase is seen in HAV infection, but is rare in HBV and HCV infections.
4. *Convalescence or recovery phase*: There is improvement in the gastrointestinal symptoms; decrease in jaundice, normalisation of stools and urine and decrease in the liver size. The clinical and biochemical recovery should be complete in 1–2 months from the onset in cases of hepatitis A and E and in 3–4 months from the onset in hepatitis B and C.

Points to Remember

Delta coinfection is indistinguishable from acute hepatitis B, but **delta super infection** appears like an acute episode in a person chronically infected with HBV.

Hepatitis B, D and E can result in **fulminant hepatic failure.** It is uncommon with hepatitis A and C. Pregnant women suffering from hepatitis E have a high incidence of fulminant hepatitis (20%).

Anicteric hepatitis is a mild illness with an anicteric course (no clinical jaundice).

Morphological Features (Fig. 28.5)

- **Hepatocyte injury** and **ballooning degeneration** (swelling of hepatocytes with empty looking cytoplasm due to clumping of the cytoplasm around the nucleus).
- **Cholestasis** (seen as canalicular bile plugs).
- **Hepatocyte necrosis** (necrosis of isolated cells or clusters); can be of three types:
  1. **Cytolysis (dropout necrosis)** - Ballooning degeneration followed by rupture of the cellular membrane leading to focal loss of hepatocytes.
  2. **Apoptosis** (formation of apoptotic or **Councilman bodies**) - Councilman bodies appear intensely eosinophilic

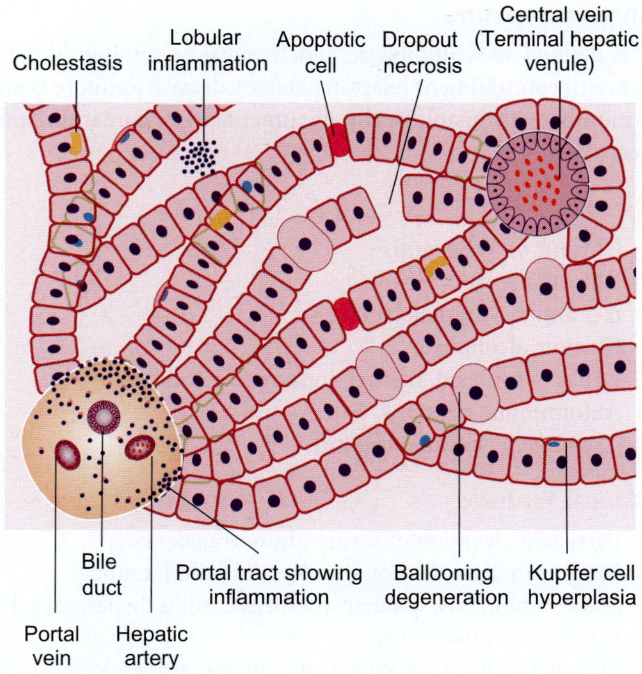

Fig. 28.5 Section from acute viral hepatitis showing hepatocyte necrosis and periportal inflammation.

with a densely staining or pyknotic nucleus, which may later fragment and get surrounded by effector T cells.

3. **Bridging necrosis** - Confluent necrosis of hepatocytes connecting portal–portal, portal–central, or central–central areas.

- **Lobular disarray** occurs due to a combination of hepatocyte necrosis, regenerative changes and inflammation and leads to loss of normal architecture.
- **Regenerative changes** including hepatocyte proliferation and reactive sinusoidal changes (Kupffer cell hyperplasia and hypertrophy) are usually seen.
- **Inflammation** - This is a prominent feature of acute hepatitis. The infiltrate is mainly mononuclear (lymphocytes and macrophages). The inflammation can be **lobular** (involving liver parenchyma away from the portal tracts or **interface** (can occur in both acute and chronic hepatitis; portal tracts show periportal inflammation with inflammatory spillover into adjacent parenchyma and hepatocyte necrosis).
- **HCV** infection is commonly associated with duct proliferation, lymphoid aggregates in the portal tracts and mild-fatty change.
- **HBV**-induced changes include development of fine granularity in the cytoplasm of liver cells or **ground glass appearance** due to the accumulation of spheres and tubules of HBsAg and **sanded nuclei** due to abundant intranuclear HBcAg.

Complications

- Fulminant hepatic failure
- Chronic hepatitis
- Cirrhosis
- Hepatocellular carcinoma
- Hepatocellular failure
- Renal failure

Chronic Hepatitis

It is defined as symptomatic, biochemical or serological evidence of continuing or relapsing hepatic disease for more than 6 months with histologically documented inflammation and necrosis.

Causes

- Chronic viral hepatitis
- Wilson disease
- α-1 antitrypsin deficiency
- Chronic alcoholism
- Drugs—isoniazid, methyl dopa and methotrexate
- Autoimmune hepatitis
- Cryptogenic chronic hepatitis

Clinical Features

- Persistent elevation of serum aminotransferases.
- Fatigue, malaise, loss of appetite and mild jaundice.
- Spider angiomas, palmar erythema, mild hepatomegaly and hepatic tenderness.
- Prolonged prothrombin time, hypergammaglobulinaemia, hyperbilirubinaemia and mild increase in alkaline phosphatase.
- In HBV and HCV disease, circulating immune complexes may cause vasculitis and glomerulonephritis.

Classification

Old classification of chronic hepatitis

1. **Chronic persistent hepatitis (CPH)**
   (a) Infiltration by chronic inflammatory cells is confined to the portal tracts.
   (b) Changes in hepatocytes are absent or slight (**'spotty necrosis'** or small foci of liver cell necrosis with inflammatory cell infiltration).
   (c) Lobular architecture is maintained.
   (d) Prognosis is excellent. Rarely, may progress to chronic active hepatitis or cirrhosis.
2. **Chronic lobular hepatitis (CLH)**
   (a) Uncommon disease with evidence of hepatitis B or hepatitis C virus infection.
   (b) Antinuclear antibodies, antismooth muscle antibodies and antimitochondrial antibodies in some patients.
   (c) Live biopsy shows features similar to acute viral hepatitis.
3. **Chronic active hepatitis (CAH)**
   (a) Both portal tracts and parenchyma are involved.
   (b) Lobular architecture is distorted.
   (c) Portal tract inflammation spills over into surrounding parenchyma.
   (d) **'Piecemeal necrosis'** and **'bridging hepatic necrosis'** seen.
   (e) Regenerative nodules develop and later progress to cirrhosis.

New classification of chronic hepatitis

The newer classification of chronic hepatitis is based on:

1. Cause of hepatitis.
2. Histological activity or grade.
3. Degree of progression or stage.

Grading of chronic hepatitis is based on the histopathological evidence of inflammation and necrosis. Proportionate to the severity of following factors, a severity score (mild, moderate or severe) is assigned.

1. *Periportal necrosis including piecemeal necrosis and/or bridging necrosis.*
2. *Intralobular necrosis.*
3. *Portal inflammation.*
4. *Fibrosis.*

Staging of chronic hepatitis is based on the degree of fibrosis (stage 0 with no fibrosis to stage 4 with cirrhosis).

Morphological Features (Fig. 28.6)

- Hepatocyte injury and regeneration.
- Reactive changes in the sinusoidal cells.
- Portal inflammation.
- Spillover of inflammation across the limiting plate into the adjacent parenchyma (causes necrosis of adjacent hepatocytes or **interface hepatitis).**
- Fibrosis **(portal, periportal and bridging)**.

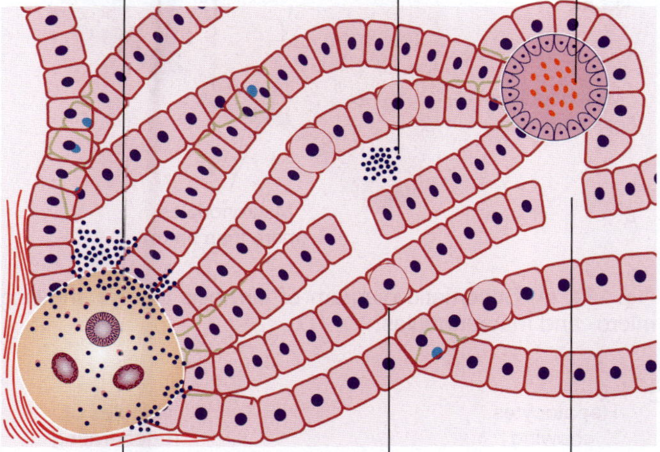

Fig. 28.6 Section from chronic hepatitis showing portal inflammation with spillover in the adjacent parenchyma.

Salient features of different types of hepatitis have been given in Table 28.3.

Q. Define fulminant hepatic failure and write briefly on its causes and clinicopathological features. (PA25.2)

Ans. Fulminant hepatic failure is defined as sudden loss of hepatic function, occurring within 4 weeks of onset of the precipitating illness, in the absence of any evidence of pre-existing liver disease. More protracted course over months is labelled **submassive** or **subacute hepatic necrosis**.

Aetiology

- Acute viral hepatitis (A, B and E; occasionally C).
- Hepatotoxic drugs (isoniazid and phenytoin).
- Poisoning, for example *Amanita phalloides*.
- Shock.
- Wilson disease.

Clinical Features

- Weakness, nausea, vomiting, right hypochondrial pain and jaundice.
- Features of hepatic encephalopathy and cerebral oedema.
- Renal failure.

Gross Pathology

- Diffuse or focal involvement of the liver.
- Shrinkage of liver with extensive parenchymal necrosis.
- Wrinkling of the capsule.

Microscopy

- Complete destruction of hepatocytic lobules leaving only preserved portal tracts.
- Collapse of reticulin framework.
- Survival beyond days is associated with influx of inflammatory cells; survival more than a week is characterised by regeneration of surviving hepatocytes.
- In case of preservation of the parenchymal framework, regeneration may completely restore the liver architecture.

Q. Write briefly on Reye syndrome.

Ans. Reye syndrome is mainly seen in children and adolescents, and is rare in adults.

- It is characterised by severe fatty degeneration of the liver and usually follows a viral illness.
- History of aspirin intake may be elicited.
- It manifests with acute encephalopathy and cerebral oedema and is a prototype of conditions called **'mitochondrial**

Table 28.3 Comparative features of different types of hepatitis

Features	Hepatitis A	Hepatitis B	Hepatitis C	Hepatitis D	Hepatitis E	Hepatitis G
Agent	Icosahedral capsid, ssRNA	Enveloped dsDNA	Enveloped ssRNA	Enveloped ssRNA	Unenveloped ssRNA	ssRNA
Incubation period	2–6 weeks	4–26 weeks	2–26 weeks	4–7 weeks	2–8 weeks	Unknown
Transmission	Faeco-oral	Parenteral, close contact	Parenteral, close contact	Parenteral, close contact	Waterborne	Parenteral
Carrier state	None	Present	Present	Present		Present
Chronic hepatitis	None	5%–10% of acute infections	>50%	<5% coinfection, 80% super infection	None	None
Hepatocellular carcinoma	No	Yes	Yes	No increase above HBV	Unknown	None
Diagnosis	Detection of serum IgM antibodies	Detection of HBsAg or antibody to HBcAg	PCR for HCV RNA; third-generation ELISA for antibody detection	Detection of IgM and IgG antibodies; HDV RNA in serum and HDAg in liver	PCR for HEV RNA; Detection of serum IgM and IgG antibodies	Not a primary hepatotropic virus; replicates in the bone marrow and spleen

hepatopathies' (associated with generalised loss of mitochondrial function).

Q. Write briefly on autoimmune (lupoid) hepatitis.

Ans. It is a chronic hepatitis with multiple immunologic abnormalities.

Salient Features

- Female preponderance; HLA association (association with HLADRB1 allelles in South Americans and DR3 in Caucasians).
- Insidious onset with fatigue, anorexia and jaundice usually secondary to triggers like viral infection, drugs, vaccination, etc.
- Signs of chronic liver disease (spider telangiectasia and hepatosplenomegaly).
- Coexistence of other autoimmune diseases (rheumatoid arthritis, thyrotoxicosis, Hashimoto thyroiditis, myxoedema, Coombs positive haemolytic anaemia).
- Absence of serologic markers of viral infections.
- Elevation of serum IgG (>2.5 g/dL) and high titres of autoantibodies, for example antinuclear antibodies (ANAs), antismooth muscle antibodies (SMAs), antibodies to actin, troponin and tropomyosin, anti-soluble liver antigen/liver pancreas antigen (SLA/LP) antibodies, antiliver cytosol 1 (ACL-1) antibodies, and liver–kidney microsomal antibody directed against cytochrome P450 (anti-LKM1 antibody).
- Two types of autoimmune hepatitis are identified – Type 1 is more common in older individuals and shows positivity for ANA, SMA, anti-SLA/LP and AMA and Type 2 which affects children and young adults and shows positivity for anti-LKM-1 antibodies and ACL-1 antibodies.
- Confluent necrosis, severe interface hepatitis, predominance of plasma cells and rosetting of hepatocytes are diagnostic histopathological features.

Q. Define cirrhosis. Enumerate its causes and consequences.

Ans. Cirrhosis is a diffuse liver disease characterised by:

1. Widespread hepatocyte necrosis with simultaneous regeneration leading to the formation of nodules of various sizes (micronodules less than 3 mm and macronodules more than 3 mm; Fig. 28.7A and Fig. 28.7B).
2. Bridging fibrous septae, which distort the hepatic architecture.
3. Destruction and distortion of hepatic vasculature by fibrosis, which eventually leads to the formation of **portosystemic shunts (portal hypertension and its sequelae; e.g. gastro-oesophageal varices)** and **splenomegaly.**
4. **Ascites** and **hepatic encephalopathy** resulting from both hepatocellular insufficiency and portal hypertension. Hepatocellular damage also leads to **jaundice, oedema, coagulopathies** and **a variety of metabolic abnormalities.**

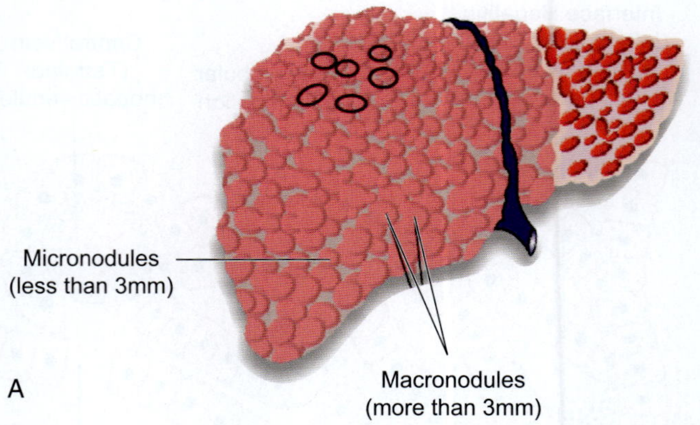

Fig. 28.7 (A) Schematic diagram of cirrhosis of liver showing micro- and macronodules.

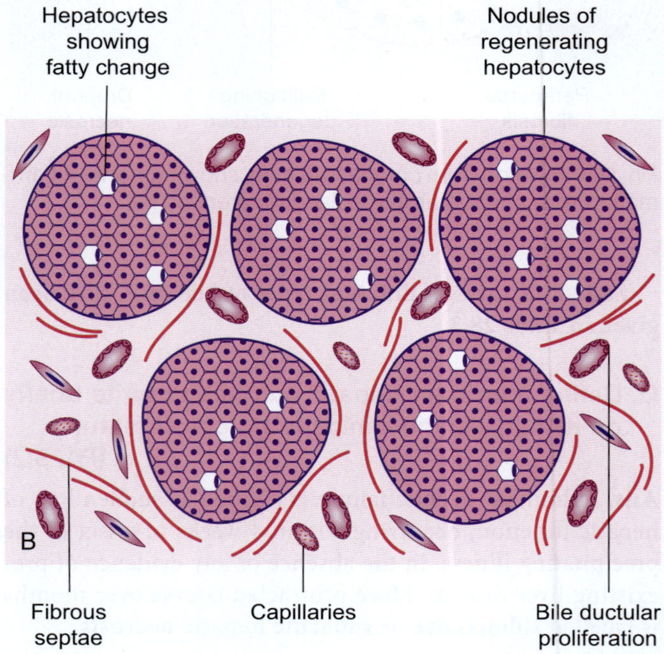

Fig. 28.7 (B) Portal cirrhosis liver.

Classification

1. ***Aetiological***
   - Alcoholic cirrhosis.
   - Non-alcoholic steatohepatitis (NASH).
   - Postnecrotic cirrhosis.
   - Biliary cirrhosis (primary and secondary).
   - Hepatitis B, C and Delta.
   - Haemochromatosis.
   - Wilson disease.
   - α-1 antitrypsin deficiency.
   - Chronic autoimmune hepatitis.
   - Drug-induced cirrhosis (methyldopa, isoniazid and methotrexate).
   - Inborn errors of metabolism (glycogen storage diseases and galactosaemia).
   - Cardiac cirrhosis.
   - Cryptogenic cirrhosis.
2. ***Morphological***
   - Micronodular cirrhosis.
   - Macronodular cirrhosis.
   - Mixed cirrhosis.

Pathogenesis

- In the **normal liver**, ECM consists of collagen Types I, III, V and XI present around central veins, in portal tracts and in the liver capsule.
- Liver does not have a true basement membrane; instead, Type IV collagen and other proteins present in the space of Disse (space between sinusoidal endothelial cells and hepatocytes) form the supporting framework.
- Collagen is synthesised by Ito cells (perisinusoidal stellate or fat-storing cells), which lie in the space of Disse. These cells normally function as storage cells for vitamin A and fat, and become activated to myofibroblast-like cells under stimulation by reactive oxygen species (ROS), growth factors and cytokines like TNF, IL-1 and lymphotoxins.
- In cirrhosis, Types I and III collagen and other ECM components are deposited in the space of Disse. This leads to loss of sinusoidal endothelial cell fenestrations, which hampers the free exchange of solutes between plasma and hepatocytes.
- Movement of proteins (albumin, clotting factors and lipoproteins) between plasma and hepatocytes is markedly impaired, leading to functional changes in the liver.

Clinical Features

1. **Compensated cirrhosis:** This is the early phase of cirrhosis where in the patient may not present with any symptoms.
2. **Decompensated cirrhosis:** The later phase of cirrhosis in which the patient presents with the following symptoms:
   - Low-grade fever, weakness, fatigue, weight loss, anorexia, nausea, vomiting, upper abdominal discomfort and abdominal distension due to ascites.
   - Menstrual irregularities like amenorrhoea and irregular menses, hypogonadism, diminished body hair and gynaecomastia (due to impaired oestrogen metabolism and resulting hyperestrogenaemia).
   - Haemorrhagic tendencies like easy bruising, purpura, epistaxis, menorrhagia and gastrointestinal bleeding (due to decreased production of coagulation factors by the liver and thrombocytopenia resulting from hypersplenism).
   - Portal hypertension and its sequelae.

Signs of Hepatocellular Failure (PA25.2)

- **Jaundice** (due to abnormal bilirubin metabolism).
- **Palmar erythema** and **spider naevi** (due to vasodilatation).
- **Parotid enlargement** (attributed to fatty infiltration since liver's ability to break down body fat is reduced in cirrhosis).
- **Ascites** (due to portal hypertension; and low levels of albumin in the blood).
- **Hepatic encephalopathy** and **flapping tremors** (associated with increased blood ammonia levels).
- **Progressive renal dysfunction** (due to decreased renal perfusion attributed to systemic vasodilatation).

Q. Outline the aetiopathogenesis and clinical features of portal hypertension. (PA25.5)

Ans. Portal hypertension is defined as a clinical condition in which there is prolonged elevation of portal venous pressure due to increased resistance to portal blood flow.

Causes

- **Prehepatic:** Portal vein thrombosis and fibrosis of bile ducts (as in schistosomiasis), massive splenomegaly with increased blood flow.
- **Intrahepatic:** Cirrhosis, schistosomiasis, massive fatty change, sarcoidosis and miliary tuberculosis.
- **Posthepatic:** Obstruction of hepatic vein by thrombosis (**Budd–Chiari syndrome**) or tumours.

Pathogenesis of Portal Hypertension in Cirrhosis (Flowchart 28.2)

- In the initial stage of portal hypertension the main factor is an increase in the vascular resistance to the portal blood flow which is not only a mechanical consequence of the disordered hepatic architectural; but also a result of the active contraction of myofibroblasts, activated stellate cells, and vascular smooth-muscle cells of the intrahepatic veins.
- The sinusoidal vascular resistance is increased as a consequence of fibrosis, scarring, and compression of sinusoids by regenerative nodules.
- Arteriovenous anastomosis develop in the fibrous septae which expose the low-pressure venous system to higher arterial pressures leading to portal hypertension.

Perivenular fibrosis and compression of sinusoids by parenchymal nodules

↓

Increased resistance to blood flow at the level of sinusoids

↓

Increased portal vascular resistance leads to:
- Reduction in the flow of portal blood to the liver
- Development of collateral vessels allowing portal blood to bypass the liver and enter systemic circulation

↓

- Collateral vessel formation occurs in the oesophagus, stomach, rectum, anterior abdominal wall and in the renal, lumbar, ovarian and testicular (spermatic) vasculature
- With the development of collateral vessels, initially some of the portal blood and later almost all of the portal blood is shunted directly to the systemic circulation, bypassing the liver

Flowchart 28.2 Pathogenesis of portal hypertension in cirrhosis.

- Factors that increase hepatic vascular resistance include endothelin-1 (ET-1), alpha-adrenergic stimulus, and angiotensin II. Factors that decrease hepatic vascular resistance include nitric oxide (NO), prostacyclin, and vasodilating drugs (e.g. organic nitrates, adrenolytics, calcium channel blockers).
- ET-1 is a powerful vasoconstrictor synthesised by sinusoidal endothelial cells that has been implicated in the increased hepatic vascular resistance of cirrhosis and in the development of liver fibrosis.
- NO is a vasodilator substance that is also synthesised by the sinusoidal endothelial cells. In the cirrhotic liver, the production of NO is decreased, and endothelial nitric oxide synthase (eNOS) activity and nitrite production by sinusoidal endothelial cells are reduced. As a result, intrahepatic vasoconstriction occurs in cirrhotic liver.
- Another major contribution to the increased portal venous pressure is the concomitant splanchnic arteriolar vasodilation causing increased portal venous inflow.

Clinical Features and Complications

- **Haematemesis** and **melena** (from variceal bleeding).
- **Fetor hepaticus** (a musty odour of breath, resulting from portal-systemic shunting of blood, which allows mercaptans to pass directly to the lungs. Mercaptans are formed by the action of GIT bacteria on methionine).
- **Caput medusae** (a number of prominent collateral vessels radiating from the umbilicus).
- **Splenomegaly** (an important diagnostic sign of portal hypertension).
- **Hypersplenism** (manifests as thrombocytopenia and leucopenia).
- **Small, contracted** and **fibrotic liver** (usually seen associated with very high portal venous pressure).
- **Haemorrhoids** (which occur from dilatation of rectal veins).
- **Ascites** (which occurs due to portal hypertension and hypoalbuminaemia due to liver cell failure).

Q. Outline the salient features of hepatorenal failure.

Ans. Hepatorenal syndrome is defined as renal failure associated with chronic liver disease. Kidneys are histologically normal and their function reverts to normal after reversal of hepatic failure. Renal failure is thought to result from **diminished renal blood flow**. In cirrhosis, circulatory changes lead to increased peripheral blood flow and decreased visceral blood flow, especially to the kidneys (this clinically manifests as a drop in urine output and rising blood urea and creatinine levels).

Q. Write briefly on alcoholic liver disease. (PA25.4)

Ans. The spectrum of alcoholic liver disease (ALD) varies from alcoholic steatosis to hepatitis (AH), to cirrhosis. The above entities do not necessarily occur sequentially and may occur independently of each other. The short-term ingestion of 80 g of ethanol/day produces mild reversible hepatic changes. Chronic intake of 50–60 g/day may cause severe injury.

Diagnosis

Distinguishing an **alcoholic basis** from a **non-alcoholic basis** for clinical and histologic steatohepatitis is difficult because of the unreliability of alcohol consumption history. The **ALD/NAFLD Index (ANI)** uses the mean corpuscular volume (MCV), the aspartate aminotransferase (AST)/alanine aminotransferase (ALT) ratio, the body mass index (BMI), and gender to identify patients with an ALD.

Risk Factors

- **Excessive weight** is a risk factor for AH, and can result in a combination of both alcoholic and non-alcoholic steatohepatitis.
- **Patients with HCV** are also more likely to develop AH and severe AH.
- **Females** are more susceptible (oestrogen increases permeability to gut derived endotoxins and increases production of proinflammatory cytokines to cause injury to hepatocytes).
- **An irregular (i.e. binge) pattern of alcohol consumption**.
- Cirrhosis is associated with **heavy alcohol use, duration greater than 15 years, and consumption greater than 200 g/day.**
- **Polymorphisms in detoxifying enzyme aldehyde dehydrogenase (ALDH)** predispose the patient to individual to ALD.
- **PNPLA3** (Patatin-like phospholipase domain-containing protein 3) is a novel risk factor for alcoholic cirrhosis and also hepatocellular carcinoma (HCC). Patients with PNPLA3 develop alcoholic cirrhosis with a shorter exposure to heavy drinking.
- **In patients with alcoholic cirrhosis, the risk factors for the development of HCC include obesity, diabetes, active alcohol consumption, and viral hepatitis.**

Pathogenesis

- Alcohol is metabolised to acetaldehyde; both alcohol and acetaldehyde have toxic effects on hepatocytes.
- Acetaldehyde is metabolised by aldehyde dehydrogenase (ALDH) in the mitochondria.
- Acetaldehyde is highly reactive and can form various protein and DNA adducts. A relative deficiency of the ALDH2 isozyme causes the accumulation of acetaldehyde.
- A minor pathway involves microsomal enzyme oxidation system (MEOS) and generates more reactive oxygen species, resulting in lipid peroxidation, mitochondrial glutathione depletion, and S-adenosylmethionine depletion.
- The cytochrome CYP2E1 of MEOS is induced in chronic alcoholism, further contributing to oxidative stress and liver injury.
- Steatosis is mediated by effects of alcohol on lipogenesis and fatty acid oxidation.
- Increased ratio of reduced nicotinamide adenine dinucleotide to oxidized nicotinamide adenine dinucleotide, has been reported to inhibit β-oxidation of fatty acids in mitochondria.
- It also inhibits fatty acid oxidation by inhibiting the transcriptional activity and DNA-binding ability of peroxisome proliferator-activated receptor alpha (PPAR-α).

- Alcohol can downregulate PPAR-α directly via its metabolite acetaldehyde, or indirectly via the cytochrome P450 2E1-derived oxidative stress.
- Alcohol is thought to stimulate lipogenesis by the upregulation of sterol regulatory element-binding transcription factor 1 c (SREBP-1c).
- Oxidative stress damages hepatocytes which in turn release Damage-Associated Molecular Patterns (DAMPs) that recruit innate and adaptive immune cells that perpetuate further liver injury. They aid in the production of proinflammatory cytokines and localization of immune cells to the site of injury.
- Alcohol also has direct effects on intestinal microbiome and gut permeability that allows bacterial products to reach liver, and further stimulate immune response and liver injury. Bacterial overload and increased gut permeability lead to an increased load of bacteria-derived LPS to the portal circulation and liver. LPS interacts with toll-like receptor 4 (TLR4) on Kupffer cells, activating the TIR-domain-containing adapter-inducing interferon-β (TRIF)/IRF-3 signalling pathway. This leads to the production of proinflammatory cytokines like tumour necrosis alpha [TNF-α], IL-1, and IL17).
- Alcohol also activates the complement system (C3, C4). The interaction between complement and Kupffer cells leads to release of proinflammatory cytokines, such as TNF-α.
- Alcohol affects multiple steps in methionine metabolism thereby impairing the metabolism of folate as well. This causes decrease in the level of glutathione which in turn sensitises the liver to oxidative stress.

Alcoholic Steatosis (Fatty Liver)

- The severity of fatty change is roughly proportional to the duration and degree of alcohol intake.
- Patient usually presents with hepatomegaly and mildly increased serum bilirubin and alkaline phosphatase.

Pathogenesis

Hepatocellular steatosis results from:

- Impaired assembly and secretion of lipoproteins.
- Increased peripheral catabolism of fat to release free fatty acids (FFA) into the circulation and increased delivery of FFA to liver.
- Generation of **excess reduced NAD (NADH)** by two major enzymes of alcohol metabolism, namely, alcohol dehydrogenase and acetaldehyde dehydrogenase. Decreased NAD^+ inhibits catabolism (oxidation) of fatty acids and leads to increased lipid synthesis and accumulation of fat in hepatocytes.

Pathology

- The liver is enlarged, soft, yellow and greasy.
- Micro- and macrovesicular fat droplets (clear vacuoles) are seen in the cytoplasm of hepatocytes (Fig. 28.8).
- Steatosis starts from the centrilobular region (acinar zone 3).
- There is minimal accompanying inflammation and absence of fibrosis.

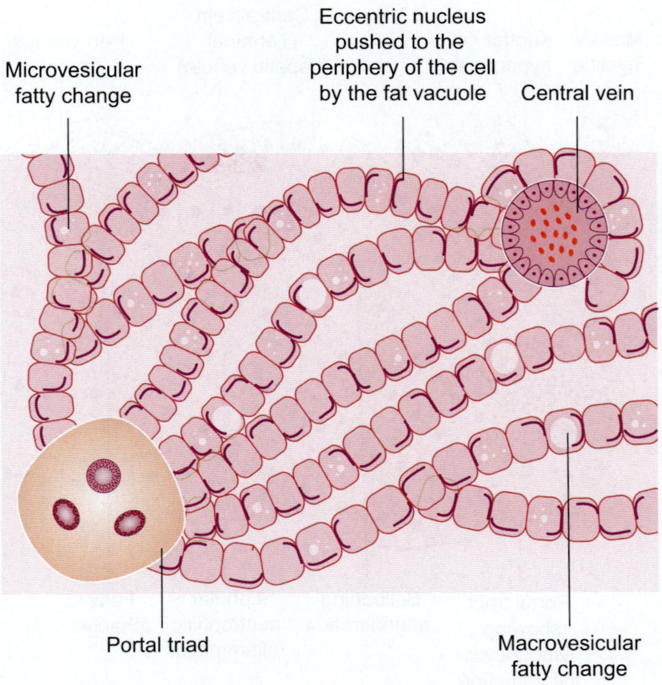

Fig. 28.8 Alcoholic steatosis showing microvesicular and macrovesicular fatty change.

Alcoholic Hepatitis

- Fifteen to twenty years of alcohol intake predispose an individual to alcoholic hepatitis. It usually presents suddenly after a bout of excessive drinking with malaise, anorexia and upper abdominal discomfort, elevated ALT and AST with AST/ALT ratio >1.
- Unlike fatty liver which reverses completely after alcohol withdrawal and proper nutrition, alcoholic hepatitis may sometimes persist and progress to cirrhosis.

Pathogenesis

- Acetaldehyde, a major metabolic intermediate of alcohol, induces lipid peroxidation and acetaldehyde–protein adduct formation, which disrupts cytoskeletal and membrane proteins.
- Alcohol directly affects microtubule organisation, mitochondrial and membrane functions.
- Reactive oxygen species (ROS) generated during oxidation of ethanol by microsomal ethanol oxidizing system can damage membrane and proteins.
- ROS are also generated by neutrophils infiltrating the liver.
- Under normal circumstances glutathione is transported from the cytoplasm to the mitochondria where it neutralizes the ROS. There is impairment of this transport in alcoholic liver disease leading to mitochondrial dysfunction by ROS.
- In the intestine, alcohol causes release of endotoxin (lipopolysaccharide or LPS) from the gram-negative flora which enters portal circulation to induce production of proinflammatory cytokines (TNF-alfa, IL-6 and TGF-alfa) from kupffer cells. This causes hepatocellular injury/damage.

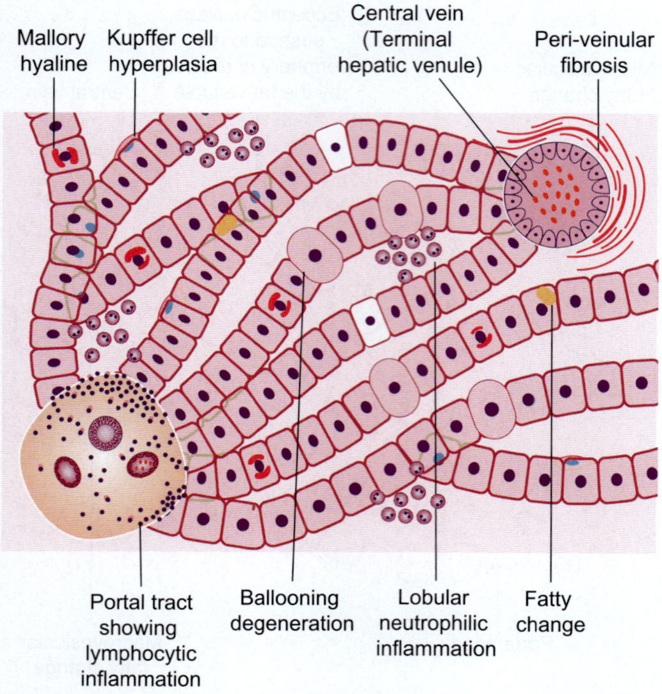

Fig. 28.9 Alcoholic hepatitis showing hepatocyte degeneration and necrosis, lobular and portal inflammation, Mallory hyaline, Kupffer cell hyperplasia and beginning of perivenular fibrosis.

Pathology (Fig. 28.9)

The liver is enlarged, yellow but firm on account of fibrosis. The following microscopic features are seen:

- **Hepatocyte swelling and necrosis:** Ballooning and necrosis of single and small groups of hepatocytes.
- **Mallory–Denk bodies or Mallory hyaline:** Tangled skeins of intermediate filaments visible as dense, eosinophilic inclusions in the perinuclear zone cytoplasm of hepatocytes. Also seen in Wilson disease, chronic cholestatic syndromes and hepatocellular tumours.
- **Neutrophil infiltration:** Present around degenerating hepatocytes particularly those with Mallory bodies.
- **Fibrosis:** Initially pericellular **(chicken wire fence pattern)**, sinusoidal and perivenular; with prolonged bouts of alcohol intake; periportal fibrosis may also be seen.

Alcoholic (Laennec or Portal) Cirrhosis

It is the irreversible end stage of alcoholic liver disease which entails a diffuse loss of architecture with fibrosis and nodule formation.

Pathogenesis

Activation of Stellate cells and portal fibroblasts eventually progresses to extensive central–central, central–portal and portal–portal fibrosis.

Clinical Classification

Clinical classification of cirrhosis is based on blood and clinical parameters:

- **Child-Pugh score/grade:** Five parameters are included, namely, albumin, bilirubin, INR/prothrombin time, ascites and hepatic encephalopathy. Each parameter is assigned a score from 1 to 3. Total score ranges from 5 to 15 and is categorised as grade A (5, 6), B (7–9) and C (10–15).
- **Model for end-stage liver disease (MELD) score:** Three parameters are included: bilirubin, creatinine and INR. Mainly used to assess a need for liver transplantation.
- **Albumin-bilirubin (ALBI) score:** Two parameters are used, namely, albumin and bilirubin.

Pathology

- Liver is yellow, fatty and enlarged in the initial stages and becomes brown, shrunken and firm in the later stages.
- Capsular surface shows nodules (hobnail appearance – initially micronodules are seen and they later coalesce to form macronodules to show a mixed pattern).
- There is diffuse loss of normal parenchymal and vascular architecture with formation of regenerating nodules.
- New vascular channels form in the fibrous septae which connect the portal vessels with the terminal hepatic veins shunting blood from the parenchyma.
- End-stage liver cirrhosis looks morphologically the same irrespective of the aetiology.

Q. Write briefly on non-alcoholic fatty liver disease (NAFLD).

Ans. NAFLD is a group of disorders which resemble alcoholic steatohepatitis but occurs in the absence of alcohol intake.

- Important risk factors for development of this entity are obesity, Type II diabetes mellitus and hyperlipidaemia (metabolic syndrome[a]). Insulin resistance increases lipid accumulation (steatosis). The lipid so formed is dysfunctional leading to decreased production of the lipid hormone 'adiponectin' with a simultaneous increase in inflammatory cytokines like IL-6 and TNF-α. This predisposes the fat-laden hepatocytes to apoptosis and oxidative injury, which in turn is responsible for hepatocellular necrosis and associated inflammation.
- NAFLD is a common incidentally discovered cause for abnormal liver tests (once other causes of liver diseases are excluded).
- NAFLD is broadly divided into two groups:
  - Patients with isolated fatty liver disease (80%): These patients are asymptomatic at the time of diagnosis; some have fatigue, malaise and hepatomegaly. They show none or minimal progression to cirrhosis.
  - Patients with non-alcoholic steatohepatitis or NASH (20%): NASH shows a histology identical and to alcoholic hepatitis. Patients with NASH have a much higher

---

[a]*Source:* WHO criteria for defining metabolic syndrome:
Any one of the following:
- Diabetes mellitus or
- Impaired glucose tolerance or
- Impaired fasting glucose or
- Insulin resistance

And two of the following:
- Blood pressure >140/90 mm Hg
- Dyslipidaemia (Triglycerides >169.5; HDL cholesterol <0.9 mmol/L in males and <1 mmol/L in females)
- Central obesity (waist -hip ratio >0.90 in males and >0.85 in females or body mass index >30 kg/m^2)
- Microalbuminuria (urinary albumin >20 mcg/min and albumin/creatinine ratio >30 mg/gm).

propensity to progress to cirrhosis and hepatocellular carcinoma. NASH is a significant contributor to the group 'cryptogenic cirrhosis'.

Q. Write briefly on the aetiology and clinicopathological features of haemochromatosis.

Ans. Iron overload is defined as excess stores of iron in the body. The most notable organs with iron deposition are the liver, heart, and endocrine glands. Resulting symptoms and disease are related to specific organ damage. Iron overload can result from numerous causes (See Table 28.4).

Haemochromatosis is a condition in which there is excessive iron absorption leading to parenchymal iron overload. It may be hereditary or acquired in nature.

Hereditary Haemochromatosis

Occurs due to mutations in genes encoding for proteins regulating hepcidin levels, for example, **haemochromatosis gene (HFE gene; located on chromosome 6), transferrin receptor (TFR) 2 gene and haemojuvenile (JJV) gene or the hepcidin gene itself**. Hepcidin, a hepatocellular protein, which has bactericidal activities, is the main regulator of iron absorption and is encoded by HAMP gene. It lowers plasma iron levels and a mutation in either hepcidin gene itself or the genes encoding for the regulatory proteins result in iron overload.

Aetiology

- Mutations in HFE gene and TFR 2 gene lead to the classic adult form of hereditary haemochromatosis.

Table 28.4 Causes of Iron overload

Causes of iron overload	

Inappropriately increased intestinal iron absorption	• Hereditary haemochromatosis
	• HFE-haemochromatosis (Type 1: mutation in HFE gene)
	• Non-HFE haemochromatosis (rare)
	  • Type 2A: mutation in haemojuvelin or HJV gene
	  • Type 2B: hepcidin mutation (mutation in HAMP gene)
	  • Type 3: transferrin receptor 2 mutation (mutation in TfR2 gene)
	  • Type 4: ferroportin mutation (mutation in FPN1 gene)

Transfusional iron overload (1 unit packed red cells ≈ 250 mg iron)	• Multiple transfusions
Anaemias associated with iron overload	• α-thalassaemia • β-thalassaemia • Congenital sideroblastic anaemia • Congenital dyserythropoietic anaemias
Chronic liver disease	• Alcoholic liver disease • NASH
Excess parenteral iron	• Excess therapeutic iron

- Mutations in the HAMP gene or HJV lead to a severe form of hereditary haemochromatosis called neonatal haemochromatosis.
- The most common form of the disease is inherited as an autosomal recessive disorder characterised by mutations in the HFE gene that regulates the levels of hepcidin, the iron hormone produced by liver, which inhibits iron absorption.
- Hepcidin levels are reduced in all known forms of haemochromatosis leading to increased absorption of dietary iron over years.
- Ninety percent of the patients are males (females are protected by the iron loss in menstruation and pregnancy).
- Excessive iron can be directly toxic to host tissues by the following mechanisms:
  - Lipid peroxidation by iron-mediated free-radical reactions.
  - Interaction of iron and reactive oxygen species generated by the iron directly with DNA leading to cell injury and predisposition to hepatocellular carcinoma.
  - Stimulation of Ito cells/hepatic stellate cells to produce more collagen.

Pathology

- The excess iron deposited in various tissues results in damage to liver, pancreas, heart, pituitary gland and skin.
- The liver appears chocolate brown in colour and may be normal or enlarged (in early stages) and contracted and small in later stages. Microscopy shows iron deposits in the periportal hepatocytes, which appear finely granular and golden-yellow and stains with Prussian blue stain. In the later stages iron can be seen in the entire lobule, within the bile duct epithelium and Kupffer cells. Fibrosis is seen in the later stages. Collagenisation starts in the peri-portal region to progress to bridging fibrosis and micro nodular cirrhosis.
- Pancreas show diffuse interstitial fibrosis and parenchymal atrophy with haemosiderin deposits in the acinar as well as islet cells (the latter causing diabetes).
- Heart is enlarged with haemosiderin deposits in the myocardial fibres (causing arrhythmias and cardiomyopathy).
- Haemosiderin deposits in the synovium leads to acute synovitis.
- Testes are small and atrophic (leading to loss of libido and infertility).

Clinical Features

- Presents in men over 40 years.
- The total body iron is increased.
- Fully developed cases show a triad of
  - Micronodular cirrhosis.
  - Diabetes mellitus **(bronze diabetes).**
  - Skin pigmentation (attributed mainly to excess melanin production and partly to haemosiderin deposits).
- Other manifestations include loss of libido, testicular atrophy, spider nevi, loss of body hair, jaundice and ascites, heart failure and cardiac arrhythmias.
- It is associated with a **high incidence of hepatocellular carcinoma.**

Acquired (Secondary) Haemochromatosis

Acquired (secondary) haemochromatosis (also called haemosiderosis) develops secondary to:

(a) Chronic anaemias:
  (i) Thalassaemia major
  (ii) Sideroblastic anaemia
(b) Exogenous iron overload:
  (i) Multiple blood transfusions
  (ii) Repeated iron injections
  (iii) Prolonged oral iron intake (including African iron overload or **Bantu siderosis**)
(c) Chronic liver diseases
(d) Porphyria cutanea tarda

Note: In secondary iron overload, iron accumulates in Kupffer cells rather than hepatocytes (accumulation in hepatocytes typically occurs in hereditary haemochromatosis).

Q. Write briefly on the aetiology and clinicopathological features of Wilson disease (hepatolenticular degeneration).

Ans. Also called hepatolenticular degeneration, Wilson disease is a disorder characterised by accumulation of toxic levels of copper in tissues / organs, usually liver, brain, eye. See Flowchart 28.3 for normal copper physiology.

Aetiology

- Hereditary disorder with autosomal recessive inheritance.
- Due to mutation in ATP7B, a gene located on chromosome 13 (encodes for ATPase metal iron transporter, localised to Golgi region of hepatocytes; the deficiency of which impairs copper excretion into bile).
- Failure of biliary copper excretion causing its accumulation in the body.
- Copper causes toxic injury by:
  - Inducing formation of free radicals by Fenton reaction.
  - Binding to sulphydryl groups of cellular proteins.
  - Displacing other metals from hepatic metalloenzymes.

Absorption of ingested copper in duodenum and jejunum

↓

Transportation to portal circulation as a complex with albumin and histidine

↓ Dissociation of free copper

Uptake by hepatocytes followed by incorporation into an α_2- globulin (apoceruloplasmin) to form ceruloplasmin

↓

Secretion of ceruloplasmin into plasma (accounts for 90–95% of plasma copper)

↓

Hepatic uptake of senescent ceruloplasmin from plasma followed by lysosomal degradation and secretion of free copper into bile

Flowchart 28.3 Normal copper physiology.

Clinical and Laboratory Work up

- Slit-lamp examination of the eyes for Kayser–Fleischer rings.
- Low-serum ceruloplasmin levels (<20 mg/dL).
- **High urinary copper excretion (>100 mcg/day; most specific test).**
- High hepatic copper content (>250 mcg/g of dry tissue; most sensitive test).
- Serum copper levels can be raised, low or normal so are of no diagnostic use.

Clinicopathological Features

- Wilson disease usually presents between 5 and 30 years.
- Deposition of excess copper in various tissues/organs damages them and may manifest as:

Liver
- Fatty change.
- Acute and chronic hepatitis with hepatocytic ballooning and presence of 'Mallory–Denk bodies'.
- Massive liver cell necrosis.
- Cirrhosis.

Brain (basal ganglia): Basal ganglia show atrophy and cavitation leading to **neuropsychiatric manifestations:**
- **Neurological manifestations:** Movement disorders, especially resting tremors. Less commonly spasticity, rigidity, chorea, dysphagia and dysarthria may be seen.
- **Psychiatric manifestations:** Bizarre behavioural disturbances similar to schizophrenia, manic-depressive psychosis and neurosis.

Eyes: Kayser–Fleischer rings (green to brown deposits of copper in the Descemet membrane in the limbus of cornea). Kayser–Fleischer rings may be associated with **'sunflower cataracts'.**

Others: RBCs show haemolysis, deposits of copper in kidneys may cause renal tubular damage and in the skeleton may cause osteoporosis.

Q. Write briefly on the aetiology and clinicopathological features of α-1 antitrypsin deficiency.

Ans. α-1 antitrypsin is an α-1 globulin produced by the liver which comprises 90% of the α-1 globulins.

- It is a serine protease inhibitor (Pi), which inhibits the protease enzymes, particularly neutrophil elastase, cathepsin G and proteinase 3, to prevent breakdown of elastin and collagen by them.
- It is encoded by a gene located on chromosome 14, which is extremely polymorphic and more than 70 forms have been identified. The most commonly encountered forms of α1-antitrypsin are:
  - PiM (medium)
  - PiS (slow)
  - PiZ (very slow)
- **PiMM** is the normal phenotype, while the phenotype **PiZZ** gives low α-1 antitrypsin concentrations (less than 10% of normal levels). α-1 antitrypsin deficiency may lead to **liver**

and **pulmonary diseases** (cirrhosis and emphysema, respectively).

Clinicopathology

- In neonates, α-1-antitrypsin deficiency produces hepatitis and cholestatic jaundice.
- In adults, the patient may present with any of the following:
  - Chronic hepatitis
  - Cirrhosis
  - Hepatocellular carcinoma (in 2%–3% patients with a PiZZ phenotype)
  - Emphysema
- Most cases of α-1-antitrypsin deficiency are characterised by presence of intrahepatic round-to-oval PAS-positive cytoplasmic globular inclusions.

Q. Name the two main autoimmune disorders of intrahepatic bile ducts. Write briefly on the clinicopathological features of both.

Ans. The two main autoimmune disorders of intrahepatic bile ducts (autoimmune cholangiopathies) are:

1. Primary biliary cholangitis (PBC).
2. Primary sclerosing cholangitis (PSC).

PBC

Occurs predominantly in **women** between **30 and 70 years**, all of who do not present with cirrhosis, indicating that the earlier name was a misnomer.

Clinical Features

- Chronic, progressive, often fatal cholestatic liver disease with destruction of small, intrahepatic bile ducts, portal inflammation and scarring leading to cirrhosis and liver failure.
- Presents with insidious onset of pruritis, malaise, jaundice, light stools and steatorrhea, hepatomegaly, xanthomas, and eyelid xanthelasmas (accumulation of cholesterol containing macrophages), osteomalacia (due to reduced absorption of Vitamin D).
- Death is usually due to cirrhosis, liver failure, bleeding varices, or infection.

Aetiopathogenesis

- PBC is thought to be autoimmune in origin and often occurs in association with other autoimmune diseases like Sjögren syndrome, scleroderma and thyroid disease.
- Genetic and environmental factors may play a role in its pathogenesis.

Laboratory Workup

- **Ninety-five percent are AMA-positive**, 20% ANA-positive and 60% ANCA-positive.
- Associated with increased serum alkaline phosphatase, cholesterol, and conjugated bilirubin (late manifestation).

Gross Pathology

- In both early and late stages, there is marked hepatomegaly, contrary to other end-stage liver diseases which show a small shrunken liver. This is probably due to the minimal hepatocytic loss and extensive regeneration, typical of PBC.
- In late stage PBC liver appears green due to extensive bile stasis.
- Capsular surface is initially smooth, then granular, and in the later stages becomes micronodular.

Microscopy

- Shows non-suppurative destruction of small- and medium-sized intrahepatic bile ducts followed by cirrhosis. Large intrahepatic ducts and the extrahepatic biliary structures are not involved.
- The histopathology varies depending on the stage:
- Stage I (Florid duct lesion): Early lesions show dense lymphocytic and plasma cell infiltrate around interlobular bile ducts (those that course alongside the hepatic artery). There is presence of poorly formed portal epithelioid granulomas, lymphocytes, plasma cells and macrophages.
- Stage II (Scarring): Inflammatory destruction of the interlobular bile ducts results in portal fibrosis and proliferation of bile ductules at the periphery of the portal tracts. This leads to impaired intrahepatic bile flow which in turn leads to more inflammation and necrosis of the peri portal parenchyma.
- Stage III (Cirrhosis): Portal tract scarring and bridging fibrosis ultimately lead to cirrhosis of the liver.

PSC

PSC is an immune-mediated chronic cholestatic disease characterised by progressive concentric periductal **(onion skin)** fibrosis and destruction of extrahepatic and large intrahepatic bile ducts.

Clinical Features

- Median age is 30 years.
- Patient presents with fatigue, pruritis, jaundice, increased ALP levels and other features of chronic cholestatic liver disease.
- Patchy involvement of the biliary tree results in characteristic **'beading'** appearance of the affected segment during a retrograde cholangiogram.
- Commonly coexists with **inflammatory bowel disease, pancreatitis** and **retroperitoneal fibrosis.**
- Sixty-five percent patients are ANCA-positive.
- Cholangiocarcinomas may develop in 10%–15% cases.

Aetiopathogenesis

- Thought to be autoimmune in origin.
- **Secondary sclerosing cholangitis** may occur due to stones, prior surgery.

Pathology

- Obstruction of intrahepatic bile ducts leads to proliferation of bile ductules, inflammation and necrosis of adjacent periportal hepatic parenchyma and cholestasis.
- Large bile ducts show periductal fibrosis that obliterates the lumen leaving a solid cord-like scar with a few inflammatory cells.

- Primary biliary cirrhosis and primary sclerosing cholangitis eventually lead to end-stage liver disease (liver becomes hard and finely granular and shows yellow-green pigmentation).

Q. Differentiate between PBC and PSC.

Ans. The differences between PBC and PSC are summarised in Table 28.5.

Q. Write briefly on the aetiology, clinical features and morphology of hepatocellular carcinoma (HCC)/ hepatoma.

Ans. Malignant tumours of the liver can be primary or metastatic. Primary tumours can arise from hepatocytes (hepatocellular carcinoma) or from the bile ductular epithelium (cholangiocarcinoma).

Salient Features

- HCC accounts for 80%–90% of all liver cancers.
- Occurs more often in men than women; presents with abdominal pain, malaise, weight loss and palpable/radiologically detected lesion.
- Most common in Africa and South-East Asia which show a high rate of chronic HBV infection. HCC in these countries occurs earlier (20–40 years) and in half the cases there is no evidence of background cirrhosis. In the Western countries, increase in the incidence of HCC is attributed to hepatitis C; it manifests after 60 years and in 90% cases shows background cirrhosis.

Predisposing Factors

- Chronic hepatitis B and C infections.
- Aflatoxin toxicity (a fungal toxin present in moulds and grains and produced by the fungus *Aspergillus flavus*).
- Alcoholic cirrhosis.
- Primary biliary cirrhosis.
- NAFLD and metabolic syndrome.
- Haemochromatosis.
- α-1 antitrypsin deficiency.
- Wilson disease.
- Tyrosinemia.
- Glycogen storage disease.
- Anabolic steroids, thorotrast and arsenic.
- Oestrogens and androgens.

Note: Aflatoxin and alcohol synergise with HBV and HCV and even cigarette smoking to increase the risk of HCC.

Pathogenesis

- Presence of structural/numerical chromosomal aberrations in HCC possibly attributed to repeated cycles of death, inflammation and active hepatocyte replication (regeneration) in chronic hepatitis induces genomic instability in hepatocytes.
  - Point mutation or overexpression of cellular protooncogenes (KRAS), β-catenin, TERT (telomerase transcriptase) gene promoter and loss of heterozygosity of tumour suppressor genes, that is P53 are seen and may be the driver mutations for oncogenesis.
  - Recent studies indicate that IL-6/JAK/STAT pathway may have a role (IL-6 is shown to suppress hepatocytic differentiation and increase their proliferation by enhancing the function of the transcription factor HNF-α).
  - Defects in DNA repair are present.
  - HBV-X gene may have some oncogenic potential. It encodes for HBVX-protein which is a transcriptional activator of numerous genes and can also inactivate tumour suppressor genes.
  - HCV core protein can interact with various cellular proteins to transform cells.
  - Aflatoxin B1 can covalently bind with hepatocytic DNA and induce mutation of TP53.
  - In haemochromatosis and Wilson's disease excessive iron and copper generate ROS and cause mutagenesis.

Table 28.5 Differences between PBC and PSC

S. No.	Feature	PBC	PSC
1	Average age affected	50 years	30 years
2	Gender	90% females	70% females
3	Evolution	Progressive	Unpredictable
4	Associated conditions	Sjögren syndrome	Inflammatory bowel disease Pancreatitis
5	Serology	95% AMA positivity 50% ANA positivity 40% ANCA positivity	5% AMA positivity 6% ANA positivity 65% ANCA positivity
6	Radiological features	Normal	Beaded appearance of the affected segment on a retrograde cholangiogram is diagnostic.
7	Pathology	Small- and medium-sized intrahepatic bile ducts are affected. Large intrahepatic ducts and the extrahepatic biliary structures are not involved.	Causes progressive sclerosing destruction of bile ducts of all sizes. Extrahepatic and large intrahepatic bile ducts are mainly involved.

Investigations

- Alpha-fetoprotein and CEA (markedly increased or rising levels).
- Ultrasonography/CT scan of abdomen.
- Hepatic artery angiography (shows 'tumour blushes')
- Aspiration (FNAC) or biopsy (for confirmation of diagnosis).

Precursor Lesions of HCC

- HCC is thought to arise from **mature hepatocytes** and **progenitor cells** called ductular cells and oval cells.
- **Hepatocellular adenoma** specially those with β-catenin activating mutations may predispose to HCC.
- Dysplasias in the liver can be classified as **small cell change** (cells show high nuclear–cytoplasmic ratio, nuclear hyperchromasia and pleomorphism) and **large cell change** (large pleomorphic cells which may show multiple nuclei). The former is thought to be directly premalignant whereas the latter is considered directly premalignant only in the presence of hepatitis B and is otherwise just identified as a marker for increased risk of HCC.
- High-grade dysplastic nodules are definitely premalignant and show cytological atypia. The premalignant potential of low-grade dysplastic nodules is uncertain though they have been shown to be clonal. They do not show cytological or architectural atypia.

Gross Pathology (Fig. 28.10A)

- HCCs can present as:
  - **A solitary (unifocal) lesion** - Large, circumscribed, solitary mass in the liver.
  - **Multi-centric (multifocal) lesions** - Multiple nodules of variable size present throughout the liver.
  - **Diffuse infiltrating lesion** - The entire liver/a large part of the liver is infiltrated by the tumour which shows indistinct margins.
- Tumour may involve the portal vein (35%–80%), hepatic vein (20%) or inferior vena cava (similar to renal cell carcinoma).
- Haemorrhage and necrosis are common.
- Liver is usually cirrhotic, often enlarged.

Morphology

- Classic HCC shows large, well-differentiated, polygonal cells with well defined cytoplasmic margins, higher N/C ratio than normal, round nuclei with coarse chromatin, thickened nuclear membrane; which may have prominent nucleoli and frequent mitotic figures. The cells are typically arranged in a trabecular pattern with 4+ cells surrounded by a layer of flattened endothelial cells. Acinar pattern (Fig. 28.10B), cord-like arrangement and nests of tumour cells (Fig. 28.10C) may also be seen.
- Variants include clear cell, giant cell, pelioid (with vascular lakes), pseudoglandular (acinar with proteinaceous material or bile in lumina, may resemble thyroid follicles), sarcomatoid, and solid (compact). Presence of sinusoidal vessels surrounding tumour cells is an important diagnostic feature. Other features which are typical include presence of bile, copper, intranuclear pseudoinclusions, Mallory hyaline, and absence of central veins.
- Based on morphology HCC can be classified into:
  - **Well differentiated:** Shows thin plates of tumour cells which are recognisable as hepatocytic in origin, plates are 1-3 hepatocytes thick, cells appear smaller than normal with minimal nuclear atypia, nuclear density is twice that seen in normal liver, cytoplasm is abundant and granular; may resemble hepatocyte adenoma. The

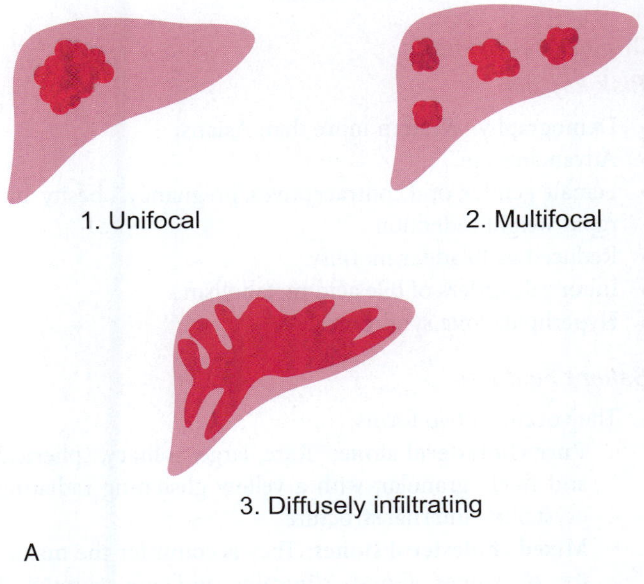

Fig. 28.10 (A) Gross patterns of hepatocellular carcinoma (HCC).

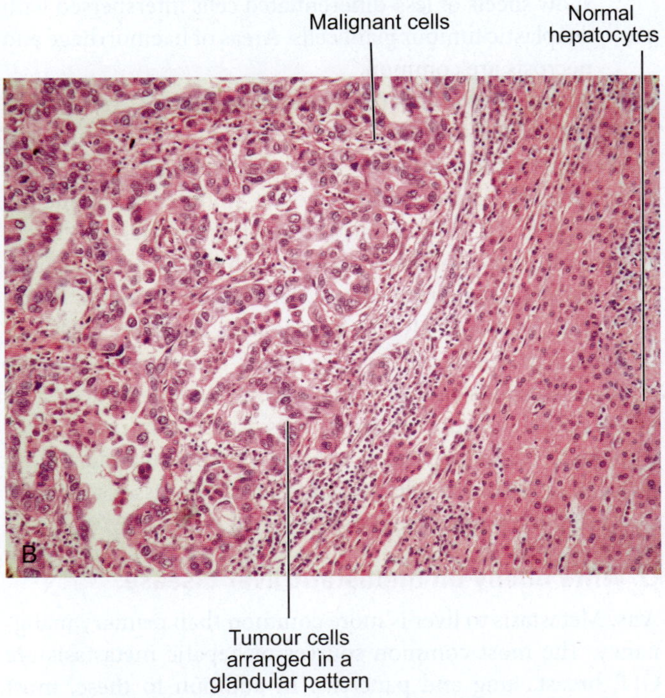

Fig. 28.10 (B) Photomicrograph of HCC showing large, well-differentiated, polygonal cells with central nuclei and frequent mitotic figures. The cells are mainly arranged in an acinar pattern (H&E; 200×).

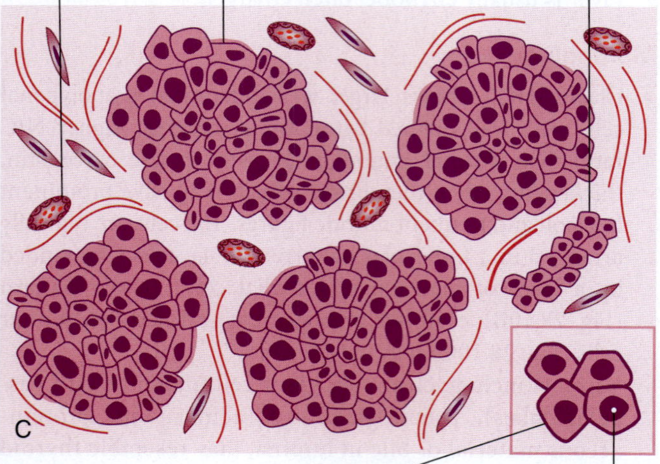

Fig. 28.10 (C) Schematic diagram of hepatocellular carcinoma.

predominant pattern is trabecular and acinar (pseudoglandular). Bile production by tumour cells is the hallmark of well differentiated HCC.
- **Moderately differentiated:** Trabecular pattern with 4+ cells thick plates are seen; tumour cells are larger than well differentiated HCC with more cellular pleomorphism, distinct nucleoli and tumour giant cells.
- **Poorly differentiated:** Poorly differentiated lesions show sheets of less-differentiated cells interspersed with anaplastic tumour giant cells. Areas of haemorrhage and necrosis are common.

- HCC can invade adjacent vascular structures (snake like extension into the portal vein) or abdominal structures and may metastasize to lungs, adrenals, lymph nodes or bone. Intrahepatic spread with satellite nodules is frequently observed. HCC may also spread to portal, perihilar, peripancreatic and para-aortic lymph nodes.
- A distinct histological variant, termed **fibrolamellar carcinoma** (5% of all HCCs) occurs with relatively high frequency in children and young adults. It presents as a single hard scirrhous nodule. This tumour subtype shows large polygonal well-differentiated cells arranged in nests, cords or large islands separated by bundles of acellular dense collagen. The fibrolamellar variant is generally associated with a more favourable prognosis.

Q. Write briefly on metastatic liver disease.

Ans. Metastasis to liver is more common than primary malignancy. The most common sources of hepatic metastasis are GIT, breast, lung and pancreas. In addition to these, most other cancers can metastasize to the liver (leukaemias, lymphomas, melanomas, etc.). The liver is enlarged with the presence of a single or multiple metastatic nodules. The nodules appear as umbilicated masses (umbilication occurs due to necrosis or haemorrhage in the centre as the tumour outgrows its blood supply).

Q. Write briefly on the clinicopathological features of pyogenic liver abscess.

Ans. Clinicopathological features of pyogenic liver abscess
- Bacteria can reach the liver by:
  - Vascular seeding (via portal blood in appendicitis, diverticulitis and perforated bowel and via hepatic artery in systemic bacteraemia).
  - Ascending cholangitis.
  - Direct extension from a contiguous focus of infection, like subphrenic abscess.
  - Penetrating injury.
- Solitary abscess is usually located in the right lobe of liver and results from direct extension of infection and trauma.
- Multiple abscesses are seen in elderly patients, and are usually due to ascending cholangitis.
- *E. coli*, *Klebsiella* species, anaerobic streptococci and Bacteroides are the common causative organisms.
- Clinical features include fever, right-upper quadrant pain and tender hepatomegaly.
- Small lesions respond to antibiotics whereas larger lesions need surgical drainage.

Q. Write briefly on the aetiopathogenesis, clinicopathological features and complications of gallstones.

Ans. Gallstones affect 10%–20% of adult males and 30%–40% of adult females.

Types

Based on the relative amount of cholesterol gall stones are classified into two main types (Fig. 28.11):

1. Cholesterol stones (contain more than 50% of crystalline cholesterol monohydrate); more common in the west.
2. Pigment stones (main constituents are bilirubin and calcium); more common in Asians.

Cholesterol Stones

Risk Factors

- Demography: Western more than Asians.
- Advancing age.
- Female gender, oral contraceptives, pregnancy, obesity and rapid weight reduction.
- Reduced gallbladder motility.
- Inborn disorders of bile acid metabolism.
- Hyperlipidaemia syndromes.

Salient Features

- They occur in two forms:
  - **Pure cholesterol stones:** Rare, large, solitary, spherical and finely granular, with a yellow glistening radiating crystalline internal structure.
  - **Mixed cholesterol stones:** They account for the majority of stones found clinically and are composed predominantly of cholesterol, but also contain variable amounts of bilirubin and calcium salts. Most often,

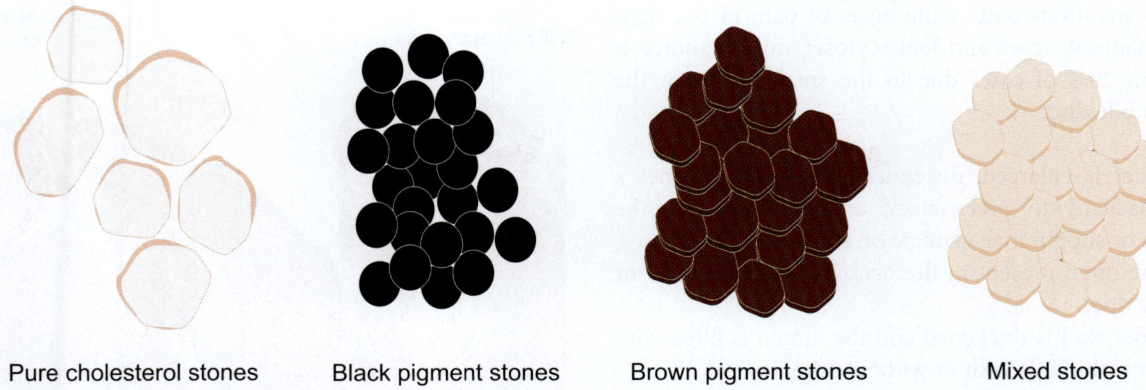

Fig. 28.11 Types of gall stones.

these stones are multiple and 85% of them are radiolucent and cannot be seen on regular X-ray films.

Pathogenesis (Flowchart 28.4)

- Cholesterol which is normally water insoluble becomes water soluble when it complexes with bile salts and lecithins secreted into bile.
- When excess cholesterol accumulates in the bile, it supersaturates (does not remain dissolved anymore and precipitates out). This results in its nucleation into solid cholesterol monohydrate crystals.

Pigment Stones

Risk Factors

- Demography: Asian more than Western.
- Chronic haemolytic syndromes.
- Biliary infection.
- Gastrointestinal disorders: Ileal disease and cystic fibrosis with pancreatic insufficiency.

Salient Features

Pigment stones are either black or brown:

- **Black stones** are composed of **calcium bilirubinate, phosphate, carbonate and very little cholesterol.** These are usually multiple, small and friable and form in chronic haemolytic anaemias, such as sickle cell anaemia or thalassaemia.
- **Brown stones** are composed of **calcium bilirubinate, calcium salts of palmitate and stearate and cholesterol but do not contain calcium phosphate or carbonate.** Usually seen in bacterial infections causing deconjugation of bilirubin and in prolonged biliary stasis and are laminated soap-like, greasy.

Supersaturation of bile with cholesterol
↓
Establishment of nucleation sites by microprecipitation of calcium salts
↓ Hypomotility of gallbladder (stasis) promotes nucleation
Mucous hypersecretion to trap crystals, enhancing their aggregation into stones

Flowchart 28.4 Pathogenesis of cholesterol stone formation.

Pathogenesis (See Flowchart 28.5)

Cholecystitis

Inflammation of gallbladder is labelled cholecystitis. It is of two types—acute and chronic.

Acute Cholecystitis

Salient features

- Females are more often affected than males.
- Associated with gallstones in 90% cases; some cases may be acalculus in origin (acalculus cholecystitis is usually encountered in severely ill patients (major trauma, surgery and burns, immunosuppression, systemic infections and sepsis). Acalculous cholecystitis in most cases is due to ischaemic injury.
- Secondary bacterial infection may follow obstruction in some cases—*Escherichia coli* is the most common pathogen.

Infection of biliary tract
↓
Release of microbial β-glucuronidase
↓
Hydrolysis of bilirubin glucuronides
↓
Formation of pigment stones
↑
Intravascular haemolysis
↓
Increased unconjugated bilirubin (→ Formation of pigment stones)

Flowchart 28.5 Pathogenesis of pigment stone formation.

- Typically manifests with acute onset of pain in the right upper quadrant, fever and leukocytosis; mild jaundice is present in 20% of cases due to the small stones in the common bile duct.

Pathology

- Gallbladder is enlarged, distended, tense and assumes a red, violaceous to green-black colour, there may be fibrinous or suppurative exudate on the serosa.
- Stones are often present in the neck of the gallbladder or the cystic duct.
- Gallbladder wall is thickened and the lumen is filled with cloudy or turbid bile with or without admixed pus.
- The mucosa may show ulceration, oedema, vascular congestion, haemorrhage and suppuration.

Complications

- When the contained exudate becomes pure pus, the condition is called **empyema.**
- In severe cases, gallbladder is transformed into a **green-black necrotic organ (gangrenous cholecystitis).**
- Infection by gas forming organisms can lead to **acute emphysematous cholecystitis.**
- Severe bacterial infection can result in **perforation.**
- Bile may release into the peritoneal cavity causing **biliary peritonitis.**
- Extension of infection can lead to formation of **pericholic** and **hepatic abscesses.**
- **Cholecystoenteric fistula** may form with small and large intestines.
- A large gall stone may pass into the bowel through the fistula causing **gall stone ileus.**

Chronic Cholecystitis

Chronic inflammation of the gall bladder, which follows repeated attacks of acute cholecystitis or develops without any history of previous attacks.

Salient features

- Clinically, it presents with recurrent attacks of colicky epigastric or right upper quadrant pain, nausea, vomiting and intolerance to fatty food.
- Usually associated with gallstones or presence of biliary gravel (thick viscous bile with micro-concretions).
- Chronic acalculus cholecystitis causes symptoms and morphological alterations similar to chronic calculus cholecystitis.

Gross Pathology

- Gallbladder may be contracted, of normal size, or enlarged.
- Serosa is dull and opaque and may show adhesions.
- The wall is thickened, indurated, opaque and grey-white.
- The lumen usually shows stones.

Microscopy

- Mucosa is oedematous and may be focally ulcerated.
- There is presence of chronic inflammatory infiltrate in the wall (Fig. 28.12A, Fig. 28.12B and Fig. 28.12C). Subepithelial and subserosal fibrosis and extension of mucosal sinuses into the muscularis **(Rokitansky–Aschoff or RA sinuses)** are commonly seen.
- Additionally, neuromatous hyperplasia, hyalinised collagen, dystrophic calcification, lymphoid aggregates, variable mucosal metaplastic changes may be seen.

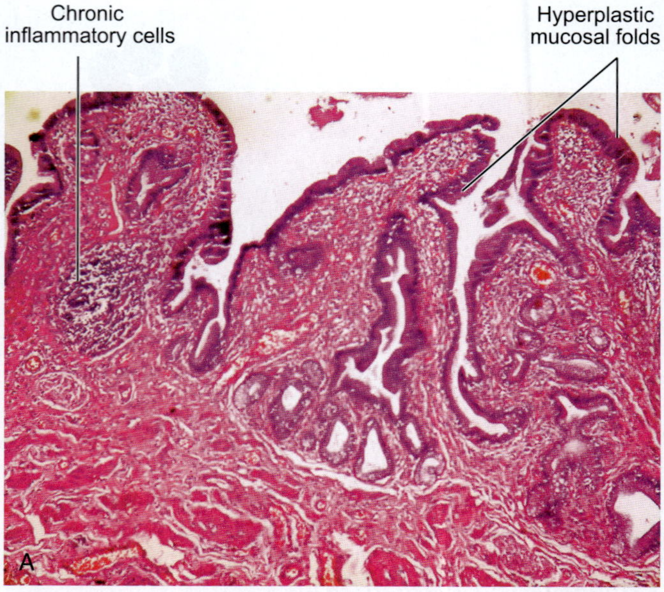

Fig. 28.12 (A) Section from chronic cholecystitis showing gall bladder wall infiltrated by chronic inflammatory cells (H&E; 100×).

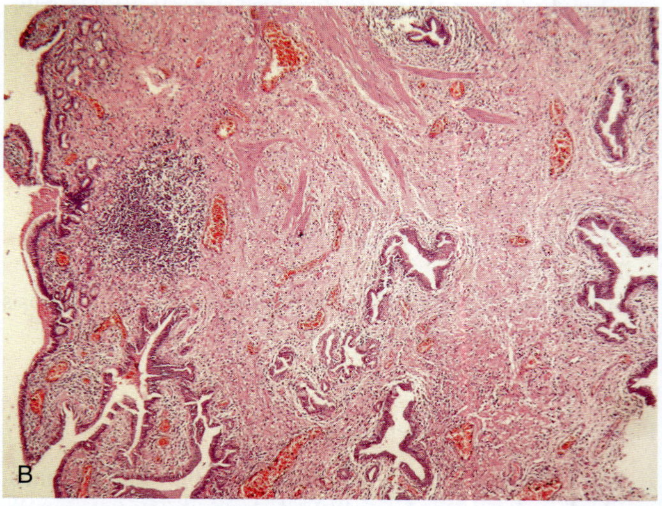

Fig. 28.12 (B) Section from chronic cholecystitis showing hyperplastic mucosal folds, and chronic mucosal inflammation with formation of lymphoid aggregates with RA sinuses (H&E; 100×).

Complications

- **Cholangitis:** Bacterial super infection leading to local spread.
- **Sepsis:** Bacterial dissemination by blood.
- **Subhepatic abscess:** Perforation leading to subhepatic abscess or bacterial peritonitis.
- **Hydrops** (obstruction due to gall stones causing distension of gall bladder with clear watery fluid) or **mucocele** (gall stones causing distension of gall bladder by cloudy, mucoid material).
- **Cholecystoenteric fistula:** Formation of a fistula between the gallbladder and the intestine.
- **Gallstone ileus:** May follow the impaction of a gallstone in the intestine.

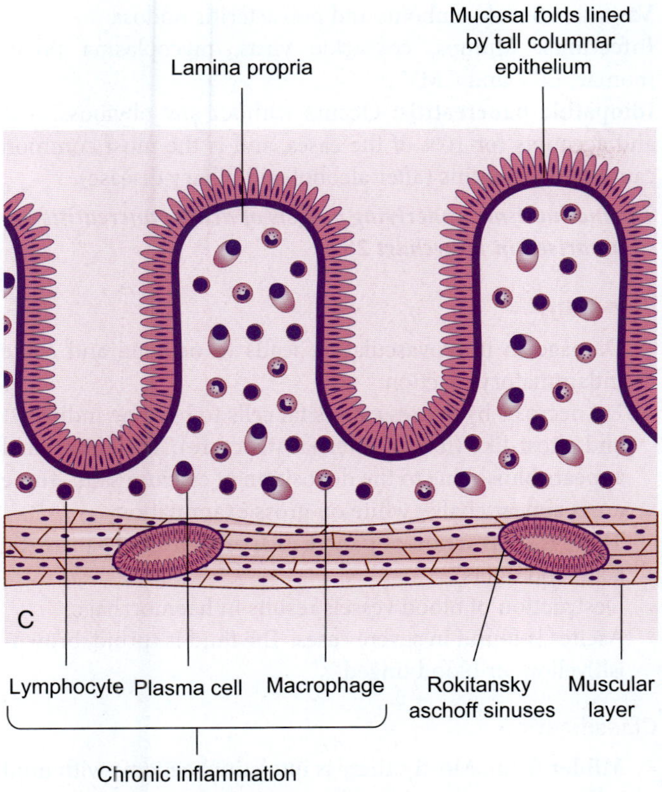

Fig. 28.12 (C) Schematic representation of chronic cholecystitis.

- **Porcelain gallbladder:** Scarring of the wall, combined with dystrophic calcification that transforms the gallbladder into a porcelain-like vessel, visible on standard X-ray films.
- **Xanthogranulomatous cholecystitis:** The gall bladder may be shrunken and show a markedly thickened wall as a result of rupture of an RA sinus. Sections from the wall show chronic inflammatory infiltrate with foamy histiocytes (xanthoma cells) and granulomas.
- **Malignancy:** Long-standing gall stones increase the risk of **carcinoma gallbladder.**

Q. Write briefly on carcinoma of gallbladder.

Ans. Carcinoma of the gallbladder clinically mimics benign gallbladder diseases and often escapes detection until advanced stage. The average age of presentation of carcinoma of gallbladder is 65 years. It has a lower incidence in Asia, where pyogenic and parasitic disease of biliary tree are more common and is more common in American Indians and Hispanics; very rare in blacks.

Aetiopathogenesis and Molecular Genetics

- Gallbladder carcinoma is associated with **gallstones** in up to 90% of cases; **porcelain gallbladder** is a high-risk condition. Calculi are thought to predispose to malignancy by causing chronic irritation and repeated epithelial damage.
- Methylation in the promotor gene is a crucial early event in gall bladder carcinogenesis.
- p16 protein over-expression, *KRAS* mutations and to a lesser extent microsatellite instability are key events in dysplastic lesions and gallbladder carcinomas.

Clinical Features

- Patient presents with abdominal pain, jaundice, anorexia, nausea and vomiting.
- Preoperative diagnosis is based on finding abnormalities in the gallbladder wall on imaging studies.
- Often invades liver, common bile duct, cystic duct, stomach, duodenum and transverse colon; may spread to peritoneal surfaces.
- 70% involve liver at diagnosis, 50% involve regional lymph nodes. The perihilar and porta-hepatic lymph nodes are involved in the initial stages. The cancer may then spread to mediastinal and supraclavicular lymph nodes.

Gross Pathology

- Most arise from the fundus and neck; few from the body.
- Grossly, carcinoma of the gallbladder may be exophytic or more commonly infiltrative in nature; the latter usually appears as diffuse thickening of the wall of the gallbladder.

Microscopy

- Most gall bladder malignancies are adenocarcinomas (90%); few are squamous or adenosquamous carcinomas (10%) that arise from areas of squamous metaplasia in chronic cholecystitis and cholelithiasis.
- Well differentiated lesions show well-formed glands and papillary architectures with wide lumina lined by atypical cuboidal cells embedded in a desmoplastic stroma.
- Poorly differentiated lesions on the other hand are difficult to recognize and may require immunohistochemistry for definite diagnosis.

Q. Write briefly on cholangiocarcinomas.

Ans. Cholangiocarcinoma, a malignancy arising from the biliary tree, is the second most common tumour of the liver after HCC. It usually presents in the fifth to seventh decades and has a male to female ratio of 1:1.

Risk Factors

Include liver fluke infestation, hepatolithiasis (intrahepatic gallstone formation), PSC, fibrocystic disease of the biliary tree (Caroli disease and choledochal cysts), hepatitis B and C, NAFLD and exposure to thorotrast.

Precursor Lesions and Classification

- **Biliary intraepithelial neoplasias (BilIN)** are known precursors of cholangiocarcinomas, which are mainly adenocarcinomas with biliary differentiation.
- May be **extrahepatic** or **intrahepatic**; extrahepatic cholangiocarcinomas (two-third of these tumours) may develop at the hilum (called **Klatskin tumours**) or more distally.
- These tumours have a poor prognosis.

Pathology

- Unencapsulated, white-tan and firm intra-hepatic mass.
- Sections show an adenocarcinoma with varying degree of atypia and differentiation, infiltrating a dense fibrous or desmoplastic stroma.
- Should be differentiated from a metastatic adenocarcinoma by thorough review of the patient's clinical history and application of an appropriate immunohistochemistry panel.

PANCREAS

The pancreas is located in the retroperitoneal space caudal to the stomach. It extends horizontally from the duodenum on the right to the spleen on the left. It has three parts:

- **The head** of the pancreas is lying in the duodenal loop in close contact with the wall of this part of the intestine.
- **The body** of the pancreas is lying over the aorta and the vena cava.
- **The tail** of the pancreas abuts onto the spleen.
- Pancreas is a mixed exocrine–endocrine organ.
- The exocrine pancreatic tissue (consists of acini and ducts) accounts for 98% of the total mass.
- Endocrine parts (islets of Langerhans) are microscopic structures that are more numerous in the tail.
- The terminal portion of the main pancreatic duct (duct of Wirsung) enters the muscular portion of the duodenal wall, where it meets with the common bile duct forming a common biliary-pancreatic duct that enters the duodenum at the ampulla of Vater.
- In some persons, the pancreatic duct enters the duodenum separately from the common bile duct.
- An accessory pancreatic duct (duct of Santorini), emptying into the duodenum, is found in many persons.

Cells Forming the Islets of Langerhans

- Alpha cells: Secrete glucagon (increases blood glucose).
- Beta cells: Secrete insulin (lowers blood glucose).
- Delta cells: Secrete somatostatin (inhibits the secretion of other islet hormones).
- Delta-1 cells: Secrete vasoactive intestinal polypeptide (VIP), which regulates and stimulates the motility of intestines.
- PP cells: Secrete pancreatic polypeptide (stimulates gastric secretion and inhibits intestinal mobility).

Q. Write briefly on the clinicopathological features of acute pancreatitis.

Ans. Acute pancreatitis is defined as acute inflammation of the pancreas usually resulting from injury to the exocrine pancreas.

Causes

Metabolic: Hyperlipoproteinaemias, hypercalcaemia, alcoholism, drugs (e.g. diuretics, azathioprine and mercaptopurine).

Genetic

- Inherited mutations in genes encoding pancreatic enzymes or their inhibitors, for example SPINK1 (serine peptidase inhibitor Kazal type 1) which is an inhibitor of trypsin.
- Hereditary pancreatitis with trypsinogen mutation is an autosomal dominant disease caused by a mutation in PRSS1 gene that affects a site on trypsinogen molecule required for cleavage of trypsin, leading to continuous activation of other digestive proenzymes and development of pancreatitis.

Mechanical: Trauma (seat-belt injury), gallstones, injury during endoscopic procedures like endoscopic retrograde cholangiopancreatography (ERCP) or perioperative injury.

Vascular: Shock, embolus and polyarteritis nodosa.

Infections: Mumps, coxsackie virus, mycoplasma pneumoniae, EBV and CMV.

Idiopathic pancreatitis: Occurs without any obvious cause and accounts for 10% of the cases, and is the most common cause of pancreatitis (after alcohol and biliary disease).

The mechanisms underlying genesis of acute pancreatitis are summarised in Flowchart 28.6.

Pathology

- Damage to microvasculature leads to oedema and acute inflammatory reaction.
- Fat necrosis by lipases causes fat cells to become indistinct and ghost-like (loss of internal structure). The entire field appears bluish due to the deposition of calcium salts. These areas appear chalky white on gross examination.
- There is destruction of pancreatic parenchyma (pancreatic acini and ducts).
- Destruction of blood vessels results in haemorrhage.
- Ascites is found in severe cases. The fluid is turbid, brownish yellow, or blood tinged.

Classification

- **Milder form:** Mostly, there is interstitial oedema with mild inflammation. Focal mild necrosis of acinar cells may sometimes be seen. This form occurs in terminally ill patients, various forms of shock and after prolonged operations. It is recognized by mild elevation of pancreatic enzymes in the blood, is self-limiting and usually resolves spontaneously.
- **Acute necrotising/haemorrhagic pancreatitis:** May be life-threatening. Caused by enzyme-mediated destruction of pancreatic and peripancreatic tissue. Neutrophils invade the necrotic tissue. In later stages, neutrophils are replaced by macrophages and the entire area undergoes fibrosis.

Clinical Features

- Sudden onset of severe abdominal pain usually in the left upper quadrant of the abdomen; may radiate to the back.
- Nausea and vomiting, fever, sweating, tachypnea and tachycardia followed by peripheral vascular collapse.

Laboratory Findings

- **Neutrophilic leukocytosis:** Increase in neutrophil count.
- **Serum amylase:** It is a sensitive marker for acute pancreatitis in the first 24 h; especially, if the elevation is four times above normal values.
- **Urinary amylase:** Amylase is excreted in urine. Amylase levels in urine become elevated from the second day onwards and may remain elevated for 7–10 days. This test has little specificity and sensitivity.
- **Serum lipase:** It appears little later than amylase in blood, but it is more specific.
- **Trypsin:** This enzyme has the highest specificity and sensitivity for pancreatic injury, but its measurement requires the use of a radioimmunoassay, which is not available in all hospitals.

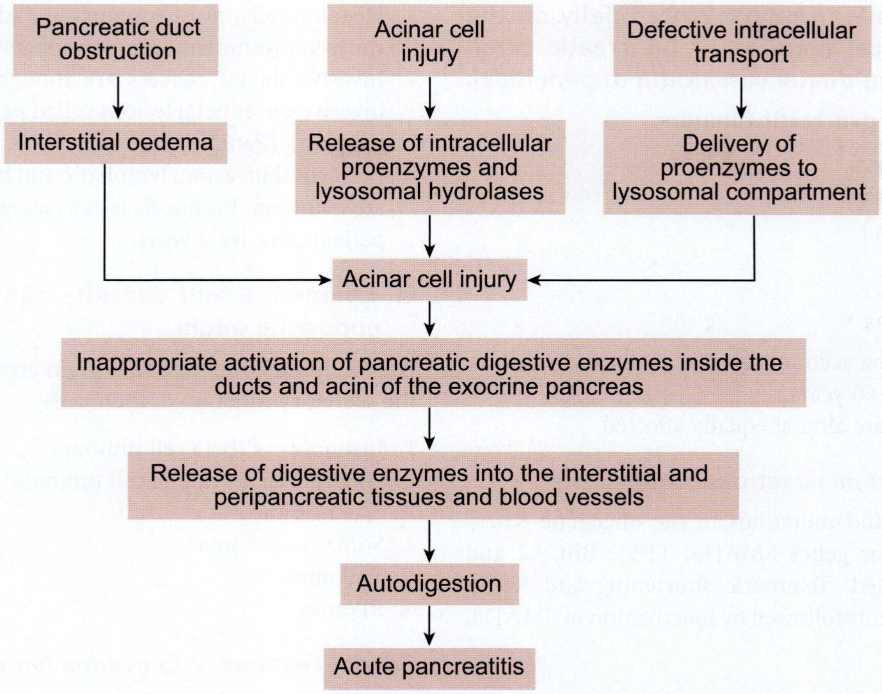

Flowchart 28.6 The mechanisms underlying the genesis of acute pancreatitis.

- **Hypocalcaemia:** Occurs due to precipitation of calcium in the areas of fat necrosis. If persistent indicates a poor prognosis.
- **X-rays:** Plain X-rays are important to exclude perforation of an ulcer (which is a close differential and can be diagnosed based on visible air under the diaphragm). **CT scan** aids in demonstrating the enlarged pancreas and ascites (ascitic fluid if analysed biochemically shows increased amount of pancreatic enzymes).

Complications

- **Shock:** It is multifactorial, but mostly due to increased vascular permeability caused by the action of pancreatic enzymes.
- **DIC:** Endothelial injury caused by pancreatic enzymes in circulation leads to the formation of platelet and fibrin thrombi in small vessels.
- **ARDS:** It is a manifestation of shock.
- **Renal failure:** It is mostly a consequence of shock.
- **Pseudocyst formation:** Massive necrosis leads to liquefactive necrosis of the tissue. The necrotic area becomes walled off by granulation tissue, which transforms later into a fibrous scar. The cyst contains fluid full of pancreatic enzymes.
- **Abscess:** Infection superimposed on pancreatic necrosis leads to abscess formation. This is associated with high mortality.
- **Haemorrhagic ascites:** Pancreatic ascites is a somewhat rare entity. It results from persistent leakage of pancreatic secretions in the peritoneum from pancreatic duct injury. Presence of bloody fluid in the peritoneal and pleural cavities is usually indicative of severe pancreatic injury and is a rare phenomenon.
- **Subcutaneous fat necrosis:** Foci of fat necrosis develop and are related to the action of lipolytic enzymes that have entered the circulation.
- **Chronic pancreatitis:** Most patients with acute pancreatitis recover, if treated appropriately. Persistence of inflammation leads to chronic pancreatitis.

Q. Write briefly on the clinicopathological features of chronic pancreatitis.

Ans. Chronic pancreatitis is characterised by chronic inflammation with fibrosis leading to a progressive loss of pancreatic function. The pancreas is reduced in size and often showed calcification.

Causes

- Chronic alcohol abuse
- Cystic fibrosis of the pancreas
- Familial chronic pancreatitis and 'tropical chronic pancreatitis'
- Idiopathic

Clinical Features

- Persistent upper abdominal pain radiating to the back, often precipitated by alcohol.
- Malabsorption due to pancreatic insufficiency—steatorrhoea, vitamins A, D, E and K deficiency.
- Diabetes mellitus.
- X-ray may show calcifications and distorted ducts can be visualised by ERCP.

Pathology

- Persistent chronic inflammation composed of lymphocytes, macrophages and plasma cells.
- Fibrosis, calcification and intraductal concretions.
- Loss and atrophy of acini, with partial preservation of ducts and islets of Langerhans.
- Cystic dilatation of ducts distal to narrowing by fibrous tissue.

Q. Classify pancreatic tumours. Write briefly on the clinicopathological features of pancreatic carcinoma (infiltrating ductal carcinoma of pancreas).

Ans. Classification of pancreatic tumours:

1. Ductal tumours (90%)
2. Islet cell tumours (5%)
3. Acinar tumours (2%)
4. Others

Pancreatic Carcinoma

- Pancreatic carcinoma accounts for 6% of all cancer deaths.
- Most patients are >60 years.
- Males and females are almost equally affected.

Molecular aspects of pancreatic carcinogenesis

Telomere shortening and mutations in the oncogene KRAS and tumour suppressor genes SMAD4, TP53, BRCA2 and CDKN2a are implicated. Telomeric shortening and KRAS mutations are early events followed by inactivation of SMAD4, TP53 and BRCA2.

Risk Factors

- Cigarette smoking.
- Chronic pancreatitis and diabetes mellitus.
- Diet high in fat and low in vegetables.

Clinical Features

- Pain (persistent and usually progressive).
- Anorexia and weight loss.
- Jaundice.
- Migratory superficial thrombophlebitis **(Trousseau sign).**

Morphology

- Indurated white mass (may be confused with chronic pancreatitis).
- Head is involved most often (60%), but it may occur in any part of the pancreas.
- Histologically, most tumours are adenocarcinomas which shows a prominent desmoplastic response.
- Invasive ductal cancers are thought to arise from non-invasive intraductal lesions called pancreatic intraepithelial neoplasia (PanIN).
- Perineural invasion, lymphatic and blood-borne metastasis are common. Prognosis is extremely poor, and only 10% of patients survive 2 years.

Q. Enumerate and describe pancreatic tumours of endocrine origin.

Ans. Tumours of endocrine origin are classified according to the secretory function of their cells:

1. Insulinomas (beta cell tumours)
2. Glucagonomas (alpha cell tumours)
3. Gastrinomas
4. Somatostatinomas
5. VIPomas
6. PPomas

Salient Features of Endocrine Tumours of Pancreas

- Endocrine tumours are rare.
- They are generally composed of cords and nests of uniform cells with round nuclei and moderate amount of cytoplasm (identical to intestinal or bronchial carcinoids).
- Most are low-grade malignant tumours (except insulinomas, which are usually benign).
- Benign tumours may show 'endocrine atypia' and cannot be distinguished from the malignant tumours on the basis of histology alone. Metastasis is the only definitive sign that a tumour is malignant.
- Endocrine tumours secrete hormones that produce typical syndromes.

Diseases of Kidney and Lower Urinary Tract

29

NORMAL STRUCTURE (PA28.1)

The kidneys are paired, bean-shaped, retroperitoneal organs, each weighing about 150 g in the adult male and 135 g in the adult female. They are typically 10–12 cm in length, 5–7 cm in width and 2–3 cm in thickness. The renal artery, vein, lymphatics and the ureters are located in the renal hilum, which is the centre of the concave area of the kidney. The upper and lower poles of each kidney lie opposite to the 12th thoracic vertebra and the 3rd lumbar vertebra, respectively. The right kidney is slightly lower because of the presence of liver. The renal capsule **is a smooth, transparent, fibrous membrane that is normally easily removable. It protects the organ and is surrounded by perirenal fat which further cushions the kidneys.**

The **cut surface** of the bisected kidney shows a pale outer region, the **cortex**, and a darker inner region, the **medulla** (Fig. 29.1). The cortex contains all the glomeruli and 85% of tubules (mainly proximal convoluted tubules). The medulla is divided into 8–18 conical masses, the **renal pyramids**, the bases of which lie along the corticomedullary junction and the apices extend into the renal pelvis (the collecting system of the kidney) to form **papillae**. The tip of each papilla has 10–25 small openings of the distal ends of the **collecting ducts (of Bellini)**. The renal cortex is about 1.5 cm in thickness and covers the base of each renal pyramid to extend downward between the individual pyramids to form the **renal columns of Bertin**. The ureter on entering the kidney dilates to form the **renal pelvis**, which is lined by transitional epithelium and forms two to three outpouchings, the **major calyces**. From each of the major calyces, several **minor calyces** extend towards the papillae of the pyramids.

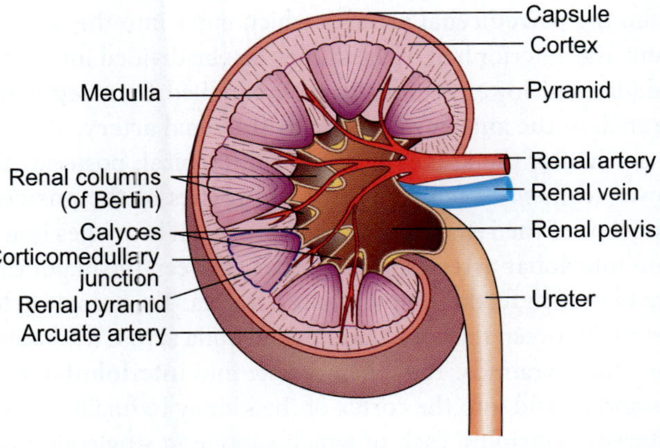

Fig. 29.1 Schematic representation of the cut surface of kidney.

The main unit of parenchyma of each kidney is the **nephron**. There are about 1–4 million nephrons in each kidney. Each nephron contains five major subunits, the dilated 'glomerulus with the Bowman's capsule', 'the proximal convoluted tubule or PCT', 'the thin and thick loop of Henle', 'the distal convoluted tubule' or DCT and the 'collecting ducts' (Fig. 29.2).

The **glomerulus** is a bulbous structure invaginated by a capillary network which is surrounded by a double-layered epithelial capsule called the **Bowman's capsule**. The inner layer enveloping the capillary tuft is called the **visceral layer** and the outer layer is called the **parietal layer**. Between the visceral and the parietal epithelial layers is a cavity called **Bowman's space**. The large area of the capillary network makes the glomerulus an efficient filtration unit. Each nephron has a **vascular pole** and a **urinary pole**. The **vascular pole** is where the afferent arteriole enters and the efferent arteriole leaves. The PCT begins at the **urinary pole**. The inner side of the glomerular capillary wall is lined by a thin layer of fenestrated endothelial cells which rest on the glomerular basement membrane (GBM). The GBM is constituted by collagen, laminin, fibronectin, proteoglycans and glycoproteins and has three layers:

(a) Lamina rara externa on the external side.
(b) Lamina densa in the middle.
(c) Lamina rara interna on the internal side.

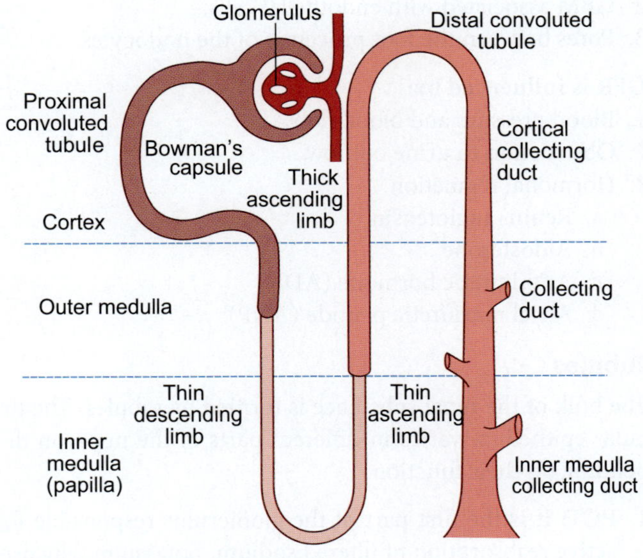

Fig. 29.2 Parts of a nephron.

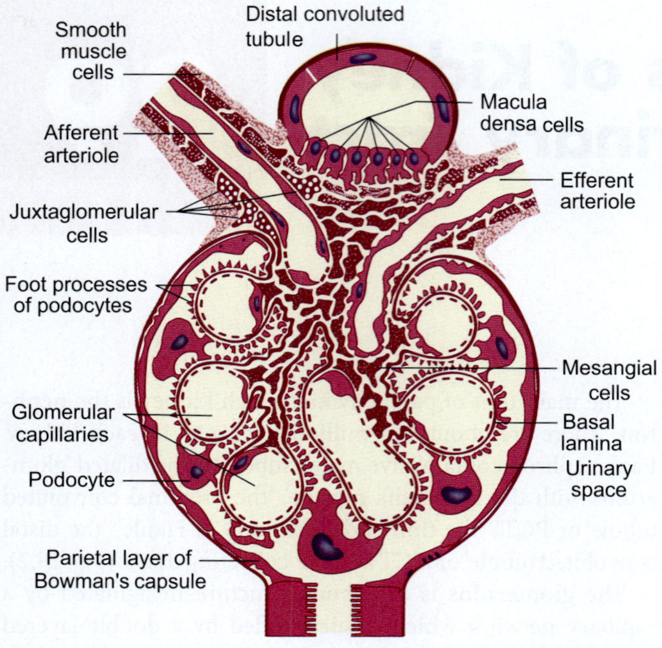

Fig. 29.3 Schematic representation of a renal glomerulus.

Any abnormality in the glomerular epithelial cells or the above-mentioned three layers may disturb the barrier to filtration of macromolecules.

The glomerulus is supported by mesangial cells with the surrounding mesangial matrix material. The external side of the capillary wall is lined by the visceral epithelial cells which rest on the lamina rara externa. These cells have foot-like extensions and are therefore also called podocytes (podo – foot). The podocytes have 20- to 30-nm-wide spaces between them to allow filtration (Fig. 29.3).

The **main function of the glomerulus** is filtration from the capillaries to the Bowman's space. Normal glomerular filtration rate (GFR) is about 125 mL/min. The glomerular filtrate is identical to plasma in composition except it lacks cells and protein.

Glomerular filtration occurs across the following barriers:

1. Fenestrated endothelial cells lining the capillaries.
2. GBM associated with endothelial cells.
3. Pores between the foot processes of the podocytes.

GFR is influenced by:

1. Blood pressure and blood flow.
2. Obstruction to urine outflow.
3. Hormonal regulation
   a. Renin–angiotensin
   b. Aldosterone
   c. Antidiuretic hormone (ADH)
   d. Atrial natriuretic peptide (ANP).

Tubules

The bulk of the renal substance is formed by tubules. The tubular epithelium varies in different parts of the nephron depending on their function.

1. **PCT:** It is the first part of the glomerulus responsible for active reabsorption of filtered sodium, potassium, glucose, amino acids and proteins, bicarbonate, phosphate, calcium and uric acid as well as passive reabsorption of water. It arises at the urinary pole and is lined by cuboidal cells with a brush border (presence of microvilli), acidophilic granular cytoplasm and central nuclei.
2. **Loop of Henle:** The PCT continues as the straight part of loop of Henle. The loop of Henle begins near the corticomedullary junction; it is U shaped and has a thin descending and a thick ascending portion. The thin portion is lined by flat epithelium with nuclei projecting into the lumen. The thick portion is identical in structure to the DCT and ends at the corticomedullary union.
3. **DCT:** The thick part of loop of Henle becomes tortuous, enters the cortex and continues as the DCT. It is lined by flatter cells which are smaller in size as compared with cells lining the PCT, are less acidophilic and do not have a brush border. The lumina of the distal tubules are larger because of the smaller size of the lining cells. DCT touches the vascular pole of the renal corpuscle of its nephron close to the point of entry of the afferent arteriole. Here, the lining epithelium gets modified to become columnar with closely packed nuclei (thereby appearing darker). This area is called the **macula densa.**
4. **Collecting tubules:** The collecting ducts join to form the larger straight ducts called the papillary ducts of Bellini. Collecting tubules form the major bulk of the medulla. The smaller ducts are lined by cuboidal epithelium; however, as they dip into the medulla, the lining epithelium becomes columnar. The cytoplasm of the cells is uniformly pale staining.

Juxtaglomerular Apparatus (JGA)

The JGA is located in the vascular pole of the glomerulus and has three parts:

1. Juxtaglomerular cells – epithelioid cells with granular cytoplasm located in the media of the afferent arteriole and secrete rennin.
2. Macula densa.
3. Extraglomerular mesangial or Lacis or Polkissen cells – lightly staining cells whose function is not clearly understood.

Vascular Supply

The kidneys receive approximately 20% of the cardiac output from the **paired renal arteries** which enter into the renal hilum. The anterior half of the kidney can be divided into upper, middle and lower segments, each supplied by a **segmental branch of the anterior division of the renal artery**. The posterior half of the kidney is divided into apical, posterior and lower segments, each supplied by **branches of the posterior division of the renal artery**. The **segmental branches** branch into **interlobar arteries**, which travel between the major calyces to branch further into **arcuate arteries**. The arcuate **arteries** run between the cortex and the medulla across the bases of the renal pyramids. They then radiate into **interlobular** arteries and extend into the cortex of the kidney to finally become **afferent arterioles**, each of which supplies a single glomerulus. From the glomerulus arise the **efferent arterioles**. The efferent arterioles supply the **peritubular capillary plexus** which anastomoses with the capillary plexus of another nephron. Some of the terminal branches of the interlobular arteries become **perforating radiate arteries**, which supply the renal capsule.

FUNCTIONS OF KIDNEY

1. Maintenance of electrolyte levels and acid–base balance.
2. Regulation of blood pressure and maintenance of salt and water balance.
3. Removal of water-soluble wastes from the blood, e.g. urea and ammonia, and reabsorption of water, glucose and amino acids.
4. Production of hormones like calcitriol, erythropoietin and rennin.

URINE FORMATION

- The kidney maintains water and electrolyte balance and contributes to acid–base homeostasis.
- Composition of urine varies with water, salt and protein intake.
- Variability in composition may create a practical problem in the timing of collection of urine specimens.
- Timed urinary collections are preferred to random specimens.
- In a normal adult, 25% of cardiac output (>1 L of blood) perfuses two kidneys each minute.
- The essential steps in formation of urine are as follows (Flowchart 29.1):
    1. Filtration of substances from blood into Bowman's capsule (glomerular filtrate formation).
    2. Reabsorption of some of the filtered substances back into the bloodstream.
    3. Secretion of substances from blood into tubule.

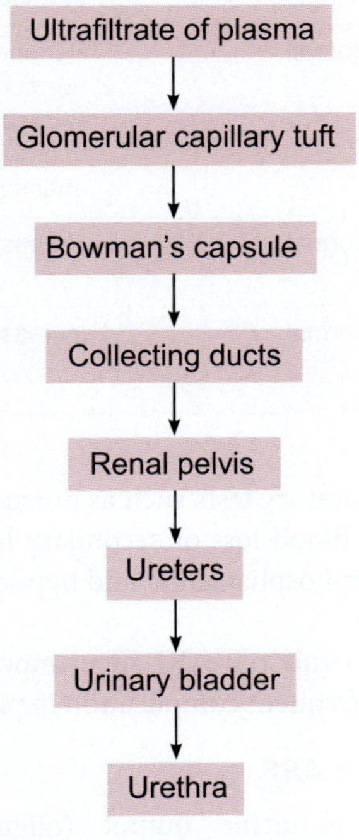

Flowchart 29.1 Formation and flow of urine.

COMPOSITION OF URINE

- Most of the solute is urea and sodium chloride.
- Protein intake affects nitrogen excretion, which is mainly as urea.
- Uric acid, creatinine, amino acids, ammonia, traces of proteins, glycoproteins, enzymes and purines account for the remaining nitrogen excreted.
- Potassium, sulphates, sulphides, cysteine, mercaptans, small amounts of sugars (pentoses), oxalic acid, citric acid, pyruvate, trace amounts of cholesterol and metals are present.
- Also present are hormones, e.g. ketosteroids, oestrogens, aldosterone, gonadotropins, catecholamines and ascorbic acid, along with trace amounts of bilirubin, haemoglobin and porphyrins seen.
- **Microscopic constituents (formed elements)** of urine include RBCs, leucocytes, renal tubular epithelium, transitional and squamous epithelium and physiological casts.

Q. Write briefly about renal failure. Differentiate between acute and chronic renal failure.

(PA28.2, 28.3, 28.4)

Ans. Renal failure, also known as **end-stage kidney disease**, is a medical condition in which the kidneys are functioning at less than 15% of normal. It is classified as either acute kidney failure, which develops rapidly and may resolve, or chronic kidney failure, which develops slowly.

Clinical Features of Renal Failure

- Nausea, vomiting and/or diarrhoea (may lead to dehydration).
- Weight loss.
- Increased urination, nocturia and pale urine.
- Haematuria.
- Itching and bone damage (due to increased phosphates).
- Muscle cramps (caused by hypocalcaemia with or without hyperphosphataemia).
- Hyperkalaemia, which may cause arrhythmias or muscle paralysis.
- Failure of kidneys to remove excess fluid, which causes oedema and shortness of breath.
- Anaemia (due to decreased erythropoietin) resulting in tiredness, impaired memory and concentration, dizziness and hypotension/hypertension.
- Loss of appetite and a bad taste in the mouth.
- Insomnia.
- Pigmentation of the skin.

Acute Renal Failure (ARF)

Causes

1. Prerenal
    - Medications (NSAIDS, ACE inhibitors, angiotensin receptor blockers, cyclosporine, penicillin analogues, cephalosporins, sulphonamides, ciprofloxacin, acyclovir, rifampin, phenytoin, interferon, proton pump inhibitors).

- Cardiorenal and hepatorenal syndrome.
- Abdominal compartment syndrome.
- Hypercalcaemia.
- Systemic vasodilation (e.g. sepsis, neurogenic shock).
- Volume depletion.
- Renal loss from diuretic overuse and osmotic diuresis in diabetic ketoacidosis.
- Extrarenal loss (vomiting, diarrhoea, burns, sweating, blood loss).

2. Renal
   - Glomerular diseases (postinfectious glomerulonephritis).
   - Infections – viruses (EBV, CMV, HIV); bacteria (*Streptococcus* and *Legionella* species); fungi.
   - Systemic disease (sarcoidosis, SLE).
   - Tubular causes – ischaemic (prolonged hypotension) and nephrotoxic (radiographic contrast agents, aminoglycosides, cisplatin, methotrexate, ethylene glycol, amphotericin, haemolysis and rhabdomyolysis, myeloma).
   - Vascular causes (renal vein thrombosis, malignant hypertension, scleroderma renal crisis, renal atheroembolic disease and renal infarction).
3. Postrenal
   - Extrarenal obstruction (prostate hypertrophy, neurogenic bladder, retroperitoneal fibrosis, bladder, prostate or cervical cancer).
   - Intrarenal obstruction (stones, clots, tumours).

History and Physical Examination

- **Prerenal azotaemia** should be suspected in the setting of vomiting, diarrhoea, glycosuria causing polyuria and medications (diuretics, NSAIDs, ACE inhibitors). Physical signs of orthostatic hypotension, tachycardia, reduced jugular venous pressure, decreased skin turgor and dry mucous membranes are often present in prerenal azotaemia.
- A history of prostatic disease, nephrolithiasis, or pelvic or para-aortic malignancy would suggest the possibility of **postrenal ARF**.
- Acute kidney injury (AKI) accompanied by palpable purpura, pulmonary haemorrhage or sinusitis raises the possibility of **systemic vasculitis with glomerulonephritis.**

Diagnostic Evaluation

- The presence of ARF or AKI is usually inferred by an elevation in the SCr (serum creatinine) concentration. AKI is currently defined by a rise from baseline of at least 0.3 mg/dL within 48 hours or at least 50% higher than baseline within 1 week, or a reduction in urine output to less than 0.5 mL/kg/h for longer than 6 hours.
- Other investigations to be done include complete blood count (CBC), urinalysis, fractional excretion of sodium and ultrasonography of the kidney.
- The distinction between AKI and chronic kidney disease (CKD) is important for proper diagnosis and treatment. Differences between ARF and chronic renal failure (CRF) are listed in Table 29.1.
- Clues suggestive of CKD can come from radiological studies (e.g. small, shrunken kidneys with cortical thinning on renal ultrasound, or evidence of renal osteodystrophy) or findings in laboratory tests such as normocytic anaemia in the absence of blood loss or secondary hyperparathyroidism with hyperphosphataemia and hypocalcaemia, consistent with CKD.
- It is difficult to rule out AKI superimposed on CKD because AKI is a frequent complication in patients with CKD.

Table 29.1 Differences between acute and chronic renal failure

Features	Acute renal failure	Chronic renal failure
Definition	• Rapid onset of renal dysfunction; may be reversible • Manifests with oliguria/anuria and increase in urea and creatinine	• Progressive and irreversible deterioration of renal function because of slow destruction of renal parenchyma • Manifests with azotaemia and acidosis
Causes	Prerenal (ischaemia and hypovolaemia), renal (vascular, glomerular and tubular disorders) and postrenal (obstruction in ureters, bladder and urethra)	All chronic nephropathies such as chronic glomerular diseases, as well as chronic tubulointerstitial diseases
Metabolic acidosis	1. Poorly tolerated	Well tolerated
Clinical presentation	Three patterns: 1. Syndrome of acute nephritis 2. Syndrome accompanying tubular dysfunction 3. Prerenal syndrome	Four stages: 1. Diminished renal reserve (50% GFR) 2. Renal insufficiency (20%–50% GFR) 3. Renal failure (5%–20% GFR) 4. End-stage renal disease (<5% GFR)
Urine output	Markedly decreased	Normal
Serum electrolytes		
Calcium	Normal/low	Low
Phosphate	Increased	Markedly increased
Sodium	Decreased	Markedly decreased
Potassium	Increased	Markedly increased
Haemoglobin	Normal	Reduced (normocytic normochromic anaemia; in case of blood loss, microcytic hypochromic anaemia)
Serum parathormone	Normal	Increased
Alkaline phosphatase	Normal	Increased

Urine Findings in ARF

- A reduction in urine output (oliguria, defined as <400 mL/24 h) usually denotes more severe AKI than when urine output is preserved. Oliguria is associated with worse clinical outcomes.

- Red or brown urine may be seen with or without gross haematuria; if the colour persists in the supernatant after centrifugation, then pigment nephropathy from rhabdomyolysis or haemolysis should be suspected.
- Myeloma light chains are not detected with conventional urine dipsticks and require the sulphosalicylic acid test or immunoelectrophoresis.
- Atheroemboli can cause a variable degree of proteinuria. Extremely heavy proteinuria ('nephrotic range', >3.5 g/day) can occasionally be seen in glomerulonephritis, vasculitis or interstitial nephritis (particularly from NSAIDs). AKI can also complicate cases of minimal change disease (MCD), a cause of the nephrotic syndrome.
- Prerenal azotaemia may present with hyaline casts or an unremarkable urine sediment exam.
- Postrenal AKI may also lead to an unremarkable sediment, but haematuria and pyuria are generally seen.
- AKI due to ischaemic injury, sepsis or certain nephrotoxins has characteristic urine sediment findings: pigmented 'muddy brown' granular casts and tubular epithelial cell casts.
- Glomerulonephritis may lead to dysmorphic red blood cells or red blood cell casts.
- Interstitial nephritis may lead to white blood cell casts.
- The urine sediment findings overlap somewhat in glomerulonephritis and interstitial nephritis, and a diagnosis is not always possible on the basis of the urine sediment alone. Urine eosinophils can be seen in interstitial nephritis.

The differences between ARF and CRF are listed in Table 29.1.

Q. Write briefly about chronic renal failure/chronic kidney disease. (PA28.4)

Ans. Chronic kidney failure also called CKD, is defined as a gradual loss of kidney function.

Stages of CKD

- Stage 1: Kidney damage with normal or increased glomerular filtration rate (GFR; >90 mL/min/1.73 m^2).
- Stage 2: Mild reduction in GFR (60–89 mL/min/1.73 m^2).
- Stage 3a: Moderate reduction in GFR (45–59 mL/min/1.73 m^2).
- Stage 3b: Moderate reduction in GFR (30–44 mL/min/1.73 m^2).
- Stage 4: Severe reduction in GFR (15–29 mL/min/1.73 m^2).
- Stage 5: Kidney failure (GFR <15 mL/min/1.73 m^2 or dialysis).

Measurement of GFR may not be sufficient for identifying stage 1 and stage 2 CKD, because in these patients the GFR may be normal. In such cases, the presence of one or more of the following markers of kidney damage can establish the diagnosis:

- Albuminuria (albumin excretion >30 mg/24 h or albumin:creatinine ratio >30 mg/g [>3 mg/mmol]).
- Urine sediment abnormalities.
- Electrolyte and other abnormalities due to tubular disorders.
- Histological abnormalities.
- Structural abnormalities detected by imaging.
- History of kidney transplantation in such cases.

Causes

The most common causes of chronic failure are long-standing diabetes mellitus (DM) and uncontrolled hypertension. Other causes include:

- Vascular disease.
- Glomerular disease (primary or secondary).
- Cystic kidney diseases.
- Tubulointerstitial disease.
- Urinary tract obstruction or dysfunction.
- Recurrent kidney stone disease.
- Congenital (birth) defects of the kidney or bladder.
- Unrecovered AKI.

Signs and Symptoms

Patients with CKD stages 1–3 are generally asymptomatic. Stages 4 and 5 may manifest with endocrine/metabolic derangements or disturbances in water or electrolyte balance.

Diagnostic Workup

- CBC and basic metabolic panel.
- Urinalysis.
- Serum albumin levels (albumin levels may be reduced due to malnutrition, urinary protein loss or chronic inflammation).
- Lipid profile (patients with CKD have an increased risk of cardiovascular disease).
- Serum calcium and phosphate, 25-hydroxyvitamin D, alkaline phosphatase and parathyroid hormone (PTH) levels.
- Serum and urine protein electrophoresis and free light chains (screening for multiple myeloma).
- Antinuclear antibodies (ANA) and double-stranded DNA antibody levels (screening for SLE).
- Serum complement levels (for glomerulonephritides).
- Cytoplasmic and perinuclear pattern antineutrophil cytoplasmic antibody (C-ANCA and P-ANCA) levels (for vasculitis).
- Anti-glomerular basement membrane (anti-GBM) antibodies (Goodpasture syndrome).
- Hepatitis B and C, HIV and Venereal Disease Research Laboratory (VDRL) serology.
- Imaging studies (renal ultrasonography, retrograde pyelography, computed tomography [CT] scanning, magnetic resonance imaging [MRI], renal radionuclide scanning).
- Percutaneous renal biopsy.

Q. Enumerate the cystic lesions of kidney. (PA28.12)

Ans. Cysts of the kidney include:

- Polycystic kidney (adult and infantile type).
- Medullary cystic disease (medullary sponge kidney and nephronophthisis).
- Localized or simple renal cyst.

- Multicystic renal dysplasia.
- Acquired (dialysis-associated) cystic disease.
- Renal cysts associated with tuberous sclerosis.
- Calyceal or pyelogenic cyst.
- Pelvic cyst.
- Perinephric cyst.
- Cystic degeneration in tumours.

Q. Differentiate between adult and childhood polycystic kidney disease.

Ans. Differences between adult and childhood polycystic kidney disease are listed in Table 29.2.

Q. Enumerate the various glomerular syndromes.

Ans. Based on clinical manifestations, renal diseases are classified into the following major glomerular syndromes:

1. **Acute nephritic syndrome:** Haematuria, azotaemia, variable proteinuria, oliguria, oedema and hypertension.
2. **Rapidly progressing glomerulonephritis (RPGN):** Acute nephritis, proteinuria and ARF.
3. **Nephrotic syndrome:** Proteinuria >3.5 g/day, hypoalbuminaemia, hyperlipidaemia and lipiduria.
4. **CRF:** Azotaemia and uraemia progressing over years.
5. **Asymptomatic haematuria/proteinuria:** Haematuria and subnephrotic proteinuria.

Table 29.2 Differences between adult and childhood polycystic kidney disease

Features	Adult	Childhood
Inheritance	Autosomal dominant, caused by a mutation in the genes encoding **polycystin 1 and 2; defective gene is PKD1 or PKD2**	Autosomal recessive with a mutation in the gene encoding **fibrocystin, i.e. PKHD1**
Frequency	More common	Less common
Presentation	• Presents after fourth decade; may be associated with a cystic liver, berry aneurysm, subarachnoid haemorrhage, colonic diverticuli and mitral valve prolapse • Large, multicystic kidney	• Presents in perinatal/neonatal age group with splenomegaly and hepatic fibrosis (oesophageal varices may be seen as a consequence of hepatic fibrosis) • External surface of the kidney is smooth; cut surface shows numerous small cysts in the cortex and medulla (dilated elongated channels at right angles to the cortical surface)
Origin of cysts	May arise from any level of nephron from tubules to collecting ducts; lining variable	Arises from collecting ducts; lined uniformly cuboidal cells
Clinical features	Haematuria, flank pain, hypertension and urinary infection	Bilateral abdominal mass
Outcome	Chronic renal failure begins at age of 40–60 years	• Young infants usually die of hepatic and renal failure • Patients who survive develop congenital hepatic fibrosis

Q. Classify glomerular diseases. (PA28.5)

Ans. Based on clinicopathological features, glomerular diseases are classified broadly into primary and secondary (Table 29.3).

Q. Write in detail about the pathogenesis of glomerular injury.

Ans. The various immune mechanisms involved in the pathogenesis of glomerular injury are as follows:

1. **Antibody-mediated injury**
   (a) **In situ immune complex deposition**
      (i) Fixed intrinsic tissue antigens.
      - *Goodpasture antigen (anti-GBM nephritis):* Antibody is directed against an intrinsic fixed antigen that is a normal component of the GBM (non-collagenous domain of the alpha-3 chain of collagen type IV). The deposits show a homogeneous, diffuse and linear pattern.
      - *Phospholipase A2 receptor (PLA2R) antigen (membranous glomerulonephritis):* Antibody is directed against M-type PLA2R located on the glomerular epithelial cell membrane. This antigen complex is partially homologous to Heymann antigen found

Table 29.3 Clinicopathological classification of glomerular diseases

Primary glomerulonephritis	Secondary (systemic diseases with glomerular involvement)	Hereditary nephritis
• Acute proliferative glomerulonephritis • RPGN • Membranous glomerulonephritis • Minimal change disease • Focal segmental glomerulosclerosis • Membranoproliferative glomerulonephritis • Dense deposit disease • IgA nephropathy • Chronic glomerulonephritis	• DM • Amyloidosis • SLE • Polyarteritis nodosa • Microscopic polyangiitis • Wegener granulomatosis • Henoch–Schönlein purpura • Bacterial endocarditis	• Alport syndrome • Fabry disease

in rats. Granular, interrupted deposits are seen along the subepithelial aspect of the GBM.

- *Mesangial antigens.*
- *Others.*

(ii) Planted antigens: These are non-glomerular antigens, which get planted in the glomerulus by interacting with various intrinsic components in the glomerulus, e.g.:

- Cationic molecules, which can bind to the glomerular capillary anionic sites.
- Larger aggregated proteins like IgG which can deposit in mesangium.
- DNA, which has affinity for GBM components.

Many exogenous (infectious agents and drugs) and endogenous (DNA, immunoglobulins and immune complexes) antigens can act as planted antigens.

(b) **Circulating immune complex deposition (immune complex glomerulonephritis)**

(i) Injury is caused by trapping of circulating antigen–antibody complexes within glomeruli because of their physicochemical properties and the prevailing haemodynamics of glomeruli (type III hypersensitivity).

(ii) Subendothelial (rarely subepithelial) granular deposits along basement membrane or mesangium or both are seen.

(iii) The antigens involved could be endogenous antigens (DNA and tumour antigens as seen in autoimmune diseases) or exogenous antigens (infectious products, e.g. bacterial, viral, spirochetal and parasitic antigens or tumour antigens).

(iv) Antibodies are produced against the antigens; antigen–antibody complexes are formed in the circulation; the complexes get trapped in the glomeruli and initiate injury by activating complement and recruiting leucocytes (by binding to their Fc receptors).

(c) **Cytotoxic antibodies:** Antibodies directed against glomerular cell components can lead to glomerular injury. For example, antibodies against endothelial cell antigen can cause endothelial injury and intravascular thrombosis. Antibody directed against visceral epithelial cell antigen can cause proteinuria.

2. **Cell-mediated glomerular injury:** Cell-mediated immune reactions in the form of delayed hypersensitivity may be involved in causing glomerular injury.
3. **Activation of alternative complement pathway**

(a) This type of injury is usually associated with 'C3 glomerulopathy', which consists of two conditions, namely dense deposit disease (DDD; earlier known as membranoproliferative glomerulonephritis [MPGN] II) and C3 glomerulonephritis or C3GN). DDD and C3GN are rare forms of glomerulonephritis that affect both children and adults and result from abnormal regulation of the alternative complement pathway.

(b) Direct activation of alternative complement pathway occurs by some polysaccharides; endotoxins or IgA aggregates deposited in glomeruli may cause glomerular injury.

(c) C3b in the presence of factors B and D generates C3bBb (alternate complement pathway convertase).

(d) C3bBb is labile and degraded by factors I and H and stabilized by properdin.

(e) Some patients with C3 glomerulopathy have an IgG autoantibody against C3 convertase named C3 nephritic factor (C3NeF).

(f) C3NeF behaves like properdin and stabilizes C3bBb and prevents its degradation resulting in persistent activation of C3 by the alternate complement pathway.

(g) In DDD, a circulating antibody termed C3NeF binds to C3 convertase, favouring persistent splitting of C3 into C3a and C3b, thus activating the alternative pathway and resulting in hypocomplementaemia.

4. **Secondary pathogenic mechanisms:** Neutrophils, macrophages, complement, platelets and mesangial cells can cause glomerular injury directly or by producing cytokines, chemokines, oxidants and enzymes.
5. **Non-immunological mechanisms**

(a) Metabolic glomerular injury (diabetic nephropathy).

(b) Haemodynamic glomerular injury (systemic hypertension).

(c) Deposition disease (amyloidosis and cryoglobulinaemia).

(d) Infectious disease (HIV and hepatitis).

(e) Inherited (Alport syndrome).

Q. Write briefly about the aetiopathogenesis and clinicopathological features of acute proliferative glomerulonephritis.

Ans. Acute proliferative (poststreptococcal/postinfectious) glomerulonephritis

- Appears 1–4 weeks after a streptococcal infection of the pharynx (pharyngitis) or skin (impetigo/pyoderma).
- Occurs most frequently in children between 6 and 10 years of age but can affect any age.
- Can also be caused by organisms other than *Streptococcus*, e.g. *Pneumococcus* and *Staphylococcus*, and viral diseases such as mumps, measles, chickenpox and hepatitis B and C.

Aetiopathogenesis

- Group A, beta-haemolytic *Streptococcus* has some nephritogenic strains (types 1, 4 and 12; typing is based on M protein of the cell wall).
- Principal antigenic determinants involved in acute poststreptococcal nephritis are thought to be nephritis-associated streptococcal plasmin receptor (NAPIr), streptococcal pyogenic exotoxin B (SpeB; most common), streptococcal glyceraldehyde-3-phosphate dehydrogenase (GAPDH) and its zymogen precursor (zSpeB).
- Immune complexes, preformed by the combination of specific antibodies against streptococcal antigens, localize on the glomerular capillary wall and activate the complement system.
- The immunological system may be activated by streptococcal antigens that adhere to the glomerular structures

and act as 'planted antigens' as well as by altered endogenous antigens (GBM proteins altered by streptococcal enzymes).

- Glomerular deposition of immune complexes leads to diffuse proliferation and swelling of glomerular cells as well as infiltration by leucocytes, especially neutrophils.

Clinical Features

- Abrupt onset of malaise and nausea with **nephritic syndrome** characterized by periorbital oedema (due to mild-to-moderate proteinuria), oliguria, azotaemia, hypertension and gross haematuria (smoky or cocoa-coloured urine), dysmorphic erythrocytes and red cell casts.
- Serum complement levels are low.
- Serum antistreptolysin O (ASO) antibody, anti-deoxyribonuclease B (anti-DNase B), antistreptokinase and antihyaluronidase levels are elevated in poststreptococcal cases.

Prognosis

- In children, recovery occurs in most cases; some children develop RPGN or chronic renal disease (incidence of chronicity is much less than in adults).
- About 15%–50% of adults, however, develop end-stage renal disease over a few years to one to two decades.

Pathology (Fig. 29.4 A and B)

- There is diffuse (involving the whole kidney) and uniform increase in cellularity of the glomerular tuft due to proliferation and swelling of endothelial and mesangial cells along with infiltration by neutrophils and monocytes.
- Rare cases show necrosis of capillary walls and formation of crescents.
- Obliteration of glomerular capillary lumina due to swelling and proliferation of endothelial and mesangial cells along with infiltration by neutrophils and monocytes leads to pale, enlarged, hypercellular glomeruli.
- Tubules may show red cell casts.
- Interstitium may show oedema and inflammatory cells.
- Blood vessels are unremarkable.

Electron Microscopy (EM)

Shows deposition of immune complexes (granular IgG and C3) as subendothelial, intramembranous and most commonly subepithelial humps. Occasionally, mesangial deposits may be seen.

Immunofluorescence (IF)

Shows granular deposits of IgG, IgM and C3 within capillary walls and mesangium.

Q. Write briefly about RPGN.

Ans. RPGN is a clinical syndrome characterized by rapid and progressive loss of renal function. It has features similar to those of nephritic syndrome but leads to death from renal failure within weeks to months of onset.

Pathogenesis

1. It is caused by systemic diseases as well as diseases localized to the kidney.
2. Regardless of cause, the histological hallmark is the formation of crescents (therefore also called crescentic glomerulonephritis [CrGN]; Fig. 29.5A, B and C). RPGN is of the following types:
   (a) **Type I (anti-GBM antibody type)**
      (i) Relatively uncommon and aggressive type of RPGN.

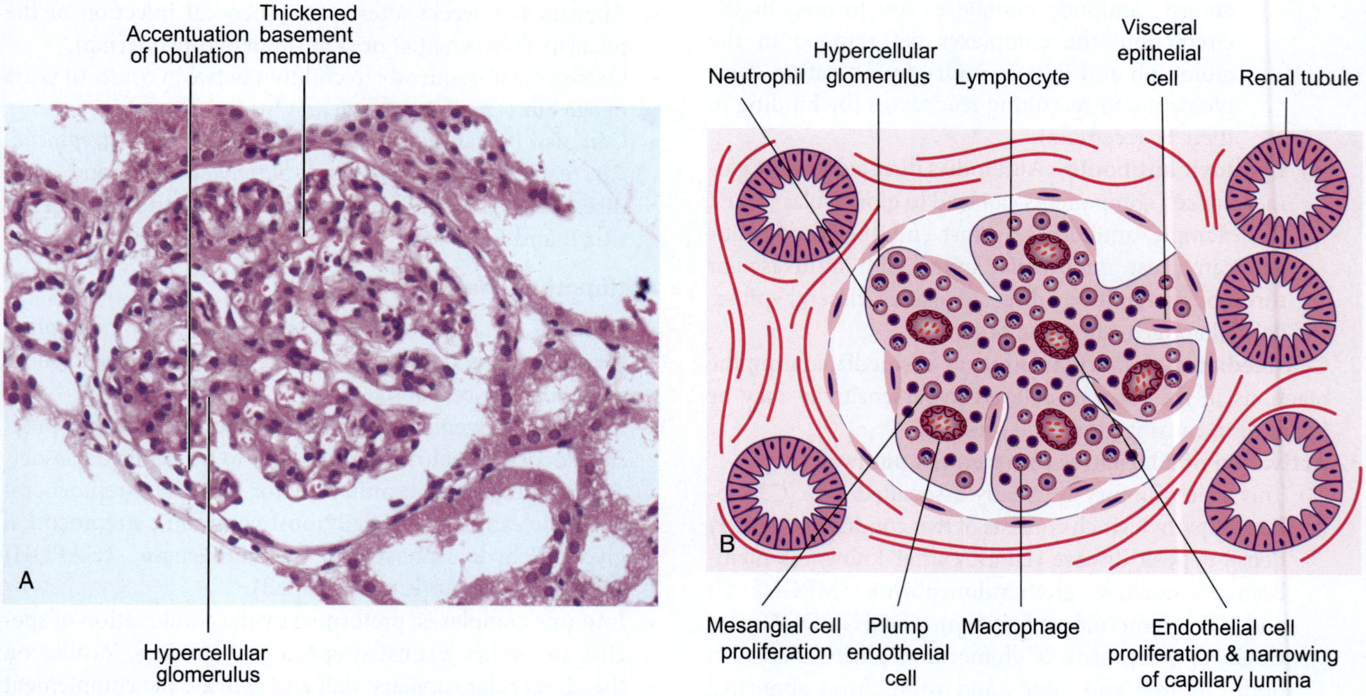

Fig. 29.4 (A) Photomicrograph of acute proliferative (postinfectious) glomerulonephritis showing proliferation of endothelial and mesangial cells along with neutrophil and monocyte infiltration (H&E; 400×). (B) Schematic representation of a hypercellular glomerulus.

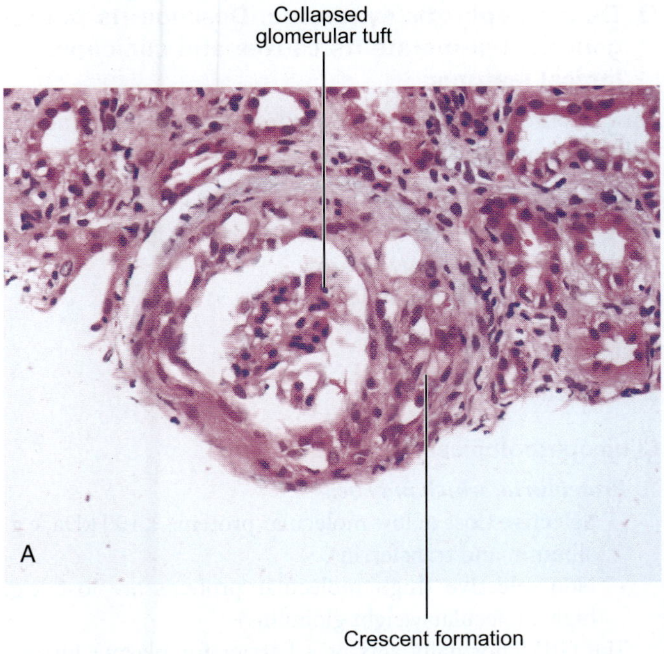

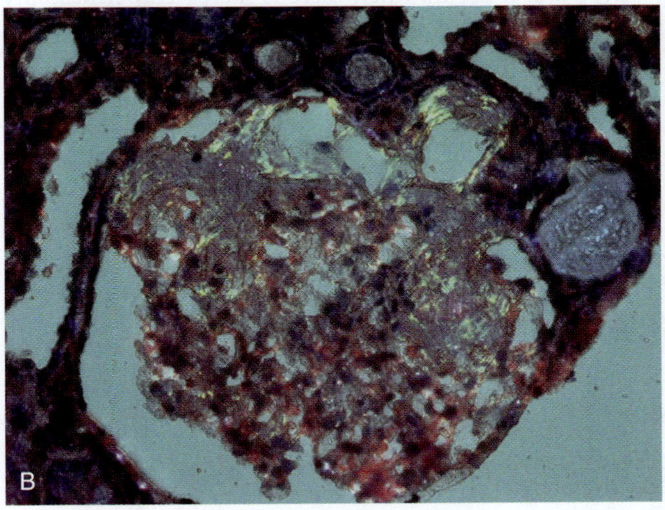

Fig. 29.5 (A) Photomicrograph of rapidly progressing glomerulonephritis (RPGN) showing crescent formation (H&E; 400×). (B) Photomicrograph showing linear immunofluorescence characteristic of RPGN.

(ii) Has two subtypes – 'renal limited' and 'Goodpasture syndrome'. The former shows linear deposits of IgG and C3 in the GBM.

(iii) In some of the affected individuals, anti-GBM antibodies also bind to the pulmonary alveolar basement membrane to clinically manifest as pulmonary haemorrhages associated with renal failure (**Goodpasture syndrome**).

(iv) Anti-GBM antibodies can also be detected in the serum and aid in the diagnosis of this disease.

(v) These individuals benefit from plasmapheresis, which removes antibodies from the circulation.

(vi) Serum C3 is normal and ANCA is negative.

Causes

- Idiopathic
- Goodpasture syndrome

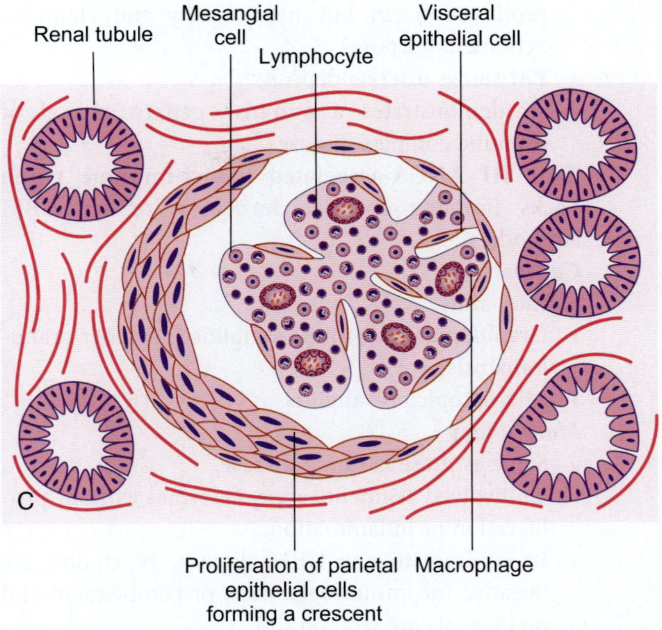

Fig. 29.5 (C) Schematic representation of RPGN showing proliferation of parietal epithelial cells resulting in formation of a crescent.

Gross morphology

Kidneys are enlarged and pale **(large white kidney)** and may show petechial haemorrhages (**flea-bitten kidney**).

Microscopy

- Segmental necrosis in glomeruli and breaks in the GBM lead to exudation of plasma proteins including fibrin in the Bowman's space.
- Fibrin acts as a stimulus for the proliferation of parietal epithelial cells and infiltration of monocytes into the Bowman's space. This results in the formation of crescents because the cells take the shape of the Bowman's space, which is crescentic.
- Uninvolved portion of the cells of the glomerulus shows no proliferation. Tubules may show red cell casts. Interstitium may show oedema and inflammatory cells. Blood vessels are unremarkable.
- ***EM*** shows breaks in the GBM.
- ***IF*** shows strong linear staining of IgG and C3 along the GBM.

(b) **Type II (immune complex type)–mediated disorder**

(i) It is characterized by granular Ig and C3 deposits.

(ii) Serum C3 is low to normal; anti-GBM antibody and ANCA are negative.

Causes

- Idiopathic
- Postinfectious
- SLE
- Henoch–Schönlein purpura
- IgA nephropathy

Morphology

- Changes are similar to those in type I disease; however, uninvolved portions of the glomerulus also show diffuse proliferation and leucocyte infiltration (in postinfectious GN and SLE) or mesangial

proliferation (in IgA nephropathy and Henoch–Schönlein purpura).
- *EM* shows discrete deposits.
- *IF* demonstrates a granular pattern typical of immune complex disease.

(c) **Type III ANCA-associated (pauci-immune type):** Lacks immune complex formation or anti-GBM antibodies.

Causes
- Idiopathic.
- Granulomatosis with polyangiitis (Wegener granulomatosis).
- Microscopic polyangiitis.

Morphology
- Same as those in type I disease.
- Uninvolved segments appear normal without proliferation or inflammation.
- In contrast to anti-GBM disease, IF studies are negative for immunoglobulins or complement and no deposits are seen on EM.

Clinical Features of RPGN

- Similar to those of nephritic syndrome except that oliguria and azotaemia are more pronounced.
- Patients with type I RPGN (Goodpasture syndrome) may present with recurrent haemoptysis and life-threatening pulmonary haemorrhages.
- Proteinuria approaches nephrotic range.
- Prognosis is related to the number of crescents.

Q. Define nephrotic syndrome. Describe its pathogenesis. Enumerate its causes and clinicopathological features.

Ans. Nephrotic syndrome is a syndrome complex having the following components:

- Daily loss of >3.5 g of protein (less in children).
- Hypoalbuminaemia with protein levels <3 g/dL.
- Generalized oedema/anasarca.
- Hyperlipidaemia and lipiduria.

Pathogenesis

See Flowchart 29.2.

Clinicopathological Manifestations

1. ***Proteinuria, which may be:***
   - **Selective** (loss of low molecular proteins <100 kDa, e.g. albumin and transferrin).
   - **Non-selective** (high molecular proteins are lost, e.g. high-molecular-weight globulins).

   The GBM normally acts as a barrier for plasma filtrate. Proteinuria occurs when there is increased permeability of the GBM. It is selective in the initial stages of injury and non-selective later or in the event of severe injury. Proteinuria results in hypoalbuminaemia, which in turn results in reduced colloidal osmotic pressure leading to accumulation of fluid in the interstitial spaces further leading to oedema. Decreased plasma volume reduces GFR and induces secretion of aldosterone. The oedema is

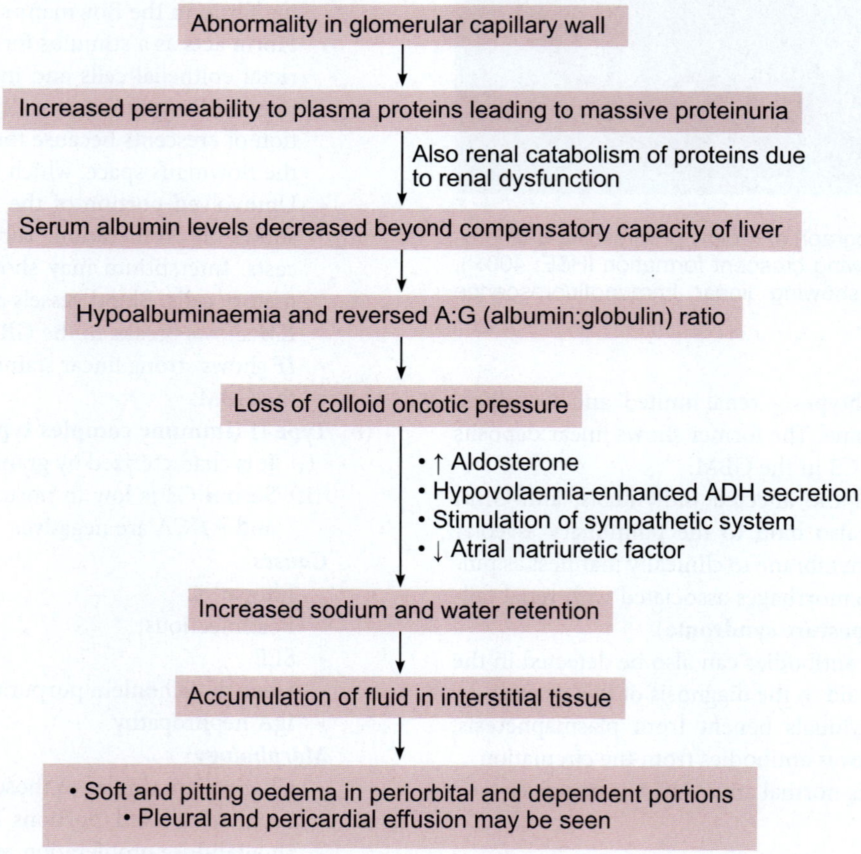

Flowchart 29.2 Pathogenesis of manifestations of nephrotic syndrome.

soft and pitting, prominent in the periorbital region and the dependent parts of the body.

2. ***Hyperlipidaemia:*** The lipid-related metabolic abnormalities seen in nephrotic syndrome are as follows:
   - Increased blood levels of cholesterol, triglycerides, VLDL, LDL, LP(a) and apoproteins.
   - Decrease in HDL (due to loss in urine).
   - Lipiduria or oval fat bodies or free fat in urine (lipoproteins are reabsorbed by the tubular epithelium and then shed with the epithelium when it gets injured and detached).
   - Causes of hyperlipidaemia include:
     i. Enhanced synthesis of lipoproteins in the liver.
     ii. Abnormal transport of circulating lipid particles.
     iii. Reduced catabolism of lipids.
3. ***Thrombotic complications:*** Renal vein thrombosis due to loss of anticoagulant factors, e.g. antithrombin III (AT III) and antiplasmins.
4. ***Increased susceptibility to infection (especially staphylococci and pneumococci):*** Due to loss of immunoglobulins in the urine.

Causes

- Primary glomerular diseases
  - Membranous glomerulonephritis.
  - Lipoid nephrosis.
  - Focal segmental glomerulosclerosis (FSGS).
  - MPGN.
  - IgA nephropathy.
- Systemic diseases
  - DM.
  - Amyloidosis.
  - SLE.
  - Drugs (gold, penicillamine and street heroin).
  - Infections (malaria, syphilis, hepatitis B, hepatitis C and AIDS).
  - Malignancy (carcinoma and melanoma).
  - Miscellaneous (bee-sting allergy and hereditary nephritis).

Membranous Glomerulonephritis (Glomerulopathy)

Primary or idiopathic membranous nephropathy is thought to be an autoimmune disease characterized by uniform diffuse thickening of the glomerular capillary wall.

Pathogenesis

- Linked to a susceptibility gene like HLA-DQ, membranous nephropathy is caused by an in situ immune reaction involving renal autoantigens (e.g. PLA2R) and, in some cases, planted antigens. The disease shows resemblance to Heymann nephritis (induced by the formation of antibodies to the megalin antigenic complex present in rat podocytes, which is the animal counterpart of PLA2R).
- Circulating immune complexes are present in 25% of cases.
- Paucity of neutrophils, monocytes and platelets in glomeruli and virtually uniform presence of complement point to direct action of C5b-9 (membrane attack complex), which is thought to activate glomerular epithelial and mesangial cells to release proteases and oxidants, which cause capillary wall injury to lead to protein leakage.

Aetiology

Idiopathic (primary) in 75% of cases; the remaining 25% are labelled **secondary** and may be caused by:

- Malignancies (carcinoma lung and colon, melanoma).
- SLE.
- Exposure to inorganic salts (gold and mercury).
- Drugs (penicillamine and captopril) and NSAIDs.
- Infections (hepatitis B and C, syphilis, schistosomiasis and malaria).
- DM and thyroiditis.

Morphology (Fig. 29.6)

Light microscopy

- The early stages show no abnormality; later, uniform and diffuse thickening of the glomerular capillary wall due to IgG deposits along the epithelial side of the basement membrane is noted.
- Glomeruli appear normocellular, and may appear sclerosed in the later stages.
- Tubules may show droplets of reabsorbed protein in the initial stage and atrophy in the later stage.

EM

- It shows irregular dense deposits of immune complexes between basement membrane and overlying epithelial cells (which have lost their foot processes).
- Basement membrane material is deposited between these immune complexes as **irregular spikes** projecting from the GBM.
- The spikes are best seen by silver stains which colour the GBM but not the deposits. They eventually cover the immune deposits and fuse over them resulting in membrane thickening.

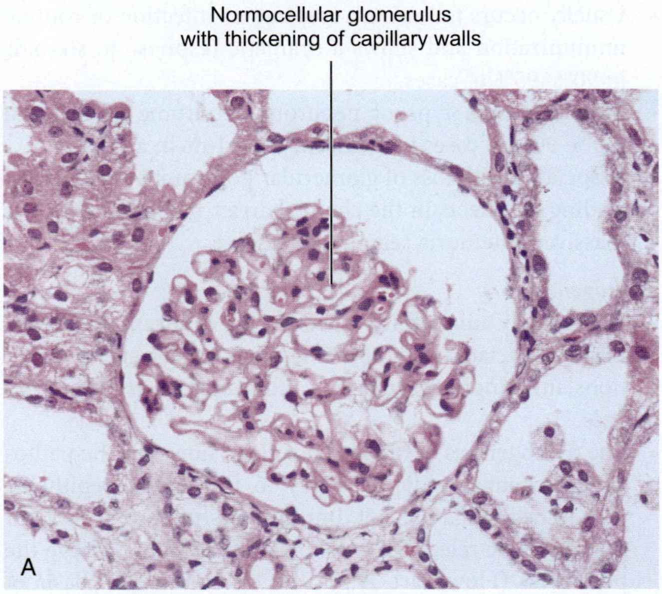

Fig. 29.6 (A) Photomicrograph of membranous glomerulopathy showing uniform and diffuse thickening of the glomerular capillary wall with a normocellular glomerulus (H&E; 400×).

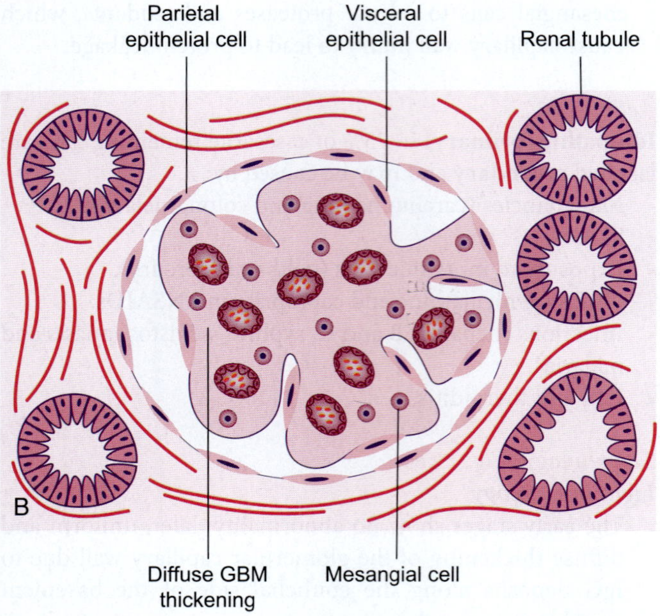

Fig. 29.6 (B) Schematic representation membranous glomerulopathy.

- In the later stage, the immune deposits may undergo lysis leaving cavities within the GBM.

IF: Granular deposits of IgG and C3 in the subepithelial region with intense staining for membrane attack complex.

Clinical Features

- Insidious onset of nephrotic syndrome in majority of patients; non-nephrotic proteinuria in a few patients.
- Proteinuria is non-selective and responds poorly to steroids (unlike MCD). It persists in >60% of patients and 10% of these go into renal failure.

Lipoid Nephrosis/Minimal Change Disease (MCD)

- Usually occurs following a respiratory infection or routine immunization and shows a dramatic response to steroids in 90%–95% of cases.
- Most common type of nephrotic syndrome in children (70%–90% of cases in children; 11%–16% in adults).
- Associated with loss of glomerular polyanions in the GBM leading to defects in the charge barrier responsible for the massive proteinuria seen in the disease.

Pathogenesis

- It is usually idiopathic, especially in children; secondary forms, associated with viral infections, drugs, allergic reactions, immunological diseases and neoplasia, are seen in all ages.
- The pathogenesis of MCD is not clear; however, the pathological changes indicate injury to the visceral epithelial cells to be the main event. Immune dysfunction is thought to induce the release of cytokines, which then damage the podocytes (Flowchart 29.3). The immunological basis of the disease is re-enforced by the following features:
  - Follows a respiratory infection or prophylactic immunization.

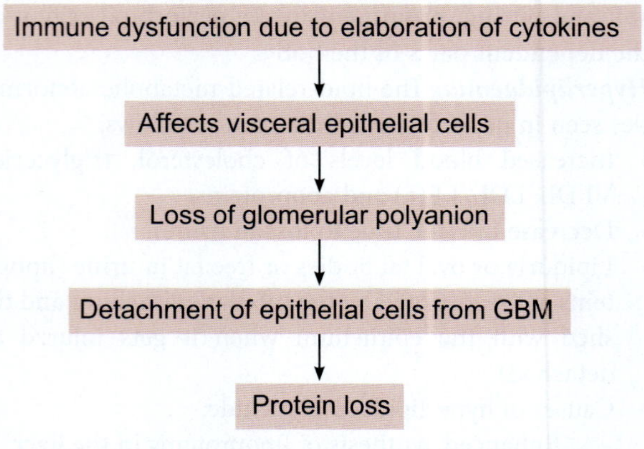

Flowchart 29.3 Pathogenesis of proteinuria in MCD.

  - Responds to therapy with immunosuppressants or corticosteroids.
  - Associated with atopy and other allergic disorders.
  - Has an increased incidence in patients with defects in T-cell-mediated immunity, e.g. Hodgkin lymphoma.
- Non-immunological mechanisms are also thought to contribute to the pathogenesis of MCD. Mutations in structural proteins such as nephrin, dysferlin and podocin (NPHS2) are known to result in structural defects in podocytes.

Morphology (Fig. 29.7)

Light microscopy is within normal limits or shows minimal changes.

EM shows effacement of foot processes of visceral epithelial cells, which show a thin rim of cytoplasm with cytoplasmic vacuolization, swelling and villous hyperplasia. No electron-dense deposits are seen. Proximal convoluted tubular cells are lipid laden (therefore, the disease is also called **lipoid nephrosis**).

IF does not show immunoglobulin or complement deposits.

Focal Segmental Glomerulosclerosis (FSGS)

- FSGS typically shows focal and segmental sclerosis. "Focal" indicates involvement of some glomeruli and "segmental" indicates involvement of only a part of a glomerulus. It has the following types:
  1. Idiopathic or primary (10%–35% of patients).
  2. FSGS superimposed on another primary glomerular lesion.
  3. Renal ablation FSGS (seen with unilateral agenesis, acquired reflux nephropathy and analgesic abuse-associated reduction in renal mass).
  4. Secondary FSGS (seen with heroin abuse/HIV/sickle cell disease/massive obesity).
  5. A rare inherited type in which the disease is caused by mutations in genes encoding for glomerular proteins, e.g. podocin and α-actinin.
- Eighty per cent of patients present with nephrotic syndrome.
- Fifty per cent convert to end-stage renal disease.
- FSGS differs from MCD in the following ways:
  - Greater incidence of haematuria and hypertension.

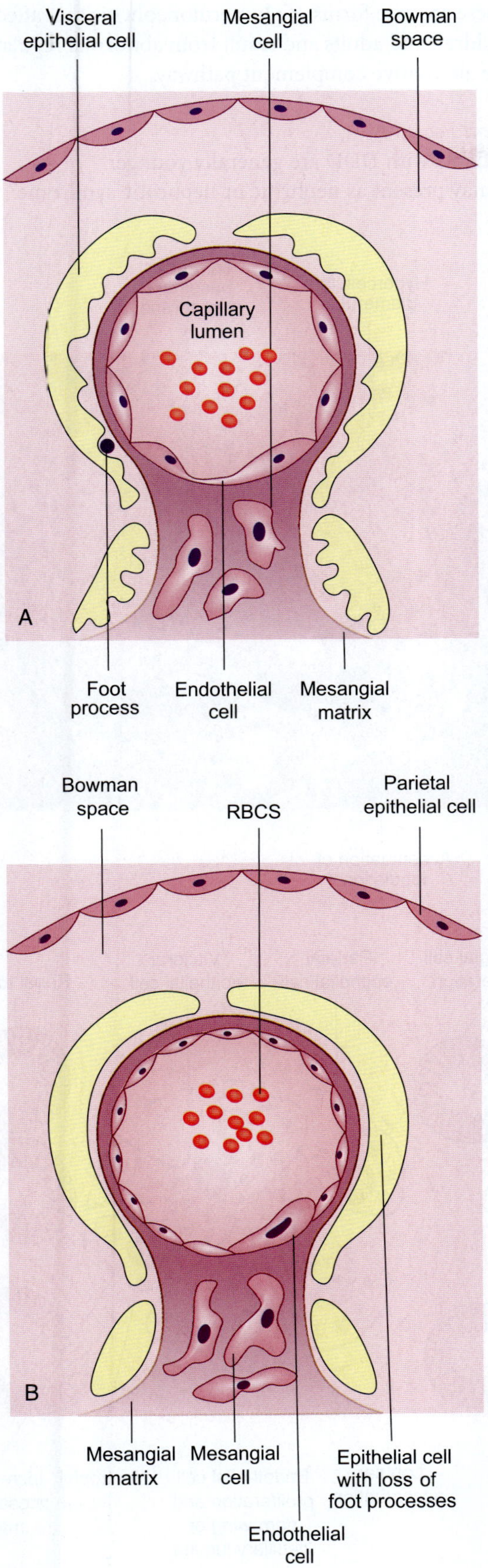

Fig. 29.7 Diagrammatic representation of electron microscopic appearance of (A) normal glomerulus and (B) glomerulus in MCD showing effacement of foot processes.

- Non-selective proteinuria.
- Poor response to steroids and progression to chronic glomerulonephritis (CGN) or end-stage renal disease in 50% of cases.

Pathogenesis

The epithelial damage, which is a hallmark of FSGS, is caused by different mechanisms:

1. Genetic mechanisms: Genetic defects that affect the integrity of the normal glomerular filtration barrier (e.g. mutations in the NPHS (nephrin, encoded by podocyte-specific) genes, NPHS1 and NPHS2, which encode for the proteins nephrin and podocin, respectively; mutations in the gene encoding the podocyte actin-binding protein, α-actinin-4; and mutation in the gene encoding transient receptor potential calcium channel-6 [TRCP6], a podocyte protein responsible for maintaining calcium flux).
2. Circulating factors: Presence of an unknown circulating factor is thought to be responsible for the epithelial damage because it is noted that the disease recurs even after transplantation.

Morphology

Light microscopy

- It shows segmental involvement (starts with involvement of the juxtamedullary glomeruli and progresses to involve all levels of the cortex).
- Affected glomeruli show increased mesangial matrix, collapse of capillary loops, hyalinosis (deposition of plasma proteins along the capillary wall), and lipid droplets in the affected segment, gradually leading to occlusion of capillary lumina and global sclerosis (sclerosis of the entire glomerulus). The sclerosis is due to entrapment of plasma proteins (a result of excessive membrane permeability) and increased ECM deposition.
- Unaffected glomeruli may show increased mesangial matrix/mesangial proliferation.

EM

- Loss of foot processes.
- Detachment of epithelial cells and denudation of the GBM.

IF: IgM and C_3 deposits in sclerotic areas.

Clinical Course

One-fourth of patients develop intractable massive proteinuria ending in renal failure within 2 years.

HIV-Associated Nephropathy

- It is seen in 5%–10% of HIV-infected patients.
- It shows features of severe collapsing FSGS with foci of cystically dilated tubules filled with proteinaceous material. Inflammation and fibrosis may be seen in later stages.
- EM shows a large number of tubuloreticular inclusions in endothelial cells. These inclusions are basically interferon-α-mediated alterations in the epithelial endoplasmic reticulum.

Membranoproliferative Glomerulonephritis

- As the name suggests, MPGN is characterized by proliferation of glomerular cells and changes in the GBM. The proliferation is predominantly mesangial; thus, the condition is also called **mesangiocapillary glomerulonephritis**.
- It is responsible for 5%–10% of cases of idiopathic nephrotic syndrome. It may sometimes arise secondary to SLE, hepatitis B and C, CLL, α_1-AT deficiency, endocarditis, systemic infections, HIV and schistosomiasis.

Clinical Features

Usually presents in adolescents and young adults with proteinuria in the nephrotic or non-nephrotic range and haematuria.

Light Microscopy (Fig. 29.8)

- **Glomeruli**
  - Glomeruli appear large and hypercellular, and show proliferation of mesangial cells, infiltration by leucocytes and increase in mesangial matrix.
  - Also seen is lobular accentuation and formation of epithelial crescents.
  - GBM is thickened and has a **double contour or tram track appearance** due to '**duplication**', which is the formation of a new basement membrane. The new membrane forms consequent to stimulation by the subendothelial deposits of immune complexes. Duplication is followed by inclusion of mesangial, endothelial or leucocytic cells between the two layers leading to splitting of GBM. This change is highlighted with **PAS** and **silver stains**).
- **Tubular epithelial cells:** These show vacuolization and droplets of hyaline.
- **Interstitium:** It may show chronic inflammation.
- **Blood vessels:** These are normal in the early stages; however, they may show changes associated with hypertension later.

EM: Discrete subendothelial electron dense deposits are seen.

IF: Granular deposits of C3 along with deposits of early complement components (C1q and C4).

Types

- ***Type I or immune complex deposit disease (more common)***
  - Characterized by subendothelial electron-dense deposits and Clq, C3, C4 and IgG granular deposits.
  - Can be seen with SLE, hepatitis B and C, schistosomiasis, α_1-AT deficiency, certain malignancies and infected arteriovenous shunts (also called secondary MPGN).
- ***Type II (now known as DDD):*** DDD belongs to a group of disorders known as **C3 glomerulopathies**.

C3 Glomerulopathy

- It encompasses two main conditions, namely **DDD** (earlier known as MPGN II) and **C3GN**.
- These are rare forms of glomerulonephritis that affect both children and adults and result from abnormal regulation of the alternative complement pathway.

Clinical Features

- Patients with DDD are generally younger.
- It may present as nephritic or nephrotic syndrome.

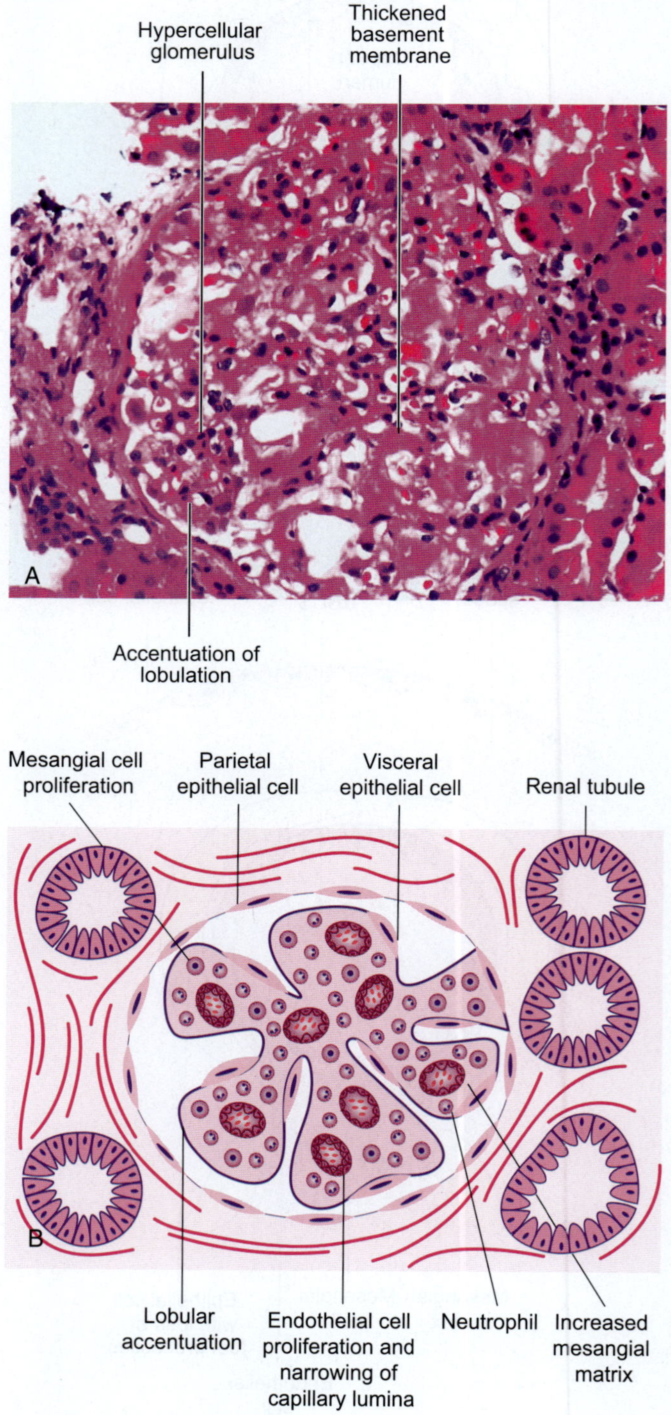

Fig. 29.8 (A) Photomicrograph of membranoproliferative glomerulonephritis showing a hypercellular glomerulus with thickened basement membrane and accentuation of lobulation (H&E; 400×). (B) Schematic representation of the same.

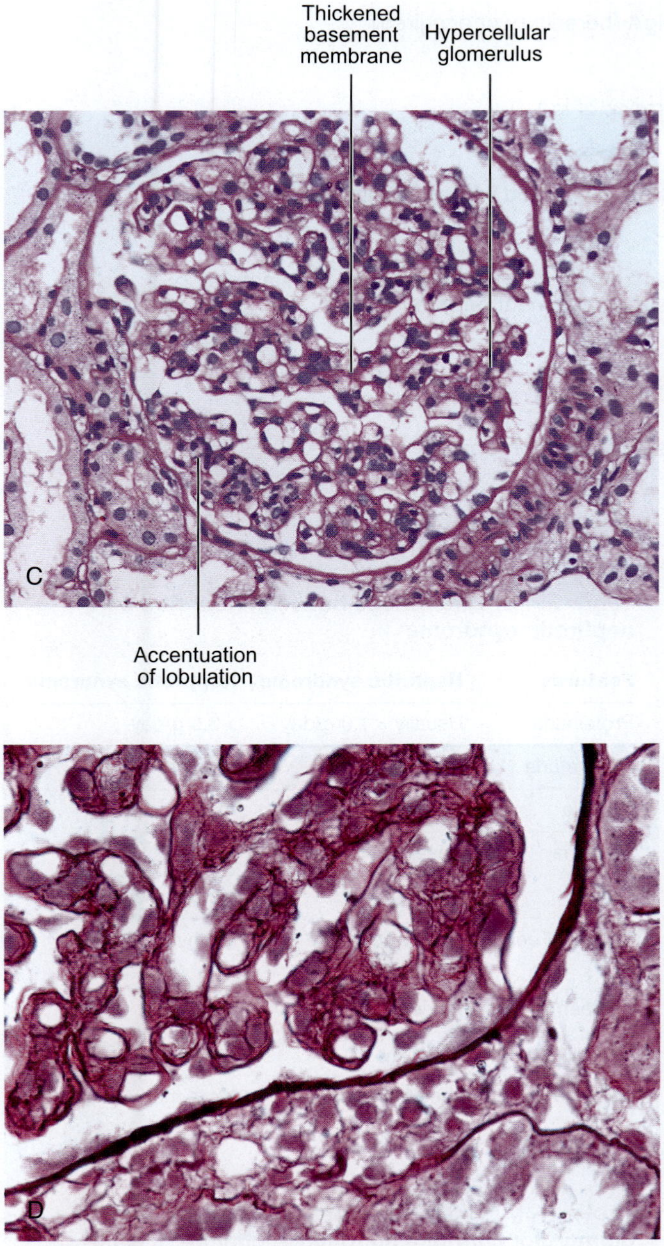

Fig. 29.8 (C) Photomicrograph of membranoproliferative glomerulonephritis showing a double contour or tram track appearance (PAS stain; 400×). (D) Photomicrograph of membranoproliferative glomerulonephritis showing splitting of the basement membrane.

- Both C3GN and DDD have poor prognosis.
- These patients usually have an increased serum C3 and normal C1 and C4.

Sequence of Events in C3 Glomerulopathy

- Direct activation of alternative complement pathway occurs by some polysaccharides, endotoxins or IgA aggregates deposited in glomeruli.
- C3b in the presence of factors B and D generates C3bBb (alternate complement pathway convertase).
- C3bBb is labile and degraded by factors I and H and stabilized by properdin.
- Some patients with C3 glomerulopathy have an IgG autoantibody against C3 convertase named C3NeF.
- C3NeF behaves like properdin and stabilizes C3bBb and prevents its degradation, resulting in persistent activation of C3 by the alternate complement pathway.
- In DDD, a circulating antibody termed C3NeF binds to C3 convertase, favouring persistent splitting of C3 into C3a and C3b, thus activating the alternative pathway and resulting in hypocomplementaemia.

Morphology

Light microscopy: The glomeruli are hypercellular with a mesangial proliferation pattern. There is increase in the mesangial matrix. Duplication of BM can be seen.

EM

- C3GN shows mesangial and subendothelial electron-dense waxy deposits. These deposits can sometimes be seen along the tubular basement membrane also.
- In DDD, the lamina densa or the central area of the GBM shows irregular ribbon-like electron-dense deposits (C3-containing material).

IF

- C3 staining is seen in the mesangium (as circular deposits called **mesangial rings**) and glomerular capillary walls in both C3GN and DDD.
- IgG, C1q and C4 are absent.

IgA Nephropathy (Berger Disease) (PA28.6)

- Typically shows prominent IgA deposits in the mesangial region.
- Most common type of glomerulonephritis seen on renal biopsy.

Clinical Features

- It affects children and adults.
- It occurs after mucosal (respiratory, gastrointestinal or urinary tract) infections (increased IgA synthesis in response to viruses, bacteria, food allergens, etc.).
- It presents with gross or microscopic haematuria and/or proteinuria.
- About to 5%–10% present as acute nephritic syndrome.
- Course of the disease is variable; many individuals maintain normal renal function for decades.
- CRF may occur in as many as 50% of cases.
- Henoch–Schönlein purpura (a systemic disorder characterized by purpura, abdominal pain and arthritis) has many similarities with IgA nephropathy.

Pathogenesis (Flowchart 29.4)

- It involves abnormality in IgA production and clearance (IgA is the main immunoglobulin in mucosal secretions).
- Normally, serum IgA levels are low and IgA exists predominantly in monomeric form. Polymeric form, which is catabolized by the liver, has a greater tendency of forming immune complexes.
- Plasma polymeric IgA levels are increased in IgA nephropathy.

Abnormality in glycosylation of IgA (hereditary or acquired)

↓

Decreased clearance of IgA

↓

IgA-containing immune complexes get entrapped in mesangium

↓

Activation of mesangial cells, release of cytokines and growth factors, recruitment of inflammatory cells and activation of alternate complement pathway

↓

Initiation of glomerular injury

Flowchart 29.4 Pathogenesis of IgA nephropathy.

- IgA nephropathy is initiated by an increase in either the production of IgA or the formation of circulating IgA-containing immune complexes (due to an abnormality of immune regulation). Increased frequency of IgA nephropathy is noted in coeliac disease (characterized by the presence of intestinal mucosal defects) and liver disease (characterized by defective hepatobiliary clearance of IgA complexes). Another key factor in the pathogenesis of IgA nephropathy is abnormal glycosylation of IgA due to hereditary or acquired defects. This abnormally glycosylated IgA may either itself deposit in the glomeruli or initiate an autoimmune response leading to the formation of IgG autoantibodies against it. This leads to the formation of circulating immune complexes which deposit in the mesangium.

Morphology

- Mesangial widening and segmental inflammation confined to certain glomeruli (focal proliferative GN) or overt crescent formation (crescentic GN) or diffuse mesangial proliferation (mesangioproliferative GN) may be seen.
- Mesangium shows electron-dense deposits.
- ***IF*** shows mesangial deposition of IgA, C3, properdin and small amounts of IgG/IgM.

Q. Differentiate between nephritic and nephrotic syndrome.

Ans. Differences between nephritic and nephrotic syndrome are listed in Table 29.4.

Q. Differentiate between membranous glomerulonephritis and minimal change disease.

Ans. Differences between membranous glomerulonephritis and MCD are listed in Table 29.5.

Q. Write briefly about the aetiopathogenesis, clinical features and pathology of tubulointerstitial nephritis (TIN). (PA28.8)

Ans. TIN is defined as inflammation of the tubules and interstitium with sparing of the glomeruli or their involvement in very late stages. It has two components:

Table 29.4 Differences between nephritic and nephrotic syndrome

Features	Nephritic syndrome	Nephrotic syndrome
Proteinuria	Usually <1.0 g/day	>3.5 g/day
Haematuria	Present	Absent
Oliguria	Present	Absent
Lipiduria	Absent	Present
Casts	Red cell casts	Lipid casts
Colour of urine	Cocoa coloured/ smoky urine	Frothy urine
Azotaemia	Present	Absent
Hyperlipidaemia	Absent	Present
Oedema	Less marked	More marked

Table 29.5 Differences between membranous glomerulonephritis and minimal change disease

Features	Membranous glomerulonephritis	Minimal change disease
Age	Adults	Children
Light microscopy	Thickening of GBM (GBM width in healthy adults is 300–400 nm)	Normal GBM
Electron microscopy	Granular subepithelial deposits	Foot process effacement and lipid-laden cells in PCT
Immunofluorescence	Granular deposits of IgG and C3	No deposition
Hypertension	Present	Absent
Haematuria	Present	Absent
Corticosteroid therapy	Minimal response	Good response

- **Pyelonephritis** (usually due to bacterial infections) is a term applied to TIN with prominent involvement of the renal pelvis in addition to tubules and interstitium.
- The term **interstitial nephritis** is reserved for cases of TIN that are non-bacterial in origin (include tubular injury due to drugs, metabolic disorders, physical and immunological injury).

Q. Write briefly about the aetiopathogenesis, clinical features and pathology of pyelonephritis. (PA28.10)

Ans. Pyelonephritis is defined as inflammation of the tubules, interstitium and renal pelvis.

Pathogenesis

Principal causative organisms: Enteric Gram-negative rods, mainly *Escherichia coli, Proteus, Klebsiella, Enterobacter, Pseudomonas, Staphylococcus* and *Streptococcus faecalis*; rarely, mycobacterial, fungal and viral organisms.

Predisposing Conditions

- Urinary tract manipulations, e.g. catheterization, urethral instrumentation and cystoscopy.
- Congenital or acquired anomalies of the urinary tract (intrarenal reflux, vesicoureteral reflux [VUR] and deranged vesicoureteric junction).
- Outflow obstruction (nodular hyperplasia prostate, uterine prolapse, calculi, strictures, tumours and neurogenic bladder).
- Immunodeficiency or immunosuppression.

Routes of Spread of Bacteria to Kidneys

- Haematogenous: Seen in septicaemia or infective endocarditis and is less common.
- Ascending infection: This is more common and occurs by the following mechanism (Flowchart 29.5):
  - In the absence of instrumentation, urinary tract infection (UTI) more commonly affects females because of the **proximity of the urethra to the rectum (colonization by enteric bacteria favoured)**.
  - Other factors aiding the development of UTI in women are the presence of **a short urethra, trauma to the urethra during sexual intercourse** and **pregnancy**.
  - **Incompetent vesicoureteric orifice** in children allows bacteria to ascend the ureters. Normally, the ureters are inserted into the bladder in a way that prevents retrograde flow of urine into the ureters, especially during micturition when the intravesical pressure rises. Incompetency of the opening allows retrograde flow of urine into the ureters and this is called VUR. This is present in 20%–40% of children with UTI.
  - **Intrarenal reflux** is a condition in which the infected bladder urine is propelled into the renal pelvis and into the renal parenchyma through the open ducts at the tips of the renal papillae.

Types

Acute Pyelonephritis

- UTI may involve the upper urinary tract (pyelonephritis) or the lower urinary tract (cystitis, prostatitis and urethritis).
- Infections of the lower urinary tract may remain localized or may spread to involve the kidney.
- Acute suppurative inflammation of the renal tubules and interstitium is called acute pyelonephritis.

Clinical Features

- Sudden onset of pain at the costovertebral angle, fever, chills and malaise.
- Signs of bladder irritation such as dysuria, frequency and urgency.
- Urine examination shows pyuria and bacteriuria (culture shows growth).
- Usually self-limiting; in the presence of predisposing conditions, it may become recurrent or chronic.

Gross Morphology

- Affects one or both kidneys.
- The affected kidney is normal in size or slightly enlarged.
- Discrete yellow, raised abscesses are seen on the renal surface.

Microscopy

- Necrosis and abscess formation in the renal parenchyma.
- Abscesses limited to the interstitium initially, moving into the tubules later.
- Large masses of neutrophils in the tubules give rise to the characteristic WBC casts.
- When obstruction is severe, it prevents the drainage of pus, leading to pus filling up the renal pelvis, calyces and ureters **(pyonephrosis)**.
- **Papillary necrosis** is a relatively rare form of pyelonephritis in which there is necrosis of the tips of the renal papillae (particularly common in diabetes and analgesic abuse). Development of papillary necrosis indicates a poor prognosis.

Attachment of bacteria to the urothelial lining by fimbriae
↓ Facilitated by genetically determined properties of the urothelium and bacterial pathogens
Colonization of distal urethra (introitus in females)
↓
Access of bacteria into the bladder due to catheterization, urethral instrumentation and cystoscopy

Flowchart 29.5 Spread of bacteria to kidneys by ascending infection.

- The pathognomonic morphological finding of papillary necrosis is a sharply defined area of yellow necrosis in the apical two-thirds of the renal pyramid.

Chronic Pyelonephritis (CPN) and Reflux Nephropathy

Morphological entity in which interstitial inflammation and scarring of renal parenchyma is associated with scarring and deformity of the pelvocalyceal system.

Types

- ***Chronic obstructive pyelonephritis.***
  - Recurrent infections occurring in a background of obstruction, which lead to repeated inflammation and scarring.
  - The disease can be bilateral as in congenital anomalies of the urethra (posterior urethral valves) or unilateral as in calculi and unilateral obstructive lesions.
- ***Chronic reflux-associated pyelonephritis:*** This more common form of CPN results from the superimposition of UTI on congenital VUR and intrarenal reflux. It may be unilateral or bilateral.

Clinical Features

- Presents as gradual onset of renal insufficiency (azotaemia); often noticed because of hypertension.
- Ultrasonography used to determine the size of the kidney and a pyelogram used to show the asymmetrical contraction of kidneys, blunting and deformity of the pelvocalyceal system.

Gross Morphology (Fig. 29.9A)

- It may be unilateral or bilateral, patchy or diffuse.
- Coarse, discrete corticomedullary scars are seen corresponding to the overlying blunted or dilated calyces.
- Asymmetrical pelvocalyceal scarring leads to blunting of papillae and deformity of calyces.

Microscopy (Fig. 29.9B)

- Uneven interstitial fibrosis with interstitial inflammatory infiltrate composed of lymphocytes, plasma cells and rarely neutrophils.
- Dilatation as well as contraction of tubules showing atrophy of lining epithelium.
- Dilated tubules contain pink PAS-positive casts called **'colloid casts'** that resemble colloid in thyroid **(thyroidization)**.
- Fibrosis of calyceal mucosa.
- Vascular changes similar to those in benign arteriosclerosis.
- Late stages may show glomerulosclerosis secondary to nephron loss.

Q. Differentiate between acute and chronic pyelonephritis.

Ans. Differences between acute and chronic pyelonephritis are listed in Table 29.6.

Q. Differentiate between chronic glomerulonephritis (CGN) and chronic pyelonephritis (CPN).

Ans. Contrasting features of CGN and CPN are given in Table 29.7.

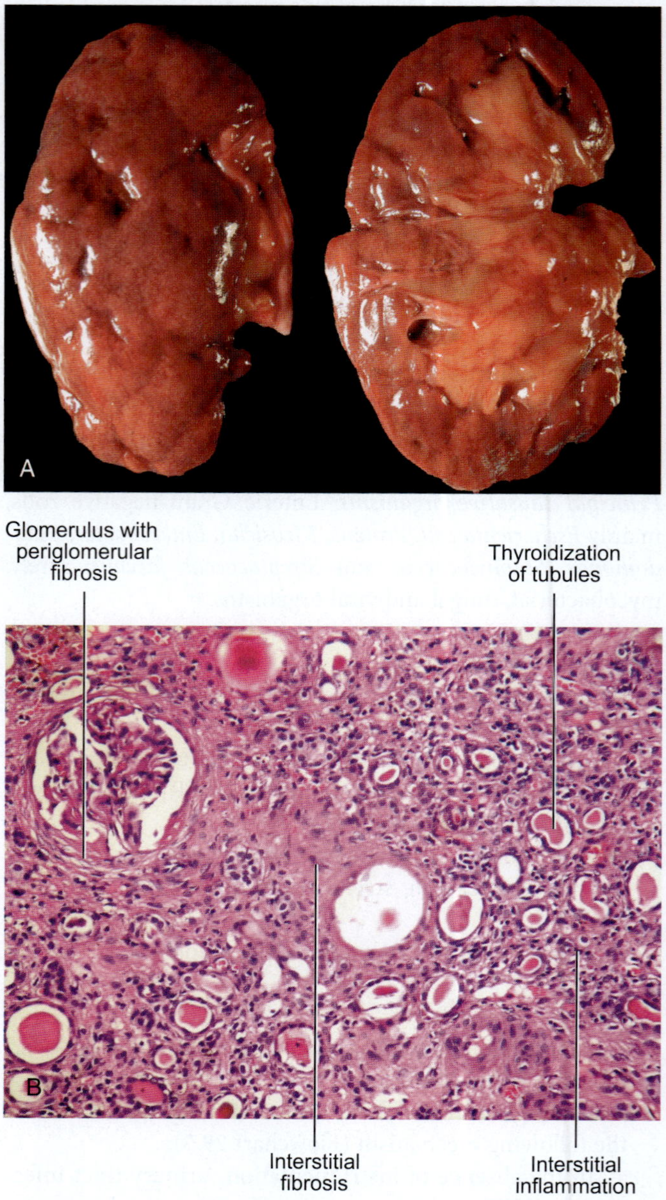

Fig. 29.9 (A) Gross picture of chronic pyelonephritis showing irregular scarring and blunted, distorted calyces. (*Source: Robbins & Cotran Pathologic Basis of Disease,* Tenth Edition: Vinay Kumar, Abul K. Abbas, Jon C. Aster, Figure 20.31(A), page 931, Elsevier Inc., 2021.) (B) Photomicrograph showing uneven interstitial fibrosis, interstitial inflammatory infiltrate, dilatation and contraction of tubules with atrophy of lining epithelium. Dilated tubules contain pink PAS-positive casts (thyroidization; H&E; 200×).

Q. Describe the aetiopathogenesis, clinical features and morphology of acute tubular injury (ATI) or acute kidney injury (AKI). (PA28.3, 28.9)

Ans. AKI is a reversible disorder characterized by destruction of tubular epithelial cells and acute suppression of renal function. It is the most common cause of ARF. Other causes of **ARF** besides AKI include:

- Severe glomerular disease, e.g. RPGN.
- Diffuse renal vascular disease, e.g. microscopic polyangiitis and TMA (Thrombotic microangiopathy).
- Acute papillary necrosis associated with acute pyelonephritis.

Table 29.6 Differences between acute and chronic pyelonephritis

Features	Acute pyelonephritis	Chronic pyelonephritis
Definition	Acute suppurative inflammation of kidney caused by bacterial infection	Chronic tubulointerstitial disease showing tubular inflammation and renal scarring with pathological involvement of calyces and pelvis
Predisposing factors	Urinary obstruction, instrumentation, catheterization, pregnancy, DM and pre-existing renal lesions	Obstructive pathology, presence of reflux
Subtypes	No subtypes	Chronic obstructive pyelonephritis and reflux-associated nephropathy
Gross	Discrete yellow, raised abscesses are seen on the renal surface	Coarse corticomedullary scars overlying blunted or dilated calyces
Microscopy	Tubules show suppurative necrosis with preserved outline	• Tubules show atrophy in some areas and dilatation in others • Dilated tubules filled with colloid-like casts (thyroidization)
Clinical features	Sudden onset with back pain, fever and malaise	Insidious (silent) onset with progressive decline in renal function

Table 29.7 Contrasting features of CGN and CPN

Features	CGN	CPN
Primary disease	Glomerular, cortical	Tubulointerstitial
Distribution	Diffuse	Patchy
Proteinuria	Marked	Mild or absent
Involvement	Symmetrical	Asymmetrical
Cortical scars	Fine	Coarse
Calyces	Normal	Distorted
Glomerulosclerosis	>50%	Occasional
Interstitial fibrosis	Mild	Marked
Periglomerular fibrosis	Mild	Marked
Tubular atrophy or loss	Mild	Marked
Thyroidization	Absent	Present

- Acute drug-induced interstitial nephritis.
- Urinary obstruction due to tumours, NHP, blood clots, etc.

Types

1. Ischaemic AKI (massive haemorrhage, dehydration, severe burns, septic shock, heart failure, real vascular disease).
2. Nephrotoxic AKI (antibiotics, heavy metal poisoning, organic solvents, radiation).
3. Combined ischaemic and nephrotoxic AKI (mismatched transfusions, haemolytic crises, myoglobinuria).

Pathogenesis

Tubular epithelial cells are particularly sensitive to anoxia and toxins. In **ischaemic AKI**, ischaemia leads to vasoconstriction induced by renin–angiotensin system, whereas in **toxic AKI** there is direct damage to tubules. Tubular cell injury is followed by the following sequence of events:

- Desquamation and detachment of tubular epithelial cells.
- Tubular obstruction by oedema, desquamated cells and casts.
- Increased intratubular pressure and decreased tubular flow.
- Tubular rupture and backleak of tubular fluid into the interstitium.
- Increased interstitial pressure and compression of tubules and blood vessels causing further ischaemia and reduced GFR leading to oliguria.

Ischaemic AKI is characterized by necrosis of short segments of tubules.

- Kidneys appear enlarged with a pale cortex and medullary congestion.
- There are multiple areas of involvement of the nephron with intervening skip areas.
- Most lesions are seen in the straight portion of the proximal tubule and ascending thick loop of Henle.
- There is blebbing of brush border, vacuolization of cells, detachment of tubular cells from their basement membrane and sloughing in the urine.
- Proteinaceous casts are present in distal tubules and collecting ducts; these casts consist of Tamm–Horsfall protein, secreted normally by tubular epithelial cells along with haemoglobin and other plasma proteins. In the later stages, disruption of tubular basement membrane (tubulorrhexis) adjacent to the casts may be seen.
- The interstitium shows oedema and inflammatory infiltrate.

Toxic AKI demonstrates a similar morphology, but tubular necrosis is most prominent in proximal tubules and tubular basement membrane is spared (Fig. 29.10). The appearance varies depending on the cause of toxic AKI. AKI due to haemoglobinuria or myoglobinuria shows reddish brown pigment casts. Epithelial regeneration is seen in the form of mitotic activity and replacement of tubular lining by cuboidal cells.

Clinical Course

AKI evolves through three stages:

1. Initial: It lasts for about 36 hours; it is dominated by the signs and symptoms of the causative event; there is an increase in BUN (blood urea-nitrogen) due to a transient decrease in renal output.
2. Maintenance: During the maintenance phase, renal tubule injury is established, the GFR stabilizes at a level well below normal and the urine output is low or absent. Although oliguria (or anuria) is one of the clinical hallmarks of AKI,

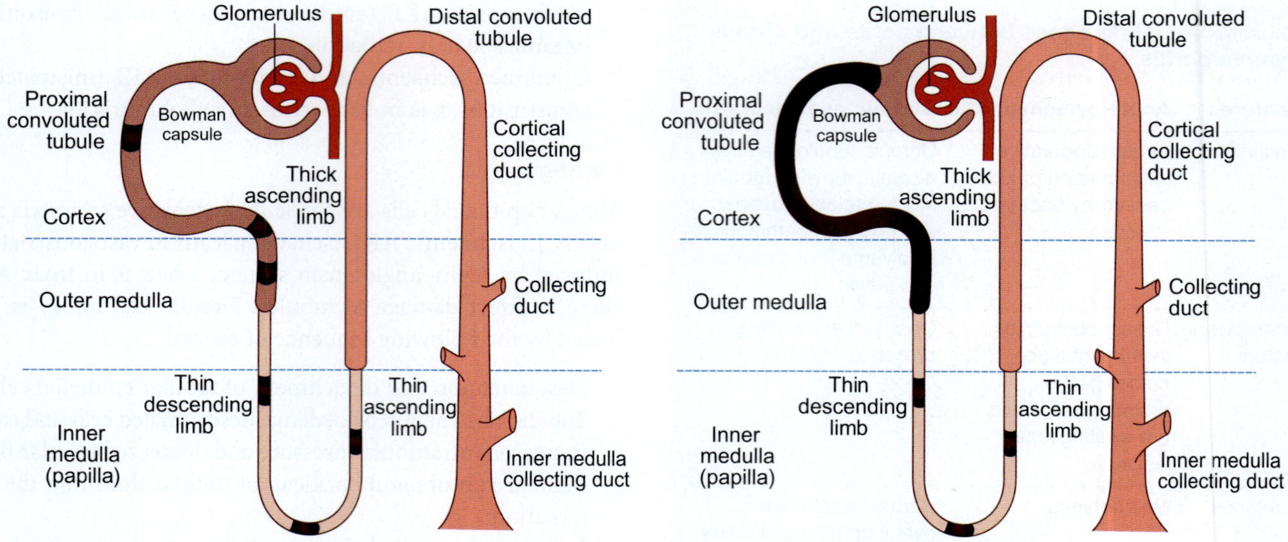

Fig. 29.10 Diagrammatic representation of acute kidney injury (AKI).

it is absent in a minority of patients (ARF due to nephrotoxins is typically non-oliguric). The second phase of AKI lasts usually for 1–2 weeks but may extend to a few months.

3. Recovery: The recovery phase of AKI is characterized by polyuria and gradual normalization of GFR; however, when there is multiorgan dysfunction, regeneration of renal tissue may be severely impaired, and renal function may not return.

Q. Differentiate between ischaemic and nephrotoxic AKI.

Ans. Differences between ischaemic and nephrotoxic AKI are listed in Table 29.8.

Table 29.8 Differences between ischaemic and nephrotoxic AKI

Features	Ischaemic AKI	Nephrotoxic AKI
Definition	AKI caused by renal ischaemia	AKI caused by toxic agents
Causes	Shock, mismatched blood transfusion, haemolytic crises, myoglobinuria, acute pancreatitis and septicaemia	Nephrotoxins like heavy metals, e.g. mercuric organic solvents, gentamicin and amphotericin B, cisplatin and radiographic contrast media
Distribution of lesions	Straight portion of proximal tubule and ascending thick loop of Henle	Proximal convoluted tubules
Pathology	Blebbing and sloughing of brush border, detachment of tubular cells from their basement membrane and their sloughing in the urine	Tubular basement membrane is spared; mercury salts cause coagulative necrosis, CCL4 causes lipoid degeneration and ethylene glycol causes hydropic degeneration of the PCT
Oliguria	Present	Typically non-oliguric
Casts	Eosinophilic and pigmented granular casts consisting of Tamm–Horsfall protein, haemoglobin, myoglobin and other plasma proteins are present	Non-specific; dependent on the causative agents, e.g. lipid casts are present in CCL4 poisoning

Q. Describe the clinicomorphological features and pathogenesis of diabetic nephropathy. (PA28.7)

Ans. Diabetic nephropathy can involve glomeruli, tubules, blood vessels as well as interstitial tissue and pelvis.

Clinical Features

Patients may present with any of the three glomerular syndromes, namely non-nephrotic proteinuria, nephritic syndrome and CRF.

Pathogenesis

- **Metabolic defects:** Insulin deficiency and recurrent hyperglycaemia.
- **Biochemical changes in GBM:** Increased collagen and fibronectin, decreased proteoglycans and heparin sulphate.
- **Non-enzymatic glycosylation** of haemoglobin and other proteins (collagen and BM material), resulting in thickening of BM.
- **Haemodynamic changes:** ↑GFR associated with glomerular hypertrophy.

Morphological Changes (Fig. 29.11)

1. **Capillary basement membrane thickening:** There is widespread thickening of GBM with mesangial widening.
2. **Diffuse glomerulosclerosis**
   (a) Overall thickening of GBM.
   (b) Diffuse increase in PAS-positive mesangial matrix with proliferation of mesangial cells.

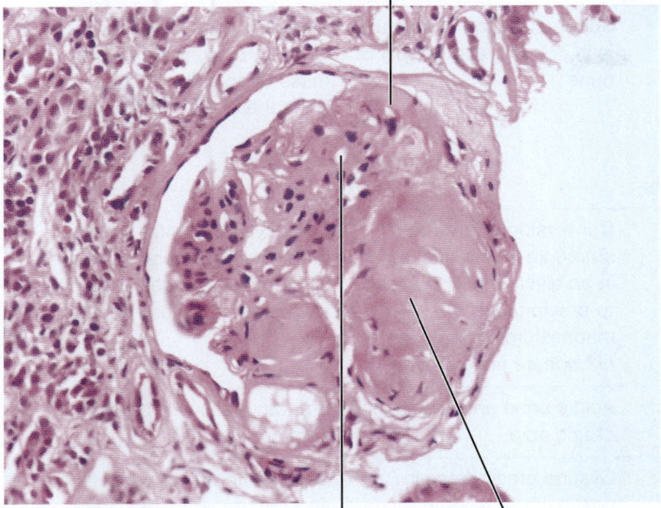

Fig. 29.11 Photomicrograph of a section of diabetic glomerulosclerosis showing mesangial nodules (KW lesions) accompanied by thickening of the basement membrane of the surrounding capillaries (H&E; 400×).

3. **Nodular glomerulosclerosis (Kimmelstiel–Wilson [KW] lesions/intercapillary glomerulosclerosis)**
   (a) KW lesions develop in 15%–30% of long-term diabetes patients.
   (b) These lesions are specific for islet cell antibody–positive DM.
   (c) One or more nodules of the mesangial matrix are seen in glomeruli (usually in the periphery) accompanied by thickening of the basement membrane of the surrounding capillaries.
   (d) Nodules are ovoid, spherical, laminated, hyaline, acellular and PAS-positive masses, which contain lipid and fibrin and compress capillaries to obliterate glomerular tufts leading to tubular atrophy and interstitial fibrosis.
4. **Vascular lesions**
   (a) Atheromas in renal arteries.
   (b) Hyaline arteriosclerosis of afferent and efferent arterioles (arteriosclerosis of efferent arterioles is rare in non-diabetes patients).
   (c) These vascular lesions are responsible for renal ischaemia, which results in tubular atrophy and interstitial fibrosis.
   (d) The above-mentioned changes may result in a small contracted kidney.
5. **Exudative lesions**
   (a) Capsular hyaline drops – eosinophilic hyaline thickening of the parietal layer of Bowman's capsule, which bulges into the glomerular space.
   (b) Fibrin caps – homogenous, brightly eosinophilic material in the wall of a peripheral capillary of a lobule.
6. **Diabetic pyelonephritis:** Poorly controlled diabetes patients are susceptible to bacterial infection and acute pyelonephritis. Papillary necrosis is an important complication.
7. **Tubular lesions (Armanni–Ebstein lesions):** In untreated diabetes patients, who have high blood sugar levels, the epithelial cells of PCT develop extensive glycogen deposits appearing as vacuoles.

EM: Thickening of lamina densa with increase in mesangial matrix and electron-dense masses.

IF: Deposits of IgG, albumin, fibrinogen and other plasma proteins seen in the GBM.

Q. Differentiate between benign and malignant nephrosclerosis. (PA28.11)

Ans. Differences between benign and malignant nephrosclerosis are listed in Table 29.9.

Q. Describe the aetiopathogenesis, gross appearance and complications of renal calculi/urolithiasis. (PA28.13)

Ans. The clinicopathological features of various renal calculi/urolithiasis are summarized in Table 29.10.

Complications of Urolithiasis

1. Loss of function in the affected kidney.
2. Obstruction of the ureter (acute unilateral obstructive uropathy) and hydronephrosis; secondary infection gives rise to pyonephrosis.
3. UTI.
4. Haematuria.

Table 29.9 Differences between benign and malignant nephrosclerosis

Features	Benign nephrosclerosis	Malignant nephrosclerosis
Cause	Benign hypertension, DM, increasing age	Malignant hypertension
Gross	Leather grain appearance	Flea-bitten appearance due to tiny petechial haemorrhages
Microscopy	• Narrowing of the lumen of arterioles caused by thickening and hyalinization of the walls (hyaline arteriosclerosis) • Fibroelastic hyperplasia of arteries and arterioles	• Hyperplastic arteriolitis (onion skinning) due to proliferation and elongation of smooth muscle cells • Necrotizing glomerulitis (neutrophilic infiltration and thrombosis of capillaries) • Fibrinoid necrosis of arterioles (necrotizing arteriolitis)
Clinical features	• Hypertension • Microscopic haematuria • Contracted kidney • Trace proteinuria	• Accelerated hypertension with renal impairment, encephalopathy and retinopathy • Enlarged kidneys • Marked proteinuria

Table 29.10 Clinicopathological features of various renal calculi/stones

Type of calculi	Incidence	Causes	Pathogenesis	Gross
Calcium stones (oxalate and phosphate)	75%–80%	• Idiopathic • Hypercalciuria • Hypercalcaemia • Hyperoxaluria • Hyperuricosuria • Primary hyperthyroidism • Distal renal tubular acidosis	Supersaturation of calcium ions in urine, alkaline pH of urine	Oxalate: Small, smooth contour, or irregular jagged mass of spicules Phosphate: Soft and pale
Struvite stones [$MgNH_4(PO)_3$] triple stone/stag-horn calculus	10%–15%	Urinary infection by urease-containing organisms like *Proteus*	Conversion of urea to ammonia (by urease) results in an alkaline pH; this leads to precipitation of magnesium, ammonium, phosphate and calcium	Large, yellow white, solitary, branching structure, sometimes fills the pelvicalyceal region to form a cast of these spaces
Uric acid stones	6%	Gout, dehydration, idiopathic and malignant tumours	Acidic urine and ↓ solubility of uric acid	Smooth, yellow to brownish, hard and multiple
Cystine stones	1%–2%	Hereditary	Cystine precipitates in acidic urine	Small, smooth yellow, multiple and round
Others	Up to 10%	Inherited abnormality of amino acid metabolism	Xanthinuria	

Q. Classify renal tumours and describe the clinicopathological features of renal cell carcinoma. (PA28.14)

Ans. See Table 29.11 for classification of renal tumours. The most common malignant neoplasm of the kidney is renal carcinoma.

Table 29.11 Classification of renal tumours

Origin	Benign	Malignant
Epithelial tumours of renal parenchyma	Adenoma, oncocytoma, adrenal rests	Renal cell carcinoma (RCC or hypernephroma)
Epithelial tumours of renal pelvis	Transitional cell papilloma	Transitional cell carcinoma (TCC), squamous cell carcinoma, adenocarcinoma of renal pelvis
Embryonal tumours	Mesoblastic nephroma, multicystic nephroma	Wilms' tumour
Non-epithelial tumours	Angiomyolipoma, fibroma, leiomyoma	Sarcoma
Miscellaneous	Reninoma	–
Metastatic tumours	–	–

Renal Cell Carcinoma (RCC)

Synonyms: nephrocellular carcinoma, **Grawitz tumour** and **hypernephroma** (due to perceived origin from the adrenal gland).

Salient Features

- Age: >60 years.
- Male:female ratio = 2:1 to 3:1.
- Constitutes up to 90% of all primary malignant tumours of the kidney, 2%–3% of all cancers.
- Called 'hypernephroma' because of resemblance to clear cells of adrenal cortex and gross yellow colour.
- Arises from the tubular epithelium (renal adenocarcinomas).

Epidemiology

- Predisposing factors: Smoking, obesity, hypertension, unopposed oestrogen therapy, exposure to asbestos, cadmium, petroleum products and heavy metals and acquired cystic disease in patients with long-standing dialysis.
- Majority of cases of RCC are sporadic; about 5% are inherited and associated with the following:
  - von Hippel–Lindau (VHL) syndrome: Predisposition to a large number of neoplasms, mainly haemangioblastomas of the cerebellum and retina, multiple bilateral renal cysts, pheochromocytomas and multicentric bilateral RCCs.
  - Hereditary leiomyomatosis and renal cell cancer syndrome: Autosomal dominant inheritance; mutation in fumarate hydratase (FH) gene; associated with uterine and cutaneous leiomyomas and an aggressive variety of papillary RCC.
  - Hereditary papillary RCC: Autosomal dominant inheritance; multiple cytogenetic abnormalities; mutation in MET proto-oncogene; associated with multiple bilateral papillary RCCs.
  - Birt–Hogg–Dube (BHD) syndrome: Autosomal dominant inheritance; mutation in BHD gene (expresses folliculin); associated with skin appendageal tumours of hair follicular origin, pulmonary cysts and renal tumours.

- Tuberous sclerosis
  - Mutations in TSC1 and TSC2 genes via an alternate pathway not involving VHL mutations.
  - Multiple, bilateral angiomyolipomas.

Clinical Features

- The three classic diagnostic clinical features of RCC are **painless intermittent haematuria, palpable abdominal mass** and **costovertebral pain** but they are rarely seen together. The most common presentation is intermittent haematuria.
- Fever and constitutional symptoms are commonly seen.
- RCC produces a number of paraneoplastic syndromes because of abnormal hormone production including **polycythaemia** (due to elaboration of erythropoietin), **hypercalcaemia** (due to secretion of PTH-rp), **hyperkalaemia, hypertension** (due to release of renin), **Cushing syndrome** (due to secretion of corticosteroids), **hepatic dysfunction** (due to release of IL-6), **leukaemoid reactions, amyloidosis, feminization and masculinization**.
- Tendency to invade renal vein where it grows as a solid column even up to inferior vena cava and right side of heart.
- Propensity for early and widespread metastases before giving rise to any local signs and symptoms. The most common sites are lungs **(cannon ball metastases)**, bones, liver, adrenal and brain.

Gross Morphology (Fig. 29.12)

- Globular, encapsulated, 3–5 cm, soft, lobulated tumour with a variegated appearance (grey-white to yellow with necrosis, haemorrhage and cyst formation); invades or grows into the pelvis.
- Polar in distribution; the upper pole more commonly involved than the lower pole.
- Renal vascular invasion common.
- Usually sharply defined; however, small satellite nodules often found in the surrounding substance.
- Enlarges → bulges into pelvis and calyces → fungates through walls of collecting system → ureters.
- Penetrates through capsule → invades perinephric fat and adrenals.

The clinicopathological features of the most common types of RCC are described in Table 29.12.

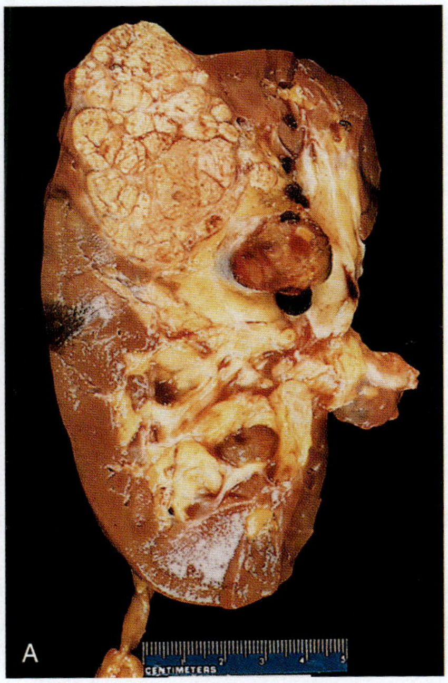

Fig. 29.12 (A) Gross specimen of kidney showing a lobulated tumour with a variegated appearance (the cut surface appearing grey-white to yellow with foci of haemorrhage, breakdown and cyst formation). (*Source: Robbins & Cotran Pathologic Basis of Disease,* Tenth Edition: Vinay Kumar, Abul K. Abbas, Jon C. Aster, Figure 20.50, page 950, Elsevier Inc., 2021.)

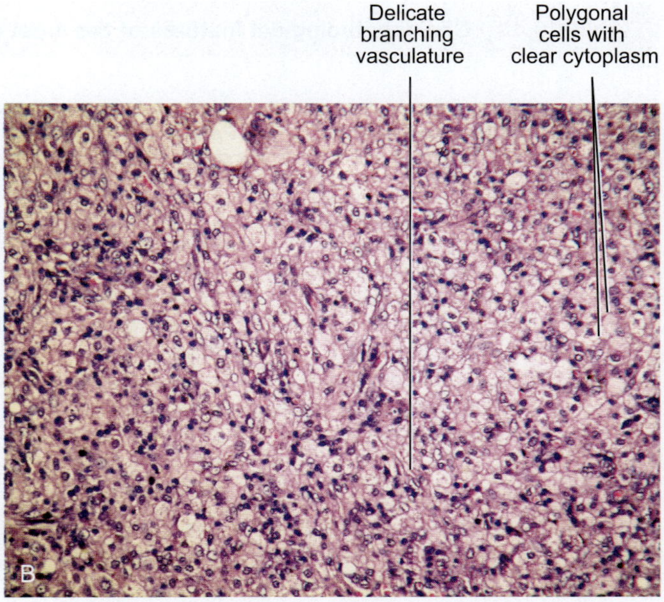

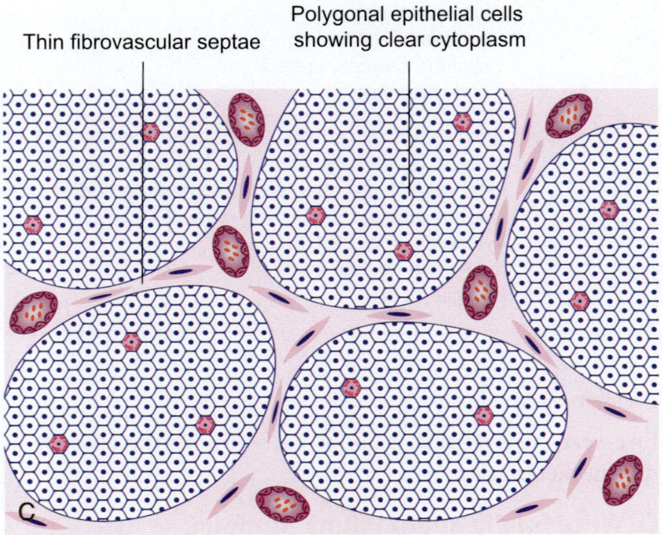

Fig. 29.12 (B) Photomicrograph of renal cell carcinoma, clear cell type, showing solid growth pattern, with round to polygonal cells having clear to granular cytoplasm. Nuclei show moderate atypia (H&E; 400×). (C) Schematic diagram of clear cell RCC.

Table 29.12 Clinicopathological features of the most common types of RCC

Features	Clear cell RCC	Papillary RCC	Chromophobe RCC	Collecting duct (Bellini duct) carcinoma	Xp11 translocation carcinoma
Incidence	70%–80%	10%–15%	5%–8%	1%	
Genetics	• Majority sporadic • 98% show loss of material on the short arm of chromosome 3 • Second allele lost by somatic mutation • Loss of both copies of VHL gene gives rise to clear cell carcinoma	• Culprit (tyrosine kinase receptor for the hepatocytic growth factor) is on chromosome 7q31 • Duplication of chromosome 7 increases gene dosage of MET oncogene leading to abnormal growth of distal tubular cells	• Multiple chromosomal loss and hypodiploidy • Arise from intercalated cells lining collecting ducts	Several chromosomal abnormalities seen but no definite pattern recognized	Seen in young patients and is associated with overexpression of TFE3 transcription factor due to translocations of TFE3 gene located at Xp11.2 with a number of other genes
Gross	• Solitary, unilateral, bright yellow to grey-white with prominent cystic change and haemorrhage • Aggressive; may infiltrate into surrounding substance, collecting system, calyces, ureters and renal vein	Multifocal, bilateral, less yellow due to lower lipid content, papillae may be seen, haemorrhagic and cystic areas present	• Tan brown • Excellent prognosis	Seen in medullary region	–
Microscopy	Solid to tubular growth pattern, round cells with clear (due to glycogen and lipid) or granular cytoplasm (Fig. 29.13); may show nuclear atypia and giant cells	Papillae lined by cuboidal to low columnar cells; psammoma bodies present	Solid sheets of cells arranged around blood vessels, individual cell is eosinophilic with well-defined cytoplasmic margins and perinuclear halo	Irregular channels lined by malignant cells with a hobnail appearance; cells enmeshed within a fibrotic stroma	Clear cytoplasm with papillary architecture

Prognosis

Five-year survival rate is about 45%–70% in the absence of distant metastasis.

Q. Write briefly about Wilms' tumour.

Ans. Wilms' tumour/nephroblastoma is the most common primary renal tumour of childhood. It has a peak age of 2–5 years and a sex ratio of 1:1. It usually occurs in the background of three syndromes:

1. WAGR syndrome, characterized by:
   (a) Aniridia.
   (b) Genital anomalies.
   (c) Mental retardation.
   (d) Germline WT1 deletion followed by a nonsense or frame shift mutation of second WT1 allele (WT1 gene is present at 11p13 and its protein product is a transcriptional factor).
2. Denys–Drash syndrome, characterized by:
   (a) Gonadal dysgenesis (male pseudohermaphroditism).
   (b) Renal abnormalities (diffuse mesangial sclerosis leading to renal failure).
   (c) Missense mutation of WT1 affecting DNA-binding properties.
3. Beckwith–Wiedemann syndrome, characterized by:
   (a) Enlargement of the body organs (organomegaly).
   (b) Hemihypertrophy, macroglossia, omphalocele, renal medullary cysts and abnormal large cells in the adrenal cortex (adrenocytomegaly).
   (c) WT-2 abnormalities (WT-2 gene is present on 11p15.5; its function is unknown; however, WT-2 mutation is known to increase the risk of Wilms' tumour).

Morphology

Gross

Large, solitary, well-circumscribed mass, rarely bilateral or multicentric; soft, homogeneous, tan to grey in colour; foci of haemorrhage and necrosis may be present (Fig. 29.13A).

Microscopic Features (Fig. 29.13B)

- Recapitulates different stages of nephrogenesis. Typically shows a classic triphasic combination of blastema (sheets of small blue cells), epithelial elements (abortive tubules or glomeruli) and stroma (fibrocystic or myxoid in nature).
- Rarely, heterologous elements are identified including squamous or mucinous epithelium, smooth muscle cells, adipose tissue, cartilage, osteoid and neurogenic tissue.

Clinical Features

Palpable abdominal mass, haematuria, pain and hypertension.

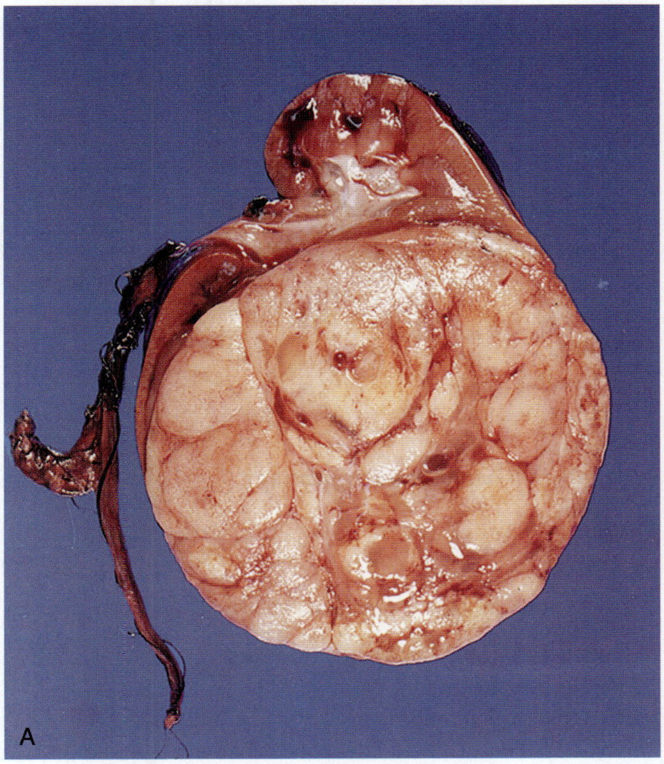

Fig. 29.13 (A) Gross specimen of Wilms' tumour showing a large, well-circumscribed mass, overwhelming the normal renal parenchyma with a homogeneous, tan to grey, fleshy cut surface. (*Source: Robbins & Cotran Pathologic Basis of Disease,* Tenth Edition: Vinay Kumar, Abul K. Abbas, Jon C. Aster, Figure 10.26, page 482, Elsevier Inc., 2021.)

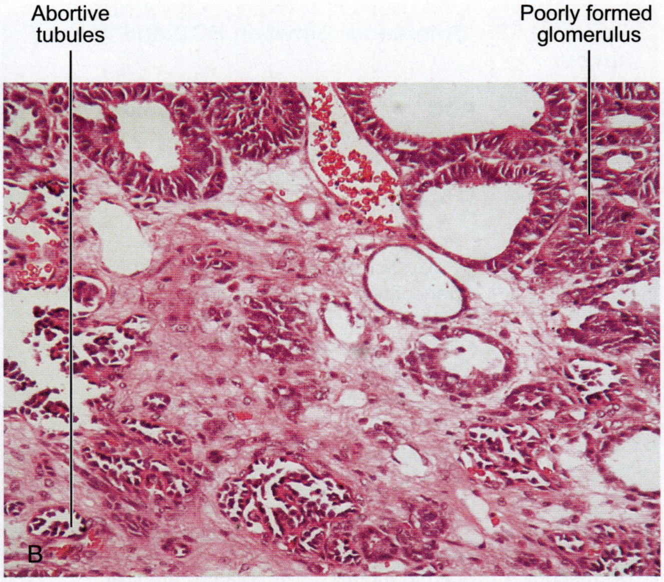

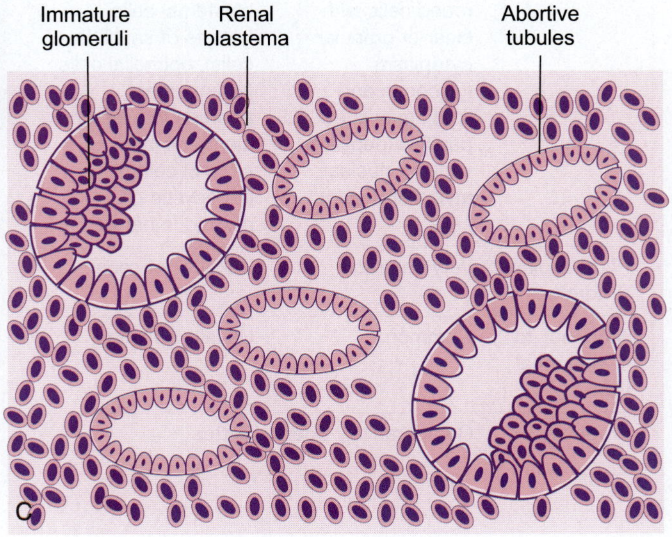

Fig. 29.13 (B) Microphotograph of Wilms' tumour showing a classic triphasic combination of blastema (sheets of small blue cells), epithelial elements (abortive tubules or glomeruli) and stroma (fibromyxoid in nature) (H&E; 200×). (C) Schematic diagram showing a classic triphasic combination of blastema, abortive tubules, glomeruli and stroma.

Metastasis

- Through blood to lung and liver.
- Renal (hilar) and para-aortic lymph nodes.

Prognosis

Five-year survival rate is above 75%.

Q. Differentiate between RCC and Wilms' tumour.

Ans. Differences between RCC and Wilms' tumour are listed in Table 29.13.

Q. Enumerate the causes of a small contracted kidney.

Ans. Causes of a small contracted kidney:

1. Nephrosclerosis: Symmetrically atrophic kidneys with fine, pale granularity (resembles grain leather).
2. CGN: Symmetrically contracted kidneys with red-brown, diffusely granular surface, corticomedullary junction (CMJ) not well made out.
3. CPN: One or both kidneys may be involved (asymmetric, diffuse or patchy involvement), coarse scars, poorly defined CMJ, thickening of pelvic mucosa with yellow tinge and pelvocalyceal deformities.
4. Late stages of diabetic nephropathy.
5. Late stages of amyloidosis.
6. Multiple myeloma.
7. Gout.
8. Senile nephritic syndrome.

A contracted kidney with large scars is most commonly the result of:

1. Old infarcts.
2. Polyarteritis nodosa.

Q. Enumerate the causes of a large white kidney.

Ans. Causes of a large white kidney (pale, soft and grey kidney which weighs more than 250 g):

- Acute diffuse GN and RPGN.
- Lipoid nephrosis.
- Early DM and amyloidosis.

Table 29.13 Differences between RCC and Wilms' tumour

Features	RCC	Wilms' tumour
Age	Adults	Children
Associated genes	VHL, MET	WT1 and WT-2
Gross	• Polar distribution • Variegated appearance • Bright yellow to grey-white with prominent cystic change and haemorrhage	• Large, rapidly growing mass, which overwhelms the kidney and can replace it entirely • Homogeneous appearance • Tan to grey • Haemorrhage and cystic change occasionally seen
Microscopy	Solid to tubular growth pattern, round cells with clear or granular cytoplasm (glycogen and lipid); may show papillae (papillary variant), nuclear atypia and giant cells	Classic triphasic combination of blastemal cells (sheets of small blue cells), epithelial cells (arranged as abortive tubules or glomeruli) and stromal cells (fibrocystic or myxoid in nature)
Paraneoplastic syndromes	Very common	Usually not seen
Tendency to invade renal vein	Common	Usually not seen
Prognosis	Comparatively poor	Better

Table 29.14 WHO grading of urothelial (transitional cell) tumours of urinary bladder

1. Urothelial papilloma (exophytic, inverted)
2. Papillary urothelial neoplasms of low malignant potential
3. Low- or high-grade papillary urothelial cancers
4. Carcinoma in situ (CIS or flat non-invasive urothelial cancers)

- SLE.
- Toxaemia.
- Leukaemia.
- Malaria.
- Irradiation nephritis/chemotherapy.

Q. Write briefly about urothelial (transitional cell) tumours. (28.16)

Ans. Tumours of urinary bladder include:

1. Urothelial (transitional cell) tumours.
   (a) Exophytic papilloma.
   (b) Inverted papilloma.
   (c) Papillary urothelial neoplasms of low malignant potential (PUNLMPs).
   (d) Low-grade and high-grade papillary urothelial cancers
   (e) Carcinoma in situ (CIS or flat non-invasive urothelial carcinoma).
2. Mixed carcinoma.
3. Adenocarcinoma.
4. Small cell carcinoma.
5. Sarcomas.

WHO grading of urothelial (transitional cell) tumours is given in Table 29.14 (also see Fig. 29.14).

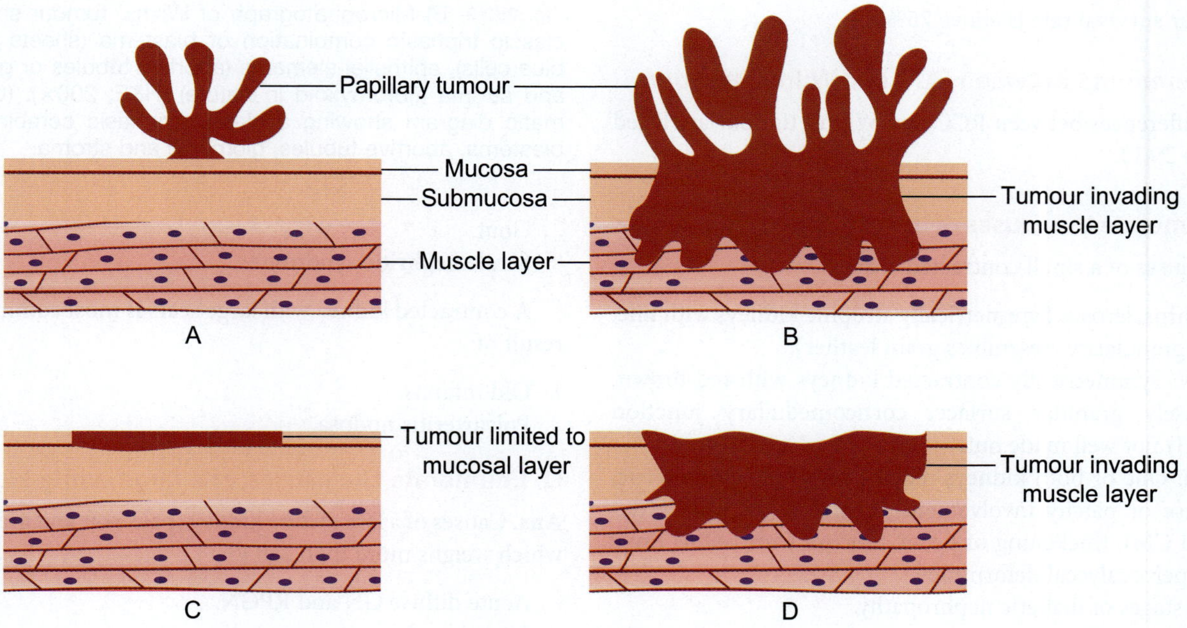

Fig. 29.14 Schematic representation of gross types of urothelial (transitional cell) tumours.

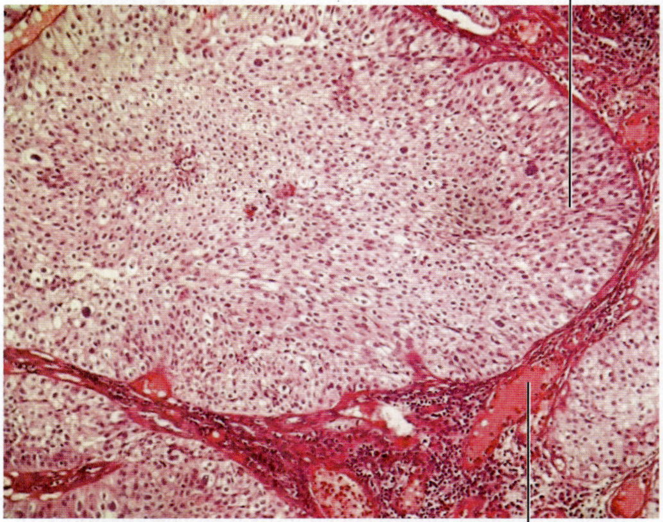

Fig. 29.15 Low grade urothelial carcinoma (H&E; 400×).

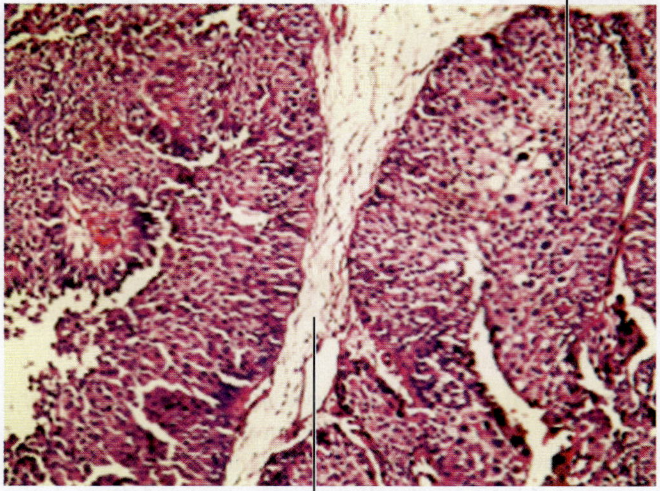

Fig. 29.16 High grade urothelial carcinoma (H&E; 400×).

Peak Age

50–80 years.

Gender Distribution

Male:female ratio = 3:1.

Pathogenesis

Tumours arising from the urothelium are known to be associated with the following:

- Cigarette smoking.
- Industrial exposure to arylamines.
- *S. haematobium* infection.
- Long-term use of analgesics.
- Long-term exposure to cyclophosphamide.
- Monosomy of chromosome 9.
- Deletions of 9p and 9q as well as deletions of 17p, 13q, 11p and 14q.
- 9p deletions (9p21) involving the tumour suppressor gene p16 (MTS 1 and INK4-alpha, which encodes an inhibitor of a cyclin-dependent kinase and also the related p15).

Morphology

- **Exophytic papillomas** are small, delicate, pedunculated/papillary lesions composed of a connective tissue stalk covered by normal-appearing urothelium.
- **Inverted papillomas** appear as nodular lesions in the trigone area and show invaginations of bland-appearing epithelium extending down into the lamina propria.
- **PUNLMPs** differ from a papilloma in having a thicker urothelial layer.
- **Low-grade papillary urothelial carcinomas** comprise branching papillae, which show mild atypia and increased mitoses but have an orderly architecture and maintain nuclear polarity. They may infrequently recur or rarely invade (Fig. 29.15).
- **High-grade papillary urothelial carcinomas** show marked atypia and increased mitoses including atypical ones. They have a disorderly architecture and show loss of nuclear polarity and dyscohesiveness (Fig. 29.16). They have major potential for recurrence and metastases.

Clinical Features

Painless haematuria, frequency, urgency and dysuria.

Complications

Stricture formation, hydronephrosis and pyonephrosis.

Prognosis

Depends on tumour grade or blood group antigens (tumour cells expressing A, B and H antigens have a better prognosis).

30 Diseases of Male Genital System

TESTIS AND EPIDIDYMIS

Normal Structure

- The **scrotal sac** lodges the **testis** and the **epididymis** along with the **lower part of the spermatic cord.**
- The testes are a pair of ovoid glandular structures that are responsible for the production of sperms and the male sex hormone testosterone.
- They are invaginated by the **tunica** which has three layers, namely the **tunica vasculosa, albuginea** and **vaginalis. Tunica vasculosa** is the innermost connective tissue layer of the tunica which carries blood vessels to the testis. It is covered by the **tunica albuginea** which encases the testis and also extends into it. Overlying this is the outer layer of the tunica, the **tunica vaginalis.**
- Each testis is divided by invaginations of the tunica albuginea into small compartments called **lobules.** Each lobule contains numerous tightly coiled **seminiferous tubules**, the walls of which contain the **germ cells, Sertoli cells** and **Leydig cells.**
- The germ cells multiply and differentiate to produce **spermatocytes** from the onset of puberty. The spermatocytes develop into **spermatids** and eventually **spermatozoa.** About 400 million sperms are released in a single ejaculation. **Sertoli cells** provide support to the developing sperm cells. The seminiferous tubules are held together by loose connective tissue called **interstitium** which lodges the Leydig cells. **Leydig cells** produce testosterone that is responsible for the secondary sex characteristics associated with males.
- The tubules become less convoluted towards the lobular apex and continue as 20–30 straight **collecting ducts.** These ducts merge to form the **rete testis** lined by flattened epithelium. The secretions from rete testis drain into the **vasa efferentia** which opens at the upper pole of the epididymis. The lower pole of the epididymis merges with the **ductus deferens.**

Q. Write briefly about cryptorchidism.

Ans. Cryptorchidism is derived from the Greek words *kryptos*, meaning hidden, and *orchis*, meaning testicle; it indicates the absence of one or both testes from the scrotum. It has the following salient features:

- It is usually seen at birth but can rarely develop later in life. About 80% of cryptorchid testes descend by the first year of life making the actual incidence about 0.8%.
- The exact cause is not known but the risk factors include intrauterine growth retardation, prematurity, perinatal asphyxia, C-section and toxaemia of pregnancy.
- An undescended testis can be found anywhere along the 'normal path of descent' from the retroperitoneum (25% of cases) to the inguinal ring (70% of cases) or any other location in the inguinal canal (5% of cases).
- It is sometimes found outside the normal pathway, e.g. the thigh, the perineum, the opposite scrotum or the femoral canal, when it is labelled **ectopic or wandering testis.** An underdeveloped, undescended testis is labelled **hypoplastic.**
- In rare cases, the testis appears to have vanished (true hidden testes or 'anorchia').
- An undescended testis is called **retractile** when it can be manipulated into scrotum where it remains without tension. On the other hand, when it can be manipulated into upper scrotum but retracts when released, it is called **gliding.**
- Cryptorchidism is unilateral in about 80% of cases and bilateral in the remaining. Most cases are clinically asymptomatic and discovered only on physical examination.
- Cryptorchid testes can be brought into the scrotum by a surgical procedure called an 'orchiopexy'.
- Untreated cases may be associated with reduced fertility and increased risk of testicular germ cell tumours, and are also more prone to torsion, infarction and inguinal hernia.
- On gross examination, the cryptorchid testis is small and fibrotic. Histologically, there is marked reduction in the number of germ cells.

Q. Write briefly about testicular atrophy.

Ans. Testicular atrophy is a regressive change which can have a varied aetiology.

Causes

- Progressive atherosclerotic narrowing of testicular blood vessels, as in old age
- End stage of all inflammatory conditions (orchitis)
- Cryptorchidism
- Hypopituitarism
- Obstruction of flow to semen
- Malnutrition and cachexia
- Prolonged administration of female sex hormones
- Exhaustion atrophy due to high level of pituitary follicle-stimulating hormone
- Klinefelter syndrome

Gross Morphology

Testes are small in size and firm in consistency because of fibrotic changes.

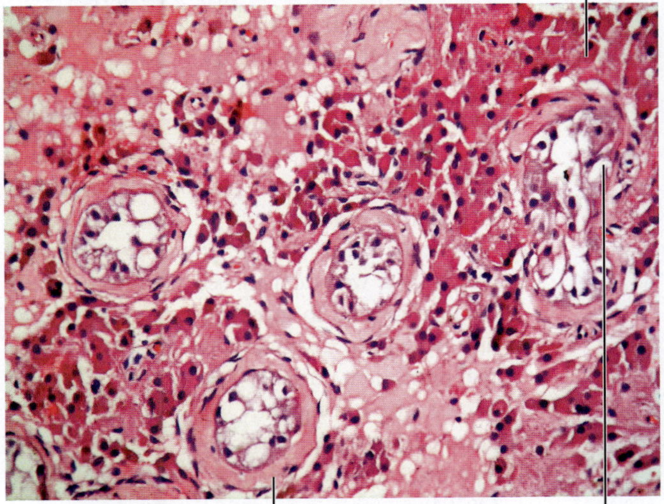

Fig. 30.1 Atrophic testis showing marked loss of germ cells within the tubules, with peritubular and interstitial fibrosis and proliferation of interstitial cells of Leydig (H&E; 100×).

Microscopy (Fig. 30.1)

- Spermatic tubules show hyalinization and thickening of the basement membrane.
- There is increased interstitial connective tissue.
- Sertoli cells are present, but there is no spermatogenesis.
- Leydig cells are prominent.

Q. Classify testicular tumours. Describe their clinicopathological features. (PA29.1)

Ans. Testicular germ cell tumours (TGCT) constitute the vast majority of testicular neoplasms and may occur in any age but >90% occur in young adult men, with the peak prevalence between 25 and 40 years of age. These tumours are derived from germ cell neoplasia in situ (GCNIS) cells, which are fetal gonocytes that failed to mature to spermatogonia. The presence of GCNIS should be suspected in men with impaired fertility and spermatogenesis or history of cryptorchidism. Many cases have been linked to the testicular dysgenesis syndrome or TDS (spectrum of disorders including cryptorchidism, hypospadias, intersex syndromes, poor sperm quality).

Classification of Testicular Tumours

1. **Germ cell tumours (95%)**
   (a) **Derived from germ cell neoplasia in situ (GCNIS)**
      (i) Seminoma
      (ii) Non-seminomatous germ cell tumours
         - Yolk sac tumour (post-pubertal)
         - Embryonal carcinoma
         - Trophoblastic tumours (choriocarcinoma, placental site trophoblastic tumour)
         - Teratoma (postpubertal) with or without malignant transformation.

   (b) **Mixed and unclassified germ cell tumours**
   (c) **Not derived from germ cell neoplasia in situ (GCNIS)**
      (i) Spermatocytic tumour
      (ii) Teratoma (prepubertal)
      (iii) Yolk sac tumour (prepubertal).
2. **Sex cord–stromal tumours** (<5% of all testicular cancers)
   (a) Leydig cell tumour
   (b) Sertoli cell tumour
   (c) Granulosa cell tumour
   (d) Mixed and unclassified sex cord–stromal tumours.
3. **Mixed germ cell and stromal tumours** (proportion of all testicular cancers not well defined)
   (a) Gonadoblastoma.
4. **Miscellaneous tumours** (proportion of all testicular cancers not well defined).

Salient Features of Testicular Tumours

- All testicular tumours are derived from totipotent germ cells, which can show progressive and retrogressive differentiation; therefore, metastatic tumours may sometimes show a different histology as compared with the primary lesion, e.g. an embryonal carcinoma may present as a teratoma in the metastatic lesion.
- In the latest classification of testicular tumours (WHO 2016) most changes have been made in the classification of germ cell tumours, including replacement of the terms intratubular germ cell neoplasia unclassified and carcinoma in situ by **germ cell neoplasia in situ (GCNIS)**; subdivision of the tumours into 2 main categories, those derived from GCNIS and those not derived from GCNIS; distinction of GCNIS from germ cells with delayed maturation; expansion of the trophoblastic tumour category to include other tumours; and substitution of spermatocytic tumour for spermatocytic seminoma and its placement in the non-germ cell neoplasia in situ group.
- Most testicular tumours are derived from GCNIS, which is also commonly seen in their vicinity. Exceptions are paediatric yolk sac tumour, teratomas and spermatocytic tumour. GCNIS is found to be present as early as intrauterine life. It remains innocuous till puberty when it progresses to seminomatous germ cell tumours (SGCTs) or non-seminomatous germ cell tumours (NSGCTs) subsequent to activating mutations, e.g. reduplication of the short arm of chromosome 12 and kit activation.
- GCNIS is histologically characterized by the presence of atypical primordial cells with large pleomorphic nuclei and clear cytoplasm (clearing is because of the presence of large amounts of glycogen). Tumour cells are larger than spermatogonia and show membranous positivity for placental alkaline phosphatase (PLAP). Seminiferous tubules show a thickened basement membrane, reduced diameter and absence of sperms. An essential feature to distinguish GCNIS from germ cells with delayed maturation is its requisite location at the base of seminiferous tubules in what has been termed the spermatogonial niche.
- Because yolk sac tumour and teratoma may either develop from GCNIS or not be derived from GCNIS, these are further designated as postpubertal type because of their marked predominance in this age group. Similarly, the

non-GCNIS related counterparts are designated prepubertal type. The GCNIS-derived tumours share certain pathophysiologic associations like an increasing incidence in heavily industrialized nations (attributed to exposure to antiandrogen additives used in the manufacture of certain plastics, phthalates, sedentary lifestyle, high calorie intake, and obesity), association with dysgenetic changes, and amplification of a segment of the short arm of chromosome 12 (often in the form of an isochromosome), The non-GCNIS derived tumours lack the epidemiologic associations seen in the GCNIS-derived germ cell tumours and have no established risk factors apart from occurrence in older men (spermatocytic tumour) or children (the prepubertal-type tumours).

- Germ cell tumours commonly present as painless enlargement of testes.
- Lymphatic spread is common; retroperitoneal para-aortic lymph nodes are the first to be involved followed by mediastinal and supraclavicular lymph nodes.
- Haematogenous spread commonly involves lungs, liver, brain and bone.
- Germ cell tumours secrete polypeptide hormones and certain enzymes that can be detected in the blood, e.g. **AFP (α-fetoprotein), hCG (human chorionic gonadotropin), PLAP (placental alkaline phosphatase), HPL (human, placental lactogen) and LDH (lactate dehydrogenase)**.
- These hormones are useful in:
  - Diagnosis and staging of testicular germ cell tumours.
  - Monitoring response to therapy.
- Elevated levels of hCG and AFP are most often associated with yolk sac tumour and choriocarcinoma.
- Non-Hodgkin lymphoma is the most common testicular tumour after the fifth decade.

Staging of Testicular Germ Cell Tumours

- Stage I: Tumours confined to the testis, epididymis or spermatic cord.
- Stage II: Spread confined to retroperitoneal lymph nodes below the diaphragm.
- Stage III: Metastasis outside the retroperitoneal lymph nodes or above the diaphragm.

1. **Germ cell tumours**
   (a) **Derived from GCNIS**
   (i) **Seminoma**

Clinical features

- Most common type of germ cell tumour.
- Peak age: Third decade; never seen in infants.
- Arises from undifferentiated germ cells.
- Extremely radiosensitive.

Gross morphology (Fig. 30.2A)

- Classical seminomas are large tumours which may replace the entire testis but the testicular shape is maintained.
- The tumour is clearly delineated from the surrounding normal testis, which appears compressed.
- Cut surface is homogeneous, rubbery, grey-white and lobulated.
- Haemorrhage and necrosis are rare.
- Tunica albuginea is generally intact; however, occasional extension to epididymis, spermatic cord and scrotal sac may be seen.

Microscopy (Fig. 30.2B and C)

- Sheets of monomorphic-looking seminoma cells are divided into poorly demarcated lobules by delicate fibrous septae. Septae are infiltrated by T lymphocytes and plasma cells; at times, granulomas may form.
- Seminoma cell is a large, round-to-polyhedral cell with a well-defined cell membrane, clear cytoplasm (due to glycogen or lipid contents) and large central vesicular nucleus with one or two prominent nucleoli.
- Mitoses are infrequent.

Immunochemistry

- Tumour cells stain positive for PLAP, KIT and OCT4.
- hCG is positive in 15% of cases where syncytial giant cells resembling syncytiotrophoblasts of placenta are present.

(ii) **Nonseminomatous germ cell tumours**

- **Yolk sac tumour**
  - Also called endodermal sinus tumour, orchioblastoma and infantile embryonal carcinoma.
  - Two biologically distinct entities:
    - Postpubertal type: GCNIS-related; usually occurs as part of a mixed tumour; associated with TDS, subfertility, single nucleotide polymorphism (SNP) variants (KITLG, SPRY4, DMRT1).

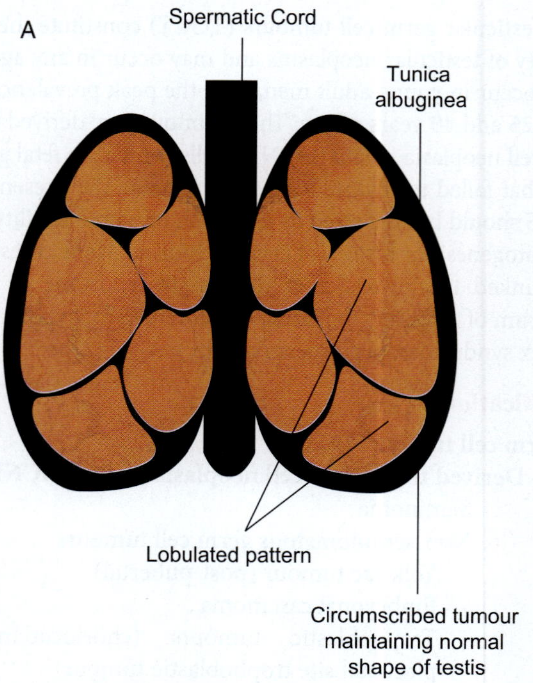

Fig. 30.2 (A) Gross image of seminomatous germ cell tumours (SGCTs).

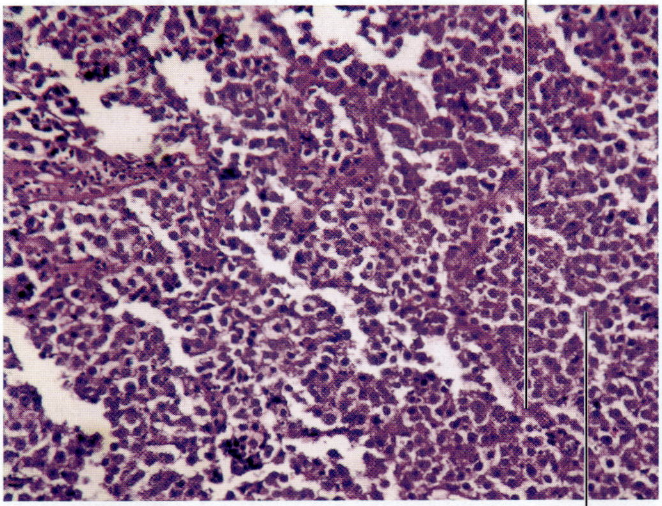

Fig. 30.2 (B) Section from seminoma testis showing sheets of large, round-to-polyhedral cells with well-defined cell membrane; clear cytoplasm, large central nucleus and one or two prominent nucleoli. The sheets are divided into poorly demarcated lobules by delicate fibrous septae which are infiltrated by T lymphocytes (H&E; 100×).

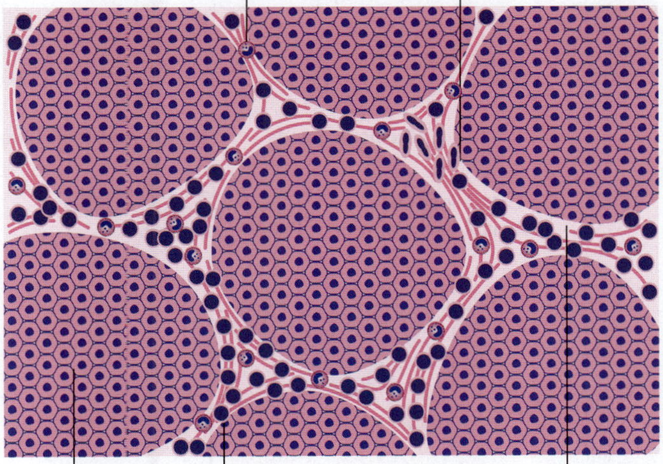

Fig. 30.2 (C) Schematic diagram of seminoma testis.

- Prepubertal type: unrelated to GCNIS; usually pure: aetiology is unknown.
- The distinction of the prepubertal-type yolk sac tumour from the post-pubertal form is important because the former is less apt to metastasize.

Clinical features

- Unilateral testicular mass, often painless; AFP level elevated in all cases.
- Postpubertal type: more aggressive (compared to prepubertal).
- Prepubertal type: Less aggressive: higher tendency to bypass retroperitoneal lymph nodes and spread haematogenously.

Gross pathology

- Postpubertal type:
  - Poorly circumscribed, unencapsulated, predominantly solid, gray-white to yellow-tan, gelatinous surface.
  - Haemorrhage, necrosis and cystic areas are common.
- Prepubertal type:
  - Relatively homogeneous, lobulated, solid to gelatinous.
  - Haemorrhage and necrosis are uncommon.

Microscopy

- Tumour cells are flattened to cuboidal with clear to vacuolated cytoplasm, arranged in a variety of patterns varying from loose, lace-like or reticular to tubular, tubulopapillary and solid.
- Cells may form distinct **perivascular structures**, i.e. a central blood vessel or mesodermal core surrounded by germ cells arranged in visceral and parietal layers such as glomeruli **(resemble yolk sac or endodermal sinus of rat placenta called Schiller–Duval bodies).**
- Intracellular and extracellular **Periodic acid–Schiff** (PAS)-positive hyaline globules may be present.
- Tumour cells may also contain AFP and α_1-antitrypsin.

- **Embryonal carcinoma**

Clinical features

- Presents in 2nd or 3rd decade with painless swelling of testis.
- More than 60% have metastases at presentation.
- Tumour secretes AFP and hCG.

Gross features

- Usually small sized, with poorly demarcated margins.
- Cut surface is variegated with areas of haemorrhage and necrosis.
- Extension into the tunica albuginea is commonly seen.

Microscopy

- Pure in 2% of the cases; most commonly part of mixed germ cell tumour.
- Variable morphological patterns with markedly pleomorphic tumour cells, arranged in tubules, acini or sheets.
- Tumour cells resemble primitive epithelial cells, have hyperchromatic nuclei with prominent nucleoli.
- Necrosis is prominent.

- **Choriocarcinoma**
  - Highly malignant form of testicular cancer.
  - May arise in placental tissue, ovaries, mediastinum and abdomen (from sequestered totipotential cells).
  - Pure form of choriocarcinoma rare; mostly mixed tumours.
  - The serum and urinary levels of hCG greatly elevated in all cases.

Gross morphology

- Most cases do not show testicular enlargement, and the tumour appears as a small palpable nodule.
- Areas of haemorrhage and necrosis are extremely common.
- Tumour may undergo extensive ischaemic necrosis to be eventually replaced by a fibrous scar leaving behind extensive metastasis.

Microscopy: Three types of cells are seen without formation of placental type villi, namely:

- ***Syncytiotrophoblasts:*** Large, multinucleated cells with irregular or lobular hyperchromatic nuclei and abundant eosinophilic cytoplasm; hCG can be localized to their cytoplasm.
- ***Cytotrophoblasts:*** Regular, polygonal cells with distinct cell borders, clear cytoplasm; single uniform nucleus; grow in cords and masses.
- ***Intermediate trophoblastic cells:*** Clear cytoplasm, larger than cytotrophoblasts with single nuclei.

- **Teratoma**
  - It is important to distinguish the prepubertal form of testicular teratoma from the postpubertal form, because the former is benign but not the latter.
  - Because prepubertal-type teratomas may occasionally be discovered in postpubertal males, age alone cannot discriminate between these lesions; a careful morphologic and molecular assessment is required for diagnosis.
  - Teratoma with somatic type malignancy is defined as a teratoma with malignant transformation that occupies at least a 4x magnification (0.5 cm).
  - Classification into mature and immature types is misleading, and is no longer accepted.

Clinical features

- Most commonly presents at age 25-35 years.
- Postpubertal teratoma more frequent that prepubertal teratoma.
- Most commonly presents with painless swelling of the testicle.

Gross description

Lobulated, variegated appearance, grey-white with solid and cystic areas; may show gelatinous foci with cartilage and bone formation.

Microscopy

- Prepubertal type (Figs 30.3A and B)
  - Absence of cytologic atypia; GCNIS; necrosis, and dysgenetic testicular parenchymal changes.
  - Organoid morphology with tissue layers visible such as epithelium, lamina propria and muscularis propria.
  - Prominent ciliated epithelium; nests of squamous epithelium and smooth muscle.
  - Hair follicles may be seen (not seen in postpubertal type).

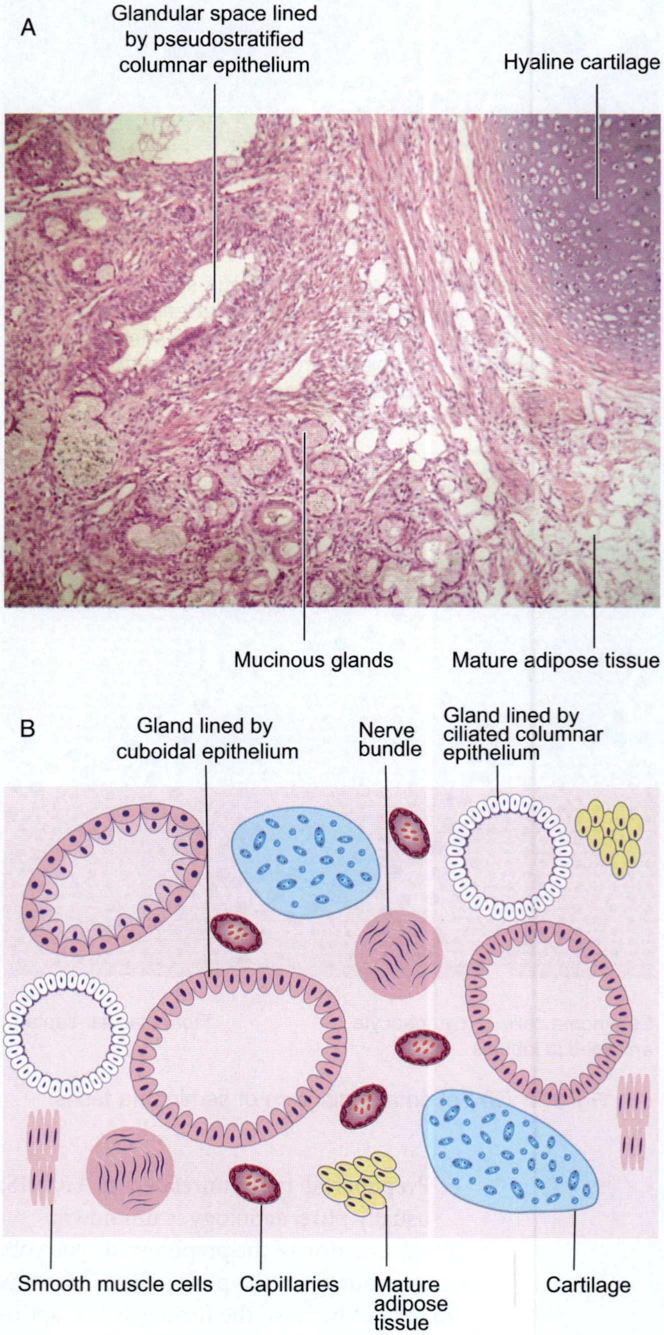

Fig. 30.3 (A and B) Photomicrograph and schematic diagram of a pre-pubertal teratoma showing organoid morphology with glandular epithelium; cartilage, mature adipose tissue, neural tissue and smooth muscle (H&E; 100×).

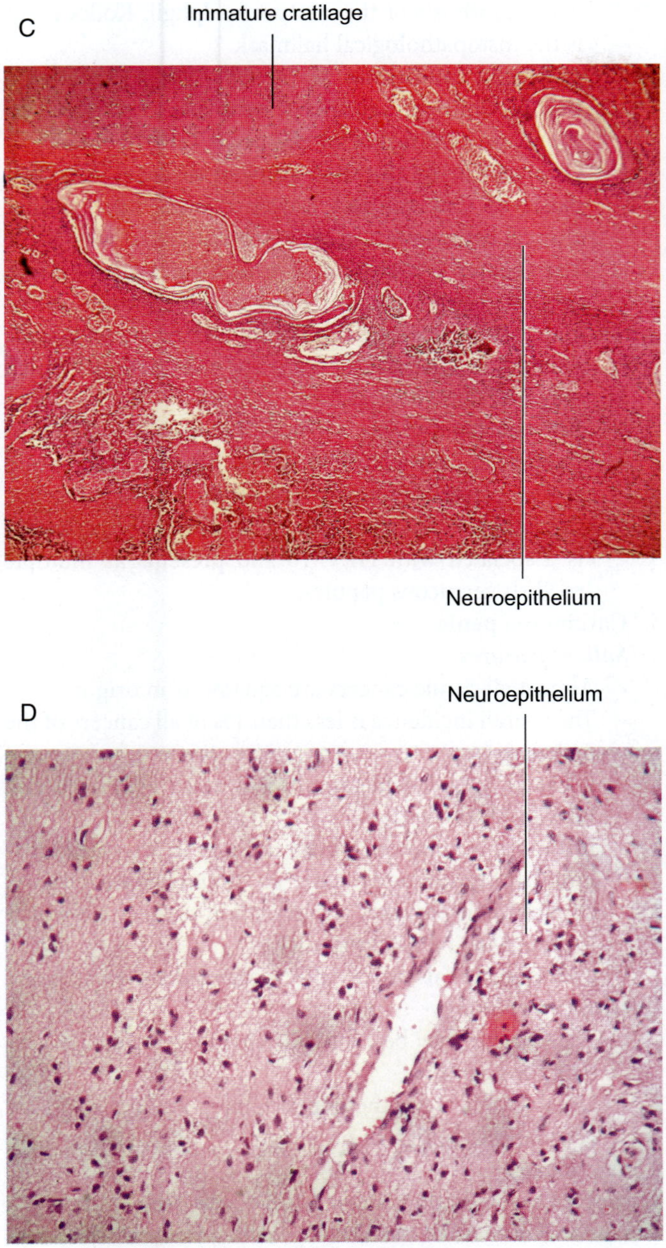

Fig. 30.3 (C and D) Postpubertal teratoma showing abundant necrosis, immature cartilage and neuroepithelium (H&E; 100×).

- Lack of chromosome 12p amplification by fluorescent in situ hybridization methodology.
- Postpubertal type (Fig. 30.3 C and D)
  - Associated with GCNIS; demonstrates varying degrees of atypia.
  - Gastrointestinal epithelium, respiratory epithelium, cartilage, bone, fat, squamous epithelium with keratinization, primitive undifferentiated spindle cells, or neuroepithelium commonly seen.
  - Chromosome 12p amplification can be demonstrated by fluorescent in situ hybridization methodology.
- Teratoma with somatic type malignancy.
  - Sarcoma is most prevalent somatic type malignancy but other tumour types including adenocarcinoma, squamous cell carcinoma and primitive neuroectodermal tumour (PNET) can occur.

2. **Germ cell tumours not derived from GCNIS**

Spermatocytic tumour

- Occurs in the sixth decade (higher mean age than seminoma).
- Does not occur together with other forms of germ cell tumour.
- Lacks the chromosome 12p amplification of the GCNIS-derived tumours, and shows a characteristic amplification of the DMRT1 gene near the telomeric end of chromosome 9p.51.
- Shows a multinodular growth pattern lacking the fibrous septa and lymphocytic infiltrate of seminoma.
- Oedema may be a striking feature in many spermatocytic tumours and is responsible for the formation of irregular to follicle-like spaces.
- Some tumours may have a predominance of intermediate-sized cells with prominent nucleoli (a finding that has been termed anaplastic, although this is a not a recognized designation as there is no difference in clinical behavior of tumours.
- OCT3/4, placental alkaline phosphatase, a-fetoprotein, human chorionic gonadotropin, CD30 are negative unlike other testicular tumours, but CD117, SALL4 and DMRT1 are positive.

3. **Sex cord-stromal tumours**
   (a) **Sertoli cell tumours**
      (i) Yellowish, homogenous cut surface
      (ii) Histologically, show small cells arranged in trabeculae or cords resembling immature seminiferous tubules
      (iii) Associated with hormonal effects
   (b) **Leydig cell tumours**
      (i) Derived from and resemble normal testicular interstitial cells
      (ii) Well-defined nodules <5 cm in diameter
      (iii) Characteristic golden brown colour due to intracytoplasmic inclusions called **Reinke's crystalloids** and **lipofuscin**.

PENIS

Normal Structure

- The penis consists of three cylindrical erectile vascular tissue bodies (two corpora cavernosa of the penis, placed dorsally, and one corpus cavernosum of the urethra, placed ventrally), all covered by skin.
- The longest part of the penis is labelled the shaft, at the end of which is the head, or glans penis. The *frenulum* or *frenum* is a connecting membrane on the underside of the penis.

- The glans has a covering, called the foreskin or prepuce. The prepuce is a retractile fold of skin containing connective tissue, smooth muscle and sebaceous glands.

Q. Write briefly about the inflammatory conditions affecting the penis.

Ans. The foreskin of the penis (prepuce) and the glans penis (the conical end of the penis) are the areas usually affected by inflammation. Inflammation of the glans and foreskin are labelled **balanitis** and **posthitis**, respectively. **Balanoposthitis** is inflammation of both the glans penis and the foreskin.

Salient Features

- Causes of penile inflammation include **infectious** and **non-infectious conditions.**
- **Common infectious causes** are yeast infections (*Candida albicans*), sexually transmitted diseases (STD–gonorrhoea, herpes and syphilis) and scabies.
- **Non-infectious causes** include *allergic reactions* (to latex condom or to contraceptive gels), *papulosquamous disorders* (lichen planus, psoriasis), *seborrhoeic dermatitis* and *balanitis xerotica obliterans* (chronic inflammation of the glans which results in the formation of white plaques on the foreskin and glans, which on histopathology show changes similar to lichen sclerosus et atrophicus and may lead to constriction of the urinary passage).
- Penile inflammation may manifest with pain, swelling, irritation, redness, erosions/ulceration and enlarged groin lymph nodes.
- Patients with balanoposthitis are predisposed to **phimosis** (narrowing of the preputial orifice resulting in non-retraction of the preputial skin over the glans) and penile cancer.
- Diagnosis and typing of inflammatory conditions of the penis entails the following steps:
  1. Physical examination
  2. Blood sugar measurement (for diabetes)
  3. KOH mount and culture for yeast infections
  4. Specific tests for STDs

Q. Write briefly about the neoplasms involving the penis. (PA29.2)

Ans. Following are the commonly encountered benign and malignant lesions involving the penis:

1. **Condyloma acuminatum**
   (a) Also known as 'anogenital wart', it is associated with HPV 6 and 11 and may present as solitary or multiple lesions. Common sites are the coronal sulcus of the penis and the perianal area.
   (b) Condyloma acuminatum has a large cauliflower-like exophytic variant labelled **'Buschke–Lowenstein tumour' (verrucous carcinoma)**.
   (c) Microscopy shows papillary projections composed of a connective tissue core lined by squamous epithelium. The epithelium shows hyperkeratosis/parakeratosis with acanthosis of the stratum malphgii. Koilocytosis is the histopathological hallmark.
2. **Premalignant conditions**
   (a) **PeIN** (penile intraepithelial neoplasia) can occur on the glans or foreskin of the penis (**erythroplasia of Queyrat**) or on the shaft (**Bowen disease**). Erythroplasia of Queyrat and Bowen disease have similar clinical behaviour and both are associated with HPV. The former is common in uncircumcised men and presents as reddish and velvety pigmentation on the glans. **Bowen disease** is characterized by well-marginated, reddish plaques over the shaft of penis which may ulcerate and crust.
   (b) **Bowenoid papulosis** is histopathologically identical to the two above-mentioned entities (Bowen disease and erythroplasia of Queyrat) and all show severe dysplastic changes on biopsy. Clinically, 'Bowenoid papulosis' is associated with HPV 16 and presents as multiple reddish verrucous papules.
3. **Carcinoma penis**
   Salient features
   - Almost all penile cancers are squamous in origin.
   - The overall incidence is less than 1% of all cancers of the male.
   - It has an established causal association with high-risk HPV types (16 and 18).
   - It is more common in blacks and rare in Jews and Muslims who customarily undergo circumcision (because circumcision prevents accumulation of smegma which is thought to be carcinogenic).
   - Carcinoma penis usually affects men older than 50 years.

   Gross morphology
   - The tumour may be exophytic (papillary or cauliflower type) or ulcerative.
   - Usual locations are the fraenum, prepuce, glans and the coronal sulcus, in that order.

   Microscopy
   In most cases, sections show a well-to-moderately differentiated squamous cell carcinoma, which commonly metastasize to the regional lymph nodes as well as viscera.

PROSTATE

Normal Structure

- The prostate weighs about 20 g in a normal adult. It surrounds the beginning of the male urethra and has three lobes – one median and two lateral.
- Histologically, it is constituted by 30–50 branched acini (tubule alveolar structures) lying in a fibromuscular stroma. The acini are lined by two layers, a basal cuboidal cell layer and an inner layer of mucus-secreting columnar cells.
- The prostate is divided into two parts depending on the hormone responsiveness, the inner periurethral part which is sensitive to oestrogen and androgens and an outer subcapsular part that is sensitive to androgen.

Q. Describe the aetiology, pathogenesis, pathology and progression of prostatitis. (PA29.5)

Ans. Prostatitis is inflammation of the prostate.

Salient Features

- Includes acute bacterial, chronic bacterial, chronic pelvic pain syndrome (CPPS) and granulomatous prostatitis.
- Clinical diagnosis should be based on quantitative bacterial cultures and microscopic examination of fractionated urine specimens (first 10 mL of urine is urethral; midstream urine is from bladder) and expressed prostatic secretions (EPS).
- CPPS, which includes prostatodynia, category III or abacterial prostatitis, is the most common urological diagnosis after 50 years.
- Prostate-specific antigen (PSA) is elevated, particularly with acute prostatitis.
- **CPPS**
  - Histopathological diagnosis is less crucial or may not be required for diagnosis.
  - Clinically similar to bacterial prostatitis, with persistent pain, especially after ejaculation but no bacteria are cultured from EPS.
  - This syndrome is subdivided into inflammatory and non-inflammatory subtypes. Inflammatory CPPS is defined by the presence of white blood cells in the semen, EPS, or voided bladder urine after prostatic massage. Non-inflammatory CPPS is defined by the absence of white blood cells.
- **Acute bacterial prostatitis**
  - Causative organisms include *Escherichia coli*, Gram-negative rods, enterococci and staphylococci; usually due to reflux; also following surgical manipulation or sexually transmitted disease.
  - Usually localized, may cause obstruction, retention and abscess.
- **Chronic bacterial prostatitis**
  - Symptoms of low back pain, dysuria, perineal and suprapubic discomfort.
  - Often have history of urinary tract infection (UTI) by same organism.
  - May have NO symptoms.
- **Granulomatous prostatitis**
  - Necrotizing or non-necrotizing granulomas may be seen in men who have undergone BCG treatment for bladder cancer.
  - It also occurs after transurethral resection.
  - Otherwise, most cases are idiopathic and do not require acid-fast stain.

Laboratory Work up

- Bacterial: Prostatic secretion cultures should have bacterial counts 10× urethral/bladder cultures.
- Non-bacterial: >10 WBC/HPF in prostatic secretions without pyuria.

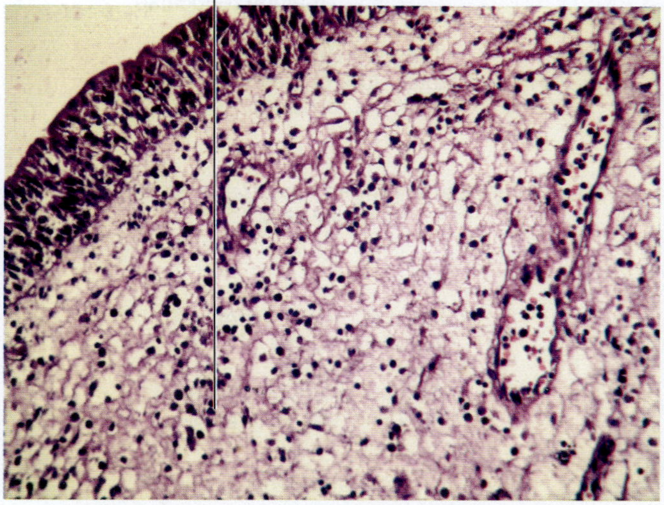

Fig. 30.4 Chronic bacterial prostatitis (H&E; 400×).

Histopathology (Fig. 30.4)

- Macrophages in stroma and neutrophils in lumen spaces are specific for acute prostatitis. When complicated by abscess formation, prostatic tissue may become necrotic.
- Lymphoid aggregates are not specific for prostatitis.

Q. Write briefly about the aetiopathogenesis, clinical features and morphology of nodular hyperplasia of prostate (NHP). (PA29.3)

Ans. NHP (benign prostatic hyperplasia) is defined as hyperplasia of prostatic stromal and epithelial cells, resulting in the formation of discrete nodules in the transitional and inner periurethral zones (prostate is divided into several zones, namely peripheral, central, transitional and periurethral).

Salient Features

- NHP was earlier called 'benign hypertrophy', which is a misnomer because the fundamental lesion is a hyperplasia and not hypertrophy.
- Age group affected is older than 50 years; incidence increases with increasing age.
- The nodules compress the prostatic urethra to produce the clinical symptoms of NHP. Over a period of time, obstruction to urinary flow leads to bladder hypertrophy, diverticulum formation, cystitis and pyelonephritis.

Pathogenesis (Flowchart 30.1)

- **Testosterone** is converted into Dihydrotestosterone **(DHT) by 5α-reductase type II enzyme specifically located in the stromal cells.**
- **DHT is 10 times more potent than testosterone**, because it dissociates slowly from androgen receptors (ARs).
- DHT thus produced acts on **nuclear receptors to produce growth factors** that are mitogenic to **epithelial and stromal cells.**

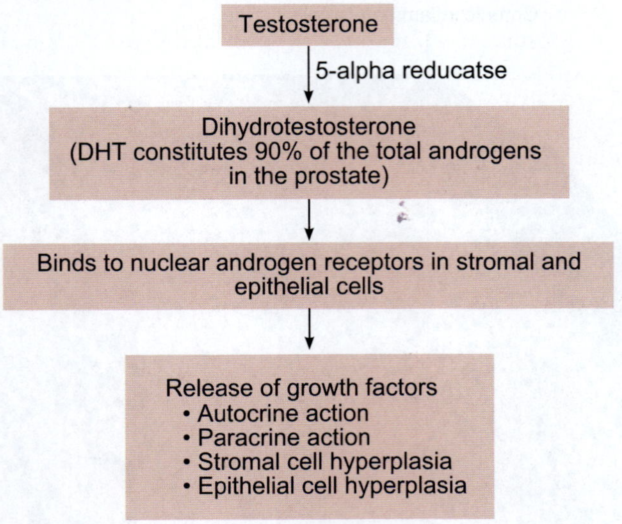

Flowchart 30.1 Pathogenesis of NHP.

- Testosterone acts similarly, but is **very weak**.
- **Oestrogen** increases the expression of ARs, thus providing DHT more sites for action. Oestrogen levels increase with age, making its role significant.

Clinical Features

- **Clinical symptoms are seen in 10% of affected patients.**
- **Early changes:** Compression of urethra leading to increased frequency, nocturia (urgency), problem in starting and stopping the stream of urine, overflow dribbling and painful micturition.
- **Late complaints:** Retention of urine in the bladder causing UTI, cystitis, hypertrophy or trabeculation and later hydronephrosis.

Gross Morphology

- The affected gland is enlarged, and may weigh up to 300 g or more.
- Cut surface shows multiple well-defined nodules that bulge from the surface.
- Two types of proliferation, **glandular** and **stromal (fibromuscular)**, are seen.
- In nodules with primarily *glandular* proliferation, the cut surface is yellow-pink; consistency is soft with milky-white fluid oozing out of it.
- In nodules with primarily *stromal (fibromuscular)* proliferation, the surface is pale-grey and tough without any fluid oozing out.
- True capsule is absent but plane of cleavage is present.

Microscopy (Fig. 30.5 A–C)

There is proliferation of acinar/glandular and ductular epithelium along with stromal proliferation resulting in the formation of five types of nodules – fibrous, fibromuscular, muscular, fibroadenomatous and fibroadenomyomatous.

Epithelial Proliferation

- There is proliferation and cystic dilatation of glands, which are lined by two layers: inner layer of columnar cells and outer layer of cuboidal or flattened epithelium.
- The basement membrane is intact.
- Multilayering and crowding of the epithelium leads to the formation of papillary infoldings.
- Eosinophilic laminated concretions (corpora amylacea) are commonly seen in the glandular lumina.
- Squamous metaplasia and small foci of infarction may be present.

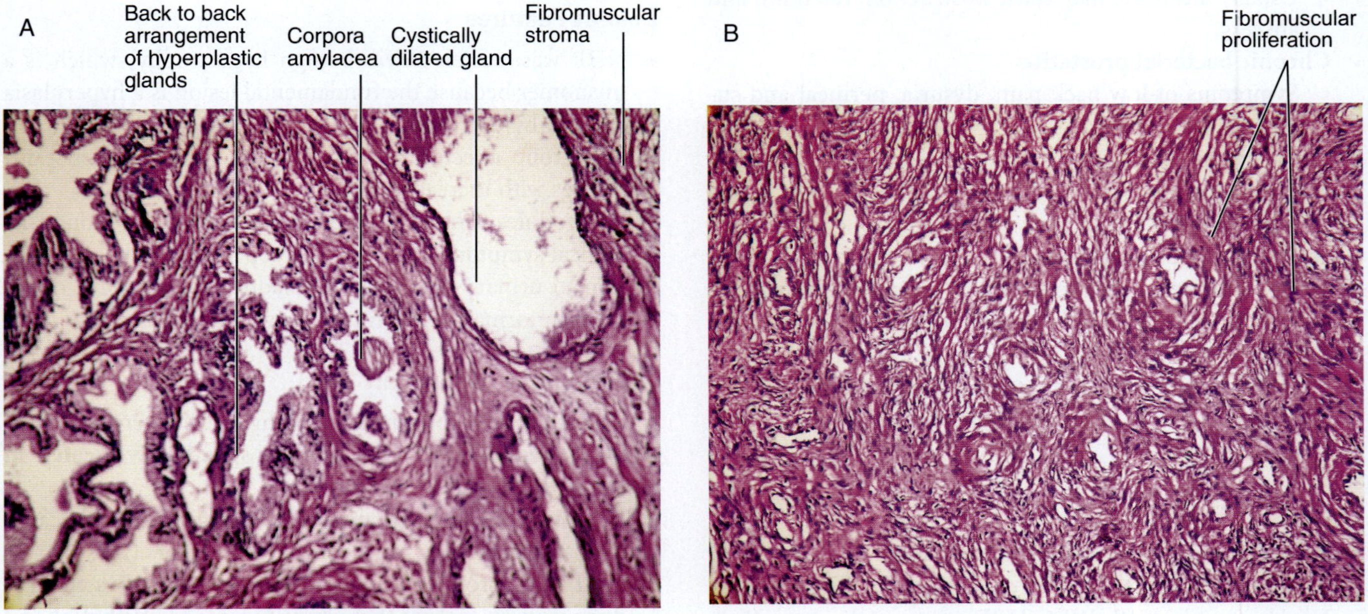

Fig. 30.5 (A) Section from NHP showing proliferation and cystic dilatation of glands lined by two layers – inner layer of columnar cells and outer layer of cuboidal or flattened epithelium. Multilayering and crowding of epithelium with formation of papillary infoldings is also seen (H&E; 100×). (B) Section from NHP showing stromal hyperplasia (H&E; 100×).

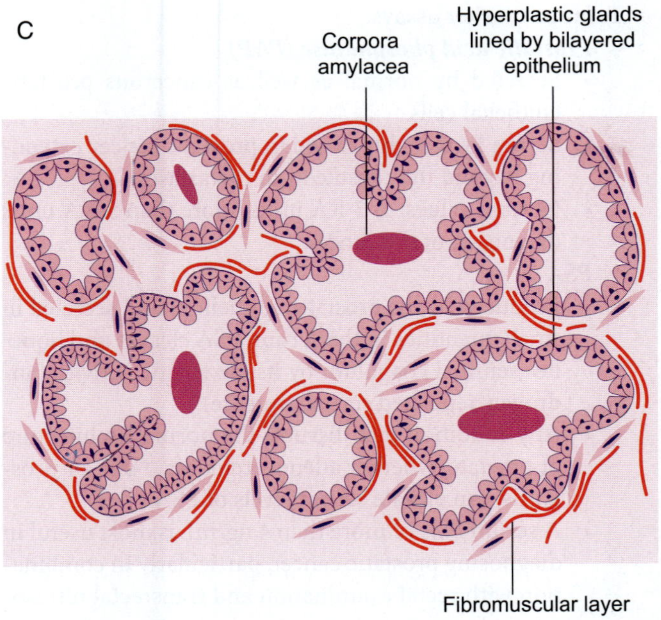

Fig. 30.5 (C) Schematic representation of nodular hyperplasia of prostate (NHP).

Stromal Proliferation

Glandular proliferation is accompanied by the fibrous and muscular proliferation.

Q. Describe the aetiopathogenesis, clinical features and morphology of the carcinoma prostrate. (PA29.4)

Ans. Carcinoma prostate is the most common form of visceral cancer (followed by lung cancer), and the second leading cause of death in males.

Clinical Features

- It usually affects men older than 50 years.
- About 70%–80% arises in the **peripheral zone**; because of its peripheral location, it is less likely to cause urethral obstruction in the early stages.
- Most cases are clinically silent; a few are discovered accidentally in the prostatic tissue removed for NHP.
- Extensive prostatic disease can produce 'prostatism' (local discomfort and lower urinary tract obstruction).
- It may come to attention because of bone metastases (may be lytic, more commonly blastic).

Factors Implicated in the Pathogenesis of Carcinoma Prostate

- **Dietary factors:** Increased consumption of fats and reduced consumption of lycopenes, selenium, soya products and vitamin D increase the risk of prostatic cancer.
- **Family history:** Men with a family history of prostatic cancer have a twofold increase in incidence and an earlier age of onset.
- **Environmental factors:** Exposure to oxidants, carcinogenic substances and exogenous oestrogens induce genetic and epigenetic changes conducive to cancer development.
- **Genetic factors**
  - Prostatic carcinoma is initially androgen dependent and relies on the AR to mediate the effects of androgens (therapy includes antiandrogens and LHRH analogues). However, all cancers eventually become androgen independent, often referred to as hormone-refractory prostate cancer. This transformation is not yet fully understood (AR amplification, overexpression or mutation and alterations in the AR signalling pathway may play a role).
  - Analyses have revealed that **hypermethylation of GSTP1 (glutathione S-transferase P) gene**, encoding the carcinogen detoxification enzyme glutathione S-transferase pi, may serve as an initiating genome lesion for prostatic carcinogenesis. Somatic mutation leading to juxtaposition of coding sequence of **ETS family transcription factor gene** next to **androgen-regulated TMPRSS2 promoter** induces overexpression of ETS transcription factors which upregulates matrix metalloproteinases to enhance invasiveness of prostatic cancer cells.
  - Germline mutations of BRCA2 are associated with a 20-fold increase in the risk.
  - Mutations and deletions which activate PI3K/AKT signalling pathway are commonly involved. There is amplification of 8q24 locus containing the MYC oncogene as well as deletions affecting the PTEN, P53 and RB tumour suppressor genes.

Gross Morphology

- The prostate is enlarged, normal sized or smaller than normal, hard and fixed.
- Cut section is homogeneous and fibrous, and may show yellowish irregular areas.
- Local invasion into seminal vesicles, adjacent soft tissue and wall of the urinary bladder may be seen.
- Invasion of rectum is less common (Denonvilliers fascia, separating the lower urinary tract structures from the rectum, prevents growth into the rectum).

Microscopy

Four common histological types:

1. Adenocarcinoma
2. Transitional cell carcinoma
3. Squamous cell carcinoma
4. Undifferentiated carcinoma

Adenocarcinoma Prostate (Fig. 30.6)

- It is the most common histological type (96% of cases).
- The tumour is composed of closely packed acini arranged in a back-to-back manner with little or no stroma between them. The acinai are "too many, too small, too crowded".
- Glands may be well differentiated to almost undifferentiated and are lined by a single layer of epithelium (basal layer seen in normal or hyperplastic glands is absent). Tumour cells may be clear, hyperchromatic or eosinophilic

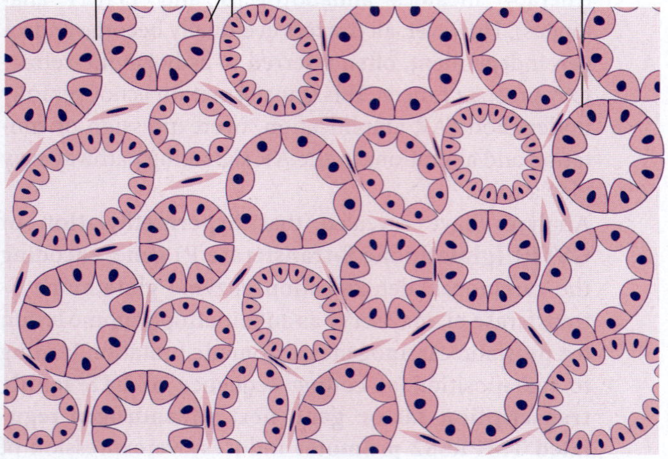

Fig. 30.6 Schematic representation of adenocarcinoma prostate.

(granular). Absence of basal cells can be demonstrated by using immunohistochemical (IHC) markers which label basal cells.

- Foci of prostatic intraepithelial neoplasia (PIN) may be seen in close association with carcinoma.
- Invasion of intraprostatic perineural spaces is a common occurrence.
- Stage, grade, surgical margins, preoperative PSA, angiolymphatic and perineural invasion are important prognostic markers.

Grading of Carcinoma Prostate

Gleason grading is the most widely used grading system for adenocarcinoma prostate. It is based on the glandular architectural patterns and the relationship of the tumour cells with the stroma.

Diagnosis and Staging of Carcinoma Prostate

- **Digital rectal examination:** Most of the prostatic tumours are located in the posterior lobe and so are easily palpable on per rectal examination.
- **Transrectal ultrasonography with guided biopsy** for early detection of tumour.
- **Computed tomography and magnetic resonance imaging scan** to evaluate the lymph node status.
- **Pelvic lymphadenectomy** to look for microscopic metastasis because metastasis to regional pelvic lymph nodes can occur.
- **Skeletal survey or radionuclide scanning** for the detection of osteoblastic metastasis.
- **Tumour marker assays.**
  - ***Prostatic acid phosphatase (PAP)***
    - Secreted by normal as well as cancerous prostatic epithelial cells.
    - Serum level highly raised in prostatic cancer extending beyond the capsule or in metastases.
    - Normal values: 1–3 KA units, more than 5 KA units diagnostic of the cancer.
  - ***PSA***
    - Produced by the prostatic epithelium and secreted in small quantities in the serum, PSA cleaves and liquefies seminal coagulum by its enzymatic activity (androgen-regulated serine protease).
    - Any condition that disrupts the normal architecture of prostate, whether adenocarcinoma, NHP or prostatitis, can elevate serum levels of PSA.
    - A serum PSA of more than 4 ng/mL is most useful in diagnosing prostatic cancer, particularly in combination with rectal examination and transrectal ultrasonography.
    - PSA levels are generally higher in cancer as compared with in nodular hyperplasia, but their values may overlap, so criteria other than simply serum levels should be looked for, namely **free PSA levels** (levels lower than 10% are indicative of prostatic cancer, whereas levels greater than 25% indicate a low risk of cancer). Other indicators include:
      - **Ratio of free and bound PSA.**
      - **PSA density** (ratio between the serum PSA levels and the volume of the prostate gland).
      - **PSA velocity** (ratio of change in PSA value with time).
    - **Uses of PSA**
      - Diagnosis of prostatic diseases.
      - To assess the response to chemotherapy in cancer.
      - To check whether radical prostatectomy is complete or not.
      - To confirm the origin of metastatic deposits as prostate.
  - ***EZH2 (enhancer of zeste 2):*** Loss of E-cadherin (adhesion protein) from prostatic cancer cells is associated with high levels of EZH2 and may contribute to prostatic cancer progression.
  - ***AMACR (α-methylacyl-CoA racemase):*** AMACR is an enzyme involved in β-oxidation of branched amino acids and is upregulated in prostatic cancer compared with in normal prostate.
  - ***PCA3:*** A gene on chromosome 9q that possibly encodes a regulatory RNA, it is overexpressed in >90% of cases of prostatic carcinoma.

Diseases of Female Genital System

31

NORMAL ANATOMY

The uterus has three anatomical and functional regions:

1. Cervix
2. Lower uterine segment
3. Corpus

Cervix

Cervix is further divided into:

- **Ectocervix (vaginal portion):** It is the part of the cervix that is visible from the vaginal canal. Ectocervix is lined by non-keratinizing stratified squamous epithelium continuous with the vagina. The squamous epithelium converges centrally at a small opening called **external os**, which is closed in nulliparous women.
- **Endocervix:** It is lined by columnar mucus-secreting epithelium, which meets the squamous epithelial covering at the **squamocolumnar junction**. The endocervical stroma contains endocervical glands.

Progressive differentiation of the subcolumnar reserve cells determines the position of the squamocolumnar junction. The portion of the columnar epithelium ultimately replaced by the squamous epithelium is termed the **transformation zone**, which is important clinically because this is where the precancerous and cancerous lesions develop.

Lower Uterine Segment and Corpus

Uterus has two main components – the **endometrium** and the **myometrium**. The endometrium is composed of glands embedded in a stroma and the myometrium is composed of interwoven smooth muscle bundles. The **endometrial cavity (internal cavity of the uterus)** is slit-like and best opened by inserting a probe and cutting along with it. The **endometrium** is 1–5 mm wide and the **myometrium** is 1–2 cm wide. From each side of the uterus, a broad ligament arises, which is inserted into the lateral wall of the pelvis. The fallopian tube travels in the free border of the broad ligament.

Ovaries

- The surface is lined by germinal epithelium and the average size is 4 cm × 1.5 cm × 1.5 cm.
- It is divided into **cortex** and **medulla**. The cortex consists of closely packed stromal cells with a thin covering of collagen.
- The outer cortex shows follicles in varying stages of maturation. In each menstrual cycle, one follicle develops into **Graafian follicle**, which is transformed into a **corpus luteum** after ovulation. Senescent corpus luteum is called **corpora albicans.**
- The medulla consists of loosely arranged mesenchymal tissue and contains remnants of **Wolffian duct** as well as round to polygonal epithelioid cells around vessels and nerves called **hilus cells**.

Fallopian Tube

- The average size is 10 cm × 1 mm; it is divided into four anatomical regions – isthmus, ampulla, fimbriae and abdominal opening.
- The mucosa is lined by three cell types – ciliated columnar, non-ciliated columnar and intercalated cells (inactive secretory cells).
- Anterior to the tubes, there is insertion of **round ligament.** The most lateral portion of the broad ligament is called **infundibulopelvic** or **suspensory ligament** and transmits ovarian vessels and nerves.

Nulliparous Uterus

- It weighs 30–40 g, with an average size of 7.5 cm × 5 cm × 2.5 cm.
- It has an inverted flattened pear appearance with the presence of a constriction called isthmus.
- Anterior peritoneal reflection is at isthmus; posteriorly, peritoneum covers the entire uterus and passes down to cover the upper portion of the vagina.
- The vaginal portion is covered by moist, smooth vaginal epithelium.
- The cervical canal is narrow and fusiform.

Multiparous Uterus

Weighs 60–70 g, with an average size of 10 cm × 5 cm × 4 cm.

Postmenopausal Uterus

- Atrophic/more fibrous.
- Cervix less prominent.
- Uterus anteflexed (sharply bent forward upon the vagina).

Q. Write briefly about cervical intraepithelial neoplasia (CIN)/Describe the role of HPV in the pathogenesis of carcinoma cervix. (PA30.1)

Ans. CIN is a precancerous lesion frequently associated with HPV infection. HPV is a sexually transmitted DNA virus which can lead to CIN as well as invasive squamous cell carcinoma (SCC) g. HPV infects the immature basal cells of the stratified squamous epithelium or the squamous metaplastic cells present at the squamocolumnar junction in areas of epithelial breaks or damage. Replication occurs in the resting non-proliferating squamous cells and this leads to the viral cytopathic effects or koilocytic atypia (nuclear atypia and perinuclear halo). The mucosa tropic types of HPV can be subdivided into low-risk and high-risk types. The low-risk types have been associated with the formation of genital warts. These include HPV types 6, 11, 40, 42, 43, 44, 54, 61, 72 and 81 (also known as HPV types with low oncogenic potential). The high-risk types are those associated with intraepithelial neoplasia and invasive malignancy. These include HPV types 16, 18, 31, 33, 35, 39, 45, 51, 52, 56, 58, 59, 68, 69 and 82 (also known as HPV types with high oncogenic potential).

HPV is found in 99% of cervical cancers, with types 16 and 18 being found in 70% of them. Almost all precancerous and cancerous lesions are associated with long-term, persistent HPV infection. About 90% of HPV infections are thought to clear within 2 years because of a cell-mediated immune response. Dysplasia and invasive malignancy occurs in patients who fail to clear the HPV infection.

All HPV subtypes contain early (E) genes and late (L) genes, which are essential to viral integration and replication. L genes encode viral capsid proteins. E genes are responsible for episomal replication. The HPV genome is maintained in a non-integrated free episomal (extrachromosomal) form in low-oncogenic-risk HPV infection, whereas it integrates into the host DNA in high-oncogenic-risk HPV infection. High-risk HPV subtypes overexpress E6 and E7 proteins that are involved in oncogenesis. Overexpression of E6 protein results in degradation of the tumour suppressor gene p53 and upregulation of telomerase-inducing immortalization of the cells. Overexpression of E7 protein results in inactivation of the RB gene and inhibition of CDK inhibitors (p21 and p27) leading to impaired repair of DNA damage and induction and progression of cell cycle.

According to the Bethesda system, precancerous lesions of the cervix are divided into two groups:

- **Low-grade squamous intraepithelial lesion (LSIL; CIN I).**
- **High-grade squamous intraepithelial lesion (HSIL; CIN II and III).**

CIN I

- Dysplasia is present in lower one-third of stratified squamous epithelium.
- It may be raised (as in condyloma acuminatum) or macular (flat condyloma).
- Abundant HPV nucleic acid of low-risk HPV type is present.
- **Koilocytic atypia** or viral cytopathic effect is seen (koilocytosis is seen as nuclear abnormalities with perinuclear halo).

CIN II

- Dysplasia is limited to basal two-thirds of stratified squamous epithelium.
- Increased number of atypical cells in lower layers (increased N/C ratio, anisokaryosis, loss of polarity, mitotic figures and hyperchromasia).
- Upper layer cells appear differentiated.
- It is associated with high-risk HPV types.

CIN III/Carcinoma in Situ

Dysplasia spreads to the entire thickness of the epithelium.

Note: A low-grade lesion does not always progress to a high-grade lesion. Most low-grade lesions regress spontaneously, whereas most high-grade lesions progress.

Q. Classify tumours of the cervix. (PA30.1)

Ans. WHO classification of tumours of cervix (abridged):

Epithelial tumours

- Squamous cell tumours and precursors
  - Squamous intraepithelial lesions
    - LSIL
    - HSIL
  - SCC, NOS
    - Keratinizing
    - Non-keratinizing
  - Benign squamous cell lesions
    - Condyloma acuminatum
    - Squamous papilloma
- Glandular tumours and precursors
  - Adenocarcinoma in situ
  - Adenocarcinoma
    - Endocervical adenocarcinoma, usual type
    - Mucinous adenocarcinoma, NOS
- Other epithelial tumours
  - Adenosquamous carcinoma
  - Adenoid cystic carcinoma
  - Adenoid basal carcinoma
  - Neuroendocrine tumours
  - Undifferentiated carcinoma

Mesenchymal tumours and tumour-like conditions

- Benign
  - Leiomyoma
  - Rhabdomyoma
  - Others
- Malignant
  - Leiomyosarcoma
  - Rhabdomyosarcoma
- Tumour-like lesions
  - Postoperative spindle cell nodule
  - Lymphoma-like lesion

Melanocytic tumours

- Malignant melanoma
- Blue nevus

Germ cell tumours

- Yolk sac tumour

Lymphoid and myeloid tumours

Secondary tumours

Q. Write briefly about predisposing factors, aetiology, morphology and diagnosis of carcinoma cervix. (PA30.1)

Ans. Carcinoma cervix is a major cause of morbidity and mortality worldover.

Predisposing Factors

- HPV infection (nearly all cervical carcinomas are HPV related).
- Early age at first intercourse.
- Multiple sexual partners or a male partner with multiple sexual partners.
- Oral contraceptives.
- Cigarette smoking.
- High parity.
- Family history.
- Associated genital infections.
- Lack of circumcision in male sexual partner.

Pathogenesis

Sequence of events that follow HPV infection is given in Flowchart 31.1.

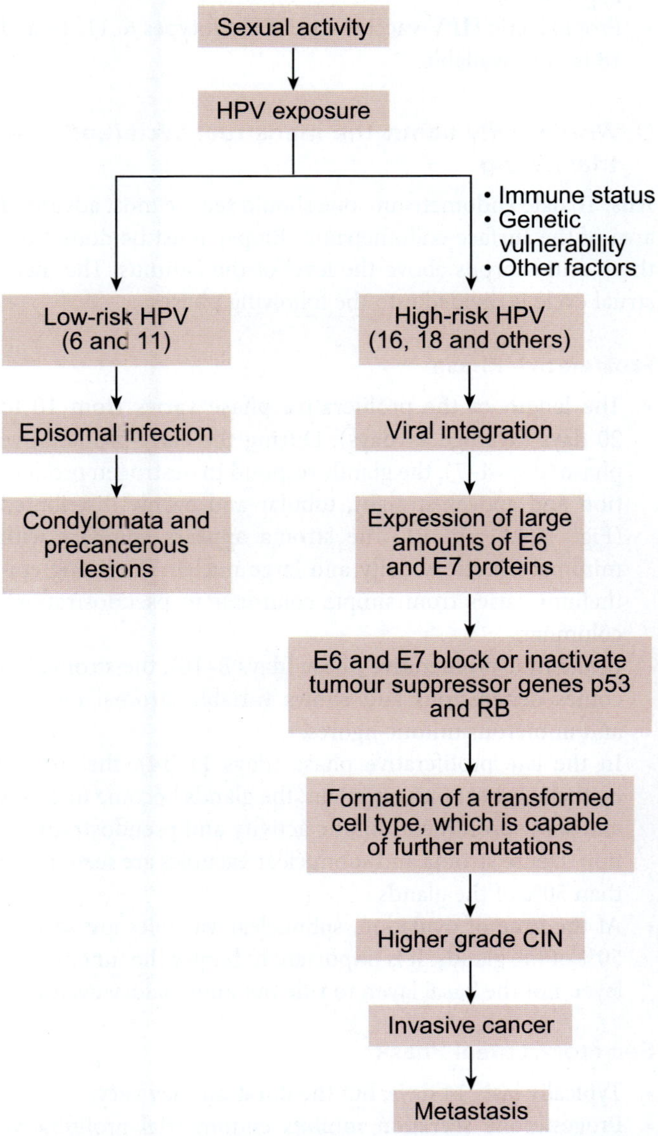

Flowchart 31.1 Mechanism of evolution of cervical cancer.

Clinical Features

- Usually affect women between fourth and sixth decades.
- Presents with unexpected vaginal bleeding, leucorrhoea, painful coitus (dyspareunia) and dysuria (due to bladder infiltration).

Gross Morphology

Arises from the transformation zone and has three main gross types:

- **Fungating or exophytic (most common):** Nodular exophytic or cauliflower-like growth projecting into the vaginal cavity.
- **Ulcerative or ulceroinfiltrative:** Granular eroded lesion with or without infiltration into the underlying stroma causing diffuse thickening of the cervix.
- **Infiltrative:** Tumour showing infiltration into the underlying stroma causing diffuse thickening of the cervix.

Microscopy

- Most (90%) are SCCs.
- Subtypes include:
  - Large cell keratinizing: Nests of keratinized cells which form concentric whorls known as keratin pearls (Fig. 31.1).
  - Large cell non-keratinizing: Nests of large malignant squamous cells which show individual cell keratinization but no keratin pearls.
  - Small cell carcinoma: tThe least common but has the most aggressive course; it is composed of small non-keratinized malignant cells.

Other Morphological Types of Carcinoma Cervix

- Adenocarcinoma: Shows malignant endocervical cells arranged in a glandular pattern.
- Adenosquamous carcinoma: Shows malignant squamous epithelium admixed with malignant endocervical cells arranged in a glandular pattern.

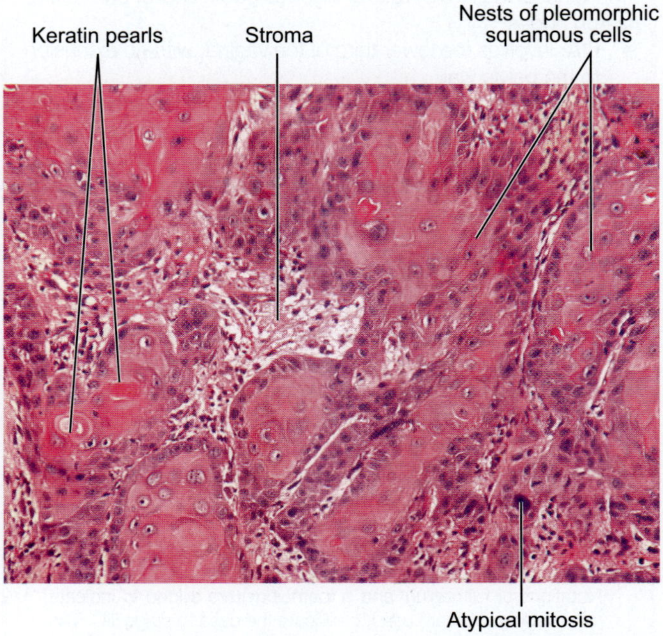

Fig 31.1 H&E-stained section from a large cell keratinizing squamous cell carcinoma cervix showing nests of pleomorphic squamous cells with keratin pearls (H&E; 200×).

- Small cell neuroendocrine carcinoma: Round/oval blue cells with minimal cytoplasm; usually small to medium sized with finely dispersed chromatin, no distinct nucleoli, moulding, smudging and high mitotic rate arranged in a thin, delicate, scant fibrovascular stroma.
- Undifferentiated carcinoma: Squamous or glandular differentiation usually not present.

Spread and Staging (The International Federation of Gynecology and Obstetrics or FIGO, 2018)

Stage I

The carcinoma is strictly confined to the cervix uteri (extension to the corpus should be disregarded).

- **IA:** Invasive carcinoma that can be diagnosed only by microscopy, with maximum depth of invasion <5 mm[a]
  - **IA1:** Measured stromal invasion <3 mm in depth
  - **IA2:** Measured stromal invasion ≥3 mm and <5 mm in depth
- **IB:** Invasive carcinoma with measured deepest invasion ≥5 mm (greater than stage IA), lesion limited to the cervix uteri[b]
  - **IB1:** Invasive carcinoma ≥5 mm depth of stromal invasion and <2 cm in the greatest dimension
  - **IB2:** Invasive carcinoma ≥2 and <4 cm in the greatest dimension
  - **IB3:** Invasive carcinoma ≥4 cm in the greatest dimension

Stage II

The carcinoma invades beyond the uterus, but has not extended onto the lower third of the vagina or to the pelvic wall.

- **IIA:** Involvement limited to the upper two-thirds of the vagina without parametrial involvement
  - **IIA1:** Invasive carcinoma <4 cm in the greatest dimension
  - **IIA2:** Invasive carcinoma ≥4 cm in the greatest dimension
- **IIB:** With parametrial involvement but not up to the pelvic wall

Stage III

The carcinoma involves the lower third of the vagina and/or extends to the pelvic wall and/or causes hydronephrosis or non-functioning kidney and/or involves pelvic and/or para-aortic lymph nodes[c]

- **IIIA:** Involves the lower third of the vagina, with no extension to the pelvic wall
- **IIIB:** Extension to the pelvic wall and/or hydronephrosis or non-functioning kidney (unless known to be due to another cause)
- **IIIC:** Involvement of pelvic and/or para-aortic lymph nodes, irrespective of tumour size and extent (with r and p notations)[c]
  - **IIIC1:** Pelvic lymph node metastasis only
  - **IIIC2:** Para-aortic lymph node metastasis

Stage IV

The carcinoma has extended beyond the true pelvis or has involved (biopsy proven) the mucosa of the bladder or rectum. A bullous oedema, as such, does not permit a case to be allotted to stage IV.

- **IVA:** Spread of the growth to adjacent organs
- **IVB:** Spread to distant organs

[a]Imaging and pathology can be used, when available, to supplement clinical findings with respect to tumour size and extent, in all stages.

[b]The involvement of vascular/lymphatic spaces does not change the staging. The lateral extent of the lesion is no longer considered.

[c]Notations of r (imaging) and p (pathology) are added to indicate the findings that are used to allocate the case to stage IIIC. The type of imaging modality or pathology technique used should always be documented. When in doubt, the lower staging should be assigned.

Q. Write a short note on diagnosis and prevention of carcinoma cervix. (PA30.1)

Ans. Diagnosis and prevention of carcinoma cervix:

- Pap smear examination is the most important tool for screening of carcinoma cervix. It entails cytological examination of exfoliated cervical cells after staining them with the Papanicolaou method. The transformation zone is scraped with an Ayer's spatula or a cytological brush to obtain the material.
- Pap smear detection of low-grade cervical dysplasia has a sensitivity of 70% and a specificity of 75%. Pap smear detection of high-grade cervical dysplasia has a sensitivity of 75% and a specificity of 95%.
- Also, HPV DNA testing can be done to assess the HPV status of the patient.
- In case of an abnormal Pap smear, colposcopic examination of the cervix and vagina is performed to determine the extent of the lesion. The lesion is then biopsied. Application of acetic acid may also highlight abnormal areas.
- LSIL is generally followed up by repeated Pap smear examination and HSIL is excised by conization and follow-up Pap smears.
- Prophylactic HPV vaccine for HPV subtypes 6, 11, 16 and 18 is now available.

Q. Write briefly about the menstrual cycle/endometrial dating.

Ans. To date endometrium, one should see the most advanced area of the surface endometrium. Biopsy must be done from the uterine corpus above the level of the isthmus. The menstrual cycle is divided into the following phases:

Proliferative Phase

- The length of the proliferative phase varies from 10 to 20 days (average 14 days). During the early proliferative phase (days 4–7), the glands respond to oestrogen production and appear straight, tubular and evenly distributed (Fig. 31.2A and B). The stroma appears compact with minimal mitotic activity and large nuclei. The lining epithelium varies from simple columnar to pseudostratified columnar.
- In the mid-proliferative phase (days 8–10), the stroma becomes oedematous and shows variable stromal oedema and numerous mitotic figures.
- In the late proliferative phase (days 11–14), the surface epithelium becomes undulant, the glands become tortuous and show prominent mitotic activity and pseudostratification. Dense stroma and subnuclear vacuoles are seen in less than 50% of the glands.
- At the time of ovulation, subnuclear vacuoles are seen in 50% of the glands. It is important to biopsy the functionalis layer, not the basal layer, to rule out anovulatory cycles.

Secretory/Luteal Phase

- Typically lasts 14 days, but the duration may vary.
- Progesterone secretion inhibits endometrial proliferative activity and induces secretory activity.

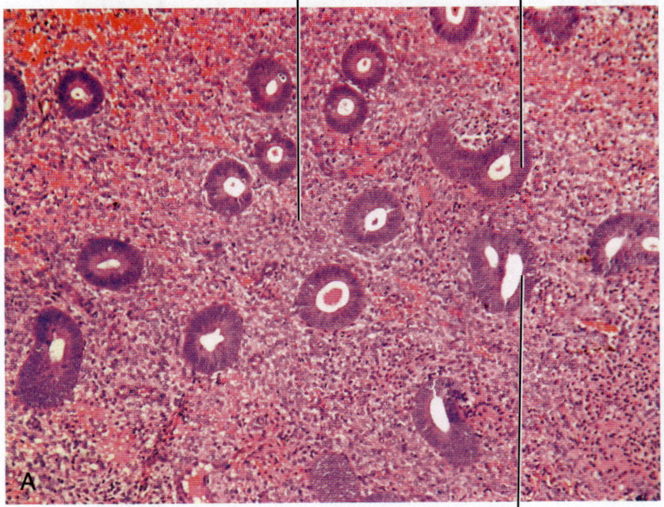

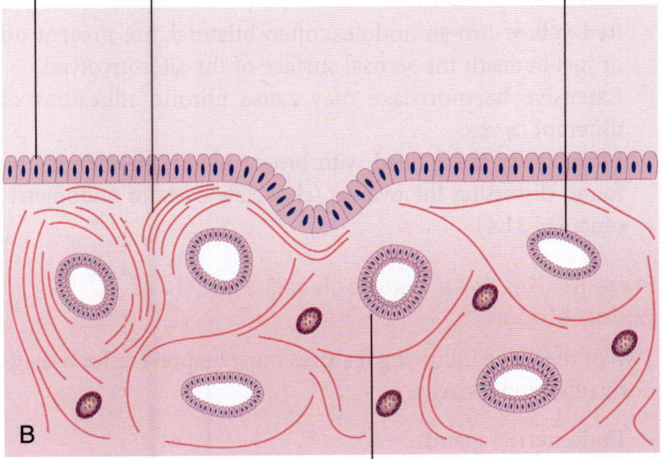

Fig 31.2 Photomicrograph (A) and schematic diagram (B) showing straight, tubular endometrial glands lined by epithelium varying from simple columnar to pseudostratified columnar. The stroma is compact showing minimal mitotic activity (H&E; 100×).

- Secretory material in glands is NOT specific for secretory epithelium; it is also seen in disordered proliferative and hyperplastic endometrium and carcinoma.
- No change from late proliferative phase is seen on day 15 (also known as interval endometrium). Scattered nuclear vacuoles are not specific for ovulation (must be 50% or more; Fig. 31.3A and B). Well-formed subnuclear vacuoles are seen subsequently.

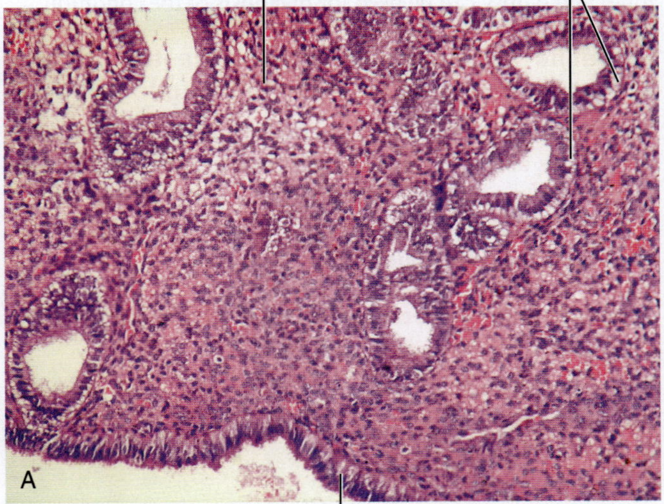

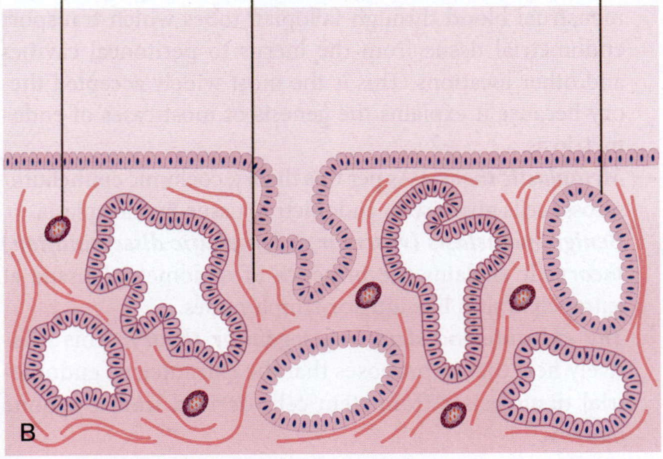

Fig 31.3 Photomicrograph (A) and schematic diagram (B) showing oedematous stroma and tortuous endometrial glands with subnuclear vacuoles (beginning of secretory phase; H&E; 100×).

- Intraluminal secretion begins at day 19.
- Day 22 shows maximal stromal oedema. This is followed by the formation of prominent spiral arterioles, perivascular predecidualization (stromal cells show abundant cytoplasm with increased cytoplasmic eosinophilia) and serrated/tortuous glands.

Q. Define adenomyosis. (PA30.8)

Ans. Invagination of the stratum basalis of the endometrial mucosa into the myometrium is called adenomyosis. Clinical features of adenomyosis include irregular, heavy menses, dysmenorrhoea and pelvic pain. Microscopy shows the presence of nests of endometrial glands and/or stroma well down in the myometrium between the muscle bundles. The endometrial tissue must be separated from the basalis by at least 2–3 mm. High-resolution ultrasound, MRI (shows a thickened junctional zone) and biopsy can be used for diagnosis of the condition.

Q. Define endometriosis. Enumerate the theories that are proposed to explain its origin. (PA30.7)

Ans. Endometriosis is the presence of functioning endometrial glands and/or stroma in abnormal locations outside the uterus. It is seen in the reproductive age group and mostly manifests in the third and fourth decades. Multifactorial inheritance has been implicated.

Sites Involved (in Decreasing Order of Frequency)

- Ovaries
- Uterine ligaments
- Rectovaginal septum
- Pelvic peritoneum
- Laparotomy scar
- Rarely, in umbilicus, vagina, vulva and appendix

Pathogenesis

Several theories have been proposed to explain endometriosis:

- ***Regurgitation/transplantation theory:*** According to this theory, endometriosis occurs because of regurgitation of menstrual blood through fallopian tubes which transport endometrial tissue from the uterus to peritoneal cavities and other locations. This is the most widely accepted theory because it explains the genesis of most cases of endometriosis.
- ***Metaplastic theory:*** As per this theory, coelomic epithelium/serosal cells give rise to endometrial tissue by metaplasia.
- ***Benign metastasis (vascular or lymphatic dissemination) theory:*** It explains the presence of endometrial tissue at extrapelvic sites like lung or lymph nodes.
- ***The extrauterine stem or progenitor theory:*** This relatively new theory proposes that the extrauterine endometrial tissue arises from stem cells derived from the bone marrow.

Molecular analysis has shown that endometriotic implants release proinflammatory factors (IL-1β, TNF-α, IL-6, IL-8, PGE2, NGF, VEGF, MCP1, MMPs and TIMPs), which increase oestrogen levels (PGE2 stimulates local synthesis of oestrogen), promote invasion and increase survival of extrauterine endometriotic tissue by reducing its immune clearance. Also, high levels of an enzyme 'aromatase' have been demonstrated in these implants which also contribute to increase oestrogen production.

Clinical Features

- Dysmenorrhoea.
- Menstrual irregularities.
- Dyspareunia.
- Infertility.
- Pelvic pain because of intrapelvic bleeding and periuterine adhesions.
- Pain on defecation or urination (because of involvement of bowel or bladder).

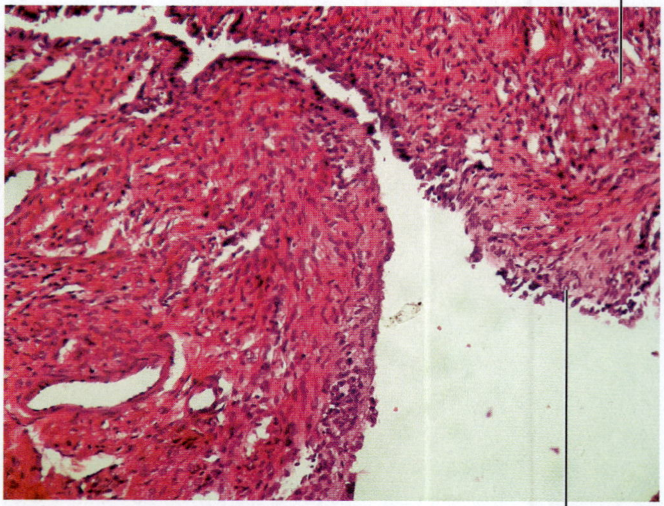

Fig 31.4 Large cystic space, lined by endometrial type epithelium (chocolate cyst or endometrioma; H&E; 100×).

Gross Morphology

- Red-yellow-brown nodules, often bilateral, are present on or just beneath the serosal surface of the sites involved.
- Extensive haemorrhage may cause fibrotic adhesions of different layers.
- Large cystic space filled with brown bloody debris may be found distorting the ovaries (chocolate cysts or endometrioma; Fig 31.4).

Prerequisites for a Histological Diagnosis of Endometriosis

Two of the three following features must be present for a diagnosis of endometriosis:

- Endometrial glands.
- Endometrial stroma.
- Haemosiderin-laden macrophages.

Scar Endometriosis

Scar endometriosis is a rare entity usually reported in women who have undergone a previous abdominal or pelvic surgery. Many theories as to the evolution of scar endometriosis have been put forward of which the most accepted theory is the iatrogenic transplantation of endometrial implants to the wound edge during an abdominal or pelvic surgery. Patients usually complain of tenderness on palpation and a raised hypertrophic scar.

Atypical Endometriosis

Endometriosis is said to be atypical if the epithelium lining the endometriotic cyst shows atypia without architectural distortion or if there is architectural distortion (glandular crowding) with atypia. Atypical endometriosis and endometrioid and clear cell types of endometrial carcinoma share PTEN and AT-rich interactive domain-containing protein (ARIDA1) mutations suggesting that endometriosis may be a precursor to carcinoma.

Q. Classify endometrial hyperplasia. Write briefly about its different types. (PA30.9)

Ans. Proliferation of glandular and stromal tissue associated with prolonged, profuse and irregular uterine bleeding in menopausal or postmenopausal women is known as endometrial hyperplasia. Endometrial hyperplasia may lead to endometrial carcinoma if left untreated.

Classification

The International Society for Gynaecological Pathology earlier classified endometrial hyperplasia into:

1. Simple hyperplasia without atypia.
2. Simple hyperplasia with atypia.
3. Complex hyperplasia without atypia.
4. Complex hyperplasia with atypia.

New WHO (2014) classification of endometrial hyperplasias:
1. Non-atypical endometrial hyperplasia (benign hyperplasia).
2. Atypical endometrial hyperplasia or endometrial intraepithelial neoplasia (EIN)/well-differentiated carcinoma.

Gross Morphology

Diffuse thickening of endometrium with a velvety appearance or focal overgrowth, which may be mistaken for a polyp.

Microscopy

Increase in endometrial glands relative to the stroma.

Non-atypical Hyperplasia (Fig. 31.5A and B)

Includes both simple and complex hyperplasia without atypia. Increase in number, size and variation in shape of the glands is seen. Even with a back-to-back arrangement of glands, some intervening stroma is visible. This type of hyperplasia results from persistent oestrogenic stimulation and rarely gives rise to endometrial cancer.

Atypical Hyperplasia (Endometrioid Intraepithelial Neoplasia Fig. 31.6A and B)

Includes both simple and complex hyperplasia with atypia and endometrioid intraepithelial neoplasia. Complex architectural patterns with cellular atypia are the hallmark. The glands are usually arranged back to back with branching and loss of polarity. There is nuclear atypia of varying degree. Atypical hyperplasia is difficult to differentiate from a well-differentiated carcinoma on biopsy. About 20%–30% of these cases show foci of endometrial carcinoma on hysterectomy.

Q. Classify uterine tumours. (PA30.2)

Ans. Uterine neoplasms may be localized at the corpus, or isthmus. They may affect the endometrium, myometrium or other supporting tissue. They are classified based on their origin mainly into epithelial and mesenchymal tumours.

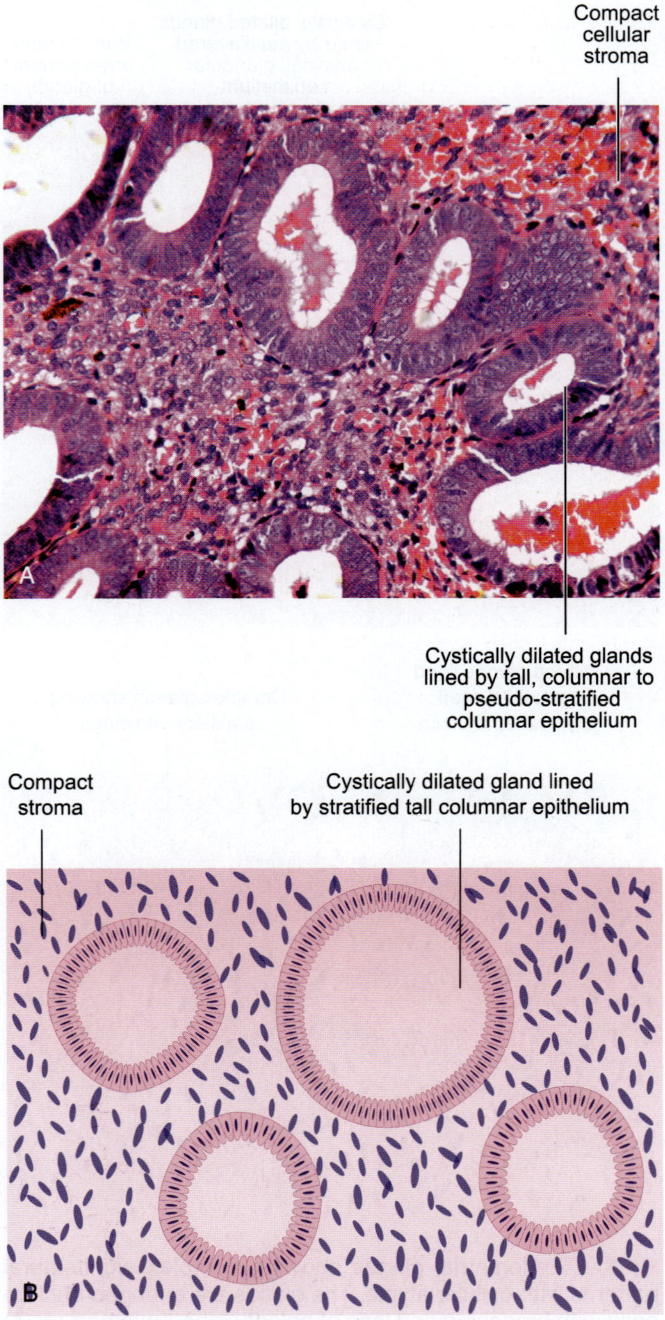

Fig 31.5 Increase in number, size and variation in shape of the endometrial glands with a back-to-back arrangement, and scant intervening stroma. The glands are lined by tall columnar stratified epithelium showing increased mitotic activity; photomicrograph (A) and schematic diagram (B) (H&E; 100×).

Tumours of the Uterine Corpus (WHO Abridged)

- **Epithelial tumours and precursors**
  Precursors
  - Hyperplasia without atypia
  - Atypical hyperplasia/endometrioid intraepithelial neoplasia

  Endometrial carcinoma
  - Endometrioid carcinoma type I
  - Serous carcinoma type II
  - Neuroendocrine tumours

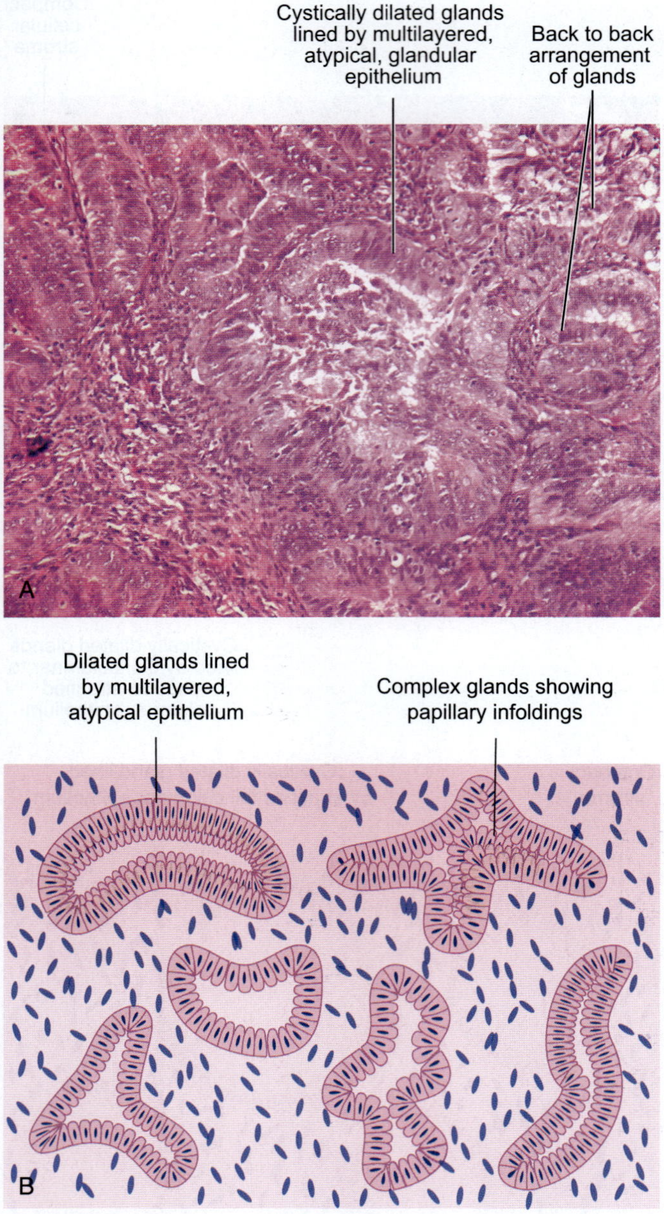

Fig 31.6 Endometrial glands showing complex architectural patterns with cellular atypia. The glands are arranged back to back with branching and loss of polarity (photomicrograph (A) and schematic diagram (B) (H&E; 100×).

- **Mesenchymal tumours**
  - Leiomyoma
  - Leiomyosarcoma
- **Mixed epithelial and mesenchymal tumours**
- **Lymphoid and myeloid tumours**
- **Secondary tumours**

Q. Write in detail about the aetiology, clinical features and morphology of endometrial carcinoma. (PA30.2)

Ans. Endometrial carcinoma (EC) is the most common cancer of the female genital tract. It presents with irregular or postmenopausal bleeding and leucorrhoea.

Table 31.1 Differences between types I and II of endometrial carcinoma

Features	Endometrial carcinoma type 1 (endometrial carcinoma)	Endometrial carcinoma type 2 (serous carcinoma)
Age	55–60 years	65–75 years
Predisposing factors	• Unopposed oestrogen stimulation • Obesity • Hypertension • Diabetes • Nulliparity/infertility • Breast carcinoma	Thin physique
Morphological type	Endometrioid carcinoma (mimics normal endometrial glands); varies from being well differentiated to poorly differentiated	Serous or clear cell type (mimics subtypes of ovarian carcinoma)
Precursor	Atypical endometrial hyperplasia	Atrophic endometrium Serous endometrial intraepithelial carcinoma
Molecular genetics	Mutations in PTEN, ARID1A (chromatin regulator), KRAS, β-catenin, p53, PIK3CA, FGF2 (growth factor), CTNNB1 (Wnt signalling) and microsatellite instability (Flowchart 31.2)	Mutations in p53, FBXW7, PPP2R1A and PIK3CA; germline BRCA1/2 mutations (Flowchart 31.3)
Outcome	Low-grade malignancy; spreads mainly via lymphatics	Aggressive; intraperitoneal and lymphatic spread is common

Types (Table 31.1)

- Type 1 (constitutes 80% of all cases; is oestrogen associated).
- Type 2 (less common; not associated with hyperoestrogenaemia).

Proliferative endometrium
↓ PTEN abnormality
Hyperplasia without atypia
↓ MLH1 and KRAS abnormalities; Microsatellite instability
Atypical hyperplasia
↓ ARID 1A, PIK3CA, CTNNB1 and FGFR2 abnormalities
Grade 1 endometrioid carcinoma

Flowchart 31.2 Mechanism of evolution of endometrial carcinoma type 1 (endometrial carcinoma).

Atrophic endometrium
↓ TP53 mutation
Serous endometrial intraepithelial carcinoma
↓ FBXW7, PPP2RIA, CCNE1 abnormalities
Serous carcinoma

Flowchart 31.3 Mechanism of evolution of endometrial carcinoma type 2 (serous carcinoma).

Gross Morphology (Fig 31.7A)

- May be exophytic or infiltrative.
- Haemorrhage and necrosis common; may give rise to a shaggy, tan-coloured endometrium.

Aetiopathogenesis

Types I and II ECs are characterized by distinctive types of genetic instability and molecular alterations. Four major genetic changes are responsible for the evolution of endometrioid (type I) carcinoma: the silencing of the *PTEN* tumour suppressor gene, the presence of microsatellite instability, a mutation of the KRAS proto-oncogene, and alteration of the β-catenin gene. On the other hand, a p53 mutation, a p16 mutation, loss of E-cadherin, and overexpression of the Her2/neu oncogene are major genetic alterations in serous and clear cell (type II) carcinomas.

Microscopy

Definitive diagnosis is made only when clear invasion of endometrial stroma or myometrium is seen (differential diagnosis is atypical hyperplasia which does not demonstrate invasion).

Criteria for Stromal Invasion

- Irregular infiltration by glands inducing stromal fibrosis (**desmoplastic response**).
- Confluent glands, merging and creating a cribriform pattern with minimal intervening stroma.
- Extensive papillary formations.
- Replacement of stroma by masses of squamous epithelium.

Histological Types

Most endometrial carcinomas are **adenocarcinomas**. Based on the degree of differentiation shown by the tumour, **endometrioid (type I) endometrial adenocarcinoma** is classified into:

- **Well-differentiated adenocarcinoma** (Fig. 31.7B) which has a back-to-back arrangement of well-formed glands showing minimal atypia (less than 5% solid growth).
- **Moderately differentiated adenocarcinoma** which shows solid sheets of tumour cells in addition to a glandular pattern (5%–50% solid growth).
- **Poorly differentiated adenocarcinoma** which is composed of solid sheets of tumour cells with marked cellular atypia and frequent mitoses; glandular pattern is difficult to find (greater than 50% of the tumour shows a solid pattern).

Type II endometrial carcinomas are most often serous carcinomas. These occur a decade later than type 1 carcinomas.

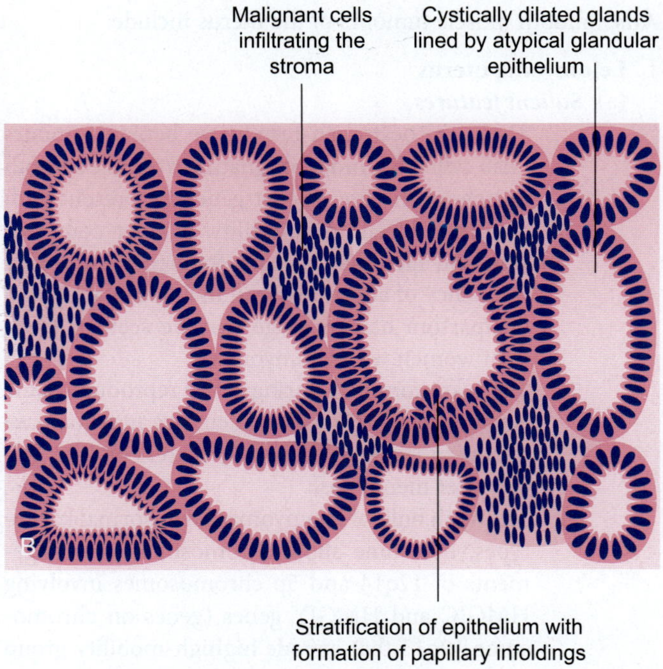

Fig 31.7 (B) Well-differentiated endometrial adenocarcinoma showing a back-to-back arrangement of well-formed glands showing minimal cytological atypia.

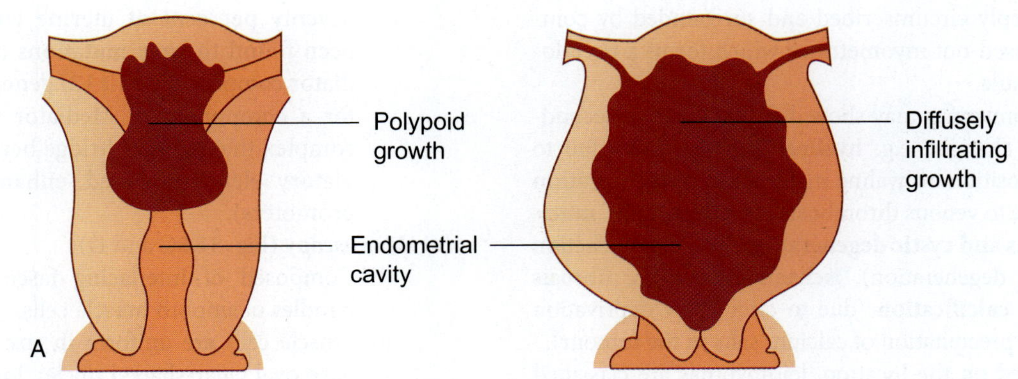

Fig 31.7 (A) Gross types of endometrial carcinoma.

Histopathology shows glandular arrangement and papillary projections lined by cuboidal to columnar cells with moderate to marked nuclear atypia. Serous adenocarcinoma is differentiated from endometrioid carcinoma based on the marked atypia seen in the former. Other less common histological subtypes include clear cell adenocarcinoma and malignant mixed Müllerian tumour (carcinosarcoma). Serous endometrial intraepithelial carcinoma is the precursor lesion that arises from atrophic endometrium or a polyp and remains confined to the endometrium. Histologically, the cells resemble a serous carcinoma.

Spread

The tumour spreads by direct invasion (extension into myometrium and periuterine structures), lymphatic spread (to regional lymph nodes) and haematogenous spread (to lungs, liver, bones and other organs).

Q. Describe the clinicopathological features of smooth muscle tumours of uterus. (PA30.3)

Ans. Smooth muscle tumours of the uterus include:

1. **Leiomyoma uterus**
   (a) ***Salient features***
   - (i) These are oestrogen-responsive benign tumours (also called **fibroids**) originating from the smooth muscle of the uterus that generally present with abnormal bleeding, infertility, bladder compression and increased urinary frequency. Increased frequency of abortions, fetal malpresentation and postpartum haemorrhage may be seen in pregnant women with leiomyomas.
   - (ii) These are common during active reproductive life (incidence of 30%–50%); their size may increase during pregnancy. These may regress or even calcify after menopause.
   - (iii) The main bulk of leiomyomas have normal karyotypes, but some show chromosomal rearrangements of 12q14 and 5p chromosomes involving HMGIC and HMGIY genes (genes on chromosome 12q15 that encode highigh-mobility group non-histone chromosomal protein isoforms I-C and I-Y, which regulate transcription).

   (b) ***Gross appearance (****Fig 31.8A and B****)***
   - (i) Variable sized, round, firm and grey-white tumours, with their cut surface showing whorling.
   - (ii) Sharply circumscribed and surrounded by compressed-out myometrium which forms a pseudocapsule.
   - (iii) Leiomyomas may show different types of secondary changes, e.g. **hyaline degeneration** (due to deposition of hyaline material), **red degeneration** (due to venous thrombosis and congestion), **mucinous and cystic degeneration** (due to liquefaction and degeneration), **ischaemic necrosis**, **fibrosis** and **calcification** (due to circulatory deprivation and precipitation of calcium salts in the tumour).
   - (iv) Based on the location, leiomyomas are classified into **subserosal** (located beneath the serosa), **submucosal** (located beneath the mucosa) or **intramural** (embedded in the myometrium).
   - (v) Seventy per cent of uterine leiomyomas have been found to have mutations in MED12 (mediator complex subunit 12) gene, which encodes for a component of Mediator (a multiprotein complex that forms a bridge between DNA regulatory elements called 'enhancers' and gene promoters).

   (c) ***Microscopy*** (Fig. 31.8C and D)
   - (i) Composed of interlacing fascicles or whorled bundles of smooth muscle cells.
   - (ii) Muscle cells are uniform in size and shape, and have oval cigar-shaped nuclei, long bipolar cytoplasmic processes and low mitotic rate.

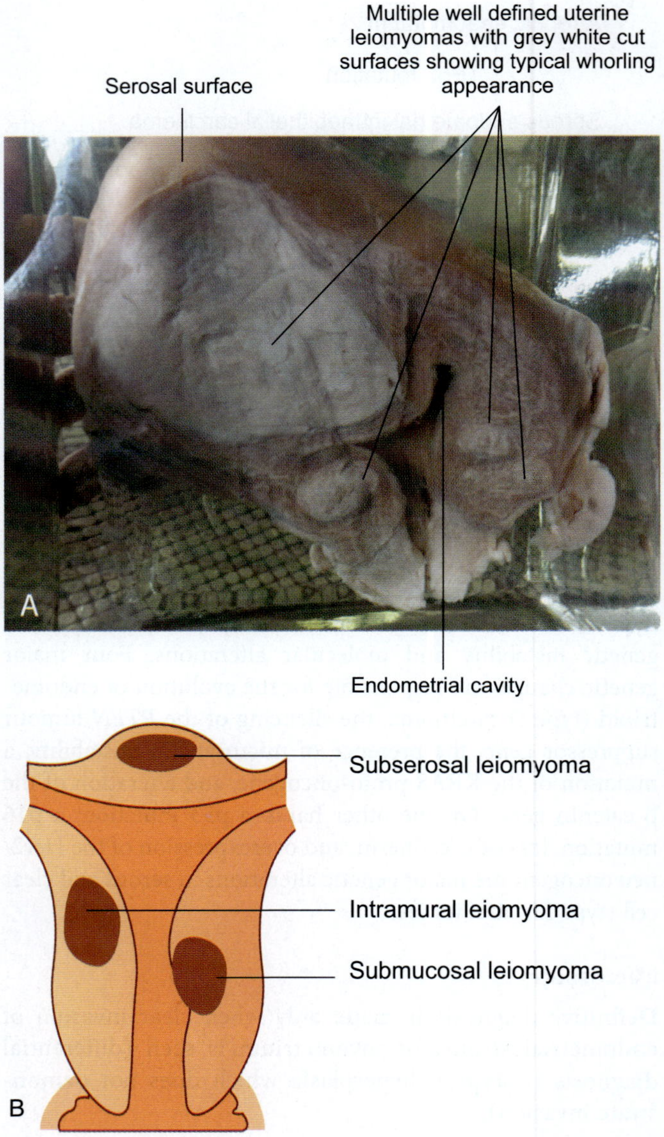

Fig 31.8 (A and B) Gross photograph and schematic diagram of uterine leiomyomata showing multiple round, grey-white tumours, variable in size and location with the cut surface showing a typical whorled pattern. The tumours are sharply circumscribed and surrounded by compressed-out myometrium which forms a pseudocapsule.

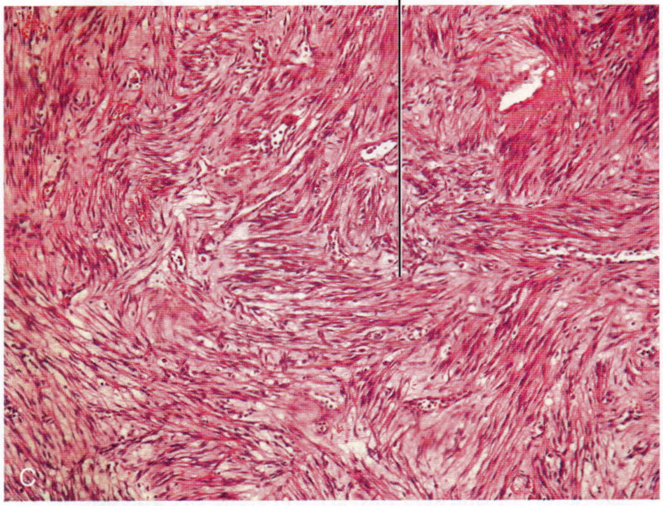

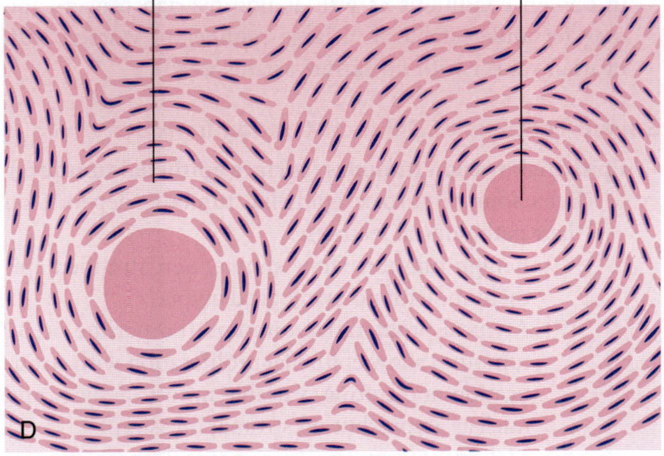

Fig 31.8 (C and D) Microphotograph and schematic representation of a leiomyoma showing intersecting fascicles of smooth muscle cells with hyaline change (H&E; 100×).

(iii) Rare variants of leiomyoma include:
- **Symplastic or bizarre leiomyoma** (cellular tumours with pleomorphic and atypical nuclei but low mitoses).
- **Benign metastasizing leiomyoma** (leiomyomas which may migrate into vessels and other organs, e.g. lungs).
- **Disseminated peritoneal leiomyomatosis** (manifesting as multiple nodules in the peritoneum).
- **Epithelioid leiomyoma** (composed of large epithelioid cells).

2. **Leiomyosarcomas**
   (a) Arise from mesenchymal cells de novo, not from pre-existing leiomyomas.
   (b) Almost always solitary unlike leiomyomas, which are usually multiple.
   (c) May present as bulky masses infiltrating the uterine wall or polypoid masses projecting into the endometrial cavity.
   (d) Usually show haemorrhage and necrosis.
   (e) Diagnostic histopathological features are cytological atypia, presence of increased (usually >10 mitoses/10 HPF) and atypical mitoses, and tumour necrosis. In the presence of cytological atypia and epithelioid cells, greater than 5 mitoses/10 HPF are enough to label the tumour as malignant.
   (f) Recurrence after removal is common, and these tumours may metastasize to lungs. Five-year survival is 40%.
3. **Smooth muscle tumours of uncertain malignant potential.**

   Lie at the interface between leiomyomas and leiomyosarcomas and are difficult to classify.

Q. Classify ovarian tumours. Write in detail about their aetiopathogenesis and clinicopathological features. (PA30.4)

Ans. The World Health Organization Histological Classification for ovarian tumours separates ovarian neoplasms according to the most probable tissue of origin: surface epithelial (65%), germ cell (15%), sex cord-stromal (10%), metastases (5%) and miscellaneous.

- **Surface epithelial-stromal tumours**
  - **Serous tumours**
    - Benign (cystadenoma, cystadenofibroma)
    - Borderline (BL) tumours (serous BL tumour)
    - Malignant (low- and high-grade serous adenocarcinoma)
  - **Mucinous tumours, endocervical-like and intestinal type**
    - Benign (cystadenoma, cystadenofibroma)
    - BL tumours (mucinous BL tumour)
    - Malignant (mucinous adenocarcinoma)
  - **Endometrioid tumours**
    - Benign (cystadenoma, cystadenofibroma)
    - BL tumours (endometrioid BL tumour)
    - Malignant (endometrioid adenocarcinoma)
  - **Clear cell tumours**
    - Benign
    - BL tumours
    - Malignant (clear cell adenocarcinoma)
  - **Transitional cell tumours**
    - Brenner tumour
    - Brenner tumour of BL malignancy/atypical proliferative Brenner tumour
    - Malignant Brenner tumour
    - Transitional cell carcinoma (non-Brenner type)
  - **Epithelial-stromal**
    - Adenosarcoma
    - Carcinosarcoma (formerly mixed Müllerian tumours)
- **Sex cord-stromal tumours**
  - **Pure stromal tumours**
    - Fibromas
    - Thecomas
    - Leydig cell tumour
  - **Pure sex cord tumours**
    - Adult granuloma cell tumour
    - Juvenile granulosa cell tumour
    - Sertoli cell tumour

    - **Sex cord tumour with annular tubules**
    - **Gynandroblastoma**
    - **Steroid (lipid) cell tumours**
- **Germ cell tumours**
    - **Teratoma**
        - Immature
        - Mature
        - Solid
        - Cystic (dermoid cyst)
        - Monodermal (e.g. struma ovarii, carcinoid)
    - **Dysgerminoma**
    - **Yolk sac tumour** (endodermal sinus tumour)
    - **Embryonal carcinoma**
    - **Non-gestational choriocarcinoma**
    - **Mixed germ cell tumours**
- **Malignant, not otherwise specified**
    - **Metastatic cancer from non-ovarian primary**
        - Colonic, appendiceal, gastric, breast

1. **Surface epithelial-stromal ovarian tumours**
   (a) Occur primarily in adults (second decade onwards).
   (b) Constitute 65%–75% of all ovarian tumours.
   (c) Thought to arise by transformation of coelomic epithelium, which may evolve into serous (tubal), endometrioid (endometrial) and mucinous (cervical) epithelium (coelomic epithelium gets incorporated into the ovaries by invagination of the surface epithelium, which later gets detached).
2. **Germ cell ovarian tumours**
   (a) Derived from the egg-producing cells within the body of the ovary.
   (b) Occur primarily in children and adolescents.
   (c) Constitute 15%–20% of all ovarian tumours and 3%–5% of all ovarian cancers.
3. **Sex cord-stromal ovarian tumours**
   Rare, constitute 2%–3% of all malignant ovarian tumours and produce steroid hormones.
4. **Cancers derived from other organs (colon, appendix, pancreas, biliary system, breast) can also spread to the ovaries (metastatic cancers).**

Aetiopathogenesis of Ovarian Cancer

- Two most important risk factors are **nulliparity** and **positive family history**.
- About 5%–10% of ovarian carcinomas are familial and may be caused by mutations in BRCA1 and BRCA2 genes (mutations in these genes may increase risk for both ovarian and breast carcinoma).
- The protein HER2/neu is overexpressed in 35% of ovarian cancers and its overexpression is associated with a poor prognosis.
- KRAS is expressed in 30% of tumours (mostly mucinous cystadenocarcinomas).
- p53 is mutated in about 50% of all ovarian cancers.
- Low-grade serous adenocarcinomas show KRAS, BRAF or ERBB2 mutations. High-grade tumours show TP53 mutations and lack KRAS or BRAF mutations.

Clinical Features of Ovarian Tumours

- Generally produce no signs or symptoms till they are advanced.
- Clinical presentation is similar despite morphological diversity.
- Functional tumours produce hormones causing endocrinopathies.
- Benign tumours generally produce pressure symptoms because of their size (pain, urinary frequency and gastrointestinal symptoms) and malignant tumours may present with weakness, weight loss and cachexia.
- Torsion of tumours on their pedicles can present as an acute emergency.
- Fibromas and malignant tumours are both associaed with ascites.

Screening Modalities for Ovarian Tumours

- Radiology.
- Elevation of markers like glycoprotein CA-125 and osteopontin is noted in 75%–90% of women with epithelial ovarian cancers (CA-125 may also be increased, however, in benign conditions as well as non-ovarian cancers and may be undetectable in a large number of women with ovarian cancer with no extraovarian spread).

Salient Features of Different Ovarian Tumours

- **Epithelial ovarian tumours (surface epithelial tumours)**
  (a) Behaviour of surface epithelial tumours depends on their pathological features:
    (i) Benign tumours show simple, non-stratified epithelium, with no cytological atypia.
    (ii) Atypical proliferative tumours (borderline or BL tumours) show epithelial proliferation with stratification and tufting, variable mitotic activity and nuclear atypia, but no stromal invasion.
    (iii) Malignant tumours (carcinomas) show stromal invasion and marked cytological atypia.
  (b) Biochemical markers of surface epithelial tumours include CA-125 and osteopontin.

  Types
    - **Serous:** Lining resembles fallopian tube epithelium.
    - **Mucinous:** Lining resembles gastrointestinal tract (GIT) or endocervical epithelium.
    - **Endometrioid:** Lining resembles proliferative endometrium.
    - **Clear cell:** Lining resembles gestational endometrium.
    - **Transitional cell (Brenner):** Lining resembles urinary tract epithelium.

  (a) **Serous tumours**
    - These are the most common ovarian tumours.
    - Sixty per cent are benign, 15% of low malignant potential and 25% malignant.
    - Twenty per cent of the benign tumours and 60% of the malignant tumours are bilateral.
    - Average size is smaller than that of mucinous tumours.

- These tumours can spread locally to opposite ovary, abdominal viscera, peritoneal surfaces and omentum and are often associated with ascites. Para-aortic and pelvic lymph nodes are frequently involved. Liver and lungs are the most common sites for metastases.
- Umbilical metastasis is labelled **'Sister Mary Joseph nodule'.**
- The cyst lining may be smooth or papillary (cauliflower-like masses composed of soft brittle tissue may be seen in malignant tumours). Cysts are filled with clear fluid and lined by cuboidal epithelium with apical mucin.
- Changes suggestive of malignancy are:
  - Predominance of papillary projections and solid areas.
  - Presence of haemorrhage and necrosis.
  - Invasion of cyst wall.
  - Irregular nodular surface due to penetration of the serosal covering by the tumour.

(i) **Benign serous cystadenomas**

Gross morphology: Unilocular cystic tumours containing clear fluid and having a smooth glistening wall. Size varies between 15 and 30 cm.

Microscopy (Fig. 31.9): Lining is mostly smooth; may occasionally show papillae which have a central fibrovascular core lined by tall columnar ciliated or non-ciliated epithelium.

(ii) ***BL serous cystadenomas***

- These constitute 15% of all serous tumours.
- Majority are limited to the ovary; some show extra-ovarian spread.

Gross morphology: Have a greater papillary component than benign serous cystadenoma.

Microscopy

- Stratification of the epithelial lining of papillae occurs with the formation of microscopic papillary tufts.
- Nuclear atypia and increased mitotic activity may be seen.
- Absence of stromal invasion even on extensive sampling (one block for every 1–2 cm of tumour diameter). Deep invaginations should not be confused with invasion.

(iii) **Frank serous carcinoma**

- Most common malignant tumour of ovary.
- Arises between the ages of 45 and 65 years.

Gross morphology

- Average size is 5–15 cm, predominantly solid with variable cystic areas.
- External surface is smooth or papillary; soft friable papillae fill the cavity.

Microscopy (Fig. 31.10)

- **Low grade:** Delicate well-formed papillary structures with prominent fibrous stalks. Papillae may be crowded together; individual stalks may not be discerned. Single cells and small nests may be seen infiltrating the stroma. The tumour cells show low-grade (mild to moderate) atypia.
- **High grade**
  - Papillary pattern obliterated; solid sheets of pleomorphic cells or complex growth patterns seen.

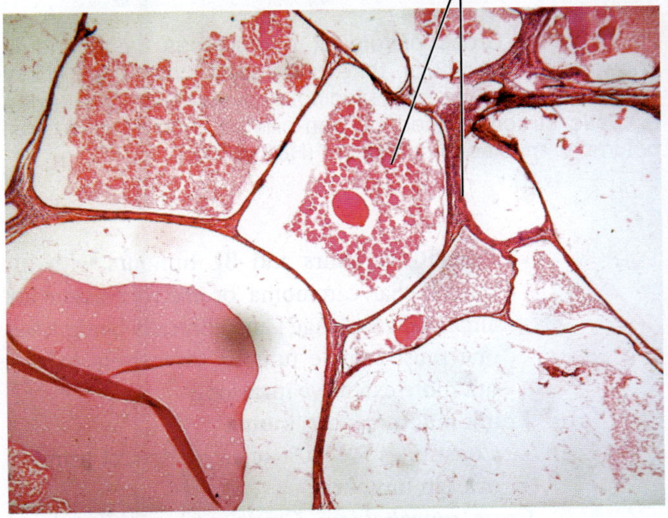

Fig 31.9 Photomicrograph of a serous cystadenoma showing multiple cystic spaces lined by simple cuboidal epithelium (H&E; 100×).

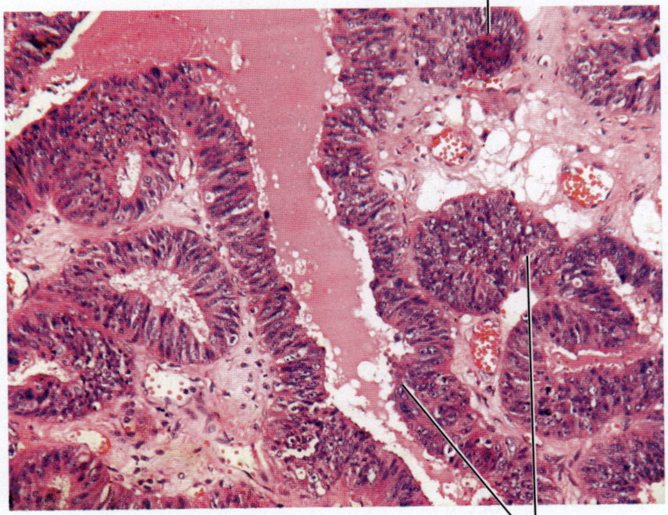

Fig 31.10 Serous cystadenocarcinoma showing crowded papillae lined by atypical, stratified columnar epithelium along with single cells and small nests infiltrating the stroma (H&E; 100×).

- Widespread stromal invasion, marked nuclear atypia with bizarre mono- or multinucleate forms and prominent mitotic activity.
- Capsular invasion present.
- Psammoma bodies in 32% of cases (thought to be associated with a better survival).
- Five-year survival <20%.

(b) **Mucinous tumours**

- Less common than serous tumours.
- Common in the reproductive age group.
- Eighty per cent benign, 10% of low malignant potential and 10% frankly malignant.
- Five per cent benign tumours and 20% malignant tumours bilateral.
- Associated with smoking and KRAS mutations.
- Larger and more multilocular than their serous counterparts.
- Papillary formations and psammoma bodies less common than their serous counterparts.
- Lined by tall columnar epithelium with a basal nucleus and abundant cytoplasmic mucin (cells similar to gastric foveolar, intestinal or endocervical mucosa).
- Multiloculated cysts filled with sticky or gelatinous mucinous material.
- Glistening, smooth and papery thin wall.
- Solid areas or papillary projections on inner wall of the cyst suggestive of malignant change.

(i) **Benign mucinous tumours**

- Include cystadenoma, cystadenofibroma and adenofibroma.
- Spectrum of benign lesions with varying amounts of cysts, glands and stroma.
- May be associated with carcinoid tumours in the same ovary, dermoid cyst, Brenner tumour and endocervical adenocarcinoma; rarely with Zollinger–Ellison syndrome.

Gross morphology (Fig. 31.11A): Multilocular thin-walled cysts containing sticky gelatinous material.

Microscopy (Fig. 31.11B)

- Cysts are lined by non-ciliated, non-stratified, tall columnar, mucinous epithelium. Small bland papillae may be present occasionally.
- These are usually endocervical type; may be gastric or intestinal type (picket fence architecture with Paneth cells) or mixed.
- Stroma may be fibrous or mimic ovarian stroma (focal luteinization or calcification can occur).

(ii) **BL mucinous malignancy**

Gross morphology: Large, multilocular, cystic, with a smooth external surface; papillary excrescences may be seen.

Microscopy:

- Stratification/multilayering of lining epithelium with budding and tufting.
- Mild nuclear atypia and increased mitotic activity, but absence of stromal invasion.

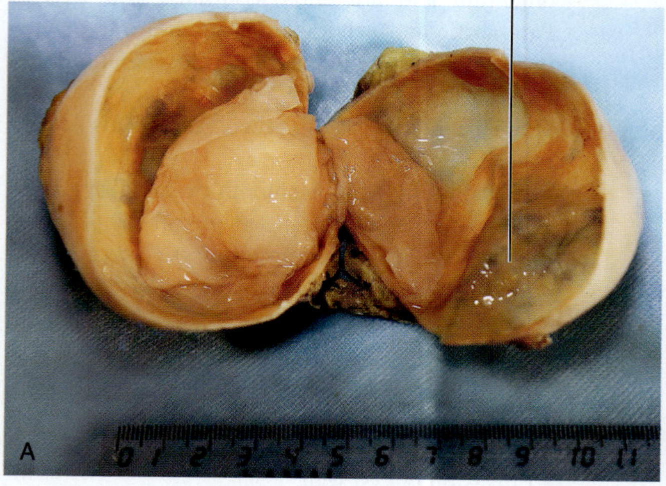

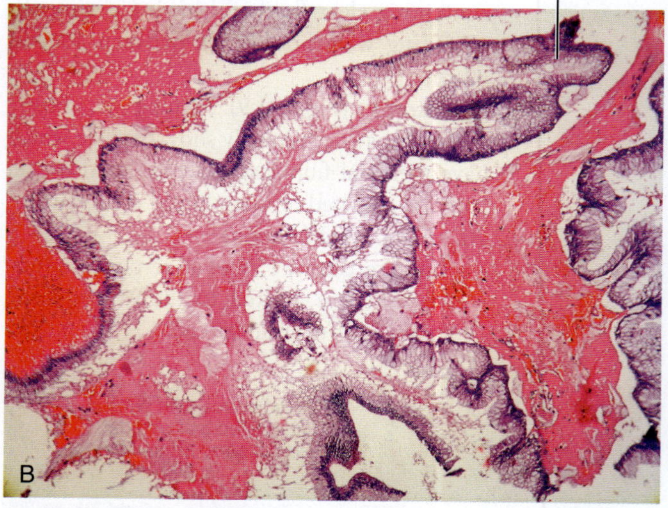

Fig 31.11 (A) Gross picture of a mucinous cystadenoma showing a multilocular thin-walled cyst containing sticky gelatinous material. (B) Mucinous cystadenoma showing a cystic structure lined by non-ciliated, non-stratified, tall columnar, mucinous epithelium (H&E; 100×).

- Pure BL tumours and BL tumours with intraepithelial carcinoma or microinvasion are almost always Stage I and clinically benign, but one must sample tumour extensively to rule out more extensive invasion.

(iii) **Frank mucinous carcinoma**

- Constitutes 6%–10% of all malignant primary ovarian tumours.

Gross morphology: Cystic and multiloculated with a size up to 50 cm. Solid areas, areas of haemorrhage and necrosis are commonly seen.

Microscopy (Fig. 31.12)

- **Well-differentiated tumours:** Predominantly composed of well-defined, gland-like structures

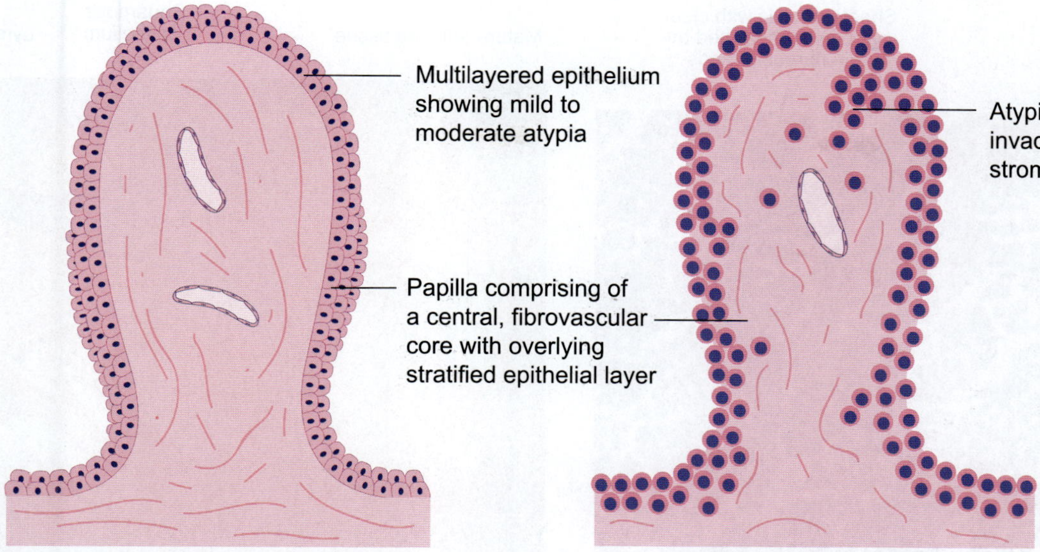

Fig 31.12 Schematic diagram to demonstrate histological differences between borderline mucinous cystadenoma and mucinous cystadenocarcinoma.

or cysts lined by stratified tall columnar mucin-producing cells with few mitoses.
- **Moderately differentiated tumours:** Loss of glandular architecture with only a few well-defined glands lined by atypical epithelium, and showing numerous mitoses.
- **Poorly differentiated tumours:** Solid nests and cords composed of highly atypical epithelium invading the stroma; infiltration of the serosa and necrosis common.

(iv) **Pseudomyxoma peritonei**
- Seen in 2%–5% of cases of ovarian mucinous tumours.
- Characterized by massive gelatinous accumulation arranged in a loculated pattern in the peritoneal cavity.
- Large amount of mucin reaches peritoneal cavity either by dissection through cyst wall or through a perforation.
- Strips of mature cells with basally arranged regular vacuoles filled with mucous or individual epithelial cells found free floating within gelatinous masses.

(c) **Endometrioid ovarian tumours**
- Ten per cent to 25% of all surface epithelial tumours.
- Thirty per cent are bilateral: 15%–30% have a concomitant endometrial carcinoma.
- Solid-cystic; may arise as a mass from an endometriotic cyst filled with chocolate-coloured fluid.
- Lined by tall columnar epithelium with a centrally located nucleus.

(d) **Brenner tumour:** Derived from coelomic epithelium of the ovary; forms the typical urothelial-like epithelial elements through a metaplastic process.

(i) **Benign Brenner tumour:** Rare ovarian neoplasm; affects individuals older than 50 years.

Gross morphology
- Usually an incidental discovery (because of a very high frequency of microscopic lesions).
- Average size 2–8 cm; may produce compression of surrounding ovarian tissue.
- Solid, encapsulated, firm and grey-white with a whorled cut surface.

Microscopy
- Solid-cystic epithelial nests surrounded by a stroma composed of bundles of tightly packed spindle-shaped cells.
- Polygonal to squamoid epithelial cells with pale eosinophilic cytoplasm and oval nucleus showing longitudinal grooving **(coffee-bean appearance).**
- No mitotic figures or atypia seen.
- Association of Brenner with other cystic neoplasms, e.g. mucinous cystadenoma and cystic teratoma, well known.

(ii) **BL malignant Brenner tumour**
- Cystic tumour with papillary fronds.
- Epithelium resembles non-invasive papillary transitional cell carcinoma of the urinary bladder or grade 3 dysplasia (SCC in situ).

(iii) **Malignant Brenner tumour:** It shows frankly malignant histological features with stromal invasion by epithelial elements. Malignant component may be:
- Transitional cell carcinoma.
- SCC.
- Undifferentiated carcinoma.

(e) **Cystadenofibroma:** In some serous neoplasms, fibroblastic stromal component is unduly prominent, appearing as a solid white nodular focus in an otherwise cystic lesion; it may be benign, BL or malignant.

(f) **Clear cell (mesonephroid) carcinoma**
Gross morphology: Spongy and cystic.

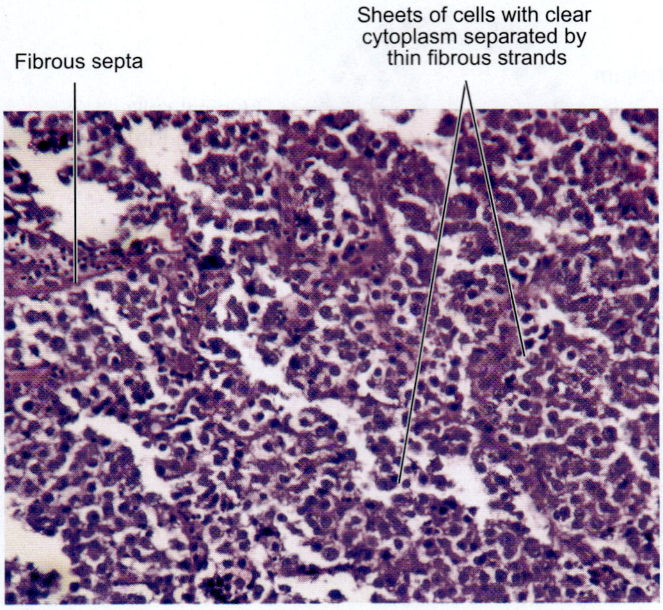

Fig 31.13 Photomicrograph of a dysgerminoma showing sheets of cells with clear cytoplasm and well-defined cytoplasmic margins, separated by thin fibrous stroma containing lymphoid cells (H&E; 100×).

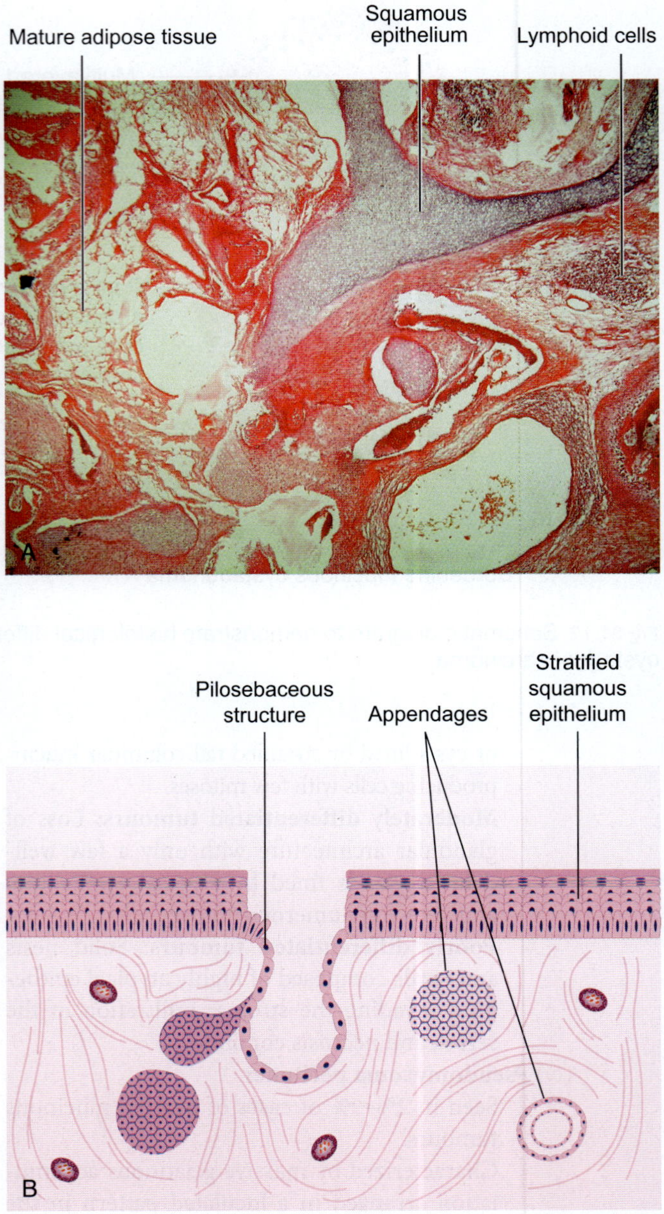

Fig 31.14 (A and B) Microphotograph and schematic representation of a cystic teratoma showing stratified squamous epithelium and appendageal structures (ectodermal differentiation; H&E; 40×).

Microscopy

- Tubular cystic, papillary or sheet-like arrangement of neoplastic epithelium.
- Tumour cells large with a clear cytoplasm and nuclei projecting into the lumina **(hob nailing).**
- Originally thought to originate from mesonephric rests but now definitely known to arise from surface epithelium.

2. **Tumours of germ cell origin**

(a) **Dysgerminoma**

- Most common malignant ovarian tumour; usually arises in second or third decade.
- It is the female counterpart of testicular seminoma.
- Associated with gonadal dysgenesis.
- Majority are unilateral and solid; cut surface of large tumours appears lobulated and fleshy.
- Histopathology shows sheets and nests of cells with clear cytoplasm and well-defined cytoplasmic margins, separated by thin fibrous strands (Fig 31.13). Stroma contains lymphoid cells and may show granulomatous inflammation.
- It is radioresponsive with 80% survival.
- Levels of serum lactate dehydrogenase (LDH) and placental alkaline phosphatase (PLAP) are usually elevated.

(b) **Teratoma:** Constitutes 15%–20% of ovarian tumours; more than 90% are benign mature cystic teratomas. Other types include immature, malignant and specialized teratomas.

(i) **Benign mature cystic teratoma**

- The most common type is a **dermoid cyst** (Fig. 31.14A and B); the cyst is filled with sebaceous secretion and matted hair and lined by stratified squamous epithelium and appendageal structures (ectodermal differentiation).
- Dermoid cysts are usually discovered accidentally in children/young women on radiographs or sonograms; they are picked up easily because they commonly show calcification and teeth formation.
- Ninety per cent are unilateral and may present with infertility or torsion (the latter is an acute surgical emergency).
- Foci of other mature/adult tissue such as bone, cartilage, bronchial and intestinal epithelium and glial tissue may sometimes be appreciated, indicating development along other germ cell layers.

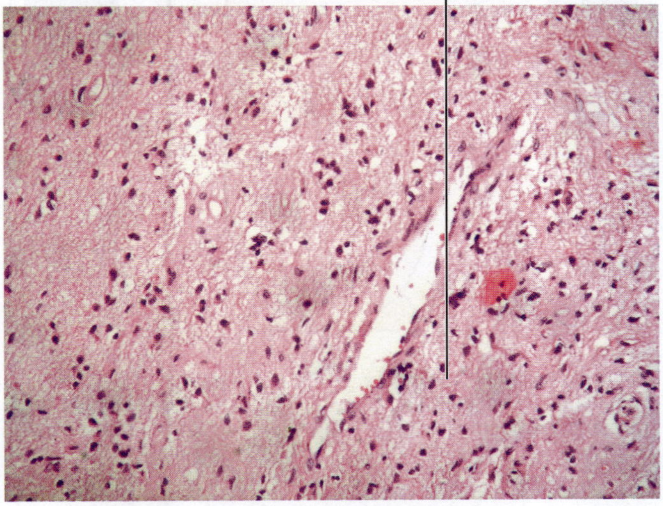

Fig 31.15 Microphotograph of an immature teratoma showing abundant neuroepithelium (H&E; 100×).

- Rarely, one of the tissue elements may undergo malignant change, most commonly a squamous cell carcinoma (the tumour is then referred to as a **teratoma with malignant transformation**).

(ii) **Immature malignant teratoma**
- Bulky, predominantly solid tumour showing foci of necrosis.
- Immature bone, cartilage, muscle, nerve and other structures are seen on microscopy.
- Also seen are areas of neuroepithelial differentiation (lesions with such areas tend to be aggressive and metastasize widely; Fig 31.15).

(iii) **Specialized (monodermal) teratomas**
Teratomas with specialized tissue, e.g. **struma ovarii** composed entirely of mature thyroid tissue that may hyperfunction and produce hyperthyroidism or the **ovarian carcinoid**, which can produce carcinoid syndrome.

(c) **Yolk sac (endodermal sinus) tumour of ovary**
- Common in children and young adults.
- Usually unilateral and presents with abdominal pain and a rapidly growing pelvic mass.
- Fatal within 2 years of diagnosis.

Morphology: See testicular neoplasms (Chapter 30).

(d) **Choriocarcinoma**
- Usually arises in the first three decades of life and is always unilateral.
- The most common symptom is vaginal bleeding.
- Untreated choriocarcinoma presents with early haematogenous metastases. Common metastatic sites include lung, brain, liver, kidney and bowel.
- Primary focus may disintegrate leaving only metastatic deposits and may be represented by a small haemorrhagic focus.
- On gross examination, the tumour appears bulky and destructive. There is presence of single to multiple dark masses in the uterus with extensive central haemorrhage and variable amount of necrosis.
- Tumour may be diffusely infiltrative or have cohesive sheets of malignant trophoblastic cells consisting of intermediate trophoblasts and cytotrophoblasts rimmed with syncytiotrophoblasts.
- There is striking cytological atypia and numerous mitotic figures.
- Lymphovascular invasion is common.

3. **Sex cord tumours**

(a) **Granulosa theca tumours**
- Majority arise in postmenopausal women, but may occur at any age.
- Unilateral small to large, yellow, with cystic spaces
- Composed of cuboidal granulosa cells in cords, sheets or strands along with spindled or plump lipid-laden theca cells, which elaborate large amounts of oestrogen.
- May recapitulate primitive ovarian follicles called **Call–Exner bodies** (Fig 31.16 A and B).

(b) **Thecoma-fibroma**
- Can affect any age.
- Mostly unilateral, solid, grey with spindled fibrous cells to plump lipid-laden theca cells.
- Most are hormonally inactive; few secrete oestrogen.
- About 40% produce ascites and hydrothorax **(Meigs syndrome)**.
- May rarely turn malignant.

(c) **Sertoli–Leydig cell tumours**
- Affect all ages.
- Unilateral, small grey to red brown, solid masculinizing tumours, which recapitulate the development of testes.
- Rarely malignant.

4. **Metastasis to the ovary**
- Seen in older age group.
- Mostly bilateral.
- Large, solid, grey-white tumours with cords, glands and individual malignant cells dispersed in the ovarian stroma, e.g. **Krukenberg tumour**.

Q. Describe the clinicopathological features of Krukenberg tumour.

Ans. Ovaries are a common site for metastases; 5%–10% of ovarian tumours are metastatic tumours. Krukenberg tumour refers to a malignancy in the ovary that has metastasized from a primary site, classically the GIT. Tumours can spread to the ovary by several pathways:

- Direct spread.
- Transcoelomic dissemination.
- Haematogenous spread.
- Lymphatic spread.

Krukenberg tumours generally affect women older than 45 years and are bilateral in more than 80% of the reported cases.

Most common ovarian metastases are from the GIT, endometrium, appendix (adenocarcinoid or mucinous adenocarcinoma), breast, carcinoid and pancreas.

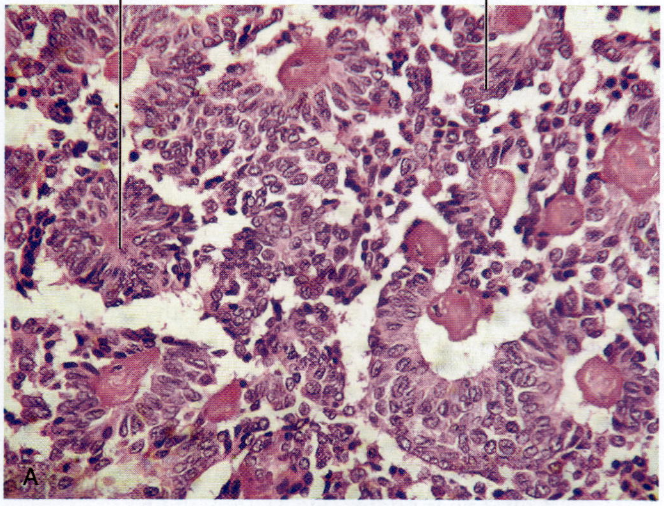

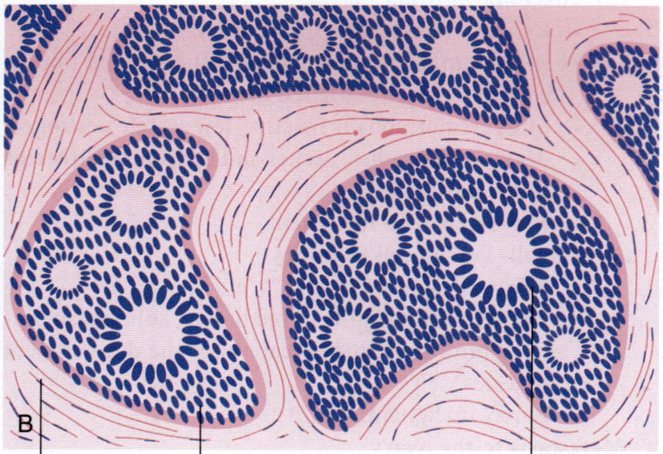

Fig 31.16 (A and B) Tumour tissue composed of cuboidal granulosa cells arranged in cords, sheets or strands recapitulating primitive ovarian follicles called Call–Exner bodies (H&E; 100×).

Pathogenesis

- Most commonly, it is a diffuse type of gastric cancer, which metastasizes to ovaries.
- Two theories have been offered to explain metastasis of tumour from the GIT to the ovary:
  - Spread due to shedding of cells into peritoneum (transcoelomic spread).
  - Lymphatic spread.

Gross Morphology

- Bilateral, symmetrically enlarged ovaries, which retain their shape and architecture (Fig 31.17A). Cut surface appears yellow-white; it is usually solid, and occasionally cystic.

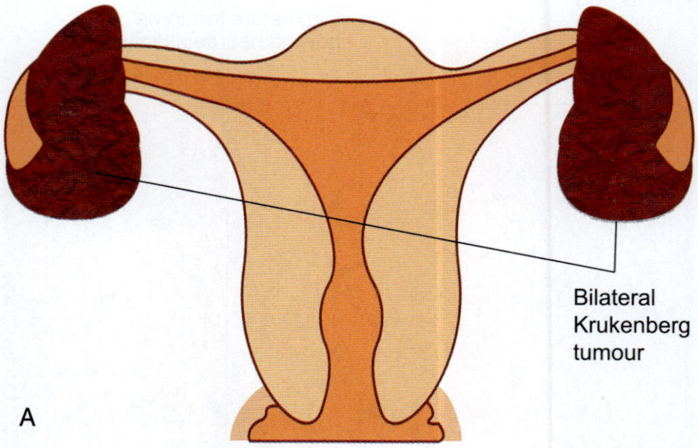

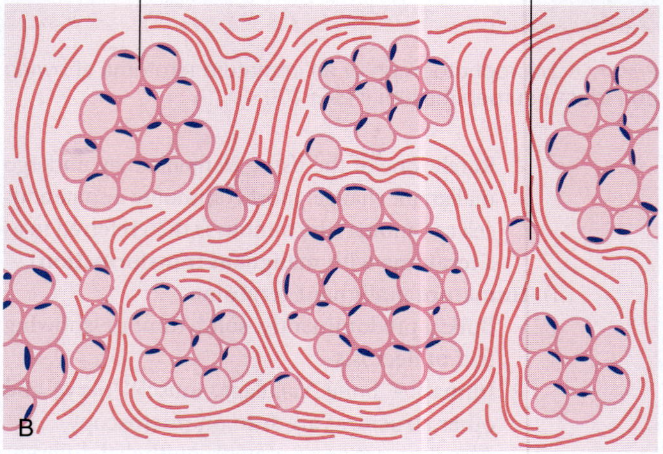

Fig 31.17 (A) Schematic representation of Krukenberg tumour showing bilateral, symmetrically enlarged ovaries, which retain their shape and architecture. (B) Signet ring cells (cells with abundant mucin, which pushes the nucleus to the periphery) are arranged in a diffusely infiltrative growth pattern, that is, cords and singly lying cells with very few glands.

- The capsular surface of the ovaries with Krukenberg tumours is typically smooth and free of adhesions or peritoneal deposits (other metastatic tumours to the ovary tend to be associated with surface implants). This may explain why the gross morphology of Krukenberg tumour can deceptively appear as a primary ovarian tumour.

Microscopy

Signet ring cells (cells with abundant mucin, which pushes the nucleus to the periphery) are arranged in a diffusely infiltrative growth pattern, that is, cords and singly lying cells with minimal gland formation (Fig. 31.17B).

Q. Differentiate between serous and mucinous ovarian tumours.

Ans. Differences between serous and mucinous ovarian tumours are listed in Table 31.2.

Table 31.2 Differences between serous and mucinous ovarian tumours

Features	Serous tumours	Mucinous tumours
Frequency	Most common ovarian tumour	Less common than serous tumours
Incidence of malignancy	Account for 60% of all malignant ovarian tumours	Account for 10% of malignant ovarian tumours
Age affected	• Benign lesions: 30–40 years • Malignant lesions: 45–65 years	Middle age; rare before puberty and after menopause
Bilateralism	Common	Less/rare
Gross	Unilocular/few cysts filled with clear serous fluid	Multilocular tumours filled with sticky gelatinous fluid rich in glycoproteins
Cell lining	Tall columnar ciliated epithelial cells	Tall columnar cells resembling endocervical or intestinal epithelium
Papillae	Very common	Less common
Psammoma bodies	Common	Not found

Q. Differentiate between mature and immature teratoma.

Ans. Differences between mature and immature teratoma are listed in Table 31.3.

Table 31.3 Differences between mature and immature teratoma

Features	Mature teratoma	Immature teratoma
Component tissue	Mature	Immature
Age affected	Young women (reproductive age group)	Adolescents and young adults (younger than 20 years)
Bilateralism	Bilateral in 10%–15% of cases	Mostly unilateral
Type	Mostly cystic (dermoid cyst)	Usually solid
Gross appearance	Unilocular cyst lined by the epidermis; cyst may have areas of calcification, teeth, matted hair and sebaceous material	Predominantly solid with areas of necrosis and haemorrhage
Microscopy	• Cyst wall lined by mature stratified squamous epithelium with appendageal structures • No immature elements/ neuroepithelium seen	• Immature structures differentiating towards cartilage, glands, muscles, bones, neuroepithelium, etc. seen; tissue resembles fetal or embryonic tissue rather than adult tissue • Proportion of immature neuroepithelium in tumour determines the prognosis

Q. Write briefly about gestational trophoblastic disease. (PA30.5)

Ans. Gestational trophoblastic disease usually develops within the uterus, but may develop at any site of ectopic pregnancy.

- It ranges in behaviour from benign hydatidiform mole (H. mole) to highly aggressive choriocarcinoma.
- All secrete human chorionic gonadotropin (hCG), which can be detected in the serum and urine.
- The fall or rise in titres of hCG can be used as an indicator of response to therapy.

Hydatidiform Mole

- It is traditionally discovered during 12–14 weeks of pregnancy.
- Uterine enlargement is more than what is anticipated for that period of gestation.
- It manifests with vaginal bleeding and passage of grape-like tissue mass.
- Elevation of hCG (particularly the beta subunit) in blood and urine and absence of fetal parts or fetal heart sound on sonography is diagnostic.
- It is of two types – complete and partial mole.

Gross Morphology (Fig 31.18A)

- Uterine cavity/ectopic site is filled with delicate, friable masses of thin-walled, translucent, cystic and grape-like structures.
- Amniotic sac is very small and collapsed.
- There are no fetal parts in complete mole; however, they may be seen in a partial mole.

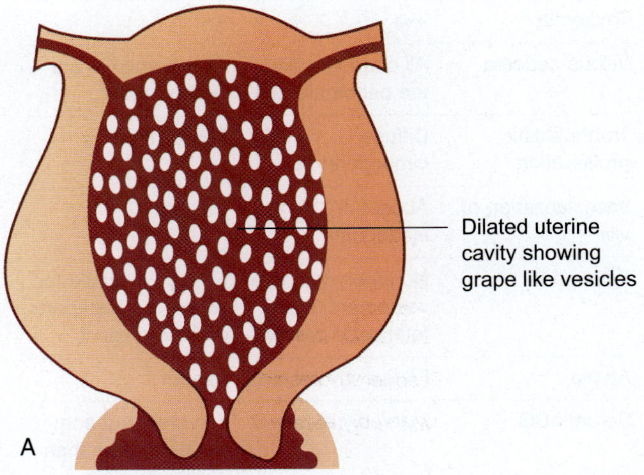

Fig 31.18 (A) Schematic diagram of uterine cavity filled with delicate, friable masses of thin-walled, translucent, cystic and grape-like structures.

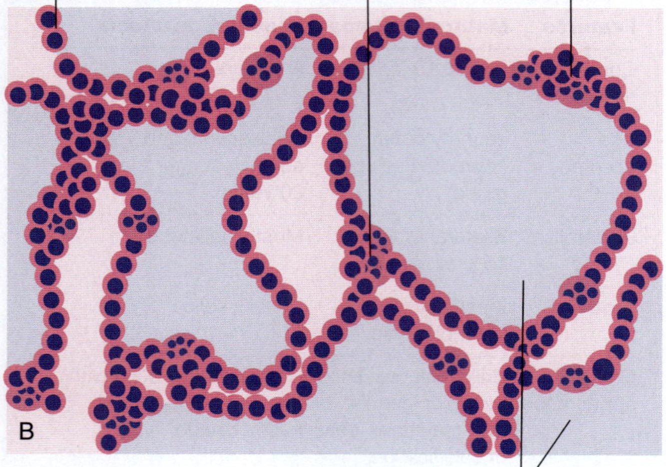

Fig 31.18 (B) Schematic diagram showing hydropic swelling and complete loss of vascularity of chorionic villi. The central substance of the villi is loose, myxomatous and oedematous, covered by a layer of chorionic epithelium (cytotrophoblast and syncytiotrophoblast). Villi show circumferential proliferation of epithelium to produce sheets and masses of the same.

Table 31.4 Differences between partial and complete mole

Features	Complete mole	Partial mole
Karyotype	46, XX (46, XY)	Triploid (69, XXY)
Incidence of missed abortion	+	+++
Heavy bleeding	+++	+
Toxaemia	+++	+/–
Villous oedema	All chorionic villi are oedematous	Only some villi are oedematous
Trophoblastic proliferation	Diffuse; circumferential	Focal; mild
Vascularization of villi	Absent or inadequate	Present
Fetal parts	No embryonic development, so no fetal parts present	Embryo is viable for weeks, so fetal parts may be present
Atypia	Frequently present	Absent
Serum hCG	Markedly elevated	Elevated, but comparatively less than complete mole
hCG in tissues	++ + +	+
Behaviour	2% incidence of choriocarcinoma	Incidence of choriocarcinoma negligible

Microscopic Examination

- **Complete mole (Fig 31. 18B)**
  - All villi show hydropic swelling and complete loss of vascularity.
  - The central substance of the villi is loose, myxomatous and oedematous, covered by a layer of chorionic epithelium (cytotrophoblast and syncytiotrophoblast).
  - Villi show circumferential proliferation of epithelium to produce sheets and masses of the same.
- **Partial mole**
  - Villous oedema is restricted to some villi.
  - Trophoblastic proliferation is mild and focal.
  - Villi have a characteristic irregular scalloped margin.

Q. Differentiate between partial and complete mole.

Ans. Differences between partial and complete mole are listed in Table 31.4.

Q. Differentiate between H. mole and choriocarcinoma.

Ans. Differences between H. mole and choriocarcinoma are listed in Table 31.5.

Table 31.5 Differences between H. mole and choriocarcinoma

Features	H. mole	Choriocarcinoma
Definition	Variable trophoblastic proliferation, mostly benign in nature; may give rise to choriocarcinoma	Choriocarcinoma is a malignant neoplasm of trophoblastic cells derived from any form of previously normal or abnormal pregnancy
Presentation	During 12–14 weeks of pregnancy, patient presents with vaginal bleeding/passage of grape-like structures	During pregnancy or after miscarriage, patient presents with bloody, brown, foul-smelling discharge
Gross	Delicate, friable mass of thin-walled, translucent, cystic and grape-like structures	Soft, fleshy, with extensive haemorrhage and areas of necrosis
Microscopy	Villous oedema with absence of vascularity, cytotrophoblast and syncytiotrophoblast cover villi	Epithelial malignancy; chorionic villi not formed; abnormal proliferation of both cytotrophoblast and syncytiotrophoblast
Uterus size	Much larger than expected for that duration of pregnancy	Mild enlargement
hCG level	↑	↑↑↑
Precedent history	None	H. mole, abortion, normal/ectopic pregnancy
Metastasis	Not seen	To lung, liver and brain
Treatment	Curettage	Curettage and chemotherapy; may be hysterectomy

Diseases of the Breast 32

- Breast is a modified apocrine gland, which is composed of 6–10 major ductal systems that can be traced from the nipple (keratinizing stratified squamous epithelium of the skin continues into the ducts and abruptly changes into double-layered cuboidal epithelium).
- The larger ducts branch successively and lead to **terminal duct lobular units** (TDLUs; Fig. 32.1).
- Terminal duct further branches into clusters of small acini to form a **lobule**.
- **Ducts** and **lobules** are lined by two cell types:
  - A basal layer of low, flattened and contractile **myoepithelial cells.**
  - A second luminal layer of **epithelial cells.**
- Majority of breast stroma consists of dense fibrous connective tissue admixed with adipose tissue **(interlobular stroma).**
- Present within the lobules is breast-specific, hormone-responsive and delicate myxomatous stroma **(intralobular stroma).**

Q. Write briefly about benign epithelial lesions of the breast. (PA31.1)

Ans. Benign epithelial lesions of the breast include the various benign alterations in its ducts and lobules. They are classified into **three types**, depending on the subsequent risk of breast cancer, namely:

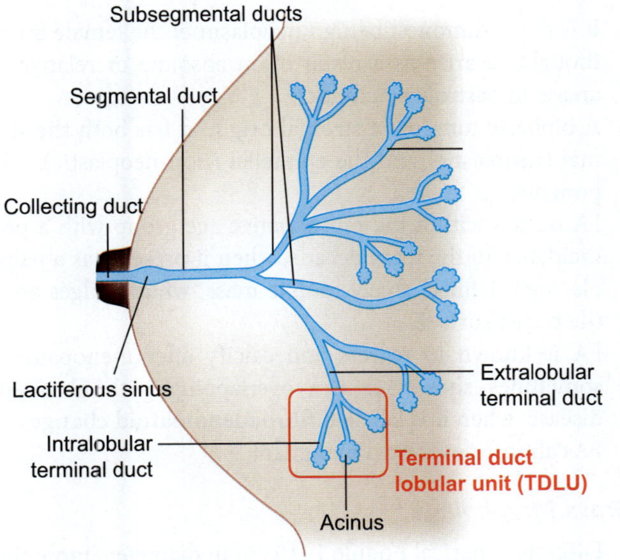

Fig. 32.1 Diagrammatic representation of normal breast parenchyma.

- **Non-proliferative breast changes** (also called fibrocystic changes).
- **Proliferative breast disease without atypia.**
- **Atypical hyperplasia.**

Non-proliferative Breast Changes

Clinically significant disease (lumpy-bumpy breast) without epithelial hyperplasia.

Clinical Features

- Presents with an ill-defined lump/nodularity, mammographic densities/calcification or nipple discharge.
- Affects women aged between 20 and 40 years; peaks at or just before menopause; is rare after menopause and before adolescence.
- Usually multiple and bilateral.
- No risk of developing cancer.
- Clue to diagnosis: Disappearance of the mass after fine needle aspiration of cyst contents.

Aetiology

Hormonal imbalance: increased oestrogen (duct epithelium is oestrogen sensitive) and decreased progesterone.

Morphology

Three main morphological changes are seen:

- **Cystic dilation of ducts and lobules**
  - Large cysts contain semitranslucent and turbid fluid, which imparts brown to blue colour to them (**blue dome cysts**).
  - Epithelium lining the cysts is flattened and atrophic; it may show **apocrine metaplasia** (large polygonal cells that have abundant granular eosinophilic cytoplasm and small, round, hyperchromatic nucleus).
- **Fibrosis**
  - Cysts release a secretory material into the stroma, which causes chronic inflammation and fibrosis with loss of the normal myxomatous appearance.
- **Adenosis**
  - Increase in the number of acini per lobule. The acini are lined by columnar epithelium which may occasionally show nuclear atypia (labelled 'flat epithelial atypia' – a clonal disorder associated with deletions of chromosome 16q which is thought to be the earliest recognizable precursor of low-grade malignancy; however, it does not

necessarily translate into an increased risk of invasive breast cancer).

- The acini are enlarged only (as in **blunt duct adenosis**) or enlarged and distorted (as in **sclerosing adenosis**).
- Calcifications may be seen in the lumens.
- A **lactating adenoma** presents as a palpable mass in pregnant or lactating women. It is composed of closely packed glands lined by cuboidal cells with foamy to finely vacuolated cytoplasm, uniform nuclei with fine chromatin and prominent nucleoli.

Proliferative Breast Disease Without Atypia

Proliferative (hyperplastic) changes may be seen in the ductules, terminal ducts and sometimes the lobules. They are classified into:

(a) **Epithelial hyperplasia**
  (i) It is defined as presence of more than two cell layers in the lining of ducts and lobules.
  (ii) It can vary from mild to florid hyperplasia.
  (iii) The ducts, ductules and lobules are filled with cuboidal cells showing small glandular pattern called fenestrations.

(b) **Sclerosing adenosis**
  (i) It is less common but significant type of proliferative breast disease because of its clinical and morphological similarity to invasive carcinoma.
  (ii) It is characterized by marked intralobular fibrosis and proliferation of small ductules and acini.
  (iii) On gross examination, sclerosing adenosis appears hard and rubbery-like invasive breast carcinoma.
  (iv) Histopathology sections show proliferation of epithelial and myoepithelial cells lining small ducts and ductules. The proliferating glands and ductules appear back to back. There is marked stromal fibrosis which compresses and distorts the proliferating epithelium leading to obliteration of the lumina of the glands so that they appear as solid cords of cells, closely mimicking an invasive carcinoma. Identification of the myoepithelial cells is an important clue to indicate the benign nature of the lesion.

(c) **Complex sclerosing lesion:** Complex sclerosing lesion may be a part of sclerosing adenosis, papillomatosis or radial sclerosing lesion (radial sclerosing lesion closely mimics invasive carcinoma, radiologically and pathologically, and is composed of a central nidus of glands entrapped in a hyalinized stroma).

(d) **Papillomas**: These grow within ducts and are composed of fibrovascular cores lined by luminal and myoepithelial cells; these may be large duct papillomas (solitary and located in lactiferous sinuses) or small duct papillomas (multiple and located in the deeper ducts). These usually present with nipple discharge.

Proliferative Breast Disease With Atypia

(a) In some cases, the cells lining ducts show hyperplasia and form a regularly spaced pattern (**atypical ductal hyperplasia [ADH]**). Micropapillae, tufts, bridges, solid and cribriform patterns of evenly distributed, monomorphic cells with rounded or ovoid nuclei are seen. ADH should be differentiated from **ductal carcinoma in situ (DCIS)** based on the fact that in the former the ductal hyperplasia is limited in extent and does not completely fill the ducts. Clinically, ADH is usually less than 2–3 mm, and may be multicentric.

(b) **Atypical lobular hyperplasia** is a term used to describe a hyperplasia that resembles lobular carcinoma in situ (LCIS), but in which the cells do not fill or distend more than 50% of the acini within a lobule. It is usually not associated with specific mammographic findings and does not from a palpable mass. Atypical lobular hyperplasia is associated with increased risk of invasive carcinoma.

Relationship Between Benign Epithelial Breast Lesions and Invasive Carcinoma

- ***Non-proliferative breast disease*** includes fibrosis, cystic change, apocrine metaplasia, mild hyperplasia, duct ectasia, adenosis and fibroadenoma (FA); it is associated with minimal or no increased risk.
- ***Slightly increased risk (1.5–2 times)*** is noted with moderate or florid hyperplasia without atypia, papillomatosis, sclerosing adenosis, radial sclerosing lesion and FA with complex features.
- ***Significantly increased risk (four to five times)*** is noted with atypical hyperplasia (ductular or lobular).
- A family history of breast cancer may increase the risk in all categories, e.g. atypical hyperplasia (ductular or lobular) associated with a family history may increase the risk 10-fold.

Q. Write briefly about stromal tumours of breast.

Ans. There are two main stromal tumours of breast – **fibroadenoma (FA)** and **phyllodes tumour**, both of which arise from the intralobular stroma.

Fibroadenoma Breast

Salient Features

- It is the commonest benign neoplasm of the female breast, thought to arise as a result of an absolute or relative increase in oestrogen activity.
- A biphasic tumour of stromal origin, it has both the stromal (neoplastic) and the epithelial (non-neoplastic) components.
- FA occurs within the reproductive age group with a peak incidence in the third decade, when it presents as a palpable, well-defined, freely mobile mass, which bulges above the breast surface.
- FA is known to regress and calcify after menopause; it sometimes shows features overlapping with fibrocystic disease, when it is labelled **fibroadenomatoid change.**
- FAs almost never turn malignant.

Gross Morphology

- Discrete spherical nodule 1–10 cm in diameter (more than 10 cm is labelled as **giant FA**).
- Freely mobile, sharply circumscribed and easily enucleated.

Microscopic Features

- Most of the tumour is composed of delicate myxoid stroma resembling interlobular stroma. Stromal overgrowth and ductal proliferation produces two patterns, which may coexist in the same tumour (Fig. 32.2A and B):
  - **Intracanalicular pattern:** Delicate myxoid stroma compresses ducts to slit-like spaces lined by ductal epithelium, which appears as cords of epithelium surrounded by abundant fibrous stroma.
  - **Pericanalicular pattern:** Abundant stroma surrounds patent or dilated ducts. The stroma may get hyalinized and the lining epithelium may become atrophic in older patients.
- Ducts are usually lined by a double-layered epithelium which may show variable hyperplasia.

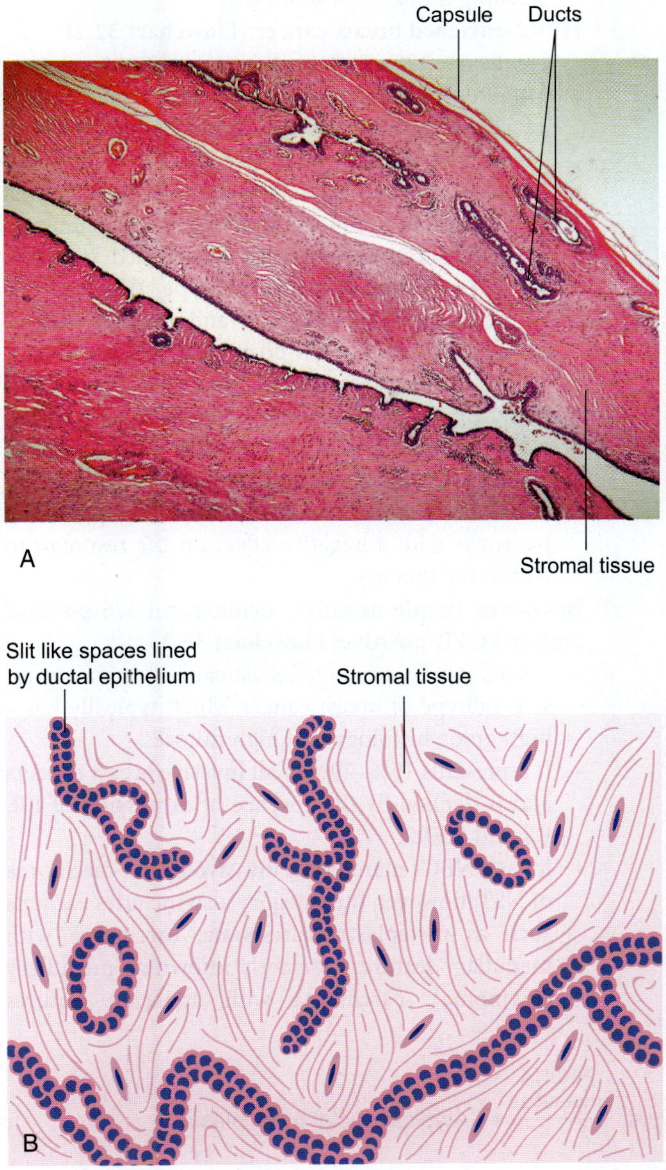

Fig. 32.2 (A and B) H&E-stained section and schematic diagram from fibroadenoma breast showing slit-like and patent ducts surrounded by stromal tissue and enveloped by a well-formed capsule (H&E; 100×).

Phyllodes Tumour

Salient Features

- 'Phyllodes tumour' is a name given to an uncommon bulky breast tumour with **leaf-like gross appearance**.
- It affects any age, but is more common in the sixth decade, 10–20 years later than FAa.
- It arises from intralobular, periductal stroma and not from a pre-existing FA.
- The term 'cystosarcoma phyllodes' is a misnomer because most of these tumours are benign and without cysts.
- They are associated with acquired clonal chromosomal aberrations like gain in chromosome 1q. High-grade tumours are associated with overexpression of HOXB13.

Gross Morphology

- May be a few centimetres to massive, involving the whole breast.
- Varies from being well defined to infiltrative (depending on whether it is low or high grade).
- Cut surface shows a solid, firm, grey-white, bulging tumour. Cystic cavities and areas of haemorrhage and necrosis may be seen. Whorling and cleft-like spaces resembling a leaf are characteristic.

Microscopic Features

- **Low-grade tumours** resemble intracanalicular FA, but cellularity and mitotic figures are increased (Fig. 32.3). Stroma resembles fibroblasts and myofibroblasts and determines the biological potential of the tumour. Epithelial component has luminal epithelial cells resting on myoepithelial layer. The epithelial cells may exhibit hyperplasia and squamous metaplasia and line bulbous/leaf-like projections.
- **High-grade tumours** are like other soft-tissue sarcomas, and are differentiated from low-grade lesions on the basis

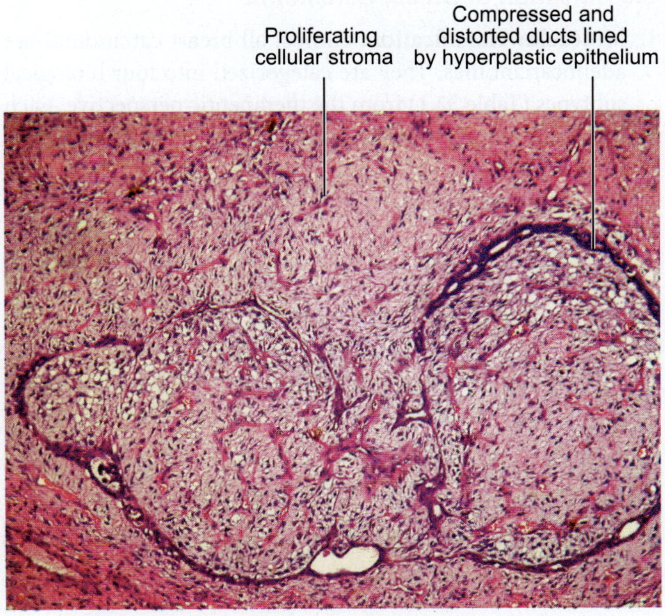

Fig. 32.3 Low-grade phyllodes tumour showing an exaggerated intracanalicular growth pattern with increased stromal cellularity (H&E; 100×).

Table 32.1 Classification of molecular subtypes and correlation with biomarker staining on immunohistochemistry

Molecular subtype	ER		PR		HER 2
Luminal A	Positive	and/ or	Positive		Negative
Luminal B	Positive	and/ or	Positive	or	Negative
			Negative[a]		
Luminal B	Positive	and/ or	Positive	or	Positive
			Negative[b]		
HER2	Negative		Negative		Positive
Triple negative or basal-like	Negative		Negative		Negative

[a]PR < 20% + Ki-67 > 14%.
[b]Any PR + any Ki-67.

of cellularity, mitotic rate, nuclear pleomorphism, stromal overgrowth and infiltrative borders.

Q. Describe the aetiopathogenesis, clinical features and morphology of breast carcinoma. (PA31.2)

Ans. All breast carcinomas arise from the TDLU and usually affect women in the third decade onwards. Invasive cancers are thought to arise through a series of molecular alterations at the cellular level, which immortalize the breast epithelial cells and result in uncontrolled growth. Genomic profiling has demonstrated the presence of discrete subsets of invasive breast cancer with distinct individual evolution and clinical behaviour. The classification is based on the presence or absence of oestrogen receptor (ER), progesterone receptor (PR) and human epidermal growth factor receptor 2 (HER2).

Classification of Breast Carcinoma

1. **Molecular classification:** Almost all breast carcinomas are adenocarcinomas. They are categorized into four biological subtypes (Table 32.1) from the therapeutic perspective. Each has its own distinct genetic and epigenetic aberrations:
   (a) Luminal A
   (b) Luminal B
   (c) Basal-like
   (d) HER2-positive

   (a) **Luminal A tumours (Flowchart 32.1)**
   - *Frequency:* 30%–40% of all invasive breast cancers.
   - *Morphology:* Grading 1 or 2; most are well differentiated carcinomas of no special type (NST), classical lobular carcinomas, tubular, mucinous, neuroendocrine and cribriform carcinomas.
   - *Immunohistochemical (IHC) profile:* ER-positive, PR high expression (≥20%), HER2-negative and low Ki-67. Several studies showed that a Ki-67 of 14% was the cut-off point to separate luminal A from luminal B subtypes. More recently, this cut-off was changed to 20%.
   - ER-positive, HER2-negative tumours are slow growing and respond well to hormonal therapy.

   (b) **Luminal B tumours**
   - *Frequency:* 20%–30% of all invasive breast cancers.
   - *Morphology:* Grading 2 or 3; less well-differentiated cancers, mostly invasive ductal carcinomas NST and also some invasive micropapillary carcinomas.
   - *IHC profile:* ER-positive, lower PR expression (<20%), HER2-negative and higher level of Ki-67 labelling index (>14% or 20%).

   (c) **HER2-enriched breast cancer (Flowchart 32.2)**
   - *Frequency:* 12%–20% of all invasive breast cancers.
   - *Mutations:* Associated with HER2 amplification, TP53 mutations, cyclin D1 amplification and high genomic instability.
   - *Morphology:* Grading 2 or 3; infiltrating carcinoma NST, apocrine and pleomorphic lobular carcinomas.
   - HER2-positive tumours can be divided into two subtypes: HER2-enriched subtype (ER- and/or PR-negative/HER2-positive) and luminal HER2 subtype (ER- and/or PR-positive, HER2-positive).
   - These are further divided into two phenotypes based on PR expression: ER-positive, PR-positive, HER2-positive and ER-positive, PR-negative, HER2-positive. There is preclinical evidence for crosstalk between the HER2 and ER signalling pathways with a negative effect on the response to endocrine therapy.

   (d) **Basal-like (triple-negative, cytokeratin 5/6-positive and/or EGFR-positive; Flowchart 32.3)**
   - TNBC (triple negative breast cancer) is an aggressive subtype of breast cancer which typically has a high grade histology and high mitoses.
   - It represents 15%–20% of all invasive breast cancers and is defined by the absence of expression of ER, PR and HER2.
   - Most TNBCs manifest as invasive ductal carcinoma of NST; however, the category also includes variants such as metaplastic carcinoma, carcinoma with medullary features (formerly known as medullary carcinoma), carcinoma with apocrine features

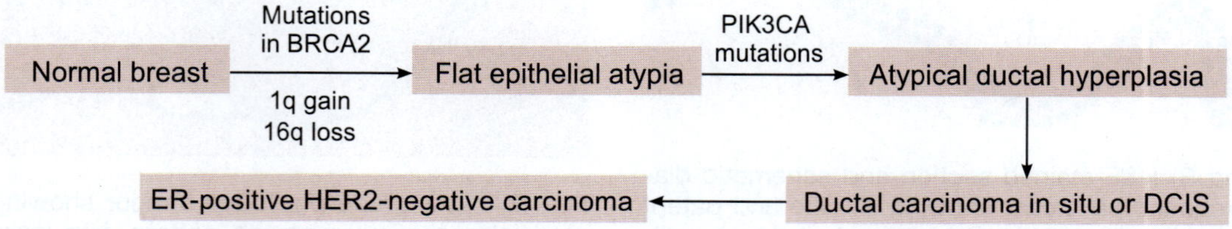

Flowchart 32.1 Pathway of development of ER-positive, HER2-negative breast carcinoma.

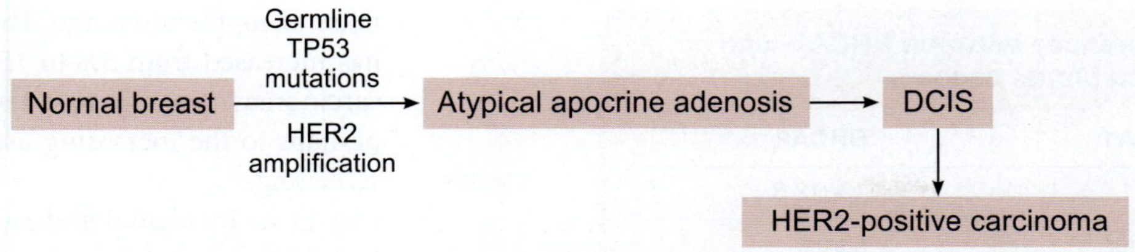

Flowchart 32.2 Pathway of development of HER2-positive breast carcinoma.

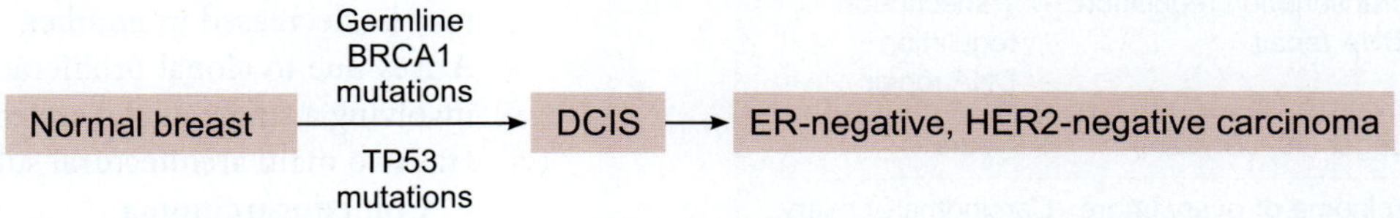

Flowchart 32.3 Pathway of development of ER-negative, HER2-negative breast carcinoma.

(formerly known as apocrine carcinoma), secretory carcinoma (formerly known as juvenile breast cancer) and adenoid cystic carcinoma.

- Gene expression profiling has enabled the subdivision of these cancers into different, prognostically significant subtypes that, in some cases, correlate with a particular pathological variant. The most common, and best characterized, molecular subtypes of TNBC are basal-like (BL breast cancers).
- BL breast cancers usually manifest clinically and pathologically as invasive ductal carcinoma NST and have high Ki-67 proliferative indices, whereas their expression profile is enriched in genes associated with basal cytokeratin genes (including *KRT5*), cell cycle and DNA replication, and DNA damage response pathways.

2. **Histological classification** (PA31.3)
   (a) **Non-invasive (precursor lesions):** Lesions that are confined to ducts and lobules and have not penetrated the limiting basement membrane. They can be further classified into:
   - DCIS
   - LCIS

   (b) **Invasive:** Lesions that have penetrated the limiting basement membrane. These include:
   - **Invasive breast carcinoma**
     - Invasive carcinoma of NST
     - Invasive lobular carcinoma (ILC)
     - Tubular carcinoma
     - Cribriform carcinoma
     - Mucinous carcinoma
     - Carcinoma with medullary features
     - Carcinoma with apocrine differentiation
     - Carcinoma with signet ring differentiation
     - Invasive micropapillary carcinoma
     - Metaplastic carcinoma of NST
     - Rare types
       - Carcinoma with neuroendocrine features
       - Secretory carcinoma
       - Invasive papillary carcinoma
       - Salivary gland/skin adnexal type tumours
   - **Epithelial-myoepithelial tumours**
     - Pleomorphic adenoma
     - Adenomyoepithelioma
     - Adenoid cystic carcinoma

Risk Factors for Breast Carcinoma

- **Age:** It is rare before 25 years, except in familial cases, peaks at 70–80 years and then declines in incidence. Menarche at age <11 years increases risk by 20% as compared with menarche at age >14 years.
- **Geography:** It has six times higher incidence in developed countries but the incidence is rising in developing countries.
- **Genetic factors**
  - Genetics involved in <10% of cases.
  - Increase in risk of breast cancer if family history of breast or ovarian cancer in a first-degree relative, especially if the disease occurred at an early age (<50 years).
  - Autosomal dominant mutations in BRCA1 (familial breast and ovarian cancer) and BRCA2 (familial breast and ovarian cancer), p53 (Li-Fraumeni syndrome) and CHEK2.
  - Family history of breast cancer (affected first-degree relatives who do not carry an established breast cancer gene mutation).
  - Overexpression of HER2/neu proto-oncogene.
  - Amplification of RAS and MYC genes.
- **Breastfeeding:** The longer the duration of breastfeeding, the less the incidence of breast carcinoma.
- **Hormonal influences:** Oestrogen excess (long duration of reproductive life, nulliparity, first child at a late age, increasing age and exogenous oestrogens). Oral contraceptives are not known to be associated with an increased incidence. Oophorectomy decreases the risk by decreasing endogenous oestrogens. Also, drugs like tamoxifen (which blocks oestrogen) and aromatase inhibitors (which decrease oestrogen synthesis) decrease the risk of ER-positive cancers.
- **Environmental factors:** Tobacco smoke, radiation exposure, organochlorine pesticides (have oestrogen-like effects) and alcohol intake increase the risk of breast carcinoma.

Table 32.2 Differences between BRCA1- and BRCA2-associated breast cancers

Features	BRCA1	BRCA2
Chromosome	17q21	13q12.3
Gene size	Smaller	Larger
Functions	- Tumour suppression - Transcription regulation - DNA repair	- Tumour suppression - Transcription regulation - DNA repair
Age at onset	Younger (40–50 years)	50 years
Risk of other tumours	Carcinoma of ovary (more than BRCA2), prostate, pancreas, fallopian tube and male breast cancer (less than BRCA1)	Carcinoma of ovary, prostate, pancreas, stomach, melanoma, biliary system, pharynx and male breast cancer
Pathology of breast cancers	Greater incidence of medullary carcinoma, poorly differentiated carcinoma, ER–PR and HER2/neu-negative carcinoma and carcinoma with P53 mutations	Similar to sporadic cancers (ER-negative cancers)

- **Proliferative breast disease and carcinoma of contralateral breast or endometrium** have several common risk factors.
- **Breast density:** High breast density on mammography has a four to five times higher risk of ER-positive and ER-negative cancers.
- **Obesity:** Obese women younger than 40 years have anovulatory cycles and lower progesterone levels, thereby reducing the risk, whereas postmenopausal obesity increases the risk attributed to oestrogen synthesis in the fat depots.

Familial Breast Cancer

Many familial cancers and 80%–90% of single-gene familial breast cancers are due to two autosomal dominant genes: BRCA1 and BRCA2 (Table 32.2).

Sporadic Breast Cancer

The main risk factors for sporadic cases of breast carcinoma include oestrogen excess, reproductive history, gender and age.

Distribution of Breast Carcinoma

Central area (20%), upper outer quadrant (50%), upper inner quadrant (10%), lower outer quadrant (10%) and lower inner quadrant (10%); left breast is more often involved than the right.

Pathology of Breast Carcinoma

1. **Non-invasive lesions**
   (a) **DCIS or intraductal carcinoma**
   (i) Presents most frequently as mammographic calcification, and less frequently as a vaguely palpable mass or nipple discharge. The incidence of DCIS has increased from 5% to 15%–30% of all breast carcinomas over the past few years, attributable perhaps to the increasing use of mammographic screening.
   (ii) May be an incidental finding on biopsy.
   (iii) Consists of a malignant population of cells limited to the ducts by the basement membrane.
   (iv) Myoepithelial cells are preserved, although they may be decreased in number.
   (v) Arises due to clonal proliferation of cells usually involving a single ductal system.
   (vi) Has two main architectural subtypes:
   - **Comedocarcinoma**
     - Characterized by solid sheets of pleomorphic cells with central necrosis.
     - Necrotic cell membranes frequently calcify and are seen on mammography as speckled microcalcifications, which may be grouped together or arranged in parallel lines.
     - Periductal concentric fibrosis and inflammation is common.
     - Extensive lesions may be palpable as vague nodularity.
   - **Non-comedo DCIS**
     - Does not show cellular pleomorphism or central necrosis.
     - May show different architectural patterns.
     - Consists of a monomorphic population of cells completely filling up the duct lumina **(solid type)**; cells may grow into the spaces lining fibrovascular cores **(papillary DCIS)**, or project into the spaces without definite fibrovascular cores forming complex intraductal patterns **(micropapillary DCIS)**. **Cribriform DCIS** has a cribriform pattern with round spaces between cell aggregates.

   (b) **LCIS**
   (i) Usually an incidental finding in breast biopsies performed for some other reason.
   (ii) Not associated with a clinically apparent mass or a mammographic abnormality (calcification or stromal reaction); so it is not readily diagnosed.
   (iii) Bilateral in up to 40% of the patients when both breasts are biopsied.
   (iv) LCIS is an intraepithelial proliferation of the TDLU. The cells of atypical lobular hyperplasia, LCIS and ILC are identical, i.e. loosely cohesive, small with oval-to-round nuclei and small nucleoli. LCIS is diagnosed when the entire lobular unit is replaced by tumour cells.
   (v) Signet ring cells containing mucin are frequently seen.
2. **Invasive carcinomas**
   - The terminology for the most common type of breast cancer has changed from invasive ductal carcinoma, not otherwise specified (NOS; 2003) to invasive carcinoma of (NST (2012). This group of breast cancers comprises

all tumours without the specific differentiating features that characterize the other specific categories of breast cancers. The name 'ductal' has been omitted because it indicates derivation of the tumours from only the ductal system. The use of 'carcinoma of NST' is the preferred term. The diagnosis is made by exclusion of recognized specific types of breast cancers. Other types of breast cancer with specific features are regarded as invasive ductal carcinomas, albeit of special type.

- The most common specific subtypes include invasive lobular, tubular, cribriform, metaplastic, apocrine, mucinous, papillary and micropapillary carcinoma, as well as carcinoma with medullary, neuroendocrine and salivary gland/skin adnexal-type features. These specific tumour types are defined by their morphology, but these are also linked to particular clinical, epidemiological and molecular features.

Invasive (infiltrating) carcinoma, NST

- Common type of invasive carcinoma; it usually has abundant fibrous stroma (therefore referred to as **scirrhous carcinoma**). Presents as a firm-to-hard lesion which makes a grating sound on cutting.
- Has irregular infiltrating borders with small pinpoint foci or streaks of **chalky-white elastosis/calcification** in the centre of the lesion.
- Well-differentiated tumours consist of tubules lined by minimally atypical cells which express hormone receptors and do not overexpress HER2/neu.
- Less-differentiated lesions are composed of cords and sheets of pleomorphic cells that do not express hormone receptors or overexpress HER2/neu (Fig. 32.4A and B).
- May be accompanied by **variable amounts of DCIS**. The grade of DCIS correlates with the grade of IDC (NOS). Large amounts of DCIS warrant wider excision.

Special subtypes of invasive breast carcinoma

(a) **ILC**

(i) Most cases present as a palpable ill-defined thickening/mass or a mammographic density.

(ii) Most common type of breast cancer to present as an occult primary.

(iii) Associated with a biallelic loss of expression of CDH1 (gene encoding for E-cadherin). Loss of E-cadherin induces a discohesiveness in the tumour because of which the tumour is seen histopathologically as single files of tumour cells infiltrating the stroma without induction of a desmoplastic response.

(iv) Tumour cells show minimal pleomorphism except in some variants (pleomorphic variant) and appear deceptively monomorphic.

(v) Variants such as solid, alveolar, pleomorphic, tubulolobular and mixed type are recognized and have differences in prognosis when compared with ILC of classic type. Among pleomorphic lobular carcinomas, apocrine, histiocytic or signet-ring cell differentiation can be observed.

(vi) Tumour grading of ILC is advocated, with the majority of classic ILCs being grade 2 in the Nottingham histological grading system and ILC of grade 3 comprising mostly a solid and pleomorphic subtype.

(vii) Immunostaining with E-cadherin can help in distinguishing ILC from NST carcinomas.

(viii) Lobular carcinomas metastasize to unusual sites. Metastasis to meninges, serosal surfaces, retroperitoneum, ovaries and GIT is more common than to lungs and pleura.

(b) **Medullary carcinoma**

(i) Although germline BRCA1 mutations are not present in most of these, hypermethylation of the

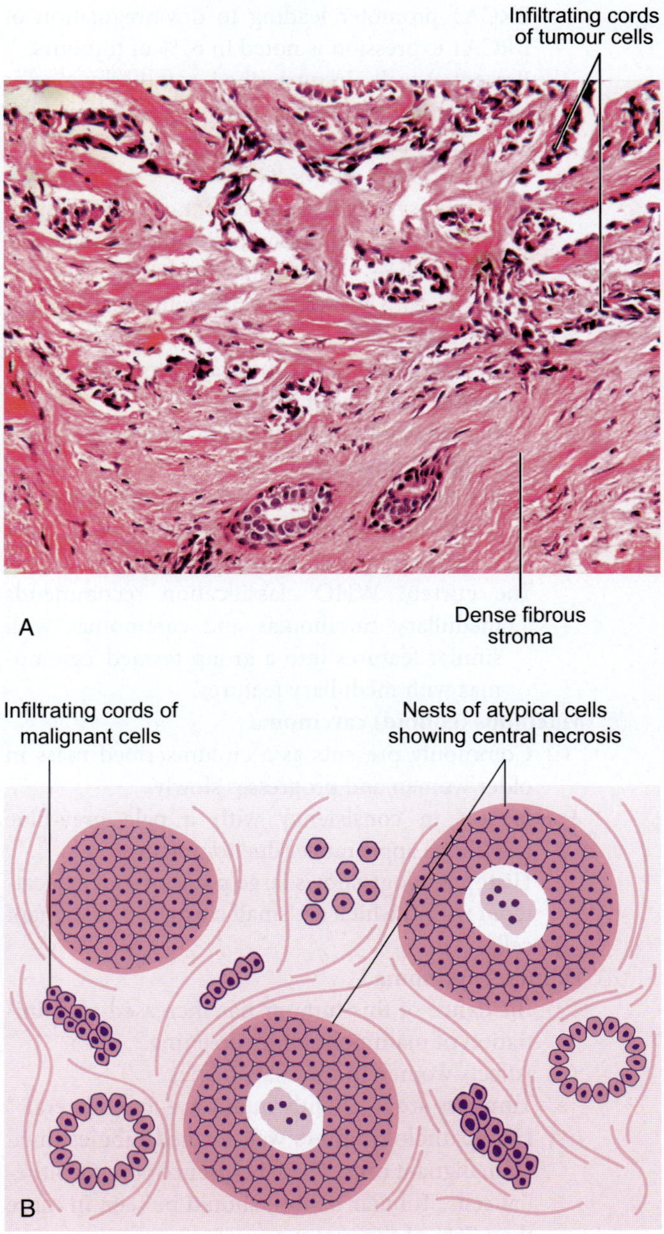

Fig. 32.4 (A and B) H&E-stained section and schematic diagram from invasive breast carcinoma (NST) showing tubules and cords of pleomorphic cells invading the fibrous stroma (H&E; 200×).

BRCA1 promoter leading to downregulation of BRCA1 expression is noted in 67% of tumours.

(ii) Present as well-circumscribed, soft, fleshy masses (*medulla* in Latin means *marrow*), which may be confused with benign lesions.

(iii) Histopathology shows:
- A solid syncytial arrangement occupying more than 75% of the tumour, with the tumour cells being large, pleomorphic, having vesicular nuclei with prominent nucleoli with frequent mitoses.
- Lymphoplasmacytic infiltrate surrounding and within the tumour nests.
- Pushing and non-infiltrative tumour margins.
- Minimal or absent DCIS.
- Absence of lymphatic or vascular invasion; lymph node involvement is rare.
- A better prognosis than NST.

The current WHO classification recommends medullary carcinomas and carcinomas with similar features into a group termed 'carcinomas with medullary features'.

(c) **Mucinous (colloid) carcinoma**

(i) Commonly presents as a circumscribed mass in older women and progresses slowly.

(ii) Is soft in consistency with a pale grey-blue gelatinous appearance (due to mucin).

(iii) Histopathology shows large pools of mucin, scattered within which are small clusters of malignant cells.

(d) **Tubular carcinoma**

(i) Incidence of this tumour has increased after initiation of mammographic screening.

(ii) Affects women in their late forties.

(iii) Tumours are frequently multifocal and bilateral.

(iv) Histopathology shows well-formed tubules lined by malignant cells. There is absence of myoepithelial cells. Tubular pattern should be seen in more than 75% of the tumour.

(v) Apocrine snouts are present and calcification is common.

(vi) Axillary metastasis is seen in fewer than 10% of the cases (excellent prognosis).

(e) **Invasive papillary carcinomas**

(i) Rare invasive carcinoma with papillary architecture.

(ii) Clinical presentation is similar to NST but prognosis is better.

(f) **Metaplastic carcinoma**

(i) Represents a group of invasive breast cancers showing differentiation of the tumour cells into squamous and mesenchymal elements (spindle, chondroid, osseous and rhabdomyoid cells) which are mixed with carcinoma of usual type.

(ii) Based on nuclear features, metaplastic carcinomas are classified into 'low-grade tumours' (e.g. low-grade adenosquamous carcinoma or low-grade spindle cell carcinoma) and 'high-grade tumours' (e.g. high-grade squamous cell carcinoma or high-grade spindle cell carcinoma).

(iii) They are triple-negative tumours, but have a worse prognosis than other forms of triple-negative breast cancers.

Prognostic or Predictive Factors of Breast Carcinoma

Major Prognostic Factors

- **Lymph node metastases:** Axillary lymph node status is the single most important prognostic factor. With no nodal involvement, 10-year disease-free survival rate is 70%–80%; with 1–3 positive nodes, it is 35%–40%; and with more than 10 positive nodes, it is 10%–15%. **Size of metastatic deposits** and **presence of invasion through the capsule** indicate poor prognosis.
- **Locally advanced disease:** Invasion into the skin and skeletal muscle indicates poor prognosis.
- **Inflammatory carcinoma:** Women presenting with a malignant breast mass with redness, oozing, inflamed appearance and skin thickening have a poor prognosis.
- **Tumour size:** It is the second most important independent factor. Five-year survival rate for tumour of size <1 cm (node-negative) is nearly 98% and it drops to 77% for tumours >2 cm.
- **Distant metastasis:** Presence of distant metastasis indicates poor prognosis.
- **Invasive carcinoma versus in situ disease:** In situ carcinoma is confined to the ductal system and does not metastasize, whereas at least half the invasive carcinomas metastasize.

Minor Prognostic Factors

- **Histological subtypes:** Special types of invasive carcinoma (tubular, colloid, medullary, lobular and papillary) have better prognosis than NST. Tubular and colloid carcinomas have an exceptionally good prognosis.
- **Tumour grade:** Most commonly used grading system is the **Nottingham histological score** or **Scarff–Bloom–Richardson** grading based on nuclear grade, tubule formation and mitotic rate. Ten-year survival for grade I tumours is 85%; grade II is 60% and grade III is 15%.
- **ER and PR:** Eighty per cent of tumours that are both ER- and PR-positive respond to hormonal therapy. Only 40% of those positive only for ER or PR receptors respond to the same. Strongly ER-positive tumours do not respond well to chemotherapy, and tumours that are neither ER-positive nor PR-positive are more likely to respond to chemotherapy than hormonal therapy.
- **HER2/neu (erb-B2):** Overexpression is associated with a bad prognosis. **Herceptin** is a monoclonal antibody to HER2/neu which targets tumour cells (**targeted therapy**).
- **Lymphovascular invasion:** Associated with a poor prognosis.
- **Proliferative rate:** Tumours with high proliferation rates have a worse prognosis.
- **Response to neoadjuvant therapy:** The degree to which the tumour responds to therapy given before surgery is an important prognostic factor. Clinical and radiological examination can be used to assess this response.

The major prognostic factors are used by the American Joint Committee on Cancer to divide breast carcinoma into the following stages:

- **Stage 0:** DCIS or LCIS (5-year survival rate, 92%).
- **Stage 1:** Invasive carcinoma 2 cm or less in diameter (including carcinoma in situ with microinvasion) without nodal involvement (5-year survival, 87%).
- **Stage 2:** Invasive carcinoma 5 cm or less in diameter with up to three involved axillary lymph nodes.

  Or invasive carcinoma more than 5 cm without nodal involvement (5-year survival, 75%).
- **Stage 3:** Invasive carcinoma 5 cm or less with four or more involved axillary lymph nodes.

  Or invasive carcinoma more than 5 cm with nodal involvement.

  Or invasive carcinoma with 10 or more involved axillary lymph nodes.

  Or invasive carcinoma with involvement of ipsilateral internal mammary lymph nodes.

  Or invasive carcinoma with skin involvement (oedema, ulceration or satellite skin nodules).

  Or chest wall fixation or clinical inflammatory carcinoma (5-year survival, 46%).
- **Stage 4:** Any breast carcinoma with distant metastasis (5-year survival, 5%–13%).

Q. Write briefly about Paget disease of breast.

Ans. Paget disease of breast is a rare form of DCIS with an incidence of 1%–4%. It presents as an erythematous eruption with scaling and crusting and may be mistaken for eczema.

Pathogenesis

Tumour cells from underlying ductal carcinoma migrate up into the lactiferous duct and invade the epidermis producing a skin lesion without invading the basement membrane.

Gross Morphology

- Skin of nipple and areola is fissured and ulcerated with or without nipple discharge.
- Inflammatory oedema and hyperaemia are seen in the surrounding tissue.
- Underlying palpable mass is present in 50%–60% of cases of Paget disease.

Microscopic Features

- **Histological hallmark** is involvement of epidermis by malignant cells **(Paget cells)**.
- Paget cells are large with abundant clear or lightly stained cytoplasm and nuclei with prominent nucleoli.
- Cells contain mucin and are positive for epithelial membrane antigens (EMA), *c-erb-B2* and low-molecular-weight keratins.

Prognosis depends on the extent of underlying carcinoma.

MALE BREAST

Q. Write briefly about gynaecomastia. (PA31.4)

Ans. Gynaecomastia is defined as enlargement of the male breast due to benign subareolar glandular proliferation. It may be unilateral or bilateral and has the following salient features:

- It may be idiopathic or due to hyperestrinism (cirrhosis and functioning testicular tumours), drugs (anabolic steroids, cimetidine, omeprazole, ketoconazole, spironolactone, digoxin, diethylstilbestrol, antipsychotics) and Klinefelter syndrome.
- Morphological features include proliferation of dense collagenous connective tissue and marked hyperplasia of the ductal and myoepithelial cells. Lobule formation is rare.

Q. Write briefly about male breast cancer.

Ans. Male breast cancer is rare and often gets diagnosed in late stages.

Salient Features

- Incidence is 1% that of females.
- Risk factors are similar to those in women; 3%–8% of cases are associated with Klinefelter syndrome and decreased testicular function.
- It usually presents between sixth and seventh decades with a subareolar mass and nipple discharge (breast epithelium in males restricted to large ducts near areola).
- It is associated with BRCA2 and BRCA1 mutations.
- Eighty-one per cent are ER-positive; prognostic factors and pathology are similar to those of female breast cancer.

33 Diseases of the Endocrine System

THYROID

- Weighs 15–20 g.
- Has a rich intraglandular capillary network from superior and inferior thyroid arteries and nerve supply from cervical sympathetic ganglia.
- The gland is divided by thin fibrous septae into lobules composed of 20–40 evenly dispersed follicles.
- Follicles are lined by cuboidal to low-columnar epithelium and contain thyroglobulin.
- Homoeostasis in the hypothalamus–pituitary–thyroid axis ensures maintenance of normal thyroid functioning (Flowchart 33.1).

Q. Enumerate the functions of thyroid.

Ans. The primary function of the thyroid is the production of iodine-containing thyroid hormones, triiodothyronine (T_3) and thyroxine (T_4), and the peptide hormone calcitonin. Thyroid hormones are created from iodine and tyrosine. T_3 contains three atoms of iodine per molecule and T_4 contains four atoms of iodine per molecule. Thyroid hormones have a wide range of effects on the human body:

- **Metabolic:** Thyroid hormones increase the basal metabolic rate (BMR; thereby increasing appetite, absorption and gut motility). They also control the synthesis of low-LDL receptors for LDL and β-adrenergic receptors for catecholamines.
- **Cardiovascular:** These hormones increase breathing rate, intake and consumption of oxygen, and the activity of mitochondria, thereby increasing blood flow and the body temperature.
- **Developmental:** Thyroid hormones contribute to normal development by increasing the growth rate and cellular regeneration. They play a crucial role in brain maturation during fetal development, and maintain normal sexual function and menstrual cycle in females.

Q. Write briefly about thyroid function tests.

Ans. Important thyroid function tests include:

1. **Thyroid-stimulating hormone (TSH) assay:** Third-generation TSH assays are readily available and are generally the most sensitive screening tool for primary hypothyroidism (reference range for normal serum TSH is 0.40–4.2 mIU/L). A decreased serum TSH is seen in thyrotoxicosis (increased T_3/T_4 decrease the serum TSH by negative feedback), hypopituitarism (decreased synthesis of TSH causes a reduced synthesis of T_3/T_4, also called secondary hypothyroidism) and hypothalamic dysfunction (decreased synthesis of thyrotropin-releasing hormone [TRH] reduces the synthesis of TSH; Table 33.1). In patients with hypothalamic or pituitary dysfunction, TSH levels do not increase proportionately to the low free T_4 levels. The absolute levels may be in the reference range or even slightly elevated while still being inappropriately low for the severity of the hypothyroid state. Hence, when secondary or tertiary hypothyroidism is suspected, measurement of serum TSH alone is inadequate; free T_4 should also be measured (see Table 33.1).
2. **Free T_3 and T_4 levels:** In cases with increased TSH levels, free thyroxine (T_4) levels are measured. T_4 is highly protein-bound (99.97%), with approximately 85% bound to thyroid-binding globulin (TBG), approximately 10% bound to transthyretin or thyroid-binding prealbumin and the remainder bound loosely to albumin. The levels of these binding proteins can vary based on genetics and hormonal status; therefore, free T_4 assays are considered more reliable. However, free T_4 assays can be unreliable in the setting of severe illness or pregnancy.
3. **Assays for anti–thyroid peroxidase (anti-TPO) and anti-thyroglobulin (anti-Tg) antibodies:** These are helpful in determining the underlying aetiology of hypothyroidism.
4. **The TRH stimulation test:** This test is rarely needed for assessing pituitary and hypothalamic dysfunction. With the improvements in TSH and free T_4 assays, TRH stimulation is now only occasionally done.
5. **Other tests:** There may be accompanying **anaemia, dilutional hyponatraemia, hyperlipidaemia and reversible increases in serum creatinine**. Elevations in transaminases and creatinine kinase have also been found. Primary hypothyroidism causes an elevation of TRH, which can cause an elevation of prolactin along with TSH. Prolactin levels in patients with hypothyroidism tend to be lower than those usually seen with prolactinomas.
6. **Imaging:** Ultrasonography of the neck and thyroid can be used to detect nodular or diffuse disease. Hashimoto thyroiditis and lymphomas are usually associated with a diffusely heterogeneous ultrasonographic imaging. Doppler scanning is used for assessment of vascularity, which aids in differentiating thyroiditis from Graves' disease (former will have decreased flow, whereas the latter will have increased flow).

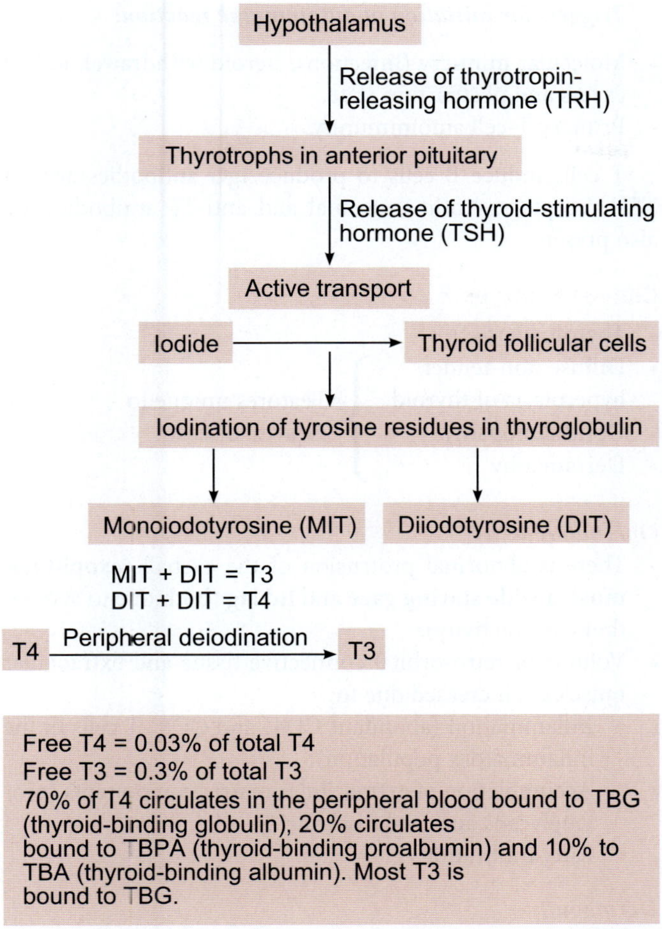

Flowchart 33.1 Mechanism of homoeostasis in the hypothalamus–pituitary–thyroid axis and release of thyroid hormones.

Table 33.1 Hormone levels in various thyroid conditions

Condition	Thyroid-stimulating hormone (TSH)	Free T_4	T_3
Hypothyroidism (clinical)	High	Low	Low
Hypothyroidism (subclinical)	High	Normal	Normal
Hyperthyroidism	Low	High	High
Subclinical hyperthyroidism	Low	Normal	Normal

7. **Radioactive iodine uptake (RAIU) and thyroid scanning:** These are not useful in hypothyroidism, because these tests require some level of endogenous thyroid function if they are to provide useful information. The test evaluates synthetic activity of the thyroid gland (iodine is used for synthesis of thyroid hormones). Increased uptake is seen in Graves' disease and toxic nodular goitre. Increased I-123 uptake is seen in 'hot thyroid nodules' and decreased uptake in 'cold thyroid nodules'. Examples of cold thyroid nodules include thyroid cysts, adenomas and thyroid cancer. Examples of hot thyroid nodules include a toxic nodular goitre.
8. **Serum thyroglobulin:** Can be used as a marker for thyroid cancer.

Q. Define thyrotoxicosis. Enumerate the disorders associated with hyperthyroidism.

(PA32.2, 32.3, IM12.1, 12.3)

Ans. Thyrotoxicosis is a hypermetabolic systemic state which occurs due to increased free T_3 and T_4 levels regardless of the cause. It is most commonly due to hyperfunctioning of the thyroid gland, also known as 'hyperthyroidism'. Hyperthyroidism indicates increased thyroid hormone synthesis and secretion from the thyroid gland, whereas thyrotoxicosis refers to the clinical syndrome of excess circulating thyroid hormones, irrespective of the source.

Disorders Associated With Hyperthyroidism

Common

- Diffuse toxic hyperplasia (**Graves' disease**).
- Toxic multinodular goitre (**Plummer disease**).
- Toxic adenoma.

Uncommon

- Acute or subacute thyroiditis.
- Hyperfunctioning thyroid carcinoma.
- Choriocarcinoma or hydatidiform mole (due to mild thyrotropic effect of hCG).
- TSH-secreting pituitary adenoma.
- Neonatal thyrotoxicosis with maternal Graves' disease.
- Struma ovarii.
- Iodide-induced hyperthyroidism.
- Iatrogenic (**Job–Basedow disease**).

Q. Write briefly about the clinical manifestations and diagnosis of hyperthyroidism. (PA32.2, 32.3)

Ans. Hyperthyroidism is a systemic state in which there is hyperfunctioning of the thyroid gland.

Clinical Manifestations of Hyperthyroidism

- Increased BMR, tachycardia, cardiomegaly, arrhythmias and congestive heart failure (due to increased cardiac contractility). Also, thyrotoxic dilated cardiomyopathy (shows lymphoeosinophilic infiltration of myocardium with fatty change and fibrosis).
- Generalized lymphoid hyperplasia and lymphadenopathy.
- Ocular changes, e.g. a wide, staring gaze and lid lag (due to sympathetic overstimulation) and true thyroid ophthalmopathy (as seen in Graves' disease).
- Increased appetite, but weight loss; increased gut motility, tremors, hyperactivity, emotional liability, anxiety, inability to concentrate, insomnia and heat intolerance (due to overactivity of sympathetic nervous system).
- Proximal muscle weakness (caused by atrophy and fatty infiltration of skeletal muscle; also called thyroid myopathy).

- Warm and moist skin showing flushing and increased sweating (due to peripheral vasodilatation).
- Bone resorption (causing osteoporosis and increased risk of fractures).
- Fatty liver.

Diagnosis of Hyperthyroidism

Hyperthyroidism is diagnosed based on findings of a low serum TSH and increased free T_4.

Q. Describe the aetiopathogenesis and clinicopathological features of Graves' disease.

Ans. Graves' disease is the most common cause of endogenous hyperthyroidism with a peak incidence between 20 and 40 years and a female to male ratio of 7:1. Its genetic basis is supported by the fact that there is a 60% concordance in monozygotic twins and an association with human leucocyte antigen (HLA)-B8 and -DR3. The genetic susceptibility is linked to polymorphisms in multiple immune regulatory genes, e.g. cytotoxic T-lymphocyte-associated antigen 4 (CTLA4) and protein tyrosine phosphatase 22 (PTPN22). Graves' disease is a triad of:

- Hyperthyroidism due to diffuse hyperplasia of follicular epithelium.
- Infiltrative ophthalmopathy with resultant exophthalmos.
- Localized infiltrative dermopathy called pretibial myxoedema.

Pathogenesis

Multiple autoantibodies have been demonstrated in Graves' disease, primarily against the TSH receptor. These include:

1. **Thyroid-stimulating immunoglobulin (TSI)**
   - TSI is an IgG immunoglobulin that binds to TSH receptor on the membrane of follicular cells and mimics the action of TSH (Flowchart 33.2).
   - Almost all patients demonstrate this antibody.
   - It is specific for Graves' disease.
2. **Thyroid growth-stimulating immunoglobulin (TGI)**
   - Also directed against TSH receptor.
   - Induces proliferation of thyroid follicular epithelium leading to diffuse hyperplasia of the gland.
3. **Thyroid binding inhibitor immunoglobulin (TBII)**
   - Also called anti-TSH receptor antibody, it prevents TSH from binding to its receptor on follicular cells.
   - Some forms of TBII mimic the action of TSH causing hyperthyroidism and others actually inhibit thyroid function leading to hypothyroidism.

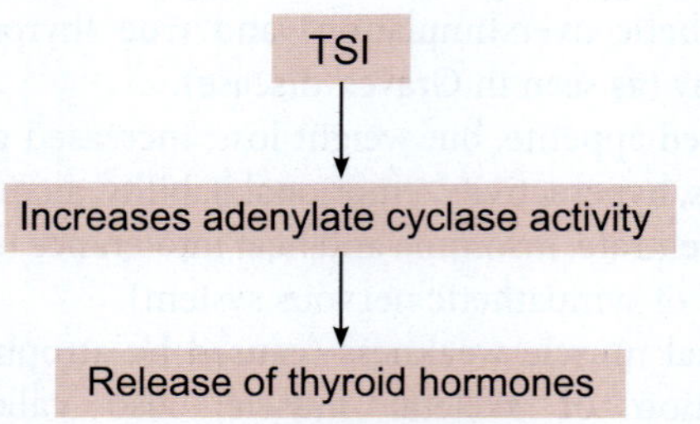

Flowchart 33.2 Mechanism of action of TSI.

Triggers for initiation of autoimmune reaction:

- Molecular mimicry (infection), steroid withdrawal, iodide excess and postpartum state.
- Primary T-cell autoimmunity.

T cells induce B cells to produce IgG antibodies against TSH receptors. Antimicrosomal and anti-Tg antibodies are also present.

Clinical Features

- Thyrotoxicosis
- Diffuse non-tender hyperplasia of thyroid
- Ophthalmopathy
- Dermopathy

} Features unique to Graves' disease (diffuse non-tender hyperplasia of thyroid, ophthalmopathy, dermopathy)

Ophthalmopathy

- There is abnormal protrusion of the eyeball (**exophthalmos**), **a wide staring gaze** and **lid lag** (both due to sympathetic overactivity).
- Volume of retro-orbital connective tissue and extraocular muscles is increased due to:
  - Inflammation (abundant $CD4^+$ and $CD8^+$ T cells in the inflammatory population).
  - Accumulation of extracellular matrix components (proteoglycans and hyaluronic acid).
  - Fatty infiltration.

Dermopathy

- Skin overlying shins shows scaly thickening and induration (**pretibial myxoedema**).
- Also seen are pigmented papules or nodules with orange peel texture.
- It is caused by excessive deposit of extracellular matrix components (proteoglycans and hyaluronic acid) in the dermis.

Other Changes

- These include clubbing of fingers, periosteal reaction of metacarpals and phalanges, lifting of nail from nail bed, normocytic normochromic anaemia, low TLC and neutropenia with relative lymphocytosis. In the elderly, Graves' disease can present with atrial fibrillation and heart failure.

Laboratory Findings

- Elevated free T_3, T_4 and TSH.
- Increased diffuse RAIU.

Gross Morphology

- The gland is diffusely enlarged, weighing more than 80 g.
- The gland is smooth and soft with an intact capsule.
- The cut surface shows a **soft meaty appearance (resembling muscle)**.

Microscopy (Fig. 33.1)

- Follicles are lined by tall columnar cells showing crowding ('too many cells'), and have pale scalloped colloid.

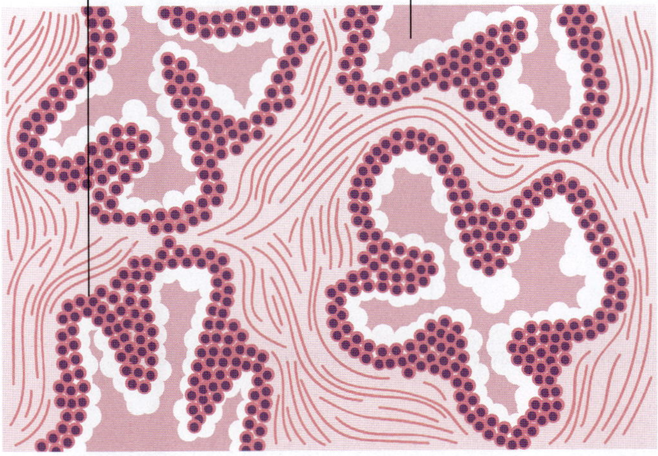

Fig. 33.1 Diagrammatic representation of histopathology of Grave's disease showing follicles lined by hyperplastic tall columnar epithelium at places thrown into papillary projections. The lumen of the follicles shows pale colloid with a scalloped appearance and the stroma is infiltrated by chronic inflammatory cells.

- Hyperplasia of the follicular lining epithelium results in the formation of hyperplastic papillae or pseudopapillae (papillae without fibrovascular cores).
- Large reactive lymphoid follicles with germinal centres may be present in the interfollicular stroma.

Q. Write briefly about the aetiopathogenesis, clinical manifestations and diagnosis of hypothyroidism. (PA32.3, IM12.1, 12.3)

Ans. Hypothyroidism is a structural or functional derangement that interferes with the production of adequate level of thyroid hormones.

Causes

Thyroidal

- **Insufficient thyroid parenchyma**
  - Developmental (thyroid dysgenesis).
  - Radiation injury.
  - Surgical ablation.
  - Hashimoto thyroiditis.
- **Interference with thyroid hormone synthesis**
  - Idiopathic primary hypothyroidism.
  - Heritable biosynthetic defects.
  - Iodine deficiency.
  - Drugs (lithium, iodides, P-aminosalicylic acid).
  - Hashimoto thyroiditis.

Suprathyroidal

- Pituitary lesions (tumours, radiation damage and surgical removal) reducing TSH.
- Hypothalamic lesions that reduce TRH delivery.

Classical Clinical Manifestations

- **Cretinism** Hypothyroidism developing in infancy and childhood which is characterized by impaired development of the skeletal system and CNS presenting as delayed milestones, delayed bone maturation, severe mental retardation, short stature, coarse facial features, protruding tongue and umbilical hernia.
- **Myxoedema:** Hypothyroidism developing in older children or adults characterized by:
  - Decreased physical and mental activity, fatigue, apathy, mental sluggishness and depression.
  - Slow speech and intellectual functions.
  - Increased weight and cold intolerance.
  - Reduced cardiac output causing shortness of breath and decreased exercise capacity.
  - Constipation and decreased sweating.
  - Oedema, broadening and coarsening of facial features, enlargement of tongue and deepening of voice.

Laboratory Findings

- Increased TSH and decreased T_3 and T_4.
- Low free T_4 and high TSH levels used for screening.

Q. Define and classify thyroiditis. Describe the aetiopathogenesis, clinical features and morphology of different types of thyroiditis.

Ans. Thyroiditis is inflammation of thyroid gland.

Types

1. **Infectious thyroiditis**
   - May be acute or chronic.
   - The patient presents with fever, tender thyroid, painful lymphadenopathy and initial thyrotoxicosis (due to destruction of the gland). Sustained hypothyroidism is rare.
   - Infection reaches thyroid by haematogenous route or through direct seeding (trauma) of the gland.
   - Common causative organisms include *Staphylococcus aureus,* mycobacteria, fungi and pneumocystis.
2. '**Other common and clinically significant thyroiditis**', **which include:**
   (a) **Hashimoto thyroiditis**
   Salient features
   - Most common cause of autoimmune thyroiditis and primary hypothyroidism.
   - May occur in children and is the main cause of non-endemic goitre in this age group.
   - Peak incidence is between 45 and 65 years; female to male ratio = 10:1.
   - Occurs in clusters in families.
   - Concordance in monozygotic twins is 30%–60%.
   - Shows HLA-DR3 and -DR5 association and increased incidence of SLE, Sjögren's syndrome, pernicious anaemia, type I diabetes mellitus (DM) and rheumatoid arthritis.
   - Patients present with painless enlargement of thyroid. There is insidious onset of hypothyroidism after a transient phase of Hashitoxicosis (thyrotoxicosis is due to inflammatory disruption of thyroid follicles leading to the release of thyroid hormones).

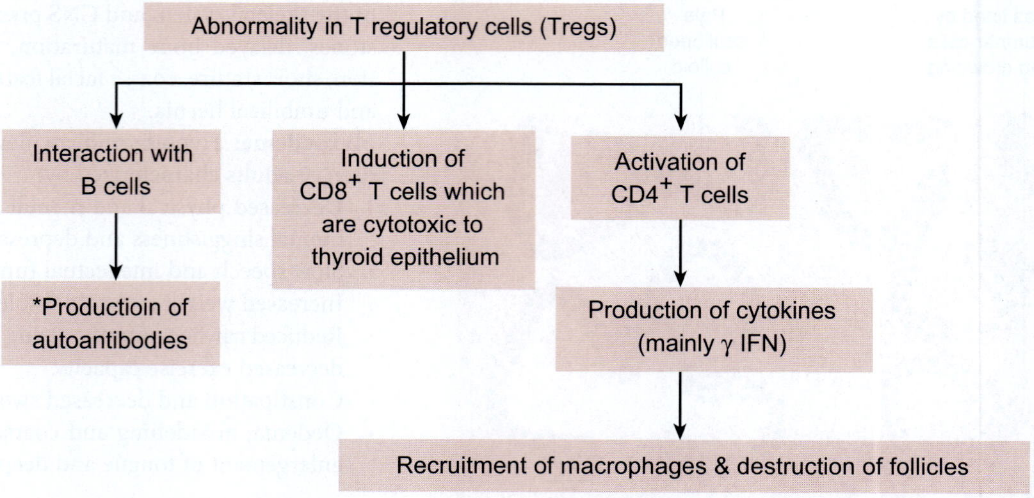

*B cells produce autoantibodies to:

- Thyroglobulin and thyroid peroxidase
  - Thyroglobulin: Follicular cells synthesize thyroglobulin, which is secreted into the lumen as colloid.
  - Thyroid peroxidase: Thyroid peroxidase is located on the luminal surface of follicular cells; catalyses both tyrosine iodination and coupling of iodotyrosyl residues to form T3 and T4. Antibodies to thyroglobulin and thyroid peroxidase are non-specific.
- TSH receptor: TSH receptor is a G protein-coupled transmembrane receptor, antibodies against which are specific in nature.
- Iodine transporter: Mediates the transport of iodine into thyroid (first step in thyroid hormone synthesis).

Note: *'Most antithyroid antibodies can fix complement'. Follicular destruction is attributed to complement-dependent, antibody-mediated cytotoxicity (ADCC). Apoptosis by Fas–Fas ligand system is also implicated in destruction of thyroid tissue.

Flowchart 33.3 Pathogenesis of Hashimoto thyroiditis.

Pathogenesis

- The genetic susceptibility is linked to polymorphisms in multiple immune regulatory genes, e.g. CTLA4 and PTPN22.
- Both cellular and humoral mechanisms are involved.
- Cellular immunity is primarily mediated by a defect in T cells (abnormalities of regulatory T cells [Tregs], exposure of normally sequestrated thyroid antigens, decreased number of suppressor T cells and emergence of thyroid-specific helper T cells, all contributing to autoimmunity).
- Abnormality in Tregs and breakdown of tolerance lead to autoimmunity (Flowchart 33.3).
- Cytotoxic T cells destroy the parenchyma via type IV hypersensitivity. Blocking antibodies are present against TSH receptor and these decrease hormone synthesis via type II hypersensitivity. $CD4^+$ T cells release cytokines which induct macrophages that damage the thyroid via type IV hypersensitivity.

Gross morphology

- Diffuse/rarely localized.
- The capsule remains intact.
- The cut surface is pale, grey-tan, firm and rubbery with accentuation of lobulation.

Microscopy (Fig. 33.2)

- There is extensive infiltration of parenchyma by a mononuclear infiltrate (lymphocytes, including well-developed germinal centres and plasma cells).
- Follicles undergo atrophy and there is formation of Hürthle cells (degenerated follicular cells with abundant granular eosinophilic cytoplasm and prominent nucleoli; also called **Askanazy cells** or **oncocytes**).
- Interstitial connective tissue is increased; however, fibrosis does not extend outside the capsule.
- Hashimoto thyroiditis has a **fibrous variant**, in which the thyroid becomes small and atrophic because of extensive fibrosis.

(b) **Granulomatous thyroiditis/de Quervain thyroiditis**

Salient features

- Peak age 30–50 years; female to male ratio = 3–5:1.
- Association with HLA-B35.
- Seasonal peak in summers.

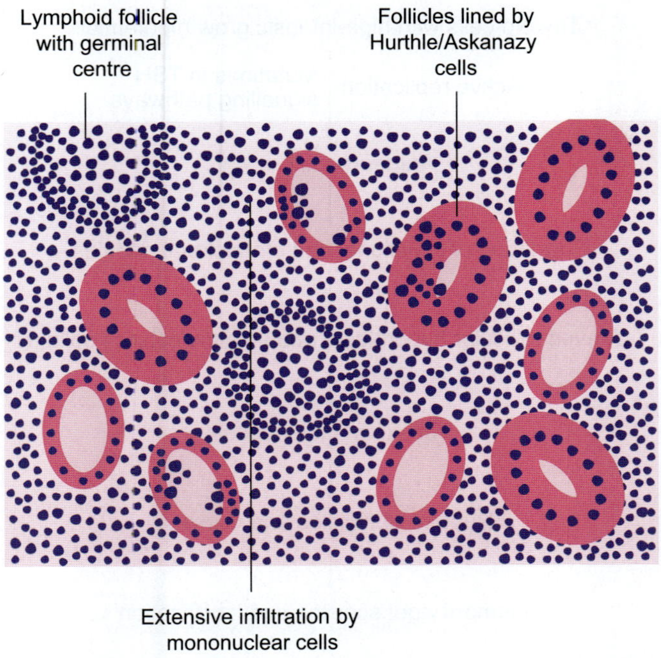

Fig. 33.2 Schematic diagram showing extensive infiltration of thyroid parenchyma by a mononuclear infiltrate (lymphocytes, including well-developed germinal centres and plasma cells). Follicular atrophy is seen with presence of Hürthle cells (degenerated follicular cells with abundant granular eosinophilic cytoplasm and prominent nucleoli; also called Askanazy cells or oncocytes).

- Usually follows an upper respiratory tract infection with coxsackievirus, mumps, measles and adenovirus.
- Presents with pain in upper neck, jaw, throat, ears, fever, fatigue, malaise, anorexia, myalgias and enlargement of the thyroid.
- The usual sequence of events: Transient hyperthyroidism (lasting approximately 2–6 weeks) followed by hypothyroidism (lasting 2–8 weeks) followed by recovery.

Pathogenesis: See Flowchart 33.4.

Viral infection
↓
Availability of antigen (viral antigen or virus-induced/altered host antigen)
↓
Antigen presentation in association with HLA-B35
↓
Formation of cytotoxic T cells
↓
Damage to thyroid follicular cells
↓
Rupture of thyroid follicles and release of thyroid hormones
↓
Transient hyperthyroidism
↓
Hypothyroidism (due to loss of thyroid substance)
↓
Recovery

Flowchart 33.4 Pathogenesis of de Quervain thyroiditis.

Gross morphology
- Unilateral or bilateral enlargement.
- The capsule is intact and may be adherent to surroundings.
- The cut surface is yellow-white, rubbery and firm.

Microscopy

Early changes
- Scattered disruption of follicles.
- Replacement by neutrophilic microabscesses.

Late changes
- Aggregates of lymphocytes, histiocytes and plasma cells.
- Presence of multinucleate giant cells around pools of colloid.
- Fibrosis.

(c) **Subacute lymphocytic (painless) thyroiditis**

Salient features
- Affects middle-aged women generally in the postpartum period.
- Associated with HLA-DR3 and -DR5.
- Thought to be a variant of Hashimoto thyroiditis.
- Patients demonstrate increased levels of antibodies to thyroglobulin and TPO.
- Manifests with hyperthyroidism followed by reversion to a euthyroid state (in a minority of patients, the disease may progress to hypothyroidism).

Gross morphology: Mild symmetric enlargement of thyroid

Microscopy
- Focal disruption of thyroid follicles.
- Multifocal inflammatory infiltrate (predominantly small lymphocytes).
- No plasma cells, germinal centres or Hürthle cell metaplasia; if present, think of Hashimoto thyroiditis.

Q. Define and classify goitre. Describe the aetiopathogenesis, clinical manifestations and morphology of the various types of goitre. (PA32.1)

Ans. Goitre is defined as enlargement of the thyroid gland.

Sequence of Events in the Development of Goitre (See Flowchart 33.5)

1. **Diffuse non-toxic (simple) goitre:** Diffuse enlargement of the thyroid gland without nodularity.

   Types

   (a) **Endemic**

   (i) Common in **Alps, Andes and Himalayas** (labelled endemic when more than 10% of the population is affected).

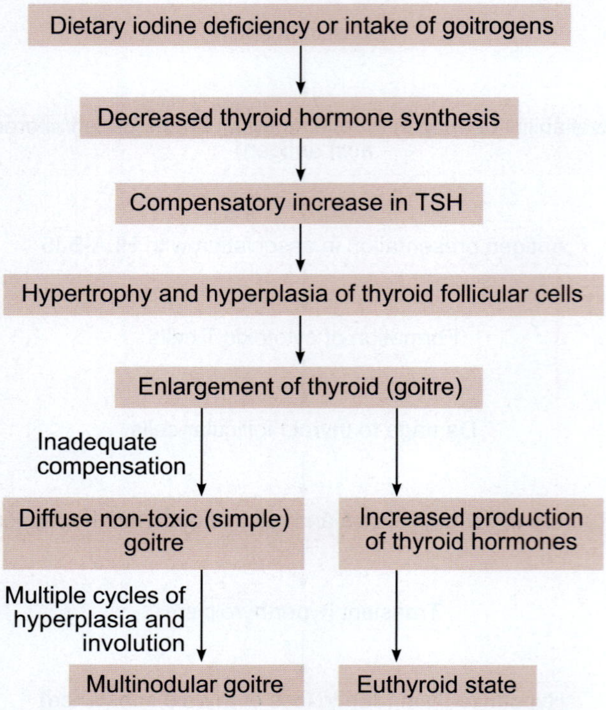

Flowchart 33.5 Sequence of events in development of goitre.

(ii) Dietary supplements decrease the incidence.

(iii) Variation in the prevalence of goitre in regions with similar levels of iodine deficiency indicates the existence of other dietary influences, called **goitrogens**, which may influence the prevalence rate.

(iv) Goitrogens, e.g. vegetables of Brassicaceae and Cruciferae families (cabbage, cauliflower, Brussels sprouts, turnip and cassava) and excessive calcium in the diet, interfere with thyroid hormone synthesis.

(b) **Sporadic**

(i) Less common than endemic goitre; females affected more often than males.

(ii) Seen at the onset of puberty or in young adults.

(iii) Associated with hereditary enzyme defects and ingestion of goitrogens; not corrected by dietary supplements. There are four major types of enzyme defects:

- Iodide transport defect.
- Organification defect **(Pendred syndrome)**.
- Dehalogenase defect.
- Iodotyrosine coupling defect.

Morphology

Two morphological stages are identified, namely:

- Stage of hyperplasia.
  - Diffuse and symmetric enlargement of the thyroid.
  - Follicles lined by crowded columnar cells with piling up of epithelium and formation of pseudopapillary projections.
  - Variable colloid content in the follicles.

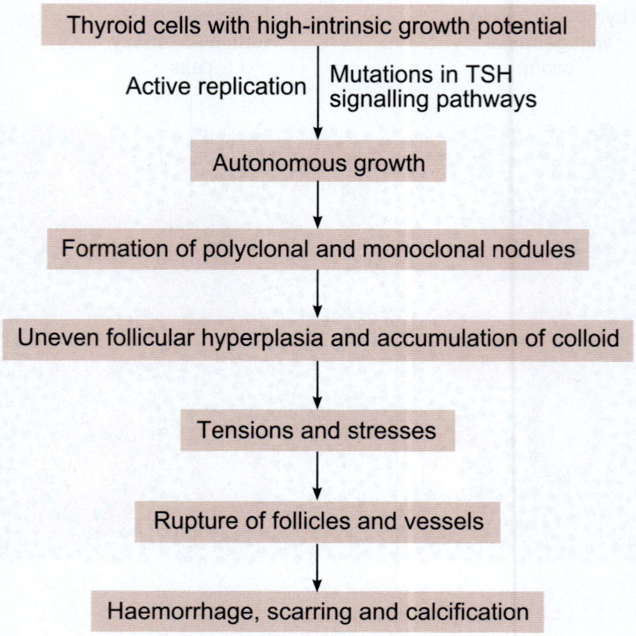

Flowchart 33.6 Evolution of a multinodular goitre.

- Stage of involution
  - It starts if the dietary iodine increases or demand for thyroid hormones decreases.
  - Follicular epithelium involutes and becomes flattened.
  - Flattened follicular epithelium with abundant colloid results in an enlarged, colloid-rich gland (**colloid goitre**).

Clinical features

- Patients are usually clinically euthyroid.
- Main symptoms are due to mass effects.

2. **Multinodular goitre (MNG)**

- Repeated episodes of hyperplasia and involution lead to irregular enlargement of thyroid with the formation of nodules.
- MNG may be non-toxic or toxic depending on the secretion of T_3 and T_4.
- Normal thyroid cells are heterogeneous with respect to response to TSH and ability to replicate. Thyroid cells with high intrinsic growth potential replicate actively.

Steps in the evolution of MNG are given in Flowchart 33.6.

Gross morphology (Fig. 33.3A)

- Multinodular, asymmetrically enlarged thyroid.
- May exert lateral pressure on midline structures (trachea and oesophagus).
- Growth behind sternum and clavicles labelled **'intrathoracic or plunging goitre'.**

Cut surface

- Irregular nodules showing a variable amount of brown gelatinous colloid.
- Regressive changes, such as haemorrhage, calcification, fibrosis and cystic change.

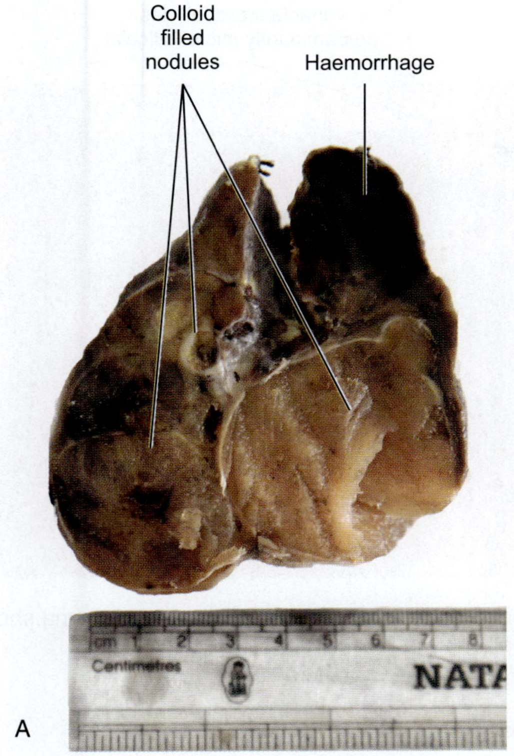

Fig. 33.3 (A) Gross picture of a multinodular goiter showing multiple nodules of variable size, some colloid filled, with areas of haemorrhage.

Microscopy (Figs. 33.3B and C)

- The nodules consist of colloid-filled follicles of varying size lined by flat to cuboidal epithelium. These follicles may fuse to form large colloid-filled cysts.
- In the background of an enlarged multinodular thyroid, a solitary dominant or hyperplastic nodule may show follicular hyperplasia and hypertrophy (called **nodular adenomatous goitre**).
- Adenomatous goitre can be confused with a follicular adenoma; however, the latter shows a prominent capsule which is lacking in an adenomatous nodule.

Clinical features

- Patients are usually euthyroid and present with an asymptomatic mass in the neck. Some patients may have subclinical hyperthyroidism and decreased TSH levels and others may develop frank hyperthyroidism or toxic MNG (**Plummer syndrome**).
- Main symptoms are due to mass effects (airway obstruction due to compression of trachea, dysphagia due to compression of the oesophagus, venous congestion of the head due to compression of superior vena cava and hoarseness due to recurrent laryngeal nerve compression).

Q. Enumerate the salient features of a solitary nodule of thyroid.

Ans. A solitary thyroid nodule is a palpable discrete swelling within an otherwise normal thyroid gland. It demonstrates the following salient features:

- It is more likely to be malignant than multiple nodules.

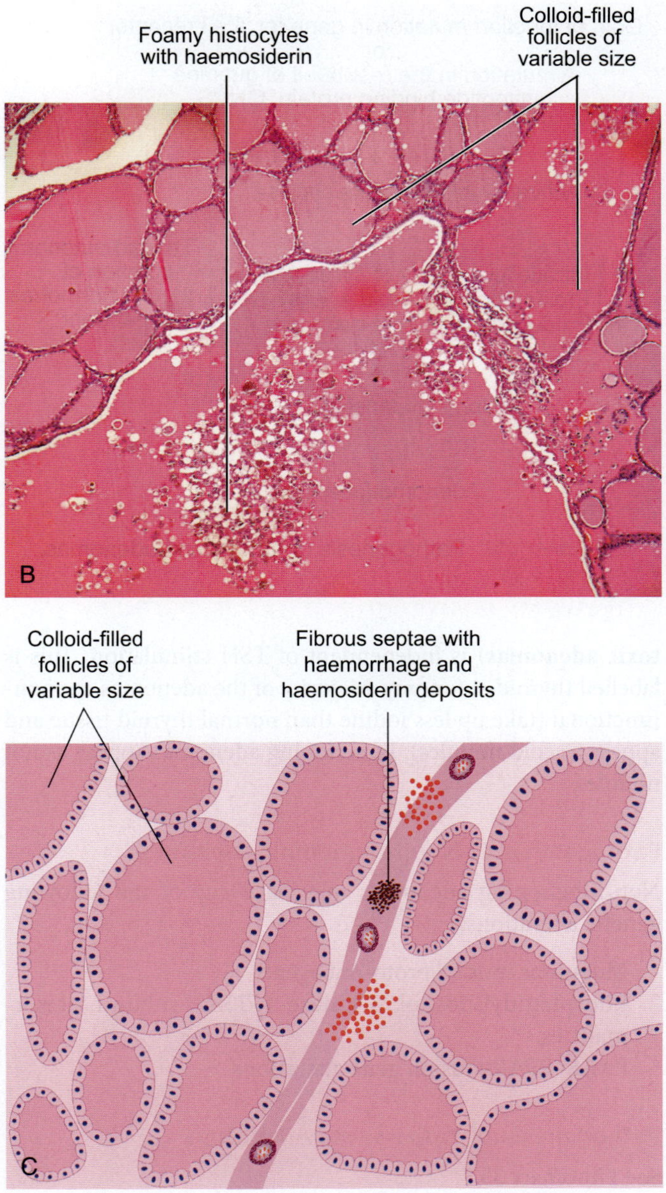

Fig. 33.3 (B and C) Photomicrograph and diagrammatic representation of a nodule showing follicles of varying size lined by flat to cuboidal epithelium. There is a focus of haemorrhage with aggregates of haemosiderin-laden macrophages (H&E; 100×).

- Nodules in younger patients and males are more often malignant than nodules in older patients and females.
- Nodules that do not take up radioactive iodine (cold nodules) are more likely to be malignant.
- Nodules that take up radioactive iodine (hot nodules) are more likely to be benign, e.g. nodular (adenomatous) goitre, thyroiditis and simple cysts.
- Causes of a solitary thyroid nodule include cysts, follicular adenoma and thyroid malignancy in that order of frequency.

Q. Write briefly about the pathogenesis and clinicomorphological features of adenomas of thyroid.

Ans. Adenomas are discrete, solitary masses derived from the follicular epithelium (thus, also called follicular adenomas). Hormone production in functional adenomas (also called

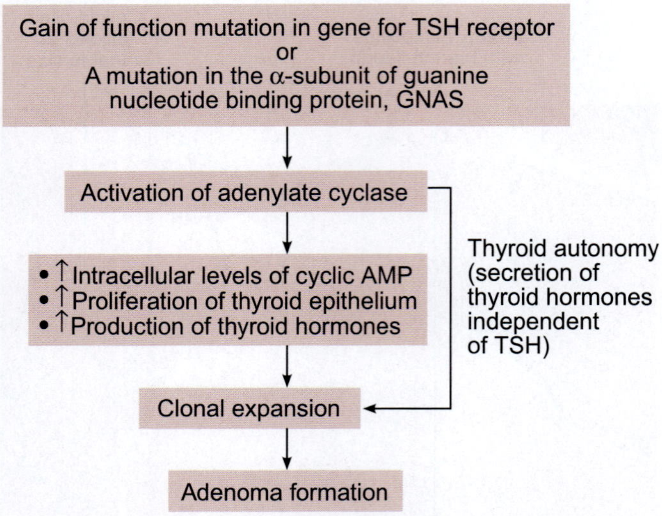

Flowchart 33.7 Pathogenesis of functioning adenomas.

toxic adenomas) is independent of TSH stimulation. This is labelled thyroid autonomy. Majority of the adenomas are non-functional (take up less iodine than normal thyroid tissue and appear as cold nodules). Functioning adenomas appear as hot nodules.

Pathogenesis of Non-functioning Adenomas

Non-functioning adenomas may have any of the following genetic alterations:

1. Mutations in RAS proto-oncogene.
2. Phosphatidylinositol 3-kinase (PI3K) subunit abnormalities.
3. PAX8–PPARγ fusion gene alterations.

Pathogenesis of Functioning Adenomas

See Flowchart 33.7.

Clinical Features

- Unilateral painless masses; variable in size.
- Larger masses produce local symptoms, e.g. difficulty in breathing and swallowing.
- On radionuclide scanning, most adenomas appear as cold nodules (non-functioning adenomas take up less radioactive iodine than normal thyroid parenchyma).
- Approximately 10% progress to follicular carcinoma. Definite exclusion of follicular carcinoma is possible only after careful histological examination of capsular integrity.

Gross Morphology

- Solitary, spherical and encapsulated lesions, varying in size from 1 to 10 cm in diameter.
- In fresh specimens, adenomas bulge above the surface and compress the adjacent thyroid.
- The cut surface is grey-white to red-brown, usually homogenous. Areas of haemorrhage, fibrosis, calcification and cystic change may sometimes be seen.

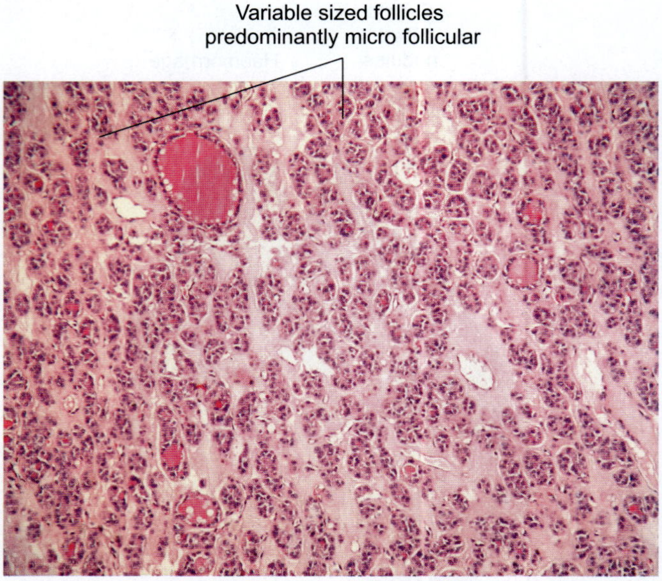

Fig. 33.4 Photomicrograph of a follicular adenoma showing a microfollicular pattern (H&E; 100×).

Microscopy (Fig. 33.4)

Classification of adenomas is based on the following:

- Presence and size of follicles.
- Degree of cellularity.
- Amount of colloid.

Types

1. Macrofollicular or colloid adenoma.
2. Microfollicular or fetal adenoma.
3. Embryonal or trabecular adenoma.
4. Hürthle cell or oxyphil (oncocytic) adenoma.
5. Atypical follicular adenoma (presence of endocrine atypia but absence of capsular invasion).
6. Adenoma with papillae.
7. Clear cell and signet-ring adenoma.

Q. Differentiate between an adenomatous nodule and a follicular adenoma.

Ans. Differences between an adenomatous nodule and a follicular adenoma are tabulated in Table 33.2.

Q. Classify malignant lesions of thyroid. Describe the pathogenesis, clinicopathological features and prognosis of various thyroid malignancies.

Ans. Malignant lesions (carcinoma) of thyroid are mostly seen in adults (papillary carcinoma [PTC] may be seen in children). Females are more commonly affected than males.

Subtypes

- PTC (>85%)
- Follicular carcinoma (5%–15%)
- Anaplastic carcinoma (5%)

} Follicular epithelium-derived malignancies

- Medullary carcinoma (<5%) — Non-follicular cancer

Table 33.2 Differences between an adenomatous nodule and a follicular adenoma

Features	Adenomatous nodule	Follicular adenoma
Nodules	Multiple	Solitary
Encapsulation	Poor	Good
Size of follicles within the nodules	Variable	Uniform
Morphology of adjacent thyroid	Similar	Architecture is different within and outside the nodule
Compression of adjacent gland	Not present	Present

Pathogenesis

Contribution from genetic and environmental factors:

1. **Genetic factors**
   - Genetic abnormalities in the follicular epithelium-derived malignancies (see the earlier text) are mainly observed in two pathways, namely mitogen-activated protein (MAP) kinase pathway and PI3K/AKT pathway.
   - In normal cells, these pathways are transiently activated by binding of soluble growth factor ligands to extracellular domain of receptor tyrosine kinases resulting in autophosphorylation of the cytoplasmic domain of the receptor allowing intracellular signal transduction.
   - In thyroid carcinoma, gain-of-function mutations along these pathways lead to continuous constitutive activation, promoting carcinogenesis. Examples include:

     (a) **Follicular carcinoma**
     - Abnormalities in PI3K/AKT signalling pathway due to:
       - Gain-of-function point mutations in RAS and PI3K.
       - Amplification of PIK3CA.
       - Mutations in PTEN tumour suppressor.
     - Formation of PAX8–PPAR (peroxisome proliferator-activated receptor) gamma 1 fusion product due to translocation (2; 3) (q13; p25), which is a nuclear hormone receptor and induces terminal differentiation of cells.

     (b) **PTC:** MAP kinase pathway is the major pathway involved in PTC and abnormalities in this pathway can occur by the following mechanisms:
     - Rearrangements of the tyrosine kinase receptors (TKRs), RET or NTRK1 (neutrophilic tyrosine kinase receptor 1) due to inversion of chromosome 10 or a reciprocal translocation between chromosomes 10 and 17 → formation of RET/PTC fusion gene or NTRK1 fusion gene → activation of MAP kinase pathway.
     - Mutations in signal transduction genes (RAS mutations and mutations in BRAF oncogene).

     (c) **Medullary carcinoma**
     - It is sporadic in 80% of cases; remainder occur in a setting of multiple endocrine neoplasia (MEN) types 2A or 2B or as familial tumours not associated with MEN syndrome.
     - Familial tumours occurring in MEN type 2 are associated with germline mutations in RET proto-oncogene which leads to constitutive activation of TKR and cellular proliferation.

2. **Environmental factors**
   - Association with ionizing radiation.
   - Pre-existing thyroid pathology, e.g. nodular goitre, adenomas and Hashimoto thyroiditis.

Papillary Thyroid Carcinoma

Clinical features

- It is the most common thyroid malignancy.
- Peak incidence is between 20 and 40 years; may be seen at any age.
- It presents as a solitary (cold) nodule (about 45% are actually found to be multicentric on histopathology).
- In most cases, primary thyroid nodule is asymptomatic and cervical lymph node metastasis is the first manifestation. Occult tumours are seen in 6% of cases at autopsy.
- Primary thyroid nodule may sometimes manifest with hoarseness, dysphagia, cough and dyspnoea.

Predisposing factors

- Previous exposure to ionizing radiation.
- Increased incidence of PTC is observed in Gardner's syndrome (familial adenomatous polyposis coli) and Cowden disease (familial goitre and skin haematomas).

Gross morphology (Fig. 33.5A)

- May be solitary or multifocal, often cystic.
- Well circumscribed/encapsulated or ill-defined/infiltrative.
- On the cut surface, papillary areas are easily identified and appear granular. Areas of fibrosis may be seen.

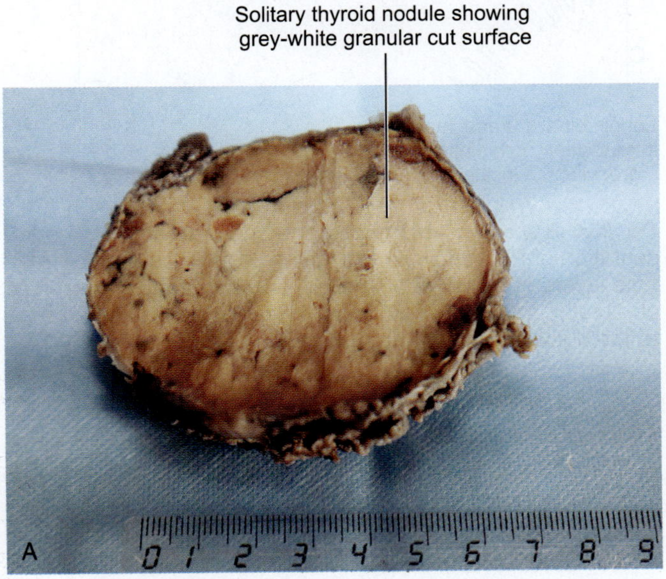

Fig. 33.5 (A) Gross picture of a circumscribed solitary thyroid nodule showing a homogenous grey-white, granular cut surface.

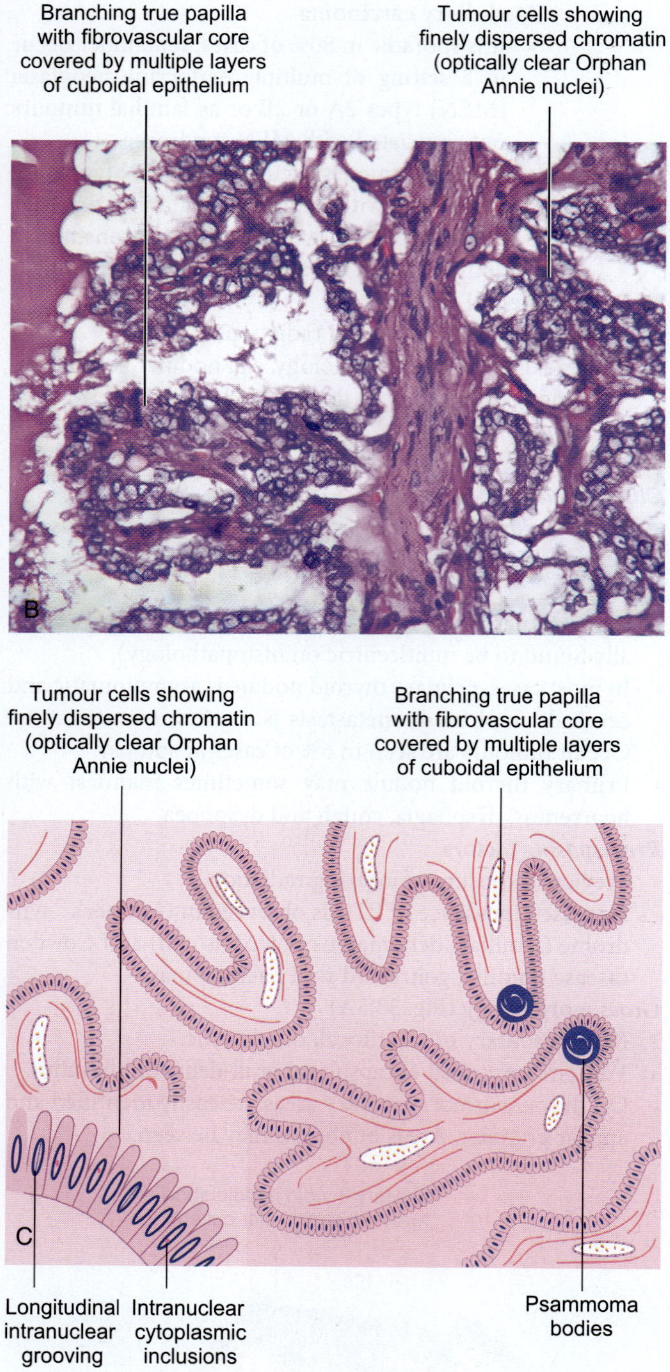

Fig. 33.5 (B and C) Photomicrograph and diagrammatic representation of PTC showing branching papillae covered by multiple layers of cuboidal epithelium showing a finely dispersed chromatin, imparting an optically clear or empty appearance to the nuclei **(Orphan Annie or ground glass nuclei; 100×)**

Microscopy (Fig. 33.5B and C)

- Branching true papillae with fibrovascular cores covered by multiple layers of cuboidal epithelium (to be differentiated from hyperplastic or pseudopapillae, which do not show true fibrovascular cores).
- Cells show finely dispersed chromatin, imparting an optically clear or empty appearance to the nuclei (**Orphan Annie** or **ground glass nuclei**).
- Invaginations of the cytoplasm may in cross-sections give an appearance of eosinophilic **intranuclear inclusions** or **pseudoinclusions** or **intranuclear grooves**.
- Concentrically calcified structures called **psammoma bodies**, usually located within cores of papillae, are often seen and are diagnostic of PTC.
- **Lymphatic invasion is common**; however, involvement of blood vessels is relatively rare.

  Note: Diagnosis of PTC is based on nuclear features irrespective of the presence or absence of papillary architecture.

Variants

- **Encapsulated variant:** It is well encapsulated, vascular or lymph node dissemination is rare and prognosis is excellent.
- **Follicular variant:** Tumours are unencapsulated with a follicular architecture, and characteristic nuclear features of PTC and psammoma bodies.
- **Tall cell variant:** Neoplastic epithelium is tall columnar with intensely eosinophilic cytoplasm. Large tumours often present with vascular invasion and local and distant metastases. Older individuals have a worse prognosis. Hürthle cell neoplasms are a close differential.
- **Diffuse sclerosing variant:** Younger individuals including children are affected; they show diffuse fibrosis, abundant psammoma bodies and squamous morules (metaplasia).
- **Hyalinizing trabecular tumour:** Growth is organoid (resembles extra-adrenal paraganglioma); both intracellular and extracellular hyalinization are seen.

Prognosis

- Ten-year survival 98%.
- Metastasis seen in 10%–15% of cases.

Follicular Carcinoma

Clinical features

- Second most common thyroid carcinoma
- Peak incidence between 40 and 50 years; females more commonly affected than males.
- Incidence higher in areas with iodine deficiency, indicating that follicular carcinoma might arise from nodular goitre.
- No definite evidence that follicular carcinoma arises from adenomas except for common RAS mutations.
- Presents as a slowly enlarging painless cold nodule.
- Regional lymph nodes rarely involved; vascular invasion common with spread to bones, lungs and liver.

Gross morphology

- Solitary nodule; may be well circumscribed or infiltrative.
- Grey-tan-pink and translucent (due to large colloid-filled follicles).
- Degenerative changes, e.g. central fibrosis and foci of calcification, common.

***Microscopy* (Fig. 33.6)**

- Most tumours show a follicular pattern; in some cases, follicular differentiation is less apparent; trabecular pattern, nests and sheets of polygonal to spindle-shaped cells and oncocytic (Hürthle) cells are more prominent.
- Anaplasia is variable (generally not marked); mitosis is increased.

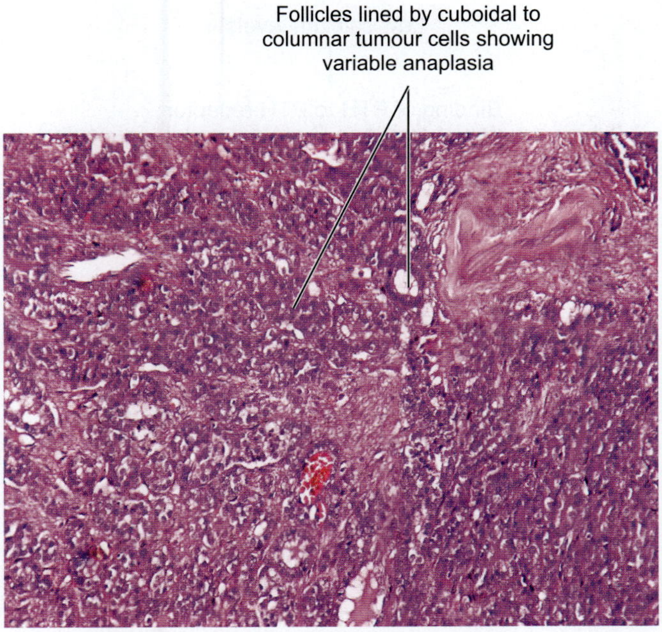

Fig. 33.6 Photomicrograph of follicular carcinoma thyroid showing variable sized follicles lined by cuboidal to columnar epithelium with moderate atypia (H&E; 100×).

- Blood vessels are preferentially invaded than lymphatics. Bones, lungs and liver are common sites of metastases.

Types

1. Minimally invasive (appear well defined and encapsulated like follicular adenomas but show capsular invasion and mitoses on histopathology).
2. Widely invasive (extensive invasion of adjacent thyroid parenchyma or extrathyroidal tissue).
3. Encapsulated angioinvasive (are encapsulated but show vascular invasion).

Prognosis

- Most follicular carcinomas are treated with total thyroidectomy followed by administration of radioactive iodine. Better differentiated lesions are treated with thyroid hormones to suppress endogenous TSH (better differentiated lesions are stimulated by TSH).
- Widely invasive tumours commonly develop metastasis, and about 50% of patients succumb to their disease within 10 years.
- Minimally invasive follicular carcinoma has a 10-year survival greater than 90%.

Anaplastic Carcinoma

Anaplastic carcinoma is an undifferentiated tumour derived from thyroid follicular epithelium which usually expresses epithelial markers on immunohistochemistry (IHC) but is negative for thyroglobulin.

Clinical features

- Presents as a rapidly enlarging bulky neck mass, which spreads to contiguous structures.
- Seen in older patients (mean age of 65 years).
- Fifty per cent of patients have a previous history of MNG.
- Twenty per cent of patients have a previous history of a differentiated carcinoma.
- Twenty per cent to thirty percent of patients have a concurrent differentiated thyroid tumour, most commonly PTC.

Differentiated tumours —(Genetic defects; Loss of P_{53})→ Anaplastic carcinoma

Morphology

Highly anaplastic tumour, which may show any of the following histological patterns:

- Giant cell pattern (large pleomorphic giant cells).
- Spindle cell (sarcomatoid) pattern.
- Mixed spindle cell and giant cell pattern.
- Small cell pattern.

Prognosis: It commonly metastasizes to lungs; is aggressive and fatal.

Medullary Carcinoma

Neuroendocrine neoplasm derived from the parafollicular 'C cells'

Clinical features

- Secrets calcitonin, which has an important role in diagnosis and postoperative follow-up of patients.
- In addition, it may secrete other polypeptide hormones, e.g. somatostatin, serotonin and vasoactive intestinal peptide (VIP).
- Medullary carcinoma is sporadic in 70% of cases and familial in 30% of cases. Sporadic lesions are common in adults (40–50 years); cases associated with MEN syndrome are seen in younger patients/childhood.
- May present as/due to:
  - A paraneoplastic syndrome, e.g. diarrhoea due to excessive VIP or hypocalcaemia due to increased serum calcitonin.
  - Mass symptoms.

Gross morphology

- Solitary/multiple lesions seen in both lobes of thyroid.
- Bilateral and multicentric in a familial setting, and solitary and unilateral in a sporadic setting.
- Firm, pale grey-tan and infiltrative.
- Foci of haemorrhage and necrosis may be seen in larger lesions.

Microscopy (Fig. 33.7A and B)

- It is composed of polygonal to spindle-shaped cells, which may form nests, trabeculae and follicles; rarely, small, more anaplastic cells are the predominant cell type.
- Acellular amyloid deposits (derived from altered calcitonin) may be seen in the stroma.
- Multicentric C-cell hyperplasia is often seen in the surrounding thyroid in familial medullary carcinoma thyroid (absent in sporadic medullary carcinoma).
- Electron microscopy shows membrane-bound, electron-dense granules and calcitonin can be demonstrated in the tumour cells and amyloid deposits on IHC.
- ***Prognosis:*** Prognosis of familial cancers is worse than sporadic (familial cancers tend to be multiple and are associated with C-cell hyperplasia or micromedullary carcinomas <1 cm).

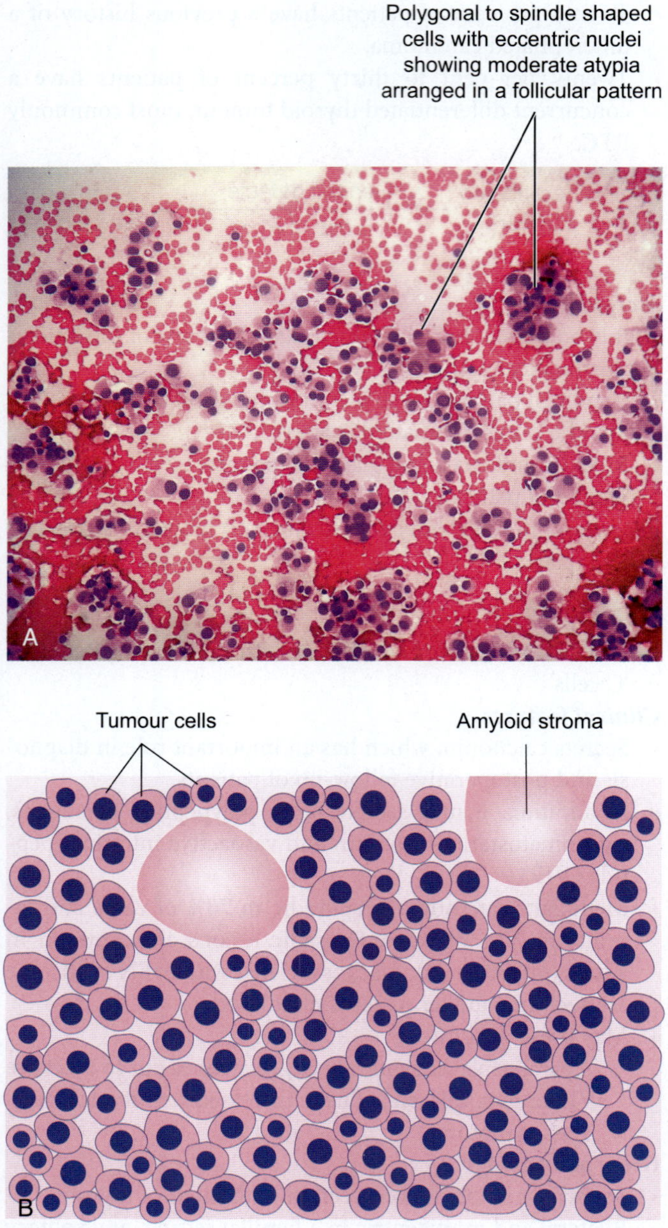

Fig. 33.7 Photomicrograph (A) of a cytology smear from medullary carcinoma thyroid showing polygonal to spindle-shaped cells with eccentric nuclei showing moderate atypia arranged in a follicular pattern and diagrammatic representation (B) of medullary carcinoma thyroid showing a dispersed population of polygonal to spindle to ovoid cells showing moderate atypia with deposits of amyloid (acellular pink material in the stroma; H&E; 100×).

PARATHYROID GLAND

- Derived from developing pharyngeal pouches that also give rise to thymus.
- Four glands (two each at upper and lower poles of thyroid).
- Yellow-brown, ovoid, encapsulated, measuring 35–40 mg.
- Composed of the following:
  - Chief cells (secrete PTH or parathormone).
  - Oxyphil cells (appear at the onset of puberty, but have no known function).

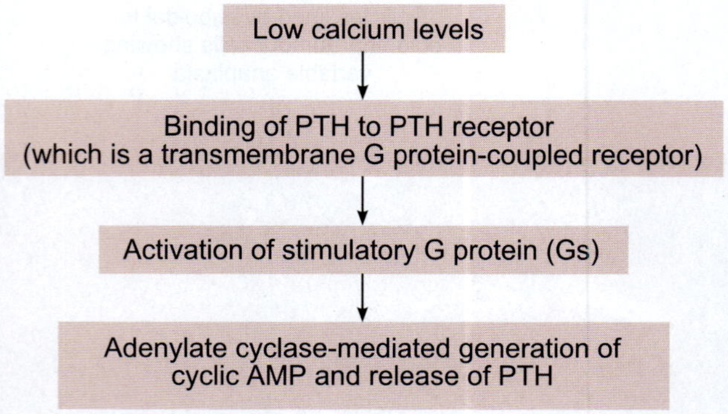

Note: Abnormalities of G protein result in hyper-or hypofunctioning of parathyroid.

Flowchart 33.8 Regulation of parathormone secretion.

Regulation of parathormone secretion (See Flowchart 33.8) Activity of parathyroid is controlled by levels of free ionized calcium in the bloodstream.

Metabolic functions of PTH

- Activates osteoclasts and mobilizes calcium from bone to blood.
- Increases renal tubular reabsorption of calcium and conserves free calcium.
- Increases conversion of vitamin D to its active form in the kidneys.
- Increases urinary phosphate excretion, lowering the serum phosphate levels.
- Enhances gastrointestinal calcium absorption.

Q. Classify hyperparathyroidism. Describe the salient clinicopathological features of the various types of hyperparathyroidism. (PA32.5)

Ans. Hyperparathyroidism is defined as excessive production and secretion of parathormone (PTH) from the parathyroid glands. It is classified into:

1. **Primary hyperparathyroidism**
   (a) One of the most common endocrine disorders associated with autonomous spontaneous overproduction of PTH and hypercalcaemia, primary hyperparathyroidism is a disease of the adults with a female to male ratio of 3-5:1.
   (b) Parathyroid lesions causing its hyperfunction include:
      (i) Adenomas (75%–85% of cases); may be familial or sporadic.
      (ii) Primary hyperplasia (10%–15% of cases).
      (iii) Parathyroid carcinoma (5%–10% of cases).
   (c) In more than 95% of cases, disorder is caused by sporadic parathyroid hyperplasia or parathyroid adenoma; less than 5% of cases are familial.

Parathyroid adenoma

Pathogenesis

- Genetic syndromes associated with familial primary hyperparathyroidism are as follows:
  - MEN-1 (**Werner syndrome**): Associated with inactivation of tumour suppressor gene on chromosome 11q13.

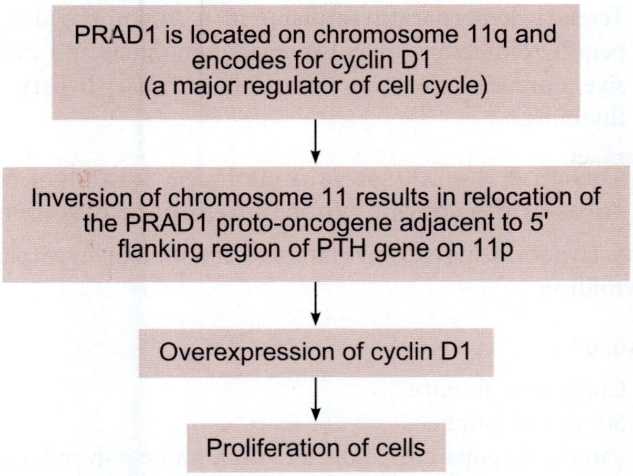

Flowchart 33.9 PRAD1-associated evolution of a sporadic parathyroid adenoma.

- MEN-2A: Mutations in tyrosine kinase receptor RET on chromosome 10q.
- Familial hypocalciuric hyperkalaemia (FHH): An autosomal dominant disorder in which the patient shows enhanced parathyroid function due to decreased sensitivity to extracellular calcium because of mutations in PTH calcium-sensing receptor (CASR) gene on chromosome 3q.

- Sporadic parathyroid adenomas are mostly monoclonal and associated with two molecular defects:
  - Parathyroid adenomatosis gene 1 (PRAD1; See Flowchart 33.9).
  - MEN-1 mutations: Mutations in both copies of MEN-1 gene seen in up to 30% of sporadic adenomas.

Gross morphology

- Parathyroid adenomas are always solitary, and lie in close proximity to thyroid or in ectopic sites, e.g. mediastinum.
- They weigh about 0.5–5.0 g and are well circumscribed, soft tan-reddish brown, with a delicate capsule.
- Gland outside the adenoma may be normal in size or shrunken due to feedback inhibition by increased serum calcium.

Microscopy (Fig. 33.8)

- Parathyroid adenomas are predominantly composed of fairly uniform, polygonal chief cells with small centrally placed nuclei. Few nests of oxyphil cells may be seen scattered.
- Pure oxyphil adenomas are rare.
- Mild endocrine atypia may be seen and should not be interpreted as a malignancy.

Primary parathyroid hyperplasia

- It occurs sporadically or as a component of MEN syndrome.
- Classically, all four glands are involved; frequent asymmetry with sparing of one or two glands may be seen.
- The most common pattern is chief cell hyperplasia, which may involve the gland in a diffuse or multinodular pattern.

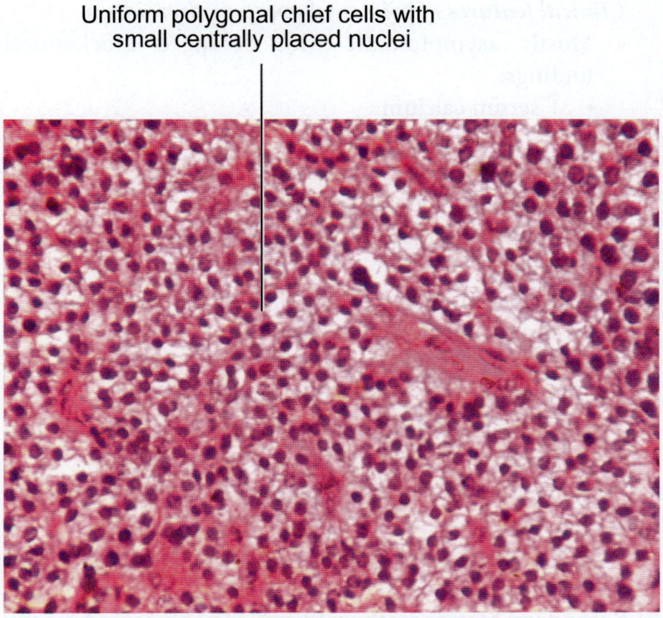

Fig. 33.8 Photomicrograph of a parathyroid adenoma composed of uniform, polygonal chief cells with small centrally placed nuclei (H&E; 200×).

- Rarely, constituent cells contain **'water clear cells'** (water clear cell hyperplasia). Chief cells appear clear due to loss of glycogen are called water clear cells.

Parathyroid carcinoma

- May be circumscribed or clearly invasive, grey-white and irregular mass.
- Nodular or trabecular arrangement of cells resembling normal parathyroid cells.
- Diagnosis of carcinoma based on invasion of adjacent tissue or metastases.

Morphological changes in other organs due to primary hyperparathyroidism

Skeletal changes

- Prominent osteoclasts (cause erosion of bone matrix).
- Increased osteoblastic activity (induces formation of new bony trabeculae).
- The cortex is grossly thinned; the marrow shows an increase in fibrous tissue with foci of haemorrhage and cyst formation **(osteitis fibrosa cystica)**.
- Radiographic findings include subperiosteal bone resorption of the phalanges and tooth sockets, resorption of distal phalanges (acro-osteolysis) and "salt and pepper" appearance of the skull.
- Aggregates of osteoclasts, reactive giant cells and haemorrhagic debris, labelled **Brown tumour of hyperparathyroidism**, are typically encountered (commonly involve the jaw).

Renal changes

Formation of urinary tract stones (nephrolithiasis). Metastatic calcification of the basement membrane of collecting tubules (nephrocalcinosis) causes refractoriness to ADH and polyuria causing nephrogenic diabetes insipidus.

Clinical features of primary hyperparathyroidism

- Mostly asymptomatic with deranged biochemical findings:
  - ↑ serum calcium.
  - ↑ PTH levels.
  - ↑ urinary excretion of both calcium and phosphate.
- Symptomatic patients may manifest with:
  - Bone pain, fractures, osteoporosis and osteitis fibrosa cystica.
  - Nephrolithiasis, pain, obstructive uropathy and chronic renal insufficiency.
  - GIT disturbances, such as nausea, constipation, peptic ulcers, pancreatitis and gallstones.
  - CNS alternations, such as depression, lethargy and seizures.
  - Neuromuscular abnormalities, such as weakness and fatigue.
  - Cardiac manifestations, such as aortic or mitral valve calcification.

2. **Secondary hyperparathyroidism:** May be caused by any condition which is associated with chronic hypocalcaemia, hypophosphatemia or decreased serum calcitriol.

Causes

- Renal failure.
- Inadequate dietary intake of calcium.
- Steatorrhoea.
- Vitamin D deficiency.

Mechanism of development of secondary hyperparathyroidism is complex, not fully understood (Flowchart 33.10).

Clinical features

- Manifestations of chronic renal failure.
- Bone abnormality **(renal osteodystrophy)** is seen but is less severe than in primary hyperparathyroidism.
- Vascular calcification leads to ischaemia **(calciphylaxis)**.

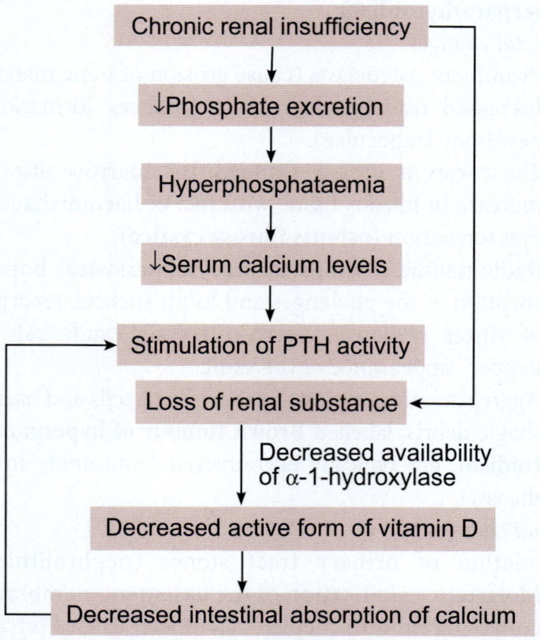

Flowchart 33.10 Mechanism of development of secondary hyperparathyroidism.

3. **Tertiary hyperparathyroidism:** In a minor population, parathyroid activity may become autonomous and excessive, a process sometimes referred to as tertiary hyperparathyroidism.

Q. Describe the causes and clinicopathological features of the various types of hypoparathyroidism.

Ans. Hypoparathyroidism is far less common than hyperparathyroidism.

Causes

- Congenital absence.
- Surgical ablation.
- Familial hypoparathyroidism (autoimmune polyendocrine syndrome, type I).
  - Mutation in the autoimmune regulator (AIRE) gene.
  - Associated with mucocutaneous candidiasis and primary adrenal insufficiency.
- Idiopathic hypoparathyroidism.
  - Autoimmune disease with isolated atrophy of the parathyroid.
  - Of these patients, 60% have antibodies against CASR.

Clinical Features

It presents mainly with manifestations of hypocalcaemia:

- Tetany, characterized by neuromuscular irritability (circumoral numbness, paraesthesias of the distal extremities, carpopedal spasm, laryngospasm and generalized seizures).
- Mental status changes including emotional instability, anxiety, depression, confusion, hallucinations and frank psychosis.
- Intracranial manifestations including calcification of basal ganglia, Parkinson-like movement disorder and increased intracranial pressure with resultant papilloedema.
- Ocular disease (calcification of the lens resulting in cataract formation).
- Cardiovascular manifestations including conduction abnormalities.
- Dental abnormalities (dental hypoplasia, failure of eruption, defective enamel and root formation and abraded carious teeth).

ADRENAL GLANDS

- Paired endocrine organs.
- Weigh about 4 g in adults.
- Acute stress leads to lipid depletion, which causes decreased weight of the gland.
- It has the following three components:
  - Capsule.
  - Cortex: Composed of:
    - Zona glomerulosa.
    - Zona fasciculata (broad middle zone comprising more than 75% of the cortex).
    - Zona reticularis.
  - Adrenal medulla: Composed of chromaffin cells, which synthesize and secrete catecholamines.

'Adrenal cortex' synthesizes three different types of steroids:

1. Glucocorticoids synthesized in zona fasciculata and zona reticularis.
2. Mineralocorticoids synthesized in zona glomerulosa.
3. Sex steroids synthesized in zona reticularis.

Q. Write briefly about the pathogenesis, clinical features and morphology of Cushing's syndrome. (PA32.8)

Ans. Cushing's syndrome is a state of hypercortisolism (increased glucocorticoid levels).

Pathogenesis

Endogenous Cushing's syndrome

- Primary hypothalamic–pituitary disease associated with hypersecretion of ACTH, also called **Cushing's disease**' (constitutes 70%–80% of cases of endogenous Cushing's syndrome).
- Hypersecretion of cortisol by an adrenal adenoma, carcinoma or nodular hyperplasia called '**ACTH-independent Cushing's syndrome**' (constitutes 10%–20% of cases of endogenous Cushing's syndrome).
- Secretion of ectopic ACTH by a neuroendocrine neoplasm called **paraneoplastic Cushing's syndrome** seen in small cell carcinoma of the lung, carcinoid tumour, medullary carcinoma thyroid and islet cell tumour of the pancreas.

Exogenous or iatrogenic Cushing's syndrome

- Because of administration of exogenous corticosteroids.

Clinical Features

- Central obesity (upper trunk and back) with moon faces and buffalo hump.
- Weakness and fatigability due to selective atrophy of fast twitch (type II) myofibrils and decreased muscle mass.
- Hirsutism and menstrual irregularities.
- Hypertension.
- Glucose intolerance/diabetes (induction of gluconeogenesis and decrease in uptake of glucose by cells with resultant hyperglycaemia, glycosuria and polydipsia).
- Osteoporosis and skin striae (catabolic effect on proteins causing loss of collagen and resorption of bone).
- Neuropsychiatric manifestations, e.g. mood swings, depression and frank psychosis.

Morphology

Main lesion of Cushing's syndrome is found in pituitary and adrenal glands.

- **Pituitary glands**
    - Changes occur regardless of the cause of Cushing's syndrome.
    - Most common alteration due to high levels of glucocorticoids is labelled **Crooke hyaline change** in which the normal granular basophilic cytoplasm of the ACTH-producing cells in the anterior pituitary is replaced by homogenous lightly basophilic material; the alteration is because of accumulation of **intermediate keratin filaments** in the cytoplasm.
- **Adrenals:** Morphology varies depending on the cause of hypercortisolism. The adrenals may have one of the following abnormalities:
    - Cortical atrophy (exogenous glucocorticoids cause suppression of endogenous ACTH).
    - Diffuse hyperplasia.
    - Nodular hyperplasia.
    - Adenoma.
    - Carcinoma.

Q. Write briefly about the pathogenesis, clinical features and morphology of hyperaldosteronism.

Ans. Hyperaldosteronism is a generic term for a group of many closely related syndromes, characterized by **excessive aldosterone secretion**. Excessive aldosterone secretion causes sodium retention and potassium excretion resulting in hypertension and hypokalaemia.

Types

- Primary.
- Secondary (due to an extra-adrenal cause).

1. **Primary hyperaldosteronism**
    (a) Autonomous overproduction of aldosterone.
    (b) Resultant suppression of renin–angiotensin system and decreased plasma renin activity.
    (c) Causes include:
        (i) Primary idiopathic adrenocortical hyperplasia, which is characterized by bilateral nodular enlargement.
        (ii) Glucocorticoid-remediable hyperaldosteronism (familial), which is caused by a chimeric gene, resulting from fusion of CYP11B1 (11 β-hydroxylase) and CYP11B2 (aldosterone synthase).
2. **Secondary hyperaldosteronism** (Flowchart 33.11): Aldosterone release occurs secondary to activation of renin–angiotensin system.

Morphology

- **Aldosterone-producing adenomas**
    - Solitary, small (less than 2 cm in diameter) and well circumscribed with yellow, cut surface.
    - Affect patients in third to fourth decades; females more commonly involved than males.
    - Composed of lipid-laden cortical cells with the presence of eosinophilic, laminated inclusions, known as **spironolactone bodies** found after treatment with the antihypertensive drug **spironolactone**.
- **Bilateral idiopathic hyperplasia**
    - Diffuse or focal hyperplasia of cells resembling those of normal zona glomerulosa.
    - Focal hyperplasia wedge-shaped extending from the periphery to the centre of the gland.

Q. Write briefly about adrenogenital syndromes.

Ans. Adrenogenital syndromes are disorders of sexual differentiation, e.g. virilization and feminization, caused by the following:

1. Primary gonadal disorders.

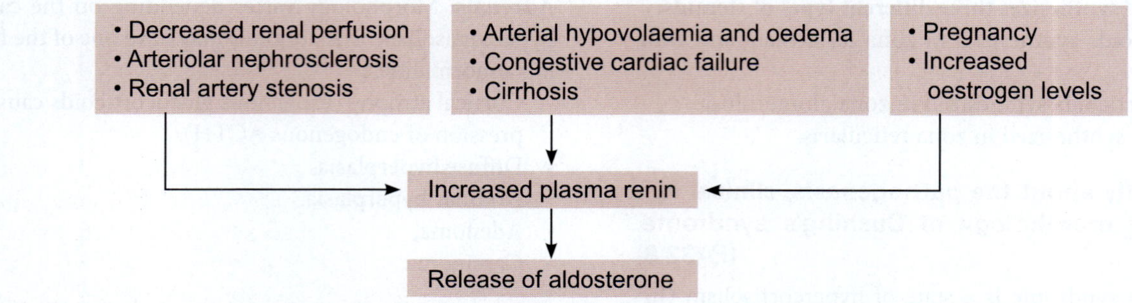

Flowchart 33.11 Pathogenesis of secondary hyperaldosteronism.

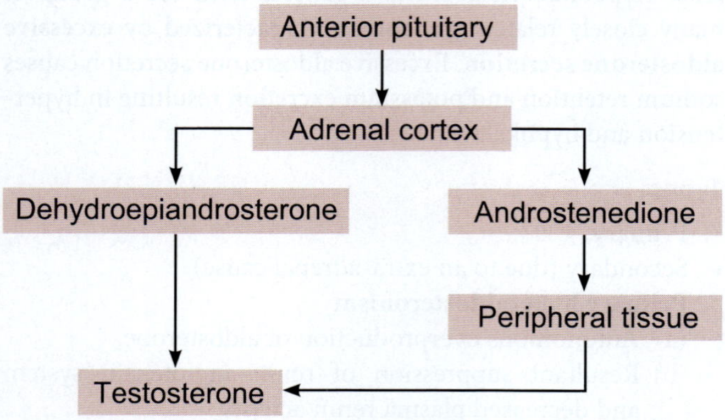

Flowchart 33.12 Regulation of testosterone secretion.

2. Several adrenal disorders.
   (a) Regulation of testosterone secretion is summarized in Flowchart 33.12. Hypersecretion of sex steroids, mainly androgens, occurs as follows:
      (i) A pure syndrome.
      (ii) Component of Cushing's syndrome.
   (b) It may occur in children or adults.
   (c) In children, it is caused by congenital adrenal hyperplasia (total lack of a particular enzyme involved in the biosynthesis of cortical steroids).
   (d) In adults, it is caused by adrenal cortical adenomas and adrenal carcinomas.

Clinical features

- In children: Distortion of external genitalia in girls and precocious puberty in boys is seen.
- In adults: Females show virilization (hirsutism, oligomenorrhoea and deepening of voice) and males show feminization.

Q. Write briefly about the causes, clinical features and morphology of adrenal insufficiency. (PA32.7)

Ans. Adrenal insufficiency is classified into:

1. **Primary and secondary insufficiency based on the underlying cause**
   (a) Causes of primary insufficiency
      (i) Congenital adrenal hyperplasia.
      (ii) Adrenoleukodystrophy.
      (iii) Autoimmune adrenal insufficiency.
      (iv) Infections (AIDS, tuberculosis, fungi and acute haemorrhagic necrosis).
      (v) Amyloidosis, sarcoidosis and haemochromatosis.
      (vi) Metastatic carcinoma.
   (b) Causes of secondary insufficiency
      (i) Hypothalamic pituitary disease, neoplasms and inflammation (sarcoidosis, tuberculosis, pyogenic and fungal).
      (ii) Hypothalamic pituitary suppression (long-term steroid administration and steroid-producing neoplasms).
2. **Acute and chronic insufficiency, based on onset and duration**
   (a) Acute adrenal insufficiency or adrenal crisis.

   Causes
   - Bilateral adrenalectomy.
   - Septicaemia, e.g. endotoxic shock and meningococcal infection.
   - Rapid withdrawal of steroids.
   - Acute stress in chronic deficiency.

   Salient features
   - Deficiency of mineralocorticoids results in salt deficiency, hyperkalaemia and dehydration.
   - Deficiency of glucocorticoids results in hypoglycaemia, increased insulin sensitivity and vomiting.

   (b) 'Chronic adrenal insufficiency' or **Addison's disease:** Clinical manifestations do not appear till 90% of the gland (adrenal cortex) is compromised.

   Causes
   - Lymphomas.
   - Amyloidosis.
   - Sarcoidosis.
   - Haemochromatosis.
   - Fungal infections.
   - Adrenal haemorrhage.
   - More than 90% of cases are due to **autoimmune adrenalitis, tuberculosis and metastatic cancer.**

   Salient features
   - Irregularly shrunken glands are difficult to identify in the suprarenal adipose tissue.
   - Cortex contains only scattered residual cortical cells in a collapsed network of connective tissue.
   - Variable lymphoid infiltrate may be seen.

Q. Write briefly about Waterhouse–Friderichsen syndrome.

Ans. It is an uncommon and catastrophic syndrome with the following characteristics:

- May affect any age group but is common in children.

- Usually follows overwhelming bacterial infection due to *Neisseria meningitidis, Pseudomonas*, pneumococci, *Haemophilus influenzae* and staphylococci.
- Presents with rapidly progressing hypotension, shock, disseminated intravascular coagulation (DIC) and widespread purpura due to rapidly progressing adrenocortical insufficiency and massive bilateral adrenal haemorrhage (adrenals converted to sacs of blood).
- Direct bacterial seeding of small vessels in adrenals may lead to DIC.
- It is thought to be endotoxin-induced or hypersensitivity-mediated vasculitis.
- Clinical course is abrupt; early recognition and institution of appropriate therapy is a must.

Q. Enumerate adrenocortical neoplasms and describe their salient features. (PA32.9)

Ans. Adrenocortical neoplasms include:

1. **Adrenocortical adenoma**
   (a) It is indistinguishable from hyperplastic nodules except that hyperplastic nodules tend to be smaller than 2 cm.
   (b) Most adenomas are slow growing and non-functional; a few larger ones may be functional.
   (c) Occasionally, it may be a part of MEN-1 syndrome.
   (d) Microscopically, tumour cells are arranged in trabeculae and resemble the cells of zona fasciculata. In a few cases, tumour cells may resemble the cells of zona glomerulosa or reticularis.
2. **Adrenocortical carcinoma**
   (a) Rare, can occur at any age including childhood.
   (b) More likely to be functional than adenomas.
   (c) Large invasive lesions, many exceeding 20 cm in diameter.

   Cut surface
   - Variegated and shows areas of haemorrhage, necrosis and cystic change.
   - Invasion of contiguous structures including adrenal vein and inferior vena cava is common. Median survival is 2 years.

   Microscopy
   Cells vary from being well differentiated (resembling adenoma cells) to bizarre monstrous giant cells.

Q. Write briefly about the clinicopathological features and laboratory diagnosis of pheochromocytoma.

Ans. Pheochromocytoma is an uncommon neoplasm composed of chromaffin cells, which synthesize and secrete catecholamines. The following are salient features:

- **Important because it is a cause of surgically correctable hypertension.**
- Associated with **rules of '10'** - 90% arise from adrenal medulla and 10% from extra-adrenal tissue (those developing in extra-adrenal paraganglia are called **paragangliomas**); is malignant in approximately 10% of cases and bilateral in 10% cases.
- Known to occur with MEN-2A, MEN-2B and von Hippel–Lindau syndromes, as well as von Recklinghausen disease and Sturge–Weber syndrome (germline mutations in RET, NF1, VHL and succinate dehydrogenase complex subunit or SDHB, SDHC and SDHD genes).

Histology

- Polygonal to spindle-shaped chromaffin cells arranged in small nests (**Zellballen pattern**) or alveoli along with their supporting cells. They are separated by a rich vascular network.
- Finely granular cytoplasm (seen better with silver stain).
- Variable cellular and nuclear pleomorphism; mitotic figures are rare.
- Capsular and vascular invasion may be seen in benign lesions also; a diagnosis of malignancy is exclusively based on the presence of metastasis.

Clinical Course

- There is abrupt increase in blood pressure with palpitations, headache, vomiting, sweating, tremors and a sense of apprehension. In two-thirds of patients, hypertension is chronic and sustained.
- Paroxysms are precipitated by stress.
- Cardiac complications include congestive cardiac failure, pulmonary oedema, myocardial infarction, cerebrovascular accidents, myocardial instability and arrhythmias.

Laboratory Diagnosis

Increased urinary excretion of free catecholamines and their metabolites, e.g. vanillylmandelic acid (VMA) and metanephrines, is typically seen.

Q. Define and classify diabetes mellitus (DM). Describe its pathogenesis, clinical features and complications. (PA32.4)

Ans. As per the WHO, DM is a heterogeneous metabolic disorder, characterized by chronic hyperglycaemia with disturbance of carbohydrate, fat and protein metabolism.

PANCREAS

Aetiological Classification of DM

1. **Type 1 DM** (10% incidence), **earlier called IDDM (insulin-dependant diabetes mellitus) or juvenile-onset diabetes:** Contrary to its earlier name, type 1 DM can manifest at any age and is associated with autoimmune β-cell destruction and absolute insulin deficiency. It is classified into two subtypes – immune-mediated type 1 DM and idiopathic type 1 DM. Patients with the latter are permanently insulinopenic but have no evidence of β-cell autoimmunity. Markers representing immune destruction of the β cells include islet cell antibodies, antibodies to insulin, antibodies to glutamic acid decarboxylase (GAD65), and autoantibodies to the tyrosine phosphatases IA-2 and IA-2β and ZnT8. At least one of these autoantibodies is present in 85%–90% of individuals affected by Type 1A DM.
2. **Type 2 DM** (80% incidence): **Earlier called NIDDM (non-insulin dependant diabetes mellitus)**, type 2 DM is

characterized by progressive loss of β-cell insulin secretion frequently in a background of insulin resistance.

3. **Gestational DM:** Diabetes diagnosed in the second and third trimesters of pregnancy that was not clearly overt diabetes in the pregestational period.
4. **Specific types of diabetes because of other causes:**
   (a) **Genetic defects in insulin secretion including monogenic diabetic syndromes** (most commonly, neonatal diabetes and maturity-onset diabetes of the young [MODY]).
      (i) Genetic defect of β-cell function due to mutations in various enzymes – hepatocyte nuclear factor 4α (HNF1-α), MODY1, glucokinase and MODY2; earlier called **MODY**.
      (ii) Neonatal diabetes (activating mutations in KCNJ11 and ABCC8 encoding Kir6.2 and SUR1, respectively).
      (iii) Maternally inherited diabetes and deafness (MIDD) due to mitochondrial DNA mutations, defects in proinsulin conversion, insulin gene mutations, type A insulin resistance and lipoatrophic diabetes.
   (b) **Exocrine pancreatic defects**
      (i) Chronic pancreatitis.
      (ii) Pancreatectomy/trauma.
      (iii) Neoplasia.
      (iv) Cystic fibrosis.
      (v) Haemochromatosis.
      (vi) Fibrocalculous pancreatopathy.
   (c) **Endocrinopathies**
      (i) Acromegaly.
      (ii) Cushing's syndrome.
      (iii) Hyperthyroidism.
      (iv) Pheochromocytoma.
      (v) Glucagonoma.
   (d) **Infections**
      (i) Cytomegalovirus.
      (ii) Coxsackie B virus.
      (iii) Congenital rubella.
   (e) **Drugs**
      (i) Glucocorticoids.
      (ii) Thyroid hormone.
      (iii) Interferon-α.
      (iv) β-Adrenergic agonists.
      (v) Thiazides.
      (vi) Nicotinic acid.
      (vii) Phenytoin.
   (f) **Genetic syndromes associated with diabetes**
      (i) Down syndrome.
      (ii) Klinefelter syndrome.
      (iii) Turner syndrome.
      (iv) Prader–Willi syndrome.

Glucose Homeostasis

Normal glucose homoeostasis regulation involves three steps:

- Glucose production by liver.
- Uptake and utilization by peripheral tissue.
- Secretion of insulin and counter-regulatory hormones – such as glucagon.

The principal hormone required for regulation of glucose metabolism and uptake of glucose from the blood into cells, especially liver, muscle, and adipose tissue, is insulin. Therefore, deficiency of insulin or the lack of responsiveness of its receptors plays a central role in all forms of DM.

Insulin

1. ***Synthesis and release*** (Flowchart 33.13)
   (a) Two factors, namely 'glucose-dependent insulinotropic polypeptide (GIP)' secreted by endocrine K cells located in the small bowel and 'glucagon-like peptide-1 (GLP-1Z)' secreted by L cells located in distal ileum and colon are released immediately after food intake.
   (b) They are called **incretins** and their stimulatory effect on secretion of insulin from β cells is labelled '**incretin effect**'. This effect is blunted in type 2 diabetes.
2. ***Signalling pathways***
   (a) Insulin receptor is a tetrameric protein composed of two α and two β chains.
   (b) The β subunit cytosolic domain possesses tyrosine kinase activity.
   (c) Insulin binds to the extracellular domain of α subunit to activate the β subunit tyrosine kinase, leading to autophosphorylation of the receptor and phosphorylation of several intracellular substrate proteins, e.g. family of insulin receptor substrate (IRS) proteins, which includes IRS1–4 and GRB2-associated-binding protein 1 (GAB1).
   (d) The substrate proteins activate multiple downstream signal cascades including PI3K and MAP kinase pathways, which mediate several actions of insulin.
   (e) Insulin aids in the docking of glucose transporter unit GLUT-4 to the plasma membrane (GLUT-4 promotes glucose uptake).
3. ***Actions*** (See Flowchart 33.14).

Pathogenesis of Type 1 DM (Flowchart 33.15) (IM11.2)

The main defect in Type 1 DM is loss of β cells. The following factors are implicated in β cell destruction:

1. **Genetic susceptibility:**
   (a) Persistent presence of two or more autoantibodies is an almost certain predictor of clinical hyperglycaemia in the first-degree relatives of patients with type 1 diabetes. The rate of progression of the disease is dependent on the age at which the antibodies are first detected, number of antibodies, antibody specificity and titre.
   (b) There is 50% concordance in identical twins.
   (c) More than 30 susceptibility genes have been identified, of which the most important locus has been identified as human leukocyte antigen or HLA-D region on chromosome 6. Approximately 95% of patients with type 1 DM have either HLA-DR3 or HLA-DR4 haplotype. A concurrent HLA-DQ8 haplotype is considered a specific marker of type 1 DM susceptibility.

A

Induction of insulin gene on β cells of pancreatic islets

↓

Synthesis of insulin mRNA

↓

Synthesis of preproinsulin in the rough endoplasmic reticulum

↓

Delivery to Golgi apparatus

↓ Proteolytic cleavage → C peptide

Mature insulin

↓

Storage in secretory granules

↓ Physiologic stimuli, eg, rise in blood glucose facilitated by an insulin-independent glucose transporter unit, GLUT-2

Release of insulin

B

Early phase to insulin release:

Intake of food and metabolism of glucose

↓

Generation of ATP

↓

*Inhibition of activity of ATP sensitive K+ channel

↓

Membrane depolarization and influx of calcium ions

↓

Increased intracellular calcium

↓

Secretion of insulin from storage granules of β cells

Delayed phase of insulin release:

↓

Persistence of secretory stimulus

↓

Active synthesis of insulin release

↓

Delayed and protracted release

*β Pancreatic cells express an ATP sensitive K+ channel on their membrane, which comprises two subunits
a) An ATP-sensitive K+ channel.
b) The sulphonyl urea receptor (binds to this class of hypoglycaemic drugs)

Flowchart 33.13 (A and B) Synthesis and release of insulin.

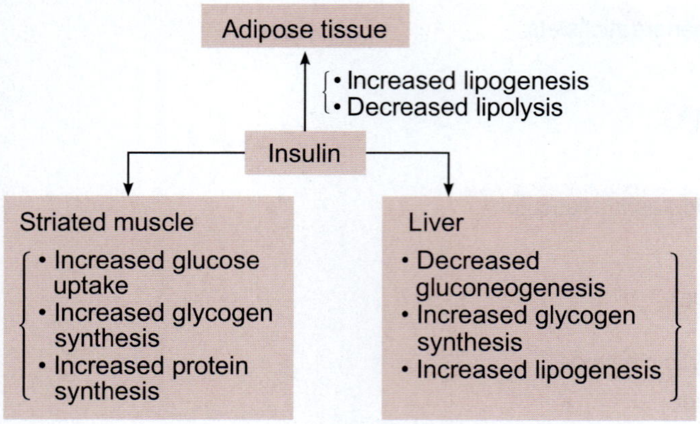

Flowchart 33.14 Actions of insulin.

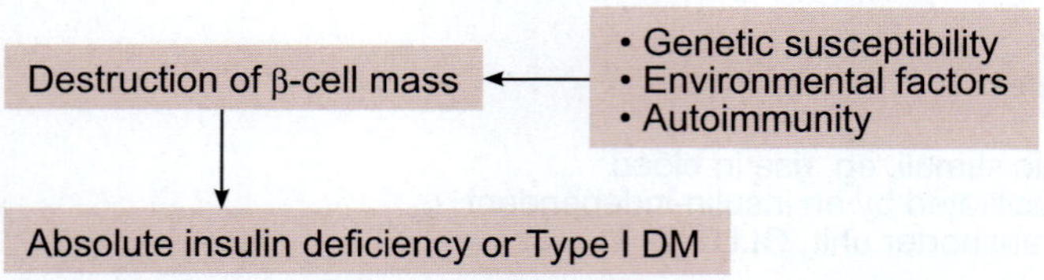

Note: Clinical features of Type I DM manifest after 80% of β-cell mass has been destroyed.

Flowchart 33.15 Pathogenesis of type 1 DM.

(d) Polymorphisms in non-MHC genes such as CTLA4, PTPN22 and CD25 (which codes for the α chain of IL-2 receptor) have been implicated in causation of type 1 DM. All three are critical for regulation of T cells.

2. **Environmental factors:** Damage to pancreatic β cells due to infectious or environmental agents are known to induce type 1 DM. Agents implicated are as follows:
   (a) Viruses (e.g. mumps, rubella, coxsackie B4): Three different mechanisms explain the role of viruses in inducing autoimmunity in type 1 DM:
      (i) Bystander damage: Viruses induce islet injury leading to release of sequestered antigens and activation of autoreactive T cells.
      (ii) Molecular mimicry: Viruses produce proteins that mimic β-cell antigens and the immune response to viral proteins cross-reacts with the self-tissue.
      (iii) Theory of predisposing and precipitating viruses: Viral infection early in life persists (predisposing virus) and a subsequent infection with a related virus (precipitating virus) that shares antigenic epitopes leads to an immune response against the infected islet cells.
   (b) Toxic chemicals and drugs like alloxan, streptozocin, and pentamidine.
   (c) Exposure to cow's milk in infancy.
   (d) Cytotoxins.
   (e) A role for vitamin D in the pathogenesis and prevention of DM suggested by recent evidence.
3. **Autoimmune factors:** Currently, autoimmunity is considered the major factor in the pathophysiology of type 1 DM. Evidence implicating autoimmunity includes:
   (a) Prominent insulitis (including cellular necrosis and lymphocytic infiltration) and circulating islet cell [glutamic acid decarboxylase (GAD)] and antiinsulin antibodies.
   (b) β-Cell damage, which can be caused by circulating autoantibodies;, cytokines (IFN-γ, TNF and IL-1),; macrophages activated by CD4⁺ T cells; and CD8⁺ T cells (direct killing).
   (c) Increased prevalence of type 1 DM in patients with other autoimmune diseases, such as Graves' disease, Hashimoto thyroiditis, coeliac disease, autoimmune hepatitis, vitiligo, myasthenia gravis, pernicious anaemia and Addison's disease.

Pathogenesis of Type 2 DM (Flowchart 33.16) (IM11.3)

Type 2 DM is characterized by insulin resistance with relative deficiency of insulin. The abnormal response of the tissue, particularly the liver and skeletal muscle, to insulin is believed to involve the insulin receptors; however, specific underlying defects are still to be figured out. Insulin resistance has also been attributed to polymorphisms in postreceptor intracellular signaling pathways. Genetics and lifestyle factors like obesity (defined by a body mass index of greater than 30), lack of physical activity, poor diet, stress, and urbanization have been implicated. Pathogenesis of type 2 DM has been depicted in Flowchart 33.16.

Insulin Resistance in Type 2 DM

Peripheral resistance to insulin in Type 2 DM results in:
- Failure to inhibit gluconeogenesis (glucose production in the liver) leading to high glucose levels.
- Failure of postprandial uptake and utilization of glucose by skeletal muscle leading to increased levels of glucose after a meal.
- Failure to inhibit lipoprotein lipase adipose tissue leading to increased levels of free fatty acids (FFAs).

Role of Obesity in Insulin Resistance

- Inverse correlation exists between fasting plasma non-esterified fatty acids (NEFA) and insulin sensitivity.
- Central fat is more lipolytic as compared to peripheral fat, therefore central obesity leads to generation of excessive circulating NEFA which gets deposited in the liver and muscle.
- Intracellular NEFA overwhelms the fatty acid oxidation pathways leading to accumulation of toxic intermediates like diacylglycerol (DAG) and ceramide. These activate the serine/threonine kinases, which cause aberrant serine phosphorylation of insulin receptor and IRS proteins.
- Adipocytes also release adipocytokines (several proteins including leptin, adiponectin, retinol-binding protein-4 and resistin, etc.) into the systemic circulation. Excessive resistin and retinol-binding protein-4 (RBP-4) are associated with insulin resistance. Adiponectin, whose levels are decreased in obesity, is insulin sensitizing. Leptin is also an insulin-sensitizing adipocytokine, which acts through central receptors in hypothalamus.

Quantitative Defects in Type 2 DM

- Decreased β-cell mass due to chronic hyperglycaemia (glucose toxicity).

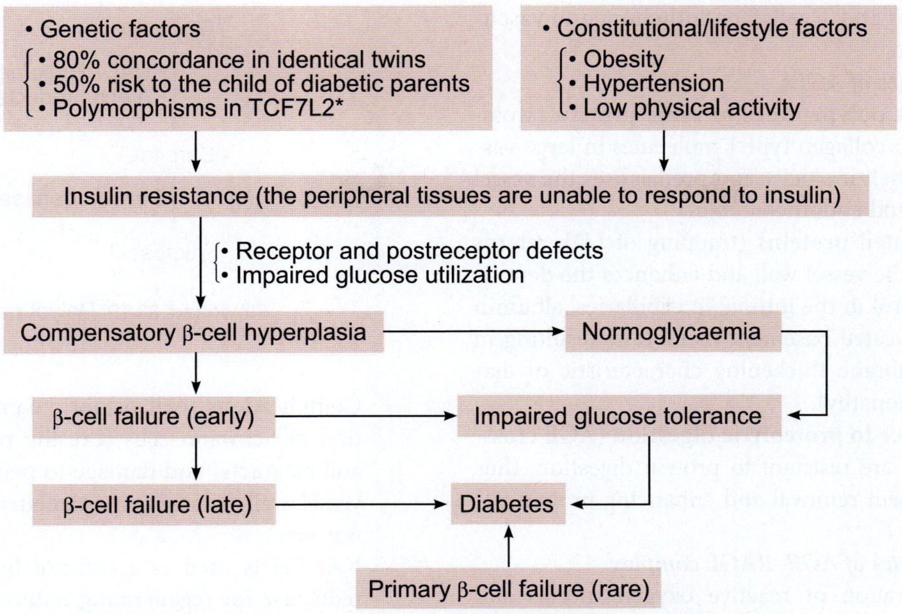

*TCF7L2 encodes a transcription factor in the WNT signalling pathway.

Flowchart 33.16 Pathogenesis of type 2 DM.

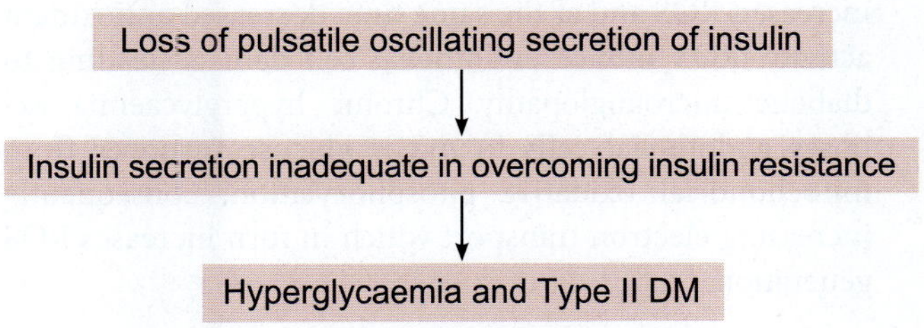

Flowchart 33.17 Qualitative defect in β cells.

- Islet degeneration and impaired function due to increased FFAs (lipotoxicity).
- Islet amyloid deposition (deposition of the protein amylin in long-standing DM also impairs islet cell function).

Qualitative Defects in Type 2 DM

Qualitative Defects in Type 2 DM are summarized in Flowchart 33.17.

Clinical Features of DM

Type 1 DM

- When hyperglycaemia exceeds the renal threshold for reabsorption, glycosuria occurs. Glycosuria induces osmotic diuresis and **polyuria** causing loss of water and electrolytes. Depletion of intracellular water because of water loss and hyperosmolarity (resulting from increased blood glucose levels) triggers osmoreceptors of the thirst centres of brain resulting in intense thirst or **polydipsia**.
- Deficiency of insulin leads to a catabolic state (because insulin is an anabolic steroid). Catabolism of proteins and fat causes a negative-energy state, which leads to increased appetite or **polyphagia**.
- The catabolic state dominates over the polyphagia and causes progressive loss of weight and muscle weakness.
- Insulin deficiency coupled with glucagon excess decreases peripheral utilization of glucose and induces abnormally high levels of blood glucose, which result in severe osmotic diuresis and dehydration as well as increased ketone synthesis leading to ketonaemia, ketonuria and ultimately diabetic ketoacidosis (DKA; presents with severe nausea, vomiting and respiratory difficulty).

Type 2 DM

- High portal insulin levels in type 2 DM prevent unrestricted hepatic fatty acid oxidation and keep ketone body production in check.
- Osmotic diuresis and resulting dehydration can induce hyperosmolar non-ketotic coma especially in case of poor fluid intake.

Complications of DM (IM11.5)

Prolonged hyperglycaemia along with other comorbidities are responsible for most of the complications in DM. Complications of DM are broadly categorized into:

- **Macrovascular disease (affects large- and medium-sized muscular arteries):** Accelerated atherosclerosis leading to increased myocardial infarction, stroke and lower extremity gangrene.
- **Microvascular disease (causes capillary dysfunction in target organs):** Most profound effects on retina, kidneys and peripheral nerves resulting in diabetic retinopathy, nephropathy and neuropathy.

Pathogenesis of Complications

1. **Formation of advanced glycation end products (AGE):** Non-enzymatic reaction between intracellular glucose and amino group of intracellular and extracellular proteins leads to the formation of AGEs. AGEs bind to a specific receptor (RAGE) expressed on inflammatory

cells (macrophages and T cells), endothelium and vascular smooth muscle.

Chemical properties of AGEs

- **AGE cross-link polypeptides of same protein** (cross-linking between collagen type I molecules in large vessels decreases their elasticity and predisposes the vessel to shear stress and endothelial injury).
- **Trap non-glycated proteins** (trapping of LDL retards its efflux from the vessel wall and enhances the deposition of cholesterol in the intima; in capillaries, albumin binds to the glycated basement membrane resulting in basement membrane thickening characteristic of diabetic microangiopathy).
- **Shows resistance to proteolytic digestion** (AGE cross-linked proteins are resistant to protein digestion, thus decreasing protein removal and enhancing protein deposition).

Biological properties of AGE–RAGE complex

- Leads to generation of reactive oxygen species and NF-κB activation.
- Induces monocyte emigration.
- Induces cytokine and growth factor secretion.
- Increases vascular permeability and procoagulant activity.
- Increases extracellular matrix (ECM) production and cellular proliferation.

2. **Activation of protein kinase C** (PKC; Flowchart 33.18)

Downstream effects of PKC

- Stimulates production of VEGF (induces neovascularization characterizing diabetic retinopathy).
- Increases activity of vasoconstrictor endothelin-1.
- Decreases activity of vasodilator nitric oxide synthase (NOS).
- Increases production of profibrogenic molecule TGF-β leading to increased deposition of extracellular matrix and basement membrane material.
- Increases production of procoagulant molecule of plasminogen activator inhibitor (PAI-1) leading to decreased fibrinolysis and vascular occlusive episodes.
- Enhances formation of proinflammatory cytokines by vascular endothelium.

3. **Polyol pathway** (Flowchart 33.19)

- Both sorbitol and fructose are osmotically active and draw water into tissues, leading to permanent damage.

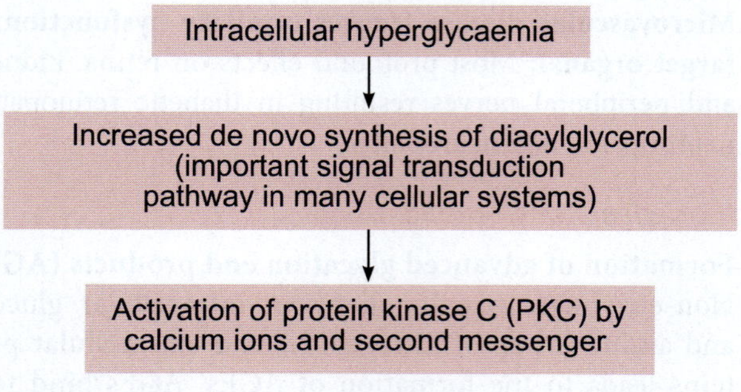

Flowchart 33.18 Activation of protein kinase C.

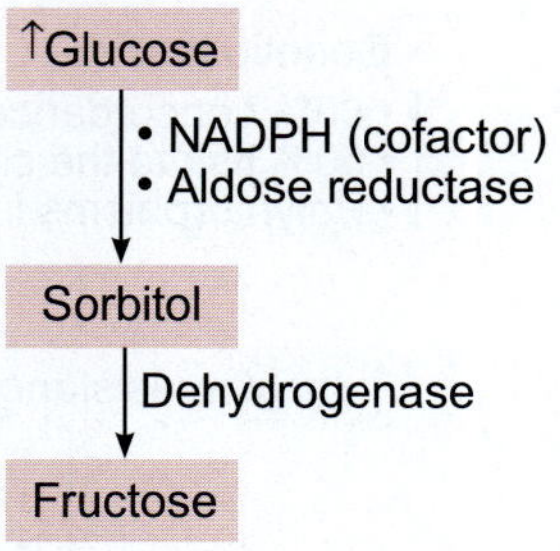

Flowchart 33.19 Polyol pathway.

- Complications with osmotic damage include destruction of Schwann cells (causing peripheral neuropathy and cataracts) and damage to pericytes, weakening the vessel wall (causing microaneurysms in diabetic retinopathy).
- NADPH is used as a cofactor by enzyme glutathione reductase for regenerating reduced glutathione (GSH). GSH is an antioxidant and reduction in GSH level increases cellular susceptibility to oxidative stress (NADPH is used as cofactor in polyol pathway).

4. **Oxidative stress**: Biochemical changes in diabetes cause an increased ROS and at the same time decreased antioxidant activity. ROS induce endothelial cell damage leading to diabetic microangiopathy. Chronic hyperglycaemia exposes endothelial cells to major glucose turnover from mitochondrial oxidative phosphorylation, consequently increasing electron transport which in turn increases ROS generation.

Morphology of Diabetes and its Late Complications

Long-standing diabetes results in morphological changes in several organs as outlined below:

Pancreas

- Reduction in number and size of islets (more in type 1 than in type 2 diabetes).
- Insulitis (leucocytic infiltration of the islets).
- Amyloid replacement of islets in long-standing type 2 diabetes.

Diabetic Vasculopathy

- Accelerated atherosclerosis (hallmark).
- Gangrene and myocardial infarction.
- Hyaline arteriolosclerosis (amorphous hyaline thickening of the wall of the arterioles causing narrowing of the lumen).
- Diabetic microangiopathy (diffuse thickening of the basement membrane, most evident in the capillaries of the skin, skeletal muscle, retina, renal glomeruli, renal tubules, peripheral nerves and placenta).

Diabetic Nephropathy

Patients may present with one of the three glomerular syndromes, namely, non-nephrotic proteinuria, nephritic syndrome, and chronic renal failure (For pathological changes in diabetic nephropathy see chapter 29).

Diabetic Ocular Complications

Ocular complications include the following:

a. Retinopathy: It can manifest with two types of lesions:
   i. Non-proliferative lesions that include capillary aneurysms, dot-and-blot hemorrhages, waxy exudates, and cotton-wool spots.
   ii. Proliferative lesions that include neovascularization, vitreous hemorrhages, and retinal detachment.
b. Cataract.
c. Glaucoma.

Diabetic Neuropathy

Both **central and peripheral nervous systems** are affected. **Distal symmetric polyneuropathy** affecting both motor and sensory functions is seen. It usually starts in the lower extremities but may later involve the upper extremities too (**glove and stocking type of polyneuropathy**). This may be accompanied by autonomic neuropathy producing disturbances in bowel, bladder and sexual function and mononeuropathies (isolated cranial nerve palsies, wrist and foot drop).

Defective Immunity

- Enhanced susceptibility to infections.
- Defects in neutrophilic function.
- Impaired cytokine production by macrophages.

Q. Enumerate the criteria for diagnosis of DM. Enlist the investigations advocated in a patient with DM.

Ans. Diagnostic criteria for DM are tabulated in Table 33.3. The work up of diabetics should include the following investigations:

Determination of Blood Glucose

- Glucose concentration is uniform in water phase of plasma and erythrocytes. Because plasma contains per unit volume 27% more water than erythrocytes, glucose levels are higher in a given volume of plasma than in an identical volume occupied by erythrocytes. For this reason, plasma glucose values are higher than whole blood glucose values.
- In the fasting state, glucose levels in arterial and venous blood are similar. However, postprandially arterial and capillary bloods have glucose levels about 20 mg/dL higher than venous blood. This is because extraction of glucose by tissues in the presence of insulin gets elevated in response to nutrient absorption in the gastrointestinal tract.
- Quantitative determinations of glucose are based on a variety of chemical and enzymatic methods. The older chemical methods are less specific. Newer enzymatic methods (glucose oxidase, hexokinase) for glucose analysis are highly specific.
- In whole blood, clotted and kept at room temperature, glucose disappears at a rate of approximately 7% per hour owing to ongoing glycolytic activity of leucocytes and red cells. It is thus preferable to collect blood in tubes containing fluoride – a strong inhibitor of glycolysis – as well as citrate (acidity) to immediately inhibit glycolysis (grey-stoppered Vacutainer tubes).

Table 33.3 Diagnostic criteria for diabetes mellitus

- HbA_{1c} >6.5% (48.0 mmol/mol).
  OR
- Fasting plasma glucose (FPG) >126 mg/dL (7.0 mmol/L); fasting is defined as no calorie intake for at least 8 hours (fasting whole blood glucose >110 mg/dL).
  OR
- Two-hour plasma glucose >200 mg/dL (11.1 mmol/L) during an oral 75 g anhydrous glucose tolerance test (whole blood >175 mg/dL).
  In the absence of unequivocal hyperglycaemia or presence of acute metabolic decompensation, these criteria should be confirmed by repeat test.
  Impaired fasting glucose (IFG)
- FPG >110 but <125 mg/dL (whole blood glucose >100 but <110 mg/dL).
  Impaired glucose tolerance (IGT)
- Plasma glucose between 140 and 200 mg/dL, 2 hours after oral glucose load (whole blood glucose between 125 mg/dL, 2 hours after oral glucose load).

Oral Glucose Tolerance Test (OGTT)

This test is intended to measure capability and timely response of the insulin-secreting cells to integrated signals provided by GI hormones and rising blood glucose levels.

Patient Preparation

Put the patient for 3 days or more on a normal diet including at least 150 g of carbohydrates per day. In morning after an overnight fast, 75 or 100 g of an aqueous solution of glucose is given.

Steps

1. The patient, who should have been taking an unrestricted carbohydrate diet for at least 3 days or more prior to the test, fasts overnight (at least 8 hours).
2. The patient should rest for at least half an hour before starting the test. A sample of blood is drawn to estimate the glucose level.
3. A glucose load of 75 g dissolved in 300 mL of water is given orally.
4. Blood samples are withdrawn at half-hourly intervals for 2 hours (0.5, 1, 1.5 and 2 hours) and glucose levels are estimated.

Interpretation

1. Normal (in non-pregnant adult).
   (a) **Fasting value:** <95 mg/dL.
   (b) **Value at 1 hour:** <180 mg/dL.
   (c) **Value at 2 hours:** <155 mg/dL.
   (d) **Value at 3 hours:** <140 mg/dL.
2. Indicative of impaired glucose tolerance (IGT).
   (a) **Fasting value:** 110–126 mg/dL.
   (b) At least one of the values at 30, 60 or 90 minutes >200 mg/dL and value at 120 minutes between 140 and 200 mg/dL.
3. Indicative of DM.
   (a) If the fasting glucose determination revealed diabetic values (>126 mg/dL), the OGTT should not be performed.

4. If the fasting glucose fell into the IGT range (110–126 mg/dL) and an OGTT is performed, the results are indicative of DM if two or more of venous plasma concentrations are reached or exceeded.
5. The criteria for the diagnosis of diabetes during pregnancy (gestational diabetes) are stricter than outlined earlier for non-pregnant adults. This is because even mild diabetes during pregnancy becomes a significant risk factor for fetal morbidity and mortality. Thus, the OGTT is performed with 100 g of glucose, and it indicates gestational diabetes when two or more of the following values (in mg/dL) are reached or exceeded: fasting, 110; 1 hour, 190; 2 hours, 165; and 3 hours, 145.

Variants of OGTT

1. **Extended GTT:** It is used for the diagnosis of reactive hypoglycaemia. Dissolve 75 g of anhydrous glucose in water. After fasting the patient from midnight, give the patient the glucose solution to drink (within 10 minutes). Take blood samples at 30, 60, 90, 120, 150, 180 and 240 minutes (total test time 4 hours). If any glucose meter readings are below 3.0 mmol/L during the test, take two further samples at 270 and 300 minutes. Record any symptoms the patient has with the times in the notes.
2. **Intravenous GTT:** This is undertaken in patients who have intestinal malabsorption or those who have had a gastrectomy.
3. **Cortisone primed GTT:** It is a provocative test used to diagnose potential diabetics.

2-Hour Postprandial Plasma Glucose

This determination has no standardized role for diagnostic purposes. It is, however, often valuable when attempting to optimize patients' treatment. Normally, 120-minute values are below 140 mg/dL.

Glycosylated Haemoglobin

During the 120-day lifespan of a red cell, haemoglobin A and other forms become glycated because of non-enzymatic, largely irreversible, post-translational attachment of glucose to the α- and β-chains. Degree of glycation is directly proportional to the level of glucose in the blood, and it has been shown that the amount of glycated haemoglobin present in blood is a reflection of average blood glucose level over the lifespan of a red cell. Thus, quantitative determination of glycated haemoglobin has become a useful adjunct in the assessment of the efficacy of long-term therapeutic control of diabetic patients. Glycated haemoglobin can be measured in several ways. The two most common methods are ion exchange and affinity chromatography. When measured by ion exchange, the results are reported as HbA_{1c}.

Reference range: 3.8%–6.3%; target for therapy is <7%.

Determination of Ketone Bodies

Ketone bodies (acetoacetate, β-hydroxybutyrate, and acetone) are produced by liver from oxidation of FFAs. Insulin deficiency accelerates both the release of FFAs from adipose tissue stores (lipolysis) and their metabolism to ketones.

Ketonemia and ketonuria can be estimated by nitroprusside tablets (Acetest) or reagent strips (Ketostix). Nitroprusside reacts with acetoacetate and acetone, but fails to react with β-hydroxybutyrate.

Glycosuria

Glycosuria appears when the blood glucose level exceeds renal threshold for reabsorption of glucose. This normally lies at about 170 mg/dL, but it may be lower in renal tubular disease or elevated in diabetics to above 300 mg/dL. Thus, glycosuria may be absent in these patients despite markedly elevated blood glucose levels.

Non-diabetic causes of glycosuria are:

- Glycosuria not associated with hyperglycaemia:
  - Pregnancy.
  - Fanconi syndrome.
  - Renal glycosuria (true renal diabetes).
  - Nephrotic syndrome.
- Glycosuria associated with hyperglycaemia:
  - Thyrotoxicosis.
  - Cushing's syndrome.
  - Damage to CNS.
  - Infections.
  - Anesthesia.
  - Excitement and stress.

Semiquantitative tests for glycosuria are based either on use of glucose oxidase as in the dipstick or on copper reduction methods as in the tablet test (Clinitest).

Proteinuria

Diabetic patients have an increased urinary excretion of proteins due to increased glomerular permeability. The proteinuria can become non-selective (excretion of proteins with high molecular weight) and may progress to several grams of protein loss per 24 h. The first sign of renal damage is appearance of microalbuminuria (albumin excretion rate of 30–300 mg/24 h). Microalbuminuria may occur at a time when there is not yet any evidence of decreased GFR or evidence of glomerular lesions. Quantitative and semiquantitative test systems are used to determine low rates of abnormal albumin excretion. For quantitative measurement, the following principles are applied:

- Radioimmunoassay.
- Enzyme-linked immunoassay.
- Immunoturbidimetric assay.
- Nephelometric assay.

Fructosamine Test

Because albumin also contains free amino groups, non-enzymatic reaction with glucose in plasma occurs. Therefore, glycated albumin can serve as a marker to monitor blood glucose. Glycated albumin provides a retrospective measure of average blood glucose concentration over a period of 1–3 weeks. Under alkaline conditions, glycated proteins (ketoamine) reduce nitroblue tetrazolium (NBT) to formazan. In the fructosamine test, absorption of formazan at 530 nm is photometrically measured and compared with appropriate standards to determine the concentration of glycated proteins in plasma, the major part being contributed by albumin.

Determination of Insulin and C-Peptide

Insulin is synthesized first as a precursor molecule, proinsulin. The A and B chains in proinsulin are held together by a connecting peptide called C-peptide. Proinsulin is then converted in the β cells to insulin, which is secreted together with C-peptide. Measurements of serum insulin and C-peptide are mostly used to verify classification and for various investigational purposes. Measurements are performed by radioimmunoassay. C-peptide assays are more sensitive than insulin assays because C-peptide levels are not affected by insulin therapy.

Islet Autoantibodies

Markers of cell-mediated autoimmune destruction of islet β cells that can be demonstrated in type 1 DM are as follows:

1. Islet cell antibodies (ICAs).
2. Autoantibodies to insulin (IAAs).
3. Autoantibodies to glutamic acid decarboxylase (GAD65).
4. Autoantibodies to tyrosine phosphatases IA-2α and IA-2β.

Population Screening for Type 2 DM

Screening is now recommended for those at risk of developing DM. ADA proposes that all asymptomatic people aged 45 years or more, particularly those with BMI ≥ 25 kg/m^2, should be screened in a health care setting. Either fasting plasma glucose (FPG) or 2-hour OGTT or both are appropriate for screening. The FPG is more convenient, more reproducible, less costly and easier to administer than the 2-hour OGTT. The FPG is, therefore, the recommended initial screening test. If FPG is <5.6 mmol/L (100 mg/dL) and/or 2-hour plasma glucose is <7.8 mmol/L (140 mg/dL), testing should be repeated at 3-year intervals.

Q. Differentiate between type 1 and type 2 DM.

Ans. General characteristics of type 1 and type 2 DM are enlisted in Table 33.4.

Q. Write briefly about diabetic emergencies.

Ans. Diabetic coma is a reversible form of a medical emergency seen in DM. Three different types of diabetic coma can occur:

1. Severe diabetic hypoglycaemia.
2. DKA.
3. Hyperosmolar non-ketotic coma.

Severe Diabetic Hypoglycaemia

- People with type 1 diabetes who take insulin in full replacement doses are most vulnerable to episodes of hypoglycaemia.
- Hypoglycaemia is usually mild and easily reversed by eating or drinking carbohydrates, but can be severe enough to produce unconsciousness before it can even be recognized.
- A person suffering from hypoglycaemia is usually pale, and may present with tachycardia, excessive sweating and twitching or convulsions. Unconsciousness due to hypoglycaemia can occur within 20 minutes to 1 hour after early symptoms.
- Hypoglycaemic episodes may also result in worsening of diabetic control and rebound hyperglycaemia – a phenomenon called Somogyi effect.

Table 33.4 General characteristics of type 1 and type 2 DM

Features	Type 1 DM	Type 2 DM
Prevalence	5%–10%	90%–95%
Age at onset	Generally <30 years (may occur at any age)	Generally >40 years
Onset	Rapid	Insidious
Body habits	Usually thin	Usually overweight
Pathogenesis	• Family history uncommon • Absolute insulin deficiency • HLA-DR3 and -DR4 association and contribution from autoimmunity (islet cell antibodies, e.g. anti-insulin, anti-GAD); environmental factors also contribute	• Strong family history • Relative insulin deficiency • No HLA association or autoimmune basis • Peripheral tissue resistance secondary to receptor and postreceptor defects (glucose transport abnormal)
Islet cells	• Early insulitis • Marked atrophy and fibrosis • Marked β-cell depletion	• No insulitis • Focal atrophy and amyloid deposits • Mild β-cell depletion
Initial symptoms	• Manifests with polydipsia, polyuria, polyphagia and weight loss	• May be symptomatic or asymptomatic
Ketoacidosis	May occur due to lack of insulin	Rare (hyperosmolar non-ketotic coma common)
Treatment	Insulin	Diet control and oral hypoglycaemics
Insulin levels	Low or immeasurable	Normal to high
Plasma glucagon	High, suppressible	High, resistant

Diabetic Ketoacidosis

DKA is a state of absolute or relative insulin deficiency aggravated by hyperglycaemia, dehydration and acidosis. The most common causes are underlying infection, disruption of insulin treatment and new onset of diabetes. Biochemically, DKA is defined as follows:

1. An increase in serum concentration of ketones greater than 5 mEq/L.
2. A blood glucose level greater than 250 mg/L.
3. A blood (usually arterial) pH less than 7.3.
4. Ketonaemia and ketonuria and a serum bicarbonate level of 18 mEq/L or less is indicative of severe DKA.

Sequence of Evolution of DKA

The combination of insulin deficiency and increased counter regulatory hormones in DKA leads to release of FFAs into circulation from adipose tissue (lipolysis) and to unrestrained hepatic-fatty acid oxidation to ketone bodies (β-hydroxybutyrate and acetoacetate), with resulting ketonemia and metabolic acidosis.

When accumulated ketones exceed body's capacity to extract them, they overflow into urine (i.e., ketonuria). If the situation is not treated promptly, a greater accumulation of organic acids leads to frank clinical metabolic acidosis (ketoacidosis; Flowchart 28.8), with a drop in pH and bicarbonate serum levels. Respiratory compensation for this acidotic condition results in rapid shallow breathing (Kussmaul respiration). Ketones—in particular, β-hydroxybutyrate—induce nausea and vomiting that consequently aggravate fluid and electrolyte loss already existing in DKA. Moreover, acetone produces the fruity breath odour, which is characteristic of ketotic patients.

Hyperglycaemia, osmotic diuresis, serum hyperosmolarity, and metabolic acidosis result in severe electrolyte disturbances. The most characteristic disturbance is the total body potassium loss. This loss is not mirrored in serum potassium levels, which may be low, within the reference range, or even high (see Flowchart 33.20).

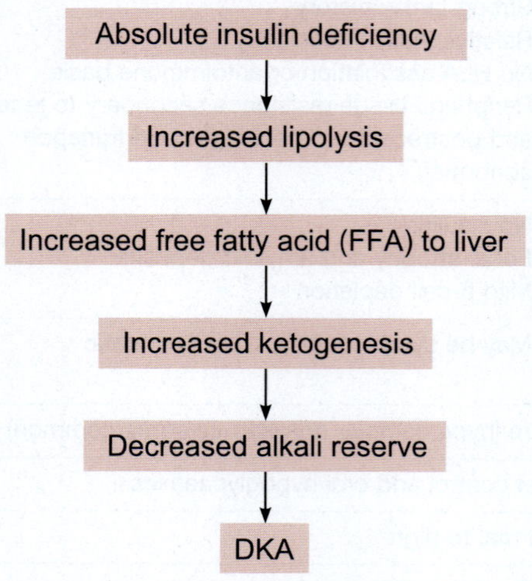

Flowchart 33.20 Sequence of evolution of DKA.

Non-ketotic Hyperosmolar Coma

- Non-ketotic hyperglycaemia is a type of diabetic coma more often associated with a type 2 DM. The preferred term used by ADA is hyperosmolar hyperglycaemic non-ketotic syndrome (HHNS).
- HHNS is due to severe dehydration resulting from prolonged hyperglycaemia-induced diuresis.
- Osmotic diuresis promotes net loss of electrolytes, including sodium, potassium, calcium, magnesium, chloride and phosphate.
- Intracellular dehydration occurs as hyperglycaemia and water loss leads to increased plasma tonicity, causing a shift of water out of cells. This is associated with movement of potassium from the cell to the extracellular compartment.

Sequence of Evolution of HHNS

See Flowchart 33.21.

Q. Differentiate between DKA and HHNS.

Ans. Differentiating features of DKA and HHNS are listed in Table 33.5.

Q. Define a prediabetic.

Ans. Prediabetics are persons with glucose levels that do not meet the criteria for diabetes but are too high to be considered normal (impaired fasting glucose [IFG] and/or IGT and/or A1C levels between 5.7% and 6.4%). Testing for prediabetes and/or type 2 diabetes should be considered in individuals who are overweight (BMI > 25 kg/m^2) or those who have one or more of the following risk factors:

- First-degree relative with diabetes.
- High-risk race/ethnicity (African Americans, Latino, Asian Americans, Native Americans).

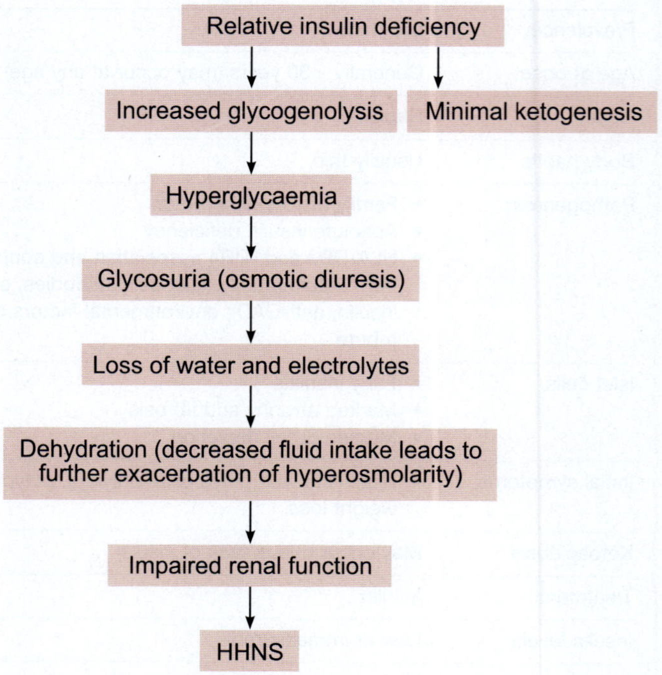

Flowchart 33.21 Sequence of evolution of HHNS.

Table 33.5 Diagnostic criteria and typical total body deficits in DKA and HHNS

Diagnostic criteria	DKA	HHNS
Plasma glucose (mg/dL)	>250	>600
Arterial pH	<7.00	>7.30
Serum bicarbonate (mEq/L)	<10	>15
Urine ketones	Marked increase	Mild increase, if any
Serum ketones	Positive	Small amounts
Effective serum osmolarity	<320	>330
Mental status	Drowsy stupor/coma	Variable
Serum sodium (mEq/L)	Usually low	Normal, increased or low
Serum potassium (mEq/L)	Normal, increased or low	Normal or increased
Serum phosphorus (mEq/L)	Normal or increased	Normal or increased
Serum magnesium (mEq/L)	Normal or increased	Normal or increased
Serum lactate (mmol/L)	2–3	1–2
Blood urea nitrogen (BUN)	Less increase	Greater increase

- History of CVD.
- Hypertension.
- HDL cholesterol <35 mg/dL and/or triglyceride levels >250 mg/dL.
- Women with PCOD.
- Physical inactivity.

Q. Define a potential diabetic.

Ans. Potential diabetics are persons with a normal glucose tolerance test, who have an increased risk of developing diabetes for genetic reasons.

Examples

- Children of two diabetic parents.
- Sibling of a diabetic.
- Non-diabetic member of a pair of monozygotic twins where the other is a diabetic.

Q. Define a latent diabetic.

Ans. Latent diabetics are persons in whom the glucose tolerance test is normal but who are known to have given an abnormal result under conditions imposing a burden on the pancreatic cells, e.g. during pregnancy, infection, severe stress (physical or mental) and treatment with corticosteroids, thiazide diuretics or other diabetogenic drugs, or when overweight.

Q. What is glycosuria?

Ans. Glycosuria occurs when blood glucose level exceeds the renal glucose threshold of 180 mg/dL. It can be secondary to hyperglycaemia (DM) or non-diabetic in origin. Non-diabetic glycosuria can be:

1. Renal glycosuria: It refers to glycosuria in the absence of hyperglycaemia due to a lowered renal threshold for glucose.
2. Alimentary (lag storage) glycosuria: There is a transient abnormal rise in blood glucose level following a meal, and the concentration exceeds the normal renal threshold. During this time, glucose spills into the urine. This may occur in patients undergoing gastric surgery resulting in rapid gastric emptying, hyperthyroidism or hepatic diseases.

Q. What is gestation diabetes?

Ans. This class of patients is defined as women in whom during pregnancy diabetes or IGT become manifest. After pregnancy, the condition usually reverses to normal, but in some patients diabetes or IGT persists. Untreated gestational diabetes can damage health of fetus or mother. Risks to baby include macrosomia (high birth weight); congenital cardiac, central nervous system and skeletal muscle malformations; respiratory distress syndrome; and red blood cell destruction leading to jaundice. Gestational diabetes should be tested at 24–28 weeks of gestation. Women with gestational diabetes should be tested at 4–112 weeks postpartum for prediabetes or diabetes.

34 Diseases of the Skin

NORMAL SKIN

Cell Types in Normal Skin

- **Squamous epithelial cells or keratinocytes:** Produce keratin, defensins and cytokines responsible for regulation of proliferation and differentiation of adjacent epidermal cells, as well as cells in the dermis.
- **Melanocytes:** Responsible for production of melanin; melanin-producing cells are located in the stratum basalis with their dendritic processes extending between keratinocytes.
- **Langerhans cells:** Epidermal dendritic cells that process antigens.
- **Merkel cells:** Reside within the basal layer and function as the neuroendocrine cells of the skin.

Layers of Skin (Fig. 34.1)

1. **Epidermis:** Composed of stratified squamous epithelium with the following layers:
   (a) Stratum basale: It is the lowermost layer of epidermis that contains actively dividing stem cells along the basement membrane. As the basal cells divide, daughter cells migrate upwards.
   (b) Stratum spinosum: Intercellular bridges called desmosomes link the cells together. The cells are polygonal and become increasingly flattened as they move upwards.
   (c) Stratum granulosum: It is constituted by one to three layers of flat cells with keratohyaline basophilic granules.
   (d) Stratum corneum: It contains anucleate cells with keratin.
2. **Dermis:** Consists of two parts:
   (a) Superficial papillary dermis: Superficial part of dermis is composed of loose connective tissue.
   (b) Deep reticular dermis: Deeper layer of dermis is composed of dense dermal collagen.
   (c) Dermis contains specialized appendages called adnexal structures, e.g. hair. Hair follicles produce hair shafts and are closely associated with sebaceous (oil-producing) glands and erector pilaris muscle. Sweat glands guard against the deleterious effects of temperature variations.

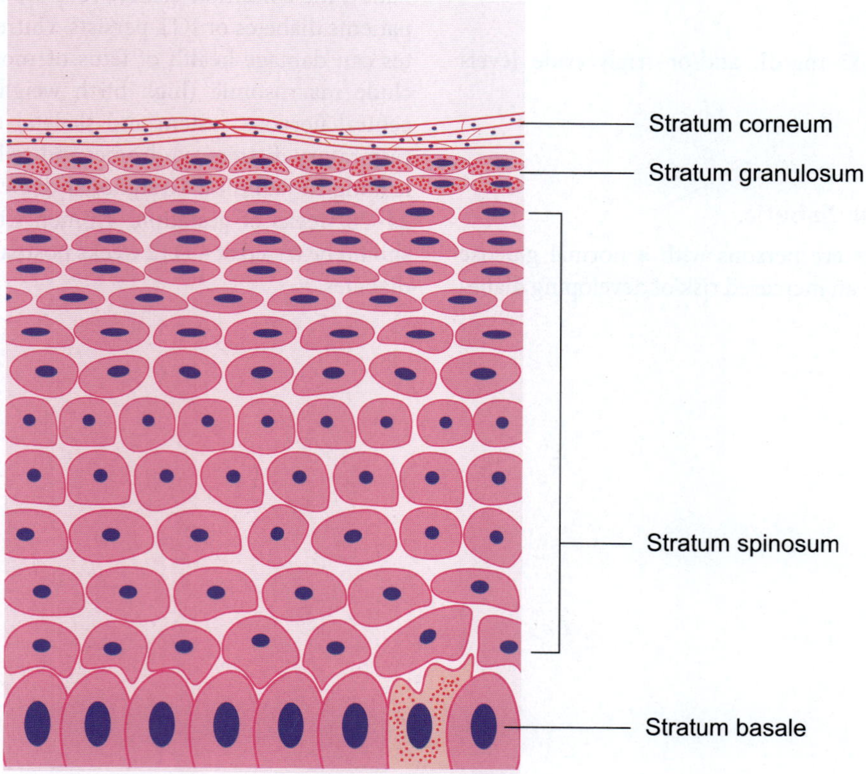

Fig. 34.1 Layers of skin.

Definitions of Macroscopic Terms

- **Macule:** Circumscribed flat lesion up to 5 mm in diameter, distinguished from the surrounding skin by its colouration, without any alteration in the texture of the skin.
- **Patch:** Circumscribed flat lesion more than 5 mm in diameter, distinguished from the surrounding skin by its colouration.
- **Papule:** Circumcised solid, dome-shaped or flat-topped lesion, 5 mm or less in size.
- **Nodule:** Solid, raised and bumpy lesion with spherical contour greater than 5 mm.
- **Plaque:** Elevated, flat-topped lesion greater than 5 mm across.
- **Vesicle:** Fluid-filled, raised lesion 5 mm or less across.
- **Bulla:** Fluid-filled, raised lesion more than 5 mm across.
- **Blister:** Common term used for vesicle or bulla.
- **Pustule:** Discrete pus-filled lesion.
- **Wheal:** Itchy, transient, elevated lesion formed as a result of dermal oedema.
- **Scale:** Dry, horny, plate-like excrescence due to imperfect cornification.
- **Lichenification:** Thickened and rough skin with prominent skin markings, usually a result of frequent rubbing.
- **Excoriation:** Raw, linear lesion due to breakage of epidermis, subsequent to trauma.

Definitions of Microscopic Terms

- **Hyperkeratosis:** Thickening of stratum corneum, which may be associated with qualitative abnormalities of keratin.
- **Parakeratosis:** Retention of nuclei in the stratum corneum.
- **Hypergranulosis:** Hyperplasia of stratum granulosum.
- **Acanthosis:** Diffuse epidermal hyperplasia.
- **Papillomatosis:** Surface elevation caused by hyperplasia and enlargement of contiguous dermal papillae.
- **Dyskeratosis:** Abnormal or premature keratinization within cells below stratum granulosum.
- **Spongiosis:** Intercellular oedema of epidermis.
- **Acantholysis:** Loss of intercellular junctions resulting in loss of cohesion between keratinocytes.
- **Hydropic swelling:** Intracellular oedema seen in keratinocytes.
- **Exocytosis:** Infiltration of the epidermis by inflammatory or circulating blood cells.
- **Erosion:** Discontinuity of the skin or incomplete loss of the epidermis.
- **Ulceration:** Discontinuity of the skin or incomplete loss of the epidermis.
- **Lentiginous:** Linear pattern of melanocyte proliferation within the epidermal basal layer.

Q. Define dermatitis.

Ans. Dermatitis is a non-specific term which indicates 'inflammation of the skin'.

Q. Write briefly about eczematous dermatitis.

Ans. Eczema (spongiotic dermatitis) is characterized by a large group of pruritic skin lesions with different aetiologies.

Stages

1. **Acute eczema** is characterized by oozing, crusting and erythematous papulovesicular eruptions with spongiosis (intercellular oedema) in the epidermis.
2. **Subacute eczema** is associated with crusts developing over ruptured vesicles in the stratum corneum.
3. **Chronic eczema** shows raised scaly plaques or lichenification (thickening because of hyperkeratosis from constant scratching) and hyperpigmentation.

Classification

1. **Atopic dermatitis** is a type I IgE-mediated disease that presents in neonates as a rash on the cheeks, trunk and extensor surfaces, and moves to the flexor creases as the child grows older.
2. **Allergic contact dermatitis** is a type IV cell-mediated hypersensitivity reaction against poison ivy, oak, nickel and chemicals found in the household cleaners, cosmetics, fabrics, dyes, medications and rubber products.
3. **Irritant contact dermatitis**, the most common type of eczematous dermatitis, is a non-immunologic reaction due to the local toxic effect of a chemical on the skin (e.g. detergents in soaps).
4. **Photoeczematous dermatitis** is a type of allergic contact dermatitis that is caused by ultraviolet (UV) light reacting with drugs that have a photosensitizing effect (e.g. tetracycline, sulphonamides and thiazides).
5. **Drug-related eczematous dermatitis** is reaction to an internal circulating antigen derived from an ingested drug.

Morphology

Spongiosis is defined as the accumulation of oedema fluid within the epidermis. Intercellular bridges are stretched and become more prominent, giving rise to a spongy appearance. This is accompanied by superficial perivascular lymphocytic infiltrate and papillary dermal oedema.

Note: There are no specific histopathological features to distinguish various causes of eczema.

Q. Write briefly about superficial mycoses.

Ans. The superficial mycoses causing fungi (dermatophytes) make up a group of fungi that is confined to the outermost layers of the skin or its appendages. Most infections present with a scaling rash. The infection is identified or named 'tinea' followed by the location of the lesion/s.

- **Tinea capitis** is most common in children, in whom it presents with circular or ring-shaped patches (thus also called 'ringworm') of alopecia (hair loss) with erythema and scaling and is usually caused by *Trichophyton tonsurans.* There is generally a visible black dot on the scalp where the hair breaks off.
- ***Trichophyton rubrum* and *T. mentagrophytes*** are responsible for many other types of tinea infections (e.g. tinea cruris, pedis, unguium and corporis). One or more lesions with an elevated, erythematous, scaly border and a clear centre are seen. **Tinea pedis** manifests with a macerated scaling rash between one or more toes. **Tinea unguium** manifests with a raised thickened nail plate which appears

crumbly and discoloured. Dermatophyte infection of the beard area is called **tinea barbae**. It presents as superficial annular lesions or as lesions similar to folliculitis.

- **Tinea versicolor** is caused by *Malassezia furfur* (a yeast) and is associated with areas of hyper- and hypopigmentation. Scrapings reveal the classic '**spaghetti (hyphae)** and **meatball (yeast)**' appearance.
- ***Candida albicans*** commonly produces disease involving the skin (common cause of diaper rash) and nails (onychomycosis).
- **Seborrhoeic dermatitis** is a chronic superficial infection of the hairy areas rich in sebaceous glands, clinically characterised by a scaly greasy dermatitis. It is caused by *Malassezia* yeast. In the newborns, it may cause 'cradle cap' lesions.

Q. Write briefly about sporotrichosis.

Ans. Sporotrichosis is caused by a dimorphic fungus *Sporothrix schenckii* that primarily produces a lymphocutaneous infection. It grows as a mould in soil and yeast in tissue. Human inoculation occurs subsequent to traumatic implantation. Clinically, it manifests as a chain of suppurating lymphocutaneous nodules in the subcutaneous tissue.

Q. Enumerate and describe chronic inflammatory dermatoses.

Ans. Chronic inflammatory dermatoses include:

Psoriasis

- Chronic inflammatory dermatosis associated with arthritis, myopathy, enteropathy and heart disease.
- Affects skin of the elbows, knees, scalp and lumbosacral areas.
- The most typical lesion is a well-demarcated, itchy, pink to salmon plaque covered by loosely adherent silvery white scales.
- Nail changes are seen in up to 30% of cases and include pitting, thickening, yellow-brown discolouration, crumbling and separation of the nail plate from the underlying bed (**onycholysis**).
- Many of these patients present with psoriatic arthritis, which may manifest as classic distal interphalangeal joint involvement, symmetric polyarthritis, asymmetric oligoarthritis (the most common type of psoriatic arthritis) or ankylosing spondylitis.
- Pathogenesis of psoriasis is multifactorial in origin with the contribution from the following:
  - Immunological status of the individual.
  - Genetic susceptibility (strong association with HLA-C, especially with HLA-Cw*0602 allele).
  - Environmental factors.
- There is accumulation of $CD4^+$ T_H1 and $CD8^+$ T cells in the epidermis, which secrete cytokines and growth factors inducing keratinocyte hyperproliferation, which results in the characteristic lesions.
- Psoriasis can be induced in susceptible individuals by local trauma (**Koebner phenomenon**), *S. pyogenes* pharyngitis, HIV and drugs such as lithium, beta-blockers and NSAIDs.

Morphology

- Marked epidermal thickening **(acanthosis).**
- Regular downward elongation of rete ridges **(psoriasiform hyperplasia).**
- Rapid epidermal cell turnover, which results in **loss of stratum granulosum with extensive parakeratotic scaling.**
- **Suprapapillary thinning** (thinning of the epidermal cell layer overlying the tips of dermal papillae).
- Bleeding of vessels on removal of the scale, giving rise to multiple bleeding points **(Auspitz sign).**
- Small aggregates formed by neutrophils within the spongiotic superficial epidermis **(pustules of Kogoj)** and the parakeratotic stratum corneum **(Munro microabscesses).**

Lichen Planus (LP)

- Presents with pruritic, purple, polygonal papules and plaques in the skin and mucosa.
- Is self-limited and may resolve spontaneously; oral lesions may persist for years.
- The papules are highlighted by white dots or lines called **Wickham's striae**.
- Pathogenesis is unknown; however, it is hypothesized that LP occurs due to cytotoxic T-cell response to an altered antigen in the basal cells.

Morphology

- **Basal keratinocytes** show degeneration and necrosis.
- Anucleate necrotic basal cells called **colloid** or **Civatte bodies** are seen in the papillary dermis.
- There is epidermal hyperplasia, hypergranulosis and hyperkeratosis.
- **Interface dermatitis** (dense continuous band-like infiltrate of lymphocytes along the dermoepidermal junction) is classically seen. The infiltrate may assume an angulated zigzag contour (sawtoothing).

Lichen Simplex Chronicus (LSC)

- LSC is characterized by roughening and gradual thickening of skin called lichenification (like lichen on a tree), because of repeated trauma or irritation (rubbing and scratching).
- Sometimes the thickening may result in the formation of nodules called **prurigo nodularis**.

Morphology

- Acanthosis, hyperkeratosis and hypergranulosis.
- Elongation of rete ridges, papillary dermal fibrosis and chronic dermal inflammatory infiltrate.

Pityriasis Rosea (PR)

- Self-limiting eruptive dermatitis of uncertain genesis.
- Common papulosquamous disease which presents as a single, large, scaly, rose-coloured plaque on the trunk **(herald patch)** which is followed by a pruritic papular rash which develops over the trunk days or weeks later. The rash is usually seen along the lines of cleavage (Christmas tree distribution) and remits spontaneously.
- Herald patch is commonly confused with tinea corporis.

Morphology

- Histopathology shows non-specific lymphohistiocytic infiltrate, mainly perivascular in location, with focal hyperkeratosis, parakeratosis and acanthosis.
- Granular cell layer is absent beneath the foci of parakeratosis and intraepidermal cytoid body may be present.
- Focal acantholytic dyskeratosis and occasional eosinophil and erythrocyte may be seen within the epidermis.

Q. Write briefly about verrucae.

Ans. Verrucae are common lesions of children and adolescents but may be encountered at any age.

- They are caused by low-risk types of human papillomavirus (HPV).
- Transmission is by direct contact and autoinoculation.
- They may regress spontaneously within 6 months to 2 years.
- **Verruca vulgaris** is the most common type of wart (found frequently on dorsum of the hands and periungual areas, seen as grey-white to tan, flat to convex papules with a pebble-like appearance).
- **Verruca plana or flat wart** is common on the face and dorsum of the hands, seen as smooth tan macules.
- **Verruca plantaris** and **palmaris** occur on the soles and palms, respectively, and are seen as rough, scaly lesions, 1–2 cm in diameter.
- **Condyloma acuminatum** occurs on the penis, female genitalia, urethra and perianal areas.
  Morphology
  - Verrucous epidermal hyperplasia and papillomatosis.
  - Viral cytopathic effect (haloes surrounding the infected nuclei).
  - Infected cells show prominent keratohyalin granules.

Q. Write briefly about blistering or bullous disorders.

Ans. Group of disorders in which blisters are the primary and the most distinguished feature:

Pemphigus

- Rare autoimmune blistering disorder resulting from loss of normal intercellular attachments.
- Three major variants:
  - Pemphigus vulgaris.
  - Pemphigus foliaceus.
  - Paraneoplastic pemphigus (pemphigus associated with internal malignancy).

Pathogenesis

- **Pemphigus vulgaris** and **foliaceus** are caused by a type II hypersensitivity reaction (antibody directed against a fixed-tissue antigen) and are linked to specific HLA types.
- Patient's sera contain pathogenic IgG antibodies to intercellular desmosomal proteins (desmoglein types I and III).
- **Pemphigus vulgaris** (most common type) involves mucosa and skin of scalp, face, axillae, groin, trunk and points of pressure.
- **Pemphigus foliaceus** results in bullae confined to skin with infrequent involvement of mucosa.

Morphology

- Histological hallmark in all forms of pemphigus is **acantholysis** (separation of individual keratinocytes due to lysis of intercellular adhesion sites); detached acantholytic cells become rounded.
- In **pemphigus vulgaris**, acantholysis involves the layer of cells just above the basal layer giving rise to a suprabasal blister.
- In **pemphigus foliaceus**, acantholysis involves the superficial epidermis at the level of stratum granulosum.
- **Variable superficial dermal infiltration** by lymphocytes, histiocytes and eosinophils accompanies the acantholysis.

Bullous Pemphigoid

- Affects elderly people, and presents with bullous lesions on normal or erythematous skin and mucosa; the bullae are tense and filled with clear fluid.
- Usual sites are inner aspect of thighs, flexor surface of forearms, axillae, groin and lower abdomen.

Pathogenesis

- Autoimmune disorder in which the characteristic finding is linear deposits of IgG antibodies and complement in the basement membrane zone.
- Area affected is the basal cell–basement membrane attachment (hemidesmosomes), where the bullous pemphigoid antigen (BPAG) is located. This protein is normally involved in dermoepidermal bonding.
- IgG autoantibodies to hemidesmosome components fixes complement with subsequent tissue injury.

Morphology

- Characterized by a subepidermal non-acantholytic blister.
- Lesions show perivascular inflammation (lymphocytes, eosinophils and occasional neutrophil), superficial dermal oedema and associated basal cell liquefaction, which eventually gives rise to the blister.

Dermatitis Herpetiformis

- Affects predominantly males in the third and fourth decades.
- May be associated with gluten-sensitive enteropathy (celiac disease).
- Urticarial plaques and vesicles seen in a bilaterally symmetrical distribution on the extensor surface of elbows, knees, upper back and buttocks.

Pathogenesis

- IgA antibodies to dietary gluten are present.
- Antibodies cross-react with reticulin (a component of fibrils that anchor the epidermal basement membrane to the superficial dermis).
- Resulting injury produces a subepidermal blister.

Morphology

- Formation of microabscesses occurs (fibrin and neutrophils at the tips of dermal papillae).

- Basal cells show vacuolization and focal dermoepidermal separation, eventually leading to formation of a subepidermal bulla.
- Direct immunofluorescence shows discontinuous, granular deposits of IgA localized in the tips of dermal papillae.

Q. Write briefly about benign epithelial tumours.

Ans. Common benign epithelial tumours include:

Seborrhoeic Keratosis

Common epidermal tumour that occurs most frequently in middle-aged and older individuals, usually on the trunk, extremities, head and neck.

Pathogenesis

- Activating mutations are present in the fibroblast growth factor (FGF) receptor 3.
- Onset of lesions may be part of a paraneoplastic syndrome **(sign of Leser–Trélat)**.
- Patients may have internal malignancies, which produce growth factors that stimulate epidermal proliferation.

Morphology

It is a raised, pigmented lesion with a verruca-like surface, which histologically exhibits hyperkeratosis, papillomatosis, entrapment of keratin in the epidermis (horn cysts) and proliferation of basaloid (basal cell-like) cells showing increased pigmentation.

Acanthosis Nigricans

- Cutaneous manifestation of a diverse group of diseases.
- May occur as an inherited disorder or as a reaction to drugs.
- Usually autosomal dominant in origin or associated with tissue resistance to insulin (metabolic syndrome, diabetes, obesity, PCOD, MEN syndromes and Cushing disease).
- Eighty per cent have a 'benign' course; 20% are associated with gastrointestinal or other visceral malignancies.

Clinical Features

- Manifests as brown, velvety and verrucous plaques in axillae, back of neck and other skin folds.
- Oral mucosa or oesophagus may be involved occasionally.

Morphology

Histopathology shows orthokeratotic hyperkeratosis and papillomatosis of stratum spinosum with increased pigmentation of basal cell layer without melanocytic hyperplasia and absence of dermal inflammation.

Keratoacanthoma

Results from proliferation of infundibular portion of hair follicle.

Clinical Features

- Males more commonly affected; usually seen in sun-exposed skin of face.
- May be associated with inflammatory dermatoses, genetic diseases, scars, etc.
- Multiple lesions associated with familial cases.

Morphology

Histopathology shows orthokeratotic hyperkeratosis and papillomatosis of stratum spinosum with increased pigmentation of basal cell layer without melanocytic hyperplasia and absence of dermal inflammation.

Fibroepithelial Polyp/Skin Tag

- Common, benign skin lesion of adults, also known as acrochordon, skin tag or soft fibroma.
- Usually occurs on intertriginous areas (i.e. axilla, groin), face, neck and eyelids.
- Associated with metabolic syndrome, diabetes, pregnancy and abnormal lipid profile. Multiple lesions can be seen in **Birt–Hogg–Dube** syndrome.

Clinical Features

Flesh coloured to dark brown, sessile to pedunculated, variable size.

Morphology

Shows fibrovascular cores covered by squamous epithelium which may vary from being hyperplastic to flattened.

Q. Describe the clinicopathological features of squamous cell carcinoma (SCC). (PA34.1)

Ans. SCC is a malignancy of the keratinocytes which may present as follows:

1. Crusted or scaly patches on the skin with a red, inflamed base.
2. Nodular lesions/proliferative growth.
3. A non-healing ulcer.

Salient Features

- SCC generally occurs in sun-exposed areas among people older than age 50.
- May also occur on the lips, inside the mouth, on the genitalia or anywhere on the body.
- Is known to be associated with long-standing inflammation of the skin.

Risk Factors

- Excessive radiological exposure (X-rays).
- Exposure to arsenic and industrial carcinogens (tar and oils).
- Exposure to UV radiation (produces DNA damage).
- Actinic (solar keratosis).
- Chronic immunosuppression by chemotherapy or organ transplantation (reduces host surveillance by epidermal Langerhans cells and increases susceptibility to infection by oncogenic viruses like HPV subtypes 5 and 8).
- Chronic non-healing ulcers and burn scars (**Marjolin ulcer**).

Pathogenesis

- Malignant transformation of normal epidermal keratinocytes is the hallmark of SCC. The critical pathogenic event is the development of apoptotic resistance through functional loss of TP53, a tumour suppressor gene.

- UV radiation causes DNA damage through the creation of pyrimidine dimers, a process known to result in genetic mutation of TP53.
- TP53 mutations are seen in a large number of skin cancers, as well as most precursor skin lesions, suggesting that loss of TP53 is an early event in the development of SCC.
- Other genetic abnormalities believed to contribute to the pathogenesis of SCC include mutations of BCL2 and RAS, alterations in intracellular signal transduction pathways involving epidermal growth factor receptor (EGFR) and cyclooxygenase (COX) and mutations in DNA repair genes.

Morphology

- Squamous cell carcinoma in situ (CIS), sometimes referred to as **Bowen disease**, is a precursor to invasive SCC. This lesion is characterized by nuclear atypia, frequent mitoses, cellular pleomorphism and a disorganized progression of cells from the basal to apical layers of the epidermis.
- **Actinic keratosis (AK)**, a similar precancerous skin lesion, is a scaly, crusty lesion in fair-skinned people, which occurs because of solar damage.
- Invasive SCC is differentiated from CIS and AK, based on invasion of the basement membrane by malignant cells seen in the former. In invasive SCC, nests of malignant cells are found in the dermis, without a definitive basment membrane, usually surrounded by an inflammatory infiltrate.
- Conventional SCCs can be divided into three histological grades, based on the degree of differentiation (resemblance to normal squamous epithelium), nuclear atypia and keratinization.
- A **well-differentiated SCC** (Fig. 34.2) is characterized by cells with near-normal-appearing nuclei and abundant cytoplasm with **extracellular keratin pearls**.
- In contrast, a **poorly differentiated SCC** shows a high degree of nuclear atypia with frequent mitoses, a greater nuclear-to-cytoplasmic ratio and less keratinization. Poorly differentiated SCCs have an increased rate of metastasis and an overall worse prognosis.
- **Moderately differentiated SCCs** exhibit features between those of well-differentiated and poorly differentiated lesions.
- Histological variants include **acantholytic (adenoid) SCC**, which is characterized by a pseudoglandular appearance due to necrosis in the centre of tumour nests, and **spindle cell SCC**, which has atypical spindle-shaped cells, resembling a sarcoma. Both the variants exhibit a more aggressive clinical course.

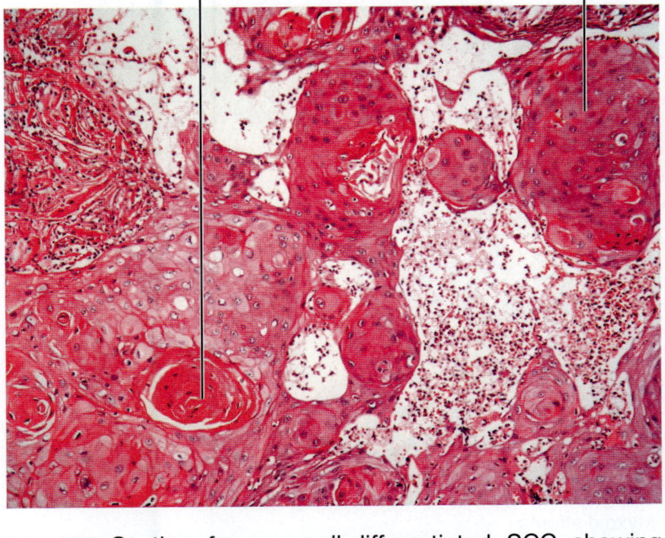

Fig. 34.2 Section from a well-differentiated SCC showing atypical squamous cells with abundant cytoplasm and extracellular keratin pearls (H&E; 200×).

Q. Describe the clinicopathological features of basal cell carcinoma (BCC). (PA34.2)

Ans. BCC arises from the basal layer of the epidermis and constitutes approximately 80% of all non-melanoma skin cancers.

- The tumour most often affects individuals aged 40–60 years; it is locally aggressive and rarely metastasizes.
- Advanced lesions may ulcerate and locally invade into the underlying bone and facial sinuses like a rodent (therefore also called rodent ulcer).
- BCC is commonly located on the face, on the inner aspect of the nose, around the orbit and on the upper lip (sun-exposed parts of the body), where it appears as an insidious, painless, non-healing ulcer or raised nodule containing a central crater.
- In patients with recurrent or deeply infiltrative tumours, involvement of the facial nerve or branches of the trigeminal nerve may be seen.

Pathogenesis

Risk is related to the skin type and the degree of exposure to sunlight, particularly UVB radiation. Mutations in protein patched homolog-1 (PCTH)-1 tumour suppressor gene are implicated in both sporadic and inherited forms of BCC. P53 mutations are seen in 40%–60% of BCCs.

Genetic Syndromes Involving BCC

1. **Xeroderma pigmentosa** is a rare, autosomal recessive disorder characterized by hypersensitivity to UV radiation. It occurs because of defects in DNA repair mechanisms and results in predisposition to cutaneous cancers (e.g. BCC, SCC and melanoma).
2. **Nevoid basal cell (Gorlin) syndrome** is an autosomal dominant disorder associated with multiple BCCs, odontogenic keratocysts, calcification of falx cerebri and rib abnormalities.
3. **Epidermodysplasia verruciformis** is an autosomal recessive disorder characterized by the development of BCC and SCC from warts.

Types

Different clinicopathological types of BCC exist, each with distinct biological behaviour:

- **Nodular or noduloulcerative BCC**
  - Constitutes more than 60% of BCCs.
  - Presents as a well-circumscribed, dome-shaped, pearly nodule with or without ulceration.

- **Superficial BCC**
  - This BCC subtype appears as a red scaly patch that resembles chronic dermatitis; it is predominantly seen in the extremities.
  - It spreads superficially and can involve a large surface area.
- **Morphoea type or sclerosing BCC**
  - Accounts for 10% of cases.
  - Presents as a flat or slightly depressed, fibrotic and firm lesion.
  - Deeply infiltrative in character and tends to extend beyond the clinically obvious margins.
- **Micronodular BCC**
  - Manifests as a plaque-like indurated lesion with poorly demarcated contours.
  - Has a high incidence of recurrence and an aggressive behaviour.
- **Other types include** keratotic BCC, infundibulocystic BCC, follicular BCC and pleomorphic BCC.

Morphology (Fig. 34.3A and B)

- Tumour cells are basaloid and predominantly arranged as islands showing prominent peripheral palisading, at places forming cords and nests.
- Cells within the centre of the epithelial islands appear syncytial (having ill-defined cytoplasmic margins).
- The stroma shows varying amounts of collagen deposition with abundant mucin. A characteristic retraction artefact or clefting is exhibited by the stroma immediately adjacent to the islands/nests of tumour cells on H&E staining.

Q. Enumerate the common cystic disorders of skin.

Ans. Common cystic disorders of skin include:

1. **Epidermal inclusion cyst:** Derived from the epidermis of a hair follicle and contains laminated keratin material.
2. **Pilar (sebaceous) cyst:** Most commonly located on the scalp, it is similar to an epidermal inclusion cyst except for the absence of a stratum granulosum layer in the cyst wall and absence of laminated keratin within the cyst.

Q. Describe the clinicopathological features of melanocytic disorders of the skin. (PA34.3)

Ans. Melanocytic disorders of the skin include:

1. **Vitiligo:** Acquired depigmentation resulting from autoimmune destruction of melanocytes.
2. **Freckles:** Pigmented macular lesions that occur in sun-exposed areas of the skin; they are not premalignant and have a normal number of melanocytes along the basal cell layer but increased melanosomes.
3. **Lentigo simplex:** Similar to a freckle, except that there are increased numbers of melanocytes along the basal layer as well as increased melanin in each melanocyte.
4. **Naevus:** Denotes any congenital lesion of the skin which has 'naevus cells'. Naevus cells are similar to melanocytes but differ from melanocytes in being arranged in clusters or nests.
5. **Melanocytic naevus:** Benign neoplastic proliferation of neural crest-derived melanocytes. It may be congenital or acquired.
6. **Junctional naevi:** Nevi containing nests of pigmented naevus cells proliferating along the epidermodermal junction (appear as flat, pigmented lesions). The naevus cells have round uniform nuclei with inconspicuous nucleoli and sparse mitoses.
7. Junctional naevi usually develop into **compound naevi**, because naevus cells extend into the underlying superficial dermis, forming cords and columns of cells, so that both a junctional and an intradermal component are present (raised, pigmented and verruca-like lesions). The extension

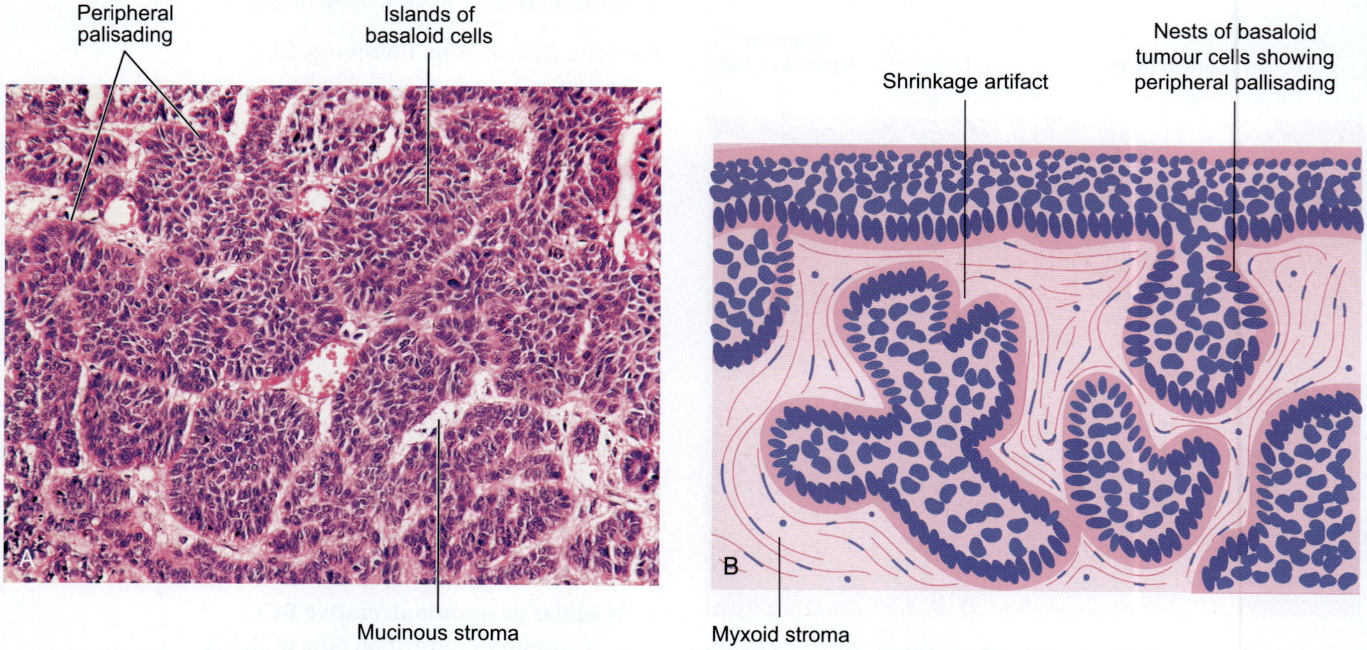

Fig. 34.3 (A and B) Photomicrograph and schematic diagram of BCC skin comprising islands of basaloid tumour cells showing prominent peripheral palisading, surrounded by a mucinous stroma (H&E; 200×).

of naevus cells in the underlying dermis occurs as a result of a process called maturation.

8. **Intradermal naevus**, which is the most common type of naevus in adults, is located in the upper dermis.
9. **Dysplastic naevi** may be a part of the **dysplastic naevus syndrome** (autosomal dominant syndrome associated with >100 naevi on the skin which invariably converts into malignant melanoma), and they may be precursor lesions of malignant melanoma. They are benign lesions that have clinical features similar to those of a malignant melanoma including asymmetry, irregular borders and colour variation.

Malignant Melanoma

- It is a malignant tumour derived from melanocytes.
- Both sexes are affected equally; it is more common in whites than in African Americans, and has a predilection for fair-skinned people.
- Exposure to excessive sunlight at an early age is the single most important predisposing risk factor. Other risk factors include a history of severe sunburn, dysplastic naevus syndrome, melanoma in a first- or second-degree relative and xeroderma pigmentosum.
- About 10%–15% of melanomas have genetic abnormalities. Most common aberrations are mutations in CDKN2A (seen in familial and sporadic melanoma), RB and PTEN genes. Activating mutations in NRAS and BRAF are also implicated. CDKN2A encodes for three different tumour suppressor genes – p15/INK4b, p16/INK4a and p14/ARF; therefore, mutations in CDKN2A lead to uncontrolled melanocyte proliferation. Normally, PTEN downregulates PI-3KAKT signalling. Epigenetic silencing of PTEN in melanomas results in activation of the signalling and induces cellular proliferation. Activating mutations in NRAS and BRAF induce RAS/RAF/MAP kinin cascade resulting in cell proliferation.
- Symptoms such as bleeding, itching, ulceration and pain in a pigmented lesion warrant evaluation. The following signs are indicative of development of malignancy in a pre-existing lesion:
  - **Asymmetry:** One-half of the lesion does not match the other half.
  - **Border irregularity:** The edges are ragged, notched or blurred.
  - **Colour variation:** Pigmentation is not uniform and may display shades of tan, brown or black; white, reddish or blue discolouration is of particular concern.
  - **Diameter:** A diameter greater than 6 mm is characteristic, although some melanomas may have smaller diameters; any growth in a naevus warrants an evaluation.
  - **Evolving:** Changes in the lesion over time are characteristic; this factor is critical for nodular or amelanotic (non-pigmented) melanoma, which may not exhibit the classic criteria mentioned earlier.
- Most variants have an initial **radial growth phase** in which malignant melanocytes proliferate laterally/horizontally within the epidermis, along the dermoepidermal junction or within the papillary dermis; metastasis cannot occur in this phase.
- There may be a **vertical growth phase** in which malignant cells penetrate the underlying reticular dermis; metastasis can occur in this phase.
- Tumour cells are polygonal to spindled, larger than normal melanocytes, and have atypical nuclei showing irregular contours and prominent eosinophilic nucleoli. Intracytoplasmic melanin is usually seen. Tumours not showing pigment are called amelanotic melanomas (Fig. 34.4A and B). Various patterns of growth of tumour cells may be seen including solid sheets, islands, glands, etc.

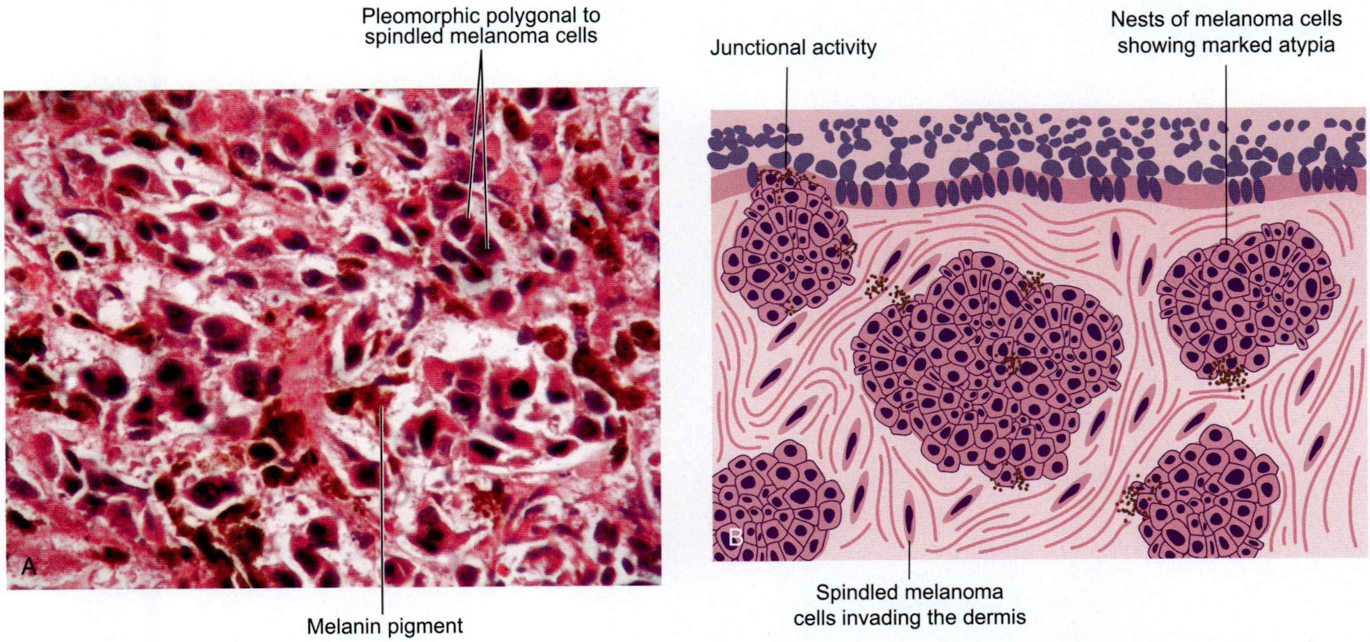

Fig. 34.4 (A and B) Photomicrograph and schematic diagram of malignant melanoma showing nets and singly lying melanoma cells. The cells vary from being polygonal to spindled and are invading the dermis. Extra and intracellular melanin pigment is seen (H&E; 400×).

- **Superficial spreading melanoma**, the most common type, primarily affects women older than 50 years. The lower extremities and back are the most common locations. Histologically, it is characterized by pagetoid infiltration of the epidermis by atypical melanocytes.
- **Lentigo maligna melanoma** is an extension of a lentigo maligna (intraepidermal lesion). It mainly occurs on the sun-exposed face of an elderly person. Histologically, it is characterized by a predominantly junctional proliferation of melanocytes and extension along adnexal structures. Solar elastosis is typically present.
- **Nodular melanomas** lack a radial growth phase and directly invade the dermis.
- **Acral lentiginous melanomas** are located on the palms, soles or subungual regions and usually affect African-Americans.
- The **Breslow system** of staging measures the depth of invasion from the outermost granular layer to the deepest margin of the tumour; lesions with <0.76 mm of invasion usually do not metastasize, whereas those >1.7 mm of invasion have the potential for lymph node metastasis. The **Clark system** subdivides invasion into levels I–V. In addition to the Breslow thickness, prognostic factors for malignant melanoma include (a) the number of mitoses, (b) presence and number of tumour-infiltrating lymphocytes and (c) location of the tumour (location on the extremities has a better prognosis).
- Most melanomas metastasize to regional lymph nodes; thus, sentinel lymph node biopsy also helps in prognosticating the tumour.

Diseases of the Musculoskeletal System

35

BONE

Bone is the basic unit of the human skeletal system which is responsible for weight bearing, protection of visceral organs, locomotion and haematopoietic cell production. Bones can be classified based on their location, size and structure.

Location

1. **Axial skeleton:** Bones of the skull, vertebral column, sternum and ribs.
2. **Appendicular skeleton:** Bones of the pectoral girdle, pelvis girdle and limbs.

Size

1. **Long bones:** They are tubular and hollow with two ends, e.g. bones of the limbs. A long bone can further be divided into several regions (Fig. 35.1):
   - **Epiphysis:** Region between the growth plate and the expanded end of bone, covered by articular cartilage.
   - **Metaphysis:** Region where the growth plate and the diaphysis meet.
   - **Diaphysis:** The shaft of long bones located between the two metaphyses.
   - **Physis (epiphyseal plate, growth plate):** Separates the epiphysis from the metaphysis and is the zone of endochondral ossification in an actively growing bone.
2. **Short bones:** They are cuboidal in shape, and located only in the foot (tarsal bones) and wrist (carpal bones).

Structure

1. **Based on texture of cross-sections, bone tissue can be classified as follows:**
   (a) **Compact bone (dense bone, cortical bone):** Compact bone is ivory-like and dense in texture without any spaces or cavities. It consists mainly of Haversian systems or secondary osteons.
   (b) **Spongy bone (trabecular bone, cancellous bone):** Spongy bone is so named because it is sponge-like with numerous cavities. It is located within the medullary cavity and consists of extensively connected bony trabeculae that form a sponge-like network. Mature trabecular bone exhibits lamellae and osteocytes between the lamellae. Inactive flattened osteocytes are also present on the bone surface.
2. **Based on matrix arrangement, bone tissue can be classified as follows:**
   (a) **Lamellar bone:** Lamellar bone is mature bone in which the constituent collagen fibres are arranged in lamellae. In contrast to spongy bone, the lamellae are arranged parallel to each other; in compact bone, the lamellae are organized concentrically around a vascular canal (Haversian canal).
   (b) **Woven bone:** Woven bone is immature bone, in which collagen fibres are arranged in irregular random arrays and contain smaller amounts of mineral substance and a higher proportion of osteocytes than in lamellar bone. Woven bone is temporary and is eventually converted to lamellar bone.

Microscopic Structure of Bone

1. **Bone cells**
   (a) **Osteoblasts:** They line the surface of bone or osteoid and synthesize collagen, proteoglycans and glycoproteins. Osteoblasts also synthesize alkaline phosphatase, an enzyme needed for the mineralization of osteoid. The cell has an eccentrically located nucleus with a prominent

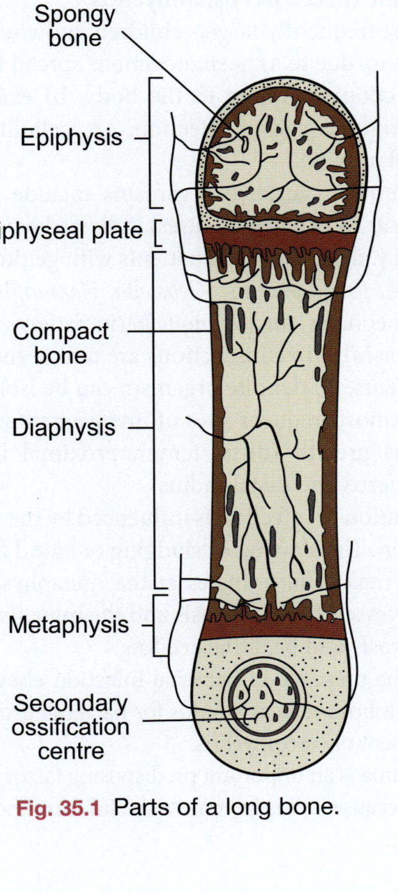

Fig. 35.1 Parts of a long bone.

nucleolus and a perinuclear halo similar to a plasma cell but lacks the cartwheel-like chromatin pattern that is typical of the latter. An inactive osteoblast has a flattened shape and low alkaline phosphatase activity.

(b) **Osteocytes:** An osteoblast gives rise to an osteocyte which lies in a lacunar space and is connected to other osteocytes by dendritic processes through tunnels called 'canaliculi'.

(c) **Osteoclasts:** Osteoclasts are thought to be derived from the monocyte–macrophage system and are responsible for bone resorption. They are multinucleated cells with fine, finger-like cytoplasmic processes. An increased number of osteoclasts may be seen in diseases with increased bone turnover.

2. **Bone matrix:** Bone matrix consists of organic and inorganic components. The association of organic and inorganic substances gives bone its hardness and resistance. The organic component or osteoid forms 35% of the bone and the inorganic or mineral component forms 65% of the bone. Osteoid is composed of collagen fibres with predominately type I collagen (95%) and amorphous material, including glycosaminoglycans that are associated with proteins like osteopontin. The inorganic part is constituted by hydroxyapatite which serves as a reservoir for calcium.

Q. Define and classify osteomyelitis.

(PA33.1, OR3.1)

Ans. Osteomyelitis is defined as infection of the bone (osteo) and marrow (myelo) by bacteria, viruses or fungi. It may be primary (when bone is the solitary focus of infection) and secondary (when bone is involved as a complication of a systemic infection).

Classification

1. **Pyogenic (bacterial) osteomyelitis**
   - Most frequently targets children and young adults.
   - Occurs due to a) haematogenous spread from a focus of infection elsewhere in the body; b) extension from a contiguous site of infection, e.g. cellulitis or c) direct implantation.
   - Common causative organisms include *Staphylococcus aureus* (80%–90% of cases), followed by *Escherichia coli* (in i.v. drug users and patients with genitourinary infection), *Pseudomonas*, *Klebsiella*, *Haemophilus influenzae* (in neonates) and *Salmonella* (in patients with sickle cell diseases). Mixed infections are also seen. In half of the patients, no definite organism can be isolated.
   - The most frequent sites of involvement are the areas of rapid growth (distal femur, proximal tibia, proximal humerus and distal radius).
   - Location of infection is influenced by the vascular circulation. The slowing or sludging of blood flow as the vessels make sharp angles at the metaphyses predisposes the vessels to thrombosis and the bone itself to localized necrosis and bacterial seeding.
   - In the presence of bacterial infection elsewhere, a site of thrombosis acts as a nidus for bacterial growth and development of osteomyelitis.
   - Trauma is an important predisposing factor for osteomyelitis because it aids in venostasis and thrombosis.

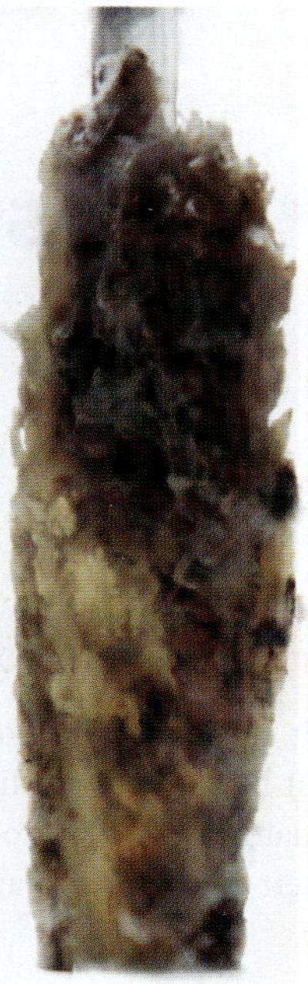

Fig. 35.2 Sequestrum or dead bone showing irregular surface and ragged margins.

Stages of infection

- **Acute:** Develops over days and weeks.
- **Chronic:** Develops over weeks to months; may persist for years.

Pathology

The dead bone (sequestrum) appears as bone with ragged brown- to black-coloured margins (Fig. 35.2). On histopathology, acute followed by chronic inflammatory cells are seen surrounding fragments of dead bone. Occasionally, foreign body giant cell reaction may be seen; the sequestrum shows empty lacunae without osteocytes (Fig. 35.3).

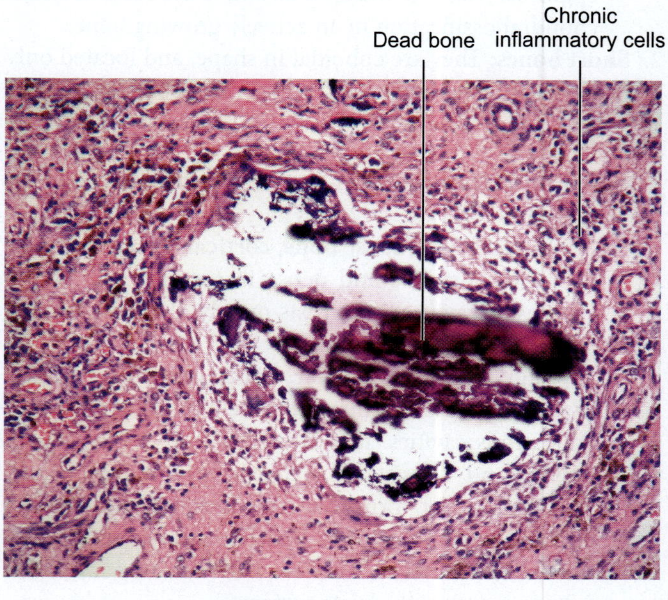

Fig. 35.3 Photomicrograph of chronic osteomyelitis showing fragments of dead bone surrounded by chronic non-specific inflammation and foreign body giant cells (H&E; 200×).

Localization of bacteria
↓
Induction of acute inflammatory reaction and cell death
↓ Influx of neutrophils which enzymatically destroy bone
Raised tissue pressure due to continuing exudation
↓
Compromise of blood vessels and ischaemia
↓
Transmission of infection via Haversian system to periosteum
↓
Subperiosteal abscess formation
↓
Lifting of the periosteum, which further impairs blood supply
↓
Segmental devitalization of bone resulting in formation of sequestrum or dead bone
↓
Rupture of periosteum and formation of a draining sinus

Flowchart 35.1 Sequence of events in osteomyelitis.

Sequence of events
See Flowchart 35.1.
Complications
1. Draining sinus tract
2. Suppurative arthritis
3. Pathological fracture
4. Secondary ankylosis (fibrosis and fusion of joint)
5. Endocarditis
6. Squamous cell carcinoma with a chronic non-healing ulcer (**Marjolin ulcer**)
7. Secondary amyloidosis

Clinical features
Fever, leucocytosis and throbbing pain over the affected region (**differential diagnosis** is Ewing sarcoma because it may have a similar clinical presentation).
X-ray
Lytic focus surrounded by sclerosis.
Clinicomorphological variants
Chronic osteomyelitis results from inadequate antibiotic treatment or incomplete surgical debridement. Extensive periosteal reactive new bone formation associated with chronic osteomyelitis is called **involucrum**.

Brodie abscess is a small devascularized osteomyelitic focus which becomes encapsulated and surrounded by dense sclerotic reactive bone. It is a manifestation of subacute osteomyelitis.

Sclerosing osteomyelitis of Garre typically develops in the **jaw**, and is associated with extensive new bone formation that obscures many of the underlying osseous structures.

2. **Tuberculous osteomyelitis** (OR4.1)

About 1%–3% of cases of pulmonary and extrapulmonary tuberculosis present with osseous involvement. Age group affected is adolescents and young adults. Skeletal tuberculosis usually presents as a solitary lesion but may be multifocal in immunodeficient state, e.g. AIDS.

Modes of spread
- Haematogenous: From active visceral disease.
- Direct extension: From a pulmonary focus into the ribs or tracheobronchial nodes into the vertebrae.

Clinical features
- Commonly affected sites are spine (lumbar and thoracic), knee and hip.
- Almost all patients present with pain, fever (typically low grade with evening rise) and weight loss.

Pathology: Epithelioid cell granulomas with or without necrosis (Fig. 35.4).
Complications
- **Pott spine (tuberculous spondylitis):** The infection breaks through the intervertebral discs to involve multiple vertebrae and drains into the soft tissue anteriorly along the spinal ligaments forming a cold abscess (an abscess without acute inflammation [**psoas abscess**]).
- **Bony deformity or fracture:** Destruction of the vertebrae can cause deformity (scoliosis, kyphosis) or fracture.
- **Neurological deficit and paraplegia:** Occurs due to extension of disease process into dural space with resultant pressure on the cord.
- **Tuberculous arthritis**
- **Sinus tract formation**
- **Ankylosis**
- **Secondary amyloidosis**

3. **Syphilitic osteomyelitis**

In skeletal syphilis, bone involvement is rare, because the disease is readily diagnosed and treated before this stage.

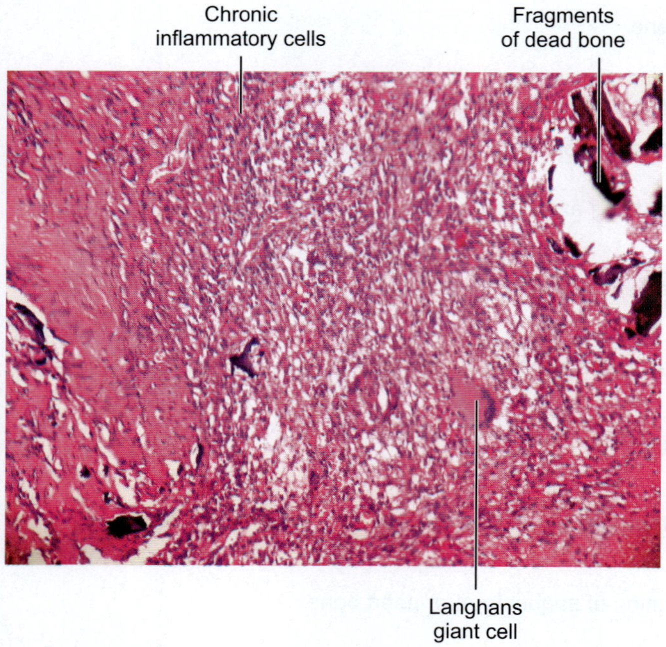

Fig. 35.4 Section from tuberculous osteomyelitis showing necrosis, fragments of dead bone (sequestrum) and granulomatous inflammation (Langhans giant cells and chronic inflammatory cells: H&E; 100×).

Clinical features

Skeletal involvement may be:

(a) Congenital: Bone involvement starts in the fifth month of gestation, and manifests with osteochondritis and periostitis because spirochetes tend to localize in areas of active endochondral ossification (osteochondritis) and the periosteum (periostitis).

(b) Acquired: Bone involvement is seen in the tertiary stage. Skull and long tubular bones are involved, e.g. tibia which shows massive reactive periosteal bone deposition on its medial and anterior surfaces (**saber shin**).

Pathology

Necrotic bone is surrounded by chronic inflammatory cells with a predominance of plasma cells.

Q. Classify primary bone tumours and describe their salient features. (PA33.2, OR10.1)

Ans. Classification of primary bone tumours is given in Table 35.1.

Salient Features

- They are predominantly seen in the first three decades of life, during the period of greatest skeletal growth.
- Benign tumours are by far more common than the malignant ones. The most common benign tumours are osteochondroma, fibro-osseous lesions and enchondroma, in that order.
- Some primary bone tumours are labelled as potentially malignant tumours because they show local aggression but only rarely metastasize, e.g. giant cell tumour (GCT) of bone.
- Among primary malignant neoplasms, multiple myeloma and osteosarcoma have the highest incidence, followed by chondrosarcoma and Ewing sarcoma.

Table 35.1 Classification of primary bone tumours (WHO 2020 abridged)

Histological types	Tumours
Haematopoietic (40%)	• Solitary plasmacytoma of bone • Myeloma • Malignant lymphoma
Chondrogenic (22%)	**Benign** Osteochondroma Enchondroma Periosteal chondroma Chondroblastoma NOS Chondromyxoid fibroma Osteochondromyxoma **Intermediate (locally aggressive)** Chondromatosis NOS Atypical cartilaginous tumour **Malignant** Chondrosarcoma grade I Chondrosarcoma grade II Chondrosarcoma grade III Dedifferentiated chondrosarcoma Mesenchymal chondrosarcoma Clear cell chondrosarcoma Periosteal chondrosarcoma
Osteogenic (20%)	**Benign** Osteoma NOS Osteoid osteoma NOS **Intermediate (locally aggressive)** Osteoblastoma NOS **Malignant** Low-grade central osteosarcoma Osteosarcoma NOS - Conventional osteosarcoma - Telangiectatic osteosarcoma - Small cell osteosarcoma Parosteal osteosarcoma Periosteal osteosarcoma High-grade surface osteosarcoma Secondary osteosarcoma
Undifferentiated round cell sarcomas of bone	Ewing sarcoma
Osteoclastic giant cell–rich tumours	**Benign** Aneurysmal bone cyst Non-ossifying fibroma **Intermediate locally aggressive, rarely metastasizing** Giant cell tumour of bone NOS **Malignant** Malignancy in giant cell tumour of bone
Fibrogenic tumours	**Internediate locally aggressive** Desmoplastic fibroma of bone **Malignant** Fibrosarcoma of bone
Notochordal tumours	**Benign** Benign notochordal tumour **Malignant** Chordoma

Table 35.1 Classification of primary bone tumours (*Cont.*)

Histological types	Tumours
Vascular tumours	**Benign** Haemangioma **Intermediate locally aggressive, rarely metastasizing** Epithelioid haemangioma **Malignant** Epithelioid haemangioendothelioma Angiosarcoma
Other mesenchymal tumours of bone	**Benign** Simple bone cyst Fibrous dysplasia **Intermediate locally aggressive** Osteofibrous dysplasia **Malignant** Adamantinoma

- The commonest sites for primary bone tumours, both benign and malignant, are distal femur and proximal tibia, which are the bones with the highest growth rate.
- Primary bone tumours have very typical radiographic appearances and a clinicoradiological correlation is a must for the correct histopathological diagnosis.
- The typical location/sites of common primary bone tumours are shown in Fig. 35.5.

Q. Describe the gross and microscopic features of the common bone-forming tumours.

Ans. Bone-forming tumours are neoplasms in which the constituent neoplastic cells produce bone.

Classification

1. **Benign**
   (a) Osteoma
   (b) Osteoid osteoma
2. **Intermediate (locally aggressive)**
   Osteoblastoma
3. **Malignant**
   Osteogenic sarcoma (OS)

Osteoma

Skeletal Distribution

- Flat bones of skull and face
- Paranasal sinuses (frontal and ethmoid)

Clinical Features

- Often asymptomatic; discovered incidentally; occur in middle age; are solitary and slow growing.
- May lead to cosmetic deformity, obstruction of sinus cavity or impinge on brain and eye.

Gross Morphology

- Sessile, round to oval, bosselated.
- Project from the subperiosteal/endosteal surface of the cortex.
- Multiple osteomas may present with intestinal polyposis and soft-tissue tumours **(Gardner syndrome).**

Microscopy

Composed of dense and mature lamellar bone.

Osteoid Osteoma

Skeletal Distribution

- Long bones (femur and tibia).
- Usually intracortical; less frequently arise from the medullary cavity.

Clinical Features

- Common in the age group between 10 and 30 years.
- Presents with intense pain which increases during night and is relieved by aspirin. The pain is attributed to excessive PGE2 produced by proliferating osteoblasts and may be accompanied by localized swelling and tenderness.

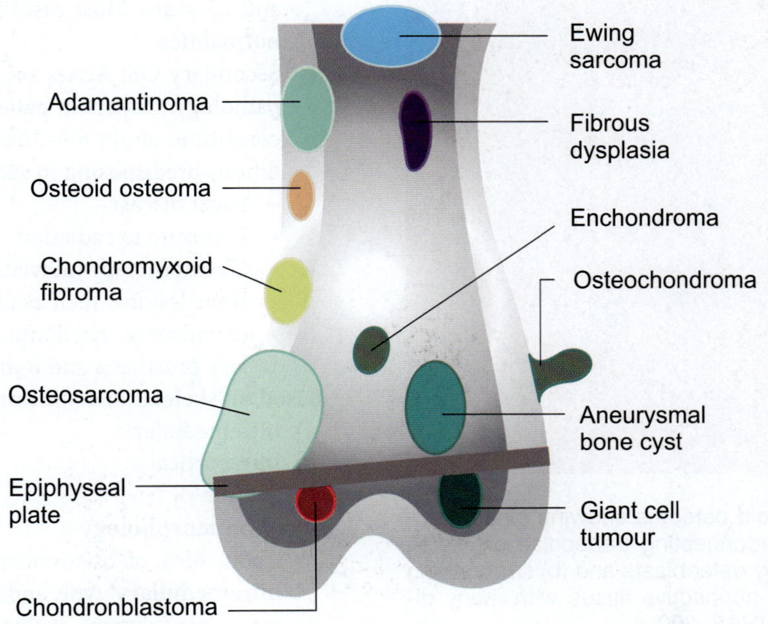

Fig. 35.5 Sites of primary bone tumours.

X-Ray

Shows a central nidus smaller than 1.5 cm that is surrounded by sclerotic bone. The nidus may be difficult to see on plain X-ray. CT is the modality of choice to identify it.

Gross Morphology

Appears as a well-defined, round-to-oval mass of gritty tissue with a size less than 2 cm.

Microscopy (Fig. 35.6)

Osteoid osteoma has two components:

- **Central nidus:** Composed of randomly interconnecting trabeculae of woven bone prominently rimmed by osteoblasts. Stroma surrounding tumour bone consists of loose connective tissue with many dilated-congested capillaries.
- **Envelope:** Sclerotic bone forms an envelope around the nidus.

Osteoblastoma

Osteoblastoma and osteoid osteoma are histologically similar, yet very different in their presentation, localization, radiographic appearance, treatment and potential for recurrence. Osteoblastoma is differentiated from an osteoid osteoma based on the following features:

- Size is larger than 2 cm (therefore also called giant osteoid osteoma).
- Affects older individuals.
- Does not cause localized night pain and when pain occurs, it is not relieved by NSAIDs.
- Does not present with an intense bony reaction unlike osteoid osteoma.

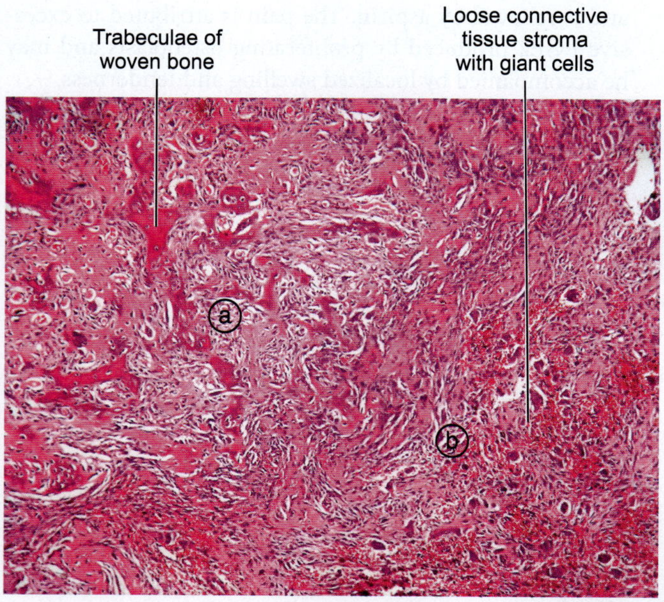

Fig. 35.6 Section from osteoid osteoma showing nidus composed of (a) randomly interconnecting trabeculae of woven bone prominently rimmed by osteoblasts and (b) surrounding stroma consisting of loose connective tissue with many dilated-congested capillaries (H&E; 200×).

- Preferentially involves posterior elements of vertebrae, spine, femur and bones of the foot.
- Less commonly involves the long bones where it is typically metaphyseal in location. May be either be intracortical or intramedullary in origin unlike osteoid osteoma, which is mostly intracortical.

Osteogenic Sarcoma (OS)

OS is a malignant mesenchymal tumour in which the neoplastic stromal cells directly lay down bone matrix or osteoid without an intervening stage of cartilage formation. It is the most common primary malignant bone tumour after myeloma and lymphoma.

Pathogenesis

1. ***Genetic contribution***
   (a) Increased incidence of OS in patients with germ line mutations in P53 gene (Li–Fraumeni syndrome).
   (b) Mutations in RB gene seen in 70% of sporadic cases of OS. Patients with hereditary retinoblastoma have up to 1000 times greater risk of developing OS.
   (c) INK4A which encodes p16 (negative regulator of CDKs) and p14 (which enhances the action of p53), is inactivated in some osteosarcomas.
   (d) CDK4 and MDM2, which are cell cycle regulators and inhibit p53 and RB genes are implicated in low-grade osteosarcomas.
   (e) Risk increased in Rothmund–Thomson syndrome (AR inheritance, mutations in RECQL4 gene, chr 8q24.3).
2. ***Environmental contribution:*** Thorotrast and therapeutic irradiation are implicated. Children treated with alkylating agents have an increased risk of OS.

Classification

1. **Based on age of involvement and presence of pre-existing bone pathology**
   (a) Primary OS: Arises de novo and occurs between 10 and 25 years. Most cases have underlying genetic abnormalities.
   (b) Secondary OS: Arises secondary to pre-existing bone pathology. Occurs in patients older than 40 years and constitutes about 6%–10% of all osteosarcomas. Conditions predisposing to secondary OS include:
   - Paget disease
   - Exposure to radiation
   - Chemotherapy (alkylating agents)
   - Bone lesions, such as fibrous dysplasia (FD), osteochondroma, enchondroma, fractures, intramedullary prosthesis and bone infarcts
2. **Based on skeletal distribution/anatomical site**
   (a) Intramedullary
   (b) Intracortical
   (c) Surface
3. **Based on morphology**
   (a) About 85% of osteosarcomas are of the **'high grade intramedullary'** type, and the other 15% consist of several other subtypes, including telangiectatic, low-grade

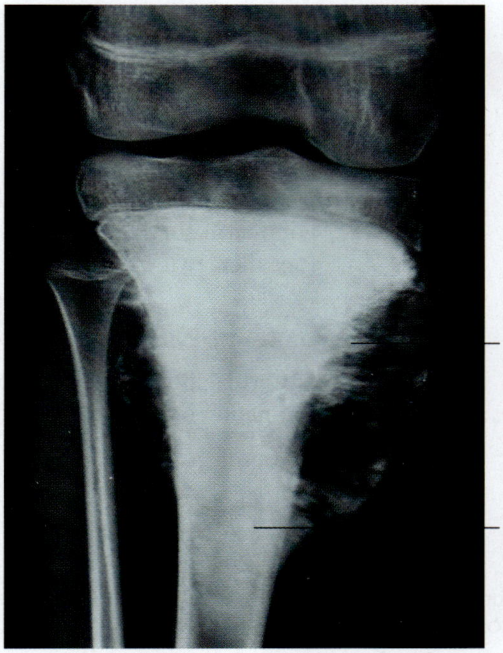

Fig. 35.7 Plain radiograph showing the typical sunray appearance of osteogenic sarcoma (periosteal reaction perpendicular to cortical surface).

intramedullary and small cell, as well as the surface subtypes parosteal, periosteal and high-grade surface osteosarcoma.

(b) Conventional intramedullary OS is mostly metaphyseal in origin and involves long bones, such as lower end of femur, upper end of tibia and upper end of humerus, in that order. It can be further classified into the following subtypes depending on the predominant constituent element:
   (i) Osteoblastic (shows a large amount of osteoid and bony trabeculae)
   (ii) Chondroblastic (malignant cartilage is the predominant matrix type)
   (iii) Fibroblastic (composed of a large spindle cell/fibroblastic component)

Clinical Features

- Presents as a painful, progressively enlarging mass with a large soft-tissue component, sometimes associated with a pathological fracture.
- Has a bimodal age distribution.
- May show markedly raised levels of serum alkaline phosphatase.

Radiological Investigations

- **X-Ray (Fig. 35.7)**
  - Conventional OS usually presents as a metaphyseal, large, permeative, destructive, mixed sclerotic–lytic lesion.
  - Tumour breaks through the cortex, induces reactive periosteal bone formation and lifts the periosteum. The triangular shadow between the cortex and the raised periosteum is radiographically called ***Codman's triangle***.
  - Typically, the periosteal new bone is laid down perpendicular to the surface of the bone (***sunray/sunburst appearance***).
- **MRI:** Required to determine
  - Soft tissue involvement
  - Neurovascular involvement
  - Presence skip metastases (if skip metastases are found, this is equivalent to metastatic (stage III) disease).
- **Bone scan:** Very hot in osteosarcoma; useful to evaluate extent of local disease and presence of bone metastases.
- **CT:** Chest CT is required to evaluate for pulmonary metastases.

Gross Morphology (Fig. 35.8)

- Bulky gritty and grey-white tumour, often containing areas of haemorrhage and necrosis.
- Destruction of cortex and soft-tissue extension are common.
- Penetration of epiphyseal plate/entry into the joint is however relatively infrequent.

Microscopy (Fig. 35.9)

- The stroma is frankly sarcomatous, composed of large atypical spindle-shaped cells with bizarre tumour giant cells and frequent mitoses.
- There is direct formation of tumour osteoid by neoplastic cells. Osteoid is arranged in a thin anastomosing lace-like pattern and appears eosinophilic, glassy and homogenous on H&E sections.
- Chondroblastic and fibroblastic elements may be present besides osteoid.
- Spontaneous necrosis and vascular invasion are frequent.

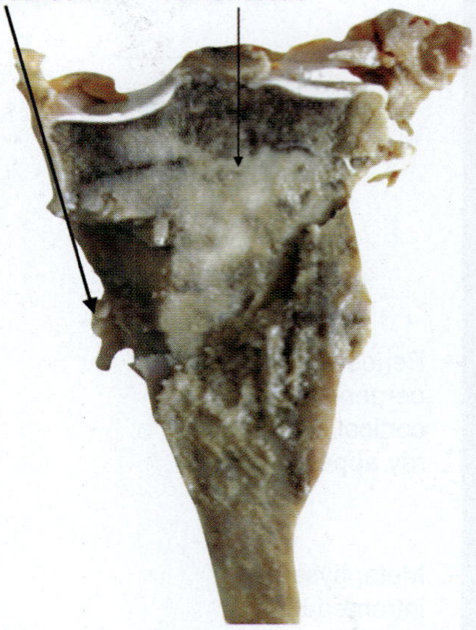

Fig. 35.8 Gritty, grey-white, metaphyseal tumour taking origin from the medullary cavity, causing destruction of cortex and soft-tissue extension.

Surface Osteosarcomas

- **Juxtacortical (parosteal)**
  - Slow growing
  - Classically, located on the posterior aspect of the lower femur
  - Appears as a lobulated mass encircling the bone
  - Low-grade tumour with a good prognosis
- **Periosteal osteosarcoma**
  - Grows on the surface of long bones
  - Occurs on the periosteal surface between the cortex and the periosteum
  - Has a prominent cartilaginous component
  - High-grade osteosarcoma; poor prognosis
- **Osteosarcoma of the jaw**
  - Affects in older age
  - Involves mandible and alveolar ridges of the maxilla
  - Prominent chondroblastic component
  - Good prognosis

Prognosis

- Lungs, other bones, pleura and heart are common sites of metastases. Regional lymph nodes are however rarely involved.
- Long-term survival rate with chemotherapy and limb salvage therapy is 60%–70%.

Q. Describe the gross and microscopic features of the common cartilage-forming tumours.

Ans. Cartilaginous neoplasms of bone are characterized by the formation of hyaline or myxoid cartilage.

Classification

- **Benign**
  - Osteochondroma
  - Enchondroma
  - Periosteal chondroma
  - Chondroblastoma NOS
  - Chondromyxoid fibroma
  - Osteochondromyxoma
- **Intermediate (locally aggressive)**
  - Chondromatosis NOS
  - Atypical cartilaginous tumour
- **Malignant**
  - Chondrosarcoma

Osteochondroma (Exostosis)

- The most frequent benign bone tumour, osteochondroma presents as a bony outgrowth capped by hyaline cartilage which is attached to the underlying bone.
- Multiple osteochondromas occur in the setting of **multiple hereditary exostoses**, an autosomal dominant condition, which is associated with inactivation of EXT-1 and -2 genes. Solitary osteochondromas are thought to arise from displacement of lateral portion of the growth plate.

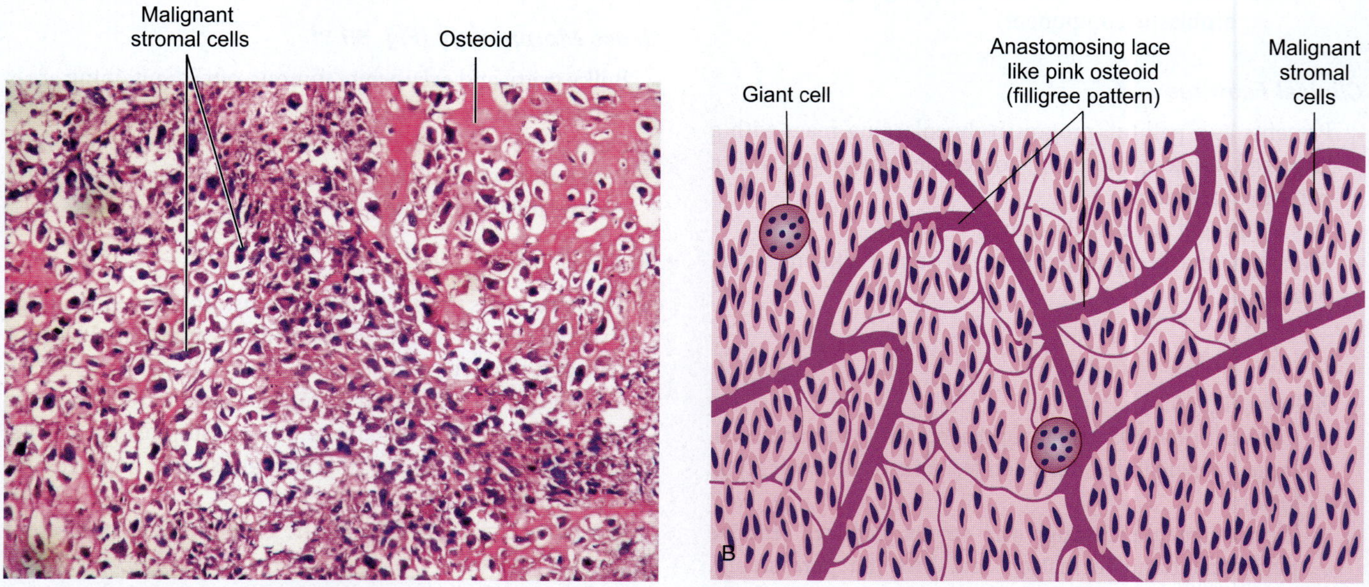

Fig. 35.9 (A and B) Photomicrograph and schematic diagram of sarcomatous stroma composed of large atypical polygonal to spindle-shaped cells showing direct formation of tumour osteoid, seen as eosinophilic, glassy, homogenous, lace like material (H&E; 400×).

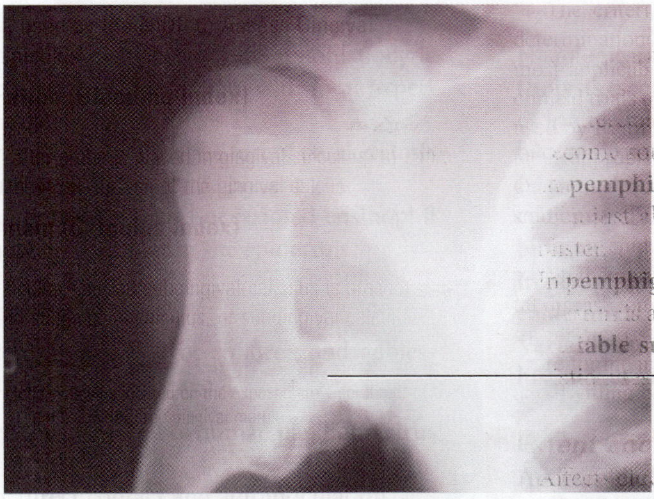

Fig. 35.10 X-ray showing a lobulated cartilaginous exostosis arising from upper humerus.

Skeletal Distribution

Metaphysis of lower femur, upper tibia and upper humerus.

Clinical Features

- Most patients are asymptomatic. The most common complaint is presence of a hard mass of long-standing duration.
- Solitary osteochondromas are diagnosed later in life as compared with multiple osteochondromas which usually manifest in childhood itself.
- Osteochondromas are mostly asymptomatic but may present with pain and deformity. They sometimes interfere with the functioning of regional tendons and blood vessels.

X-Ray (Fig. 35.10)

Seen as metaphyseal lesions which grow in a direction opposite to the adjacent joint. The cortex and medullary cavity of the lesion are continuous with those of the native bone. Cartilage cap is usually radiolucent and involutes at skeletal maturity.

Gross Morphology (Fig. 35.11)

May be sessile or pedunculated, mushroom shaped, with an average size of 4–10 cm.

Microscopy (Fig. 35.12)

- The outermost layer is a fibrous membrane (perichondrium) continuous with the periosteum of the adjacent bone.
- Under the fibrous membrane is cartilage cap (which is formed by mature hyaline cartilage).
- Cross-section through the lesion demonstrates mature trabecular bone.

Complications

- Bursitis (development of bursa around the head of a long-standing osteochondroma).
- Formation of osteocartilaginous loose bodies.
- Infarction/fracture of the stalk.
- Impingement of adjacent vascular and neural structures
- Pseudoaneurysm of an overlying vessel.

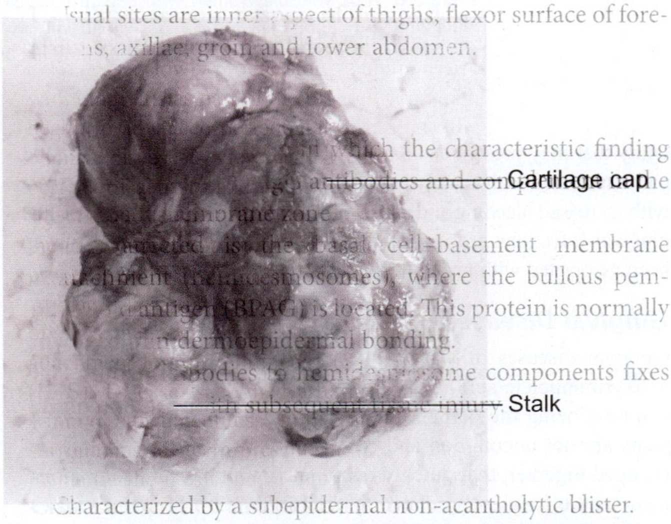

Fig. 35.11 Gross picture of an osteochondroma showing the stalk of the exostosis with an overlying cartilage cap.

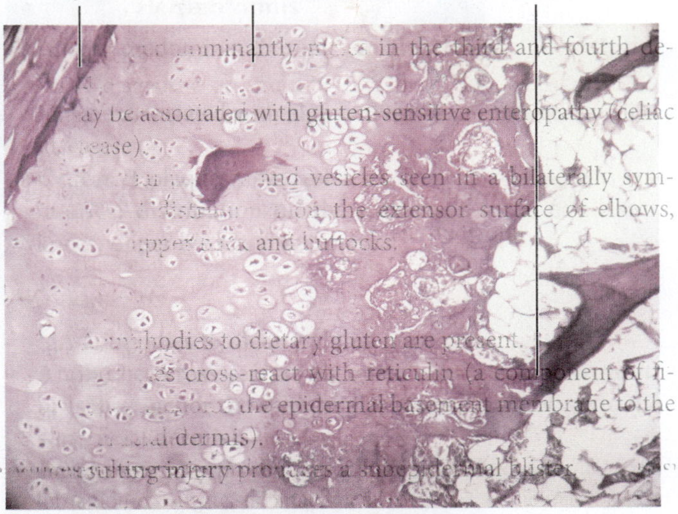

Fig. 35.12 Osteochondroma composed of outermost fibrous layer, with underlying cartilage cap, and mature trabecular bone (H&E; 100×).

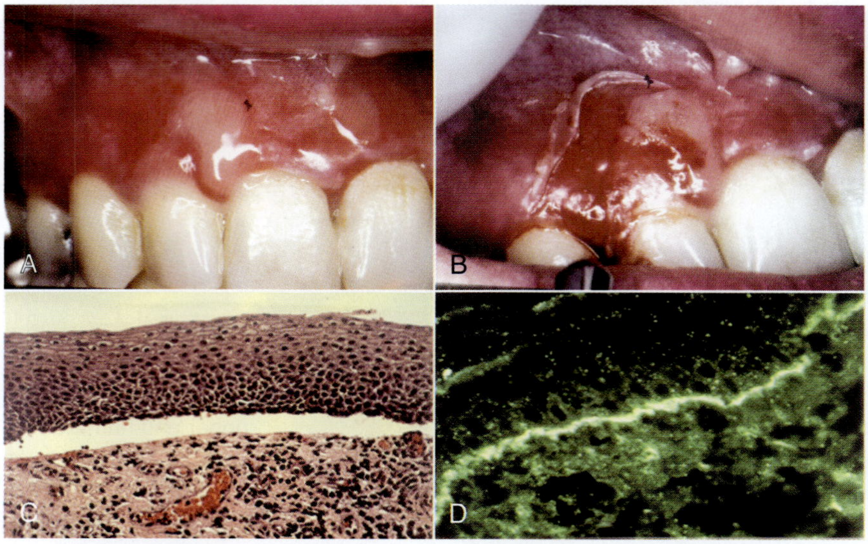

Fig. 5.8 A 62-year-old woman with benign mucous membrane pemphigoid. A and B, Clinical images with sloughing of the epithelial surface. C, Hematoxylin–eosin stain depicting the separation of the epithelium from the connective tissue. D, Immunofluorescent-labeled antibodies in the basement membrane.

entity that may present as an acute condition with fever, malaise, and pain associated with acutely inflamed, diffuse, red, and swollen gingiva with increased bleeding and occasional gingival abscess formation. The gingival infections are usually preceded by tonsillitis and they have been associated with group A β-hemolytic Streptococcal infections.

Gingival Diseases of Viral Origin

Gingival diseases of viral origin may be caused by a variety of deoxyribonucleic acid- and ribonucleic-acid viruses, with the most common being the herpes viruses (Figs. 5.9A and B). Herpetic lesions are not uncommon and develop as intraoral blisters, usually grouped together, that quickly burst, leaving minuscule ulcerations. Lesions are frequently related to the reactivation of latent viruses, especially as a result of reduced immune function. The oral manifestations of viral infection have been comprehensively reviewed. Viral gingival diseases are treated with topical or systemic antiviral drugs (Figs. 5.9C and D).

Gingival Diseases of Fungal Origin

Gingival diseases of fungal origin are relatively uncommon in immunocompetent individuals, but they occur more frequently in immunocompromised individuals and in those with normal oral flora that has been disturbed by the long-term use of broad-spectrum antibiotics. The most common oral fungal infection is candidiasis, which is caused by infection with *Candida albicans*; it can also be seen under prosthetic devices, in individuals using topi-

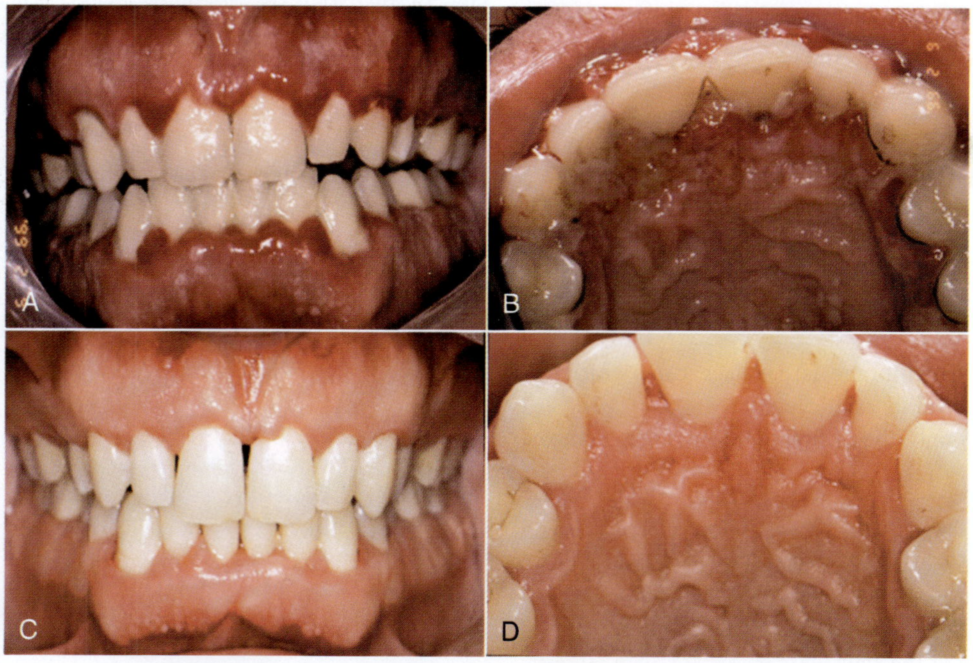

Fig. 5.9 A and B, A 29-year-old man with primary herpetic infection and severe gingival inflammation. C and D, Six weeks after treatment with systemic acyclovir.

cal steroids, and in individuals with decreased salivary flow, increased salivary glucose, or decreased salivary pH. A generalized candidal infection may manifest as white patches on the gingiva, tongue, or oral mucous membrane that can be removed with gauze and that leave a red, bleeding surface. In individuals with human immunodeficiency virus (HIV), candidal infection may present as erythema of the attached gingiva; this has been referred to as *linear gingival erythema* or *HIV-associated gingivitis*.

The diagnosis of candidal infection can be made by culture, smear, or biopsy. Less common fungal infections have also been described.

Gingival Diseases of Genetic Origin

Gingival diseases of genetic origin may involve the tissues of the periodontium and have been described in detail. One of the most clinically evident conditions is *hereditary gingival fibromatosis,* which exhibits autosomal-dominant or (rarely) autosomal recessive modes of inheritance. The gingival enlargement may completely cover the teeth, delay eruption, and present as an isolated finding; alternatively, it may be associated with several more generalized syndromes.

Gingival Manifestations of Systemic Conditions

Gingival manifestations of systemic conditions may appear as desquamative lesions, ulcerations of the gingiva, or both. Allergic reactions that manifest with gingival changes are uncommon but have been observed in association with several restorative materials (Fig. 5.10A), toothpastes, mouthwashes, chewing gums (Fig. 5.11), and foods (Box 5.2). The diagnosis of these conditions may prove difficult and may require an extensive history and the selective elimination of potential causes. Conjoint assessment with an allergologist is indicated, and percutaneous tests are often recommended. Histologic traits of biopsies from gingival allergic reactions include a dense infiltrate of eosinophilic cells (Figs. 5.10B and C).

Traumatic Lesions

Traumatic lesions may be self-inflicted and *factitious* in origin, which means that they are produced by intentional or unintentional

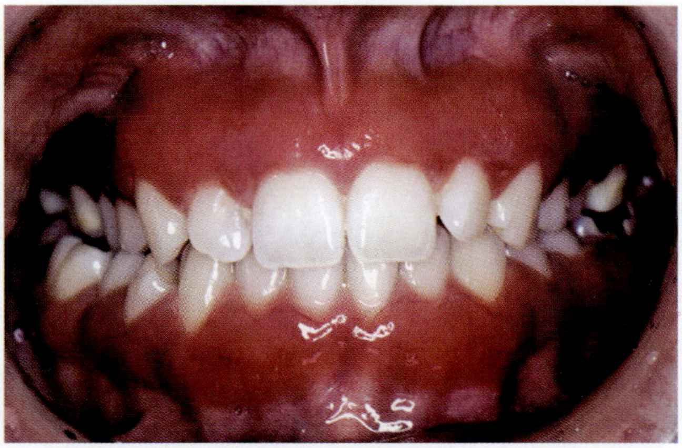

Fig. 5.11 A generalized severe allergic response of the gingiva in response to an additive in chewing gum.

artificial means (Fig. 5.12). Other examples of traumatic lesions include toothbrush trauma that results in gingival ulceration, recession, or both. *Iatrogenic trauma* (i.e., induced by the dentist or health professional) to the gingiva can be caused by the induction of orthodontic cement or preventive or restorative materials (Fig. 5.13A). Peripheral ossifying fibroma may develop in response to the embedment of a foreign body, (Figs. 5.13B and C) and the complete resolution after 4 weeks after excisional biopsy (Fig. 5.13D). Alternatively, *accidental damage* to the gingiva may occur as a result of minor burns from hot foods and drinks.

Foreign-Body Reactions

Foreign-body reactions lead to localized inflammatory conditions of the gingiva and are caused by the introduction of foreign material into the gingival connective tissues through breaks in the epithelium. Common examples include the introduction of amalgam into the gingiva during the placement of a restoration, the extraction of a tooth, or an endodontic apicoectomy with retrofill leaving an amalgam tattoo (Fig. 5.14A), with resultant metal fragment observed during biopsies (Fig. 5.14B); abrasives may also be introduced during polishing procedures.

Periodontitis

Periodontitis is defined as "an inflammatory disease of the supporting tissues of the teeth caused by specific microorganisms or groups of specific microorganisms, resulting in progressive destruction of the

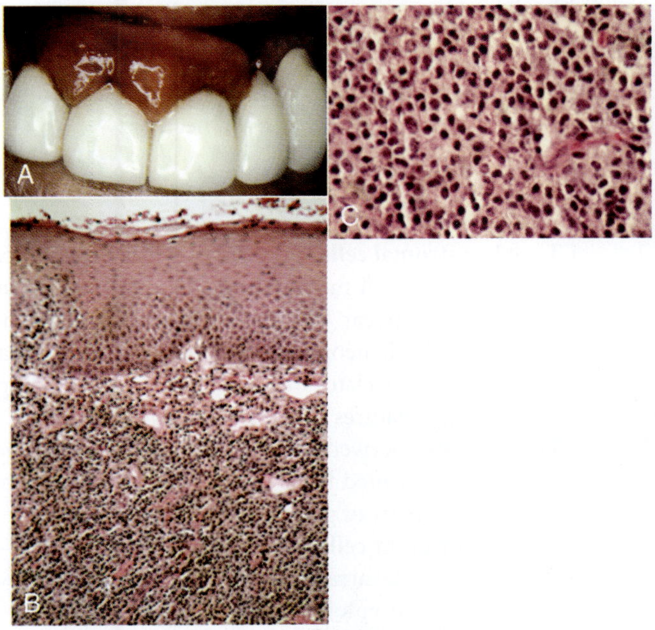

Fig. 5.10 A, Localized pronounced gingival inflammation in response to a nickel allergy. B and C, Biopsy of a dense infiltrate of plasma cells.

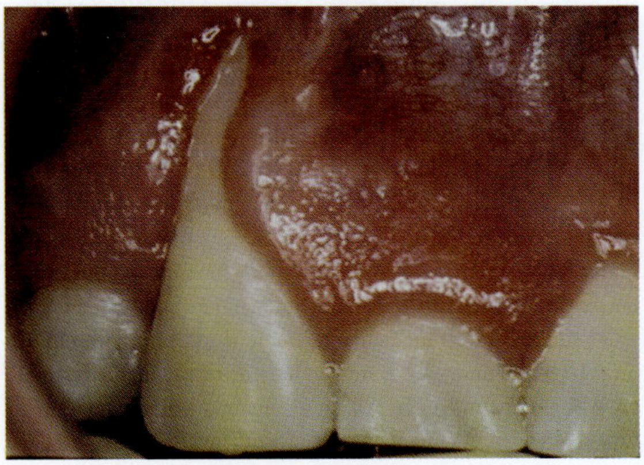

Fig. 5.12 Self-inflicted gingival dehiscence induced via the patient's fingernail.

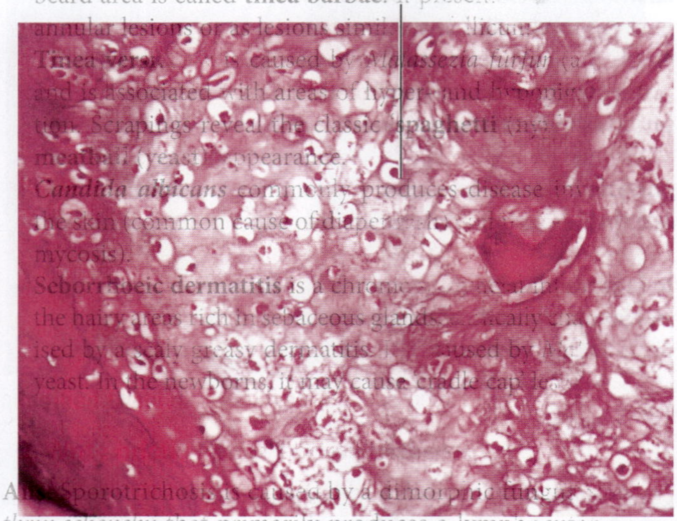

Fig. 35.17 Section from a chondrosarcoma showing cartilaginous lobules composed of atypical chondrocytes (H&E; 200×).

3. **Based on morphology**
   (a) Conventional (which is further subtyped as hyaline or myxoid)
   (b) Clear cell
   (c) Dedifferentiated
   (d) Mesenchymal

Gross Morphology

They are grey-white, lobulated, bulky, translucent masses with a gelatinous consistency. Erosion/destruction of the cortex is frequently seen. Calcification and ossification are not uncommon.

Microscopy (Fig. 35.17)

- Histologically, chondrosarcoma is composed of invasive lobules of anaplastic cartilage and is differentiated from benign cartilaginous tumours based on the following features:
  - Presence of two or more cells per lacuna, binucleate cells, enlarged, plump and hyperchromatic nuclei, nuclear pleomorphism and abundant mitoses
  - Infiltrating margins
- Chondrosarcoma is classified into central atypical cartilaginous tumour (ACT)/grades I, II and III, based on cellularity, pleomorphism, mitoses and necrosis. ACT/chondrosarcoma grade I (CS1) is a locally aggressive hyaline cartilage producing tumour which arises in the medulla of long bone. Tumours in the appendicular skeleton are termed ACTs and tumours in the axial skeleton are usually labelled CS1.
- A chondrosarcoma shows endochondral ossification unlike osteosarcoma in which the osteogenesis is directly from malignant stromal cells without an intervening phase of cartilage formation.

Q. Describe the gross and microscopic features of giant cell tumour of bone (GCT).

Ans. Also known as osteoclastoma, GCT is the most common tumour of epiphyses in skeletally mature individuals with closed growth plates. It often shows metaphyseal extension.

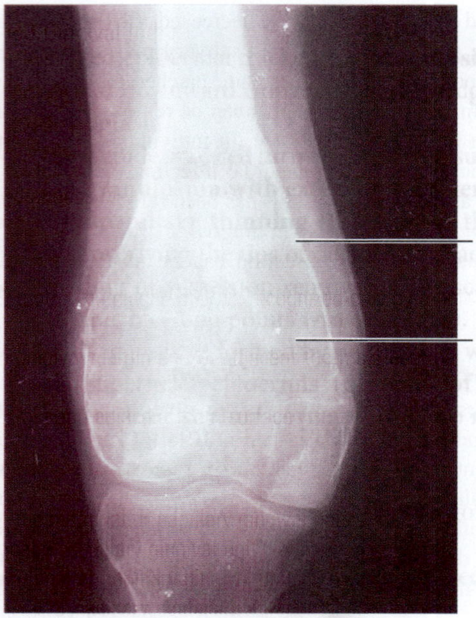

Fig. 35.18 Plain radiograph of GCT arising from the distal end femur showing a large lytic, expansile lesion with thinning of the cortex, well-defined margins without any periosteal reaction. This type of destruction is typically referred to a "geographic destruction".

Common sites include lower end of femur, upper end of tibia and lower end of radius. 10% occur in sacrum (sacral ala) and vertebrae (vertebral body). Phalanges of the hand is also a common location.

X-Ray (Fig. 35.18)

Radiographs show a lytic, expansile lesion which usually does not show any peripheral sclerosis or periosteal reaction. There is thinning and destruction of cortex with frequent extension of the tumour into intermuscular septae and joint space. Because of pockets of lysis, a typical soap-bubble appearance may be seen.

Gross Morphology (Fig. 35.19)

The tumour is variable sized, solid, tan brown and trabeculated with abundant haemorrhage and necrosis.

Microscopy (Fig. 35.20A and B)

- GCT has three histopathological components:
  - **Type I or stromal cells:** Uniform oval mononuclear cells with indistinct cell membranes arranged in a syncytial pattern (cells appear to merge with each other). These cells are the basic neoplastic element of the tumour and their number correlates with its clinical evolution. Type I cells have the features of mesenchymal stem cells.
  - **Type II cells:** Derived from the monocyte/macrophage family and recruited from peripheral blood, these cells are the precursors of giant cells.
  - **Type III or giant cells:** They are large cells with 20–30 (up to 100) nuclei arranged towards the centre (believed to form via receptor activator of nuclear factor-κB [RANK]/RANKL signalling pathway). They have similar characteristics as osteoclasts, resorb bone and possess

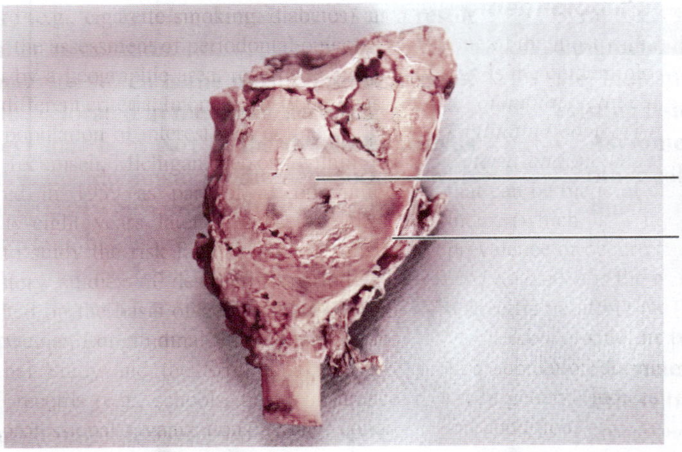

Fig. 35.19 Gross picture of a giant cell tumour arising from the epiphysis. The cut surface shows a variegated appearance with grey-white to yellow to tan-brown areas (areas of haemorrhage and degeneration). There is thinning of the cortex without sclerosis or periosteal reaction.

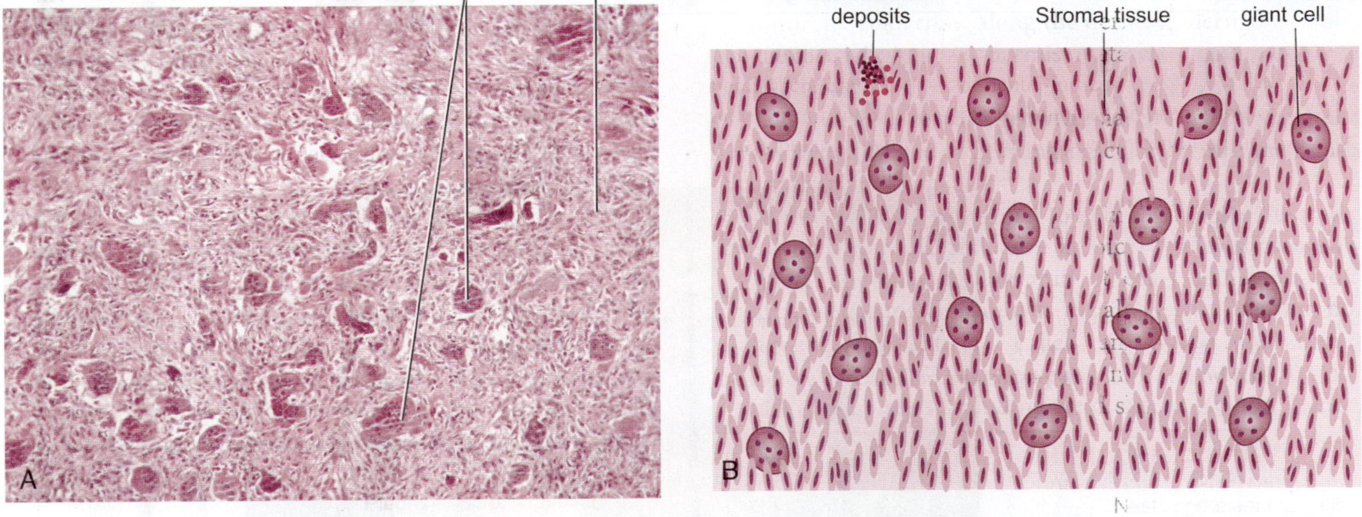

Fig. 35.20 (A and B) Photomicrograph and schematic diagram of a giant cell tumour of bone showing a biphasic population comprising stromal cells (uniform oval mononuclear cells with indistinct cell membrane, arranged in a syncytial pattern) and giant cells (large cells with upto 100 nuclei); (H&E; 200×).

same enzymes (tartrate resistant acid phosphatase, carbonic anhydrase II, cathepsin K, vacuolar ATPase).

- Focal deposition of osteoid or bone may occasionally be seen, especially in cases presenting with pathological fracture. A secondary degenerative ABC component is not uncommon.
- All GCTs should be regarded as *potentially malignant* (approximately 4% give rise to distant metastasis). Metastatic lesions often noted to have altertions in *c-myc* oncogene or p53.
- H3.3 pGly34Trp is a reliable diagnostic marker on immunohistochemistry and molecular analysis.

Q. Enumerate the other giant cell–containing lesions of bone. How is GCT of bone differentiated from these?

Ans. Other giant cell–containing lesions:

1. Metaphyseal fibrous defect
2. Non-ossifying fibroma
3. CMF
4. Chondroblastoma
5. Eosinophilic granuloma
6. Solitary bone cyst (SBC)
7. Osteitis fibrosa cystica (OFC)
8. Aneurysmal bone cyst (ABC)
9. Osteoid osteoma
10. Osteoblastoma

Features differentiating GCT of bone from other giant cell–containing lesions are as follows:

- Giant cells in other giant cell–containing lesions have fewer nuclei as compared with GCT bone. The nuclei in GCT bone are similar in morphological characteristics as the nuclei of the stromal cells, unlike other giant cell–containing lesions.
- There is a uniform and diffuse distribution of giant cells in GCT bone, unlike other giant cell lesions wherein giant cells are focally aggregated.

BOX 5.1 Classification of Periodontal Diseases and Conditions

1. Gingival Diseases
   Plaque-induced gingival diseases[a]
   Nonplaque-induced gingival lesions
2. Chronic Periodontitis[b]
   Localized
   Generalized
3. Aggressive Periodontitis
   Localized
   Generalized
4. Periodontitis as a Manifestation of Systemic Disease
   1. Necrotizing Periodontal Diseases
      Necrotizing ulcerative gingivitis
      Necrotizing ulcerative periodontitis
5. Abscesses of the Periodontium
   Gingival abscess
   Periodontal abscess
   Pericoronal abscess
6. Periodontitis Associated With Endodontic Lesions
   Endodontic–periodontal lesion
   Periodontal–endodontic lesion
   Combined lesion
7. Developmental or Acquired Deformities and Conditions
   Localized tooth-related factors that predispose an individual to plaque-induced gingival diseases or periodontitis
   Mucogingival deformities and conditions around the teeth
   Mucogingival deformities and conditions on edentulous ridges
   Occlusal trauma

[a]These diseases may occur on a periodontium with no attachment loss or on a periodontium with attachment loss that is stable and not progressing.
[b]Chronic periodontitis can be further classified on the basis of its extent and severity. As a general guide, extent can be characterized as localized (<30% of sites involved) or generalized (>30% of sites involved). Severity can be characterized on the basis of the amount of clinical attachment loss (CAL) as follows: slight, 1 or 2 mm CAL; moderate, 3 or 4 mm CAL; and severe, ≥5 mm CAL.
Data from Armitage GC: *Ann Periodontol* 4:1, 1999.

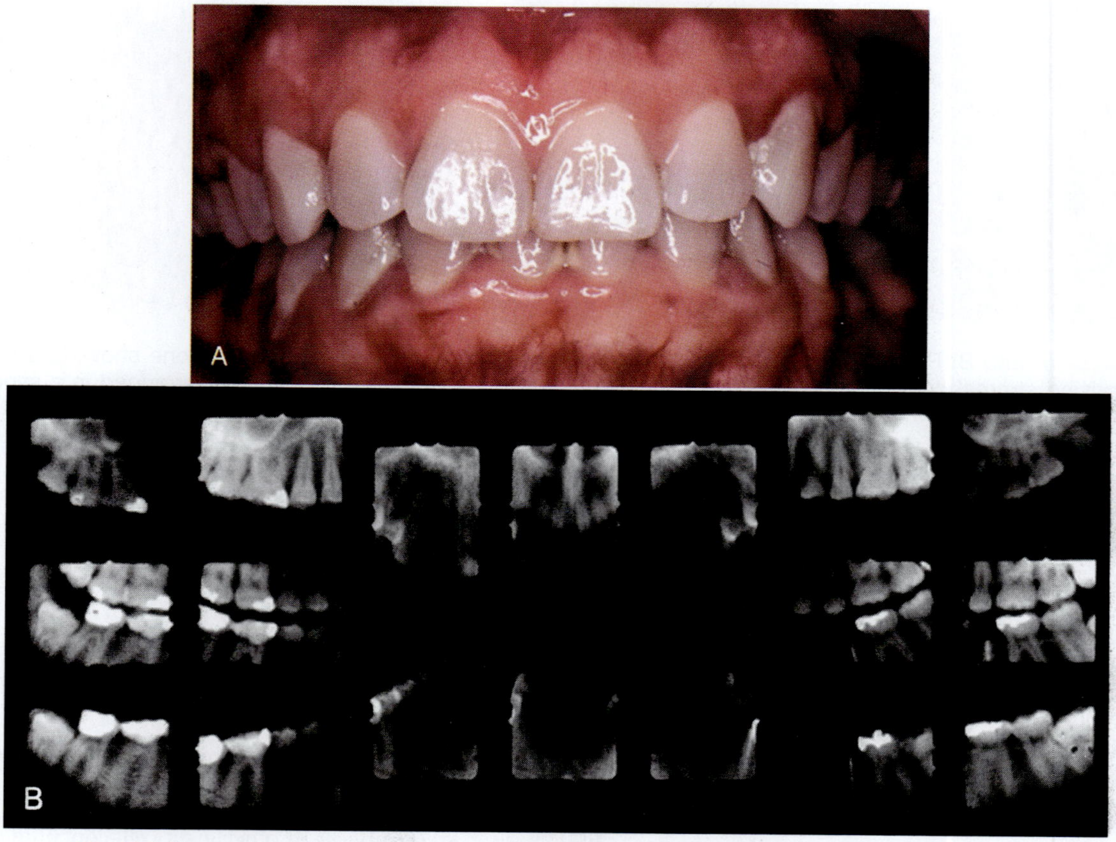

Fig. 5.1 Plaque-related gingivitis and marginal and papillary inflammation, with 1–4 mm probing depths and generalized zero clinical attachment loss, except for the recession seen with mandibular right first premolar.

BOX 5.2 Gingival Diseases

Dental-Plaque-induced Gingival Diseases

These diseases may occur on a periodontium with no attachment loss or on a periodontium with attachment loss that is stable and not progressing.

I. Gingivitis associated with dental plaque only
  A. Without local contributing factors
  B. With local contributing factors (see Box 5.4)
II. Gingival diseases modified by systemic factors
  A. Associated with the endocrine system
    1. Puberty-associated gingivitis
    2. Menstrual cycle-associated gingivitis
    3. Pregnancy-associated conditions
      a. Gingivitis
      b. Pyogenic granuloma
    4. Diabetes mellitus-associated gingivitis
  B. Associated with blood dyscrasias
    1. Leukemia-associated gingivitis
    2. Other
III. Gingival diseases modified by medications
  A. Drug-influenced gingival diseases
    1. Drug-influenced gingival enlargements
    2. Drug-influenced gingivitis
      a. Oral contraceptive-associated gingivitis
      b. Other
IV. Gingival diseases modified by malnutrition
  A. Ascorbic acid-deficiency gingivitis
  B. Other

Nonplaque-induced Gingival Lesions

I. Gingival diseases of specific bacterial origin
  A. *Neisseria gonorrhoeae*
  B. *Treponema pallidum*
  C. *Streptococcus* species
  D. Other
II. Gingival diseases of viral origin
  A. Herpes virus infections
    1. Primary herpetic gingivostomatitis
    2. Recurrent oral herpes
    3. Varicella zoster
  B. Other
III. Gingival diseases of fungal origin
  A. *Candida* species infections: generalized gingival candidiasis
  B. Linear gingival erythema
  C. Histoplasmosis
  D. Other
IV. Gingival lesions of genetic origin
  A. Hereditary gingival fibromatosis
  B. Other
V. Gingival manifestations of systemic conditions
  A. Mucocutaneous lesions
    1. Lichen planus
    2. Pemphigoid
    3. Pemphigus vulgaris
    4. Erythema multiforme
    5. Lupus erythematosus
    6. Drug-induced conditions
    7. Other
  B. Allergic reactions
    1. Dental restorative materials
      a. Mercury
      b. Nickel
      c. Acrylic
      d. Other
    2. Reactions attributable to the following:
      a. Toothpastes or dentifrices
      b. Mouth rinses or mouthwashes
      c. Chewing-gum additives
      d. Foods and additives
    3. Other
VI. Traumatic lesions (factitious, iatrogenic, or accidental)
  A. Chemical injury
  B. Physical injury
  C. Thermal injury
VII. Foreign-body reactions
VIII. Not otherwise specified

Data from Holmstrup P: *Ann Periodontol* 4:20, 1999; and Mariotti A: *Ann Periodontol* 4:7, 1999.

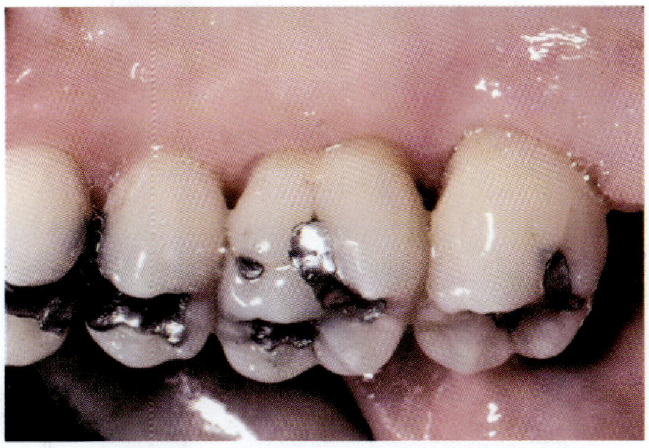

Fig. 5.2 The maxillary second molar exhibits mild inflammation at the mesial–palatal surface. However, the clinical attachment loss has been stable for 15 years after the placement of an apically positioned flap and periodontal maintenance. The diagnosis is a history of moderate periodontitis, but the case is in remission.

Gingivitis Associated with Dental Plaque Only

Plaque-induced gingival disease is the result of an interaction between the microorganisms found in the dental-plaque biofilm, the tissues, and inflammatory cells of the host. The plaque–host interaction can be altered by the effects of local factors, systemic factors, medications, and malnutrition, all of which can influence the severity and duration of the response. Local factors may contribute to gingivitis formation in addition to plaque-retentive calculus formation on the crown and root surfaces. These factors are contributory because of their ability to retain plaque microorganisms and to inhibit the removal of those microorganisms via patient-initiated plaque-control techniques.

A cause-and-effect relationship between microbial plaque and gingivitis has been elegantly demonstrated by a classic experiment demonstrating that the cessation of oral hygiene consistently leads to the manifestation of gingivitis within 2 to 3 weeks in healthy adults. Clinical gingivitis is histologically characterized by

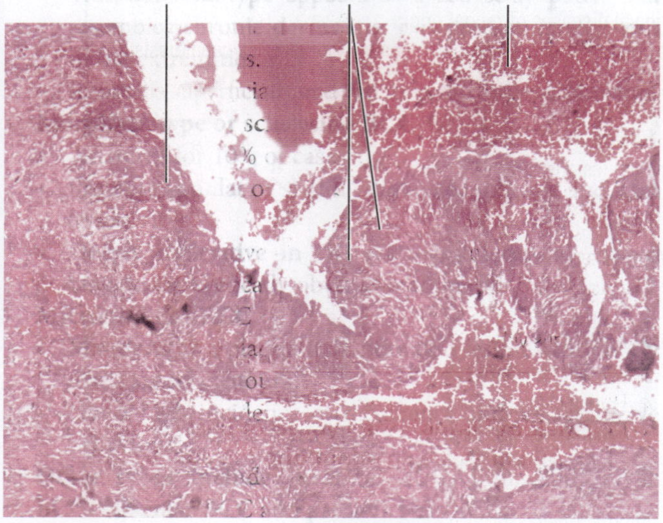

Fig. 35.23 Photomicrograph of ABC showing blood-filled cystic spaces separated by connective tissue septae which contain osteoid and numerous osteoclast-like multinucleate giant cells (H&E; 100×).

- **Osteomalacia and rickets:** Qualitative abnormality due to impaired bone mineralization because of deficiency of vitamin D in adults and children.
- **Scurvy:** Defect in collagen formation caused by the deficiency of vitamin C.
- **Hyperparathyroidism:** Condition in which increased parathyroid hormone (PTH) leads to OFC.
- **Renal osteodystrophy:** Condition associated with chronic renal failure which results in OFC, osteomalacia and focal osteosclerosis.

Q. Enlist the salient clinicopathological features of osteoporosis.

Ans. Osteoporosis, also known as osteopenia, is a common clinical syndrome which affects multiple bones. It is characterized by quantitative reduction of bone tissue mass (both organic matrix and mineralized bone) resulting in a fragile skeleton associated with increased risk of fractures and consequent pain and deformity.

Types

1. **Primary osteoporosis:** Commonly seen in elderly and postmenopausal women. May be asymptomatic or may manifest with chronic backache; more extensive involvement is associated with fractures, particularly of distal radius, femoral neck and vertebral bodies. It is further subclassified into idiopathic, type I (seen in postmenopausal women due to deficiency of oestrogen) and type II (involutional or senile type, involving both men and women; because of defective differentiation of bone marrow stem cells into adipocytes rather than osteoblasts).
2. **Secondary osteoporosis:** This refers to osteoporosis secondary to other disease processes, e.g. bone marrow infiltrative disorders (leukaemia/lymphoma/myeloma), endocrine disorders (hypercortisolism), connective tissue disorders (Marfan syndrome) and GIT causes (malabsorption syndrome).

Predisposing Factors

- **Genetic** (60%–80% contribution, variation in bone density genetically determined; associated genes are RANKL, OPG and RANK, which are the key regulators of osteoclasts).
- **Sex** (more common in females).
- **Ageing** (decreased replicative and biosynthetic activity of osteoprogenitor cells and osteoblasts with ageing results in senile osteoporosis).
- **Reduced physical activity** (decreases replicative and biosynthetic activity of osteoprogenitor cells and osteoblasts)
- **Starvation** (decreased nutritional intake causes deficiencies).
- **Intake of systemic steroids, anticonvulsants and heparin** (interferes with calcium metabolism).
- **Deficiency of sex hormones** (oestrogen in females and androgen in males), **deficiency of vitamin D** and **hyperparathyroidism.**

Radiology

- Radiological evidence becomes apparent only after more than 30% of bone mass is lost.
- Levels of serum calcium, inorganic phosphorus and alkaline phosphatase are usually within normal limits.

Pathology

- Osteoporotic trabeculae thinned out with loss of their interconnections.
- Cortex thinned out by subperiosteal and endosteal resorption (decreased thickness of cortical and trabecular bone).
- Haversian system widened, sometimes so much that the cortex mimics cancellous bone.

Q. Enlist the salient clinicopathological features of hyperparathyroidism.

Ans. Hyperparathyroidism may be:

- **Primary:** Because of autonomous hyperplasia and a neoplastic growth (usually adenoma).
- **Secondary:** Caused by a prolonged state of hypocalcaemia.

Manifestations

See Flowchart 35.2.

Biochemical Abnormalities

Excessive circulating levels of PTH, hypercalcaemia, hypophosphataemia and hypercalciuria.

X-Ray

- Cortical bone is affected more severely than cancellous bone; focal areas of erosion of cortical bone (subperiosteal resorption) are frequently seen along the radial surface of phalanges of index and middle fingers.
- Loss of lamina dura at the roots of teeth is another diagnostic feature.

Severe hyperparathyroidism of primary or secondary (chronic renal failure) type

↓

Oversecretion of parathyroid hormone

↓

Increased osteoclastic resorption of bone

↓

- Susceptibility to fractures, skeletal deformities and joint pains
- Dysfunction as a result of deranged weight bearing
- Osteitis fibrosa cystica

Note: The bony changes may disappear after cure of primary hyperparathyroidism (removal of functioning adenoma).

Flowchart 35.2 Clinicopathological manifestations of hyperparathyroidism.

Pathology

- There is a minor degree of generalized bone rarefaction to prominent areas of bone destruction (lytic lesion) with cyst formation.
- There occur an increased number of bizarre osteoclasts at the surface of moth-eaten trabeculae and cortex.
- Bone and bone marrow are replaced by fibrosis.
- In cancellous bone, osteoclasts tunnel in and dissect along the length of trabeculae to create the appearance of railroad tracks **(dissecting osteitis)**.
- Microfractures and microhaemorrhages occur in the marrow cavity inducing an influx of macrophages and repair tissue. There is formation of masses of reactive tissue called **Brown tumours** (highly vascular tissue with abundant haemosiderin; Fig. 35.24), which may undergo cystic degeneration (**OFC** or **von Recklinghausen disease of bone**).

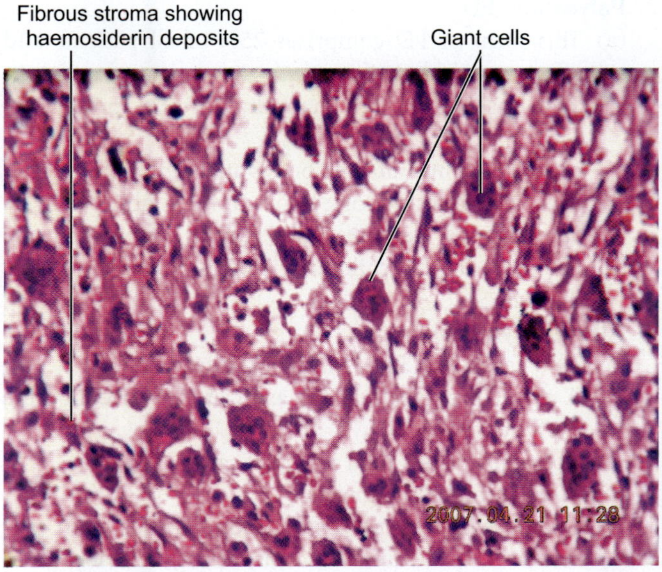

Fig. 35.24 Photomicrograph of a lesion of hyperparathyroidism showing well vascularized stromal tissue with microhaemorrhages, abundant haemosiderin deposits and osteoclastic giant cells (H&E; 200×).

Q. Enlist the salient clinicopathological features of renal osteodystrophy.

Ans. Renal osteodystrophy (metabolic bone disease) encompasses a number of skeletal abnormalities appearing in patients with chronic renal failure or patients on long-term dialysis. It is more common in children. Clinical symptoms of bone disease in advanced renal failure appear in less than 10% of the patients. Radiological and histological changes are observed in fairly large proportion of cases.

Pathogenesis

See Flowchart 35.3.

Manifestations

- Osteomalacia in adults and rickets in children.
- Secondary hyperparathyroidism and OFC.
- Osteosclerosis (enhanced bone density in the upper and lower margins of vertebrae).
- Metastatic calcification (in medium-sized blood vessels, periarticular tissue, myocardium, eyes, lungs and gastric mucosa).

Dialysis-Related Metabolic Bone Disease

Long-term dialysis using an aluminium-containing solution is a major cause of metabolic bone lesions (aluminium interferes with the deposition of calcium hydroxyapatite in bone and results in osteomalacia, secondary hyperparathyroidism and OFC). Also, in such cases, accumulation of β_2-microglobulin amyloid causes dialysis-related amyloidosis.

Q. Describe in brief Paget disease of bone (osteitis deformans). (PA33.4)

Ans. First described by Sir James Paget in 1877; Paget disease of bone is an osteolytic and sclerotic bone disease of uncertain aetiology. It has the following salient features:

- May involve one (monostotic) or more (polyostotic) bones.
- Mainly affects males older than 50 years.
- Thought to be a slow virus infection caused by a paramyxovirus. The virus-infested osteoclasts release IL-6 which induces osteoclastic recruitment leading to resorption of bone.

Clinical Features

- Monostotic Paget disease mainly involves the pelvis, femur, skull and vertebrae.
- Order of involvement in polyostotic Paget disease is: vertebrae, pelvis, femur, skull, sacrum and tibia.
- Monostotic form of the disease usually remains asymptomatic (discovered incidentally on radiological examination).
- Polyostotic form, however, is more widespread and may produce pain, fractures, skeletal deformities, bone overgrowth (**leontiasis ossea:** overgrowth of the craniofacial skeleton) and, occasionally, sarcomatous transformation.
- It may also manifest with platybasia (flattening of the base of the skull because of weakened bone), chalkstick type of fractures in the long bones or severe secondary osteoarthritis with marked elevation of serum alkaline phosphatase and normal-to-high serum calcium level.

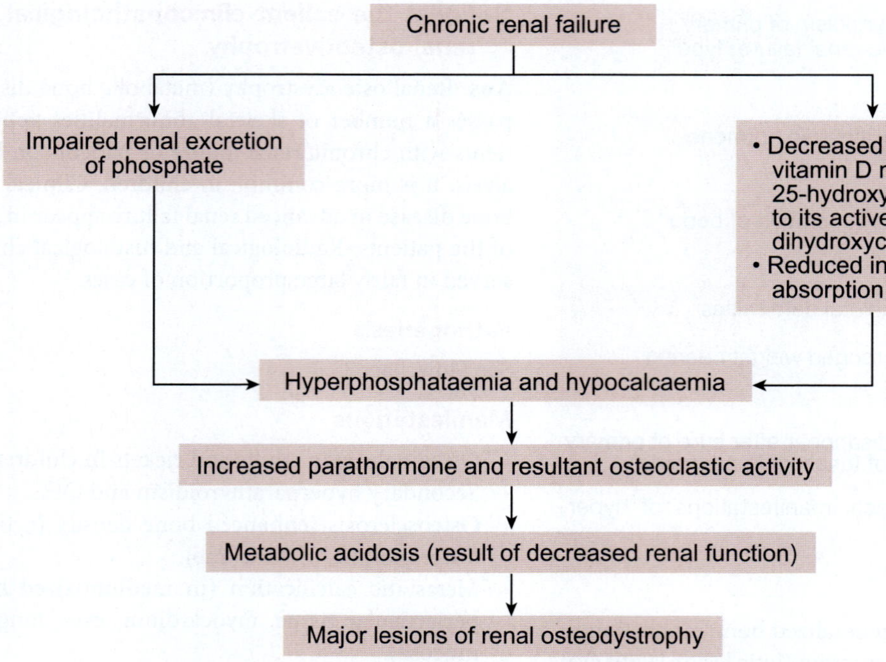

Flowchart 35.3 Clinicopathological features of renal osteodystrophy.

Pathology

Three sequential stages have been identified in Paget disease:

- **Initial osteolytic stage:** Large areas of osteoclastic resorption produced by increased number of osteoclasts are seen.
- **Mixed osteolytic–osteoblastic stage:** Imbalance between osteoblasts laying down new bone and osteoclastic resorption occurs so that mineralization of the newly laid matrix lags behind, resulting in the development of a characteristic **mosaic pattern of osteoid seams** or **cement lines**.
- **Quiescent osteosclerotic stage:** After many years, excessive bone formation results so that the bone becomes more compact and dense, producing **osteosclerosis**. However, newly formed bone is poorly mineralized, soft and susceptible to fractures. **Radiologically**, this stage produces characteristic **cotton-wool appearance** of the affected bone.

Q. Classify fibro-osseous lesions of bone. Outline the salient clinicopathological features of the different types.

Ans. Fibro-osseous lesions of bone include the following:

Fibrous Dysplasia

- It is a **benign condition**, possibly of **developmental origin** characterized by the presence of localized area of replacement of bone by fibroconnective tissue with a characteristic whorled pattern containing trabeculae of woven bone.
- **Radiologically**, the typical focus of FD is well demarcated and has a **ground-glass appearance**.
- FD has three subtypes:

1. **Monostotic FD**
   (a) Monostotic FD usually affects a solitary bone.
   (b) It is the most common type of FD and comprises about 70% of all cases.
   (c) Most patients are between 20 and 30 years of age.
   (d) Bones most often affected, in descending order of frequency, are ribs, craniofacial bones (especially maxilla), femur, tibia and humerus.
   (e) The condition generally remains asymptomatic, and is discovered incidentally, but infrequently may produce tumour-like enlargement of the affected bone.
2. **Polyostotic FD**
   (a) This form of FD comprises 25% of all patients and affects several bones.
   (b) The onset is earlier than that of the monostotic form.
   (c) Most frequently affected bones are craniofacial bones, ribs, vertebrae and long bones of the limbs.
   (d) Spontaneous fractures and skeletal deformities are common in the childhood polyostotic form of the disease.
3. **Albright syndrome**
   (a) Also called McCune–Albright syndrome.
   (b) A form of polyostotic FD associated with endocrine dysfunction.
   (c) Accounts for less than 5% of all cases.
   (d) More common in females.
   (e) Characterized by polyostotic bone lesions, skin pigmentation (café-au-lait macular spots), sexual precocity and infrequently other endocrinopathies.

Gross Pathology

- Lesions appear as sharply demarcated localized defects measuring 2–5 cm in diameter.

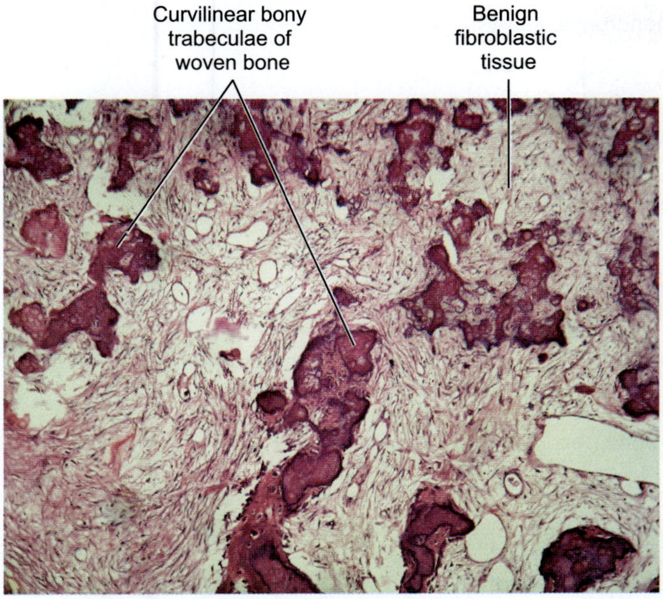

Fig. 35.25 Section shows benign-looking fibroblastic tissue arranged in a loose, whorled pattern in which irregular and curved trabeculae of woven (non-lamellar) bone are embedded (H&E; 100×).

- Thin, smooth overlying cortex with the cut section of the lesion showing replacement of normal cancellous bone of the marrow cavity by gritty, grey-pink, rubbery soft tissue, which may have areas of haemorrhage, myxoid and cystic degeneration.

Microscopy (Fig. 35.25)

- Characteristic benign-looking fibroblastic tissue arranged in a loose, whorled pattern in which irregular and curved trabeculae of woven (non-lamellar) bone are laid down.
- Numerous osteoclasts in relation to bony trabeculae.
- Rarely, secondary malignant change, most often OS.

Fibrous Cortical Defect (Metaphyseal Fibrous Defect, Non-ossifying Fibroma)

Salient Features

- Occurs in the metaphyseal cortex of long bones in children.
- Most commonly involves tibia or femur; usually resolves spontaneously; no malignant or metastatic potential is seen.
- Generally solitary, but may be multiple and bilaterally symmetrical.

X-Ray

Eccentric, bubbly lesion in the metaphysis with a sharply delimited border. As the as bone grows the lesion migrates to diaphysis and becomes sclerotic.

Pathogenesis

- Possibly due to abnormal osteoclastic resorption at the subperiosteal level during remodeling of the metaphysis.
- Associated conditions include Jaffe-Campanacci syndrome, congenital syndrome of multiple non-ossifying fibromas, cafe au lait pigmentation, mental retardation, neurofibromatosis, and ABC.

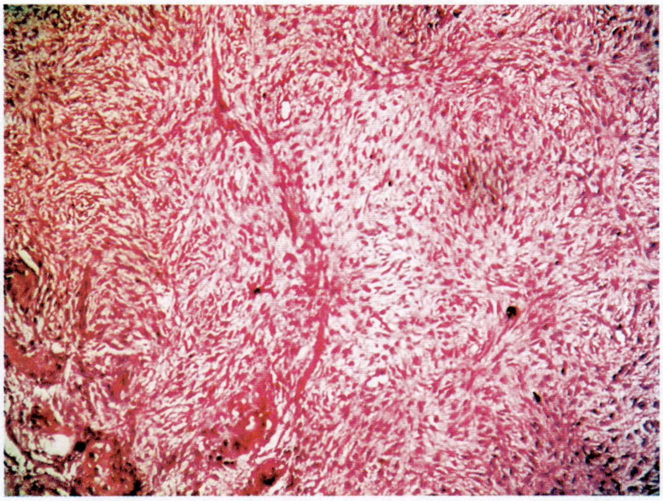

Fig. 35.26 Cellular masses of fibrous tissue showing storiform pattern interspersed with numerous multinucleate osteoclast-like giant cells along with focal areas of haemosiderin deposits (H&E; 100×).

Gross Pathology

- Lesion is generally small, less than 4 cm in diameter, granular and brown.
- Larger lesion (5–10 cm) is referred to as **non-ossifying fibroma**.

Microscopy (Fig. 35.26)

- Cellular masses of fibrous tissue showing storiform pattern interspersed with numerous multinucleate osteoclast-like giant cells.
- Focal areas showing haemosiderin-laden macrophages and foam cells.

JOINTS

Functions of Joints

- They enable movement and provide mechanical support.
- Solid joints provide structural integrity.
- Cavitated joints are lined by synovial cells and aid in movement.

Components of Synovial Lining

- Type A cells: Macrophage-like; synthesize hyaluronic acid.
- Type B cells: Fibroblast-like; produce various proteins.

Functions of Articular Cartilage

- Friction-free movement in joints.
- Spreading the load evenly in weight-bearing joints, so that the underlying bones absorb shock and weight without being crushed.

Q. Outline the aetiopathogenesis, clinical and pathological features of osteoarthritis (OA).

Ans. OA or degenerative joint disease is characterized by age- and mechanical stress–dependent progressive erosion of the articular cartilage. It is more common in females and may be

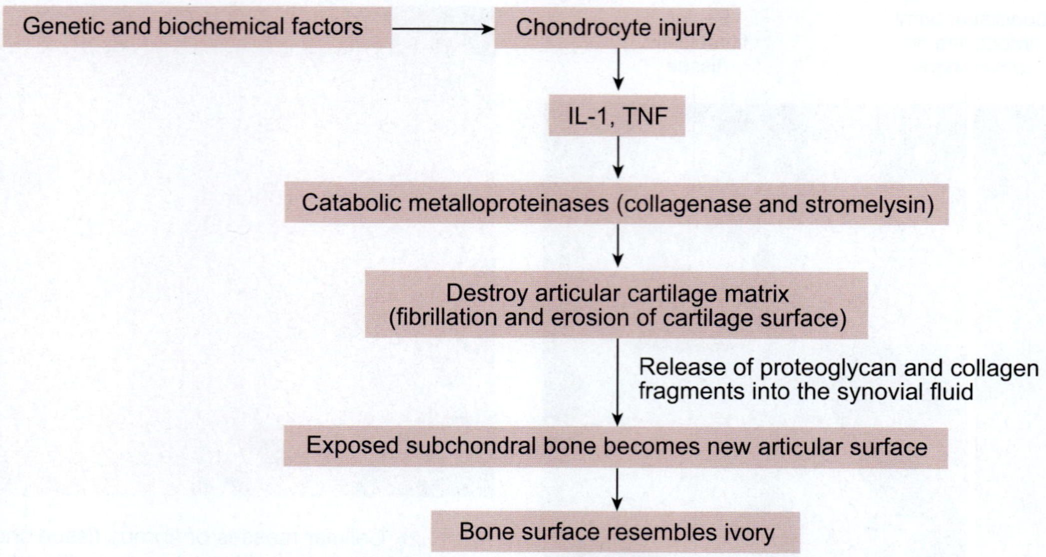

Flowchart 35.4 Pathogenesis of osteoarthritis.

primary or secondary in origin. Secondary OA usually follows endocrine or metabolic disorders (ochronosis, haemochromatosis, acromegaly, chondrocalcinosis), deformity, trauma, fracture, obesity, severe mechanical stress and diabetes.

Clinical Features

- OA primarily targets weight-bearing joints (hip, knee, distal interphalangeal [IP] joints of hands and lower lumbar vertebrae).
- It may be asymptomatic or present with the following manifestations:
  - Deep aching pain which worsens with movement.
  - Stiffness and limitation of movement with crepitus (crackling sound).
  - Bone eburnation (when cartilaginous protection is reduced, subchondral bone may be exposed and damaged; this is followed by regrowth leading to a proliferation of ivory-like, dense, reactive bone in central areas of cartilage).
  - Small fractures in articular bones.
  - Atrophy of regional muscles and laxity of ligaments (consequent to decreased movement because of the pain).
  - Degenerative changes (result in the formation of hard, bony, painless enlargements called ***Heberden's nodes*** at the base of the distal IP joint of the fingers and ***Bouchard's nodes*** on the proximal IP joints).
- Reactive bone formation at the margins of the joints **(osteophytes).** Osteophytes in the spine may cause compression of cervical/lumbar nerve roots causing pain, muscle spasms and neurological deficit.

Pathogenesis (Flowchart 35.4)

Genetic and biochemical factors lead to chondrocytes injury. In early OA, chondrocytes proliferate and release inflammatory mediators which result in injury to the synovium and subchondral bone (cytokines cause activation of metalloproteinases that degrade normal cartilage components such as proteoglycans and type II collagen). In late OA, repeated/persistent inflammation leads to chondrocyte dropout, loss of cartilage and subchondral bone alterations. Cartilage breakdown leads to the formation of **loose bodies (joint mice)**.

Diagnosis

There is no specific laboratory test for OA; however, plain radiographs and MRI are good for evaluating bony and synovial abnormalities. ESR and CRP are within normal range and synovial fluid appears non-inflammatory.

Q. Outline the aetiopathogenesis and clinicopathological features of rheumatoid arthritis (RA). (PA33.5)

Ans. RA is a chronic, non-suppurative, autoimmune, multisystem disease which involves three or more joints and has an insidious onset.

Clinical Features

- It usually starts between 40 to 70 years and shows female preponderance.
- There is symmetrical involvement of metacarpophalangeal (MCP) and proximal IP joints of hands (with sparing of distal IP joints) along with larger joints such as wrists, elbows, ankles and knees.
- Morning stiffness lasting longer than 1 hour before improvement is a classic feature (unlike OA in which the pain and stiffness gets worse with progressive use of the joint during the day).
- Advanced disease produces ulnar deviation at the MCP joints, radial deviation at the wrist, flexion of the distal interphalangeal joint (DIP) joint and extension of the proximal interphalangeal joint (PIP) joint (**swan neck deformity**) or extension of the DIP joint and flexion of the PIP joint (**Boutonniere deformity**).
- **Carpal tunnel syndrome** (compression of median nerve) is a common manifestation.
- Also seen are general malaise, weakness, fever of unknown origin, weight loss, myalgias and inflammation of tendons and bursae.

Extra-Articular Manifestations of RA

- **Anaemia** (because of anaemia of chronic disease and autoimmune mechanisms).
- **Subcutaneous (rheumatoid) nodules,** which occur on the extensor surface of limbs, occiput and sacrum.
- **Cardiac involvement** (fibrinous/constrictive pericarditis) and medium-to-small vessel vasculitis.
- **Skin ulceration, gangrene and obliterative endarteritis** (associated with high titres of RA).
- **Peripheral neuropathy.**
- **Pulmonary involvement** (pleuritis, intrapulmonary nodules, interstitial fibrosis in the form of Caplan syndrome – restrictive lung disease with rheumatoid nodules and coal workers' pneumoconiosis).
- **Hepatitis.**
- **Ocular involvement** (scleritis, episcleritis and dryness of the eye).
- **Secondary amyloidosis** and Sjögren syndrome.

Pathogenesis

Susceptibility depends upon **inherited genes,** most importantly those in the human leukocyte antigen (HLA) major histocompatibility complex (MHC). Association with HLA-DR4 and HLA DW4 influences intracellular signalling as well as certain types of synovial citrullinated proteins . Several minor genes that include cytokine promoters, T cell-signaling genes, etc., also contribute to disease susceptibility. Concordance rate for identical twins is about 15 percent. The **environmental stimuli** that contribute, include smoking and infections (EBV, parvovirus B19, HSV 6 and Mycoplasma species). Epigenetic influences, such as abnormal DNA, dysregulated histone, or expression of microRNAs, aid to the development of the disease by increasing proinflammatory gene expression. The environmental component is thought to induce repeated activation of innate immunity, especially at mucosal surfaces.

There are two major subtypes of RA according to the presence or absence of anti-citrullinated protein antibodies (ACPAs). Citrullination is catalyzed by the calcium-dependent enzyme peptidyl-arginine-deiminase (PAD), changing a positively charged arginine to a neutral citrulline as the result of a post-translational modification. ACPA occurs as a result of an abnormal antibody response to a range of citrullinated proteins, including fibrin, vimentin, fibronectin, Epstein-Barr Nuclear Antigen 1 (EBNA-1), α-enolase, type II collagen, and histones. ACPAs can be detected in approximately 67% of RA patients. The protein tyrosine phosphatase non-receptor type 22 (PTPN22), which is a lymphoid specific protein tyrosine phosphatase, has also drawn much attention because of polymorphisms associated with ACPA-positive RA.

Activation of CD4+ T-helper cells (CMI type IV reaction) leads to release of proinflammatory cytokines. Inflamed synovial cells express an antigen that induces local stimulation of B cells, which produces IgM autoantibodies directed against the Fc receptor for IgG (**rheumatoid factor** [RF]). RF and IgG join to form immune complexes (type III hypersensitivity reaction), which activate complement to produce C5a, a chemotactic factor for neutrophils which enter the joint space followed by other leukocytes. Pannus is formed. Pannus proliferation also releases cytokines which lead to articular cartilage damage. Pathogenesis of RA has been depicted in Flowchart 35.5.

Morphology (Fig. 35.27)

- Synovial hyperplasia (multilayering of synovial cells).
- Infiltration of synovium by dense perivascular inflammatory infiltrate composed of B cells and CD4+ T cells (at places forming lymphoid aggregates), plasma cells and macrophages.
- Increased vascularity due to vasodilatation and telangiectasia.
- Deposition of fibrin in the synovium and accumulation of neutrophils in the synovial fluid.
- Osteoclastic activity in the underlying bone.
- Pannus formation (pannus is a combination of neovascularization, inflammation and fibrinoid deposits, which progressively destroys the underlying cartilage and subchondral bone).

X-Ray

- Joint effusion.
- Juxta-articular osteopenia with bone erosions and narrowing of joint spaces because of loss of articular cartilage.

Diagnosis

At least four of the following should be present for the diagnosis of RA:

- Morning stiffness of 1 hour for at least 6 weeks.
- Arthritis and soft-tissue swelling of three joints, present for at least 6 weeks.
- Arthritis of hand joints, present for at least 6 weeks.
- Symmetric arthritis, present for at least 6 weeks.
- Subcutaneous nodules in specific places.
- Positive serum RF (IgM-RF has a 60%–80% sensitivity and IgG-RF has a 80%–90% sensitivity).
- Positive serum antinuclear antibody (ANA) (30% of cases).
- Presence of anticyclic citrullinated peptide (anti-CCP) has a specificity of 95%–98% and a sensitivity of 70%–80%.
- Radiological changes suggestive of joint erosion.

Q. Enlist the salient clinicopathological features of juvenile rheumatoid arthritis (JRA).

Ans. Salient features of JRA:

- It is a chronic inflammatory condition that begins in patients younger than 16 years.
- It manifests with abrupt onset of spiking fever, transient skin rash, hepatosplenomegaly and serositis and affects knees, wrists, elbows and ankles (large joints affected more than small joints).
- It is typically RA-negative, rheumatoid nodule-negative and ANA-positive.

Q. What is infectious arthritis? Enlist its important clinicopathological features.

Ans. Salient features of infectious arthritis:

- Infectious arthritis is defined as arthritis caused by infection with a microbial pathogen.
- It may occur secondary to haematogenous spread and osteomyelitis, and as a complication of intra-articular infection or surgery.

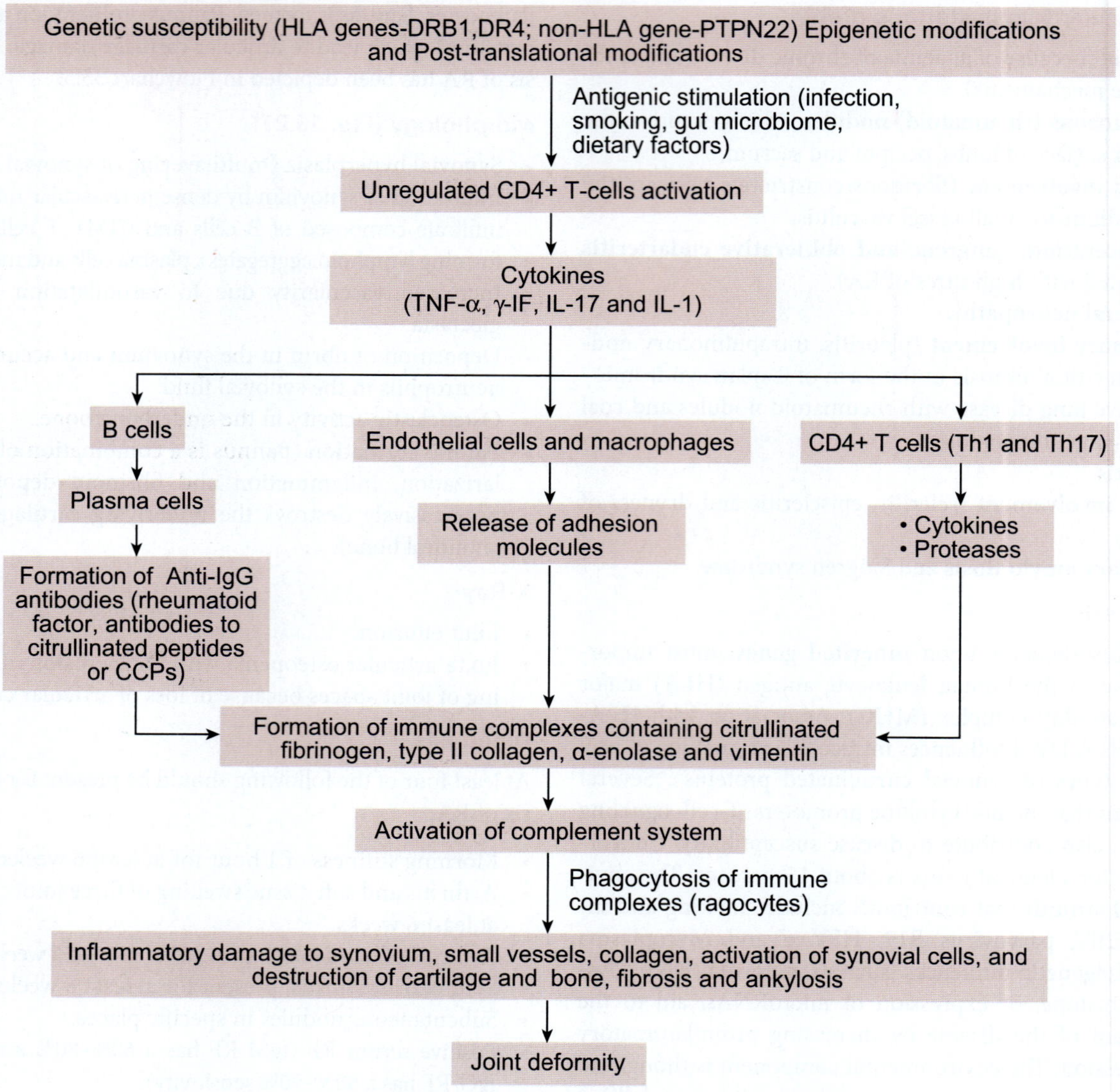

Flowchart 35.5 Pathogenesis of rheumatoid arthritis.

- Common causative organisms are *gonococci, meningococci, pneumococci, staphylococci, streptococci, H. influenzae*, Gram-negative bacilli and *M. tuberculosis*.
- The patient presents with sudden onset of pain, swollen joints, restricted mobility, fever, leucocytosis and increased ESR. Commonly involved joints include knees, hips, shoulders, elbows and wrists.
- Predisposing conditions include immune deficiency, debilitating illness, joint trauma and intravenous drug abuse.
- *Tuberculous arthritis* is a chronic progressive monoarticular arthritis, which mainly affects the weight-bearing joints, e.g. hips, knees and ankles. Systemic symptoms may or may not be present.

Q. Enumerate the various crystallopathies.

Ans. Articular crystal deposits include:

- **Endogenous crystals:** Monosodium urate (MSU), calcium pyrophosphate dihydrate and calcium phosphate.
- **Exogenous crystals:** Corticosteroids, talc, polyethylene and silicone.

Q. Write briefly about gouty arthritis.

Ans. Gouty arthritis is a male-dominant disease, characterized by hyperuricaemia with plasma urate level more than 7 mg/dL (upper limit of solubility of MSU in serum at 37 °C and blood pH).

It involves the metatarsophalangeal joints followed by ankles and knees; wrists may be affected later.

Typical manifestations include recurrent attacks of acute arthritis, deposits of MSU tophi (meaning *porous stones*) in soft tissue and renal disease affecting interstitium and blood vessels (uric acid nephrolithiasis).

Types

- **Metabolic gout (10% of cases):** Because of disorder in metabolism of uric acid (a product of purine metabolism) leading to its overproduction.
- **Renal gout (90% of cases):** Because of reduced renal excretion of uric acid secondary to diabetes mellitus, leukaemia,

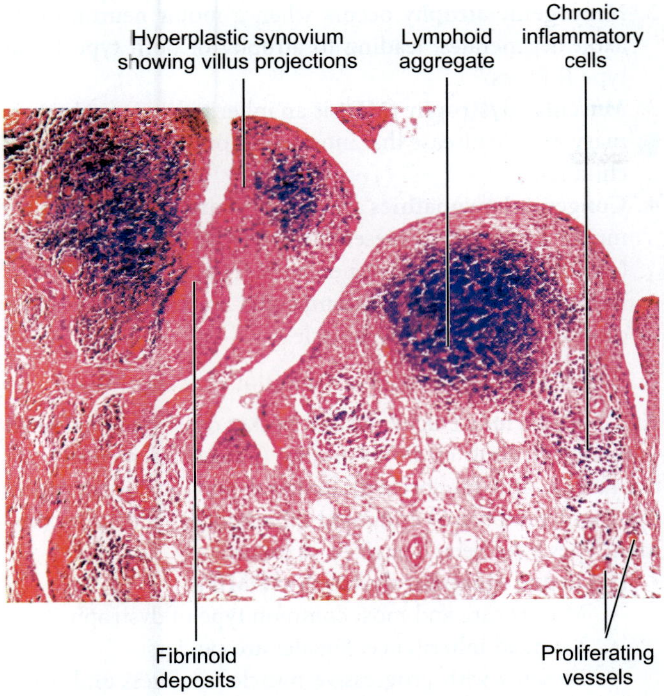

Fig. 35.27 Section showing synovial hyperplasia (multilayering of synovial cells) with infiltration by dense inflammatory infiltrate composed of lymphocytes (at places forming lymphoid aggregates), plasma cells and macrophages. Increased vascularity and fibrinoid deposits are also seen (H&E; 100×).

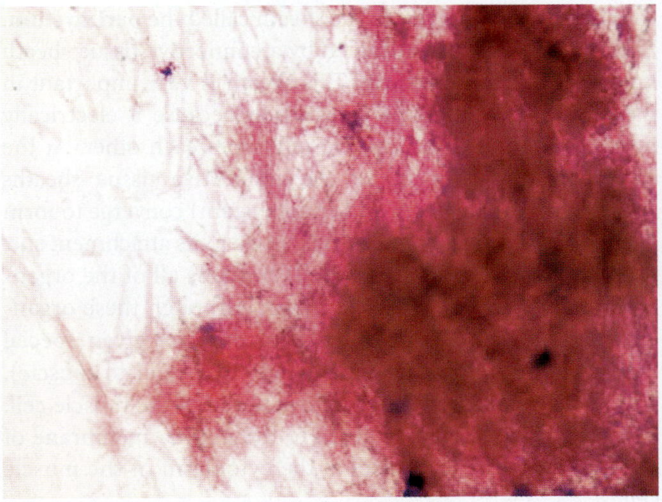

Fig. 35.28 FNAC smears from gouty tophus showing needle-shaped MSU crystals (H&E; 100×).

diuretic therapy, treatment of disseminated cancer and drugs such as aspirin, pyrazinamide, nicotinic acid, ethambutol and ethanol.

Pathogenesis

See Flowchart 35.6.

X-Ray

Juxta-articular bone erosion by crystal deposits with loss of joint space.

Pathology

- **Acute gout:** Predominantly a disease of lower extremities, acute gout most commonly affects the great toe. It is triggered by precipitation of needle-shaped crystals of MSU from serum or synovial fluid (Fig. 35.28), which leads to an intensely painful joint effusion containing crystals, polymorphs and macrophages, lasting for hours to weeks.
- **Chronic gout:** This is characterized by the presence of tophi, which usually develop after approximately 10 years of disease. Tophi represent deposits of MSU that occur in tissue most commonly in and around the affected joints. Sections through a tophus exhibit an exuberant granulomatous reaction complete with foreign body multinucleated giant cells surrounding a central core of amorphous MSU crystals.
- **Pseudogout:** Characterized by deposition of calcium pyrophosphate dihydrate crystals in the joint cavities, pseudogout can be sporadic (idiopathic), hereditary or secondary. The knee joint is affected in more than 50% of cases and the age of the patients is more than 50 years. The crystals are rhomboid in shape and deposit in the articular cartilage (chondrocalcinosis). It may be asymptomatic or manifest as acute, subacute or chronic arthritis.

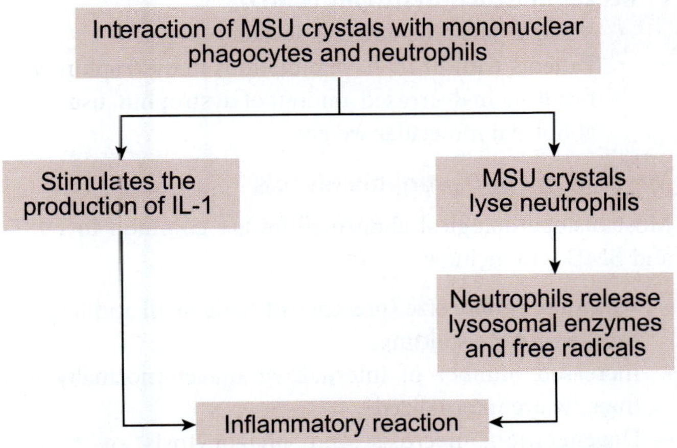

Flowchart 35.6 Pathogenesis of gouty arthritis.

MUSCLE

Muscle Terminology

- Myofibre or myocyte: A muscle cell.
- Sarcolemma: The plasma membrane of a muscle cell.
- Sarcoplasm: The cytoplasm of the muscle cell.
- Sarcoplasmic reticulum: The endoplasmic reticulum of a muscle cell.
- Sarcosome: The mitochondria of a muscle cell.
- Sarcomere: The contractile or functional unit of muscle.

The entire muscle is surrounded by connective tissue called the **epimysium** and is made up of smaller bundles known as **fascicles**. Fascicles are actually bundles of individual muscle cells (**myofibres or myocytes**). Each of these bundles is surrounded by a connective tissue sheath called the **perimysium**. Each muscle cell is surrounded by a connective tissue sheath known as the **endomysium**. This sheath is very important in the physiology of muscle contraction because it electrically insulates the individual muscle cells from each other. At the ends of the muscle, all of the connective tissue sheaths (epimysium, perimysium and endomysium) converge to form a tendon, which will connect the muscle to its attachment site.

Each muscle fibre (muscle cell) contains all of the organelles that we find in other cell types. Although these organelles are the same as in other cells, they are given special names (both the prefixes 'sarco' and 'myo' refer to muscle). The nucleus contains the genetic material of the muscle cell. **Sarcolemma** is the name given to the plasma membrane of the muscle cell. The **cytosol** is the cytoplasm of the muscle cell.

The **sarcoplasmic reticulum** is the endoplasmic reticulum of the muscle cell. There are sac-like regions of the sarcoplasmic reticulum known as **terminal cisternae**. The terminal cisternae act as calcium storage sites. The calcium ions stored in the terminal cisternae are essential in muscle contraction. A myofibril is a cylindrical bundle of contractile proteins found within the muscle cell. Myofibrils are composed of individual contractile proteins called **myofilaments**. These myofilaments are generally divided into thick and thin myofilaments. The thin myofilaments are composed mainly of a protein known as actin. Actin filaments are anchored into the Z line of a sarcomere. The thick myofilaments are composed mainly of the protein myosin.

It is the orderly overlapping of the actin and myosin filaments that give cardiac and skeletal muscle their striated appearance (light and dark bands).

Each muscle is supplied by a motor nerve originating from neurons in the spinal cord or brain stem.

Types of Fibres in Human Skeletal Muscle

- **Type I** are slow-twitch fibres (red muscle) that are rich in mitochondria and oxidative enzymes and have a great capacity for long, sustained contraction without fatigue (e.g. soleus muscle).
- **Type II** are fast-twitch fibres (white muscle) that are poor in mitochondria, use both oxidative metabolism and anaerobic glycolysis and are quicker to fatigue (e.g. biceps muscle).

Reactions of Muscle Fibres

- Segmental necrosis (only a portion of myocyte is destroyed, undergoes myophagocytosis and replacement by collagen and fat).
- Vacuolization, alteration in structural proteins and accumulation of intracytoplasmic deposits.
- Regeneration.
- Hypertrophy.

Q. Classify disorders of muscle.

Ans. Muscle disorders include:

1. **Muscle weakness** secondary to diseases involving the motor neuron pathways, neuromuscular synapse (e.g. myasthenia gravis).
2. **Neurogenic atrophy** occurs when a motor neuron or its axon degenerates, leading to atrophy of both type I and type II fibres.
3. **Muscular dystrophy (MD)** is an inherited progressive primary muscle disease that most commonly presents in early childhood.
4. **Congenital myopathies** are rare, primary, non-progressive muscle diseases that present at birth with poor muscle tone (e.g. central core disease, nemaline [rod] myopathy).
5. **Polymyositis** and **dermatomyositis** are connective tissue disorders which involve muscle.

Q. Classify and describe muscular dystrophies.

Ans. MDs include Duchenne and Becker dystrophy (X-linked inheritance), limb girdle dystrophy (autosomal recessive inheritance), and fascioscapulohumeral and oculopharyngeal dystrophy (autosomal dominant inheritance). The most common types have been described as follows:

- **Duchenne muscular dystrophy (DMD)**
  - Most severe and most common type of dystrophy.
  - X-linked inheritance; females are carriers.
  - Presents with progressive muscle weakness and wasting, which manifests by 5 years.
  - Paralysis and death by second to third decade.
  - Weakness begins in the pelvic girdle muscles, and then shoulder girdle is affected.
  - Characterized by a positive Gower manoeuvre (requiring the assistance of upper extremities to stand up) and pseudohypertrophy (enlargement of calf muscles with weakness).
  - May affect cardiac muscle resulting in arrhythmias and heart failure.
  - May be associated with intellectual impairment.
  - Death from respiratory insufficiency, pulmonary infection and cardiac failure.

  Pathogenesis
  - Abnormalities in a gene encoding dystrophin located in the Xp21 region.
  - Deletion (most common); point mutation also seen.
  - Dystrophin and dystrophin-associated protein complex anchors actin to membrane glycoprotein; absence of dystrophin causes transfer of the force of contraction to connective tissue and myocyte degeneration.
- **Becker muscular dystrophy (BMD)**
  - It is less common and less severe.
  - Patients with BMD have mutations in dystrophin gene resulting in decreased amount of dystrophin, usually of abnormal molecular weight.

Morphology of Dystrophic Muscle

Most histopathological abnormalities are common to DMD and BMD and include:

- Variation in fibre size (presence of both small and large fibres) with fibre splitting.
- Increased number of internalized nuclei (normally less than 3% are internalized).
- Degeneration, necrosis and phagocytosis of muscle fibres.

- Regeneration of muscle fibres and proliferation of endomysial connective tissue; patients with DMD also show enlarged, rounded hyaline fibres with loss of cross-striations (hypercontracted fibres) – a finding rare in BMD.

Laboratory Findings

- Antenatal diagnosis of dystrophin defect using recombinant DNA technology.
- Serum CK (creatinine kinase) levels decline as muscle tissue is progressively replaced by fat and fibrous tissue.

Q. Write briefly about myasthenia gravis.

Ans. Myasthenia gravis is an autoimmune disease characterized by reduction in acetylcholine receptors because of the presence of an autoantibody against them.

- Acetylcholine receptor antibody accelerates degradation of the receptor aided by complement activation and blocks receptor function.
- Myasthenia gravis may be associated with thymic hyperplasia as well as thymomas.
- Ptosis and diplopia are the most common initial presentations.
- Histopathology is not diagnostic; type II fibre atrophy may be observed in late stage.
- Treatment includes anticholinesterase drugs, thymectomy, immunosuppression and plasmapheresis.

Q. Write briefly about Lambert–Eaton myasthenic syndrome.

Ans. Lambert–Eaton myasthenic syndrome develops as a paraneoplastic process, commonly with small cell carcinoma of the lung.

- Patients develop proximal muscle weakness with autonomic dysfunction.
- No improvement is found with anticholinesterase agents.
- Content of anticholinesterase is normal in neuromuscular junction synaptic vesicles, but fewer vesicles are released.

SOFT TISSUE

Q. Summarize the clinicopathological features of soft-tissue tumours.

Ans. Clinicopathological features of soft-tissue tumours are summarized in Table 35.2.

Table 35.2 Clinicopathological features of common soft tissue tumours

Tumour type	Salient features
Lipomatous tumours	
Lipoma	• *Most common benign soft tissue tumour.* • Arises in subcutaneous tissue—trunk, neck, proximal extremities, and back, of middle-aged individuals; more commonly affects females. • It is solitary, soft, and mobile on examination. • Conventional lipoma (Fig. 35.29) is a well-encapsulated mass of lobules of mature adipocytes which are separated by fibrous septae. • *Generalized lipomatosis **(Dercum disease)*** is characterized by multiple lipomas in subcutaneous tissue, which on rare occasions, may transform into liposarcoma. • Other variants of lipoma include *fibrolipoma* (containing fibrous tissue), *angiolipoma* (containing blood vessels), *spindle cell lipoma* (containing spindle cells), *myelolipoma* (containing marrow material), *infiltrating* or *intramuscular lipoma*, and *pleomorphic lipoma* (Fig. 35.30). Pleomorphic lipomas are neoplasms of mature fat containing atypical cells, restricted in location to the dermis or subcutis of the posterior neck, upper back or shoulders. If located in other sites, they are considered to be atypical lipomatous tumours (well differentiated liposarcomas). Pleomorphic lipomas contain hyperchromatic enlarged nuclei and mutinucleate cells with wreath-like arrangement of nuclei (floret cells). Bundles of dense ropey collagen and myxoid stroma may be seen. Vessels if prominent are arborizing and thick walled. Mast cells may be numerous. • Lipoblasts and prominent vascularity are not prominently seen contrary to a *liposarcoma* (malignant tumour of lipocytes).
Liposarcoma	• Most common soft tissue sarcoma of adults (constitutes 20% of all sarcomas); most commonly affect males in the 5th to 7th decade. • May rarely be associated with lipomatosis. • Located in the deep soft tissue (thigh, retroperitoneum, popliteal fossa); they are very rarely superficial or intramuscular in location. • Tumour size and histologic type are important predictors of prognosis. • They are large, well-circumscribed but unencapsulated tumours. • Liposarcomas are classified into the following subtypes: – Well-differentiated liposarcomas (also called atypical lipomatous tumour; resemble lipoma but have lipoblasts).

(Continued)

Table 35.2 Clinicopathological features of common soft tissue tumours (*Cont.*)

Tumour type	Salient features
	– Myxoid liposarcoma (stellate to spindled cells with cytoplasmic processes lying in mucoid ground substance and capillary network with a typical chickenwire pattern. – Pleomorphic liposarcomas (contain cells showing marked anaplasia). – Dedifferntiated liposarcomas are biphasic neoplasms with one component of atypical lipomatous tumour and a second component of high-grade sarcoma. • Diagnostic hallmark are lipoblasts (uni- or multivacuolated cells which are smaller than mature adipocytes and resemble fetal fat cells; have sharply demarcated cytoplasmic membranes and lipid vacuoles which scallop the nucleus; may resemble signet ring cells or have central nuclei with small indentations by multiple fat vacuoles). • They are positive for S100 and calretinin and show cytogenetic translocation t(2;16) q(13; p11).
Fibrous tumours	
Fibroma	• Pure fibroma is an uncommon, benign, well-circumscribed, lobulated fibrous tumour. • Affects 30–50-year olds and presents as nodules on fingers, hands, or wrist. • Histopathology shows well-defined nodules of dense hyperplastic fibrous tissue containing occasional spindle- or stellate-shaped cells having scant cytoplasm and elongated nuclei and uniformly distributed fine chromatin. • Fibromas vary from being cellular to paucicellular and may occasionally demonstrate bizarre tumour cells or extravasated red blood cells.'
Nodular fasciitis	• Most commonly seen in young adults; is located in the fascia and subcutis; and has an average size of 2–3 cm. • Typically presents as a rapidly growing mass on the flexor aspect of forearm, chest, and back. • Exhibits benign behavior, but is sometimes misdiagnosed as sarcoma due to its cellularity, mitotic figures, and rapid growth. • It is tan-white-gray in colour, myxoid, relatively well-circumscribed, and unencapsulated. • Histopathology shows zonation effect with a hypocellular center and a hypercellular periphery. The lesion is composed of plump, spindled to stellate cells with minimal atypia, and abundant ground/myxoid substance which at times gives rise to mucin pools or microcysts. • Cellular areas may have storiform or fascicular patterns. • Nodular fasciitis usually has prominent vasculature; and appears reactive and granulation tissue like. • Inflammatory cells (mainly lymphocytes and macrophages) are sprinkled in the tumour. • Extravasated red blood cells may be seen. • May sometimes show metaplastic bone and ganglion type cells.
Fibromatosis	• Infiltrative growth characterized by proliferation of histologically benign appearing myofibroblasts and fibroblasts in the background of a collagenous stroma. • The lesion exhibits low to moderate mitotic activity, repeated local recurrences (aggressive clinical behavior), but no metastases. • It is broadly divided into adult and pediatric types. • *Adult type* includes *deep* (located deep to the fascia; also called desmoid fibromatosis) and *superficial* (limited to fascia; includes palmar, plantar, penile fibromatosis). • Examples of *pediatric (juvenile, infantile) fibromatosis* include congenital solitary fibromatosis, fibrous hamartoma of infancy, inclusion body (or infantile digital), myofibromatosis, fibromatosis coli, juvenile nasopharyngeal angiofibroma, juvenile aponeurotic fibroma, etc. • *Desmoid (musculoaponeurotic) fibromatosis* may be *abdominal* or *extraabdominal*. Both types are clinically aggressive and close differentials of STS. Hormones (estrogen), genetic predisposition, and trauma have all been implicated in their pathogenesis. On gross examination they appear as large, gray-white, firm, infiltrative tumours. On microscopy they seem to be composed of uniform, benign appearing fibroblasts and myofibroblasts, arranged in fascicular pattern, and showing minimal pleomorphism and mitoses. As the lesion ages, hypocellular collagenized or hyalinized areas increase. • *Palmar fibromatosis* ***(Dupuytren contracture)*** is the most common type of fibromatosis characterized by a nodular proliferation of palmar aponeurosis and adjacent dermis and subcutaneous fat in elderly. It causes flexion contracture of the digits (usually 4th and 5th); is superficial and does not involve deep structures, such as tendons or skeletal muscle. It is bilateral in 50% cases. • *Plantar fibromatosis* ***(Ledderhose disease)*** is a nodular proliferation of plantar aponeurosis and surrounding adipose tissue. It is common in young boys and may be associated with palmar and penile fibromatosis. It is also seen with phenobarbital therapy for epilepsy. It is important to differentiate these clinically from melanoma, synovial sarcoma, and KS. • *Penile fibromatosis* ***(Peyronie disease)*** is a fibrous thickening of dermis and Buck fascia between corpora cavernosa and tunica albuginea, causing curvature toward side of lesion and restricting movement of these structures during erection. Microvascular trauma, urethritis, and sclerosing inflammatory process have all been implicated in the pathogenesis. It may be idiopathic in origin. Histopathology shows disorganized arrangement of the collagen of tunica albuginea with formation of nodules. Fibrosis, perivascular lymphocytic infiltrate, and linear bands of calcification may also be seen.

Table 35.2 Clinicopathological features of common soft tissue tumours (*Cont.*)

Tumour type	Salient features
Fibrosarcoma	• Usually seen in retroperitoneum and extremities. • They are unencapsulated, infiltrative, fleshy masses, varying from slow growing lesions, which are better differentiated to cellular lesions characterized by a "herring bone" (interlacing) pattern. • Have 40%–50%, 5-year survival rate; may arise secondary to irradiation.
Fibrohistiocytic tumours	
Benign fibrous histiocytoma	• Usually seen in lower extremities, a fibrous histiocytoma presents as a solitary, slow growing, unencapsulated, reddish nodule. • Overlying epidermis may show hyperplasia. • Histopathology shows a benign proliferation of spindle cells confined to the dermis and subcutis. • Cells are arranged in a storiform pattern, and may show foam cells, hemosiderin, and multinucleate giant cells (Fig. 35.31). • Tumours arising from the dermis are called *dermatofibromas*. • Other benign fibrohistiocytic tumours include *juvenile xanthogranuloma*, *epithelioid histiocytoma*, and *reticulohistiocytoma*.
Dermatofibrosarcoma propuberans (DFSP)	• Low-grade malignant dermal tumour that may show overlying ulceration and satellite lesions. • It is commonly located in the chest wall and trunk and can have multiple recurrences. • Histopathology shows a characteristic "cartwheel" pattern of spindle cells with increased mitotic activity and numerous giant cells (Fig. 35.32).
Undifferentiated/ unclassified sarcoma	• Most common soft tissue sarcoma, preferentially located in extremities and retroperitoneum; affects older adults (5th to 6th decade). • It usually arises in relation to adipose tissue, skeletal muscle, and deep fascia. • On gross examination it appears multilobated and fleshy. • Histopathology shows markedly pleomorphic spindled (fibroblast-like), cells, myofibroblasts and mononuclear polygonal to rounded (histiocyte-like) cells. Phagocytosis, bizarre multinucleate cells, markedly increased mitoses including atypical mitoses are frequent findings (Fig. 35.33). Undifferentiated sarcomas are well-vascularized tumours which show presence of inflammatory cells and are positive for vimentin, chymotrypsin, CD 68, and factor VIII antigen.
Skeletal muscle tumours	
Rhabdomyoma	• Rare, benign tumour of skeletal muscle origin associated with tuberous sclerosis (AD inheritance) and typically located in the head and neck (tongue, larynx, and pharynx). • Histopathology shows large glycogen containing, round to polygonal cells having abundant, vacuolated to granular, eosinophilic cytoplasm. Cross striations can be demonstrated by PTAH stain. Rhabdomyomas may be divided into fetal and adult types.
Rhabdomyosarcomas	• Most common sarcoma in children and most common striated muscle malignancy. • Can be divided into five types based on its differentiation, growth pattern, and histological appearance - alveolar, anaplastic, embryonal, pleomorphic and sclerosing. The cell of origin is a rhabdomyoblast which on H&E-stained sections demonstrates an eccentric eosinophilic granular cytoplasm, rich in thick and thin filaments. These may appear rounded to elongated, when they are called strap cells or tadpole cells. The important subtypes are described below.
Embryonal rhabdomyosarcoma	• Most common type of rhabdomyosarcoma, usually located in the head and neck, vagina, paratesticular region, and urinary bladder. • Botryoid type presents as a grape-like mass protruding from the walls of hollow mucosa-lined structures (vagina or male urethra). Histopathologically the tumour grows under the mucosa forming the typical "cambium" layer which has prominent cellularity of small round and strap cells. The remaining tumour is myxoid and paucicellular. • Embryonal rhabdomyosarcoma may range from highly differentiated neoplasms containing large rhabdomyoblasts with abundant eosinophilic cytoplasm to poorly differentiated tumours containing round cells and spindle-shaped strap cells. Myxoid areas and mitoses are frequently seen (Fig. 35.34). • Rhabdomyoblasts stain positive for desmin and myogenin.
Alveolar rhabdomyosarcoma	• Occurs between 10 and 25 years of age in the distal extremities. • Second most common type of skeletal muscle malignancy, and has the worst prognosis. • Fibrous septae divide the cells into clusters. Cells in the center are discohesive, while those at the periphery adhere to the septae giving rise to an alveolar pattern.
Pleomorphic rhabdomyosarcoma	• Presents as a rapidly growing painful mass, with a behavior similar to other pleomorphic sarcomas. Located in the deep soft tissue of adults, it comprises numerous large, sometimes multinucleated pleomorphic tumour cells. • It is the least common type of skeletal muscle malignancy.

(*Continued*)

Table 35.2 Clinicopathological features of common soft tissue tumours (*Cont.*)

Tumour type	Salient features
Smooth muscle tumours	
Leiomyoma	• Commonly located in the uterus (myometrium, serosal surface, and mucosal surface in that order), cervix, broad ligament, genitals, skin (erector muscle), extremities, and retroperitoneum, this tumour is also called a fibromyoma or a fibroid. • It is the most common benign GI tumour. • Affects women more commonly than men (thought to be estrogen dependent). • On gross examination it appears well circumscribed and has a gray-white whorled cut surface. • Histopathologically the tumour is composed of fascicles of spindle cells that intersect each other at right angles (whorled appearance). The tumour cells have blunt-ended cigar-shaped nuclei. • Secondary changes are common and include hyaline degeneration, cystic degeneration, infarction, calcification, and necrosis. Sarcomatous change is rare (<0.5%).
Leiomyosarcoma	• Most commonly arises from wall of blood vessels, extremities, and retroperitoneum in the 4th to 6th decade. • On gross examination they appears bulky, soft, and fleshy. • Increased mitotic count (>10 mitoses/10 HPF with or without cellular atypia or 5–10 mitoses/10 HPF with cellular atypia) and atypical mitoses differentiate it from a cellular leiomyoma (Fig. 35.35). • The *most common sarcoma in the GI tract and uterus*; it is composed of fascicles of malignant spindle-shaped cells with cigar-shaped nuclei.
Neural tumours	
Benign nerve sheath tumours (Fig. 35.36)	• Arise sporadically or in association with neurofibromatosis I. • Common locations include skin and peripheral nerves. • They are well-circumscribed unencapsulated lesions comprising spindle-shaped cells with wavy nuclei. • Stroma may be collagenized to myxoid. • Some of these tumours (schwannomas) may show Antoni A regions (lining up of delicate wavy nuclei in bands separated by eosinophilic cytoplasm), rows of nuclei (called Verocay bodies), and Antoni B regions (hypocellular areas showing less organization) (Fig. 35.36).
Plexiform neurofibroma	• Most arise in conjunction with Type I neurofibromatosis in the major nerve trunks. • Nerve affected is irregularly expanded.
MPNST	• Arise de novo or from transformation of a plexiform neurofibroma. An MPNST has an association with NF I. • Its a poorly defined infiltrative tumour mass comprising spindled cells with elongated wavy nuclei showing extreme pleomorphism. Mitoses and necrosis are common. Tumour cells show positivity for CD99/O13, S100 and CD57.
Tumours of unknown origin	
Synovial sarcoma	• Misnomer; not derived from synovial tissue. • Less than 10% intraarticular. • Located around rather than in the joint in the extremities. • Exhibit male predominance, with peak incidence between 25 and 35 years of age. • They may be monophasic, biphasic or poorly differentiated. • Monophasic tumours are composed of spindled cells alone or rarely epithelial cells alone, whereas biphasic tumours (Fig. 35.37) are composed of both, with the epithelial cells arranged in a gland-like pattern.

DFSP, Dermatofibrosarcoma protuberans; KS, Kaposi sarcoma; KSHV, KS-associated herpes virus; MPNST, malignant peripheral nerve sheath tumour; RBC, red blood cell; VWF, von Willebrand factor.

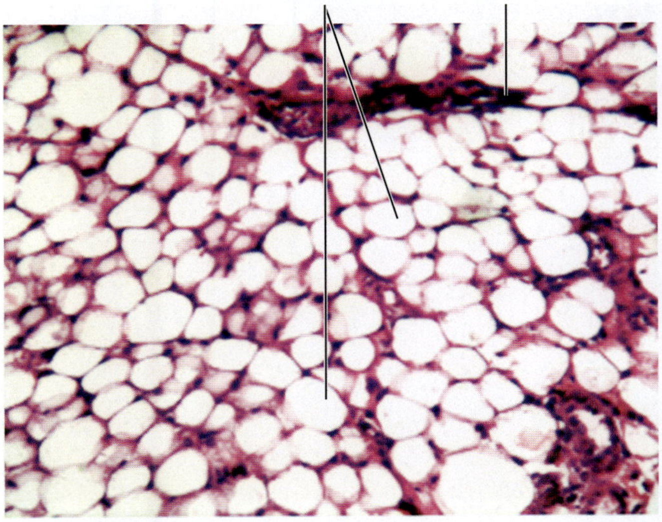

Fig. 35.29 Section from a lipoma showing a well-encapsulated mass of mature adipocytes (H&E; 100×).

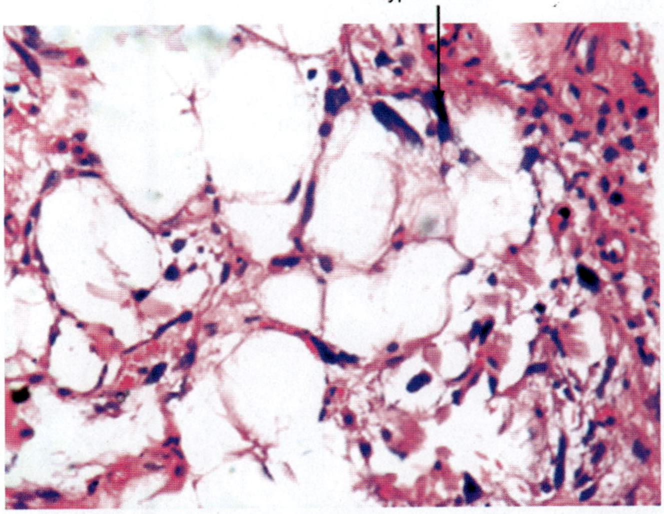

Fig. 35.30 Section from a pleomorphic lipoma shows a lipomatous component, spindle cell component, and floret-like giant cells with nuclear pleomorphism (H&E; 400×).

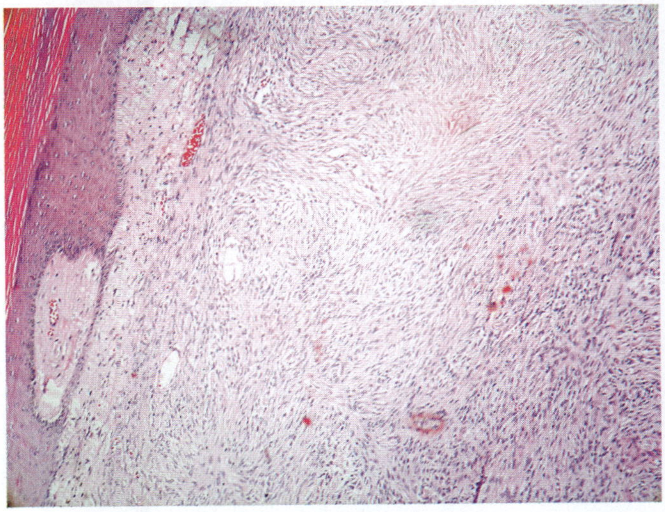

Fig. 35.31 Section from a benign fibrous histiocytoma showing focal storiform pattern (H&E; 200×).

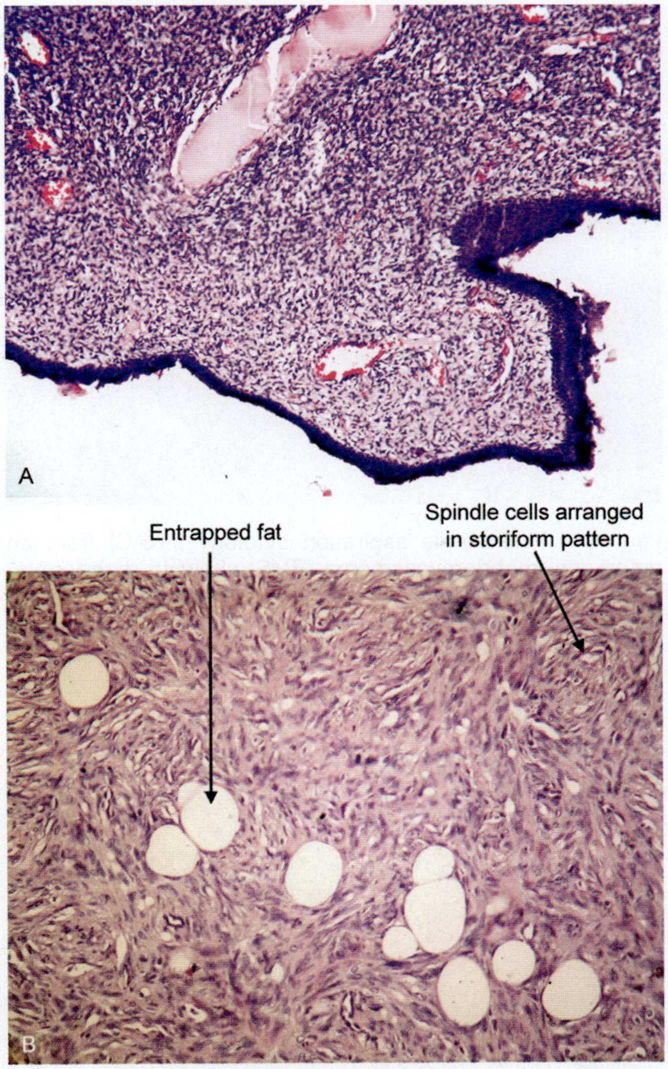

Fig. 35.32 Section from a DFSP showing (A) dermal tumour composed of interwoven bundles of spindle cells (H&E; 100×) and (B) Spindle cells arranged in a storiform or cartwheel pattern entrapping normal fat (H&E; 200×).

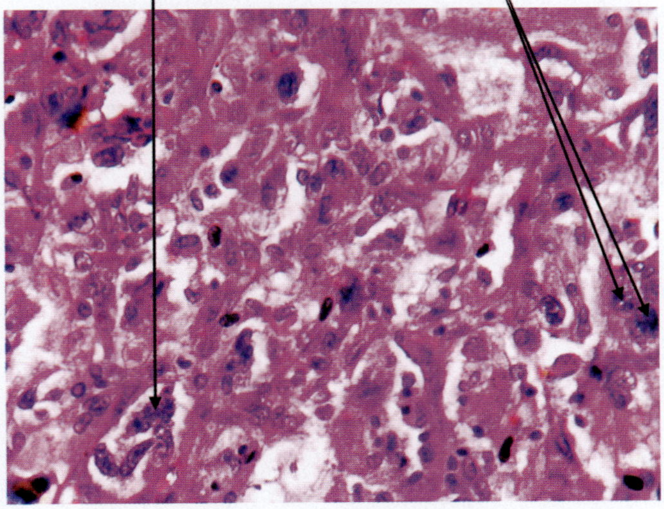

Fig. 35.33 Section from an undifferentiated pleomorphic sarcoma, showing an admixture of highly pleomorphic spindle-shaped cells and histiocytic cells with numerous bizzare tumour giant cells (H&E; 400×).

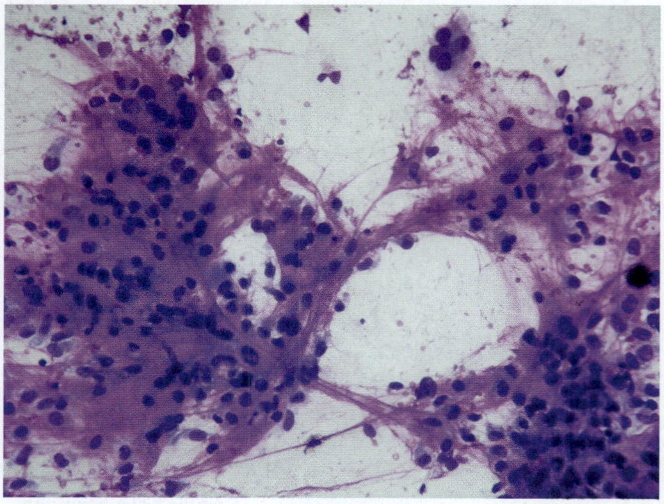

Fig. 35.34 Fine-needle aspiration cytology (FNAC) from an embryonal rhabdomyosarcoma (RMS) showing rhabdomyoblasts with abundant eosinophilic cytoplasm, along with round cells and spindle-shaped strap cells in a myxoid background (MGG; 100×).

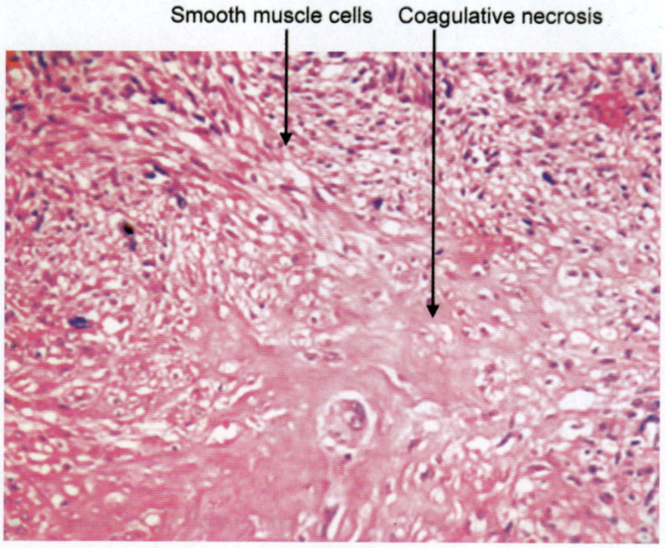

Fig. 35.35 Section from a leiomyosarcoma comprising smooth muscle cells with eosinophilic fibrillary cytoplasm, cigar-shaped, blunt-ended nuclei showing variable atypia, palisading around a central area of coagulative necrosis (H&E; 400×).

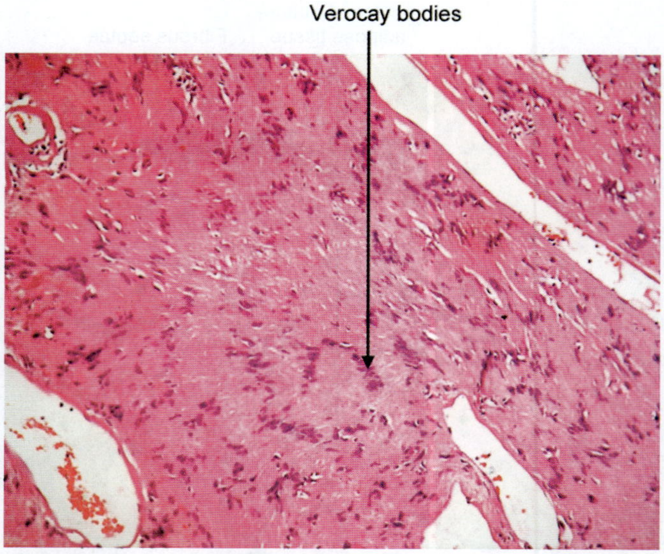

Fig. 35.36 Section from a schwannoma showing Antoni A regions (lining up of delicate wavy nuclei in bands separated by eosinophilic cytoplasm), rows of nuclei (called Verocay bodies), and Antoni B regions (showing less organization) (H&E; 100×).

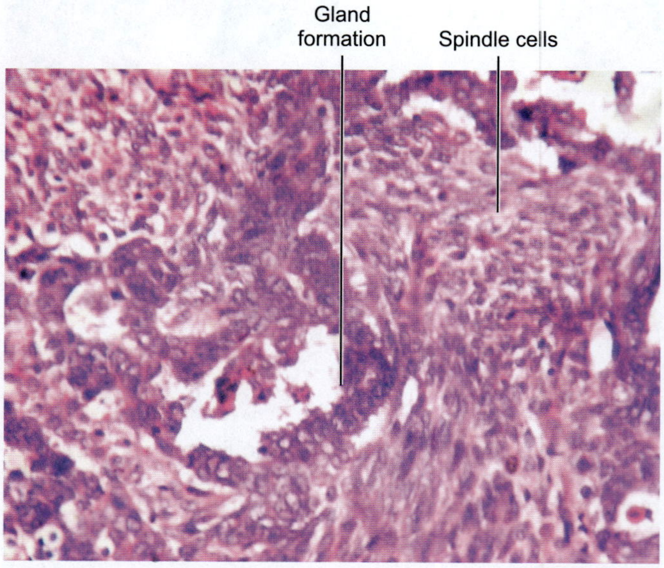

Fig. 35.37 Section from a synovial sarcoma showing a typical biphasic appearance with both fibrous and glandular elements (H&E; 400×).

Diseases of the Central Nervous System

36

The nervous system has the following components:

1. **Central nervous system (CNS):** Consists of the brain and the spinal cord.
2. **Peripheral nervous system (PNS):** Composed of nerve fibers and aggregates of nerve cells called ganglia.

CNS

The brain and the spinal cord are composed of 'grey' and 'white' matter. The former contains nerve bodies and neuroglia and a network of nerve cell processes, whereas the latter contains neuronal processes and neuroglia and no nerve cell bodies. The brain has four main functional and anatomical regions—the cerebrum, cerebellum, pons and medulla. Neurons and neuroglial cells are the two main histological elements.

Normal Cells of Central Nervous System (CNS) and Their Cellular Morphology (Fig. 36.1)

Neurons

- They are organized as aggregates (nuclei and ganglia) or elongated columns/layers (e.g. grey column of spinal cord or six-layered cerebral cortex).
- They have a cell body (perikaryon), a large eccentric nucleus, prominent nucleolus and abundant Nissl substance.

Glial Cells

- They form the supporting system for neurons and their dendritic and axonal processes.
- They play a role in inflammation, repair, fluid balance and energy metabolism.

Types of glial cells

1. **Macroglia**

   These are derived from neuroectoderm and are further classified into three main types:

   (a) **Astrocytes**

   (i) These are star shaped glial cells with long, highly branched processes.

   (ii) Astrocytic processes can be demonstrated by **PTAH (Phosphotungstic Acid Haematoxylin)** stain. Ultrastructurally, these processes are composed of abundant intermediate filaments, mostly vimentin.

   (iii) Astrocytes act like fibroblasts in response to injury (undergo hyperplasia and hypertrophy, termed **'gliosis'**).

   (iv) Long-standing gliosis results in development of **'Rosenthal fibres'**, which are eosinophilic elongated globular bodies present on astrocytic processes.

   (v) They occupy most of the interneuronal space and mediate metabolic exchange and have the following sub-types:

   - Fibrillary astrocyte: Long, thin processes; present mainly in the white matter.
   - Protoplasmic astrocyte:
     - Well-defined cytoplasmic margins and pyknotic nucleus.
     - Few cytoplasmic processes separated by minute spaces.
   - Pilocytic astrocyte: Glial fibrillary acidic protein (GFAP)-positive bipolar cells with long, thin, hair like processes.
   - Gemistocytic astrocyte:
     - Soft, grey and swollen cell with eccentric nucleus/prominent nucleolus.
     - Abundant bright eosinophilic cytoplasm with stout cytoplasmic processes.

   (b) **Oligodendrocytes**

   (i) Predominant glial element in white matter responsible for myelination of axons.

   (ii) Moderate sized cells with small darkly staining nucleus and a clear halo around it.

   (iii) Small number of short-branched processes.

   (iv) Oligodendrocytes tend to aggregate closely around neurons in the grey matter for support function (satellite cells).

   (c) **Ependymal cells**

   (i) 'Epithelial-like' cuboidal to columnar cells.

   (ii) Ciliated luminal surface (cilia aid in circulation of cerebrospinal fluid).

   (iii) Bases of the cells taper and breakdown into fine ramifying processes.

2. **Microglia**

   (a) Small mobile cells of mesenchymal origin found throughout the brain, predominantly in perivascular location.

   (b) Irregular nuclei with little cytoplasm and tiny, highly branched processes.

   (c) In response to inflammation, they are transformed into amoeboid cells for phagocytosis.

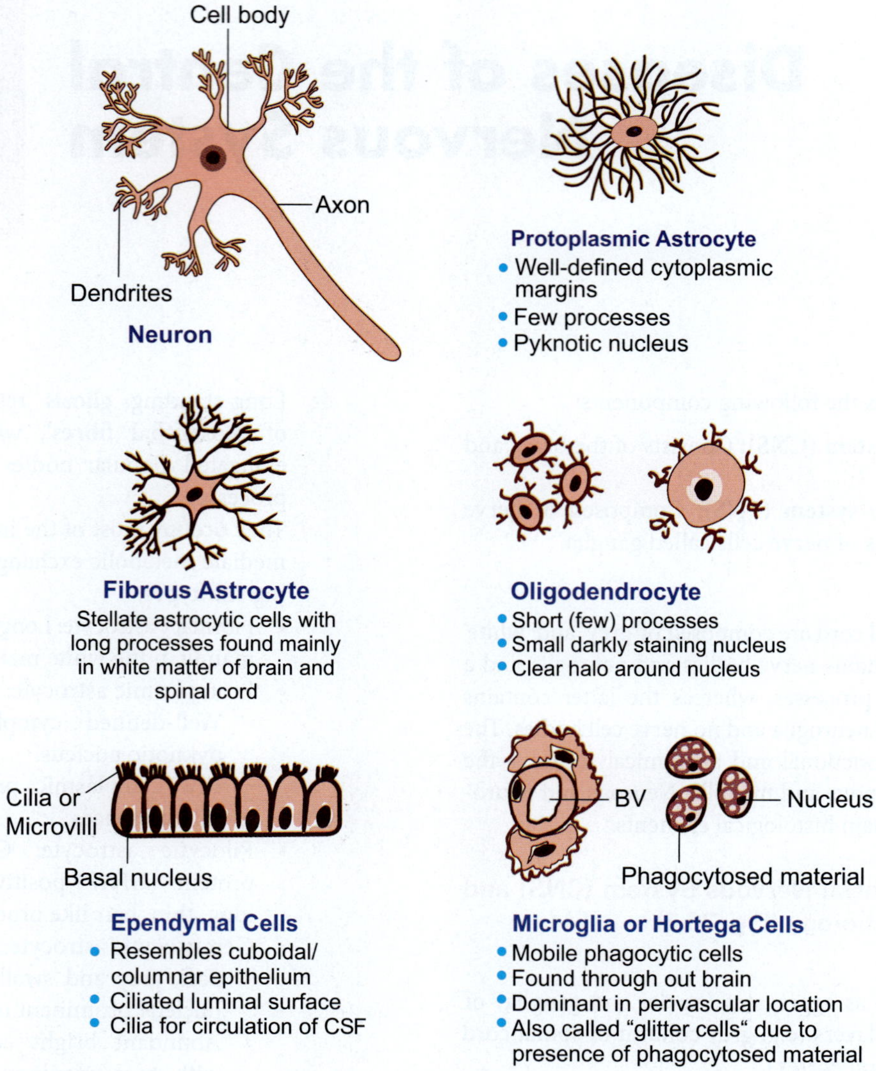

Fig. 36.1 Normal cells constituting CNS and their cellular morphology.

(d) Also called **'glitter cells'** (due to the presence of phagocytosed material).

Meninges

Leptomeninges

The arachnoid and the pia mater together form the leptomeninges (lepto = slender).

- ***Piamater***: The pia is a delicate membrane that closely covers the brain surface (due to which pathological processes, like some brain tumours, can easily spread along the subpial space). In the spinal canal, piamater forms the denticulate ligaments and the filum terminale. The pia is closely related to the peripheral layer of astrocytic end feet. Together, they form the pia-glial limiting membrane of the central nervous system. It is composed of fibroblasts, collagen and processes of underlying astrocytes.
- ***Arachnoid***: The arachnoid, a thin membrane, is connected to the underlying pia via wispy connective tissue fibers that resemble spider webs; these give the arachnoid ('spider-like') its name. The arachnoid is loosely applied to the brain and is normally almost transparent. It is lined by a layer of flattened mesothelial cells.
- ***Subarachnoid space***: It is the space between the two leptomeninges; and contains **cerebrospinal fluid (CSF)** and major blood vessels.

Dura

This is the tough fibrous covering of brain, lined on the inside by mesothelium and suspended from calvarium by denticulate ligament. The space between the dura and bone is labelled the **'epidural space'**. **'Subdural space'** on the other hand is the space between the dura and arachnoid membrane that contains a minute amount of fluid.

CSF

- Seventy percent of CSF is formed in the ventricular choroid plexus by a combined process of active secretion and ultrafiltration.
- Thirty percent of CSF is formed as interstitial fluid elaborated within intercellular spaces of the brain and spinal cord (Choroid plexus → Lateral ventricle → Foramen of

Monro → 3rd ventricle → Cerebral aqueduct of Sylvius → 4th ventricle → Two lateral foramina of Luschka and one median foramen of Magendie → Sub-arachnoid space → Arachnoid granulations → Dural sinus → Venous drainage).

- CSF cushions the brain and the spinal cord; is important for autoregulation of cerebral blood flow, delivers nutrients and removes waste products from the brain.
- Total volume of CSF in adults ranges between 90 and 150 mL.
- Two morphologically distinct blood-brain barriers prevent passage of plasma constituents into CSF, namely:
  1. Capillary endothelium.
  2. Fenestrated choroidal capillaries enclosed by specialized ependyma found in choroid plexus epithelium.
- Cell content of normal CSF is low (0–4/μL), comprising mainly lymphocytes and monocytes.
- Normal pressure of CSF is 90–180 mm of CSF (60–150 mm of water). It is measured by allowing CSF to rise in a sterile, graduated manometer tube.
- Normal CSF is crystal clear with an appearance and viscosity comparable to water.

Q: Write briefly on hydrocephalus.

Ans. Hydrocephalus is defined as excessive accumulation of CSF within the ventricular system. This may be secondary to overproduction (as in tumours, e.g. choroid plexus papilloma) or impaired flow and resorption (as in aqueduct stenosis, Arnold-chiari malformation and meningitis). Risk factors for hydrocephalus include intrauterine infection or intracranial infections resulting from trauma at the time of birth or due to prematurity in infants and infections like meningitis, otitis media, CNS tumours and intracranial haemorrhage in children and adults. Increased intraventricular volume of CSF may lead to increased intracranial pressure. If this occurs before closure of cranial sutures (in infancy) it causes enlargement of head, whereas after closure of the cranial sutures the intracranial pressure increases without increase in the head circumference. The scalp appears thin and shiny and shows distended scalp veins. The orbital roof is depressed with downward displacement of eyes and bulging sclera. There is abnormal muscle tone (due to neurological compression), high-pitched shrill cry and irritability. In *communicating* hydrocephalus, the entire ventricular system is enlarged, while in the *non-communicating* type there is localized expansion of the ventricular system. Pathological changes include dilatation of ventricles with presence of excessive fluid, compression of brain and open fontanel.

Q. Describe the aetiology, types, pathogenesis, differentiating factors, and CSF findings in meningitis. (PA35.1)

Ans. Inflammation of meninges is called meningitis. It is of two types:

- **Inflammation of dura (pachymeningitis):** This is usually due to extension of infection from chronic suppurative otitis media (CSOM) or a fractured skull.
- **Inflammation of pia-arachnoid (leptomeningitis):** The common causes of leptomeningitis include:

Infection

1. **Acute pyogenic (bacterial/purulent) meningitis.**
   (a) Infection of pia-arachnoid and of CSF enclosed in subarachnoid space.
   (b) May extend to brain, spinal cord, optic nerves and ventricles.

   Causative organisms
   (a) *Escherichia coli* (infects neonates, particularly with neural tube defects).
   (b) *Haemophilus influenzae* (infects infants and children).
   (c) *Neisseria meningitides* (infects adolescents and young adults).
   (d) *Streptococcus pneumoniae* (infects extremes of age; common following trauma).

   Routes of infection
   (a) Blood stream.
   (b) Adjacent focus.
   (c) Iatrogenic (during operation/lumbar puncture).

   Gross pathology
   Normally clear CSF becomes turbid or frankly purulent due to pus accumulating in the subarachnoid space. Pus may interfere with normal flow of CSF leading to obstructive hydrocephalus. The meninges appear opaque. The exudate is generally basal with *H. influenzae* infection and located over the cerebral convexities in Pneumococcal meningitis.

   Microscopy
   (a) Numerous polymorphonuclear leukocytes, prominent around blood vessels are seen.
   (b) Gram staining is done to demonstrate specific organisms.

   Clinical features
   (a) Medical emergency; presents with fever, severe headache, vomiting, drowsiness, stupor, coma and convulsions.
   (b) Stiffness of neck on forward bending, positive **Kernig sign** (hip flexion causes pain in the knee) and positive **Brudzinski's sign** (neck flexion causes flexion of knee and hip).

   CSF findings
   (a) Cloudy/frankly turbid CSF.
   (b) Elevated CSF pressure (above 180 mm water).
   (c) Presence of polymorphs (10–10,000/μL).
   (d) Raised CSF protein (>50 mg/dL).
   (e) Decreased sugar (<40 mg/dL).
   (f) Positive bacteriologic examination (Gram stain or culture).

   Complications
   (a) Cerebral abscess formation.
   (b) Obstructive hydrocephalus.
   (c) Subdural empyema.
   (d) Cerebral infarction.
   (e) Epilepsy.
   (f) Waterhouse-Friderichsen syndrome (may result from meningitis associated septicaemia leading to haemorrhagic infarction of the adrenal gland).

2. **Acute lymphocytic (viral, aseptic) meningitis:** Mostly affects children and young adults.
   Causative viruses: Enteroviruses, mumps, ECHO virus, coxsackie virus, EBV and HSV II.
   Gross pathology: No distinctive change; sometimes swelling of brain.
   Microscopy: Mild lymphocytic infiltrate in the leptomeninges.
   Clinical features
   (a) Acute meningeal symptoms and fever.
   (b) Benign and self-limiting, usually ends in complete recovery.
   (c) Life-threatening complications of bacterial meningitis usually not seen.
   CSF findings
   (a) Clear or slightly turbid fluid.
   (b) CSF protein normal or slightly raised.
   (c) CSF sugar normal.
   (d) CSF bacteriologically sterile.
3. **Chronic tuberculous/cryptococcal meningitis**
   Tuberculous meningitis
   (a) Affects children and adults.
   (b) Usually due to haematogenous spread (miliary tuberculosis).
   (c) Less commonly, spreads directly from tuberculosis of the vertebral body.
   Cryptococcal meningitis
   (a) Seen in debilitated or immunocompromised persons (e.g. with AIDS).
   (b) Usually due to haematogenous dissemination from a pulmonary lesion.
   Gross pathology of chronic meningitis
   (a) Thick exudate in subarachnoid space, more abundant in sulci and base of brain.
   (b) Tubercles are 1–2 mm in diameter, and located adjacent to blood vessels.
   (c) Exudate in cryptococcal meningitis is scanty, translucent and gelatinous.
   Microscopic findings in chronic meningitis
   (a) Acute and chronic inflammatory cells.
   (b) Granulomas (with or without caseation).
   (c) AFB/capsulated cryptococci.
   Clinical features of chronic meningitis
   (a) Headache, confusion, malaise and vomiting.
   (b) May have a fulminant (few weeks) or an indolent (months or years) course.
   CSF findings in chronic meningitis
   (a) Mild turbidity; may form fibrin web on standing (due to increased protein including fibrinogen).
   (b) Raised CSF pressure (>300 mm of water).
   (c) Mononuclear leucocytosis (100–1000 cells/μL); mainly lymphocytes and macrophages.
   (d) Increased protein.
   (e) Decreased glucose.
   (f) Demonstration of AFB/*cryptococcus*.
   Complications and late sequelae
   (a) Exudate and fibrous adhesions leading to obstructive hydrocephalus.
   (b) Tuberculous encephalitis.
   (c) Tuberculosis of the spine.

Note: Tuberculosis of CNS can also result in tuberculoma formation. Tuberculomas are single or multiple well circumscribed intraparenchymal masses which present as space occupying lesions. Histologically they show epithelioid cell granulomas with or without caseous necrosis.

The differentiating features of different types of meningitis are shown in Table 36.1.

Q. Write briefly on neurosyphilis.

Ans. Neurosyphilis is syphilis affecting the central nervous system (CNS). Involvement of CNS is generally seen in the tertiary stage of the disease, in approximately 10% of untreated patients.

Table 36.1 Differentiating features of different types of meningitis (PA35.3)

Features	Normal	Acute pyogenic (bacterial) meningitis	Acute lymphocytic (viral) meningitis	Chronic (tuberculous) meningitis
Naked eye appearance	Clear and colourless	Cloudy or frankly purulent	Clear or slightly turbid	Clear or slightly turbid, forms fibrin coagulum on standing
CSF pressure	60–150 mm water	Elevated (>180 mm of water)	Elevated	Elevated
Cells	0–4 lymphocytes/μL	10–10,000 neutrophils/μL	10–100 lymphocytes/μL	100–1000 lymphocytes/μL
Proteins	15–45 mg/dL	Markedly raised due to • Increased permeability of blood–CSF barrier • Decreased removal of protein molecules at arachnoid level	Raised	Raised
Glucose	50–80 mg/dL	Markedly reduced due to • Impaired glucose transport • Increased glycolysis in CNS • Increased glucose utilization by WBCs and microorganisms	Normal	Reduced
Bacteriology	Sterile	Causative organism isolated	Sterile	Tubercular bacilli present

Major Patterns of CNS Involvement in Neurosyphilis

1. **Meningovascular**
   (a) Causes chronic meningitis.
   (b) Histopathology shows obliterative endarteritis (**Heubner arteritis**) with perivascular inflammation rich in plasma cells.
   (c) Occasionally gummas (masses rich in plasma cells) may be seen in the brain parenchyma and meninges.
2. **Paretic neurosyphilis (general paresis of the insane due to invasion of brain by *Treponema pallidum*)**
   (a) Insidious and progressive loss of mental and physical functions with mood alterations and dementia.
   (b) Widespread individual cell death and brain atrophy.
   (c) Loss of cortical neurons and glial proliferation.
3. **Tabes dorsalis**
   (a) Damage of dorsal root resulting in impaired position and vibration sense, ataxia and loss of pain sensation.
   (b) Loss of both axons and myelin in the dorsal roots.

Q. Write briefly on encephalitis.

Ans. Encephalitis is infection of the brain parenchyma, which is invariably associated with meningeal inflammation (Meningoencephalitis). It manifests with fever, headache, impaired mental status and drowsiness. The most common cause of encephalitis is viral infection.

Characteristic histological features

- Perivascular and parenchymal mononuclear cell infiltrate.
- Multiple foci of necrosis; in particular, single cell necrosis with phagocytosis of the debris **(neuronophagia).**
- Formation of glial nodules (due to glial proliferation).

Diagnosis

- Direct evidence: Presence of inclusion bodies or demonstration of organism.
- Indirect evidence: Occurrence of congenital malformations (due to intrauterine viral infections) and postencephalitis Parkinsonism.

Types

1. **Arbovirus-induced viral encephalitis**
   Geographic distribution
   (a) Eastern and Western equine, Venezuelan and St. Louis encephalitis (seen in Western hemisphere).
   (b) Japanese B encephalitis (seen in Far East).
   (c) Tick-borne encephalitis (seen in Russian and Eastern European regions).
   Pathology
   (a) Colourless CSF with increased pressure.
   (b) Initially, neutrophilic pleocytosis followed by lymphocytosis.
   (c) Increased CSF protein.
   (d) Normal CSF sugar.
2. **Herpes simplex virus-1-associated viral encephalitis**
   Salient features
   (a) Affects children and young adults.
   (b) Ten percent patients have history of prior herpes labialis.
   (c) Causes encephalitis with mainly temporal lobe involvement.
   Pathology
   (a) Necrosis and haemorrhage.
   (b) Perivascular inflammation.
   (c) Cowdry Type A intranuclear viral inclusions found in both neurons and glia.
3. **Herpes simplex virus-2 (HSV-2) or herpes genitalis–associated viral encephalitis**
   (a) Causes viral meningitis and encephalitis.
   (b) Seen in 50% neonates born by vaginal delivery to women with active primary HSV infection.
4. **Varicella zoster-associated viral encephalitis:** Causes granulomatous arteritis and acute encephalitis.
5. **Cytomegalovirus (CMV)-associated viral encephalitis:** Most common viral CNS infection in AIDS. Two patient populations affected:
   (a) **Fetal:** Severe periventricular necrosis, brain damage, microcephaly and periventricular calcification.
   (b) **Immunosuppressed adults:** Subacute encephalitis.
   Histopathological examination shows presence of intranuclear eosinophilic inclusion bodies.
6. **Rabies-associated viral encephalitis**
   Salient features
   (a) Transmitted by the bite of a rabid animal usually a dog.
   (b) Virus enters CNS from the wound site via peripheral nerves.
   (c) Incubation period: 1–3 months.
   (d) Nonspecific symptoms like malaise, headache and fever.
   (e) Paraesthesias around wound, extraordinary CNS excitability, violent motor responses (convulsions), contracture of pharyngeal muscles, meningismus and flaccid paralysis.
   Pathology
   (a) Intense oedema and vascular congestion.
   (b) Widespread neuronal degeneration and inflammation (most severe in the mid-brain and floor of the fourth ventricle).
   (c) **Negri bodies** (round to oval eosinophilic intracytoplasmic inclusion bodies in pyramidal neurons of the hippocampus and Purkinje cells of the cerebellum).
7. **HIV-associated viral encephalitis**
   Clinical features
   (a) Insidious, presents with mental slowing and mood disturbances.
   (b) Motor abnormalities, ataxia and seizures may also be seen.
   Pathology
   (a) Aseptic (lymphocytic) meningitis.
   (b) Myelin loss.
   (c) Meningoencephalitis.
   (d) A very classical histological finding is fusion of microglial cells to form multinucleated giant cells, usually located perivascularly. Also seen is white matter injury and vacuolar myelopathy.

Q. Write briefly on Lyme disease.

Ans. Caused by ***Borrelia burgdorferi*** (a spirochaete).

Clinical features: May manifest with any of the following:

- Aseptic meningitis
- Facial nerve palsy
- Encephalopathy
- Polyneuropathies

Pathology

Focal proliferation of microglia with scattered organisms.

Q. Write briefly on cerebrovascular accidents.

Ans. Cerebrovascular accidents (CVAs) can be due to the following:

1. Ischaemic damage (thrombosis or embolism).
2. Intracranial haemorrhage (rupture of a blood vessel).

Ischaemic brain injury may be caused by occlusive thrombi (most commonly due to atherosclerosis), emboli from the heart, vasculitis, or external compression of the cerebral vessels by tumours.

Intracranial haemorrhage can be classified as *intracerebral* or *subarachnoid*. Causes of intracranial haemorrhage include hypertension, aneurysmal rupture, arterio-venous malformations, or trauma. Traumatic haemorrhage generally leads to the formation of a subdural or epidural haematoma.

CVAs can cause global cerebral ischaemia leading to diffuse ischaemic/hypoxic encephalopathy or focal cerebral ischaemia.

Q. Write in detail on cerebral infarcts.

Ans. Cerebrovascular injury leads to the formation of infarcts, which could be **'anaemic or pale infarcts'** (associated with thrombosis) or **'haemorrhagic or red infarcts'** (associated with embolic events). Cerebral infarction is defined as focal brain necrosis due to total prolonged ischaemia.

Causes of Ischaemic Infarction

Atherosclerosis with or without superimposed thrombus
Small vessel disease (hyaline arteriosclerosis due to hypertension and diabetes)
Embolism from the heart or major vessels
Vasculitis
Arterial dissection
Haematological disorders (Polycythemia, thrombocythemia, haemoglobinopathies like sickle cell disease, deficiencies of anticoagulant factors, thrombotic thrombocytopenic purpura)
Systemic lupus erythematosus
Sickle cell disease
Vascular spasm
Meningitis and fungal vasculitis
Hypercoagulability (Factor V Leiden, Prothrombin 20210A mutation, antiphospholipid antibody syndrome)
Inherited metabolic disorders (Fabry disease, homocystinuria, mitochondrial disorders)

Clinical Manifestations of Cerebral Infarcts

- Infarcts could be ischaemic or embolic.
- Atherothrombotic infarcts are often preceded by **transient ischaemic attacks** (TIAs).
- A TIA is defined as a focal neurological deficit that lasts less than 24 hours and resolves. It is caused by critical reduction of blood supply that impairs neurological function but falls short of causing permanent tissue damage, or by emboli that break up soon after they occlude vessels.
- Most emboli are fragments of blood clots that originate in the heart or major vessels. Conditions causing cardiac emboli include myocardial infarcts, atrial fibrillation and other arrhythmias, rheumatic heart disease, bacterial and non-bacterial endocarditis, prosthetic valves, mitral valve prolapse, atrial myxoma, calcified mitral annulus and cardiomyopathy.
- Pathologically an embolus cannot be distinguished from a locally formed thrombus. An infarct is assumed to be embolic if it is haemorrhagic, there is a source of emboli, there are multiple infarcts of the brain and other organs (kidney, spleen), and there is no atherosclerosis or other vascular disease.
- Some emboli consist of atheromatous material that is detached from ulcerated atheromas of the aorta or carotid arteries. Vascular manipulation (angiography, carotid endarterectomy) may cause atheromatous embolism. Rarer causes of embolism are fat, air, and tumour emboli. Unlike atherothrombotic infarcts, which may evolve within hours or days, embolic infarcts have an abrupt onset.

Pathology of Ischaemic Infarcts

- In the first 24 hours the infarct appears as a poorly demarcated area of softening. CT imaging at this stage may be negative, especially in brain stem infarcts. MRI is much more sensitive. The infarcted tissue later becomes sharply demarcated and soft.
- In the second week it begins to disintegrate to gradually get replaced by a cavity. The size and location of infarcts follows the anatomy of vascular territories.

Microscopic Findings

- In the first 24–48 hours, the white matter appears pale and vacuolated due to axonal swelling and damage to myelin.
- Perivascular and meningeal inflammatory reaction is seen in the first week, due to release of arachidonic acid.
- Neovascularization (which shows as contrast enhancement) peaks at 2 weeks. Blood monocytes infiltrate the infarct through damaged vessels. After ingesting the products of degradation of neurons and myelin they are transformed into lipid-laden macrophages.
- Astrocytes from the surrounding area proliferate to form a glial scar to replace the infarct in about 2 months.
- Neurons do not regenerate resulting in loss of brain tissue.

Pathology of a Haemorrhagic Infarct

A haemorrhagic infarct shows haemorrhage due to leakage of blood from collateral vessels or through damaged capillaries in the event of re-perfusion after breakdown of the culprit thrombus or embolus.

Lacunar Infarcts

These are small infarcts in the deeper parts of the brain (basal ganglia, thalamus, white matter) and in the brain stem. They are responsible for about 20% of all strokes. They are caused by occlusion of deep penetrating branches of major cerebral arteries and are particularly common in hypertension and diabetes, which are associated with atherosclerosis of small vessels and small vessel disease.

Q. Write briefly on intracranial haemorrhage.

Ans. Based on their location intracranial haemorrhages are classified into:

1. Epidural haemorrhage—Accumulation of blood between skull bone and duramater secondary to trauma.
2. Subdural haemorrhage—Accumulation of blood in the subdural space secondary to trauma causing tears in vessels at their point of entry into the dura mater.
3. Subarachnoid haemorrhage—Accumulation of blood in the subarachnoid space secondary to a ruptured aneurysm (berry aneurysm) or other vascular malformations, haematological disorders, tumours, etc.
4. Intraparenchymal haemorrhage—Occurs secondary to rupture of intraparenchymal vessels, most common causes being hypertension and cerebral amyloid angiopathy.

Q. Classify and describe the etiology, genetics, pathogenesis, pathology, presentation, sequelae and complications of CNS tumours. (PA35.2)

Ans. Neoplastic lesions of CNS and their clinicopathological features:

Epidemiology

- Intracranial tumours are more common than intraspinal.
- More than half are primary; rest are metastatic.
- Constitute 20% of all cancers of childhood.
- In children, majority occur in the posterior fossa, whereas in adults, the cerebral hemispheres are most commonly involved.
- In adults, Glioblastomas are most common followed by meningioma and astrocytoma in that order. In children, Medulloblastoma is most common followed by pilocytic astrocytoma and glioblastoma.
- Most primary CNS tumours are sporadic. Only 5% are associated with hereditary syndromes.
- Risk factors include Neurofibromatosis, VHL syndrome, Li Fraumeni syndrome, Turcot syndrome, tuberous sclerosis, Gorlin syndrome and exposure to ionizing radiation.

Unique Features

- Benign and malignant tumours are difficult to differentiate based on morphology alone.
- Anatomic site can have lethal consequences irrespective of morphology.
- Accessibility to surgical resection is limited.
- Pattern and mode of spread are different from other malignancies (spread through CSF).

Clinical Presentation

- Headache.
- Nausea and vomiting.
- Seizures.
- Manifestations of increased intracranial pressure.
- Focal neurological signs like sensory changes, visual abnormalities, muscle weakness, memory and personality changes.

Classification

- In 2016 WHO update on CNS tumours the definition of new entities has been based on molecular characteristics for the first time.
- Focus is on the use of an 'integrated' diagnosis that incorporates both phenotypic and genotypic information.
- Astrocytomas and oligodendrogliomas are now in the same category ('diffuse astrocytic and oligodendroglial tumours'), which are further defined by the presence or absence of IDH mutations.
- Molecular characteristics have been included to define entities that determine prognostic categories under the heading of Medulloblastomas.
- NOS (not otherwise specified) terminology has been used when molecular information is insufficient.
- The term **gliomatosis cerebri** (now considered a pattern instead of an entity) and 'primitive neuroectodermal tumour' (PNET) terminology for embryonal tumours has been deleted.
- Brain invasion is added as a criterion for atypical meningioma, WHO grade II.

Terminology

- Diffuse astrocytic and oligodendroglial tumours.
- Other astrocytic tumours.
- Ependymal tumours.
- Other gliomas.
- Choroid plexus tumours.
- Neuronal and mixed neuronal glial tumours.
- Tumours of the pineal region.
- Embryonal tumours.
- Tumours of the cranial and paraspinal nerves.
- Meningiomas.
- Mesenchymal, nonmeningothelial tumours.
- Melanocytic tumours.
- Lymphomas.
- Histiocytic tumours.
- Germ cell tumours.
- Tumours of the sellar region.
- Metastatic tumours.

Grading

Histological grading is still used based on morphology, despite the very important prognostic significance of the molecular characteristics.

- According to the 2016 WHO classification, diffuse astrocytomas are graded using a three tiered system (II, III and IV); there are no grade I infiltrating astrocytomas.

- WHO grading scheme is based on the presence or absence of four histological parameters:
  1. Nuclear atypia: defined as nuclear pleomorphism and hyperchromasia.
  2. Mitoses
     (a) Solitary mitosis in a large specimen does not justify the WHO grade III designation.
     (b) Ki67 proliferation index aids in the separation of grade II from grade III tumours.
  3. Microvascular proliferation: two forms are recognized:
     (a) Glomeruloid type, which is more common but prognostically less significant since it is also commonly encountered in low grade gliomas such as pilocytic astrocytoma.
     (b) Endothelial proliferation within the lumen of larger vessels, which is less common but is more closely associated with high grade gliomas.
  4. Necrosis: two types are recognized:
     (a) Coagulative necrosis.
     (b) Pseudopalisading necrosis.

WHO Histological Grading of Diffuse Astrocytic Tumours

- WHO grade II tumours (diffuse astrocytoma): show only nuclear atypia.
- WHO grade III tumours (anaplastic astrocytoma): show focal or dispersed anaplasia, significant proliferative activity and mitoses.
- WHO grade IV tumours (glioblastoma): show nuclear atypia, mitoses, microvascular proliferation or necrosis.

WHO Histological Grading of Localized Astrocytic Tumours

Pilocytic astrocytoma corresponds to WHO grade I.

Diffuse Astrocytic and Oligodendroglial Tumours

- Most common tumour of CNS and PNS.
- Three main types of gliomas are seen in the CNS, namely, astrocytomas, ependymomas and oligodendrogliomas.
  1. **Astrocytomas:** Gliomas derived from a progenitor cell with differentiation towards the astrocytic lineage are labelled astrocytomas. They are further classified into 'Diffusely Infiltrating Astrocytomas' and 'Localized Astrocytomas'. Diffuse Astrycytomas, based on their histological differentiation and clinical evolution are divided into the following subtypes:
     (a) **Diffuse astrocytomas (Grade II/IV)**
        (i) Constitute 10%–15% of all astrocytic brain tumours and 80% of all primary brain tumours.
        (ii) Usually supratentorial but can arise from any part of CNS (preferred sites: frontal and temporal lobes, brain stem, spinal cord; uncommon in cerebellum).
        (iii) Peak affected age is 3rd to 4th decades.
        (iv) They show a spectrum of histological features depending on the predominant cell type (fibrillary, protoplasmic, gemistocytic, etc.).
        (v) Ill defined with blurred margins, may have spongy or gelatinous appearance, microcysts, calcification.
        (vi) Show hypercellular areas as compared to the normal white matter, which merge imperceptibly with the surrounding brain; background is fibrillary. There is variable atypia. No mitotic figures, vascular proliferation and necrosis, is seen. Tumour cells are positive for GFAP and Vimentin.
     (b) **Anaplastic astrocytomas (Grade III/IV)** are tumours, which show increased cellular pleomorphism, proliferation of blood vessels, necrosis and numerous mitoses.
     (c) **Glioblastoma multiforme or GM (WHO Grade IV/IV tumours)** have the following salient features:
        (i) They are the commonest gliomas in adults; usually seen in 3rd to 5th decades.
        (ii) Cerebrum is the most frequent location. Also involve septum pellucidum, basal ganglia, hypothalamus and corpus callosum **(butterfly tumours).**
        (iii) Prior to the introduction of molecular advances in CNS tumours, Glioblastomas were classified into *"De novo glioblastoma"* and *"Secondary glioblastoma"*. In the adult setting, the most recent WHO guidelines distinguish between GBMs that are IDH-mutant and those that are not. The former arise often in clinically evident fashion as a progression from a lower-grade glioma and are traditionally termed "secondary glioblastoma." In contrast, those GBMs that are IDH–wild-type are classically termed "de novo glioblastoma" or "primary glioblastoma". Primary GBMs develop quickly, have no clinically evident lower-grade precursor, and are in fact molecularly distinct from secondary GBM.
        (iv) GBM has been classified into at least four molecular subgroups namely proneural (PN), neural (NL), classical (CL) and mesenchymal (MES). The MES subtype is the most aggressive and strongly associated with a poor prognosis compared to PN subtype. The molecular events driving this transition are similar to those driving the epithelial-mesenchymal transition (EMT) in carcinomas cells. EMT has been described as a crucial mechanism by which carcinoma cells enhance their invasive capacity by losing cell polarity and intercellular adhesions acquiring a mesenchymal and more motile phenotype, thus promoting cancer metastasis.
        (v) CL forms the bulk of primary GMs and is associated with mutations of PTEN tumour suppressor gene, amplification of EGFR and deletions of chromosome 10. MES subtype is associated with deletions of NF1 on chromosome 17 and increased expression of genes

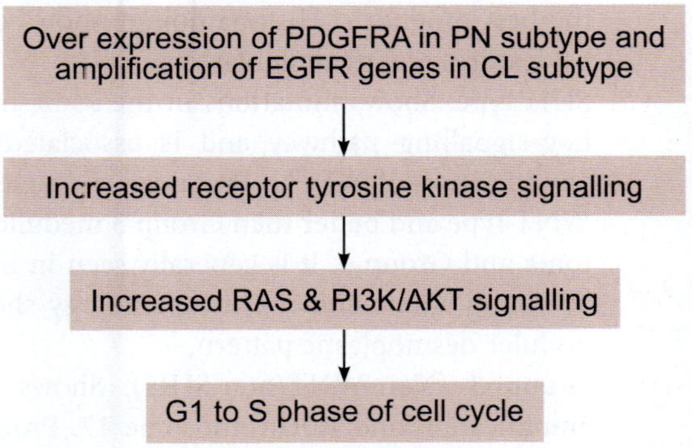

Flowchart 36.1 Pathogenesis of glioblastoma multiforme.

involved in TNF and NK-kB pathway. NL subtype typically demonstrates high levels of neuronal markers like NEFL, GABRAI, and SLC12A5. PN subtype is the most common type of secondary GM characterized by mutations of TP53, Isocitrate Dehydrogenase (IDH 1 and IDH2) genes along with over expression of PDGFRA alfa.

(vi) Common to all molecular subtypes is the loss of growth suppression and uncontrolled proliferation (Flowchart 36.1).

(vii) On gross examination the tumour appears poorly demarcated, pale yellow to salmon pink with presence of haemorrhage and necrosis (variegated appearance). Multiple foci are seen in 7% cases (gliomatosis cerebri). Cortex and leptomeninges may be infiltrated; the tumour may invade and spread through CSF.

(viii) Histopathologically tumour cells show marked cellular pleomorphism. Cellular areas, which may have a serpentine pattern, alternating with necrosis are seen. There is presence of primitive glial cells and multinucleate tumour giant cells. Prominent endothelial proliferation with piled up endothelial cells bulging into vascular lumina, at times; forming ball-like (glomeruloid) structures is seen. Regimentation/pseudopalisading of nuclei at the edges of necrotic foci can be demonstrated. Perivascular necrosis is common (differential diagnosis—metastatic carcinoma in which perivascular areas are spared unlike GM).

(ix) Prognosis is bad; mean duration of survival after diagnosis is 8–10 months.

(d) **Pilocytic astrocytomas (WHO grade I/IV tumours)**

(i) Slow growing; affect children and young adults.

(ii) Involve cerebellum, 3rd ventricle and optic nerves.

(iii) Usually cystic with a mural nodule; may be solid.

(iv) Composed of bipolar cells with long thin hair-like processes (low cellularity, low mitoses, and no infiltration of surrounding tissue).

(v) 'Rosenthal fibres' (amorphous aggregates of GFAP) and thick-walled blood vessels can be seen.

2. **Oligodendrogliomas (WHO grade II/IV tumours)**

(a) Constitute 5%–10% of all gliomas and are commonly located in cerebral white matter (frontal lobes); thalamus frequent location in children.

(b) Usually seen in adults (4th to 5th decade); less frequent in children.

(c) Slow growing; present for years, however, anaplastic oligodendrogliomas may grow into and destroy the cortex and penetrate leptomeninges.

(d) Most common genetic alterations are mutations of IDH genes (IDH 1 and 2). These are seen in 90% cases and are associated with a better prognosis. Progression to anaplastic oligodendroglioma is associated with loss of 9p10q and mutations in CDKN2A.

Gross pathology: Well-circumscribed, pink-to-red, gelatinous with foci of calcification (seen in up to 90% cases).

Microscopy

- Round cells with clear cytoplasm, well-defined cytoplasmic membranes and dark nucleus (**fried-egg appearance**); grouped together in a honeycomb-like pattern.
- Anastomosing network of blood vessels (chicken wire appearance).
- Endothelial proliferation unusual (unless undergoing malignant change).
- Grade II/IV lesions. Better prognosis than astrocytomas (average survival rate is 5–10 years).

3. **Ependymomas**

(a) Develop from lining of blood vessels and ventricles

(b) Based on location they are classified into:

(i) ***Intraneural***: located in the ventricles (common location during childhood), lumbosacral spine (common location in adults) and filum terminale.

(ii) ***Extraneural***: located in the soft tissue of sacrococcyx.

(c) Spinal ependymomas are associated with NF2 gene.

(d) Most are well differentiated and behave like WHO Grade II/IV lesions.

(e) ***Gross pathology***

(i) Well-circumscribed, typically solid papillary, friable; may show cystic areas.

(ii) Arise from the roof or floor of 4th ventricle; fill the ventricular cavity and may invade the cerebellum and medulla.

(iii) Calcification is seen in 15% of the cases.

(f) ***Microscopy***

(i) 'Epithelial-like cells' with regular round to oval nuclei and granular chromatin, dispersed in a fibrillary background (GFAP-positive). PTAH stains the basal bodies of cilia of ependymal cells (blepharoblasts).

(ii) Gland-like/round/elongated structures called rosettes/canals.

(iii) Perivascular pseudorosettes (tumour cells arranged around vessels with thin ependymal processes directed towards the wall of the blood vessel).

(iv) Prognosis poor despite slow growth and lack of anaplasia (attributed to frequent dissemination in CSF and poor surgical accessibility).

(g) ***Variants***

(i) Anaplastic ependymoma: Shows increased cell density, high mitotic rate, areas of necrosis, dedifferentiation (Grades III/IV histology).

(ii) Myxopapillary ependymoma: Arises from filum terminale:

- Composed of papillae with a core of dilated blood vessels covered by 1–2 layers of cuboidal cells. The fibrovascular stroma may show mucoid degeneration.
- Prognosis depends on completeness of surgical resection.

(iii) Subependymoma:

- Diffuse proliferation of subependymal fibrillary astrocytes and ependymal cells.
- Small, multiple and symptomless.
- Usually arise in the 4th ventricle.
- Solid, sometimes calcified; if large, may lead to hydrocephalus.

Choroid Plexus Papilloma

1. In adults, usually arise from the 4th ventricle and cerebellopontine angle. In children, lateral ventricles are a common location.
2. May cause generalized enlargement of ventricular system and subarachnoid space. Ventricular obstruction may lead to hydrocephalus.
3. On gross examination appears cauliflower-like (soft, friable and crumbling pink mass).
4. Histopathology shows specialized ependymal cells recapitulating structure of normal choroid plexus.
5. They are difficult to remove and commonly recurrent.

Neuronal Tumours

These are tumours containing mature-appearing neurons (ganglion cells). **Gangliocytomas** contain only neurons and **gangliogliomas** contain neurons admixed with glial cells.

Poorly Differentiated or Embryonal Neoplasms

Thought to be neuroectodermal in origin; however, rarely express, if any, phenotypic markers of mature cells of nervous system, e.g. medulloblastoma and atypical teratoid/rhabdoid neoplasm.

1. **Medulloblastoma**

(a) Constitutes 20%–25% of all intracranial tumours in children.

(b) Exclusively located in the cerebellar midline or vermis in children. Cerebellar hemispheres are in involved in adults. Also occurs along the cerebellopontine angle.

(c) ***Molecular genetics:*** Based on the molecular genetics medulloblastoma is classified into four types:

(i) WNT type: Shows mutations in the WNT signalling pathway. It is seen in older children and has the best prognosis. Histopathology shows classical features of a medulloblastoma.

(ii) SHH type: Shows mutations in the sonic hedgehog-signalling pathway and is associated with amplification of MYCN. Prognosis is worse than WNT type and better than Group 3 medulloblastoma and Group 4. It is generally seen in infants or young adults and on histopathology shows a nodular desmoplastic pattern.

(iii) Group 3 (Non-WNT/non-SHH): Shows MYC amplification and isochromosome 17. Prognosis is worst amongst the various subtypes. It is generally seen in infants or children and on histopathology shows a classic or large cell pattern.

(iv) Group 4: (Non-WNT/non-SHH) Shows isochromosome 17. Prognosis is intermediate. It is not associated with MYC amplification and on histopathology; it shows a classic or large cell pattern.

(d) ***Gross examination:*** Fourth ventricle appears compressed or invaded by an unencapsulated, grey white, soft, haemorrhagic and friable mass without cystic change, leading to hydrocephalus.

(e) ***Microscopy***

(i) Cellular tumour composed of round to oval carrot-shaped nuclei with ill-defined scanty cytoplasm (GFAP positive).

(ii) Tumour cells have a tendency to form linear chains, which infiltrate through cerebellar cortex and aggregate beneath pia-subarachnoid space and eventually disseminate through CSF.

(iii) Rosettes may be centred by delicate argyrophillic fibrils of tumour cells.

(iv) Tumour may show a prominent desmoplastic response (nodular/desmoplastic variant) or large cells (large cell variant).

(f) ***Prognosis***

(i) Highly malignant but exquisitely sensitive to radiotherapy.

(ii) Spread through CSF is common. Extraneural metastasis to bone and lymph nodes may be seen.

2. **Atypical Teratoid/Rhabdoid Neoplasm**

(a) Malignant tumour of childhood (WHO grade IV/IV).

(b) Common locations include posterior fossa and supratentorial compartment.

(c) Shows divergent differentiation into epithelial, mesenchymal, neuronal and glial components.

(d) Often shows rhabdoid cells as seen in rhabdomyosarcoma.

Tumours of Meningeal Origin

Most common tumour of meningeal origin is a meningioma.

Meningioma

(a) Constitutes 15% of all CNS tumours in adults and 3% of childhood tumours.

(b) Peak incidence in 4th to 6th decade; females are more commonly affected than males.

(c) Slow growing; develops from specialized arachnoid cells of villi that project into the lumen of dural venous sinuses.

(d) Common locations: Superior sagittal sinus, sphenoid ridge, tuberculum sellae, olfactory grooves, posterior cranial fossa and ventricles.
(e) Molecular genetics: Most common abnormality is loss of chromosome 22. Also seen are deletions in the region close to but different from 22q12 that harbours NF2 gene.
(f) ***Gross pathology***
  (i) Well demarcated/unencapsulated.
  (ii) Fixes to dura and buries itself in a cup-like bed; cerebrum practically never invaded.
  (iii) Cut surface is whorled; haemorrhage and necrosis may be seen.
  (iv) Rarely, calcification, ossification and cyst formation are observed.
  (v) Extends into muscles, air sinuses and orbit; may be associated with reactive hyperostosis of bone.
(g) ***Histological types***
  (i) **Syncytial:** Poorly defined polygonal cells arranged in sheets and tight groups; whorling present (Fig. 36.2).
  (ii) **Fibroblastic:** Elongated cells arranged in interlacing bundles with abundant collagen.

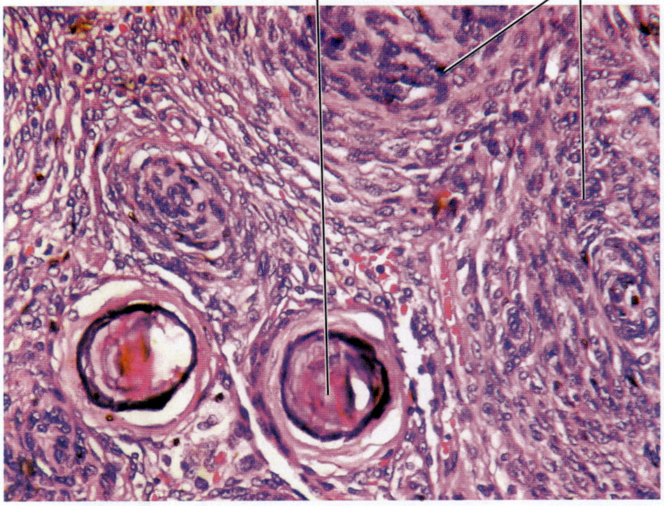

Fig. 36.2 Section from a meningioma shows polygonal cells with ill-defined cytoplasmic margins arranged in sheets and tight groups with presence of whorling and psammoma bodies (H&E; 200×).

  (iii) **Transitional/mixed:** Overlapping features of syncytial and fibroblastic type. Show a whorled pattern around a central vessel. The centre of the whorls may demonstrate psammoma bodies.
  (iv) **Psammomatous:** Numerous psammoma bodies due to calcification of syncytial nests of meningothelial cells.
  (v) **Secretory:** Characteristic PAS-positive intracytoplasmic droplets present.
  (vi) **Microcystic:** Loose spongy appearance with microcyst formation.
  (vii) **Papillary:** Papillary appearance (fibrovascular cores with pleomorphic cells around them); high rate of recurrence.
  (viii) **Angiomatous:** Vascular variant of meningioma.

Note: Xanthomatous degeneration, osseous metaplasia and moderate nuclear pleomorphism are common and usually of no prognostic significance in meningiomas.

Atypical meningioma (WHO grade II/IV) are locally aggressive and have a higher rate of recurrence. Histologically they show >4 mitoses/10HPF or at least three of the following features:
(a) Increased cellularity
(b) High N/C ratio
(c) Presence of small cells
(d) Prominent nucleoli
(e) Necrosis

Meningioma with Malignant Change: Features indicating/suggesting malignant change (Anaplastic or grade III/IV meningioma) are:
(a) Infiltration of underlying brain by a tumour with the appearance of a high-grade sarcoma with some diagnostic features of a meningioma.
(b) Abundant mitoses (>20 mitoses/10 HPF).
(c) Multifocal microscopic foci of necrosis.

Metastatic Tumours

- Most common intracranial neoplasms.
- Most common primary sites include lung, breast, skin, kidney, GIT.
- Dissemination usually through haematogenous route.
- Presents as multiple sharply demarcated nodules at the junction of grey and white matter unlike the solitary lesion seen in a primary glioma.

Normal Laboratory Values

APPENDIX

HAEMATOLOGY

Absolute neutrophil count	2–8 × 10^9/L
Activated partial thromboplastin time	20–40 s
Bleeding time	2–9 min
Erythrocyte count	4.2–5.9 x 10^{12}/L
Erythrocyte sedimentation rate • Male • Female	 • 0–15 mm/h • 0–20 mm/h
Erythropoietin	<30 mU/mL (30 units/L)
D-Dimer	<0.5 mg/L
Ferritin, serum	15–200 μg/L
Ferritin, serum	500–1500 mg/L
Haematocrit • Male • Female	 • 40%–52% • 36%–47%
Haemoglobin, blood • Male • Female	 • 4–17 g/dL (140–170 g/L) • 12–16 g/dL (120–160 g/L)
Leukocyte alkaline phosphatase	13–130/100 polymorphonuclear neutrophils and band forms
Leukocyte count	4–11 x 109/L
Mean corpuscular haemoglobin	28–32 pg
Mean corpuscular haemoglobin concentration	32–36 g/dL (320–360 g/L)
Mean corpuscular volume	80–100 fL
Platelet count	150–350 x 10^9/L
Prothrombin time	11–13 s
Reticulocyte count	0.5%–1.5% of erythrocytes; absolute 23–90 × 10^9/L

BLOOD, PLASMA AND SERUM CHEMISTRY

Albumin, serum	35–55 g/L
Alkaline phosphatase, serum	36–92 units/L
Alpha 1-antitrypsin	20–50 μmol/L
Aminotransferase, alanine (ALT)	0–35 units/L
Aminotransferase, aspartate (AST)	0–35 units/L
Ammonia, plasma	40–80 μg/dL (23–47 μmol/L)
Amylase, serum	0–130 units/L
Angiotensin-converting enzyme	23–57 U/L
Bicarbonate, serum	23–28 mEq/L (23–28 mmol/L)
Bilirubin, serum • Total • Direct	 • 0.3–1.2 mg/dL • 0–0.3 mg/dL
Blood urea nitrogen	8–20 mg/dL
C-reactive protein	<5.0 mg/L
Calcium, serum	9–10.5 mg/dL
Chloride, serum	98–106 mEq/L
Cholesterol, plasma • Total • Low-density lipoprotein (LDL) • High-density lipoprotein (HDL)	 • 150–199 mg/dL • ≤130 mg/dL • ≥40 mg/dL
Complement, serum C3	55–120 mg/dL
Creatine kinase, serum	30–170 units/L
Creatinine, serum	0.7–1.3 mg/dL (61.9–115 μmol/L)
Electrolytes, serum • Sodium • Potassium • Chloride • Bicarbonate	 • 136–145 mEq/L • 3.5–5.0 mEq/L • 98–106 mEq/L • 23–28 mEq/L
Fibrinogen, plasma	150–350 mg/dL
Folate, red cell	160–855 ng/mL
Folate, serum	2.5–20 ng/mL
Glucose, plasma fasting	70–100 mg/dL
γ-Glutamyltransferase, serum	0–30 units/L
Homocysteine, plasma • Male • Female	 • 0.54–2.16 mg/L • 0.41–1.89 mg/L
Immunoglobulins globulins, total	25–35 g/L
Iron studies • Ferritin, serum • Iron, serum • Iron-binding capacity, total, serum • Transferrin saturation	 • 15–200 μg/L • 60–160 μg/dL • 250–460 μg/dL • 20%–50%
Lactate dehydrogenase, serum	60–100 units/L

Lactic acid, venous blood	6–16 mg/dL
Lipase, serum	<95 units/L
Magnesium, serum	1.5–2.4 mg/dL
Methylmalonic acid, serum	150–370 nmol/L
Osmolality, plasma	275–295 mOsm/kg H_2O
Phosphatase, alkaline, serum	36–92 units/L
Phosphorus, serum	3–4.5 mg/dL
Prostate-specific antigen, serum	<4 ng/mL
Protein, serum • Total • Albumin • Globulins, total	 • 6.0–7.8 g/dL (60–78 g/L) • 3.5–5.5 g/dL (35–55 g/L) • 2.5–3.5 g/dL (25–35 g/L)
Rheumatoid factor	<25 IU/mL
Triglycerides	<150 mg/dL
Troponins, serum • Troponin I • Troponin T	 • 0–0.5 µg/L • 0–0.10 µg/L
Urea nitrogen, blood	8–20 mg/dL
Uric acid, serum	2.5–8 mg/dL
Vitamin B12, serum	200–800 pg/mL

ARTERIAL VALUES

pH	7.35–7.45
$PaCO_2$	35–45 mm Hg
HCO_3	22–26 mEq/L
O_2 saturation	96–100%
PaO_2	85–100 mm Hg

VENOUS VALUES

pH	7.31–7.41
$PaCO_2$	41–51 mm Hg
HCO_3	22–29 mEq/L
O_2 saturation	60–85%
PaO_2	30–40 mm Hg

HORMONES

Adrenocorticotropic hormone (ACTH), serum	4.5–20 pmol/L
Aldosterone, serum • Supine • Standing	 • 2–5 ng/dL • 7–20 ng/dL
Catecholamines • Epinephrine, plasma (supine) • Norepinephrine, plasma (supine) • Catecholamines, 24-hour, urine	 • <75 ng/L • 50–440 ng/L • <100 µg/m²/24 h
Cortisol, free, urine	<50 µg/24 h
Dehydroepiandrosterone sulphate (DHEA), plasma • Male • Female	 • 1.3–5.5 µg/mL • 0.6–3.3 µg/mL
Oestradiol, serum • Male • Female	 • 1.5–5 ng/dL • 2–14 ng/dL (follicular); 2–16 ng/dL (female, luteal), <3.5 ng/dL (postmenopausal)
Follicle-stimulating hormone, serum • Male (adult) • Female	 • 5–15 units/L • Follicular or luteal phase, 5–20 units/L; midcycle peak, 30–50 units/L; postmenopausal, >35 mIU/mL
Growth hormone, plasma	0–5 ng/mL
Parathyroid hormone, serum	10–65 ng/L
Progesterone, blood	70–280 ng/dL (ovulation)
Thyroid function tests • Thyroid iodine (131I) uptake • Thyroid-stimulating hormone (TSH)	 • 10%–30% of administered dose at 24 h • 0.5–5.0 mIU/mL
Thyroxine (T4), serum • Total • Free • Free T4 index	 • 5–12 µg/dL • 0.9–2.4 ng/dL • 4–11
Triiodothyronine, free (T3)	3.6–5.6 ng/L
Vanillylmandelic acid, urine	<8 mg/24 h
Vitamin D 1,25-dihydroxy, serum	25–65 pg/mL

TUMOUR MARKERS

Alpha fetoprotein	0–44 ng/mL
Beta human chorionic gonadotropin (HCG)	<5 IU/l
CA 19-9	<40 U/mL
Carcinoembryonic antigen (CEA)	<4 ug/L
Prostatic acid phosphatase (PAP)	0–3 U/dL
Prostate-specific antigen (PSA)	<4 ug/L

URINE

Albumin–creatinine ratio	<30 mg/g
Calcium	100–300 mg/24 h
Creatinine	15–25 mg/kg per 24 h
Glomerular filtration rate (GFR) • Normal Male • Female	 • 130 mL/min/1.73 m² • 120 mL/min/1.73 m²
Osmolality	80–1300 mOsm/L
pH	4.6–8.0
Protein–creatinine ratio	≤0.2 mg/mg

Protein	1–15 mg/dL
Sodium	100–260 mEq/24 h
Specific grav ty	1.003–1.040
Stages of chronic kidney disease • Stage 1 • Stage 2 • Stage 3 • Stage 4 • Stage 5	 • ≥90 mL/min/1.73 m^2 • 60–89 mL/min/1.73 m^2 • 30–59 mL/min/1.73 m^2 • 15–29 mL/min/1.73 m^2 • <15 mL/min/1.73 m^2
Uric acid	250–750 mg/24 h

CEREBROSPINAL FLUID

Appearance	Clear
Cell count	0–5 x 10^6/L
Glucose	40–80 mg/dL
Pressure (opening)	70–200 mm H_2O
Protein	15–60 mg/dL

CARDIAC PARAMETERS

Cardiac index	2.5–4.2 L/min/m^2
Cardiac output	4–8 LPM
Left ventricular ejection fraction	>55%
Pressures • Pulmonary artery ▪ Systolic ▪ Diastolic ▪ Mean • Pulmonary capillary wedge • Right atrium • Right ventricle ▪ Systolic ▪ Diastolic • Systolic arterial pressure • Diastolic arterial pressure • Central venous pressure	 20–25 mm Hg 5–10 mm Hg 9–16 mm Hg 6–12 mm Hg Mean 0–5 mm Hg 20–25 mm Hg 0–5 mm Hg 90–140 mm Hg 60–90 mm Hg 2–6 mm Hg; 2.5–12 cm H_2O

Index